PETERSON'S NURSING PROGRAMS 2012

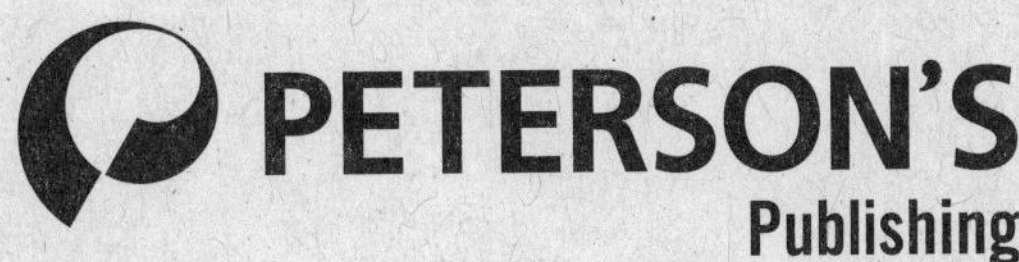

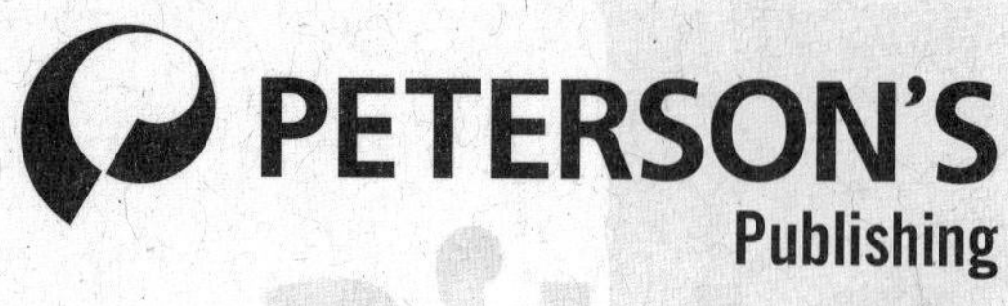

About Peterson's Publishing

To succeed on your lifelong educational journey, you will need accurate, dependable, and practical tools and resources. That is why Peterson's is everywhere education happens. Because whenever and however you need education content delivered, you can rely on Peterson's to provide the information, know-how, and guidance to help you reach your goals. Tools to match the right students with the right school. It's here. Personalized resources and expert guidance. It's here. Comprehensive and dependable education content—delivered whenever and however you need it. It's all here.

For more information, contact Peterson's Publishing, 2000 Lenox Drive, Lawrenceville, NJ 08648; 800-338-3282 Ext. 54229; or find us on the World Wide Web at www.petersonspublishing.com.

Bernadette Webster, Director of Publishing; Jill C. Schwartz, Editor; Christine Lucas, Research Project Manager; Amy Weber, Research Associate; Phyllis Johnson, Programmer; Ray Golaszewski, Manufacturing Manager; Linda M. Williams, Composition Manager; Karen Mount, Shannon White, Client Relations Representatives

ISSN 1552-7743
ISBN-13: 978-0-7689-3277-5
ISBN-10: 0-7689-3277-7

Printed in the United States of America

10 9 8 7 6 5 4 3 2 1 13 12 11

Seventeenth Edition

By producing this book on recycled paper (40% post-consumer waste) 63 trees were saved.

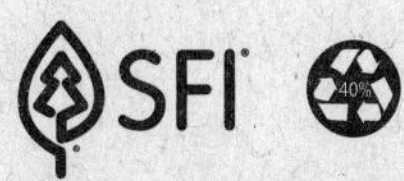

Certified Chain of Custody

60% Certified Fiber Sourcing and
40% Post-Consumer Recycled

www.sfiprogram.org

*This label applies to the text stock.

Sustainability—Its Importance to Peterson's Publishing

What does sustainability mean to Peterson's? As a leading publisher, we are aware that our business has a direct impact on vital resources—most especially the trees that are used to make our books. Peterson's Publishing is proud that its products are certified by the Sustainable Forestry Initiative (SFI) and that all of its books are printed on paper that is 40% post-consumer waste using vegetable-based ink.

Being a part of the Sustainable Forestry Initiative (SFI) means that all of our vendors—from paper suppliers to printers—have undergone rigorous audits to demonstrate that they are maintaining a sustainable environment.

Peterson's Publishing continuously strives to find new ways to incorporate sustainability throughout all aspects of its business.

CONTENTS

FOREWORD

The American Association of Colleges of Nursing (AACN) is proud to collaborate on *Peterson's Nursing Programs 2012.*

According to the Bureau of Labor Statistics, more than 1 million new and replacement registered nurses will be needed by the year 2012 to fill new positions and vacancies. Nursing schools are working hard to find creative solutions to expand capacity and recruit new students during this nursing shortage.

As registered nurses find employment beyond hospitals in such areas as home care, community health, and long-term care, newly licensed RNs must have the proper education and training to work in these settings. It is vital that those seeking to enter or advance in a nursing career find the appropriate nursing program. This guide allows readers to find the program that best fits their needs, whether beginning a new career in nursing or attempting to advance one.

According to AACN's most recent annual institutional survey, enrollment in entry-level B.S.N. programs continues to climb. Gains were reported in all parts of the country in 2010, with an overall 6.1 percent increase in enrollments nationwide.

Although the health-care environment is complex and dynamic, there continues to be a significant demand for professional-level nurses. The primary route into professional-level nursing is the four-year baccalaureate degree. The professional nurse with a baccalaureate degree is the only basic nursing graduate prepared to practice in all health-care settings, including critical care, public health, primary care, and mental health. In addition, advanced practice nurses (APNs) deliver essential services as nurse practitioners, certified nurse-midwives, clinical nurse specialists, and nurse anesthetists. APNs typically are prepared in master's degree programs, and the demand for their services is expected to increase substantially.

Higher education in nursing expands the gateway to a variety of career opportunities in the health-care field. In addition to providing primary care to patients, graduates can work as case managers for the growing numbers of managed-care companies or can assume administrative or managerial roles in hospitals, clinics, insurance companies, and other diverse settings.

The Nursing School Adviser section of this guide is instructive and invaluable. Whether you are a high school student looking for a four-year program, an RN returning to school, or a professional in another field contemplating a career change, this section will address your concerns. This information presents various nursing perspectives to benefit students from diverse backgrounds.

Peterson's effort in making this guide well organized and convenient to read cannot be overstated. Peterson's has worked with AACN in producing a publication that is comprehensive and user-friendly. Like the previous editions, this edition is a genuine collaborative work, as AACN provided input from start to finish.

AACN's dedication and achievements in advancing the quality of baccalaureate and graduate nursing education are appreciated by Peterson's. We at AACN are fortunate to work with an organization that prides itself on being the leading publisher of education search and selection.

Furthermore, this publication would not be possible without the cooperation of the institutions included in this guide. We acknowledge the time and effort of those who undertook the task of completing and returning the surveys regarding their programs. We certainly appreciate their contribution.

Peterson's Nursing Programs 2012 is the only comprehensive and concise guide to baccalaureate and graduate nursing education programs in the United States and Canada. We hope its contents will serve as the impetus for those looking for a rewarding and satisfying career in health care. AACN is proud to present this publication to the nursing profession and to those who seek to enter it.

—Kathleen Potempa, DNSc, RN, FAAN
President, AACN

—Geraldine D. Bednash, Ph.D., RN, FAAN
Chief Executive Officer and Executive Director, AACN

A Note from the Peterson's Editors

For more than forty years, Peterson's has given students and parents the most comprehensive, up-to-date information on undergraduate and graduate institutions in the United States, Canada, and abroad.

Peterson's Nursing Programs 2012 provides prospective nursing students with the most comprehensive information on baccalaureate and graduate nursing education in the United States and Canada. Our goal is to help students find the best nursing program for them.

To this end, Peterson's has joined forces with the American Association of Colleges of Nursing (AACN), the national voice for America's baccalaureate-and higher-degree nursing education programs. AACN's educational, research, governmental advocacy, data collection, publications, and other programs work to establish high-quality standards for bachelor's- and graduate-degree nursing education, assist deans and directors to implement those standards, influence the nursing profession to improve health care, and promote public support of baccalaureate and graduate education, research, and practice in nursing—the nation's largest health-care profession.

For those seeking to enter the nursing profession or to further their nursing careers, *Peterson's Nursing Programs 2012* includes information needed to make important nursing program decisions and to approach the admissions process with knowledge and confidence.

The Nursing School Adviser section contains useful articles to help guide nursing education choices, with information on nursing careers today, selecting a nursing program, financing nursing education, returning to school, and more. It also includes listings that provide valuable contact information for financial aid resources and specialty nursing organizations. And if you are one of the many people interested in accelerated nursing programs, there is an article that offers an in-depth look at this increasingly popular approach to nursing education. It is a must-read for those wishing to enter an accelerated baccalaureate or generic master's degree program.

At the end of **The Nursing School Adviser** is the "How to Use This Guide" article, which explains some of the key factors to consider when choosing a nursing program. In addition, it explains how the book is organized and shows you how to maximize your use of *Peterson's Nursing Programs 2012* to its full potential.

If you already have specifics in mind, such as a particular program or location, turn to the **Quick-Reference Chart.** Here you can search through "Nursing Programs At-a-Glance" for particular degree options offered by schools, listed alphabetically by state.

In the **Profiles of Nursing Programs** section you'll find expanded and updated nursing program descriptions, arranged alphabetically by state. Each profile provides all of the need-to-know information about accredited nursing programs in the United States and Canada.

If you are looking for additional information, you can turn to the **Two-Page Descriptions** section. Here you will find in-depth narrative descriptions, with photos, of those nursing programs that chose to provide additional information.

When you turn to the back of the book, you'll find eight **Indexes** listing institutions offering *baccalaureate, master's degree, concentrations within master's degree, doctoral, post-doctoral, online,* and *continuing education* programs. The last index lists every college and university contained in the guide along with its corresponding page reference.

At the end of the book, don't miss the special section of ads placed by our preferred clients. Their financial support helps make it possible for Peterson's Publishing to continue to provide you with the highest-quality test-prep, educational exploration, and career-preparation resources you need to succeed on your educational journey.

Peterson's publishes a full line of resources to help guide you and your family through the admission process. Peterson's publications can be found at high school guidance offices, college and university libraries and career centers, and your local bookstore or library.

Peterson's guides are also available as e-books. Continue to check our Web site, www.petersonspublishing.com for more information about our e-book program.

We welcome any comments or suggestions you may have about this publication.

Publishing Department
Peterson's, a Nelnet company
2000 Lenox Drive
Lawrenceville, NJ 08648

Your feedback will help us make your educational dreams possible. The editors at Peterson's wish you great success in your nursing program search.

THE NURSING SCHOOL ADVISER

NURSING FACT SHEET

Misconceptions about nursing have contributed to misinformation about the profession in the media. Here are the real facts:

- **Nursing is the nation's largest health-care profession, with more than 2.9 million registered nurses nationwide.** Of all licensed RNs, 2.42 million, or 83.2 percent, are employed in nursing.[1]
- **Nursing students account for more than one half (52 percent) of all health profession students in the United States.**[2]
- **Registered Nurses compose one of the largest segments of the U.S. workforce as a whole, and nursing is among the highest-paying large occupations**. Nearly 59 percent of RNs worked in general medical and surgical hospitals where RN salaries averaged $58,550 per year. With 2.5 million nurses in the workforce in 2007, RNs composed the largest segment of professionals (28 percent) working in the health-care industry.[3]
- **Nurses compose the largest single component of hospital staff.** They are the primary providers of hospital patient care, and they deliver most of the nation's long-term care.
- **Most health-care services involve some form of care by nurses.** In 1980, 66 percent of all employed RNs worked in hospitals. By 2004, that number had declined to 56.2 percent as more health care moved to sites outside of hospitals and nurses increased their ranks in a wide range of other settings, including private practices, health maintenance organizations, public health agencies, primary-care clinics, home health care, nursing homes, outpatient surgicenters, nursing-school–operated nursing centers, insurance and managed care companies, schools, mental health agencies, hospices, the military, industry, nursing education, and health-care research.[4]
- **Though often working collaboratively, nursing does not "assist" medicine or other fields.** Nursing operates independent of—not as an auxiliary to—medicine and other disciplines. Nurses' roles range from direct patient care and case management to establishing nursing practice standards, developing quality assurance procedures, and directing complex nursing care systems.
- **With more than four times as many RNs in the United States as physicians, nursing delivers an extended array of health-care services.** These services include primary and preventive care by advanced nurse practitioners in such areas as pediatrics, family health, women's health, and gerontological care. Nursing's scope also includes services by certified nurse-midwives and nurse anesthetists, as well as care in cardiac, oncology, neonatal, neurological, and obstetric/gynecological nursing and other advanced clinical specialties.
- **The primary pathway to professional nursing, as compared to technical-level practice, is the four-year Bachelor of Science in Nursing (B.S.N.) degree.** Registered nurses are prepared through a B.S.N. program, a three-year associate degree in nursing, or a three-year hospital training program, receiving a hospital diploma. All take the same state licensing exam. *(The number of diploma programs has declined steadily, to less than 10 percent of all basic RN education programs, as nursing education has shifted from hospital-operated instruction into the college and university system.)*
- **To meet the more complex demands of today's health-care environment, the National Advisory Council on Nurse Education and Practice recommended that at least two thirds of the basic nurse workforce hold baccalaureate or higher degrees in nursing by 2010.**[5] Aware of the need, RNs are seeking the B.S.N. degree in increasing numbers. In 1980, almost 55 percent of employed registered nurses held a hospital diploma as their highest educational credential, 22 percent held a bachelor's degree, and 18 percent an associate degree. By 2004, a diploma was the highest educational credential for only 17.5 percent of RNs, while the number with bachelor's degrees had climbed to 34.2 percent (with 33.7 percent holding an associate degree as their top academic preparation).[6] In 2005, 13,232 RNs with diplomas or associate degrees graduated from B.S.N. programs.[7]
- **In 2004, 13 percent of the nation's registered nurses held either a master's or doctoral degree as their highest educational credential.**[8] The current demand for master's-prepared and doctorally prepared nurses for advanced practice, clinical specialties, teaching, and research roles far outstrips the supply.
- **According to the U.S. Bureau of Labor Statistics, registered nursing is among the occupations with the greatest job growth from 2006–16.**[9] Other federal projections indicate that by 2020, the U.S. nursing shortage will expand to more than 800,000 registered nursing positions.[10] Even as health care continues to shift beyond the hospital to more community-based primary care sites and other outpatient sites, federal projections say the rising complexity of acute care will cause demand for RNs in hospitals to climb by 36 percent by 2020.[11]

---

1. Health Resources and Services Administration. (February 2007). *The Registered Nurse Population: Findings From the March 2004 National Sample Survey of Registered Nurses*. Washington, DC: U.S. Department of Health and Human Services.
2. Health Resources and Services Administration. (September 1992). *Health Personnel in the United States,*

1991: Eighth Report to Congress. Washington, DC: U.S. Department of Health and Human Services, p. 215 and other tables.

3. U.S. Bureau of Labor Statistics. (May 2008). Occupational Employment and Wages for 2007. Access online at http://www.bls.gov/news.release/pdf/ocwage.pdf.
4. Ibid.
5. Health Resources and Services Administration. (February 2007). *The Registered Nurse Population.*
6. National Advisory Council on Nurse Education and Practice. (October 1996). *Report to the Secretary of the Department of Health and Human Services on the Basic Registered Nurse Workforce.* Washington, DC: U.S. Department of Health and Human Services, Division of Nursing.
7. Health Resources and Services Administration. (February 2007). *The Registered Nurse Population.*
8. American Association of Colleges of Nursing (2007). *2006–07 Enrollment and Graduations in Baccalaureate and Graduate Programs in Nursing.* Washington, DC.
9. U.S. Bureau of Labor Statistics. (May 2008). *Occupational Employment and Wages for 2007.*
10. Hecker, D.E. (2004). *Occupational Employment Projections to 2012.* Washington, DC: U.S. Department of Labor, Bureau of Labor Statistics.
11. Health Resources and Services Administration, Bureau of Health Professions. (2002). *Projected Supply, Demand and Shortages of Registered Nurses: 2000–2020.* Washington, DC: U.S. Department of Health and Human Services.

COUNSELORS OF CARE IN THE MODERN HEALTH-CARE SYSTEM

Geraldine Bednash, Ph.D., RN, FAAN
Executive Director
American Association of Colleges of Nursing

A Different Era

The nursing profession is alive and reshaping itself. The role of nurses as those who minister exclusively to a patient's basic-care needs has changed. Much of the effectiveness and productivity of the future health-care industry will derive from the training of and services provided by nurses.

Modern nurses take a proactive role in health care by addressing health issues before they develop into problems. They oversee the continued care of patients who have left the health-care facility. Nurses are expected to make complex decisions in areas ranging from patient screening to diagnosis and education. They explore and document the effects of alternative therapies (e.g., guided imagery) and address public health problems, such as teen pregnancy. They explore and understand new technology and how it relates both to patient care and to their own job performance. They work in a variety of settings and are held accountable for their decisions. In today's health-care environment, health-care administrators must recruit nurses with a broad, well-rounded education.

Health-care providers must change the way they administer care. Instead of focusing on the treatment of illness, they must promote wellness. Nurses will oversee patient treatment and medication and must understand the repercussions of these health-care processes for the patient and his or her family.

Cost is the driving force behind this industry-wide transformation. Insurance companies have, for the most part, instigated changes in the way health-care benefits are paid. The old fee-for-service system is no longer the only option. The trend toward managed care, in which a fixed amount of money is allocated for the care of each patient, is changing the way care is provided. It seems that employers of the future will recruit nurses who understand the overall structure of the health-care industry, who possess highly developed critical-thinking skills, and who bring to their positions a well-rounded understanding of the risks and benefits of every health-care decision.

Counselors of Care

Job prospects for graduates of nursing programs are positive. Although many graduates receive associate degrees as registered nurses (RNs), hospital administrators and other employers want applicants with at least a Bachelor of Science in Nursing degree.

To practice in a fast-changing health system, entry-level RNs must understand community-based primary care and emphasize health promotion and cost-effective coordinated care—all hallmarks of baccalaureate education. In addition to its broad scientific curriculum and focus on leadership and clinical decision-making skills, a Bachelor of Science in Nursing degree education provides specific preparation in community-based care not typically included in associate degree or hospital diploma programs. Moreover, the nurse with a baccalaureate degree is the only basic nursing graduate prepared for all health-care settings—critical care, outpatient care, public health, and mental health—and so has the flexibility to practice in outpatient centers, private homes, and neighborhood clinics where demand is fast expanding as health care moves beyond the hospital to more primary and preventive care throughout the community.

Health-care administrators realize that patients are becoming more sophisticated about the care they receive, requiring an explanation and understanding of their health needs. Nurses will have to be knowledgeable care providers, working with physicians, pharmacists, and public health officials in interdisciplinary settings to satisfy these requirements.

Broader training enables graduates of baccalaureate programs to provide improved and varying types of care, and ensures stability and security in an industry now noted for its instability.

Promising Opportunities

One of the rewards of a baccalaureate education can be a competitive salary. Graduates of four-year degree programs can expect salaries starting around $37,000 per year, a figure that might fluctuate depending on geographic area and, more specifically, by the demand in that area. Obviously, the greater the need for nurses, the higher their salaries.

The baccalaureate degree also serves as a foundation for the pursuit of a master's degree in nursing, which prepares students for the role of advanced practice nurse (APN). Students can earn degrees as clinical nurse specialists in neonatology, oncology, cardiology, and other specialties or as nurse practitioners, nurse-midwives, or nurse anesthetists. Master's-prepared nurses can also enjoy rewarding careers in nursing administration and education.

These programs generally span one to two years. Graduates can expect starting salaries of approximately $50,000 annually in advanced practice nursing settings, and demand for these graduates is expected to be high over the next fifteen years. In some localities, for example, the nurse practitioner may be the sole provider of health care to a family.

Overall Transformation

The nursing field must be transformed to be compatible with the overall changes in the health-care industry. According to 2008 statistics, the average age of nurses was 46, with only 16.6 percent of nurses under the age of 35. It is projected that over the next ten years much of the nursing population will retire. Employment is projected to increase 23 percent by 2020.

The traditional career path of nurses is expected to change. More nurses will enter master's programs directly from baccalaureate programs, and more master's degree graduates will pursue doctoral degrees at a younger age. Since nurses will play a critical role in providing health care, a four-year baccalaureate degree is a crucial first step in preparing nurses to assume increased patient responsibilities within the health-care system.

RNs Returning to School: Choosing a Nursing Program

Marilyn Oermann, Ph.D., RN, FAAN, ANEF
Professor and Adult/Geriatric Health Chair
College of Nursing
The University of North Carolina at Chapel Hill

If you are thinking about returning to school to complete your baccalaureate degree or to pursue a graduate degree in nursing, you are not alone. Registered nurses (RNs) are returning to school in record numbers, many seeking advancement or transition to new roles in nursing. Over the last two decades, the number of RNs prepared initially in diploma and associate degree in nursing programs who have graduated from baccalaureate nursing degree programs has more than doubled, according to the AACN. There are expanded opportunities for nurses with baccalaureate degrees in nursing. Although the decision to return to school means considerable investment of time, financial resources, and effort, the benefits can be overwhelmingly positive.

Higher education in nursing opens doors to many opportunities for career growth not otherwise available. By continuing your education, you can do the following:

- Update your knowledge and skills, critical today in light of rapid advances in health care
- Move more easily into a new role within your organization or in other health-care settings
- Pursue a different career path within nursing

Moreover, returning to school brings personal fulfillment and satisfaction gained through learning more about nursing and the changing health-care system and using that knowledge in the delivery and management of patient care.

More Skills and Flexibility Needed

If you are contemplating returning to school, here are some facts to consider. The health-care system continues to undergo dramatic changes. These changes include hospitalized patients who are more acutely ill; an aging population; technological advances that require highly skilled nursing care; a greater role for nurses in primary care, health promotion, and health education; and the need for nurses to care for patients and families in multiple settings, such as schools, workplaces, homes, clinics, and outpatient facilities, as well as hospitals. With the nursing shortage, nurses are in great demand in hospitals. Moreover, as hospitals continue to become centers for acute and critical care, the nurse's role in both patient care and management of other health-care providers in the hospital has become more complex, requiring advanced knowledge and skills.

Because of the complexity of today's health-care environment, AACN and other leading nursing organizations have called for the baccalaureate degree in nursing as the minimum educational requirement for professional nursing practice. In fact, nurse executives in hospitals have indicated their desire for the majority of nurses on staff to be prepared at least at the baccalaureate level to handle the increasingly complex demands of patient care and management of health-care delivery. The baccalaureate nursing degree is essential for nurses to function in different management roles, move across employment settings, have the flexibility to change positions within nursing, and advance in their career. Baccalaureate nursing degree programs prepare the nurse for a broad role within the health-care system and for practice in hospitals, community settings, home health care, neighborhood clinics, and other outpatient settings where opportunities are expanding. Continuing education provides the means for nurses to prepare themselves for a future role in nursing.

The demand for nurses with baccalaureate and more advanced degrees will continue to grow. There is an excess of nurses prepared at the associate degree level, a mounting shortage of baccalaureate-prepared nurses, and only half as many nurses prepared at master's and doctoral levels as needed. Nurses with baccalaureate nursing degrees are needed in all areas of health care, and the demand for nurses with master's and doctoral preparation for advanced practice, management, teaching, and research will continue.

Identifying Strategies

The decision to return to school marks the beginning of a new phase in your career development. It is essential for you to plan this future carefully. Why are you thinking about returning to school, and what do you want to accomplish by doing so? Understanding why you want to go back to school will help you select the best program for you. Knowing what you want to accomplish will help you to focus on your goals and overcome the obstacles that could prevent you from achieving your full potential.

Even if you decide that additional education will help you reach your professional goals, you may also have a list of reasons why you think you cannot return to school—no time, limited financial resources, fear of failure, and concerns about meeting family responsibilities, among others. If you are concerned about the demands of school combined with existing responsibilities, begin by identifying strategies for incorporating classes and study time into your present schedule or consider taking an online course. Remember, you can start your program with one course and reevaluate your time at the end of the term.

Research and anecdotal evidence from adults returning to college indicate that, despite their need to balance school work with a career and often with family responsibilities, these adult learners experience less stress and manage their lives better than they had thought possible. Many of these adult learners report that the satisfaction gained from their education more than compensates for any added stress. Furthermore, studies of nurses who have returned to school suggest that while their education may create stress for them, most nurses cope effectively with the demands of advanced education.

If costs are of concern, it is best to investigate tuition-reimbursement opportunities where you are employed, scholarships from the nursing program and other nursing organizations, and loans. The financial aid officer at the program you are considering is probably the best available resource to answer your financial assistance questions.

If you are unsure of what to expect when returning to school, remember that such feelings are natural for anyone facing a new situation. If you are motivated and committed to pursuing your degree, you will succeed. Most nursing programs offer resources, such as test-taking skills, study skills, and time-management workshops, as well as assistance with academic problems. You can combine school, work, family, and other responsibilities. Even with these greater demands, the benefits of education outweigh the difficulties.

Clarifying Career Goals

Nursing, unlike many other professions, has a variety of educational paths for those who return for advanced education. You should decide if baccalaureate- or graduate-level work is congruent with your career goals. The next step in this process is to reexamine your specific career goals, both immediate and long-term, to determine the level and type of nursing education you will need to meet them. Ask yourself what you want to be doing in the next five to ten years. Discuss your ideas with a counselor in a nursing education program, nurses who are practicing in roles you are considering, and others who are enrolled in a nursing program or who have recently completed a nursing degree.

Baccalaureate degree nursing programs prepare nurses as generalists for practice in all health-care settings. Graduate nursing education occurs at two levels— master's and doctoral. Master's programs vary in length, typically between one and two years. Preparation for roles in advanced practice as nurse practitioners, certified nurse midwives, clinical nurse specialists, certified registered nurse anesthetists, nursing administrators, and nursing educators requires a master's degree in nursing. Many programs meet the needs of RNs by offering options such as accelerated course work, advanced placement, evening and weekend classes, and distance learning courses.

A trend in education for RNs is accelerated programs that combine baccalaureate and master's nursing programs. These combined programs are designed for RNs without degrees whose career goals involve advanced nursing practice and other roles requiring a master's degree. Nurses who complete these combined programs may be awarded both a baccalaureate and a master's degree in nursing or a master's degree only.

At the doctoral level, nurses are prepared for a variety of roles, including research and teaching. Doctoral programs generally consist of three years of full-time study beyond the master's degree, although some programs admit baccalaureate graduates and include the master's-level requirements and degree within the doctoral program.

Matching a Program to Your Needs

Once you have defined your career goals and the level of nursing education they will require, the next step is matching your needs with the offerings and characteristics of specific nursing programs. Some of the criteria you may want to consider in evaluating potential schools of nursing include the types of programs offered, the length of the program and its specific requirements, the availability of full-and part-time study and number of credits required for part-time study, the flexibility of the program, whether distance education courses are available, and the days, times, and sites at which classes and clinical experiences are offered as they relate to your work schedule. Take into consideration the program's accreditation status; faculty qualifications in terms of research, teaching, and practice; and the resources of the school of nursing and of the college/university, such as library holdings, computer services, and statistical consultants. You should also consider the clinical settings used in the curriculum and their relationship to your career goals, as well as the availability of financial aid for nursing students.

Carefully review the admission criteria, including minimum grade point average requirements; scores required on any admission tests, such as the Graduate Record Examinations (GRE) for master's and doctoral programs; and any requirements in terms of work experience. For students returning for a baccalaureate degree, prior nursing knowledge may be validated through testing, transfer of courses, and other mechanisms. Review these options prior to applying to a program.

While the intrinsic quality and characteristics of the program are important, your own personal goals and needs have to be included in your decision. Consider commuting distance, whether courses are offered online, costs in relation to your financial resources, program design, and flexibility of the curriculum in relation to your work, family, and personal responsibilities. While the majority of nursing programs offer part-time study, many programs also schedule classes to accommodate work situations.

Many schools offer nursing courses online, and in some places, the entire baccalaureate and master's programs are available through distance learning. The largest enrollment in nursing distance learning is in baccalaureate programs for

RNs. Distance learning allows RNs to further their education no matter where they live. Many nurses prefer online courses because they can learn at times convenient for them, especially considering competing demands associated with their jobs, families, and other commitments.

Ensure Your Success

Once you have made the decision to return to school and have chosen the program that best meets your needs, take an additional step to ensure your success. Identify the support you will need, both academic and personal, to be successful in the nursing program. Academic support is provided by the institution and may include tutoring services, learning resource centers, computer facilities, and other resources to support your learning. You should take advantage of available support services and seek out resources for areas in which you are weak or need review. Academic support services, however, need to be complemented by personal support through family, friends, and peers. With a firm commitment to pursuing advanced education, a clear choice of a nursing program to meet your goals, and support from others, you are certain to find success in returning to school.

BACCALAUREATE PROGRAMS

Linda K. Amos, Ed.D., RN, FAAN
Former Associate Vice President for Health Sciences
Dean Emerita
University of Utah

The health-care industry has continued to change dramatically over the past few years, transforming the roles of nurses and escalating their opportunities. The current shortage of nurses is caused by an increasing number of hospitalized patients who are older and more acutely ill, a growing elderly population with multiple chronic health problems, and expanded opportunities in HMOs, home care, occupational health, surgical centers, and other primary-care settings. Expanding technological advances that prolong life also require more highly skilled personnel.

The increasing scope of nursing opportunities will grow immensely as nurses become the frontline providers of health care. They are assuming important roles in the provision of managed care, and they will be responsible for coordinating and continuing the care outside traditional health-care facilities. Nurses will play a major role in educating the public and addressing the social and economic factors that impact quality of care.

Worldwide Standards

Nursing students of the future will receive a wealth of information. Understanding the technology used to manage that information will be essential to their ability to track and assess care. In this area, nurses will be able to provide care over great distances. In some areas, care is being managed by the nurse via tele-home health over the Internet. Use of the Internet and other computer-oriented systems is now an integral tool used by nurses. Nurses of the future, therefore, will have to become aware of worldwide standards of care. Nevertheless, the primary job of a nurse will be making sure that the right person is providing the right care at the right cost.

This goal will be accomplished as the industry turns away from the hospital as the center of operation. Nurses will work in a broad array of locations, including clinics, outpatient facilities, community centers, schools, and even places of business.

Much of the emphasis in health care will shift to preventive care and the promotion of health. In this system, nurses will take on a broader and more diverse role than they have in the past.

Unlimited Opportunities, Expanded Responsibilities

The four-year baccalaureate programs in today's nursing colleges provide the educational and experiential base not only for entry-level professional practice, but also as the platform on which to build a career through graduate-level study for advanced practice nursing, including careers as nurse practitioners, nurse-midwives, clinical specialists, and nurse administrators and educators. Nurses at this level can be expected to specialize in oncology, pediatrics, neonatology, obstetrics and gynecology, critical care, infection control, psychiatry, women's health, community health, and neuroscience. The potential and responsibilities at this level are great. Increasingly, many families use the nurse practitioner for all health-care needs. In almost all U.S. states, the nurse practitioner can prescribe medications and provide health care for the management of chronic non-acute illnesses and preventive care.

The health-care system demands a lot from nurses. The education of a nurse must transcend the traditional areas of study, such as chemistry and anatomy, to include health promotion, disease prevention, screening, genetic counseling, and immunization. Nurses should understand how health problems may have a social cause, such as poverty and environmental contamination, and they must develop insight into human psychology, behavior, and cultural mores and values.

The transformation of the health-care system offers unlimited opportunities for nurses at the baccalaureate and graduate levels as care in urban and rural settings becomes more accessible. According to the U.S. Bureau of Labor Statistics, employment of RNs will grow more quickly than the average employment for all occupations through 2012, due largely to growing demand in settings such as health maintenance organizations, community health centers, home care, and long-term care. The increased complexity of health problems and increased management of health problems outside of hospitals require highly educated and well-prepared nurses at the baccalaureate and graduate levels. It is an exciting era in nursing that holds exceptional promise for nurses with a baccalaureate nursing degree.

The compensation for new nurses is once again becoming competitive with that of other industries. Entry-level nurses with baccalaureate degrees in nursing can expect a salary range of about $31,000 to $46,000 per year, depending on geographic location and experience. Five years into their careers, the national average for nurses with four-year degrees is more than $50,000 per year, with many earning more than $65,000. The current shortage has prompted some employers to offer sign-on bonuses and other incentives to attract and retain staff.

Applying to College

Meeting your chosen school's general entrance requirements is the first step toward a university or college degree in nursing. Admission requirements may vary, but a high school diploma or equivalent is necessary. Most accredited colleges consider SAT scores along with high school grade point average. A strong preparatory class load in science and mathematics is generally preferred among nursing schools. Students may obtain specific admission information by writing to a school's nursing department.

To apply to a nursing school, contact the admission offices of the colleges or universities you are interested in and request the appropriate application forms. With limited spaces in nursing schools, programs are competitive, and early submission of an application is recommended.

Accreditation

Accreditation of the nursing program is very important, and it should be considered on two levels—the accreditation of the university or college and the accreditation of the nursing program itself. Accreditation is a voluntary process in which the school or the program asks for an external review of its programs, facilities, and faculty. For nursing programs, the review is performed by peers in nursing education to ensure program quality and integrity.

Baccalaureate nursing programs in the United States undergo two types of regular systematic reviews. First, the school must be approved by the state board of nursing. This approval is necessary to ensure that the graduates of the program may sit for the licensing examinations offered through the National Council of State Boards of Nursing, Inc. The second is accreditation administered by a nursing accreditation agency that is recognized by the U.S. Department of Education.

Although accreditation is a voluntary process, access to federal loans and scholarships requires it, and most graduate schools accept only students who have earned degrees from accredited schools. Further, accreditation ensures an ongoing process of quality improvement based on national standards. Canadian nursing school programs are accredited by the Canadian Association of University Schools of Nursing, and the Canadian programs listed in this book must hold this accreditation. There are two recognized accreditation agencies for baccalaureate nursing programs in the United States: the Commission on Collegiate Nursing Education (CCNE) and the National League for Nursing Accrediting Commission (NLNAC).

Focusing Your Education

Academic performance is not the sole basis of acceptance into the upper level of the nursing program. Admission officers also weigh such factors as student activities, employment, and references. Moreover, many require an interview and/or essay in which the nursing candidate offers a goal statement. This part of the admission process can be completed prior to a student's entrance into the college or university or prior to the student's entrance into the school of nursing itself, depending on the program.

In the interview or essay, students may list career preferences and reasons for their choices. This allows admission officers to assess the goals of students and gain insights into their values, integrity, and honesty. One would expect that a goal statement from a student who is just entering college would be more general than that of a student who has had two years of preprofessional nursing studies. The more experienced student would be likely to have a more focused idea of what is to be gained by an education in nursing; there would be more evidence of the student's values and the ways in which she or he relates them to the knowledge gained from preprofessional nursing classes.

Baccalaureate Curriculum

A standard basic or generic baccalaureate program in nursing is a four-year college or university education that incorporates a variety of liberal arts courses with professional education and training. It is designed for high school graduates with no previous nursing experience.

Currently, there are more than 700 baccalaureate programs in the United States. Of the 683 programs that responded to a 2009 survey conducted by the American Association of Colleges of Nursing, total enrollment in all nursing programs leading to a baccalaureate degree was 214,533.

The baccalaureate curriculum is designed to prepare students for work in the growing and changing health-care environment. As nurses take a more active role in all facets of health care, they are expected to develop critical thinking and communication skills in addition to receiving standard nurse training in clinics and hospitals. In a university or college setting, the first two years include classes in the humanities, social sciences, basic sciences, business, psychology, technology, sociology, ethics, and nutrition.

In some programs, nursing classes begin in the sophomore year; others begin in the junior year. Many schools require satisfactory grade point averages before students advance into professional nursing classes. On a 4.0 scale, admission into the last two years of the nursing program may require a minimum GPA of 2.5 to 3.0 in preprofessional nursing classes. The national average is about 2.8, but the cutoff level varies with each program.

In the junior and senior years, the curriculum focuses on the nursing sciences, and emphasis moves from the classroom to health facilities. This is where students are exposed to clinical skills, nursing theory, and the varied roles nurses play in the health-care system. Courses include nurse leadership, health promotion, family planning, mental health, environmental and occupational health, adult and pediatric care, medical and surgical care, psychiatric care, community health, management, and home health care.

This level of education comes in a variety of settings: community hospitals, clinics, social service agencies, schools, and health-maintenance organizations. Training in diverse settings is the best preparation for becoming a vital player in the growing health-care field.

Reentry Programs

Practicing nurses who return to school to earn a baccalaureate degree will have to meet requirements that may include possession of a valid RN license and an associate degree or hospital diploma from an accredited institution. Again, it is best to check with the school's admissions department to determine specifics.

Nurses returning to school will have to consider the rapid rate of change in health care and science. A nurse who passed an undergraduate-level chemistry class ten years ago would probably not receive credit for that class today because of the growth of knowledge in that and all other scientific fields. The need to reeducate applies not only to practicing nurses returning to school, but also to all nurses throughout their careers.

In the same vein, nurses with diplomas from hospital programs who want to work toward a baccalaureate degree must meet the common requirements for more clinical practice, and must develop a deeper understanding of community-based nursing practices such as health prevention and promotion.

Colleges and universities available to the RN in search of a baccalaureate give credit for previous nurse training. These programs are designed to accommodate the needs and career goals of the practicing nurse by providing flexible course schedules and credit for previous experience and education. Some programs lead to a master's-level degree, a process that can take up to three years. Licensed practical nurses (LPNs) can also continue their education through baccalaureate programs.

Nurses considering reentering school may also consider other specialized programs. For example, some programs are aimed at enabling nurses with A.D.N. degrees or LPN/LVN licenses to earn B.S.N.'s. Also, accelerated B.S.N. programs are available for students with degrees in other fields.

RN-to-Baccalaureate Programs Fact Sheet

More than 630 RN-to-baccalaureate programs are available nationwide, including programs offered in a more intense, accelerated format. Program length varies from one to two years depending upon the school's requirements, program type, and the student's previous academic achievement.

Concerns about the limited availability of RN-to-baccalaureate programs are unfounded. In fact, there are more RN-to-baccalaureate programs available than there are four-year nursing programs or accelerated bachelor's degree programs for non-nursing college graduates. Access to RN-to-baccalaureate programs is further enhanced when programs are offered completely online or on-site at various health-care facilities.

Enrollment in RN-to-baccalaureate programs is increasing in response to calls for a more highly educated nursing workforce. From 2009 to 2011, enrollments increased by 20.6 percent, marking the sixth year of increases in RN-to-baccalaureate programs.

Hundreds of articulation agreements between A.D.N. and diploma programs and four-year institutions exist nationwide (including some statewide agreements), to help students who are seeking baccalaureate-level nursing education. Before enrolling in diploma and A.D.N. programs, students are encouraged to check with school administrators to see what articulation agreements exist with baccalaureate degree–granting schools and to determine which course work will be transferable.

Choosing a Program

With more than 700 baccalaureate programs in the United States, the prospective student must do research to determine which programs match his or her needs and career objectives.

If you have no health-care experience, it might be best to gain some insight into the field by volunteering or working part-time in a care facility such as a hospital or an outpatient clinic. Talking to nurse professionals about their work will also help you determine how your attributes may apply to the nursing field.

When considering a nursing education, consider your personal needs. Is it best for you to work in a heavily structured environment or one that offers more flexibility in terms of, say, integrating a part-time work schedule into studies? Do you need to stay close to home? Do you prefer to work in a large health-care system such as a health maintenance organization or a medical center, or do you prefer smaller, community-based operations?

As for nursing programs, ask the following questions: How involved is the faculty in developing students for today's health-care industry? How strong is the school's affiliation with clinics and hospitals? Is there assurance that a student will gain an up-to-date educational experience for the current job market? Are a variety of care settings available? How much time in clinics is required for graduation? What are the program's resources in terms of computer and science laboratories? Does the school work with hospitals and community-based centers to provide health care? How available is the faculty to oversee a student's curriculum? What kind of student support is available in terms of study groups and audiovisual aids? Moreover, what kind of counseling from faculty members and administrators is available to help students develop well-rounded, effective progress through the program?

Visiting a school and talking to the program's guidance counselors will give you a better understanding of how a particular program or school will fit your needs. You can get a closer look at the faculty, its members' credentials, and the focus of the program. It's also not too early to consider what each program can offer in terms of job placement.

Master's Programs

Kathleen Dracup, D.N.Sc., RN, FNP, FAAN
Endowed Professor in Nursing Education and Former Dean
School of Nursing
University of California, San Francisco

The transformation of the health-care system is taking place as you read this, and it can be seen even today in the most common areas:

- A mother brings her child into a clinic for treatment of an earache. Instead of a physician, a nurse practitioner provides the care.
- A patient is readied for surgery. A variety of specialists move around the surgery room, but it's not a specially trained physician administering the anesthetic—it's a certified nurse anesthetist.
- During a patient's recovery from an acute illness, it's decided that the patient no longer needs to stay in the hospital but isn't well enough to return home. The best place to continue the recovery is an intermediate-care facility. Who makes that decision? A clinical nurse specialist. Who oversees the physical and emotional rehabilitation programs at this facility? Another clinical nurse specialist.

These health-care professionals are all advanced practice nurses (APNs). All have graduate-level degrees, and they serve as proof that the demand for nurses with master's and doctoral degrees for advanced practice, clinical specialties, teaching, and research will double the supply.

Another study estimated that the U.S. could save as much as $8.75 billion annually if APNs were used appropriately in place of physicians. As more and more of the restrictions on APNs succumb to legislative or economic forces, the demand for graduate-level nurses is expected to remain high.

Educational Core for APN

A master's degree in nursing is the educational core that allows advanced practice nurses to work as nurse practitioners, certified nurse-midwives, clinical nurse specialists, and certified nurse anesthetists.

Nurse practitioners conduct physical exams, diagnose and treat common acute illnesses and injuries, administer immunizations, manage chronic problems such as high blood pressure and diabetes, and order lab services and X-rays.

Nurse-midwives provide prenatal and gynecological care, deliver babies in hospitals and private settings such as homes, and follow up with postpartum care.

Clinical nurse specialists provide a range of care in specialty areas, such as oncology, pediatrics, and cardiac, neonatal, obstetric/gynecological, neurological, and psychiatric nursing.

Nurse anesthetists administer anesthesia for all types of surgery in operating rooms, dental offices, and outpatient surgical centers.

Master's degrees in nursing administration or nursing education are also available.

There are more than 340 master's degree programs accredited by the Commission on Collegiate Nursing Education (CCNE) or by the National League for Nursing Accrediting Commission (NLNAC). The wide spectrum of programs includes the Master of Science in Nursing (M.S.N.) degree, Master of Nursing (M.N.) degree, Master of Science (M.S.) degree with a nursing major, or Master of Arts (M.A.) degree with a nursing major. The specific degrees depend on the requirements set by the college or university or by the faculty of the nursing program. There are accelerated programs for RNs, which allow the nurse with a hospital diploma or associate degree to earn both a baccalaureate and a master's degree in a condensed program. Some schools offer accelerated master's degree programs for nurses with non-nursing degrees and for non-nursing college graduates. There are joint-degree programs, such as a master's in nursing combined with a Master of Business Administration, Master of Public Health, or Master of Hospital Administration.

Master's Curriculum

The master's degree builds on the baccalaureate degree to enable the student to develop expertise in one area. That specialty can range from running a hospital to providing care for prematurely born babies, from researching the effectiveness of alternative therapies to tackling social and economic causes of health problems. It is an opportunity for the student who has assessed his or her personal career goals and matched them to individual, community, and industry needs. What students can do with their APN degrees is limited only by their imagination.

Full-time master's programs consist of eighteen to twenty-four months of uninterrupted study. Many graduate school students, however, fit their master's-level studies around their work schedules, which can extend the time it takes to graduate.

Master's-level study incorporates theories and concepts of nursing science and their applications, along with the management of health care. Research provides a foundation for the improvement of health-care techniques. Students also have the opportunity to develop the knowledge, leadership skills, and interpersonal skills that will enable them to improve the health-care system.

Classroom and clinical work are involved throughout the master's program. In class, students spend less time listening to lectures and taking notes and more time participating in student-and faculty-led seminars and roundtable discussions. Extended clinical work is generally required.

Graduate-level education in many programs includes courses in statistics, research management, health economics, health policy, health-care ethics, health promotion, nutrition, family planning, mental health, and the prevention of family and social violence. When students begin to concentrate their study in their clinical areas, any number of courses that support their chosen specialty may be included. For example, a nurse wanting to specialize in pediatrics may take courses in child development.

A clinical nurse specialist can focus on acute care, geriatrics, adult health, community health, critical care, gerontology, rehabilitation, and cardiovascular, surgical, oncology, maternity/newborn, pediatric, mental/ psychiatric, and women's health nursing. Areas of specialization in nurse practitioner programs include acute care, adult health, child care, community health, emergency care, geriatric care, neonatal health, occupational health, and primary care.

Admission Requirements

The admission requirements for master's programs in nursing vary greatly. Generally, a bachelor's degree from a school accredited by the Commission on Collegiate Nursing Education or by the National League for Nursing Accrediting Commission and a state RN license are required. Scores from the Graduate Record Examinations (GRE) or the Miller Analogies Test (MAT), college transcripts, letters of reference, and an essay are also typically required. Non-nurses and nurses with non-nursing degrees have special requirements. The profiles and in-depth descriptions of colleges and universities in this publication will give you an idea of each school's specific requirements.

It is important to remember that admissions officers look at a student's transcripts, clinical work, and letters of reference together. A low grade point average is not an automatic knockout—admissions officers are after a composite package. Also, some specialties require specific courses. Students in the nurse anesthetist program, for instance, must have taken an upper-level college course in biochemistry.

A Master's That's Best for You

Most nurses who think of entering a master's program are already practicing nurses. They have a good idea of what they want to specialize in before they apply for admission. It is crucial to know what you want to study before you enter a master's program.

The best way to ensure success in a master's program is to understand your individual strengths and career desires and then find the faculty and college setting that are best suited to help you develop those strengths. Students must make an effort to educate themselves as to the strength of the faculty in each college's master's program. That's the best thing to look for: a strong faculty in one specialty.

This can be tricky. One university's master's program may be rated reasonably high in all fields. Another program might not be rated as high overall, but its cardiovascular program, for example, may be one of the best because of its access to facilities or the fact that its faculty is in the process of developing an innovative new treatment.

This type of information is not hard for the master's candidate to discover; it just takes time. Such information is available from each school's admissions office, which should be more than happy to promote its nursing faculty and support its opinion with proof, such as the research papers that faculty members have published in journals or the number of degrees each faculty member holds.

This type of research is the best way to find a program that meets your needs. The profiles of master's nursing programs in this book should help. If you can, narrow the list to three or four graduate schools, and then write each school's admissions department for catalogs and other information. Visit the schools and take time to talk to a guidance counselor from the nursing program in each one.

Other key questions to consider when applying for a master's program are: Does the school offer financial aid, such as loans, scholarships, fellowships, or teaching posts? How much clinical work is needed? Does the clinical work meet your needs, and does the type of clinical work involved match what you understand the health-care system will be using when you graduate? Is the course work flexible? Can you work part-time and still progress toward a master's degree? This is important to know. A majority of master's program students continue to work while they pursue the degree. Therefore, master's degree programs may present a flexible offering of short courses to meet the student's schedule demands.

Some programs require a thesis, whereas others provide another type of culminating experience, such as a comprehensive examination.

The Master's Trends

Today's master's programs have increased the amount of clinical practice required by students so that graduates enter the job market ready for certification. There is also a greater emphasis on applying new research findings to methods of patient care. This might involve students' reading literature about new treatments and then incorporating the appropriate changes.

All master's program candidates should consider courses in cost-benefit analysis. As managed-care systems become more predominant in the industry, health-care workers will be asked to justify the expense of each treatment, as well as its effectiveness. This leads to the crucial issue of quality. There will always be a strong effort to minimize costs in every health-care procedure, but that cannot compromise the quality of care. It's safe to say that discharging a newborn too soon from a hospital due to shortsightedness can be quite costly.

Depending on the specialty, master's candidates entering the job market may be expected to oversee auxiliary-care providers, such as nurse aides or other unlicensed employees. They may work in a team structure, and in this capacity, the nurse specialist may be expected to manage, motivate, and steer the group. This requires team-building and other management techniques.

While everyone in the health-care facility will have a part in ensuring patient satisfaction, nurses—particularly advanced

RN-to-Master's Degree Programs Fact Sheet

Currently, there are 161 programs available nationwide to transition RNs with diplomas and associate degrees to the master's degree level. These programs prepare nurses to assume positions requiring graduate preparation, including the advanced practice roles of nurse practitioner, clinical nurse specialist, certified nurse-midwife, and certified registered nurse anesthetist. Master's degree-prepared nurses are in high demand as expert clinicians, nurse executives, clinical educators, health policy consultants, and research assistants.

RN-to-master's degree programs generally take about three years to complete; specific requirements vary by institution and the student's previous course work. Although the majority of these programs are offered in traditional classroom settings, some RN-to-master's programs are offered largely online or in a blended classroom/online format.

The baccalaureate-level content missing from diploma and A.D.N. programs is built into the front end of the RN-to-master's degree program. Mastery of this upper-level basic nursing content is necessary for students to move on to graduate study. Upon completion, programs award both a baccalaureate and a master's degree.

The number of RN-to-master's degree programs in the United States has doubled within the past ten years. According to AACN's 2009 survey of nursing schools, twenty-seven new RN-to-M.S.N. programs are in the planning stages.

practice nurses—will shoulder a great deal of this load. Developing interpersonal and communication skills and having an understanding of human behavior will make it easier for the advanced practice nurse to help patients to understand modern health-care procedures, which will no doubt improve their feelings of satisfaction.

Finally, nurses at all levels should be aware of the need for flexibility. Many health-care organizations are reducing the number of beds in hospitals and transferring the care of a growing number of patients to other types of facilities or settings. In light of this trend, it's best for the master's program student to gain experience in a variety of settings, including homes, clinics, and community-based facilities.

The demand for high-quality care will continue to grow. Medical innovations and technological advances will continue. The quality and effectiveness of health care will continue to improve, and nurses with graduate degrees will play an active role in this trend.

The Hot Employment Spots

The health-care industry has undergone such radical transformation in the last five years that administrators feel they cannot predict whether any one geographic region will have more hirings than another. Generally, nurses with master's degrees will be in demand in all regions of the country, in both the United States and Canada.

Industry trends indicate that, along with continuing opportunities in hospitals, more and more nurses will also work outside the hospital in outpatient clinics and community settings—and even in businesses. As patients spend less time in hospitals, the need grows for nurse specialists to oversee home-care settings and ensure that the quality of care is high. In this vein, some nurses are taking the initiative and running their own businesses as health-care providers, offering services as they see fit in whatever locations are appropriate.

Immediate Rewards

Advanced practice nurses right out of school can expect annual salaries ranging from $60,000 to $90,000, depending on geographic location and previous experience. However, some rural county health clinics start their nurse practitioners at salaries as low as $40,000 per year.

Certified nurse anesthetists and certified nurse-midwives, however, draw higher salaries. Nurse-midwives, for example, can draw first-year salaries as high as $90,000 per year. Areas such as the Northeast and the West Coast tend to have nurses in these fields at the higher end of the salary scale. After five years of practice, the salary range for APNs stretches from $60,000 to $100,000 a year. Again, it depends on location. After five years, nurse-midwives earn salaries ranging from $65,000 to $120,000 annually.

THE CLINICAL NURSE LEADER

The Clinical Nurse Leader or CNL® is a rapidly emerging nursing role developed by the American Association of Colleges of Nursing (AACN) in collaboration with leaders from the nursing education and practice arenas. The national movement to advance the CNL is fueled by the critical need to improve the quality of patient care and better prepare nurses to thrive across the health-care system. The CNL role was developed following research and discussion with stakeholder groups as a way to engage highly skilled clinicians as leaders in outcome-based practices.

CNL provide lateral integration at the point of care and combine evidence-based practice with the following:

- Microsystems-level advocacy
- Centralized care coordination
- Outcomes measurement
- Risk assessment
- Quality improvement
- Interprofessional communication

In practice, the CNL oversees the care coordination of a distinct group of patients and actively provides direct patient care in complex situations. CNLs have master's degrees and are advanced generalists, evaluating patient outcomes, assessing risks, and using their authority to change care plans when necessary. CNLs are leaders in the health-care delivery system; the implementation of their roles will vary across settings.

Connecting Nursing Practice and Education

To support the creation of this new nursing role, AACN launched a national initiative involving more than 100 education-practice partnerships across the nation. Partners from schools of nursing and nursing practice sites are working together to transform care delivery by educating new CNLs and integrating them into the health delivery system.

More than seventy schools of nursing are now preparing CNLs for advanced generalist programs offered at the graduate level. Students may choose from traditional post-baccalaureate master's programs, degree completion programs for registered nurses (RNs), and accelerated programs for those seeking to make the transition into nursing. Most CNL programs are directly connected with practice sites interested in employing graduates to enhance care delivery, patient safety, and quality outcomes.

The Veterans Health Administration, the nation's largest employer of RNs, has embraced the CNL role and is planning to introduce it into all Veterans Affairs hospitals nationwide. Support for the clinical role is gaining momentum as many practice sites are reporting on the pioneering outcomes of the CNL staff.

The Key to Positive Patient Outcomes

CNLs provide efficient and cost-effective patient care services, as well as the leadership needed to repair fragmented health-care delivery systems. CNLs are having a measurable impact on the quality of nursing services with practice sites reporting that CNLs are

- quickly making significant progress on raising patient, nurse, and physician satisfaction; improving care outcomes; and realizing sizable cost-savings.
- elevating the level of practice for all nurses on the unit by promoting critical thinking and innovation in nursing care.
- constructively managing change and promoting a team-based approach to care.
- understanding the bigger picture, including outcomes and patient satisfaction, when considering next steps, needed changes, and improvements to the practice setting.

The CNL Mark of Excellence

The CNL Mark of Excellence certification is a unique credential that recognizes graduates of master's and post-master's CNL programs who have demonstrated accepted standards of practice. The CNL Mark of Excellence promotes safe, quality practice through its ongoing requirements for personal and professional growth. In 2007, AACN established a new certification commission—the Commission on Nurse Certification (CNC)—to oversee all aspects of the CNL certification program.

Becoming a CNL

Those interested in becoming a CNL are encouraged to visit the AACN Web site, www.aacn.nche.edu/CNL, to find out more about this nursing career option. Detailed information is available online, including frequently asked questions, the white paper on the CNL role, and a directory of Web links for related programs.

ACCELERATED PROGRAMS

With the Bureau of Labor Statistics projecting the need for more than one million new and replacement registered nurses by the year 2016, nursing schools across North America are exploring creative ways to increase student capacity and reach out to new student populations. The challenge inherent in these efforts is to quickly produce competent nurses while maintaining the integrity and quality of the nursing education provided.

One innovative approach to nursing education that is gaining momentum nationwide is the accelerated degree program for non-nursing graduates. Offered at the baccalaureate and master's degree levels, these programs build on previous learning experiences and transition individuals with undergraduate degrees in other disciplines into nursing.

Shifts in the economy and the desire of many adults to make a post–September 11 difference in their work have increased interest in the nursing profession among "second-degree" students. For those with a prior degree, accelerated baccalaureate programs offer the quickest route to becoming a registered nurse, with programs generally running twelve to eighteen months. Generic master's degrees, also accelerated and geared to non-nursing graduates, generally take three years to finish. Students in these programs usually complete baccalaureate-level nursing courses in the first year, followed by two years of graduate study.

Though not new to nursing education, accelerated programs have proliferated over the past twenty years. In 1990, thirty-one accelerated baccalaureate (B.S.N.) programs and twelve generic master's (M.S.N.) programs were offered around the country.

Today, 205 accelerated baccalaureate nursing programs are operating, and the number of generic master's programs has increased to fifty-six. According to AACN's database on enrollment and graduations, which is based on responses from 645 of 751 institutions (86 percent), thirty-seven new accelerated B.S.N. programs are now in the planning stages. This number far outpaces all other types of entry-level nursing programs currently being considered at four-year nursing schools. Thirteen new generic master's programs are also taking shape.

Graduates of accelerated programs are prized by nurse employers, who value the many layers of skill and education these graduates bring to the workplace. Employers report that these graduates are more mature, possess strong clinical skills, and are quick studies on the job. Many practice settings are partnering with schools and offering tuition repayment to graduates as a mechanism to recruit highly qualified nurses.

Changing Gears: Second-Degree Students

The typical second-degree nursing student is motivated, older, and has higher academic expectations than high school–entry baccalaureate students. Accelerated students excel in class and are eager to gain clinical experiences. Faculty members see them as excellent learners who are not afraid to challenge their instructors.

"Our accelerated students are a remarkable group," said Nancy DeBasio, Ph.D., RN, Dean of the Research College of Nursing in Kansas City. "Their mean GPA is 3.3, they come from a wide array of backgrounds, and the experiences they bring with them enrich their nursing." The compressed program format is a key motivator for this group of students. "Our exit surveys indicate that the one-year program completion time is a primary reason for enrollment in our program," Dr. DeBasio explained.

Second-degree students bring new dimensions to nursing and a rich history of prior learning. "We are seeing a steady increase in applicants to our accelerated program this year, and those accepted come with backgrounds that are varied and impressive," said Janet B. Younger, Ph.D., RN, CPNP, Professor and Associate Dean of the School of Nursing at Virginia Commonwealth University. "We welcomed several Ph.D.'s, some M.D.'s from other countries, and a few fine arts majors. These students excel in class and perform very well post-graduation."

Students in accelerated programs are competitive, maintain high grade point averages, and almost always pass the NCLEX-RN licensure exam on the first attempt. "Second-degree candidates are excellent students and are very likely to see the program through to graduation," said Afaf Meleis, Ph.D., RN, FAAN, Dean of the University of Pennsylvania School of Nursing. "These students are committed to their studies, actively engaged in research, and very often involved in university organizations."

Susan M. Di Biase, M.S.N., CRNP, a faculty member at Jacksonville State University in Alabama, knows a thing or two about second-degree students. She was one. "As a nurse educator, I have taught dozens of second-degree students who often distinguish themselves as class leaders," explained Di Biase. "When I was taking classes, I thought the students were strong academically, and many said nursing was harder than their first degree. My first employer made a custom of hiring second-degree students because she thought they were good thinkers and strong patient advocates."

Accelerated Baccalaureate Programs

Accelerated baccalaureate programs accomplish programmatic objectives in a shorter time frame than traditional four-year programs, usually through a combination of bridge courses and core content. Instruction is intense, with courses offered full-time with no breaks between sessions. Students receive the same number of clinical hours as their counterparts in traditional programs. Admission standards are high, with programs typically requiring a minimum of a 3.0 GPA and a thorough prescreening process. Typically, students with a prior degree are not required to take the liberal arts content included in a four-year B.S.N. program. Accelerated programs do have prerequisites, many of which may have been completed during the student's initial degree program. "Before students can begin our program, their college transcripts are reviewed to assure that all prerequisites are met," stated Maureen C. Creegan, Ed.D., RN, Nursing Program Director at Dominican College (NY). "Almost all students meet the arts and social sciences requirements; most do not meet the natural sciences requirements, including anatomy and microbiology. To assist students, we offer back-to-back prerequisite courses just prior to the start of the accelerated program."

Accelerated programs require a heavy credit load and intense clinical experiences. Identifying students who will flourish in this environment is a priority for administrators. "Due to the intensity of the program, an interview was added to the admission process to better screen students," explained Maryann O. Forbes, Ph.D., RN, Associate Professor at Adelphi University. "Faculty members feel that the interview and ongoing mentoring are key components to student success. The most successful accelerated students are bright, inquisitive, and sophisticated consumers of higher education who actively pursue learning opportunities," said Harriet Feldman, Ph.D., RN, FAAN, Dean and Professor at the Lienhard School of Nursing at Pace University (NY), whose Combined Degree Program (B.S.N./M.S.) has been in existence since 1984. "As adults, these students tend to know what they need and aggressively pursue programs that best meet their needs: fast-tracked, competitive, and well respected. While some students do attend part-time, most are full-time students who want to reach their career objective as quickly and efficiently as possible."

"Our accelerated B.S.N. program attracts second-career seekers who are unable to make the time and financial commitment to a generic master's program," explained Elizabeth F. McGann, D.N.Sc., RN, BC, Professor and Former Chair of the Department of Nursing at Quinnipiac University (CT). "Our program gives students the option of entering basic nursing practice now with graduate education as a potential future step."

Generic Master's Degree Programs

Having already completed a degree at the baccalaureate or graduate level, many second-degree students are attracted to the generic master's program as the natural next step in their higher education. "Why would a bachelor's-prepared applicant, thinking about a career in health care, want to get a second bachelor's in nursing when they can get a professional master's or doctorate in every other health-care field?," asked Melanie Dreher, Ph.D., RN, FAAN, Dean of the Rush University College of Nursing. Recently approved by the state board, Iowa's professional Master's Degree in Nursing and Healthcare Practice may be completed in four semesters, including a semester-long clinical internship that occurs five days a week for three months.

"In 1974, Yale University was the first school to open its door to college graduates who were not yet nurses and instituted the Graduate Entry Prespecialty in Nursing (GEPN)," explained Sharon Sanderson, Director of Student Recruitment for Yale's School of Nursing. "We recognized that bright, committed people without a background in nursing could be prepared as advanced practice nurses." At Marquette University in Wisconsin, students admitted into the direct-entry M.S.N. program are high achievers. "Our students are self-motivated, have definite goals, demonstrate good study habits, and succeed," explained Judith Fitzgerald Miller, Ph.D., RN, FAAN, former Interim Dean of the College of Nursing.

"Our generic M.S.N. students bring a wonderful expertise to the class," said Arlene Lowenstein Ph.D., RN, Professor Emerita, and former Director of the Graduate Program in Nursing at MGH Institute of Health Professions in Boston. "We run the gamut from a 53-year-old male lawyer, students holding Ph.D.'s and master's degrees in other fields, and students fresh out of a liberal arts program. One of my past students was a horticulture major who wrote a paper on therapeutic gardens for health-care settings. As they learn from us, we also learn from them, and they learn from each other. Second-degree students are a challenging, exciting group with the potential to make significant contributions to nursing as well as to their patients, families, and communities."

Interest in generic M.S.N. programs is running high. In Chicago, the DePaul University program grew from 20 students two years ago to 48 students last fall with a minimal amount of advertising. "With little more than a one-sentence notice about the program on the school's Web site when the program was announced, we received more than 100 inquiries and more than forty applications in short order," said Kathryn Anderson, Ph.D., RN, Graduate Program Director at the Seattle University School of Nursing. "Based on this initial response, it's obvious that the most effective marketing tool is the program itself."

Many universities offer both accelerated baccalaureate and generic master's programs with opportunities for students to apply credits to both degree programs. New York University, for example, offers a dual-degree program that enables B.S.N. students to take a maximum of 9 credits at the graduate level while completing the bachelor's degree, thus accelerating the completion of an M.S.N.

Education-Practice Setting Partnerships

Nurse employers recognize the value and skills that second-degree students bring to the work setting, as evidenced by the growing number of partnerships forming to support these graduates. "Our cooperative relationship with Poudre Valley Hospital brings the educational and practice settings closer together with clinical nurses at the hospital serving in faculty roles," explained Sandra Baird, Ed.D., B.S.N., Director of the School of Nursing at the University of North Colorado. The school is working to branch out and establish cooperative relationships with a wider network of health-care settings. "Second-degree students are a very attractive catch for any health-care institution and many are willing to fund them in exchange for work commitments after graduation," said Donna

Ayers Snelson, M.S.N., D.Ed., RN, Associate Professor and Director of Center for Nursing History at College Misericordia (PA). Although Creighton University (NE) is a private institution with a significantly higher tuition than that of public institutions, the reputation of its program led two Omaha health systems and four rural hospitals to offer full-tuition scholarships to accelerated nursing students in exchange for employment commitments. "More than half of the students in the accelerated baccalaureate program accepted tuition scholarships from area hospitals in return for a commitment to work in basic practice prior to going on for a master's degree," added Linda Cronenwett, Ph.D., RN, FAAN, Professor at the School of Nursing at University of North Carolina–Chapel Hill. Research College of Nursing uses grant-funded initiatives and clinical connections to build student capacity. "Recently we received a $100,000 grant from the Helene Fuld Health Trust to support financial aid for our accelerated students," said Dean Nancy DeBasio. "Fuld had never supported this type of student before, but we were able to demonstrate that these students were economically disadvantaged, not always eligible for traditional undergraduate funding, and unable to work due to the program's intensity." The school also partners with a local health-care system to secure educational debt repayment for accelerated students in exchange for work commitments. It is projected that this arrangement will save the health system more than $3 million in nurse recruitment costs over three years.

Nursing Education in the Fast Lane

Although accelerated programs have proven to produce highly qualified nurses, the programs do present some unique challenges to nursing education. "Teaching accelerated students can be challenging because of their experience, age, and high level of inquiry," said Mary E. Pike, M.S.N., RN, faculty member at Bellarmine University (KY). "Some students struggle with the transition from being a competent, worldly adult to returning to life as an undergraduate student." One key to facilitating this transition and encouraging student success is using experienced faculty members who are comfortable teaching adults. In instances where employers are not repaying educational debt, the cost of an accelerated program can be prohibitive. "I receive many inquiries about our accelerated program, but the lack of financial aid is the major deterrent," said Arlene G. Wiens, Ph.D., RN, Nursing Department Chair at Eastern Mennonite University (VA). Some find the pace of accelerated programs too intense, and they opt for more regularly paced programs offered for second-degree nursing students. "The accelerated format is taxing, and some find it too difficult to assimilate into their daily routines," said Louann Zinsmeister, Ph.D., RN, Associate Professor at Messiah College (PA). "These students often transfer into a more traditionally paced two-year B.S.N. program that permits them to continue working and attend to family responsibilities while completing a nursing degree." For students who cannot accommodate full-time study, schools are looking for creative alternatives. "We are opening a part-time evening program so second-degree students and adult learners can obtain a degree while working full-time," added Donna Ayers Snelson of College Misericordia. "Students attend classes two nights a week and are still able to obtain a nursing degree in two years and one semester."

Post-Graduation Success

In addition to nursing skills, second-degree students bring additional layers of education and significant work experience to their role as nurses, which enhances their clinical practice. "Initially when we began our program in 1991, our clinical partners were quite doubtful about what we could produce in one year," explained Dr. DeBasio of the Research College of Nursing. "Now they are at our doorstep each year to snap up students as they graduate." The college has tracked students through their careers and found that accelerated students move into management positions more quickly and generally excel in their roles." Employers of advanced practice nurses (APN) are equally pleased with graduates from both our traditional and generic M.S.N. programs," stated Linda D. Norman, D.S.N., RN, FAAN, Senior Associate Dean for Academics at Vanderbilt University School of Nursing. Employers rated Vanderbilt's M.S.N. graduates who did not have a nursing background equally high in terms of level of preparation for APN positions as those who entered with a B.S.N. degree. "We know that employers love hiring accelerated graduates because they are bright, have a track record of success, and possess an understanding of the work world not always found in younger students," said Patricia Ladewig, Ph.D., RN, Former Dean of the School of Health Care Professions at Regis University in Denver. "We have found that second-degree students are readily accepted by employers who understand that these graduates lacked only vacation during their academic program," confirmed Sandra S. Angell, M.L.A., RN, Associate Dean for Student Affairs at The Johns Hopkins University School of Nursing.

Growing Demand for Accelerated Programs

With a greater number of second-degree students turning to nursing, the demand for accelerated programs is growing. "Within two weeks of the program's approval by the state board and without any public announcement, we received more than fifty requests for applications almost immediately," explained Marianne W. Rogers, Ed.D., RN, former Chairperson for Nursing at the University of Southern Maine. "Our program is growing very quickly, and we have seen almost a 100 percent increase in applications compared to last year," said Linda A. Bernhard, Ph.D., RN, Associate Professor, Graduate Studies and Research at The Ohio State University. The 16-month Second Career/Second Degree program in nursing at Wayne State University in Michigan is one of the school's most popular degree offerings. Enrollment in the University of Virginia's second-degree program has doubled since it was introduced. "At this time, we are seeing an enormous increase in the numbers of applicants with bachelor's degrees applying for our new 12-month accelerated pathway to the B.S.N.," reports Christena Langley, Ph.D., RN, Assistant Dean for Undergraduate Programs at the College of Nursing and Health Science at George Mason University (VA). "Many of them are recent college graduates who are looking for the quickest route to the B.S.N. They are confident that they can adapt to the accelerated pace given their past success in college."

Supporting Accelerated Nursing Programs

Second-degree students bring a wealth of knowledge, experience, and energy to the nursing workforce and are highly skilled clinicians. With calls for nursing schools to produce more graduates in response to the nursing shortage, a similar call should go out to employers and legislators to increase support for accelerated nursing programs. Hospitals, health-care systems, and other practice settings are encouraged to form partnerships with schools offering accelerated programs to remove the student's financial burden in exchange for a steady stream of new nurse recruits. Legislators on the state and federal levels are encouraged to increase scholarship and grant funding for these programs that produce entry-level nurses faster than any other basic nursing education program. These programs are ideal career transition vehicles for those segments of the labor force impacted by recent fluctuations in the economy." The overwhelming response to our accelerated programs demonstrates the existence of a deep pool of career changers available to nursing," said Gloria F. Donnelly, Ph.D., RN, FAAN, Dean of the College of Nursing and Health Professions at Drexel University (PA). "We need to do more to remove barriers and attract more second-degree students to the nursing profession."

"Accelerated Programs: The Fast-Track to Careers in Nursing," updated April 2008. Reprinted with permission of the American Association of Colleges of Nursing.

The Doctor of Nursing Practice

In October 2004, the American Association of Colleges of Nursing (AACN) endorsed the Position Statement on the Practice Doctorate in Nursing, which called for moving the level of preparation necessary for advanced nursing practice roles from the master's degree to the doctorate level by the year 2015. The AACN position statement calls for educating advanced practice nurses (APNs) and other nurses seeking top clinical positions in Doctor of Nursing Practice (DNP) programs. The following points explain this evolutionary step forward for nursing education.

The Need for Change in Graduate Nursing Education

- The changing demands of the nation's complex health-care environment require that nurses serving in specialty positions have the highest level of scientific knowledge and practice expertise possible. Research from Drs. Linda Aiken, Carole Estabrooks, and others have established a clear link between higher levels of nursing education and better patient outcomes.
- Some of the many factors that are emerging to build momentum for change in nursing education at the graduate level include the rapid expansion of knowledge underlying practice, increased complexity of patient care, national concerns about the quality of care and patient safety, shortages of nursing personnel that demand a higher level of preparation for leaders who can design and assess care, shortages of doctorally prepared nursing faculty, and increasing educational expectations for the preparation of other health professionals.
- The Institute of Medicine, Joint Commission on the Accreditation of Healthcare Organizations, and other authorities have called for reconceptualizing health professions education to meet the needs of the health-care delivery system. Nursing is answering that call by moving to prepare APNs for an evolving practice.
- In a 2005 report titled "Advancing the Nation's Health Needs: NIH Research Training Programs," the National Academy of Sciences called for nursing to develop a non-research clinical doctorate to prepare expert practitioners who can also serve as clinical faculty. AACN's work to advance the DNP is consistent with this call to action.
- Nursing is moving in the direction of other health professions in the transition to the DNP. Medicine (MD), Dentistry (DDS), Pharmacy (PharmD), Psychology (PsyD), Physical Therapy (DPT), and Audiology (AudD) all offer practice doctorates.

Impact on Nursing Education and Practice

- Currently, advanced practice nurses, including nurse practitioners, clinical nurse specialists, nurse midwives, and nurse-anesthetists, are typically prepared in master's degree programs, some of which carry a credit load equivalent to doctoral degrees in the other health professions.
- DNP curricula build on current master's programs by providing education in evidence-based practice, quality improvement, and systems thinking, among other key areas.
- Transitioning to the DNP will not alter the current scope of practice for APNs. State Nurse Practice Acts describes the scope of practice allowed, and it differs from state to state. (These requirements would likely remain unchanged.) The transition to the DNP will better prepare APNs for their current roles, given the calls for new models of education and the growing complexity of health care.
- The DNP is designed for nurses seeking a terminal degree in nursing practice and offers an alternative to research-focused doctoral programs. DNP-prepared nurses will be well-equipped to fully implement the science developed by nurse researchers prepared in PhD, DNSc, and other research-focused nursing doctorates.
- The title of doctor is common to many disciplines and is not the domain of any one health profession. Many APNs currently hold doctoral degrees and are addressed as doctors, which is similar to the way in which clinical psychologists, dentists, podiatrists, and other experts are addressed. Like other providers, DNPs would be expected to display their credentials to insure that patients understand their preparation as a nursing provider.
- Nursing and medicine are distinct health disciplines that prepare clinicians to assume different roles and meet different practice expectations. DNP programs will prepare nurses for the highest level of nursing practice.

THE NURSE PH.D.: A VITAL PROFESSION NEEDS LEADERS

Carole A. Anderson, Ph.D., RN, FAAN
Dean of the College of Dentistry
The Ohio State University

There is no doubt that education is the path for a nurse to achieve greater clinical expertise. At the same time, however, the nursing profession needs more nurses educated at the doctoral level to replenish the supply of faculty and researchers. The national shortage of faculty will soon reach critical proportions, making a significant impact on educational programs and their capacity to educate future generations of nursing students.

Although the number of doctorate programs has continued to increase, the total enrollment of students in these programs has remained fairly constant, resulting in a shortage of newly trained Ph.D.'s to renew faculty ranks. As a result, approximately 50 percent of nursing faculty possess the doctorate as a terminal degree. Furthermore, with many advances being made in the treatment of chronic illnesses, there is a continuing need for research that assists patients in living with their illness. This research requires individual investigators who are prepared on the doctoral level.

One reason there is a lack of nurses prepared at the doctoral level is that, compared to other professions, nurses have more interruptions in their careers. Many in the profession are women who work as nurses while fulfilling responsibilities as wives and mothers. As a result, many pursue their education on a part-time basis. Also, the nursing profession traditionally has viewed clinical experience as being a prerequisite to graduate education. This career path results in fewer individuals completing the doctorate at an earlier stage in their career, thereby truncating their productivity as academics, researchers, and administrators. To reverse this trend, many nursing schools have developed programs that admit students into graduate (doctoral and master's) programs directly from their undergraduate or master's programs.

Nursing Research

When nurses do research for their doctorates, many people tend to think that it focuses primarily on nurses and nursing care. In reality, nurses carry out clinical research in a variety of areas, such as diabetes care, cancer care, and eating disorders.

In the last twenty years advances in medicine have involved, for the most part, advancing treatment, not cures. In other words, no cure for the illness has been discovered, but treatment for that illness has improved. However, sometimes the treatment itself causes problems for patients, such as the unwelcome side effects of chemotherapy. Nurses have opportunities to devise solutions to problems like these through research, such as studies on how to manage the illness and its treatment, thereby allowing individuals to lead happy and productive lives.

The Curricula

Doctoral programs in nursing are aimed at preparing students for careers in health administration, education, clinical research, and advanced clinical practice. Basically, doctoral programs prepare nurses to be experts within the profession, prepared to assume leadership roles in a variety of academic and clinical settings, course work, and research. Students are trained as researchers and scholars to tackle complex health-care questions. Program emphasis may vary from a focus on health education to a concentration on policy research. The majority of doctoral programs confer the Doctor of Philosophy (Ph.D.) degree, but some award the Doctor of Nursing Science (D.N.S. or D.N.Sc.), the Doctor of Science in Nursing (D.S.N.), the Nursing Doctorate (N.D.), and the Doctor of Education (Ed.D.).

Doctoral nursing programs traditionally offer courses on the history and philosophy of nursing and the development and testing of nursing and other health-care techniques, as well as the social, economic, political, and ethical issues important to the field. Data management and research methodology are also areas of instruction. Students are expected to work individually on research projects and complete a dissertation.

Doctoral programs allow study on a full-or part-time basis. For graduate students who are employed and therefore seek flexibility in their schedules, many programs offer courses on weekends and in the evenings.

Admission Requirements

Admission requirements for doctoral programs vary. Generally, a master's degree is necessary, but in some schools a master's degree is completed in conjunction with fulfillment of the doctoral degree requirements. Standard requirements include an RN license, Graduate Record Examinations (GRE) scores, college transcripts, letters of recommendation, and an essay. Students applying for doctoral-level study should have a solid foundation in nursing and an interest in research. Programs are usually the equivalent of three to five years of full-time study.

Selecting a Doctoral Program

Selecting a doctoral program comes down to personal choice. Students work closely with professors, and thus the support and mentoring you receive while pursuing your degree is as vital as the quality of the facilities. The most important question is whether there is a "match" between your research interest and faculty research. Many of the same questions you would ask about baccalaureate and master's degree programs apply to doctoral programs. However, in a doctoral program, the contact with professors, the use of research equipment and facilities, and the program's flexibility in allowing you to choose your course of study are critical.

Other questions to consider include: Does the university consider research a priority? Does the university have adequate funding for student research? Many nurses with doctoral degrees make the natural transition into an academic career, but there are many other career options available for nurses prepared at this level. For example, nurses prepared at the doctoral level are often hired by large consulting firms to work with others in designing solutions to health-care delivery problems.

Others are hired by large hospital chains to manage various divisions, and some nurses with doctoral degrees are hired to manage complex health-care systems at the executive level. On another front, they conduct research and formulate national and international health-care policy. In short, because of the high level of education and a shortage of nurses prepared at this level, there are a number of options.

Needless to say, a doctoral education does provide individuals with a wide range of opportunities, with salaries commensurate with the type and level of responsibilities. Are there opportunities to present research findings at professional meetings? Is scholarship of faculty, alumni, and students presented at regional and national nursing meetings and subsequently published? Has the body of research done at a university enhanced the knowledge of nursing and health care?

Salaries are related to the various positions. Faculty salaries vary by the type of institution and by faculty rank, typically ranging from approximately $50,000 at the assistant professor level to above $100,000 at the professor level. Salaries of nurse executives also vary, with the lowest salaries being in small rural hospitals and the highest being in complex university medical centers. In the latter, average salaries are well above $100,000 and often reach close to $200,000 annually. Consultant salaries are wide-ranging but often consist of a base plus some percentage of work contracted. Clinical and research positions vary considerably by the type of institution and the nature of the work.

AACN Indicators of Quality in Research-Focused Doctoral Programs in Nursing

Schools of nursing must consider the indicators of quality in evaluating their ability to mount research-focused doctoral programs. High-quality programs require a large number of increasingly scarce resources and a critical mass of faculty members and students. The "AACN Indicators of Quality in Research-Focused Doctoral Programs in Nursing" represent those indicators that should be present in a research-focused program.

There is considerable consensus within the discipline that while there are differences in the purpose and curricula of Ph.D. and Doctor of Nursing/Doctor of Nursing Science programs; most programs emphasize preparation for research. Therefore, AACN recommends continuing with a single set of quality indicators for research-focused doctoral programs in nursing, whether the program leads to a Ph.D. or to a Doctor of Nursing or Doctor of Nursing Science degree.

The following indicators apply to the Doctor of Philosophy (Ph.D.) in nursing, Doctor of Nursing Science (D.N.S. or D.N.Sc.), and Doctor of Nursing (N.D.) degrees.

Faculty

I. Represent and value a diversity of backgrounds and intellectual perspectives.

II. Meet the requirements of the parent institution for graduate research and doctoral education; a substantial proportion of faculty hold earned doctorates in nursing.

III. Conceptualize and implement productive programs of research and scholarship that are developed over time and build upon previous work, are at the cutting edge of the field of inquiry, are congruent with research priorities within nursing and its constituent communities, include a substantial proportion of extramural funding, and attract and engage students.

IV. Create an environment in which mentoring, socialization of students, and the existence of a community of scholars is evident.

V. Assist students in understanding the value of programs of research and scholarship that continue over time and build upon previous work.

VI. Identify, generate, and utilize resources within the university and the broader community to support program goals.

VII. Devote a significant proportion of time to dissertation advisement. Generally, each faculty member should serve as the major adviser/chair for no more than 3 to 5 students during the dissertation phase.

Programs of Study

The emphasis of the program of study is consistent with the mission of the parent institution, the discipline of nursing, and the degree awarded. The faculty's areas of expertise and scholarship determine specific foci in the program of study. Requirements and their sequence for progression in the program are clear and available to students in writing. Common elements of the program of study are outlined below.

I. Core and related course content—the distribution between nursing and supporting content is consistent with the mission and goals of the program, and the student's area of focus and course work are included in the following:

   A. Historical and philosophical foundations to the development of nursing knowledge

   B. Existing and evolving substantive nursing knowledge

   C. Methods and processes of theory/knowledge development

   D. Research methods and scholarship appropriate to inquiry

   E. Development related to roles in academic, research, practice, or policy environments

II. Elements for formal and informal teaching and learning focus on the following:

   A. Analytical and leadership strategies for dealing with social, ethical, cultural, economic, and political issues related to nursing, health care, and research

   B. Progressive and guided student scholarship

research experiences, including exposure to faculty's interdisciplinary research programs

C. Immersion experiences that foster the student's development as a nursing leader, scholarly practitioner, educator, and/or nurse scientist

D. Socialization opportunities for scholarly development in roles that complement students' career goals

III. Outcome indicators for the programs of study include the following:

A. Advancement to candidacy requires faculty's satisfactory evaluation (e.g., comprehensive exam) of the student's basic knowledge of elements I-A through I-E identified above

B. Dissertations represent original contributions to the scholarship of the field

C. Systematic evaluation of graduate outcomes is conducted at regular intervals

D. Within three to five years of completion, graduates have designed and secured funding for a research study, or, within two years of completion, graduates have utilized the research process to address an issue of importance to the discipline of nursing or health care within their employment setting

E. Employers report satisfaction with graduates' leadership and scholarship at regular intervals

F. Graduates' scholarship and leadership are recognized through awards, honors, or external funding within three to five years of completion

Resources

I. Sufficient human, financial, and institutional resources are available to accomplish the goals of the unit for doctoral education and faculty research.

A. The parent institution exhibits the following characteristics:

1) Research is an explicit component of the mission of the parent institution

2) An office of research administration

3) A record of peer-reviewed external funding

4) Postdoctoral programs

5) Internal research funds

6) Mechanisms that value, support, and reward faculty and student scholarship and role preparation

7) A university environment that fosters interdisciplinary research and collaboration

B. The nursing doctoral program exhibits the following characteristics:

1) Research-active faculty as well as other faculty experts to mentor students in other role preparations

2) Provide technical support for the following:

(a) Peer review of proposals and manuscripts in their development phases

(b) Research design expertise

(c) Data management and analysis support

(d) Hardware and software availability

(e) Expertise in grant proposal development and management

3) Procure space sufficient for the following:

(a) Faculty research needs

(b) Doctoral student study, meeting, and socializing

(c) Seminars

(d) Small-group work

C. Schools of exceptional quality also have the following:

1) Centers of research excellence

2) Endowed professorships

3) Mechanisms for financial support to allow full-time study

4) Master teachers capable of preparing graduates for faculty roles

II. State-of-the-art technical and support services are available and accessible to faculty, students, and staff for state-of-the-science information acquisition, communication, and management.

III. Library and database resources are sufficient to support the scholarly endeavors of faculty and students.

Students

I. Students are selected from a pool of highly qualified and motivated applicants who represent diverse populations.

II. Students' research goals and objectives are congruent with faculty research expertise and scholarship and institutional resources.

III. Students are successful in obtaining financial support through competitive intramural and extramural academic and research awards.

IV. Students commit a significant portion of their time to the program and complete the program in a timely fashion.

V. Students establish a pattern of productive scholarship, collaborating with researchers in nursing and other disciplines in scientific endeavors that result in the presentation and publication of scholarly work that continues after graduation.

Evaluation

The evaluation plan includes the following:

I. Is systematic, ongoing, comprehensive, and focuses on the university's and program's specific mission and goals.

II. Includes both process and outcome data related to these indicators of quality in research-focused doctoral programs.

III. Adheres to established ethical and process standards for formal program evaluation, e.g., confidentiality and rigorous quantitative and qualitative analyses.

IV. Involves students and graduates in evaluation activities.

V. Includes data from a variety of internal and external constituencies.

VI. Provides for comparison of program processes and outcomes to the standards of its parent graduate school/university and selected peer groups within nursing.

VII. Includes ongoing feedback to program faculty, administrators, and external constituents to promote program improvement.

VIII. Provides comprehensive data in order to determine patterns and trends and recommend future directions at regular intervals.

IX. Is supported with adequate human, financial, and institutional resources.

Approved by AACN Membership, November 2001.

What You Need to Know About Online Learning

Rosalee C. Yeaworth, Ph.D., RN, FAAN
Professor and Dean Emerita
College of Nursing
University of Nebraska Medical Center

Sue Schmidt, M.A. in Education and Human Development
Instructional Chair
Colorado Mountain College

Half a century ago, young women who graduated from high school and chose to enter a nursing program were expected to move into a "nurses' home," which housed not only dormitory-style rooms but also classrooms and faculty offices. Most of the clinical learning was done in apprenticeship style in a single hospital setting. There was no such thing as distance learning.

However, over the course of the past half-century, nursing education, like health care and education in general, has changed dramatically, creating a need for educators to implement distance education programs. The demographics of nursing students have changed. Not only is the nursing student far more likely to be a man than fifty years ago, but also the student who once was referred to as "nontraditional" is now becoming the traditional student. These students are mature, employed individuals who have complex family responsibilities and often live or work some distance from the university offering the courses they wish to take. The rapid advances in health-care knowledge and technology have increased the demand for nurses with graduate degrees. All nurses are faced with the need to enhance their knowledge through lifelong education as their roles and expectations change. In addition, a much greater effort is being made to provide education and training to residents in rural settings in the hope that they will continue to live and work in these areas.

Universities are addressing these changing educational needs by using advanced technologies and new communication capabilities. Distance learning offerings are continually enhanced by using new technologies and delivery systems such as the Internet and desktop videoconferencing. These technologies enable universities to reach beyond the boundaries imposed on them by traditional classrooms to deliver educational material to students located in different, noncentralized locations, thus allowing instruction and learning to occur independently of time and place. This model, known as "distributive learning," can be used in combination with traditional classroom-based courses and with traditional distance learning courses, or to create wholly virtual classrooms.

Tools used for distance education include the following:

E-mail: This is one of the most commonly used communication tools. It allows for a one-to-one exchange of information between the sender and receiver of the e-mail message. Course papers and draft materials may be sent, commented on, and returned as attached documents.

Listservs: This is a one-to-many communication exchange. People subscribe to listservs based on discussion topics that interest them. When a participant on a listserv sends an e-mail to the listserv, the message is copied and sent to all people who have subscribed to it. Listservs are generally free; there is no charge to subscribe.

Discussion Groups: This is a many-to-many communication exchange. E-mail and listservs deliver the messages directly to your electronic mailbox. Discussion groups, on the other hand, are retained in a specified area on the Internet. You must go to the discussion group to post your comments and read and reply to the comments of others. The advantage of a discussion group over e-mail or listservs is that the comments can be viewed easily by all and the sequence of comments and replies posted is readily apparent in its structure.

Chat Rooms: Chat is synchronous communication; the participants are online at the same time talking to each other. E-mail, listservs, and discussion groups, on the other hand, are asynchronous communication. With moderated chat, a moderator views the questions and comments posed by the participants and selects those that will be seen by all participants. After posting the comment or question, the moderator answers it. In a regular chat room, there is no management over what is or is not posted.

Streaming Video: Entire lectures can be delivered using streaming video technology. Even students accessing the material with slower modems can receive clear audio and good video images.

Desktop Videoconferencing: With a small camera mounted on top of the computer, students and faculty members are able to see and talk with each other using desktop videoconferencing software.

Virtual Reality: Student lounges can be constructed visually using virtual reality software. When students want to have a discussion with other students, they literally walk into the lounge as an avatar (a visual image of themselves they have selected) and hold live chat sessions with their fellow classmates.

Web Sites: Components of or the entire course content can be delivered via the Internet through the creation of a Web site. Any or all of the technology tools noted above can be linked through an educational Web site. Among other things, a Web site includes the syllabus, discussion groups, assignments, student lounges, faculty information, resources (including links to Web documents that enrich the course content), lecture notes, and other course components. Traditional distance education tools, such as satellite transmission, videotapes, telephone conferences, correspondence material, and CD-ROM interactive instruction, are also frequently used in conjunction with Web-delivered course material.

The key to using technology successfully is to define your goals and objectives and then decide which technology or combination of technologies will be most effective. Keep in mind that faculty members and students must have the appropriate computer equipment and user knowledge to participate in distance learning.

Even though computers today are much more user-friendly, it is important to allot some time for students to become accustomed to using the new technologies necessary for transmitting their course material. Campus information technology services should work closely with the faculty to prepare introductory manuals or self-help materials for students. Information technology specialists should be available to answer technology questions or solve problems so that faculty members can concentrate on the course content questions. Enthusiasm can be dampened if too much time must be devoted to learning the technology or dealing with technology problems.

When deciding to take distance-learning courses, other factors must be considered. What you need to participate in distance learning varies with the sophistication of the tools used by the course instructor. Sending and receiving e-mail, participating in discussion groups, and viewing online syllabi require fairly simple technology. You need a computer with a modem and an Internet service provider (ISP). When selecting an ISP, participants should consider cost, reliability of access, and speed. World Wide Web access provided through your cable provider is generally more expensive but provides significantly faster access to documents.

Video streaming and desktop videoconferencing require more sophisticated computer systems. Sometimes, in rural areas, the local telephone company or the Internet or TV provider may provide only limited services. Students may find, for example, that they have to use a teleconference line for sound with desktop videoconferencing. It is important to investigate the technology issues in your area before undertaking a course, because technical limitations can add to the cost and decrease your satisfaction and learning.

Access to the campus bookstore and library may also be a concern for students who are at considerable distance from the school offering the course. Books and supplies may be ordered online from the bookstore, and journal articles can be made available from the library through electronic reserve. Courses that use electronic reserve usually require a fee to cover copyright costs.

Some advantages of distance learning are the following:

Student-Centered versus Instructor-Directed Learning: Students take an active role in their own learning experience. They are able to select what material they need to cover more extensively and are given the opportunity for exploration through accessing linked material provided by their instructor. They are also given more opportunity to learn at their own pace and select the time when they are more prepared to effectively view the course material.

Flexibility: Students may work at their own computers on a weekend or the middle of the night, without having to worry about library hours or driving in bad weather. Valuable time can be focused on learning rather than on the logistics of getting to class.

Accessibility: Students who would not be able to attend classes because of geographic proximity or time constraints are now able to participate.

Student Interaction Increases: Interaction increases in a distance learning environment. Students not only listen and take notes, but they also pose ideas to and ask questions of the instructor as well as other students in discussion groups. Interaction is encouraged, and the instructor has a better understanding of what and how the student is learning. In most classroom settings, it is very difficult to get students to discuss a topic. They may ask a question of or make a comment to the instructor, but they seldom interact with classmates about course topics.

Collaboration and Team Problem Solving: Using asynchronous and synchronous communication tools, students can work together on projects much more easily. It has always been difficult to bring a group together face-to-face to discuss what needs to be done. Through these new communication channels, information can be easily passed among a group, and resources such as research documents and drafts of works in progress can be distributed instantly.

Increased Sharing of Knowledge: In the traditional classroom, the instructor is the primary source of information. In distance learning, using tools such as a discussion group, students have a greater opportunity to share their knowledge and experience, allowing the members of the group to learn from each other. In addition, access to the Internet allows students to access the experience and knowledge of others outside their immediate classroom setting.

Immediate Access to Updated Material: Any material or announcements that have been changed can be distributed instantly, reducing distribution costs and providing students with access to the most current information.

Developing Needed Technology Skills: Students are learning technology skills that they can apply later in their work setting.

Some important factors should be considered when deciding whether a distance education model is right for you. It has been shown that students can learn course content by distance methods as well as or better than in the traditional classroom setting. Less information is available on socialization issues related to the nurse generalist, specialist, or practitioner roles. Socialization involves internalizing attitudes, values, and norms. The role modeling, mentoring, and collegial friendships may or may not be as adaptable to distance methods. Careful selection of clinical settings for experience, on-site preceptors, requirements for certain on-campus experiences, and group attendance of students and faculty members at regional or national meetings are some methods used to assist socialization.

Distance learning will not suffice for the "college experience" of joining sororities and fraternities and of participating in athletic and social activities that many young undergraduate students desire. On the other hand, for the adult learner with job and family responsibilities, the distance education methodologies can provide the opportunity to participate in educational experiences that might otherwise have been beyond consideration.

When selecting your educational program, you should clearly define your goals for your educational experiences. If you want to have clinical experience in a particular setting, to be a research or teaching assistant to a certain person, or to be mentored by a selected expert, then your choice would be an on-site educational environment in a particular setting. However, if you want a degree from a particular institution but do not want to move or travel there, explore the distance learning opportunities offered. You need to remember that it is not an either-or proposition. You may be able to combine traditional classroom-based courses with distance learning for selected courses to optimize your overall educational program.

Distance learning is used by more and more educational institutions to provide both degree and continuing education. Many schools collaborate to offer students a selection of courses taught by different colleges and universities. A recent collaborative effort is the Western Governors University, a virtual university that is a partnership involving eighteen states and approximately 100 participating colleges and universities.

As noted above, the world is changing and so is the way we deliver nursing education. Distance education has opened a world of opportunities to students and faculty members. Students now have the ability to further their education by removing many of the time and access barriers they previously faced. Faculty members are presented with new and exciting challenges as they begin to use innovative technologies in their course delivery. With careful consideration and planning, the outcome will enhance the overall learning experience of both learner and teacher.

THE INTERNATIONAL NURSING STUDENT

For many international students completing baccalaureate, master's, or doctoral nursing programs, their choice of learning institutions is obvious. U.S. and Canadian colleges and universities are thought to offer the finest programs of nursing education available anywhere in the world. U.S. and Canadian nursing programs are renowned for their breadth and flexibility, for the excellence of their basic curriculum structure, and for their commitment to extensive on-site clinical training. Nursing study in the United States and Canada also affords students the opportunity for hands-on learning and practice in the world's most technologically advanced health-care systems. For many international nursing students, and especially for students from countries that are medically underserved, these features make U.S. and Canadian nursing programs unsurpassed.

Applying to Nursing School

The application process for international students often involves the completion of two separate written applications. Many colleges screen international candidates with a brief preliminary application requesting basic biographical and educational information. This document helps the admission officer determine whether the student has the minimum credentials for admission before requiring him or her to begin the lengthy process of completing and submitting final application forms.

Final applications to U.S. and Canadian colleges and universities vary widely in length and complexity, just as specific admission requirements vary from institution to institution. However, international nursing students must typically have a satisfactory scholastic record and demonstrated proficiency in English. To be admitted to any postsecondary institution in the United States or Canada, you must have satisfactorily completed a minimum of twelve years of elementary and secondary education. The customary cycle for this education includes a six-year elementary program, a three-year intermediate program, and a three-year postsecondary program, generally referred to as high school in the United States. In addition, nursing school programs generally require successful completion of several years of high school-level mathematics and science.

The documentation of satisfactory completion of secondary schooling (and university education, in the case of graduate-level applicants) is achieved through submission of school reports, transcripts, and teacher recommendations. Because academic records and systems of evaluation differ widely from one educational system to the next, request that your school include a guide to grading standards. If you have received your secondary education at a school in which English is not the language of instruction, be certain to include official translations of all documents.

International students who have completed some university-level course work in their native country may be eligible to receive credit for equivalent courses at the U.S. or Canadian institution in which they enroll. Under special circumstances, practical nursing experience may also qualify for university credit. Policies regarding the transfer of or qualification for credits based on education or nursing experience outside the United States (or Canada for Canadian schools) vary widely, so be certain to inquire about these policies at the universities or colleges that interest you.

Language skills are a key to scholastic success. "The ability to speak, write, and understand English is an important determinant of success," says Joann Weiss, former Director of the Nursing and Latin American Studies dual-degree programs at the University of New Mexico in Albuquerque. Her advice for potential international applicants is simple: "Develop a true command of written and spoken English." English proficiency for students who have not received formal education in English-speaking schools is usually demonstrated via the Test of English as a Foreign Language (TOEFL); minimum test scores of 550 to 580 are commonly required. This policy, as well as the level of proficiency required, varies from school to school, so be sure to investigate each college's policies.

In addition, most universities offer some form of English language instruction for international students, often under the rubric ESL (English as a second language). Students who require additional language study to meet admission requirements or students who wish to deepen their skills in written or verbal English should inquire about ESL program availability.

Many colleges and universities also require that all undergraduate applicants take a standardized test—either the SAT and three SAT Subject Tests or the ACT. Like their U.S. and Canadian counterparts, international applicants to graduate-level nursing programs are required by most institutions to take the standardized Graduate Record Examinations (GRE).

Applicants should also be aware that financial assistance for international students is usually quite limited. To spare international students economic hardship during their schooling in the United States or Canada, many colleges and universities require them to demonstrate the availability of sufficient financial resources for tuition and minimum living expenses and supplies. As with so many admission requirements, policies regarding financial aid vary considerably; find out early what the policies are at the colleges that interest you.

Attending School in the United States or Canada

Once you are accepted by the college or university of your choice, take full advantage of the academic and personal advising systems offered to international students. Most institutions of higher education in the United States and Canada maintain an international student advisory office staffed with trained counselors. In addition to general academic counseling and planning, an international adviser can assist in a broad range of matters ranging from immigration and visa concerns to employment opportunities and health-care issues.

With few exceptions, all university students also obtain specialized academic counseling from an assigned faculty adviser. Faculty advisers monitor academic performance and progress and try to ensure that students meet the institutional requirements for their degree. Faculty advisers are excellent sources of information regarding course selection, and some advisers offer tutorials or special language or educational support to international students.

Although all university students face academic challenges, international students often find life outside the classroom equally demanding. Suddenly introduced into a new culture where the way of life may be dramatically different from that of their native country, international students often face a variety of social, domestic, medical, religious, or emotional concerns. Questions about social conventions, meal preparation, or other personal concerns can often be addressed by your international or faculty adviser.

Lorraine Rudowski, Assistant Professor and Coordinator of the International Health Program at the College of Health and Human Services at George Mason University in Fairfax, Virginia, emphasizes the benefits of a strong relationship with your advisers: "My job as an adviser is to provide comprehensive support to my students—from academic counseling and opportunities for language development to emotional support and guidance to attending parties or other informal social events to ease the sense of social and personal isolation often experienced by foreign students."

Dr. Rudowski says that international students would do well to find a sponsor or confidant within the university who understands the conventions of the student's native country. "A culturally sensitive sponsor is better equipped to understand the unique needs of each international student and is much more likely to help students obtain the assistance they need, whether we're talking about religious issues, help with study methods or social skills, or simply knowing how to deal with such everyday chores as cooking and cleaning. All of these matters can be sources of deep concern to international students."

Yet for all the academic, social, and personal challenges facing international nursing students, there is good news. Deans of nursing, professors, and advisers typically praise the motivation and determination of their international students, and international nursing students often boast matriculation rates that match or exceed those of their U.S. and Canadian counterparts.

For more information about the rules and regulations governing international students' entrance to U.S. schools, log on to educationUSA, part of the U.S. Department of State's Web site, at http:// educationusa.state.gov.

SPECIALTY NURSING ORGANIZATIONS

Academy of Medical-Surgical Nurses
East Holly Avenue
Box 56
Pitman, NJ 08071-0056
866-877-AMSN (2676) (toll-free)
E-mail: amsn@ajj.com
www.medsurgnurse.org

Air & Surface Transport Nurses Association
7995 East Prentice Avenue
Suite 100
Greenwood Village, CO 80111
800-897-NFNA (6362) (toll-free)
Fax: 303-770-1614
E-mail: astna@gwami.com
www.astna.org

American Academy of Ambulatory Care Nursing
East Holly Avenue
Box 56
Pitman, NJ 08071-0056
800-262-6877 (toll-free)
E-mail: aaacn@ajj.com
www.aaacn.org

American Association of Critical-Care Nurses
101 Columbia
Aliso Viejo, CA 92656-4109
949-362-2000
800-899-2226 (toll-free)
E-mail: info@aacn.org
www.aacn.org

American Association of Diabetes Educators
200 West Madison Street
Suite 800
Chicago, IL 60606
800-338-3633 (toll-free)
Fax: 312-424-2427
E-mail: aade@aadenet.org
www.aadenet.org

The American Association of Legal Nurse Consultants
401 North Michigan Avenue
Chicago, IL 60611
877-402-2562 (toll-free)
Fax: 312-673-6655
E-mail: info@aalnc.org
www.aalnc.org

American Association of Neuroscience Nurses
4700 West Lake Avenue
Glenview, IL 60025
847-375-4733
888-557-2266 (toll-free in the U.S. only)
Fax: 847-375-6430
E-mail: info@aann.org
www.aann.org

American Association of Nurse Anesthetists
222 South Prospect Avenue
Park Ridge, IL 60068-4001
847-692-7050
Fax: 847-692-6968
E-mail: info@aana.com
www.aana.com

American Association of Nurse Attorneys
P.O. Box 14218
Lenexa, KS 66285-4218
877-538-2262 (toll-free)
Fax: 913-895-4652
E-mail: taana@taana.org
www.taana.org

American Association of Occupational Health Nurses, Inc.
7794 Grow Drive
Pensacola, FL 32514
800-241-8014 (toll-free)
Fax: 850-484-8762
E-mail: aaohn@aaohn.org
www.aaohn.org

American College of Nurse-Midwives
8403 Colesville Road
Suite 1550
Silver Spring, MD 20910
240-485-1800
Fax: 240-485-1818
www.midwife.org

American College of Nurse Practitioners (ACNP)
1501 Wilson Boulevard
Suite 509
Arlington, VA 22209
703-740-2529
Fax: 703-740-2533
E-mail: acnp@acnpweb.org
www.acnpweb.org

American Holistic Nurses Association
323 N. San Francisco Street
Suite 201
Flagstaff, AZ 86001
800-278-2462 (toll-free)
928-526-2196
Fax: 928-526-2752
E-mail: info@ahna.org
www.ahna.org

American Nephrology Nurses' Association
East Holly Avenue
Box 56
Pitman, NJ 08071-0056
856-256-2320
888-600-2662 (toll-free)
E-mail: anna@ajj.com
www.annanurse.org

American Psychiatric Nurses Association
1555 Wilson Boulevard
Suite 530
Arlington, VA 22209
866-243-2443 (toll-free)
703-243-2443
Fax: 703-243-3390
E-mail: inform@apna.org
www.apna.org

American Public Health Association
800 I Street, NW
Washington, DC 20001-3710
202-777-APHA
Fax: 202-777-2534
E-mail: comments@apha.org
www.apha.org

American Society for Pain Management Nursing
P.O. Box 15473
Lenexa, KS 66285-5473
888-342-7766 (toll-free)
913-895-4606
Fax: 913-895-4652
E-mail: aspmn@goamp.org
www.aspmn.org

American Society of Ophthalmic Registered Nurses
P.O. Box 193030
San Francisco, CA 94119-3030
415-561-8513
Fax: 415-561-8531
E-mail: asorn@aao.org
http://webeye.ophth.uiowa.edu/ASORN

American Society of PeriAnesthesia Nurses
90 Frontage Road
Cherry Hill, NJ 08034-1412
877-737-9696 (toll-free)
856-616-9600
Fax: 856-616-9601
E-mail: aspan@aspan.org
www.aspan.org

American Society of Plastic Surgical Nurses
7794 Grow Drive
Pensacola, FL 32514
850-473-2443
800-272-0136 (toll-free)
Fax: 850-484-8762
E-mail: aspsn@dancyamc.com
www.aspsn.org

Association for Death Education and Counseling
111 Deer Lake Road
Suite 100
Deerfield, IL 60015
847-509-0403
Fax: 847-480-9282
E-mail: info@adec.org
www.adec.org

Association for Professionals in Infection Control and Epidemiology, Inc.
1275 K Street, NW
Suite 1000
Washington, DC 20005-4006
202-789-1890
Fax: 202-789-1899
E-mail: apicinfo@apic.org
www.apic.org

Association for Radiologic & Imaging Nurses (ARIN)
7794 Grow Drive
Pensacola, FL 32514
866-486-2762 (toll-free)
850-474-7292
Fax: 850-484-8762
E-mail: arin@dancyamc.com
www.arinursing.org

Association of Nurses in AIDS Care
3538 Ridgewood Road
Akron, OH 44333-3122
800-260-6780 (toll-free)
330-670-0101
Fax: 330-670-0109
E-mail: anac@anacnet.org
www.anacnet.org

Association of Pediatric Hematology/Oncology Nurses
4700 West Lake Avenue
Glenview, IL 60025-1485
847-375-4724
Fax: 847-375-6478
E-mail: info@aphon.org
www.aphon.org

Association of Perioperative Registered Nurses
2170 South Parker Road
Suite 400
Denver, CO 80231
800-755-2676 (toll-free)
303-755-6304
E-mail: custsvc@aorn.org
www.aorn.org

Association of Rehabilitation Nurses
4700 West Lake Avenue
Glenview, IL 60025
800-229-7530 (toll-free)
E-mail: info@rehabnurse.org
www.rehabnurse.org

Association of Women's Health, Obstetric, and Neonatal Nurses
2000 L Street, NW
Suite 740
Washington, DC 20036
202-261-2400
800-673-8499 (toll-free in the U.S.)
800-245-0231 (toll-free in Canada)
Fax: 202-728-0575
E-mail: customerservice@awhonn.org
www.awhonn.org

Dermatology Nurses' Association
15000 Commerce Parkway
Suite C
Mount Laurel, NJ 08054
800-454-4362 (toll-free)
E-mail: dna@dnanurse.org
www.dnanurse.org

Developmental Disabilities Nurses Association
P.O. Box 536489
Orlando, FL 32853-6489
800-888-6733 (toll-free)
407-835-0642
Fax: 407-426-7440
www.ddna.org

Emergency Nurses Association
915 Lee Street
Des Plaines, IL 60016-6569
800-900-9659 (toll-free)
Fax: 847-460-4001
E-mail: enainfo@ena.org
www.ena.org

Hospice and Palliative Nurses Association
One Penn Center West
Suite 229
Pittsburgh, PA 15276-0100
412-787-9301
Fax: 412-787-9305
E-mail: hpna@hpna.org
www.hpna.org

Infusion Nurses Society
315 Norwood Park South
Norwood, MA 02062
781-440-9408
Fax: 781-440-9409
E-mail: ins@ins1.org
www.ins1.org

International Nurses Society on Addictions
P.O. Box 14846
Lenexa, KS 66285-4846
877-646-8672 (toll-free)
Fax: 913-895-4652
E-mail: intnsa@intnsa.org
www.intnsa.org

National Association for Home Care & Hospice
228 Seventh Street, SE
Washington, DC 20003
202-547-7424
Fax: 202-547-3540
E-mail: exec@nahc.org
www.nahc.org

National Association of Clinical Nurse Specialists
100 North 20th Street
4th Floor
Philadelphia, PA 19103
215-320-3881
Fax: 215-564-2175
E-mail: nacnsorg@nacns.org
www.nacns.org

National Association of Directors of Nursing Administration/Long Term Care
11353 Reed Hartman Highway
Suite 210
Cincinnati, OH 45241
800-222-0539 (toll-free)
513-791-3679
Fax: 513-791-3699
www.nadona.org

National Association of Neonatal Nurses
4700 West Lake Avenue
Glenview, IL 60025-1485
800-451-3795 (toll-free)
Fax: 888-477-6266
E-mail: info@nann.org
www.nann.org

National Association of Nurse Practitioners in Women's Health
505 C Street, NE
Washington, DC 20002
202-543-9693, Ext. 1
Fax: 202-543-9858
E-mail: info@npwh.org
www.npwh.org

National Association of Orthopaedic Nurses
401 North Michigan Avenue
Suite 2200
Chicago, IL 60611
800-289-6266 (toll-free)
Fax: 312-673-6941
E-mail: naon@smithbucklin.com
www.orthonurse.org

National Association of Pediatric Nurse Practitioners
20 Brace Road
Suite 200
Cherry Hill, NJ 08034-2634
856-857-9700
Fax: 856-857-1600
E-mail: info@napnap.org
www.napnap.org

National Association of School Nurses
8484 Georgia Avenue
Suite 420
Silver Spring, MD 20910
240-821-1130
E-mail: nasn@nasn.org
www.nasn.org

National Gerontological Nursing Association
1020 Monarch Street, Suite 300B
Lexington, KY 40513
800-723-0560 (toll-free)
859-977-7453
Fax: 859-977-7441
www.ngna.org

National Organization of Nurse Practitioner Faculties
900 19th Street, NW
Suite 200B
Washington, DC 20006
202-289-8044
Fax: 202-384-1444
E-mail: nonpf@nonpf.org
www.nonpf.com

Oncology Nursing Society
125 Enterprise Drive
Pittsburgh, PA 15275
866-257-4ONS (4667) (toll-free)
412-859-6100
Fax: 877-369-5497 (toll-free)
E-mail: customer.service@ons.org
www.ons.org

Preventive Cardiovascular Nurses Association
613 Williamson Street
Suite 200
Madison, WI 53703
608-250-2440
Fax: 608-250-2410
E-mail: info@pcna.net
www.pcna.net

Respiratory Nursing Society
c/o Anne Boyle, Secretary
P.O. Box 980567
Richmond, VA 23298
E-mail: aboyle@vcu.edu
www.respiratorynursingsociety.org

Society for Vascular Nursing
100 Cummings Center
Suite 124A
Beverly, MA 01915
888-536-4SVN (4786) (toll-free)
978-927-7800
Fax: 978-927-7872
www.svnnet.org

Society of Gastroenterology Nurses and Associates, Inc.
401 North Michigan Avenue
Chicago, IL 60611-4267
800-245-7462 (toll-free)
312-321-5165 (in Illinois)
Fax: 312-673-6694
E-mail: sgna@smithbucklin.com
www.sgna.org

Society of Otorhinolaryngology and Head-Neck Nurses, Inc.
207 Downing Street
New Smyrna Beach, FL 32168
386-428-1695
Fax: 386-423-7566
E-mail: info@sohnnurse.com
www.sohnnurse.com

Society of Urologic Nurses and Associates
East Holly Avenue
Box 56
Pitman, NJ 08071-0056
888-827-7862 (toll-free)
E-mail: suna@ajj.com
www.suna.org

Wound, Ostomy and Continence Nurses Society
15000 Commerce Parkway, Suite C
Mt. Laurel, NJ 08054
888-224-WOCN (9626) (toll-free)
E-mail: wocn_info@wocn.org
www.wocn.org

PAYING FOR YOUR NURSING EDUCATION

Whether you are considering a baccalaureate degree in nursing or have completed your undergraduate education and are planning to attend graduate school, finding a way to pay for that education is essential.

The cost to attend college is considerable and is increasing each year at a rate faster than most other products and services. In fact, the cost of a nursing education at a public four-year college can be more than $14,000 per year, including tuition, fees, books, room and board, transportation, and miscellaneous expenses. The cost at a private college or university, at either the graduate or undergraduate level, can be more than $30,000 per year.

This is where financial aid comes in. Financial aid is money made available by the government and other sources to help students who otherwise would be unable to attend college. More than $143 billion in aid is provided to students each year (College Board, *Trends in Student Aid 2008*). Most college students in this country receive some form of aid, and all prospective students should investigate what may be available. Most of this aid is given to students because neither they nor their families have sufficient personal resources to pay for college. This type of aid is referred to as need-based aid. Recipients of need-based aid include traditional students just out of high school or college and older, nontraditional students who are returning to college or graduate school.

There is also merit-based aid, which is awarded to students who display a particular ability. Merit scholarships are based primarily on academic merit, but may include other special talents. Many colleges and graduate schools offer merit-based aid in addition to need-based aid to their students.

Types and Sources of Financial Aid

There are four types of aid:

1. Scholarships
2. Grants
3. Loans
4. Student employment (including fellowships and assistantships)

Scholarships and grants are outright gifts and do not have to be repaid. Loans are borrowed money that must be repaid with interest, usually after graduation. Student employment provides jobs during the academic year for which students are paid. For graduate students, student employment may include fellowships and assistantships in which students work, receive free or reduced tuition, and may be paid a stipend for living expenses.

Most of the aid available to students is need-based and comes from the federal government through nine financial aid programs. Four of these programs are grant-based and are only available to undergraduate students:

1. Federal Pell Grants
2. Academic Competitive Grants
3. SMART Grants
4. Federal Supplemental Educational Opportunity Grants

Four are loan programs:

1. Federal Perkins Loan
2. Federal Stafford Student/Direct Loans (subsidized and unsubsidized)
3. Federal Graduate PLUS loans
4. Federal PLUS Loans

The final program is a student employment program called the Federal Work-Study Program, which is also awarded to undergraduate and graduate students based on financial need.

The federal government also offers a number of programs especially for nursing students. For example, the U.S. Department of Health and Human Services offers Nursing Student Scholarships, Nursing Student Loans, the Nursing Education Loan Repayment Program, and the Scholarship for Disadvantaged Students (SDS) program. Some of these programs require that the student work in a designated nursing shortage area for a period of time. These programs are administered by the nursing school's financial aid office. For more information, log on to http://bhpr.hrsa.gov/dsa.

The second-largest source of aid is from the colleges and universities themselves. Almost all colleges have aid programs from institutional resources, most of which are grants, scholarships, and fellowships. These can be either need-or merit-based.

A third source of aid is from state governments. Nearly every state provides aid for students attending college in their home state, although most only have programs for undergraduates. Most state aid programs are scholarships and grants, but many states now have low-interest loan and work-study programs. Most state grants and scholarships are not "portable," meaning that they cannot be used outside of your home state of residence.

A fourth source of aid is from private sources such as corporations, hospitals, civic associations, unions, fraternal organizations, foundations, and religious groups that give scholarships, grants, and fellowships to students. Most of these are not based on need, although the amount of the scholarship may vary depending upon financial need. The compe-

Federal Financial Aid Programs

Program	Who Benefits?	Maximum/Year
Federal Pell Grants	Undergraduate students	$5550
Federal Supplemental Educational Opportunity Grants (FSEOG)	Undergraduate students	$4000
Academic Competitivess Grants	Undergraduate students who are eligible for Federal Pell Grants	$750 (first-year students) $1300 (second-year students)
SMART Grants	Undergraduate students who are eligible for Federal Pell Grants	$4000 (third- and fourth-year students)
Federal Perkins Loans	Undergraduate students	$5500
	Graduate students	$8000
Federal Direct Loans (subsidized)	Undergraduate students	$3500 (first-year students) $4500 (second-year students) $5500 (third-year students and above)
	Graduate students	$8500
Federal Direct Loans (unsubsidized)	Dependent undergraduate students	$2000
	Independent undergraduate students	$6000 (first- and second-year students) $7000 (third-year students and above)
	Graduate students	$12,000
Federal PLUS Loans	Dependent undergraduate students	Up to cost of attendance (less other financial aid received)
Federal Graduate PLUS loans	Graduate and professional students	Up to cost of attendance (less other financial aid received)

The unsubsidized Federal Direct Loan amounts provided are in addition to the subsidized Federal Direct Loan amounts.

tition for these scholarships can be formidable, but the rewards are well worth the process. Many companies also offer tuition reimbursement to employees and their dependents. Check with the personnel or human resources department at your or your parents' place of employment for benefit and eligibility information.

Eligibility for Financial Aid

Since most of the financial aid that college students receive is need-based, colleges employ a process called "need analysis" to determine student awards. For most applicants, the student and parents (if the student is a dependent) fill out one form on which family income, assets, and household information are reported. This form is the Free Application for Federal Student Aid (FAFSA). The end result of this need analysis is the student's "Expected Family Contribution," or EFC, representing the amount a family should be able to contribute toward education expenses.

Dependent or Independent

The basic principle of financial aid is that the primary responsibility for paying college expenses resides with the family. In determining your EFC, you will first need to know who makes up your "family." That will tell you whose income is counted when the need analysis is done.

Graduate Students: By definition, all graduate nursing students are considered independent for federal aid purposes. Therefore, only your income and assets (and your spouse's if you are married) count in determining your expected family contribution.

Undergraduate Students: If you are financially dependent upon your parents, their income and assets, as well as yours, are counted toward the family contribution. If you are financially independent of your parents, only your income (and your spouse's if you are married) counts in the calculation.

According to the U.S. Department of Education, in order to be considered independent for financial aid for 2011–12, you must meet any ONE of the following:

- You were born before January 1, 1987.
- You are or will be enrolled in a master's or doctoral program (beyond a bachelor's degree) during the 2011–12 school year.

- You are married on the day you apply (even if you are separated but not divorced).
- You have children who receive more than half their support from you.
- You have dependents (other than your children or spouse) who live with you and who receive more than half of their support from you and will continue to receive more than half their support from you through June 30, 2011.
- Both your parents are deceased, or you are an orphan or ward of the court (or were a ward of the court until age 18).
- You are engaged in active duty in the U.S. Armed Forces or are a National Guard or Reserves enlistee and are called to active duty for purposes other than training.
- You are a veteran of the U.S. Armed Forces. ("Veteran" includes students who attended a U.S. service academy and who were released under a condition other than dishonorable. Contact your financial aid office for more information.)
- You were verified on or after the start of the award year for which the FAFSA is filed, as either an unaccompanied youth who is homeless or at risk of being homeless and self-supporting.

If you meet any one of these conditions, you are considered independent and only your income and assets (and your spouse's if you are married) count toward your family contribution. Remember, if you are attending school as a graduate student, you are automatically independent for federal aid consideration.

If there are extraordinary circumstances, the financial aid administrator at the college you will be attending has the authority to make a change to your dependency status. You will need to provide extensive documentation of your family situation.

Determining Cost and Need

Now that you know approximately how much you and your family will be expected to contribute toward your college expenses, you can subtract the EFC from the total cost of attending a college or graduate school to determine the amount of need-based financial aid for which you will be eligible. The average cost listed assumes that you will be attending nursing school full-time. If you will be attending part-time, you should adjust costs accordingly. For a more accurate estimate of the cost of attendance at a particular college, check the financial aid information usually available on the college's Web site or in its publications.

Applying for Financial Aid

After you have subtracted your EFC from the cost of your education and determined your financial need, you will have a better understanding of how much assistance you will need. Even if you do not demonstrate financial need, you are still encouraged to file the FAFSA, as you may be eligible for assistance that is not based on need. The process for applying for aid can be confusing if you are not familiar with completing these types of applications. If you need assistance, you should contact the financial aid office for help.

Undergraduate and graduate students applying for aid must fill out the FAFSA. This application is available in high school guidance offices, college financial aid offices, state education department offices, and many local libraries. You are strongly encouraged to file the FAFSA online at www.fafsa.ed.gov. If you file online, you will need to have a Personal Identification Number (PIN). The PIN can easily be obtained at www.pin.ed.gov. Dependent students will need a PIN for themselves and one parent. When you file online, your application is processed more rapidly, and you are far less likely to make major errors. The FAFSA, whether you file a paper application or online, becomes available in November or December, almost a year before the fall term in which you will enroll, but you cannot complete it until after January 1.

If you file a paper application, you and your parents (if appropriate) must sign your completed FAFSA and mail it to a processing center in the envelope provided. Do not send any additional materials, but do make copies of everything you filled out.

The processing center enters the data into a computer that runs the federal methodology of need analysis to calculate your EFC. This center then distributes the information to the schools and agencies you listed on the FAFSA. The actual determination of need and the awarding of aid are handled by each college financial aid office.

It is generally recommended that you complete the FAFSA as soon as possible after January 1. You should check with each college to which you are applying to determine its filing deadline. It is important to meet all college deadlines for financial aid, since there is a limited amount of funds available. However, students who procrastinate can still file for federal aid any time during the year.

What Happens After You Submit the FAFSA?

Two to four weeks after you send in your completed FAFSA, you will receive a Student Aid Report (SAR) that shows the information you reported and your official EFC. This is an opportunity for you to make corrections or to have the information sent to any new school you are considering that you did not list on the original FAFSA. The SAR contains instructions on how to make corrections or to designate additional schools. If you provided an e-mail address on the FAFSA, this information will be sent to this address rather than through conventional mail.

At the same time that you receive the SAR, the college(s) you specified also receive the information. The financial aid office at the school may request additional information from you or may ask you to provide documentation verifying the information you reported on the FAFSA. For example, they may ask you for a copy of your (and your parents') income tax return or official forms verifying any untaxed income you or your parents received (e.g., Social Security, disability, or welfare benefits).

Once the financial aid office is satisfied that the information is correct, you will receive a financial aid offer. Many colleges like to make this offer in the spring prior to the fall enrollment so that students have ample opportunity to make their plans. However, some colleges will wait until summer to notify you.

Other Applications

The FAFSA is the required form for applying for federal and most state financial aid programs. Most schools also use the FASFA to determine eligibility for institutional aid; however, some colleges and graduate schools require additional information to determine eligibility for institutional aid. Nearly 500 colleges and universities, plus more than 200 private scholarship programs, employ a form called the Financial Aid PROFILEt from the College Scholarship Service (CSS). While the form is similar to the FAFSA, several additional questions must be answered for colleges that award their own funds. You begin the process in October or November by completing a PROFILE Registration form on which you designate the schools to which you are applying. A few weeks later, you will receive a customized, individualized application that you complete and send back to CSS, which, in turn, forwards your application information to the schools you selected. There is a fee charged for each school listed on the application.

Financial Aid Offer

If you qualify for need-based aid, a college will typically offer a combination of different types of assistance— scholarship, grant, loan, and work-study—to meet this need. An offer of aid usually is made after you have been admitted to the college or program. You may accept all or part of the financial aid package. If you will be enrolling part-time (fewer than 12 credits per term), be sure to contact the financial aid office in advance since this may have impact on your overall aid eligibility.

If you are awarded Federal Work-Study Program aid, the amount you are awarded represents your earnings limit for the academic year under the program. In general, schools assume you will earn this money on an hourly basis, so it cannot be used to pay your term bill charges. On most campuses there are many jobs available for students. Not all of these are limited to students in the Federal Work-Study Program. Check with your placement office or financial aid office for more information.

Keep in mind that the student budget used to establish eligibility for financial aid is based on averages. It may not reflect your actual expenses. Student budgets usually reflect most expenses for categories of students (for example, single students living in their parents' home, campus-provided housing, or living in an apartment or house near campus, etc.). But if you have unusual expenses that are not included, you should consult with your school's financial aid office regarding a budget adjustment.

If Your Family or Job Situation Changes

Because a family contribution is based on the previous year's income, many nursing students find they do not qualify for need-based aid (or not enough to pay their full expenses). This is particularly true of older students who were working full-time last year but are no longer doing so or who will not work during the academic year. If this is your situation, you should speak to a counselor in the financial aid office about making an adjustment in your family contribution need analysis. Financial aid administrators may make changes to any of the elements that go into the need analysis if there are conditions that merit a change. Contact the financial aid office for more information.

Don't Qualify for Need-Based Aid?

If you don't qualify for need-based aid but feel you do not have the resources necessary to pay for college or graduate school, you still have several options available.

First, there is a student loan program for which need is not a consideration. This is the Federal Direct Loan (unsubsidized) program. There are also non-need-based loan programs for parents of dependent students or for graduate or professional students called the Federal PLUS Loans and the Direct PLUS Loan program. If you or your parents are interested in borrowing through one of these programs, you should check with the financial aid office for more information. There are also numerous private or alternative loan sources available. For many students, borrowing to pay for a nursing education can be an excellent investment in one's future. At the same time, be sure that you do not overburden yourself when it comes to paying back the loans. Before you accept a federal student loan, the financial aid office will schedule a counseling session to make certain that you know the terms of the loan and that you understand the ramifications of borrowing. If you can do without, it is often suggested that you postpone student loans until they are absolutely necessary.

For graduate nursing students, Federal PLUS Loans are now available to graduate and professional students. Students who are looking into alternative loan programs should be sure to compare any terms and conditions with this federal program. Students should borrow through the Federal Graduate PLUS loans (or other alternative loan) program only after they have used the Federal Stafford Student Loan or Direct Loan program. You can borrow Federal Graduate PLUS loans and alternative loan funds up to the cost of attendance less any other financial aid received.

A second option if you do not qualify for need-based aid is to search for scholarships. Be wary of scholarship search companies that promise to find you scholarships but require you to pay a fee. There are many resources that provide lists of scholarships, including the annually published *Peterson's Scholarships, Grants & Prizes,* which are available in libraries, counselors' offices, and bookstores. Non-need scholarships require application forms and are extremely competitive; only a handful of students from thousands of applicants receive awards.

Another option is to work more hours at an existing job or to find a paying position if you do not already have one. The student employment or placement office at your college should be able to help you find a job, either on or off campus. Many colleges have vacancies remaining after they have placed Federal Work-Study Program eligible students in their jobs.

You should always contact the financial aid office at the school you plan to attend for advice concerning sources of college-based and private aid.

Employer-Paid Financial Aid

Robert Atwater is a certified personnel consultant and certified medical staff recruiter and founder of Atwater Consulting in Lilburn, Georgia, a consulting firm for the employment and recruitment of physician assistants, nurse practitioners, certified nurse midwives, nurses, and nursing managers.

Health-care administrators, Atwater says, have coined a phrase to characterize their efforts to meet the growing demand for nurses with better skills and training: "Grow your own."

"Constant training through the course of a nursing career is the only way to keep pace with the technological and medical advances, but it can be a financial burden on the nurse," Atwater says.

That is why many employers now give qualified employees a benefits package that includes a continuing education allowance.

For the employer, this type of benefits package can help to recruit candidates willing to further their careers through education. Administrators feel it is the best way to build a staff of nurses with up-to-date certifications in all areas.

In a constantly expanding field, nurses should be required to continue and update their education. The nurses get a paid education, can keep their job, and work flexible hours while they are going to school. Inquiries about these allowances should be made during an interview with the company's human resources department. Additional information can be obtained from the nursing school, local hospitals in the area, or from other health-care professionals. There are many attractive options available because of the nationwide shortage of qualified nurses. Check with a number of potential employers before agreeing to any long-term contract.

Sources of Financial Aid for Nursing Students

The largest proportion of financial aid for college expenses comes from the federal government and is given on the basis of financial need. Beyond this federal need-based aid—which should always be the primary source of financial aid that a prospective student investigates and which is given regardless of one's field of study—a sizable amount of scholarship assistance specifically meant to help students in nursing programs is also available from government agencies, associations, civic or fraternal organizations, and corporations. These sources of aid can be particularly attractive for students who may not be eligible for need-based aid. The following list presents some of the major sources of financial aid specifically for nursing students. Not listed are scholarships that are specific to individual colleges and universities or are limited to residents of a particular place or to individuals who have relatively unusual qualifications. Students seeking financial aid should investigate all appropriate possibilities, including sources not listed here. You can find this information in libraries, bookstores, and guidance offices guides, including two of Peterson's annually updated publications: *Peterson's How to Get Money for College: Financing Your Future Beyond Federal Aid,* for information about undergraduate awards given by the federal government, state governments, and specific colleges, and *Peterson's Scholarships, Grants & Prizes,* for information about awards from private sources.

Air Force Institute of Technology
Award Name: Air Force Active Duty Health Professions Loan Repayment Program
Program Description: Program provides up to $40,000 (2009) to repay qualified educational loans in exchange for active duty service in the U.S. armed forces.
Application Contact:
Air Force Institute of Technology
AFIT/ENEM
Attn: Ms. Patricia Faustman
2950 Hobson Way
Wright Patterson AFB, OH 45433-7765
800-543-3490, Ext. 3015 (toll-free)
E-mail: enem.adhplrp@afit.edu
www.afit.edu/adhplrp

American Association of Colleges of Nursing (AACN)
Award Name: AfterCollege/AACN Scholarship Fund
Program Description: This scholarship program supports students who are seeking a baccalaureate, master's, or doctoral degree in nursing. Special consideration is given to students enrolled in a master's or doctoral program with the goal of pursuing a nursing faculty career, completing an RN to baccalaureate program (B.S.N.), or enrolled in an accelerated baccalaureate or master's degree nursing program.
Application Contact:
American Association of Colleges of Nursing
One Dupont Circle, NW
Suite 530
Washington, DC 20036
202-463-6930
Fax: 202-785-8320
E-mail: scholarship@aacn.nche.edu
http://bit.ly/aftercollege_AACN

American Association of Critical-Care Nurses
Award Name: AACN Educational Advancement Scholarships
Program Description: Nonrenewable scholarships for AACN members who are RNs currently enrolled in undergraduate or graduate NLNAC-accredited programs. The undergraduate award is for use in the junior or senior year. Minimum 3.0 GPA.
Application Contact:
American Association of Critical-Care Nurses
Scholarships
101 Columbia
Aliso Viejo, CA 92656-4109
800-899-2226 (toll-free)
E-mail: info@aacn.org
www.aacn.nche.edu/education/financialaid.htm

American Cancer Society
Award Name: Scholarships in Cancer Nursing
Program Description: Renewable awards for graduate students in nursing pursuing advanced preparation in cancer nursing: research, education, administration, or clinical practice. Must be U.S. citizen.
Application Contact:
American Cancer Society
Extramural Grants Program
250 Williams Street
Atlanta, GA 30303-1002
800-ACS-2345 (toll-free)
Fax: 404-321-4669
E-mail: grants@cancer.org
www.cancer.org

American Holistic Nurses' Association (AHNA)
Award Name: Charlotte McGuire Scholarship Program
Program Description: Open to any licensed nurse or nursing student pursuing holistic education. Experience in holistic health care or alternative health practices is preferred. Must be an AHNA member with a minimum 3.0 GPA.

Application Contact:
Charlotte McGuire Scholarships
American Holistic Nurses' Association
323 N. San Francisco Street
Suite 201
Flagstaff, AZ 86001
800-278-2462 Ext. 10 (toll-free)
E-mail: info@ahna.org
www.ahna.org/edu/assist.html

American Indian Graduate Center (AIGC)

Award Name: AIGC Fellowships

Program Description: Graduate fellowships available for American Indian and Alaska Native students from federally recognized U.S. tribes. Applicants must be pursuing a postbaccalaureate graduate or professional degree as a full-time student at an accredited institution in the U.S., demonstrate financial need, and be enrolled in a federally recognized American Indian tribe or Alaska Native group or provide documentation of Indian descent.

Application Contact:
American Indian Graduate Center Fellowships
American Indian Graduate Center
4520 Montgomery Boulevard, NE
Suite 1B
Albuquerque, NM 87109
800-628-1920 (toll-free)
505-881-4584
E-mail: web@aigcs.org
www.aigc.com

Association of Perioperative Registered Nurses (AORN)

Award Name: AORN Foundation Scholarships

Program Description: Applicant must be an active RN and a member of AORN for twelve consecutive months prior to application. Reapplication for each period is required. For baccalaureate, master's of nursing, or doctoral degree at an accredited institution. Minimum 3.0 GPA required.

Application Contact:
AORN Foundation Scholarship Program
2170 South Parker Road
Suite 400
Denver, CO 80231-5711
800-755-2676 (toll-free)
E-mail: foundation@aorn.org
www.aorn.org/AORNFoundation/Scholarships

Bethesda Lutheran Homes and Services, Inc.

Award Name: Nursing Scholastic Achievement Scholarship

Program Description: Award for college nursing students with a minimum 3.0 GPA who are Lutheran and have completed their sophomore year of a four-year nursing program or one year of a two-year program. Must be interested in working with people with developmental disabilities.

Application Contact:
Bethesda Lutheran Homes and Services, Inc.
Coordinator, Outreach Programs and Services
600 Hoffmann Drive
Watertown, WI 53094
800-369-4636, Ext. 4449 (toll-free)
E-mail: bethesda.institute@mailblc.org
www.blhs.org/youth/scholarships

Foundation of the National Student Nurses' Association, Inc.

Award Names: Scholarship Program

Program Description: One-time awards available to nursing students in various educational situations: enrolled in programs leading to an RN license, RNs enrolled in programs leading to a bachelor's or master's degree in nursing, enrolled in a state approved school in a specialty area of nursing, and minority students enrolled in nursing or prenursing programs. High school students are not eligible. Funds for graduate study are available only for a first degree in nursing. Based on financial need, academic ability, and health-related nursing and community activities. Application fee of $10. Send self-addressed stamped envelope with two stamps along with application request.

Application Contact:
Scholarship Chairperson
Foundation of the National Student Nurses' Association, Inc.
45 Main Street
Suite 606
Brooklyn, NY 11201
718-210-0705
E-mail: nsna@nsna.org
www.nsna.org/foundation

Heart and Stroke Foundation of Canada

Award Name: Nursing Research Fellowships

Program Description: In-training awards for study in an area of cardiovascular or cerebrovascular nursing. Award is directed toward preparing nurses who have completed their doctoral degree and who intend to undertake independent research programs. For master's degree candidates, the programs must include a thesis or project requirement.

Application Contact:
Heart and Stroke Foundation of Canada
1402-222 Queen Street
Ottawa, Ontario K1P-5V9
Canada
613-569-4361, Ext. 275
E-mail: research@hsf.ca
www.hsf.ca/research/en/general/home.html

International Order of the King's Daughters and Sons, Inc.

Award Name: International Order of King's Daughters and Sons Health Scholarships

Program Description: For study in the health fields. B.A./B.S. students are eligible in junior year. Application must be for at least third year of college. RN students must have completed first year of schooling. Send #10 self-addressed stamped envelope for application and information.

Application Contact: Director
Health Careers Scholarship Department
P.O. Box 1040
Chautauqua, NY 14722-1040
716-357-4951
E-mail: iokds5@windstream.net
www.iokds.org/scholarship.html

March of Dimes
Award Name: Graduate Scholarships
Program Description: Scholarships for registered nurses enrolled in graduate programs in maternal-child nursing. Must be a member of the Association of Women's Health, Obstetric and Neonatal Nurses; the American College of Nurse-Midwives; or the National Association of Neonatal Nurses (NANN).
Application Contact: Education Services
March of Dimes
1275 Mamaroneck Avenue
White Plains, NY 10605
914-997-4555
E-mail: mlavan@marchofdimes.com
www.marchofdimes.com/professionals/grants.html

National Alaska Native American Indian Nurses
Association (NANAINA)
Award Name: NANAINA Merit Awards
Program Description: Annual $500 awards presented to NANAINA members who are enrolled in a U.S. federally or state-recognized tribe and are enrolled as a full-time undergraduate or graduate nursing student in an accredited or state-approved school of nursing.
Application Contact:
John Lowe
NANAINA
1100 N. Stonewall, Room 465
Oklahoma City, OK 73117
888-566-8773 (toll-free)
E-mail: scholarships@nanainanurses.org
www.nanainanurses.org/Scholarships

National Association of Hispanic Nurses (NAHN)
Award Name: National Scholarship Awards
Program Description: One-time award to an outstanding Hispanic nursing student. Must have at least a 3.0 GPA and be a member of NAHN. Based on academic merit, potential contribution to nursing, and financial need.
Application Contact:
Juan F. Perez, RN-B.S.N., Chair
Awards/Scholarship Committee
1455 Pennsylvania Avenue, NW
Suite 400
Washington, DC 20004
202-387-2477
E-mail: info@thehispanicnurses.org
www.thehispanicnurses.org

National Black Nurses Association, Inc. (NBNA)
Award Names: NBNA Scholarships
Program Description: Scholarships available to nursing students who are members of NBNA and are enrolled in an accredited school of nursing. Must demonstrate involvement in African-American community and present letter of recommendation from local chapter of NBNA.
Application Contact:
National Black Nurses Association, Inc.
Scholarship Committee
8630 Fenton Street, Suite 330
Silver Spring, MD 20910-3803
301-589-3200
E-mail: contact@nbna.org
www.nbna.org/scholarship.htm

National Student Nurses' Association (NSNA)
Award Name: Educational Advancement Scholarships
Program Description: Scholarships are awarded based on academic achievement and demonstrated commitment to nursing through involvement in student organizations and school and community activities related to health care.
Application Contact:
National Student Nurses' Association Foundation
45 Main Street
Suite 606
Brooklyn, NY 11201
718-210-0705
E-mail: nsna@nsna.org
www.nsna.org

Nurses' Educational Funds, Inc.
Award Name: Nurses' Educational Fund Scholarships
Program Description: Awards for full-time students at master's level, full-time or part-time at doctoral level, or RNs who are U.S. citizens and members of a national professional nursing association. Application fee: $10.
Application Contact:
Nurses' Educational Funds, Inc.
304 Park Avenue South
11th Floor
New York, NY 10010
212-590-2443
E-mail: info@n-e-f.org
www.n-e-f.org

Oncology Nursing Society
Award Name: Scholarships
Program Description: ONF offers nearly a dozen one-time scholarships and awards at all levels of study, with various requirements and purposes, to nursing students who are interested in pursuing oncology nursing. Contact the foundation for details about appropriate awards. Application fee: $5.
Application Contact:
Oncology Nursing Society
Development Coordinator
125 Enterprise Drive
Pittsburgh, PA 15275-1214

866-257-4667 (toll-free)
E-mail: customer.service@ons.org
www.ons.org/awards

United States Air Force Reserve Officer Training Corps
Award Name: Air Force ROTC Nursing Scholarships
Program Description: One- to four-year programs available to students of nursing and high school seniors. Nursing graduates agree to accept a commission in the Air Force Nurse Corps and serve four years on active duty after successfully completing their licensing examination. Must have at least a 2.5 GPA for one- and four-year scholarships or at least a 2.65 GPA for two- and three-year scholarships. Two exam failures result in a four-year assignment as an Air Force line officer.
Application Contact:
Air Force ROTC
551 East Maxwell Boulevard
Maxwell AFB, AL 36112-6106
866-423-7682 (toll-free)
www.afrotc.com/scholarships

United States Army Reserve Officers' Training Corps
Award Name: Army ROTC Nursing Scholarships
Program Description: Two- to four-year programs available to students of nursing and high school seniors. Nursing graduates agree to accept a commission in the Army Nurse Corps and serve in the military for a period of eight years. This may be fulfilled by serving on active duty for two to four years, followed by service in the Army National Guard or the United States Army Reserve or in the Inactive Ready Reserve for the remainder of the eight-year obligation.
Application Contact:
Army ROTC Cadet Command
Army ROTC Scholarship
Fort Monroe, VA 23651-1052
800-USA-ROTC (toll-free)
www.goarmy.com/rotc/scholarships.html

United States Department of Health and Human Services, Bureau of Health Professions
Award Names: Nursing Scholarship
Program Description: Awards for U.S. citizens enrolled or accepted for enrollment as a full- or part-time student in an accredited school of nursing in a professional registered nurse program (baccalaureate, graduate, associate degree, or diploma)
Application Contact:
Division of Nursing
U.S. Dept. of Health and Human Services
5600 Fishers Lane, Room 8-37
Parklawn Building
Rockville, MD 20857
800-221-9393 (toll-free)
CallCenter@hrsa.gov
www.hrsa.gov/loanscholarships/scholarships/Nursing

How to Use This Guide

The following includes an overview of the various components of *Peterson's Nursing Programs 2012,* along with background information on the criteria used for including institutions and nursing programs in the guide, and explanatory material to help users interpret details presented within the guide.

Profiles of Nursing Programs

The **Profiles of Nursing Programs** section contains detailed profiles of schools that responded to our online survey and the nursing programs they offer. This section is organized geographically; U.S. schools are listed alphabetically by state or territory, followed by Canadian schools listed alphabetically by province.

The profiles contain basic information about the colleges and universities, along with details specific to the nursing school or department, the nursing student body, and the nursing programs offered.

Schools that are members of a consortium appear with an abbreviated profile. The abbreviated profile lists only the school heading and the specific college or university information, followed by a reference line that refers readers to the consortium profile, which contains detailed program information.

An outline of the profile follows. The items of information found under each section heading are defined and displayed. Any item discussed below that is omitted from an individual profile either does not apply to that particular college or university or is one for which no information was supplied. Each profile begins with a heading with the name of the institution (the college or university), the nursing college or unit, the location of the nursing facilities, the school's Web address, and the institution's founding date, specifically the year in which it was chartered or the year when instruction actually began, whichever date is earlier. In most cases, the location is identical to the main campus of the institution. However, in a few instances, the nursing facilities are not located in the same city or state as the main campus of the college or university.

Basic information about the college follows:

Nursing Program Faculty: The total number of full-time and part-time faculty members, followed by, if provided, the percentage of faculty members holding doctoral degrees.

Baccalaureate Enrollment: The total number of matriculated full-time and part-time baccalaureate program students as of fall 2010 is given. This snapshot of the nursing student body indicates the total number of matriculated students, both full-time and part-time, in the baccalaureate-level nursing program; the school's estimate of the percentage of nursing students in each of the following categories is provided, if applicable: Women, Men, Minority, International, and Part-time.

Graduate Enrollment: The total number of matriculated full-time and part-time students in graduate programs in fall 2010 and the percentages of **Women, Men, Minority, International,** and **Part-time** students are given.

Distance Learning Courses: This section appears if distance learning courses are available.

Nursing Student Activities: This section lists organizations open only to nursing students, including nursing clubs, Sigma Theta Tau (the international honor society for nursing), recruiter clubs, and Student Nurses' Association.

Nursing Student Resources: This section lists special learning resources available for nursing students within the nursing school's (or unit's) facilities.

Library Facilities: Figures are provided for the total number of bound volumes held by the college or university, the number of those volumes in health-related subjects, and the number in nursing and the number of periodical subscriptions held and the number of those in health-related subjects.

BACCALAUREATE PROGRAMS

Degree: Baccalaureate degree or degrees awarded are specified.

Available Programs: If, in addition to a generic baccalaureate program in nursing, a school has other baccalaureate nursing programs (e.g., accelerated programs or programs for RNs, LPNs, or college graduates with non-nursing degrees) they are specified here.

Site Options: Locations other than the nursing program's main campus at which baccalaureate programs may be taken are listed. Off-campus classes generally are held in health-care facilities or other educational facilities that are part of or affiliated with the college or nursing school.

Study Options: Lists full-time and part-time options.

Online Degree Options: This section appears if online baccalaureate degrees are available. It also specifies if the distance learning options are only available online.

Program Entrance Requirements: Lists special requirements typically required to enter a program of nursing leading to a baccalaureate degree, including completion of a specific program of prerequisite courses, sometimes called prenursing courses. These are specific course credits that must be earned by students who wish to enter the generic baccalaureate program. Students entering into other tracks may be required to prove that they have completed analogous courses. Often the minimum GPA requirement for prerequisite courses differs from that expected for general college courses. Other requirements are generally self-explanatory. This paragraph also indicates if transfer students are accepted into the program. Special tracks will require appropriate proof of experience, diplomas, or other credentials. Finally, application deadlines and fees are given.

Advanced Placement: This entry indicates that program credits may be granted on the basis of examinations or evaluations of earned credits at other facilities by the program's faculty and administrators.

Expenses: In this section, figures are provided for tuition, mandatory and other fees, and room and board, as well as an estimate of costs for books and supplies, based on the 2010–11 academic year. If a school did not return a survey, expenses for the 2008–09 or 2009–10 academic year are listed. Unless otherwise indicated, tuition is for one full academic year. If applicable, distinct tuition figures are given for state residents and nonresidents. Part-time, summer, and evening tuition is expressed in terms of the per-unit rate (per credit, per semester hour, etc.) specified by the institution. The tuition structure at some institutions is very complex, with different rates for freshmen and sophomores than for juniors and seniors or with part-time tuition prorated on a sliding scale according to the number of credit hours taken. Mandatory fees include such items as activity fees, health insurance, and malpractice insurance.

Financial Aid: This section combines data from our online nursing survey with data received on available financial aid programs. It provides information on college-administered aid for baccalaureate-level students, including the percentage of undergraduate nursing students receiving financial aid, all types of aid offered, and application deadlines. Financial aid programs are organized into these categories: gift aid (need-based), awards based on a student's formally designated inability to pay some or all of the cost of education; gift aid (non-need-based), scholarships given on the basis of a student's special achievements, abilities, or personal characteristics; loans, subsidized low-interest student loans that can be need-based or not; and work-study, a need-based program of part-time work offered to help pay educational expenditures. The application deadline is the deadline by which application forms and need calculations, such as the FAFSA, must be submitted to the institution in order to qualify for need-based and institutional aid.

Contact: This section lists the name, title, mailing address, telephone number, and, if available, fax number and e-mail address of the person to contact for admission information about the baccalaureate program.

GRADUATE PROGRAMS

The first three paragraphs provide information that is common to the college's graduate programs in nursing.

Expenses: In this section, figures are provided for tuition, room and board, and required fees based on the 2010–11 academic year. If a school did not return a survey, expenses for the 2008–09 or 2009–10 academic year are listed. Unless otherwise indicated, tuition is for one full academic year. If applicable, distinct tuition figures are given for state residents and nonresidents. Part-time, summer, and evening tuition is expressed in terms of the per-unit rate (per credit, per semester hour, etc.) specified by the institution.

Financial Aid: This section combines data from our online nursing survey with data received on available financial aid programs. It provides information on college-administered aid including the percentage of graduate nursing students receiving financial aid, all types of aid offered, and application deadlines. The major kinds of aid available are listed, including traineeships, low-interest student loans, fellowships, research assistantships, teaching assistantships, and full and partial tuition waivers. If aid is available to part-time students, this is indicated. The application deadline is the deadline by which application forms must be submitted to the college's financial aid office.

Contact: Lists the name, title, mailing address, telephone number, and, if available, fax number and e-mail address of the person to contact for admission information about graduate programs.

MASTER'S DEGREE PROGRAM

Degree(s): Master's degree or degrees awarded are specified. Joint degrees specify which two degrees are given, e.g., M.S.N./Ed. D., M.S.N./M.B.A., M.S./M.H.A., M.S.N./M.P.H., in programs that combine a master's degree (or doctorate) in nursing with a master's degree in another discipline, such as business administration, hospital administration, or public health.

Available Programs: If a college has special tracks that give credit, accelerated programs, or advanced courses designed for students with previous nursing experience or higher education credentials that enable students to complete programs in less time than regularly required, these are specified here in three categories:

1. For RNs—programs that admit registered nurses with associate degrees or diplomas in nursing and award a master's degree. These include RN-to-master's programs that combine the baccalaureate and master's degrees into one program for nurses who are graduates of associate or hospital diploma programs and programs that admit registered nurses with non-nursing baccalaureate degrees.
2. For LPNs—programs that admit licensed practical nurses and award a master's degree.
3. For College Graduates with Non-Nursing Degrees—programs that admit students with baccalaureate or master's degrees in areas other than nursing and award a master's degree in nursing.

Concentrations Available: Specific areas of study and concentrations offered by the school are listed. Areas of specialization in case management, health-care administration, legal nurse consultant, nurse anesthesia, nurse-midwifery, nursing administration, nursing education, and nursing informatics are noted. Clinical nurse specialist and nurse practitioner programs and areas of specialization within them are noted.

Site Options: Locations other than the nursing program's main campus at which the master's degree programs are offered are listed. Off-campus classes generally are held in health-care facilities or other educational facilities that are part of or affiliated with the nursing school.

Study Options: Lists full-time and part-time options.

Online Degree Options: This section appears if online master's degrees are available. It also specifies if the distance learning options are only available online.

Program Entrance Requirements: Lists generally self-explanatory requirements.

Advanced Placement: Indicates that program credits may be granted on the basis of examinations or evaluations of earned credits at other facilities by the program's faculty and administrators.

Degree Requirements: Indicates the number of master's program credit hours required to earn the master's degree and the need for a thesis or qualifying score on a comprehensive examination.

POST-MASTER'S PROGRAM

Areas of Study: Listed here are the specific areas of clinical nurse specialist programs, nurse practitioner programs, and other specializations offered as postmaster's programs.

DOCTORAL DEGREE PROGRAM

Degree: Doctoral degree awarded is specified.

Areas of Study: Lists specific areas of study and concentration offered by the school.

Program Entrance Requirements: Lists generally self-explanatory requirements.

Degree Requirements: Indicates the number of program credit hours required to earn the doctorate and the need for a dissertation, oral examination, written examination, or residency.

POSTDOCTORAL PROGRAM

Areas of Study: Lists areas of study currently reported. These may change, dependent upon the individuals in the program.

Postdoctoral Program Contact: Lists the name, title, mailing address, telephone number, and, if available, fax number and e-mail address of the person to contact for information about postdoctoral programs.

CONTINUING EDUCATION PROGRAM

Contact: The appearance of this heading indicates that the nursing school has a program of continuing education. If provided, the name, title, mailing address, telephone number, fax number, and e-mail address of the person to contact regarding the program are given.

Display Ads

Display ads, which appear near some of the institutions' profiles, have been provided by those colleges or universities that wished to supplement the profile data with information about their institutions or nursing programs.

Two-Page Descriptions

The **Two-Page Descriptions** section is an open forum for nursing schools to communicate their particular message to prospective students. The absence of any college or university from this section does not constitute an editorial decision on the part of Peterson's. Those who have chosen to write these inclusions are responsible for the accuracy of the content. Statements regarding a school's objectives and accomplishments represent its own beliefs and are not the opinions of the editors. The **Two-Page Descriptions** are arranged alphabetically by the official institution name.

Indexes

Indexes at the back of the book provide references to profiles by baccalaureate, master's, doctoral, postdoctoral, online, and continuing education programs offered; for master's-level programs, by area of study or concentration; and by institution name.

Abbreviations Used in This Guide

AACN	American Association of Colleges of Nursing
AACSB	AACSB International—The Association to Advance Collegiate Schools of Business
AAHC	Association of Academic Health Centers
AAS	Associate in Applied Science
ABSN	Accelerated Bachelor of Science in Nursing
ACT	American College Testing, Inc.
ACT ASSET	American College Testing Assessment of Skills for Successful Entry and Transfer
ACT COMP	American College Testing College Outcomes Measures Program
ACT PEP	American College Testing Proficiency Examination Program
AD	Associate Degree
ADN	Associate Degree in Nursing
AHNP	Adult Health Nurse Practitioner
ALE	American Language Exam
AMEDD	Army Medical Department
ANA	American Nurses Association
ANP	Adult Nurse Practitioner
APN	Advanced Practice Nurse
ARNP	Advanced Registered Nurse Practitioner
AS	Associate of Science
ASN	Associate of Science in Nursing
BA	Bachelor of Arts
BAA	Bachelor of Applied Arts
BN	Bachelor of Nursing
BNSc	Bachelor of Nursing Science

BRN	Baccalaureate for the Registered Nurse
BS	Bachelor of Science
BScMH	Bachelor of Science in Mental Health
BScN	Bachelor of Science in Nursing
BSEd	Bachelor of Science in Education
BSN	Bachelor of Science in Nursing
CAI	computer-assisted instruction
CAUSN	Canadian Association of University Schools of Nursing
CCNE	Commission on Collegiate Nursing Education
CCRN	Critical-Care Registered Nurse
CFNP	Certified Family Nurse Practitioner
CGFNS	Commission on Graduates of Foreign Nursing Schools
CINAHL	Cumulative Index to Nursing and Allied Health Literature
CLAST	College-Level Academic Skills Test
CLEP	College-Level Examination Program
CNA	Certified Nurse Assistant, Certified Nursing Assistant, Certified Nurses' Aide
CNAT	Canadian Nurses Association Testing
CNL	Clinical Nurse Leader
CNM	Certified Nurse-Midwife
CNS	Clinical Nurse Specialist
CODEC	coder/decoder
CPR	cardiopulmonary resuscitation
CRNA	Certified Registered Nurse Anesthetist
CS	Certified Specialist
CSS	College Scholarship Service
DNP	Doctor of Nursing Practice
DNS	Doctor of Nursing Science
DNSc	Doctor of Nursing Science
DOE	U.S. Department of Education
DrPH	Doctor of Public Health
DSN	Doctor of Science in Nursing
EdD	Doctor of Education
EFC	expected family contribution
ERIC	Educational Resources Information Center
ESL	English as a second language
ETN	Enterostomal Nurse
FAAN	Fellow in the American Academy of Nursing
FAF	Financial Aid Form
FAFSA	Free Application for Federal Student Aid
FC	family contribution
FNP	Family Nurse Practitioner
FSEOG	Federal Supplemental Educational Opportunity Grants
GED	General Educational Development test
GMAT	Graduate Management Admission Test
GPA	grade point average
GPO	Government Printing Office
GRE	Graduate Record Examinations
Gyn	gynecology
HIV	human immunodeficiency virus
HMO	health maintenance organization
ICEOP	Illinois Consortium for Educational Opportunities Program
ICU	intensive care unit
ISP	Internet service provider
ITV	interactive television
LD	Licensed Dietician
LPN	Licensed Practical Nurse
LVN	Licensed Vocational Nurse
MA	Master of Arts
MAEd	Master of Arts in Education
MAT	Miller Analogies Test
MBA	Master of Business Administration
MCSc	Master of Clinical Science
MDiv	Master of Divinity
MEd	Master of Education
MEDLINE	MEDLARS On-Line
MELAB	Michigan English Language Assessment Battery
MHA	Master of Hospital Administration Master of Health Administration
MHD	Master of Human Development
MHSA	Master of Health Services Administration
MN	Master of Nursing
MNSc	Master of Nursing Science
MOM	Master of Organizational Management
MPA	Master of Public Affairs
MPH	Master of Public Health
MPS	Master of Public Service
MS	Master of Science
MSBA	Master of Science in Business Administration
M Sc	Master of Science
MSc(A)	Master of Science (Applied)
MScN	Master of Science in Nursing
MTS	Master of Theological Studies
MSEd	Master of Science in Education
MSN	Master of Science in Nursing
MSOB	Master of Science in Organizational Behavior
NCAA	National Collegiate Athletic Association
NCLEX-RN	National Council Licensure Examination for Registered Nurses
ND	Doctor of Nursing
NLN	National League for Nursing
NNP	Neonatal Nurse Practitioner
NP	Nurse Practitioner
NSNA	National Student Nurses' Association
OB	Organizational Behavior
OB/GYN	obstetrics/gynecology
OCLC	Online Computer Library Center
OM	Organizational Management
PEP	Proficiency Examination Program
PhD	Doctor of Philosophy
PHEAA	Pennsylvania Higher Education Assistance Agency
PHS	Public Health Service
PLUS	Parents' Loan for Undergraduate Students
PNNP	Perinatal Nurse Practitioner
PNP	Pediatric Nurse Practitioner
PSAT	Preliminary SAT
RD	Registered Dietician

RN	Registered Nurse
RN, C	Registered Nurse, Certified
RN, CAN	Registered Nurse, Certified in Nursing Administration
RN, CNAA	Registered Nurse, Certified in Nursing Administration, Advanced
RN, CS	Registered Nurse, Certified Specialist
ROTC	Reserve Officers' Training Corps
RPN	Registered Psychiatric Nurse
SAR	Student Aid Report
SAT	SAT and SAT Subject Tests
SLS	Supplemental Loans to Students
SNA	Student Nurses' Association
SNAP	Student Nurses Acting for Progress
SNO	Student Nurses Organization
SUNY	State University of New York
TAP	Tuition Assistance Program
TB	tuberculosis
TOEFL	Test of English as a Foreign Language
TSE	Test of Spoken English
TWE	Test of Written English
USIS	United States Information Service
WHNP	Women's Health Nurse Practitioner

Data Collection Procedures

The data contained in the preponderant number of nursing college profiles, as well as in the indexes to them, were collected through *Peterson's Survey of Nursing Programs* during winter 2010–11. Questionnaires were posted online for more than 800 colleges and universities with baccalaureate and graduate programs in nursing. With minor exceptions, data for those colleges or schools of nursing that responded to the questionnaires were submitted by officials at the schools themselves. All usable information received in time for publication has been included. The omission of a particular item from a profile means that it is either not applicable to that institution or was not available or usable. In the handful of instances in which no information regarding an eligible nursing program was submitted and research of reliable secondary sources was unable to elicit the desired information, the name, location, and some general information regarding the nursing program appear in the profile section to indicate the existence of the program. Because of the extensive system of checks performed on the data collected by Peterson's, we believe that the information presented in this guide is accurate. Nonetheless, errors and omissions are possible in a data collection and processing endeavor of this scope. Also, facts and figures, such as tuition and fees, can suddenly change. Therefore, students should check with a specific college or university at the time of application to verify all pertinent information.

Criteria for Inclusion in This Book

Peterson's Nursing Programs 2012 covers accredited institutions in the United States, U.S. territories, and Canada that grant baccalaureate and graduate degrees. The institutions that sponsor the nursing programs must be accredited by accrediting agencies approved by the U.S. Department of Education (USDE) or the Council for Higher Education Accreditation (CHEA) or be candidates for accreditation with an agency recognized by the USDE for its preaccreditation category. Canadian schools may be provincially chartered instead of accredited.

Baccalaureate-level and master's-level nursing programs represented by a profile within the guide are accredited by the National League for Nursing Accrediting Commission (NLNAC) or the Commission on Collegiate Nursing Education (CCNE). Canadian nursing schools are members of the Canadian Association of University Schools of Nursing (CAUSN).

Doctoral, postdoctoral, continuing education, and other nursing programs included in the profiles are offered by nursing schools or departments affiliated with colleges or universities that meet the criteria outlined above.

QUICK REFERENCE CHART

NURSING PROGRAMS AT-A-GLANCE

	Baccalaureate	Master's	Accelerated	Joint Degree	Post-Master's	Doctoral	Postdoctoral	Continuing Education
UNITED STATES								
Alabama								
Auburn University	•	•						•
Auburn University Montgomery	•	•						
Jacksonville State University	•	•						•
Oakwood University	•							
Samford University	•	•		•	•	•		•
Spring Hill College	•	•	M					
Stillman College	•							
Troy University	•	•			•	•		
Tuskegee University	•							
The University of Alabama	•	•			•	•		
The University of Alabama at Birmingham	•	•	M	•	•	•		
The University of Alabama in Huntsville	•	•			•	•		•
University of Mobile	•	•						•
University of North Alabama	•	•						•
University of South Alabama	•	•	B,M		•	•		
Alaska								
University of Alaska Anchorage	•	•						
Arizona								
Arizona State University at the Downtown Phoenix Campus	•	•	B	•	•	•		•
Chamberlain College of Nursing	•	•	B					
Grand Canyon University	•	•		•	•			•
Northern Arizona University	•	•	B		•			
The University of Arizona	•	•	M		•	•		
University of Phoenix	•	•	B	•	•	•		•
University of Phoenix–Phoenix Campus	•	•	B	•	•			•
University of Phoenix–Southern Arizona Campus	•	•	B		•			•
Arkansas								
Arkansas State University - Jonesboro	•	•						
Arkansas Tech University	•	•						
Harding University	•							•
Henderson State University	•							
Southern Arkansas University–Magnolia	•							
University of Arkansas	•	•						•
University of Arkansas at Fort Smith	•							
University of Arkansas at Little Rock	•							
University of Arkansas at Monticello	•							
University of Arkansas at Pine Bluff	•							
University of Arkansas for Medical Sciences	•	•	B			•	•	•
University of Central Arkansas	•	•			•			

B = Baccalaureate; M = Master's

	Baccalaureate	Master's	Accelerated	Joint Degree	Post-Master's	Doctoral	Postdoctoral	Continuing Education
California								
Azusa Pacific University	•	•	B,M		•	•		•
Biola University	•							
California Baptist University	•	•	M					
California State University, Bakersfield	•							•
California State University Channel Islands	•							
California State University, Chico	•	•			•			•
California State University, Dominguez Hills	•	•			•			•
California State University, East Bay	•		B					
California State University, Fresno	•	•	M		•			•
California State University, Fullerton	•	•	M					•
California State University, Long Beach	•	•	B,M	•	•			
California State University, Los Angeles	•	•	M		•			
California State University, Northridge	•		B					
California State University, Sacramento	•	•						
California State University, San Bernardino	•	•						
California State University, San Marcos	•		B					
California State University, Stanislaus	•							
Concordia University	•		B					
Dominican University of California	•	•						
Fresno Pacific University	•							
Holy Names University	•	•		•	•			
Humboldt State University	•							
Loma Linda University	•	•	B		•	•		
Mount St. Mary's College	•	•	B					
National University	•		B					
Pacific Union College	•							•
Point Loma Nazarene University	•	•			•			•
Samuel Merritt University	•	•	B		•			
San Diego State University	•	•			•			•
San Francisco State University	•	•	B,M		•			•
San Jose State University	•	•						
Sonoma State University	•	•	M		•			
University of California, Irvine	•	•			•			
University of California, Los Angeles	•	•		•	•	•	•	•
University of California, San Francisco		•			•	•	•	
University of Phoenix–Bay Area Campus	•	•	B	•				
University of Phoenix–Central Valley Campus	•							
University of Phoenix–Sacramento Valley Campus	•	•	B,M		•			•
University of Phoenix–San Diego Campus	•	•	B					
University of Phoenix–Southern California Campus	•	•	B	•	•			•
University of San Diego		•	M			•		
University of San Francisco	•	•	M			•		
Vanguard University of Southern California	•							

B = Baccalaureate; M = Master's

	Baccalaureate	Master's	Accelerated	Joint Degree	Post-Master's	Doctoral	Postdoctoral	Continuing Education
West Coast University	•		B					
Western University of Health Sciences		•	M		•	•		
Colorado								
Adams State College	•							
American Sentinel University	•	•						
Colorado State University–Pueblo	•	•	B		•			
Denver College of Nursing	•							
Mesa State College	•							
Metropolitan State College of Denver	•							
Platt College	•		B					
Regis University	•	•	B					
University of Colorado at Colorado Springs	•	•	B		•	•		•
University of Colorado Denver	•	•			•	•	•	•
University of Northern Colorado	•	•	B		•	•		
University of Phoenix–Denver Campus	•	•	B					
University of Phoenix–Southern Colorado Campus								
Connecticut								
Central Connecticut State University	•							
Fairfield University	•	•	B		•	•		•
Quinnipiac University	•	•	B					•
Sacred Heart University	•	•			•	•		
Saint Joseph College	•	•			•			
Southern Connecticut State University	•	•	B		•			
University of Connecticut	•	•	M	•	•	•		•
University of Hartford	•	•		•	•			•
Western Connecticut State University	•	•			•			
Yale University		•		•	•	•	•	
Delaware								
Delaware State University	•							
University of Delaware	•	•	B		•			
Wesley College	•	•	M		•			•
Wilmington University	•	•	B,M	•	•			
District of Columbia								
The Catholic University of America	•	•	B	•	•	•		
Georgetown University	•	•	B		•			
The George Washington University	•	•	B		•	•		
Howard University	•	•	B		•			
Trinity (Washington) University	•							
University of the District of Columbia	•							
Florida								
Barry University	•	•	B	•	•	•		
Bethune-Cookman University	•							
Florida Agricultural and Mechanical University	•	•			•	•		•

B = Baccalaureate; M = Master's

	Baccalaureate	Master's	Accelerated	Joint Degree	Post-Master's	Doctoral	Postdoctoral	Continuing Education
Florida Atlantic University	•	•	B	•	•	•		•
Florida Gulf Coast University	•	•			•			•
Florida Hospital College of Health Sciences	•							
Florida International University	•	•	B,M		•	•		
Florida Southern College	•	•	M	•	•			
Florida State College at Jacksonville	•							
Florida State University	•	•	B		•	•		
Indian River State College	•							
Jacksonville University	•	•	B	•	•			
Kaplan University Online	•	•						
Miami Dade College	•		B					
Northwest Florida State College	•		B					
Nova Southeastern University	•	•		•				
Palm Beach Atlantic University	•							
Remington College of Nursing	•		B					
St. Petersburg College	•							•
South University	•	•						
South University	•	•						
University of Central Florida	•	•	B		•	•		
University of Florida	•	•	B	•	•	•		
University of Miami	•	•	B		•	•		•
University of North Florida	•	•	B		•			
University of Phoenix–Central Florida Campus	•	•	B					
University of Phoenix–North Florida Campus	•	•	B					
University of Phoenix–South Florida Campus	•	•		•				
University of Phoenix–West Florida Campus	•		B					
University of South Florida	•	•	B	•	•	•		•
The University of Tampa	•	•			•			•
University of West Florida	•							
Georgia								
Albany State University	•	•	B,M		•			
Armstrong Atlantic State University	•	•		•	•			•
Augusta State University	•							
Brenau University	•	•	M		•			•
Clayton State University	•	•						
College of Coastal Georgia	•							
Columbus State University	•							
Emory University	•	•	B	•	•	•		
Georgia Baptist College of Nursing of Mercer University	•	•			•	•		
Georgia College & State University	•	•		•	•			
Georgia Health Sciences University	•	•	M		•	•		
Georgia Southern University	•	•			•	•		
Georgia Southwestern State University	•		B					
Georgia State University	•	•			•	•		
Gordon College	•							

B = Baccalaureate; M = Master's

	Baccalaureate	Master's	Accelerated	Joint Degree	Post-Master's	Doctoral	Postdoctoral	Continuing Education
Kennesaw State University	•	•	B					•
LaGrange College	•							
Macon State College	•							
North Georgia College & State University	•	•			•			
Piedmont College	•							
Thomas University	•	•	B,M	•	•			
University of Phoenix–Atlanta Campus								
University of West Georgia	•	•			•			
Valdosta State University	•	•						•
Guam								
University of Guam	•							
Hawaii								
Hawai`i Pacific University	•	•		•	•			
University of Hawaii at Hilo	•							
University of Hawaii at Manoa	•	•	M	•	•	•		
University of Phoenix–Hawaii Campus	•	•	B					
Idaho								
Boise State University	•	•	B					
Brigham Young University–Idaho	•							
Idaho State University	•	•	B,M		•			
Lewis-Clark State College	•							
Northwest Nazarene University	•	•						
Illinois								
Aurora University	•	•						
Benedictine University	•	•	B,M					
Blessing–Rieman College of Nursing	•	•	B					
Bradley University	•	•	B,M					
Chicago State University	•							
DePaul University	•	•	B		•			
Eastern Illinois University	•							
Elmhurst College	•	•		•				
Governors State University	•	•			•			
Illinois State University	•	•	B		•	•		
Illinois Wesleyan University	•							
Lakeview College of Nursing	•		B					
Lewis University	•	•	B,M	•	•			•
Loyola University Chicago	•	•	B	•		•		
MacMurray College	•							
McKendree University	•	•			•			
Methodist College of Nursing	•		B					
Millikin University	•	•	M					
Northern Illinois University	•	•		•	•			
North Park University	•	•		•	•			

B = Baccalaureate; M = Master's

	Baccalaureate	Master's	Accelerated	Joint Degree	Post-Master's	Doctoral	Postdoctoral	Continuing Education
Olivet Nazarene University	•	•	B					•
Resurrection University	•	•	B,M		•			
Rockford College	•							
Rush University		•			•	•		•
Saint Anthony College of Nursing	•	•			•			
Saint Francis Medical Center College of Nursing	•	•	M			•		
St. John's College	•							
Saint Xavier University	•	•		•	•			•
Southern Illinois University Edwardsville	•	•	B		•	•		•
Trinity Christian College	•							
Trinity College of Nursing and Health Sciences	•		B					
University of Illinois at Chicago	•	•		•	•	•	•	•
University of St. Francis	•	•	B		•	•		
Western Illinois University	•							
Indiana								
Anderson University	•	•		•	•			
Ball State University	•	•	B		•	•		
Bethel College	•	•			•			
Goshen College	•							
Huntington University	•							
Indiana State University	•	•			•	•		•
Indiana University Bloomington	•							
Indiana University East	•							
Indiana University Kokomo	•		B					•
Indiana University Northwest	•							
Indiana University–Purdue University Fort Wayne	•	•			•			•
Indiana University–Purdue University Indianapolis	•	•	B	•	•	•	•	•
Indiana University South Bend	•	•	B					
Indiana University Southeast	•							
Indiana Wesleyan University	•	•	B		•			
Marian University	•		B					
Purdue University	•	•	B		•	•		•
Purdue University Calumet	•	•	B		•			
Purdue University North Central	•							
Saint Mary's College	•		B					
University of Evansville	•		B					
University of Indianapolis	•	•	B,M	•	•			
University of Saint Francis	•	•			•			
University of Southern Indiana	•	•			•	•		•
Valparaiso University	•	•	B	•	•			•
Vincennes University	•							
Iowa								
Allen College	•	•	B		•			•
Briar Cliff University	•	•						•

B = Baccalaureate; M = Master's

	Baccalaureate	Master's	Accelerated	Joint Degree	Post-Master's	Doctoral	Postdoctoral	Continuing Education
Clarke University	•	•			•			•
Coe College	•							
Dordt College	•							
Grand View University	•	•						•
Iowa Wesleyan College	•							
Luther College	•							•
Mercy College of Health Sciences	•							
Morningside College	•							
Mount Mercy University	•	•	B					•
Northwestern College	•							
St. Ambrose University	•	•						•
University of Dubuque	•							
The University of Iowa	•	•	M	•	•	•	•	•
Upper Iowa University	•							
Kansas								
Baker University	•							
Bethel College	•							
Emporia State University	•							
Fort Hays State University	•	•			•			
Kansas Wesleyan University	•							
MidAmerica Nazarene University	•		B					•
Newman University	•							
Pittsburg State University	•	•			•			•
Southwestern College	•		B					
Tabor College	•		B					
The University of Kansas	•	•		•	•	•	•	•
University of Saint Mary	•							
Washburn University	•	•			•			•
Wichita State University	•	•	B	•	•	•		
Kentucky								
Bellarmine University	•	•	B	•	•	•		•
Berea College	•							
Eastern Kentucky University	•	•	B					
Frontier School of Midwifery and Family Nursing		•	M			•		
Kentucky Christian University	•							•
Kentucky State University	•							
Midway College	•		B					•
Morehead State University	•							
Murray State University	•	•			•			•
Northern Kentucky University	•	•	B		•			•
Spalding University	•	•	B,M		•			•
Thomas More College	•							
University of Kentucky	•	•			•	•		•
University of Louisville	•	•	B		•	•	•	•
Western Kentucky University	•	•			•			•

B = Baccalaureate; M = Master's

	Baccalaureate	Master's	Accelerated	Joint Degree	Post-Master's	Doctoral	Postdoctoral	Continuing Education
Louisiana								
Dillard University	•							
Grambling State University	•	•			•			
Louisiana College	•							
Louisiana State University Health Sciences Center	•	•	B			•		•
Loyola University New Orleans	•	•			•	•		
McNeese State University	•	•			•			•
Nicholls State University	•							•
Northwestern State University of Louisiana	•	•			•			•
Our Lady of Holy Cross College	•							
Our Lady of the Lake College	•	•						•
Southeastern Louisiana University	•	•	B					
Southern University and Agricultural and Mechanical College	•	•			•	•		
University of Louisiana at Lafayette	•	•	B		•			•
University of Louisiana at Monroe	•		B					•
University of Phoenix–Louisiana Campus	•		B					
Maine								
Husson University	•	•			•			
Saint Joseph's College of Maine	•	•						•
University of Maine	•	•						
University of Maine at Fort Kent	•		B					
University of New England	•		B					•
University of Southern Maine	•	•	B	•	•	•		•
Maryland								
Bowie State University	•	•	B					
College of Notre Dame of Maryland	•		B					
Coppin State University	•	•	B		•			
The Johns Hopkins University	•	•	B	•	•	•	•	•
Salisbury University	•	•	B		•			
Stevenson University	•		B					
Towson University	•	•						
University of Maryland, Baltimore	•	•	M	•	•	•		•
Washington Adventist University	•		B					
Massachusetts								
American International College	•	•						
Anna Maria College	•							•
Atlantic Union College	•							
Boston College	•	•	M	•	•	•		•
Curry College	•	•	B					
Elms College	•	•						
Emmanuel College	•	•						
Endicott College	•	•						•
Fitchburg State University	•	•			•			

B = Baccalaureate; M = Master's

	Baccalaureate	Master's	Accelerated	Joint Degree	Post-Master's	Doctoral	Postdoctoral	Continuing Education
Framingham State University	•	•						•
Massachusetts College of Pharmacy and Health Sciences	•		B					•
MGH Institute of Health Professions	•	•	B		•	•		
Northeastern University	•	•	M	•	•	•		•
Regis College	•	•	B,M		•	•		•
Salem State University	•	•	B,M	•				•
Simmons College	•	•	B,M		•	•		
University of Massachusetts Amherst	•	•	B			•		•
University of Massachusetts Boston	•	•	B		•	•	•	•
University of Massachusetts Dartmouth	•	•			•	•		•
University of Massachusetts Lowell	•	•	M			•		
University of Massachusetts Worcester		•	M		•	•		•
Worcester State College	•	•						
Michigan								
Andrews University	•	•			•			
Calvin College	•							
Davenport University	•							
Davenport University	•							
Eastern Michigan University	•	•						
Ferris State University	•	•	B,M	•				
Finlandia University	•							
Grand Valley State University	•	•	B			•		•
Hope College	•							
Lake Superior State University	•							
Madonna University	•	•		•	•	•		•
Michigan State University	•	•	B		•	•		•
Northern Michigan University	•	•	B		•			•
Oakland University	•	•			•			•
Saginaw Valley State University	•	•	B		•			•
Siena Heights University	•							
Spring Arbor University	•	•		•				
University of Detroit Mercy	•	•	B,M		•			
University of Michigan	•	•	B,M	•	•	•	•	
University of Michigan–Flint	•	•	B,M			•		
University of Phoenix–Metro Detroit Campus	•	•	B					
University of Phoenix–West Michigan Campus								
Wayne State University	•	•	B		•	•	•	•
Western Michigan University	•	•						•
Minnesota								
Augsburg College	•	•						
Bemidji State University	•							•
Bethel University	•	•						
College of Saint Benedict	•							
The College of St. Scholastica	•	•	B		•	•		

B = Baccalaureate; M = Master's

	Baccalaureate	Master's	Accelerated	Joint Degree	Post-Master's	Doctoral	Postdoctoral	Continuing Education
Concordia College	•	•	B					
Crown College	•							
Globe University	•							
Gustavus Adolphus College	•							
Metropolitan State University	•	•			•			
Minnesota Intercollegiate Nursing Consortium	•							
Minnesota State University Mankato	•	•	B,M		•	•		•
Minnesota State University Moorhead	•	•				•		
St. Catherine University	•	•			•	•		
St. Cloud State University	•							
St. Olaf College	•							
University of Minnesota, Twin Cities Campus	•	•		•		•		•
Walden University	•	•			•			
Winona State University	•	•			•	•		
Mississippi								
Alcorn State University	•	•			•			
Delta State University	•	•	M		•			
Mississippi College	•							
Mississippi University for Women	•	•			•			
University of Mississippi Medical Center	•	•	B,M		•	•		•
University of Southern Mississippi	•	•			•	•		
William Carey University	•	•						
Missouri								
Avila University	•							
Central Methodist University	•	•						
Chamberlain College of Nursing	•		B					
College of the Ozarks	•							
Cox College	•		B					•
Goldfarb School of Nursing at Barnes-Jewish College	•	•	B		•	•		
Graceland University	•	•	B		•			
Grantham University	•	•						
Lincoln University	•							
Maryville University of Saint Louis	•	•	B,M			•		
Missouri Southern State University	•	•	B					
Missouri State University	•	•	B,M		•			•
Missouri Western State University	•	•						
Research College of Nursing	•	•	B					
Saint Louis University	•	•	B,M		•	•		•
Saint Luke's College	•							
Southeast Missouri State University	•	•	B		•			
Southwest Baptist University	•							
Truman State University	•							
University of Central Missouri	•	•			•			
University of Missouri	•	•	B	•	•	•		•

B = Baccalaureate; M = Master's

	Baccalaureate	Master's	Accelerated	Joint Degree	Post-Master's	Doctoral	Postdoctoral	Continuing Education
University of Missouri–Kansas City	•	•	B		•	•		•
University of Missouri–St. Louis	•	•	B		•	•		•
Webster University	•	•						
William Jewell College	•		B					
Montana								
Carroll College	•							
Montana State University	•	•	B		•			
Montana State University–Northern	•							
Salish Kootenai College	•							
Nebraska								
BryanLGH College of Health Sciences	•	•						
Clarkson College	•	•	B		•			•
College of Saint Mary	•							
Creighton University	•	•	B		•	•		
Midland Lutheran College	•							
Nebraska Methodist College	•	•	B		•			•
Nebraska Wesleyan University	•	•	B,M		•			
Union College	•							
University of Nebraska Medical Center	•	•	B		•	•	•	•
Nevada								
Great Basin College	•							
Nevada State College at Henderson	•		B					
Touro University	•	•	B		•	•		•
University of Nevada, Las Vegas	•	•	B		•	•		•
University of Nevada, Reno	•	•	B	•	•			
University of Southern Nevada	•		B					
New Hampshire								
Colby-Sawyer College	•							
Franklin Pierce University	•	•						
Rivier College	•	•			•			
Saint Anselm College	•							•
University of New Hampshire	•	•			•			
New Jersey								
Bloomfield College	•							
The College of New Jersey	•	•			•			
College of Saint Elizabeth	•		B					•
Fairleigh Dickinson University, Metropolitan Campus	•	•	B,M		•	•		•
Felician College	•	•	B,M	•	•			
Kean University	•	•	M	•				
Monmouth University	•	•			•			•
New Jersey City University	•		B					
Ramapo College of New Jersey	•	•			•			•
The Richard Stockton College of New Jersey	•	•						

B = Baccalaureate; M = Master's

	Baccalaureate	Master's	Accelerated	Joint Degree	Post-Master's	Doctoral	Postdoctoral	Continuing Education
Rutgers, The State University of New Jersey, Camden College of Arts and Sciences	•		B					
Rutgers, The State University of New Jersey, College of Nursing	•	•	B	•	•	•		•
Saint Peter's College	•	•			•			
Seton Hall University	•	•	B,M	•	•	•		
Thomas Edison State College	•	•						
University of Medicine and Dentistry of New Jersey	•	•	B		•	•		•
William Paterson University of New Jersey	•	•	B		•	•		
New Mexico								
Eastern New Mexico University	•							
New Mexico Highlands University	•							
New Mexico State University	•	•	B					•
University of New Mexico	•	•	B	•	•	•		
University of Phoenix–New Mexico Campus	•	•	B					
Western New Mexico University	•							
New York								
Adelphi University	•	•	B	•	•	•		•
The College at Brockport, State University of New York	•							
College of Mount Saint Vincent	•	•			•			
The College of New Rochelle	•	•	B		•			
College of Staten Island of the City University of New York	•	•			•			
Columbia University	•	•	B,M	•	•	•	•	•
Concordia College–New York	•		B					
Daemen College	•	•	B,M		•	•		
Dominican College	•	•	B					
D'Youville College	•	•			•			
Elmira College	•							•
Excelsior College	•	•			•			
Farmingdale State College	•							
Hartwick College	•		B					
Hunter College of the City University of New York	•	•		•	•			•
Keuka College	•		B					
Lehman College of the City University of New York	•	•	B		•	•		•
Le Moyne College	•	•			•			
Long Island University, Brooklyn Campus	•	•	B		•			
Long Island University, C.W. Post Campus	•	•			•			
Medgar Evers College of the City University of New York	•		B					
Mercy College	•	•	B,M		•			
Molloy College	•	•	B		•	•		•
Mount Saint Mary College	•	•	B		•			
Nazareth College of Rochester	•	•			•			•
New York City College of Technology of the City University of New York	•							
New York Institute of Technology	•							
New York University	•	•	B	•	•	•		•
Niagara University	•							

B = Baccalaureate; M = Master's

	Baccalaureate	Master's	Accelerated	Joint Degree	Post-Master's	Doctoral	Postdoctoral	Continuing Education
Pace University	•	•	B		•	•		
Roberts Wesleyan College	•	•	B,M		•			
The Sage Colleges	•	•	B,M	•	•	•		•
St. Francis College	•							
St. John Fisher College	•	•	B		•	•		
St. Joseph's College, New York	•	•						
State University of New York at Binghamton	•	•	B		•	•		•
State University of New York at Plattsburgh	•							
State University of New York College of Agriculture and Technology at Morrisville	•							
State University of New York College of Technology at Delhi	•							
State University of New York Downstate Medical Center	•	•	B	•	•			•
State University of New York Empire State College	•							
State University of New York Institute of Technology	•	•	B,M		•			•
State University of New York Upstate Medical University	•	•	M		•			•
Stony Brook University, State University of New York	•	•	B		•	•		•
University at Buffalo, the State University of New York	•	•	B		•	•		
University of Rochester	•	•	B,M	•	•	•	•	•
Utica College	•							
Wagner College	•	•			•			
York College of the City University of New York	•							
North Carolina								
Appalachian State University	•							
Barton College	•							
Cabarrus College of Health Sciences	•							
Duke University	•	•	B	•	•	•		
East Carolina University	•	•	M		•	•		
Fayetteville State University	•							
Gardner-Webb University	•	•		•				
Lees-McRae College	•							
Lenoir-Rhyne University	•							
North Carolina Agricultural and Technical State University	•							
North Carolina Central University	•							
Queens University of Charlotte	•	•	B	•				•
The University of North Carolina at Chapel Hill	•	•	B		•	•	•	•
The University of North Carolina at Charlotte	•	•			•			
The University of North Carolina at Greensboro	•	•		•	•	•		
The University of North Carolina at Pembroke	•							
The University of North Carolina Wilmington	•	•			•			•
Western Carolina University	•	•	B		•			
Winston-Salem State University	•	•	B					•
North Dakota								
Dickinson State University	•							
Jamestown College	•							
Medcenter One College of Nursing	•							

B = Baccalaureate; M = Master's

	Baccalaureate	Master's	Accelerated	Joint Degree	Post-Master's	Doctoral	Postdoctoral	Continuing Education
Minot State University	•							
North Dakota State University	•	•				•		
University of Mary	•	•		•				
University of North Dakota	•	•	B		•	•		
Ohio								
Ashland University	•		B					
Capital University	•	•	B	•	•			
Case Western Reserve University	•	•	M	•	•	•	•	•
Cedarville University	•							
Chamberlain College of Nursing	•	•	B					
Cleveland State University	•	•	B	•	•			•
College of Mount St. Joseph	•	•	B,M					
Defiance College	•							
Franciscan University of Steubenville	•	•						
Hiram College	•							
Kent State University	•	•	B,M	•	•	•		•
Kettering College of Medical Arts	•							
Lourdes College	•							
Malone University	•	•						
Mercy College of Northwest Ohio	•							•
Miami University	•							
Miami University Hamilton	•							
Mount Carmel College of Nursing	•	•	B		•			
Mount Vernon Nazarene University	•							
Muskingum University	•							
Notre Dame College	•							
Ohio Northern University	•							
The Ohio State University	•	•	M	•	•	•		•
Ohio University	•	•						
Otterbein University	•	•	B		•			•
Shawnee State University	•							•
The University of Akron	•	•	B		•	•		•
University of Cincinnati	•	•	B,M	•	•	•		•
University of Phoenix–Cleveland Campus	•	•	B					
University of Rio Grande	•							
The University of Toledo	•	•			•	•		•
Urbana University	•	•						
Ursuline College	•	•	B,M		•	•		
Walsh University	•		B					
Wright State University	•	•	B	•	•	•		•
Xavier University	•	•		•				
Youngstown State University	•	•						
Oklahoma								
Bacone College	•		B					

B = Baccalaureate; M = Master's

	Baccalaureate	Master's	Accelerated	Joint Degree	Post-Master's	Doctoral	Postdoctoral	Continuing Education
East Central University	•							
Langston University	•							
Northeastern State University	•	•	B					
Northwestern Oklahoma State University	•		B					
Oklahoma Baptist University	•	•						
Oklahoma Christian University	•							
Oklahoma City University	•	•	B	•		•		•
Oklahoma Panhandle State University	•							
Oklahoma Wesleyan University	•		B					
Oral Roberts University	•							
Rogers State University	•							
Southern Nazarene University	•	•	M					
Southwestern Oklahoma State University	•							
University of Central Oklahoma	•							
University of Oklahoma Health Sciences Center	•	•	B		•	•		•
University of Phoenix–Oklahoma City Campus								
University of Phoenix–Tulsa Campus								
University of Tulsa	•							
Oregon								
Concordia University	•							
George Fox University	•							
Linfield College	•		B					•
Oregon Health & Science University	•	•	B,M	•	•	•	•	•
University of Portland	•	•				•		
Pennsylvania								
Alvernia University	•							•
Bloomsburg University of Pennsylvania	•	•		•	•			•
California University of Pennsylvania	•							
Carlow University	•	•	B,M		•			•
Cedar Crest College	•	•						
Chatham University		•				•		
Clarion University of Pennsylvania	•	•			•			
DeSales University	•	•	B,M	•	•			•
Drexel University	•	•			•	•		•
Duquesne University	•	•	B		•	•		•
Eastern University	•		B					
East Stroudsburg University of Pennsylvania	•							
Edinboro University of Pennsylvania	•		B					
Gannon University	•	•	B,M		•			
Gwynedd-Mercy College	•	•	B		•			
Holy Family University	•	•	B					•
Immaculata University	•	•	B					
Indiana University of Pennsylvania	•	•				•		
La Roche College	•	•	B					•

B = Baccalaureate; M = Master's

	Baccalaureate	Master's	Accelerated	Joint Degree	Post-Master's	Doctoral	Postdoctoral	Continuing Education
La Salle University	•	•		•	•			•
Mansfield University of Pennsylvania	•	•						
Marywood University	•	•		•				•
Messiah College	•							
Millersville University of Pennsylvania	•	•			•			•
Misericordia University	•	•	B		•			
Moravian College	•	•						•
Mount Aloysius College	•		B					•
Neumann University	•	•			•			
Penn State University Park	•	•		•	•	•	•	•
Pennsylvania College of Technology	•							
Robert Morris University	•	•				•		
Saint Francis University	•							
Slippery Rock University of Pennsylvania	•							
Temple University	•	•			•	•		•
Thomas Jefferson University	•	•	B,M		•	•		•
University of Pennsylvania	•	•	B,M	•	•	•	•	•
University of Pittsburgh	•	•	B		•	•	•	•
University of Pittsburgh at Bradford	•							
The University of Scranton	•	•	M		•			
Villanova University	•	•	B,M		•	•		•
Waynesburg University	•	•	B,M	•		•		
West Chester University of Pennsylvania	•	•	B					
Widener University	•	•		•	•	•		•
Wilkes University	•	•	B,M		•			•
York College of Pennsylvania	•	•			•			
Puerto Rico								
Inter American University of Puerto Rico, Arecibo Campus	•							
Inter American University of Puerto Rico, Metropolitan Campus	•		B					
Pontifical Catholic University of Puerto Rico	•							
Universidad Adventista de las Antillas	•							•
Universidad del Turabo	•							
Universidad Metropolitana	•							
University of Puerto Rico at Arecibo	•							
University of Puerto Rico at Humacao	•							
University of Puerto Rico, Mayagüez Campus	•							•
University of Puerto Rico, Medical Sciences Campus	•	•						•
University of the Sacred Heart	•	•						
Rhode Island								
Rhode Island College	•	•						
Salve Regina University	•							•
University of Rhode Island	•	•			•	•		
South Carolina								
Charleston Southern University	•	•						

B = Baccalaureate; M = Master's

	Baccalaureate	Master's	Accelerated	Joint Degree	Post-Master's	Doctoral	Postdoctoral	Continuing Education
Clemson University	•	•			•			•
Francis Marion University	•							
Lander University	•		B					
Medical University of South Carolina	•	•	B		•	•	•	•
South Carolina State University	•							
University of South Carolina	•	•			•	•		•
University of South Carolina Aiken	•							
University of South Carolina Beaufort	•							
University of South Carolina Upstate	•							
South Dakota								
Augustana College	•							
Dakota Wesleyan University	•							
Mount Marty College	•		B					
National American University	•							
Presentation College	•							
South Dakota State University	•	•	B		•	•		•
Tennessee								
Aquinas College	•							
Austin Peay State University	•							
Baptist College of Health Sciences	•							
Belmont University	•	•	B		•			
Bethel University	•							
Carson-Newman College	•	•	B		•			
Cumberland University	•		B					
East Tennessee State University	•	•	B		•	•		•
King College	•	•	B,M	•				
Lincoln Memorial University	•							
Lipscomb University	•							
Martin Methodist College	•							
Middle Tennessee State University	•	•	M		•			
Milligan College	•							
South College	•							
Southern Adventist University	•	•	M	•				•
Tennessee State University	•	•			•			•
Tennessee Technological University	•	•						
Tennessee Wesleyan College	•							
Union University	•	•	B		•			•
University of Memphis	•	•	B,M		•			
The University of Tennessee	•	•	B,M		•	•		•
The University of Tennessee at Chattanooga	•	•			•	•		•
The University of Tennessee at Martin	•							•
The University of Tennessee Health Science Center		•	M		•	•		
Vanderbilt University		•	M	•	•	•	•	

B = Baccalaureate; M = Master's

	Baccalaureate	Master's	Accelerated	Joint Degree	Post-Master's	Doctoral	Postdoctoral	Continuing Education
Texas								
Angelo State University	•	•	B					
Baylor University	•	•	B		•	•		
East Texas Baptist University	•							
Houston Baptist University	•							
Lamar University	•	•		•	•			•
Lubbock Christian University	•							
Midwestern State University	•	•			•			•
Patty Hanks Shelton School of Nursing	•	•			•			•
Prairie View A&M University	•	•			•			
Southwestern Adventist University	•							
Stephen F. Austin State University	•							
Tarleton State University	•							•
Texas A&M Health Science Center	•		B					
Texas A&M International University	•	•						
Texas A&M University–Corpus Christi	•	•	B,M		•			•
Texas A&M University–Texarkana	•	•						
Texas Christian University	•	•	B		•	•		•
Texas Tech University Health Sciences Center	•	•	B		•	•		•
Texas Woman's University	•	•	B		•	•		
University of Houston–Victoria	•	•	B					
University of Mary Hardin-Baylor	•	•						•
The University of Texas at Arlington	•	•	B	•	•	•		•
The University of Texas at Austin	•	•		•	•	•	•	
The University of Texas at Brownsville	•	•						
The University of Texas at El Paso	•	•	B		•			
The University of Texas at Tyler	•	•	B,M	•	•	•		•
The University of Texas Health Science Center at Houston	•	•	B	•	•	•		•
The University of Texas Health Science Center at San Antonio	•	•	B	•	•	•		•
The University of Texas Medical Branch	•	•	B		•	•		
The University of Texas–Pan American	•	•			•			
University of the Incarnate Word	•	•	M		•			
Wayland Baptist University	•							
West Texas A&M University	•	•			•			
Utah								
Brigham Young University	•	•			•			
Dixie State College of Utah	•							
Southern Utah University	•							
University of Phoenix–Utah Campus								
University of Utah	•	•	B	•	•	•	•	
Utah Valley University	•							
Weber State University	•	•	B					
Western Governors University	•	•						
Westminster College	•	•			•			

B = Baccalaureate; M = Master's

	Baccalaureate	Master's	Accelerated	Joint Degree	Post-Master's	Doctoral	Postdoctoral	Continuing Education
Vermont								
Norwich University	•							
Southern Vermont College	•							
University of Vermont	•	•			•			
Virgin Islands								
University of the Virgin Islands	•							
Virginia								
Eastern Mennonite University	•	•						
ECPI College of Technology	•							
George Mason University	•	•	B		•	•		•
Hampton University	•	•	B			•		
James Madison University	•	•	B		•			
Jefferson College of Health Sciences	•	•						•
Liberty University	•	•						
Lynchburg College	•	•	B	•				
Marymount University	•	•	B		•	•		
Norfolk State University	•		B					
Old Dominion University	•	•	B		•	•		•
Radford University	•					•		
Shenandoah University	•	•	B		•			•
University of Virginia	•	•		•	•	•	•	
The University of Virginia's College at Wise	•							
Virginia Commonwealth University	•	•	B,M		•	•	•	
Washington								
Gonzaga University	•	•	M		•			
Northwest University	•							
Olympic College	•							
Pacific Lutheran University	•	•	M	•				•
Seattle Pacific University	•	•			•			
Seattle University	•	•	M		•			
University of Washington	•	•	B	•	•	•	•	•
Walla Walla University	•							
Washington State University College of Nursing and Consortium	•	•	M		•	•		•
West Virginia								
Alderson-Broaddus College	•							
Bluefield State College	•							
Fairmont State University	•		B					•
Marshall University	•	•	B		•			
Mountain State University	•	•			•			
Shepherd University	•							•
University of Charleston	•							
West Liberty University	•		B					
West Virginia University	•	•	B,M		•	•		•

B = Baccalaureate; M = Master's

	Baccalaureate	Master's	Accelerated	Joint Degree	Post-Master's	Doctoral	Postdoctoral	Continuing Education
West Virginia Wesleyan College	•	•						
Wheeling Jesuit University	•	•	B		•			
Wisconsin								
Alverno College	•	•						•
Bellin College	•	•	B					
Cardinal Stritch University	•	•	M					
Carroll University	•							
Columbia College of Nursing/Mount Mary College Nursing Program	•							
Concordia University Wisconsin	•	•			•	•		
Edgewood College	•	•	B	•				
Maranatha Baptist Bible College	•							
Marian University	•	•			•			
Marquette University	•	•		•	•	•		
Milwaukee School of Engineering	•							
Silver Lake College	•							
University of Phoenix–Milwaukee Campus	•	•				•		
University of Wisconsin–Eau Claire	•	•	B		•	•		•
University of Wisconsin–Green Bay	•							
University of Wisconsin–Madison	•					•	•	•
University of Wisconsin–Milwaukee	•	•		•		•		
University of Wisconsin–Oshkosh	•	•	B		•			•
Viterbo University	•	•			•			•
Wisconsin Lutheran College	•							•
Wyoming								
University of Wyoming	•	•	B		•			
CANADA								
Alberta								
Athabasca University	•	•		•	•			
University of Alberta	•	•	B		•	•		
University of Calgary	•	•	B		•	•		
University of Lethbridge	•	•	B					
British Columbia								
British Columbia Institute of Technology	•							•
Kwantlen Polytechnic University	•							
Thompson Rivers University	•							•
Trinity Western University	•	•	M					
The University of British Columbia	•	•	B	•		•	•	
University of Northern British Columbia	•	•					•	
University of Victoria	•	•				•		
Vancouver Island University	•							

B = Baccalaureate; M = Master's

	Baccalaureate	Master's	Accelerated	Joint Degree	Post-Master's	Doctoral	Postdoctoral	Continuing Education
Manitoba								
Brandon University	•							
University of Manitoba	•	•				•		•
New Brunswick								
Université de Moncton	•	•						•
University of New Brunswick Fredericton	•	•	B					•
Newfoundland and Labrador								
Memorial University of Newfoundland	•	•	B		•			
Nova Scotia								
Dalhousie University	•	•	B		•	•		
St. Francis Xavier University	•		B					•
Ontario								
Brock University	•							
Lakehead University	•		B					
Laurentian University	•							•
McMaster University	•	•		•		•		
Nipissing University	•							
Queen's University at Kingston	•	•	B			•		
Ryerson University	•	•						•
Trent University	•		B					
University of Ottawa	•	•				•	•	
University of Toronto	•	•	B		•	•		•
The University of Western Ontario	•	•	B			•	•	
University of Windsor	•	•						•
York University	•							•
Prince Edward Island								
University of Prince Edward Island	•							
Quebec								
McGill University	•	•	B			•	•	
Université de Montréal	•	•			•	•	•	•
Université de Sherbrooke	•	•				•	•	
Université du Québec à Chicoutimi	•	•	B,M	•				
Université du Québec à Rimouski	•	•						•
Université du Québec à Trois-Rivières	•	•						
Université du Québec en Abitibi-Témiscamingue	•							
Université du Québec en Outaouais	•	•						
Université Laval	•	•	B,M		•	•	•	•
Saskatchewan								
University of Saskatchewan	•	•	B		•	•		•

B = Baccalaureate; M = Master's

PROFILES OF NURSING PROGRAMS

U.S. AND U.S. TERRITORIES

ALABAMA

Auburn University

School of Nursing
Auburn University, Alabama

http://www.auburn.edu/academic/nursing/au_nursing.html
Founded in 1856

DEGREES • BSN • MSN

Nursing Program Faculty 15 (90% with doctorates).
Baccalaureate Enrollment 171 **Women** 90% **Men** 10% **Minority** 3%
Graduate Enrollment 38 **Women** 95% **Men** 5% **Minority** 7% **Part-time** 65%
Nursing Student Activities Nursing Honor Society, Sigma Theta Tau, Student Nurses' Association, nursing club.
Nursing Student Resources Academic advising; academic or career counseling; assistance for students with disabilities; bookstore; campus computer network; career placement assistance; computer lab; computer-assisted instruction; e-mail services; employment services for current students; interactive nursing skills videos; Internet; library services; nursing audiovisuals; placement services for program completers; remedial services; resume preparation assistance; skills, simulation, or other laboratory; tutoring.
Library Facilities 3.1 million volumes; 275,732 periodical subscriptions.

BACCALAUREATE PROGRAMS

Degree BSN
Available Programs Generic Baccalaureate.
Study Options Full-time.
Program Entrance Requirements Minimum overall college GPA of 2.5, transcript of college record, CPR certification, health exam, health insurance, immunizations, interview, minimum GPA in nursing prerequisites of 2.5, professional liability insurance/malpractice insurance, prerequisite course work. Transfer students are accepted. *Application deadline:* 2/1 (fall), 5/1 (spring).
Financial Aid 75% of baccalaureate students in nursing programs received some form of financial aid in 2009-10. *Gift aid (need-based):* Federal Pell, FSEOG, state, private, college/university gift aid from institutional funds. *Loans:* Federal Nursing Student Loans, Federal Direct (Subsidized and Unsubsidized Stafford PLUS), Perkins, college/university. *Work-study:* Federal Work-Study. *Financial aid application deadline (priority):* 3/1.
Contact Pam Hennessey, Academic Advisor, School of Nursing, Auburn University, 118 Miller Hall, Auburn University, AL 36849. *Telephone:* 334-844-5665. *Fax:* 334-844-4177. *E-mail:* hennepp@auburn.edu.

GRADUATE PROGRAMS

Contact Dr. Anita All, Director, MSN Program, School of Nursing, Auburn University, 118 Miller Hall, Auburn University, AL 36849. *Telephone:* 334-844-5665. *E-mail:* aca0001@auburn.edu.

MASTER'S DEGREE PROGRAM

Degree MSN
Available Programs Master's.
Concentrations Available Nursing education. *Clinical nurse specialist programs in:* adult health, gerontology, pediatric.
Study Options Full-time and part-time.
Program Entrance Requirements Minimum overall college GPA of 3.0, transcript of college record, nursing research course, statistics course.
Degree Requirements 51 total credit hours, thesis or project.

CONTINUING EDUCATION PROGRAM

Contact Dr. Stuart Pope, Outreach Coordinator, School of Nursing, Auburn University, Miller Hall, Auburn University, AL 36849-5505. *Telephone:* 334-844-5665. *Fax:* 334-844-4177.

Auburn University Montgomery

School of Nursing
Montgomery, Alabama

http://www.aum.edu/nursing
Founded in 1967

DEGREES • BSN • MSN

Nursing Program Faculty 20 (70% with doctorates).
Baccalaureate Enrollment 650 **Women** 80% **Men** 20% **Minority** 33%
International 1% **Part-time** 20%
Graduate Enrollment 30
Nursing Student Activities Nursing Honor Society, Sigma Theta Tau, Student Nurses' Association.
Nursing Student Resources Academic advising; academic or career counseling; assistance for students with disabilities; bookstore; campus computer network; career placement assistance; computer lab; computer-assisted instruction; daycare for children of students; e-mail services; housing assistance; interactive nursing skills videos; Internet; learning resource lab; library services; nursing audiovisuals; remedial services; resume preparation assistance; skills, simulation, or other laboratory; tutoring.
Library Facilities 367,620 volumes (9,568 in nursing); 349,120 periodical subscriptions (273 health-care related).

BACCALAUREATE PROGRAMS

Degree BSN
Available Programs Generic Baccalaureate; RN Baccalaureate.
Study Options Full-time.
Program Entrance Requirements Transcript of college record, CPR certification, health exam, high school transcript, immunizations, interview, minimum GPA in nursing prerequisites of 2.5, professional liability insurance/malpractice insurance, prerequisite course work. Transfer students are accepted. *Application deadline:* 2/1 (fall), 5/1 (spring).
Expenses (2010-11) *Tuition, state resident:* part-time $214 per credit hour. *Tuition, nonresident:* part-time $626 per credit hour. *Required fees:* full-time $1600.
Financial Aid 75% of baccalaureate students in nursing programs received some form of financial aid in 2009-10. *Gift aid (need-based):* Federal Pell, FSEOG, state, college/university gift aid from institutional funds. *Loans:* Federal Direct (Subsidized and Unsubsidized Stafford PLUS), Perkins. *Work-study:* Federal Work-Study. *Financial aid application deadline (priority):* 3/1.
Contact Mrs. Lorinda Brewer Stutheit, Admissions Chair/Coordinator, Advising/Recruiting, School of Nursing, Auburn University Montgomery, PO Box 244023, Montgomery, AL 36124-4023. *Telephone:* 334-244-3431. *Fax:* 334-244-3243. *E-mail:* lorinda.stutheit@aum.edu.

GRADUATE PROGRAMS

Expenses (2010-11) *Tuition, state resident:* part-time $241 per credit hour. *Tuition, nonresident:* part-time $741 per credit hour. *Required fees:* full-time $300.
Financial Aid 10% of graduate students in nursing programs received some form of financial aid in 2009-10.
Contact Dr. Anita C. All, Professor and Director, School of Nursing, Auburn University Montgomery, 213 Miller Hall, Auburn University, AL 36849-5055. *Telephone:* 334-844-5613. *Fax:* 334-844-4177. *E-mail:* msnnurse@auburn.edu.

MASTER'S DEGREE PROGRAM

Degree MSN
Available Programs Master's.
Concentrations Available Nursing education. *Clinical nurse specialist programs in:* adult health, gerontology, pediatric. *Nurse practitioner programs in:* primary care.
Study Options Full-time and part-time.
Program Entrance Requirements Clinical experience, minimum overall college GPA of 3.0, written essay, 3 letters of recommendation, resume, statistics course.
Advanced Placement Credit given for nursing courses completed elsewhere dependent upon specific evaluations.

Degree Requirements 42 total credit hours, thesis or project, comprehensive exam.

Jacksonville State University
College of Nursing and Health Sciences
Jacksonville, Alabama

http://www.jsu.edu/depart/nursing
Founded in 1883

DEGREES • BSN • MSN

Nursing Program Faculty 31 (42% with doctorates).
Baccalaureate Enrollment 473 **Women** 84% **Men** 16% **Minority** 30% **International** 1% **Part-time** 20%
Graduate Enrollment 76 **Women** 93% **Men** 7% **Minority** 25% **International** 1% **Part-time** 62%
Distance Learning Courses Available.
Nursing Student Activities Sigma Theta Tau, Student Nurses' Association.
Nursing Student Resources Academic advising; academic or career counseling; campus computer network; computer lab; computer-assisted instruction; e-mail services; Internet; learning resource lab; nursing audiovisuals; remedial services; skills, simulation, or other laboratory; tutoring.
Library Facilities 685,991 volumes (27,787 in health, 1,873 in nursing); 14,376 periodical subscriptions (1,479 health-care related).

BACCALAUREATE PROGRAMS

Degree BSN
Available Programs Generic Baccalaureate; RN Baccalaureate.
Study Options Full-time and part-time.
Online Degree Options Yes.
Program Entrance Requirements Transcript of college record, CPR certification, health exam, health insurance, high school transcript, immunizations, minimum GPA in nursing prerequisites, professional liability insurance/malpractice insurance, prerequisite course work. Transfer students are accepted. *Application deadline:* 6/1 (fall), 10/1 (spring).
Expenses (2010-11) *Tuition, area resident:* full-time $5424; part-time $226 per credit hour. *Tuition, state resident:* full-time $6720; part-time $280 per credit hour. *Tuition, nonresident:* full-time $10,848; part-time $452 per credit hour. *Room and board:* $6162; room only: $2950 per academic year.
Financial Aid 70% of baccalaureate students in nursing programs received some form of financial aid in 2009-10.
Contact Mr. David Hofland, Student Services Coordinator, College of Nursing and Health Sciences, Jacksonville State University, 700 Pelham Road North, Jacksonville, AL 36265-1602. *Telephone:* 256-782-5276. *Fax:* 256-782-5406. *E-mail:* hofland@jsu.edu.

GRADUATE PROGRAMS

Expenses (2010-11) *Tuition, state resident:* full-time $6354; part-time $353 per credit hour. *Tuition, nonresident:* full-time $6354; part-time $353 per credit hour. *Room and board:* $6162; room only: $2950 per academic year.
Financial Aid 60% of graduate students in nursing programs received some form of financial aid in 2009-10.
Contact Dr. Beth Hembree, Director, Graduate Studies, College of Nursing and Health Sciences, Jacksonville State University, 700 Pelham Road North, Jacksonville, AL 36265-1602. *Telephone:* 256-782-5431. *Fax:* 256-782-5406. *E-mail:* bhembree@jsu.edu.

MASTER'S DEGREE PROGRAM

Degree MSN
Available Programs Master's.
Concentrations Available *Clinical nurse specialist programs in:* community health.
Study Options Full-time and part-time.
Online Degree Options Yes (online only).
Program Entrance Requirements Minimum overall college GPA of 3.0, transcript of college record, written essay, interview, 3 letters of recommendation, nursing research course, physical assessment course, statistics course. *Application deadline:* Applications may be processed on a rolling basis for some programs.
Advanced Placement Credit given for nursing courses completed elsewhere dependent upon specific evaluations.
Degree Requirements 36 total credit hours, thesis or project, comprehensive exam.

CONTINUING EDUCATION PROGRAM

Contact Mr. David Hofland, Student Services Coordinator, College of Nursing and Health Sciences, Jacksonville State University, 700 Pelham Road North, Jacksonville, AL 36265-1602. *Telephone:* 256-782-5276. *Fax:* 256-782-5406. *E-mail:* hofland@jsu.edu.

Oakwood University
Department of Nursing
Huntsville, Alabama

http://www.oakwood.edu/nursing/
Founded in 1896

DEGREE • BS

Nursing Program Faculty 9 (33% with doctorates).
Baccalaureate Enrollment 73 **Women** 87% **Men** 13% **Minority** 100% **International** 2%
Nursing Student Activities Nursing club.
Nursing Student Resources Academic advising; academic or career counseling; assistance for students with disabilities; bookstore; campus computer network; career placement assistance; computer lab; computer-assisted instruction; e-mail services; employment services for current students; externships; interactive nursing skills videos; Internet; learning resource lab; library services; nursing audiovisuals; paid internships; placement services for program completers; remedial services; resume preparation assistance; skills, simulation, or other laboratory; tutoring; unpaid internships.
Library Facilities 133,106 volumes (5,147 in health, 3,474 in nursing); 726 periodical subscriptions (47 health-care related).

BACCALAUREATE PROGRAMS

Degree BS
Available Programs Generic Baccalaureate; RN Baccalaureate.
Study Options Full-time and part-time.
Program Entrance Requirements Minimum overall college GPA of 3.00, transcript of college record, written essay, health exam, health insurance, high school transcript, immunizations, 3 letters of recommendation. Transfer students are accepted. *Application deadline:* 11/16 (fall).
Expenses (2010-11) *Tuition:* full-time $6521; part-time $563 per credit hour. *Room and board:* $5000; room only: $2500 per academic year. *Required fees:* full-time $30; part-time $15 per term.
Financial Aid 95% of baccalaureate students in nursing programs received some form of financial aid in 2009-10.
Contact Mrs. Denise Finley, Secretary, Department of Nursing, Oakwood University, 7000 Adventist Boulevard, Huntsville, AL 35896. *Telephone:* 256-726-7287. *Fax:* 256-726-8338. *E-mail:* dfinley@oakwood.edu.

Samford University
Ida V. Moffett School of Nursing
Birmingham, Alabama

http://www.samford.edu
Founded in 1841

DEGREES • BSN • DNP • MSN • MSN/MBA

Nursing Program Faculty 33 (54% with doctorates).
Baccalaureate Enrollment 300 **Women** 97% **Men** 3% **Minority** 5% **International** 2% **Part-time** 10%
Graduate Enrollment 125 **Women** 88% **Men** 12% **Minority** 32% **Part-time** 5%
Nursing Student Activities Sigma Theta Tau, Student Nurses' Association, nursing club.
Nursing Student Resources Academic advising; academic or career counseling; assistance for students with disabilities; bookstore; campus computer network; career placement assistance; computer lab; computer-assisted instruction; e-mail services; externships; interactive nursing skills videos; Internet; learning resource lab; library services; nursing audiovisuals; paid internships; placement services for program completers; remedial services; resume preparation assistance; skills, simulation, or other laboratory; tutoring; unpaid internships.
Library Facilities 439,760 volumes (7,000 in health, 2,500 in nursing); 3,724 periodical subscriptions (100 health-care related).

BACCALAUREATE PROGRAMS

Degree BSN
Available Programs Baccalaureate for Second Degree; Generic Baccalaureate.
Study Options Full-time and part-time.
Program Entrance Requirements Minimum overall college GPA of 2.7, transcript of college record, CPR certification, written essay, health exam, health insurance, high school biology, high school chemistry, 2 years high school math, 2 years high school science, high school transcript, immunizations, minimum high school GPA of 3.0, minimum GPA in nursing prerequisites of 2.0, professional liability insurance/malpractice insurance, prerequisite course work. Transfer students are accepted.
Advanced Placement Credit given for nursing courses completed elsewhere dependent upon specific evaluations.
Contact ***Telephone:*** 205-726-2872 Ext. 2746. *Fax:* 205-726-4269.

GRADUATE PROGRAMS

Contact ***Telephone:*** 205-726-2047. *Fax:* 205-726-4269.

MASTER'S DEGREE PROGRAM

Degrees MSN; MSN/MBA
Available Programs Master's; RN to Master's.
Concentrations Available Nurse anesthesia; nursing administration; nursing education. *Nurse practitioner programs in:* family health, primary care.
Study Options Full-time and part-time.
Program Entrance Requirements Clinical experience, computer literacy, minimum overall college GPA of 3.0, transcript of college record, CPR certification, immunizations, interview, 3 letters of recommendation, nursing research course, physical assessment course, professional liability insurance/malpractice insurance, prerequisite course work, statistics course, GRE General Test or MAT. *Application deadline:* 7/7 (fall), 11/1 (spring), 4/15 (summer). Applications may be processed on a rolling basis for some programs. *Application fee:* $35.
Advanced Placement Credit given for nursing courses completed elsewhere dependent upon specific evaluations.
Degree Requirements 38 total credit hours.

POST-MASTER'S PROGRAM

Areas of Study Nurse anesthesia; nursing administration; nursing education. *Nurse practitioner programs in:* family health, primary care.

DOCTORAL DEGREE PROGRAM

Degree DNP
Available Programs Doctorate.
Areas of Study Advanced practice nursing, faculty preparation, family health, health-care systems, nursing administration, nursing education.
Program Entrance Requirements Minimum overall college GPA of 3.5, interview by faculty committee, interview, 3 letters of recommendation, MSN or equivalent, statistics course, vita, writing sample. Application deadline: 1/31 (spring). Application fee: $35.
Degree Requirements 38 total credit hours.

CONTINUING EDUCATION PROGRAM

Contact ***Telephone:*** 205-726-2045. *Fax:* 205-726-2219.

Spring Hill College

Division of Nursing
Mobile, Alabama

http://faculty.shc.edu/nursing
Founded in 1830

DEGREES • BSN • MSN
Nursing Program Faculty 8 (84% with doctorates).
Baccalaureate Enrollment 124 **Women** 86% **Men** 14% **Minority** 12%
Graduate Enrollment 62 **Women** 95% **Men** 5% **Minority** 45% **Part-time** 40%
Distance Learning Courses Available.
Nursing Student Activities Nursing Honor Society, Sigma Theta Tau, Student Nurses' Association.
Nursing Student Resources Academic advising; academic or career counseling; assistance for students with disabilities; bookstore; campus computer network; career placement assistance; computer lab; computer-assisted instruction; e-mail services; employment services for current students; externships; interactive nursing skills videos; Internet; learning resource lab; library services; nursing audiovisuals; placement services for program completers; resume preparation assistance; skills, simulation, or other laboratory; tutoring; unpaid internships.
Library Facilities 193,638 volumes (330 in health, 300 in nursing); 988 periodical subscriptions (58 health-care related).

BACCALAUREATE PROGRAMS

Degree BSN
Available Programs Baccalaureate for Second Degree; Generic Baccalaureate.
Study Options Full-time.
Program Entrance Requirements Minimum overall college GPA of 2.75, transcript of college record, CPR certification, written essay, health exam, health insurance, high school transcript, immunizations, 1 letter of recommendation, minimum GPA in nursing prerequisites of 2.75, prerequisite course work. Transfer students are accepted. *Application deadline:* 3/1 (spring).
Advanced Placement Credit by examination available.
Contact ***Telephone:*** 334-380-4492. *Fax:* 334-380-4495.

GRADUATE PROGRAMS

Contact ***Telephone:*** 251-380-3067. *Fax:* 251-460-2190.

MASTER'S DEGREE PROGRAM

Degree MSN
Available Programs Accelerated AD/RN to Master's; Master's; RN to Master's.
Concentrations Available Clinical nurse leader.
Study Options Full-time and part-time.
Online Degree Options Yes (online only).
Program Entrance Requirements Clinical experience, minimum overall college GPA of 3.0, transcript of college record, immunizations, professional liability insurance/malpractice insurance, prerequisite course work, resume, statistics course. *Application deadline:* Applications may be processed on a rolling basis for some programs.
Advanced Placement Credit by examination available. Credit given for nursing courses completed elsewhere dependent upon specific evaluations.
Degree Requirements 36 total credit hours, thesis or project.

Stillman College

Nursing Major
Tuscaloosa, Alabama

Founded in 1876

DEGREE • BSN
Library Facilities 117,500 volumes; 6,300 periodical subscriptions.

BACCALAUREATE PROGRAMS

Degree BSN
Available Programs RN Baccalaureate.
Contact Information, Nursing Major, Stillman College, 3600 Stillman Boulevard, Tuscaloosa, AL 35403-9990. *Telephone:* 205-349-4240. *Fax:* 205-366-8996.

Troy University

School of Nursing
Troy, Alabama

http://troy.troy.edu/nursing
Founded in 1887

DEGREES • BSN • DNP • MSN
Nursing Program Faculty 39 (49% with doctorates).
Baccalaureate Enrollment 800 **Women** 88% **Men** 12% **Minority** 35% **International** 4% **Part-time** 10%
Graduate Enrollment 200 **Women** 97% **Men** 3% **Minority** 23% **Part-time** 29%
Distance Learning Courses Available.
Nursing Student Activities Sigma Theta Tau, Student Nurses' Association.

Nursing Student Resources Academic advising; academic or career counseling; assistance for students with disabilities; bookstore; campus computer network; career placement assistance; computer lab; computer-assisted instruction; e-mail services; employment services for current students; externships; housing assistance; interactive nursing skills videos; Internet; learning resource lab; library services; nursing audiovisuals; placement services for program completers; resume preparation assistance; skills, simulation, or other laboratory; tutoring; unpaid internships.
Library Facilities 571,172 volumes (45,006 in health, 3,843 in nursing); 3,309 periodical subscriptions (703 health-care related).

BACCALAUREATE PROGRAMS

Degree BSN
Available Programs Generic Baccalaureate; RN Baccalaureate.
Site Options Montgomery, AL; Phenix City, AL; Dothan, AL.
Study Options Full-time.
Program Entrance Requirements Minimum overall college GPA of 2.5, transcript of college record, CPR certification, health exam, health insurance, immunizations, professional liability insurance/malpractice insurance, prerequisite course work. Transfer students are accepted. *Application deadline:* 3/15 (fall), 9/15 (spring). *Application fee:* $20.
Advanced Placement Credit by examination available. Credit given for nursing courses completed elsewhere dependent upon specific evaluations.
Expenses (2010-11) *Tuition, area resident:* part-time $216 per credit hour. *Tuition, nonresident:* part-time $432 per credit hour. *Room and board:* $2840; room only: $2620 per academic year. *Required fees:* full-time $400.
Financial Aid 90% of baccalaureate students in nursing programs received some form of financial aid in 2009-10. *Gift aid (need-based):* Federal Pell, FSEOG, state, private, college/university gift aid from institutional funds. *Loans:* Perkins. *Work-study:* Federal Work-Study. *Financial aid application deadline (priority):* 3/1.
Contact Ms. Amy Owens, Departmental Secretary I, School of Nursing, Troy University, 400 Pell Avenue, Troy, AL 36082. *Telephone:* 334-670-3428. *Fax:* 334-670-3744. *E-mail:* acowens@troy.edu.

GRADUATE PROGRAMS

Expenses (2010-11) *Tuition, state resident:* part-time $420 per credit hour. *Tuition, nonresident:* part-time $420 per credit hour. *Required fees:* full-time $200.
Financial Aid 40% of graduate students in nursing programs received some form of financial aid in 2009-10.
Contact Dr. Patsy Riley, Director, Graduate Nursing Programs, School of Nursing, Troy University, 340 Montgomery Street, Montgomery, AL 36104. *Telephone:* 334-834-2320. *Fax:* 334-241-8627. *E-mail:* priley@troy.edu.

MASTER'S DEGREE PROGRAM

Degree MSN
Available Programs Master's.
Concentrations Available Nursing administration; nursing education; nursing informatics. *Clinical nurse specialist programs in:* adult health, maternity-newborn. *Nurse practitioner programs in:* family health.
Site Options Montgomery, AL; Phenix City, AL.
Study Options Full-time and part-time.
Online Degree Options Yes.
Program Entrance Requirements Minimum overall college GPA of 3.0, transcript of college record, CPR certification, immunizations, 3 letters of recommendation, physical assessment course, professional liability insurance/malpractice insurance. *Application deadline:* Applications may be processed on a rolling basis for some programs. *Application fee:* $20.
Advanced Placement Credit given for nursing courses completed elsewhere dependent upon specific evaluations.
Degree Requirements 39 total credit hours, thesis or project, comprehensive exam.

POST-MASTER'S PROGRAM

Areas of Study *Nurse practitioner programs in:* family health.

DOCTORAL DEGREE PROGRAM

Degree DNP
Available Programs Doctorate; Post-Baccalaureate Doctorate.
Areas of Study Advanced practice nursing.
Site Options Montgomery, AL; Phenix City, AL.
Online Degree Options Yes (online only).
Program Entrance Requirements Clinical experience, minimum overall college GPA of 3.0, interview by faculty committee, 2 letters of recommendation, MSN or equivalent, vita, writing sample. Application deadline: 2/1 (fall). Application fee: $75.
Degree Requirements 74 total credit hours, oral exam, residency.

Tuskegee University
Program in Nursing
Tuskegee, Alabama

http://www.tuskegee.edu/Global/Category.asp?C=52456
Founded in 1881

DEGREE • BSN

Nursing Program Faculty 6 (50% with doctorates).
Baccalaureate Enrollment 131 **Women** 98% **Men** 2% **Minority** 100%
Nursing Student Activities Nursing Honor Society, Student Nurses' Association, nursing club.
Nursing Student Resources Academic advising; academic or career counseling; assistance for students with disabilities; bookstore; campus computer network; career placement assistance; computer lab; computer-assisted instruction; e-mail services; interactive nursing skills videos; Internet; learning resource lab; library services; nursing audiovisuals; placement services for program completers; remedial services; resume preparation assistance; skills, simulation, or other laboratory; tutoring; unpaid internships.
Library Facilities 623,824 volumes (3,500 in health); 81,157 periodical subscriptions (250 health-care related).

BACCALAUREATE PROGRAMS

Degree BSN
Available Programs ADN to Baccalaureate; Generic Baccalaureate; RN Baccalaureate.
Study Options Full-time.
Program Entrance Requirements Minimum overall college GPA of 3.0, transcript of college record, CPR certification, written essay, health exam, health insurance, high school biology, high school chemistry, 2 years high school math, 1 year of high school science, high school transcript, immunizations, interview, minimum high school GPA of 3.0, minimum GPA in nursing prerequisites of 3.0, professional liability insurance/malpractice insurance, prerequisite course work. Transfer students are accepted. *Application deadline:* 3/30 (fall), 10/30 (spring), 4/30 (summer). Applications may be processed on a rolling basis for some programs. *Application fee:* $35.
Advanced Placement Credit given for nursing courses completed elsewhere dependent upon specific evaluations.
Expenses (2010-11) *Tuition:* full-time $16,100; part-time $1780 per credit hour. *Room and board:* $10,920 per academic year. *Required fees:* full-time $1320.
Financial Aid 96% of baccalaureate students in nursing programs received some form of financial aid in 2009-10.
Contact Dr. Doris S. Holeman, Associate Dean and Director, Program in Nursing, Tuskegee University, 209 Basil O'Connor Hall, Tuskegee, AL 36083. *Telephone:* 334-727-8382. *Fax:* 334-727-5461. *E-mail:* dholeman@tuskegee.edu.

The University of Alabama
Capstone College of Nursing
Tuscaloosa, Alabama

http://nursing.ua.edu/
Founded in 1831

DEGREES • BSN • DNP • MSN • MSN/ED D • MSN/MA

Nursing Program Faculty 52 (74% with doctorates).
Baccalaureate Enrollment 1,452 **Women** 88% **Men** 12% **Minority** 16% **International** .3% **Part-time** 7%
Graduate Enrollment 232 **Women** 90% **Men** 10% **Minority** 25% **Part-time** 68%
Distance Learning Courses Available.
Nursing Student Activities Sigma Theta Tau, Student Nurses' Association.
Nursing Student Resources Academic advising; academic or career counseling; assistance for students with disabilities; bookstore; campus computer network; career placement assistance; computer lab; computer-assisted instruction; e-mail services; interactive nursing skills videos; Internet; learning resource lab; library services; nursing audiovisuals;

paid internships; placement services for program completers; skills, simulation, or other laboratory; tutoring; unpaid internships.

Library Facilities 3.3 million volumes (21,000 in health, 400 in nursing); 79,938 periodical subscriptions (1,500 health-care related).

BACCALAUREATE PROGRAMS

Degree BSN

Available Programs Baccalaureate for Second Degree; Generic Baccalaureate; RN Baccalaureate.

Study Options Full-time and part-time.

Program Entrance Requirements Minimum overall college GPA of 3.0, transcript of college record, CPR certification, health exam, health insurance, 4 years high school math, 4 years high school science, high school transcript, immunizations, minimum high school GPA of 2.5, minimum GPA in nursing prerequisites of 3.0, professional liability insurance/malpractice insurance, prerequisite course work. Transfer students are accepted. *Application deadline:* 6/15 (fall), 3/15 (summer). *Application fee:* $25.

Expenses (2010-11) *Tuition, state resident:* full-time $7900; part-time $600 per credit hour. *Tuition, nonresident:* full-time $20,500; part-time $1125 per credit hour. *Room and board:* $8100; room only: $7500 per academic year. *Required fees:* full-time $1200.

Financial Aid 31% of baccalaureate students in nursing programs received some form of financial aid in 2009-10.

Contact Ms. Rebekah Welch, Director of Nursing Student Services, Capstone College of Nursing, The University of Alabama, Box 870358, Tuscaloosa, AL 35487-0358. *Telephone:* 205-348-6639. *Fax:* 205-348-5559. *E-mail:* rebekah.welch@ua.edu.

GRADUATE PROGRAMS

Expenses (2010-11) *Tuition, state resident:* full-time $10,640; part-time $312 per credit hour. *Tuition, nonresident:* full-time $10,640; part-time $312 per credit hour.

Financial Aid 70% of graduate students in nursing programs received some form of financial aid in 2009-10.

Contact Dr. Mariettta Stanton, Assistant Dean, Graduate Program, Capstone College of Nursing, The University of Alabama, Box 870358, Tuscaloosa, AL 35487-0358. *Telephone:* 205-348-1020. *Fax:* 205-348-5559. *E-mail:* mstanton@ua.edu.

MASTER'S DEGREE PROGRAM

Degrees MSN; MSN/Ed D; MSN/MA

Available Programs Master's; RN to Master's.

Concentrations Available Clinical nurse leader; nurse case management; nursing administration; nursing education.

Study Options Full-time and part-time.

Online Degree Options Yes (online only).

Program Entrance Requirements Minimum overall college GPA of 3.0, transcript of college record, written essay. *Application deadline:* 7/1 (fall), 12/1 (spring), 3/1 (summer). Applications may be processed on a rolling basis for some programs. *Application fee:* $25.

Degree Requirements 35 total credit hours.

POST-MASTER'S PROGRAM

Areas of Study Clinical nurse leader; nurse case management.

DOCTORAL DEGREE PROGRAM

Degree DNP

Available Programs Doctorate.

Areas of Study Advanced practice nursing, nursing administration.

Online Degree Options Yes (online only).

Program Entrance Requirements Minimum overall college GPA of 3.0, interview, 2 letters of recommendation, MSN or equivalent, writing sample. Application deadline: 7/1 (fall). Applications may be processed on a rolling basis for some programs. Application fee: $25.

Degree Requirements 34 total credit hours, residency.

The University of Alabama at Birmingham

School of Nursing
Birmingham, Alabama

http://www.uab.edu/son/

Founded in 1969

DEGREES • BSN • MSN • MSN/MPH • PHD

Nursing Program Faculty 48 (100% with doctorates).

Baccalaureate Enrollment 552 **Women** 82% **Men** 18% **Minority** 24% **International** 2% **Part-time** 36%

Graduate Enrollment 1,186 **Women** 91% **Men** 9% **Minority** 21% **International** 1% **Part-time** 78%

Distance Learning Courses Available.

Nursing Student Activities Sigma Theta Tau, Student Nurses' Association, nursing club.

Nursing Student Resources Academic advising; academic or career counseling; assistance for students with disabilities; bookstore; campus computer network; career placement assistance; computer lab; computer-assisted instruction; e-mail services; housing assistance; interactive nursing skills videos; Internet; learning resource lab; library services; nursing audiovisuals; paid internships; placement services for program completers; resume preparation assistance; skills, simulation, or other laboratory; tutoring.

Library Facilities 1.4 million volumes (318,000 in health, 6,862 in nursing); 67,902 periodical subscriptions (2,566 health-care related).

BACCALAUREATE PROGRAMS

Degree BSN

Available Programs Baccalaureate for Second Degree; Generic Baccalaureate; RN Baccalaureate.

Study Options Full-time.

Program Entrance Requirements Minimum overall college GPA of 2.75, transcript of college record, CPR certification, written essay, health exam, health insurance, high school biology, high school transcript, immunizations, minimum high school GPA of 2.0, minimum GPA in nursing prerequisites of 2.75, prerequisite course work. Transfer students are accepted. *Application deadline:* 4/22 (fall), 9/2 (spring).

Expenses (2010-11) *Tuition, state resident:* full-time $6838; part-time $271 per credit hour. *Tuition, nonresident:* full-time $15,622; part-time $637 per credit hour. *Room and board:* $9470; room only: $5000 per academic year.

Financial Aid 59% of baccalaureate students in nursing programs received some form of financial aid in 2009-10. *Gift aid (need-based):* Federal Pell, FSEOG, state, private, college/university gift aid from institutional funds, United Negro College Fund. *Loans:* Federal Direct (Subsidized and Unsubsidized Stafford PLUS), Perkins, state, college/university. *Work-study:* Federal Work-Study. *Financial aid application deadline (priority):* 3/1.

Contact Mr. Peter Tofani, Interim Assistant Dean for Student Affairs, School of Nursing, The University of Alabama at Birmingham, Nursing Building, 1530 3rd Avenue South, Room 208A, Birmingham, AL 35294-1210. *Telephone:* 205-975-7529. *Fax:* 205-934-5490. *E-mail:* tofanip@uab.edu.

GRADUATE PROGRAMS

Expenses (2010-11) *Tuition, state resident:* full-time $6418; part-time $338 per credit hour. *Tuition, nonresident:* full-time $14,626; part-time $794 per credit hour. *Room and board:* $9470; room only: $5000 per academic year.

Financial Aid 3 fellowships (averaging $12,833 per year), 1 research assistantship, teaching assistantships (averaging $6,760 per year) were awarded; Federal Work-Study also available.

Contact Mr. Peter Tofani, Interim Assistant Dean for Student Affairs, School of Nursing, The University of Alabama at Birmingham, NB 208A, 1530 3rd Avenue South, Birmingham, AL 35294-1210. *Telephone:* 205-975-7529. *Fax:* 205-934-5490. *E-mail:* tofanip@uab.edu.

MASTER'S DEGREE PROGRAM

Degrees MSN; MSN/MPH

Available Programs Accelerated Master's for Non-Nursing College Graduates; Master's.

Concentrations Available Clinical nurse leader; health-care administration; nursing administration; nursing education; nursing informatics. *Clinical nurse specialist programs in:* adult health. *Nurse practitioner programs in:* acute care, adult health, family health, gerontology, neo-

natal health, occupational health, pediatric, primary care, psychiatric/mental health, women's health.
Study Options Full-time and part-time.
Online Degree Options Yes (online only).
Program Entrance Requirements Clinical experience, minimum overall college GPA of 3.0, transcript of college record, CPR certification, written essay, immunizations, 3 letters of recommendation, prerequisite course work, statistics course, GRE General Test. *Application deadline:* 5/27 (fall), 9/23 (spring). *Application fee:* $45.
Advanced Placement Credit given for nursing courses completed elsewhere dependent upon specific evaluations.
Degree Requirements 30 total credit hours, comprehensive exam.

POST-MASTER'S PROGRAM

Areas of Study *Nurse practitioner programs in:* acute care, adult health, family health, gerontology, neonatal health, pediatric, psychiatric/mental health.

DOCTORAL DEGREE PROGRAM

Degree PhD
Available Programs Doctorate; Post-Baccalaureate Doctorate.
Areas of Study Nursing research, nursing science.
Program Entrance Requirements Clinical experience, minimum overall college GPA of 3.0, interview by faculty committee, interview, 3 letters of recommendation, scholarly papers, statistics course, vita, writing sample, GRE General Test. Application deadline: 1/14 (fall). Application fee: $45.
Degree Requirements 66 total credit hours, dissertation, oral exam, written exam, residency.

The University of Alabama in Huntsville

College of Nursing
Huntsville, Alabama

http://www.uah.edu/nursing
Founded in 1950

DEGREES • BSN • DNP • MSN

Nursing Program Faculty 46 (30% with doctorates).
Baccalaureate Enrollment 662 **Women** 90% **Men** 10% **Minority** 14% **International** 1% **Part-time** 22%
Graduate Enrollment 106 **Women** 92% **Men** 8% **Minority** 15% **International** 1% **Part-time** 65%
Distance Learning Courses Available.
Nursing Student Activities Sigma Theta Tau, Student Nurses' Association.
Nursing Student Resources Academic advising; academic or career counseling; assistance for students with disabilities; bookstore; campus computer network; career placement assistance; computer lab; computer-assisted instruction; e-mail services; employment services for current students; housing assistance; interactive nursing skills videos; Internet; learning resource lab; library services; nursing audiovisuals; placement services for program completers; remedial services; resume preparation assistance; skills, simulation, or other laboratory; tutoring.
Library Facilities 323,637 volumes (13,004 in health, 3,480 in nursing); 655 periodical subscriptions (3,200 health-care related).

BACCALAUREATE PROGRAMS

Degree BSN
Available Programs Baccalaureate for Second Degree; Generic Baccalaureate; RN Baccalaureate.
Study Options Full-time and part-time.
Program Entrance Requirements Minimum overall college GPA of 2.0, transcript of college record, CPR certification, health exam, health insurance, immunizations, minimum GPA in nursing prerequisites of 2.0, professional liability insurance/malpractice insurance, prerequisite course work. Transfer students are accepted. *Application deadline:* 3/1 (fall), 9/1 (spring).
Advanced Placement Credit by examination available. Credit given for nursing courses completed elsewhere dependent upon specific evaluations.
Financial Aid 75% of baccalaureate students in nursing programs received some form of financial aid in 2008-09. *Gift aid (need-based):* Federal Pell, FSEOG, state, private, college/university gift aid from institutional funds, Federal Nursing. *Loans:* Federal Direct (Subsidized and Unsubsidized Stafford PLUS). *Work-study:* Federal Work-Study. *Financial aid application deadline:* 7/31(priority: 4/1).
Contact Mrs. Laura Mann, Director, Nursing Undergraduate Programs, College of Nursing, The University of Alabama in Huntsville, 207 Nursing Building, Huntsville, AL 35899. *Telephone:* 256-824-6742. *Fax:* 256-824-2850. *E-mail:* laura.mann@uah.edu.

GRADUATE PROGRAMS

Financial Aid 65% of graduate students in nursing programs received some form of financial aid in 2008-09. 11 teaching assistantships with full and partial tuition reimbursements available (averaging $9,996 per year) were awarded; career-related internships or fieldwork, Federal Work-Study, institutionally sponsored loans, scholarships, traineeships, and unspecified assistantships also available. Aid available to part-time students. *Financial aid application deadline:* 4/1.
Contact Mr. Charles Davis, Director of Nursing Graduate Program Student Affairs, College of Nursing, The University of Alabama in Huntsville, Huntsville, AL 35899. *Telephone:* 256-824-6742. *Fax:* 256-824-6026. *E-mail:* charles.davis@uah.edu.

MASTER'S DEGREE PROGRAM

Degree MSN
Available Programs Master's; RN to Master's.
Concentrations Available Clinical nurse leader; health-care administration. *Clinical nurse specialist programs in:* adult health. *Nurse practitioner programs in:* acute care, family health.
Study Options Full-time and part-time.
Online Degree Options Yes.
Program Entrance Requirements Minimum overall college GPA of 3.0, transcript of college record, CPR certification, immunizations, 3 letters of recommendation, professional liability insurance/malpractice insurance, statistics course, MAT or GRE. *Application deadline:* 4/15 (fall).
Advanced Placement Credit given for nursing courses completed elsewhere dependent upon specific evaluations.
Degree Requirements 42 total credit hours, thesis or project, comprehensive exam.

POST-MASTER'S PROGRAM

Areas of Study Nursing education. *Nurse practitioner programs in:* family health.

DOCTORAL DEGREE PROGRAM

Degree DNP
Available Programs Doctorate.
Areas of Study Advanced practice nursing, nursing administration.
Online Degree Options Yes (online only).
Program Entrance Requirements interview by faculty committee, letters of recommendation, MSN or equivalent, vita, writing sample. Application deadline: 4/15 (fall). Application fee: $40.
Degree Requirements 34 total credit hours, oral exam, written exam.

CONTINUING EDUCATION PROGRAM

Contact Mrs. Ina Warboys, Director of Continuing Education, College of Nursing, The University of Alabama in Huntsville, Huntsville, AL 35899. *Telephone:* 256-824-2456. *Fax:* 256-824-6026. *E-mail:* ina.warboys@uah.edu.

University of Mobile

School of Nursing
Mobile, Alabama

http://www.umobile.edu
Founded in 1961

DEGREES • BSN • MSN

Nursing Program Faculty 14 (22% with doctorates).
Baccalaureate Enrollment 84 **Women** 89% **Men** 11% **Minority** 25%
Graduate Enrollment 22 **Women** 91% **Men** 9% **Minority** 45% **Part-time** 50%
Nursing Student Activities Sigma Theta Tau, Student Nurses' Association.
Nursing Student Resources Academic advising; academic or career counseling; assistance for students with disabilities; bookstore; campus computer network; career placement assistance; computer lab; computer-assisted instruction; e-mail services; employment services for current students; interactive nursing skills videos; Internet; learning resource lab;

library services; nursing audiovisuals; remedial services; resume preparation assistance; skills, simulation, or other laboratory; tutoring; unpaid internships.
Library Facilities 111,285 volumes (7,846 in health, 6,500 in nursing); 323 periodical subscriptions (109 health-care related).

BACCALAUREATE PROGRAMS

Degree BSN
Available Programs ADN to Baccalaureate; Generic Baccalaureate; RN Baccalaureate.
Study Options Full-time.
Program Entrance Requirements Minimum overall college GPA of 2.75, transcript of college record, CPR certification, health exam, health insurance, high school transcript, immunizations, minimum GPA in nursing prerequisites of 2.75, prerequisite course work. Transfer students are accepted.
Advanced Placement Credit given for nursing courses completed elsewhere dependent upon specific evaluations.
Contact ***Telephone:*** 251-442-2337. *Fax:* 251-442-2520.

GRADUATE PROGRAMS

Contact ***Telephone:*** 251-442-2446. *Fax:* 251-442-2520.

MASTER'S DEGREE PROGRAM

Degree MSN
Available Programs Master's.
Concentrations Available Nursing administration; nursing education.
Study Options Full-time and part-time.
Program Entrance Requirements Minimum overall college GPA of 3.0, transcript of college record, CPR certification, immunizations, 3 letters of recommendation, statistics course.
Advanced Placement Credit given for nursing courses completed elsewhere dependent upon specific evaluations.
Degree Requirements 39 total credit hours, thesis or project, comprehensive exam.

CONTINUING EDUCATION PROGRAM

Contact ***Telephone:*** 251-442-2227. *Fax:* 251-442-2520.

University of North Alabama
College of Nursing and Allied Health
Florence, Alabama

http://www2.una.edu/nursing/
Founded in 1830

DEGREES • BSN • MSN
Nursing Program Faculty 37 (22% with doctorates).
Baccalaureate Enrollment 390 **Women** 87% **Men** 13% **Minority** 20.5% **International** 1% **Part-time** 31%
Graduate Enrollment 36 **Women** 97% **Men** 3% **Minority** 17% **Part-time** 25%
Distance Learning Courses Available.
Nursing Student Activities Sigma Theta Tau, Student Nurses' Association.
Nursing Student Resources Academic advising; academic or career counseling; assistance for students with disabilities; bookstore; campus computer network; career placement assistance; computer lab; e-mail services; employment services for current students; housing assistance; interactive nursing skills videos; Internet; learning resource lab; library services; nursing audiovisuals; remedial services; resume preparation assistance; skills, simulation, or other laboratory; tutoring.
Library Facilities 393,457 volumes; 3,742 periodical subscriptions.

BACCALAUREATE PROGRAMS

Degree BSN
Available Programs Generic Baccalaureate; RN Baccalaureate.
Study Options Full-time and part-time.
Online Degree Options Yes (online only).
Program Entrance Requirements Transcript of college record, CPR certification, health exam, health insurance, high school transcript, immunizations, minimum GPA in nursing prerequisites of 2.5, professional liability insurance/malpractice insurance, prerequisite course work. Transfer students are accepted.
Contact ***Telephone:*** 256-765-4984. *Fax:* 256-765-4935.

GRADUATE PROGRAMS

Contact ***Telephone:*** 256-765-4931. *Fax:* 256-765-4701.

MASTER'S DEGREE PROGRAM

Degree MSN
Available Programs Master's.
Concentrations Available Nursing administration; nursing education.
Study Options Full-time and part-time.
Online Degree Options Yes (online only).
Program Entrance Requirements Clinical experience, minimum overall college GPA of 3.0, transcript of college record, written essay, 3 letters of recommendation, professional liability insurance/malpractice insurance.
Degree Requirements 42 total credit hours, thesis or project.

CONTINUING EDUCATION PROGRAM

Contact ***Telephone:*** 256-765-4787. *Fax:* 256-765-4872.

University of South Alabama
College of Nursing
Mobile, Alabama

http://www.southalabama.edu/nursing/
Founded in 1963

DEGREES • BSN • MSN
Nursing Program Faculty 57 (30% with doctorates).
Baccalaureate Enrollment 316 **Women** 82% **Men** 18% **Minority** 24% **International** 3% **Part-time** 11%
Graduate Enrollment 368 **Women** 86% **Men** 14% **Minority** 19% **Part-time** 22%
Nursing Student Activities Sigma Theta Tau, Student Nurses' Association.
Nursing Student Resources Academic advising; academic or career counseling; assistance for students with disabilities; bookstore; campus computer network; career placement assistance; computer lab; learning resource lab; library services; nursing audiovisuals; resume preparation assistance.
Library Facilities 1.1 million volumes (2,406 in health, 2,300 in nursing); 1,244 periodical subscriptions (299 health-care related).

BACCALAUREATE PROGRAMS

Degree BSN
Available Programs ADN to Baccalaureate; Accelerated Baccalaureate; Generic Baccalaureate; RN Baccalaureate.
Site Options Fairhope, AL.
Study Options Full-time and part-time.
Program Entrance Requirements Minimum overall college GPA of 2.5, transcript of college record, CPR certification, health exam, health insurance, immunizations, minimum GPA in nursing prerequisites of 2.5, professional liability insurance/malpractice insurance, prerequisite course work. Transfer students are accepted.
Advanced Placement Credit given for nursing courses completed elsewhere dependent upon specific evaluations.
Contact ***Telephone:*** 251-434-3410. *Fax:* 251-434-3413.

GRADUATE PROGRAMS

Contact ***Telephone:*** 251-434-3410. *Fax:* 251-434-3413.

MASTER'S DEGREE PROGRAM

Degree MSN
Available Programs Accelerated Master's; Master's; Master's for Nurses with Non-Nursing Degrees.
Concentrations Available Nursing administration; nursing education. *Clinical nurse specialist programs in:* acute care, community health, family health, gerontology, maternity-newborn, pediatric, psychiatric/mental health, women's health. *Nurse practitioner programs in:* acute care, family health, gerontology, neonatal health, pediatric, psychiatric/mental health, women's health.
Study Options Full-time and part-time.
Program Entrance Requirements Computer literacy, minimum overall college GPA of 3.0, transcript of college record, immunizations, nursing research course, physical assessment course, resume.
Advanced Placement Credit given for nursing courses completed elsewhere dependent upon specific evaluations.
Degree Requirements 30 total credit hours, thesis or project.

POST-MASTER'S PROGRAM

Areas of Study Nursing administration; nursing education. *Clinical nurse specialist programs in:* acute care, community health, family health, gerontology, maternity-newborn, pediatric, psychiatric/mental health, women's health. *Nurse practitioner programs in:* acute care, family health, gerontology, neonatal health, pediatric, psychiatric/mental health, women's health.

ALASKA

University of Alaska Anchorage

School of Nursing
Anchorage, Alaska

http://www.son.uaa.alaska.edu
Founded in 1954

DEGREES • BS • MS

Nursing Program Faculty 26 (42% with doctorates).

Baccalaureate Enrollment 224 **Women** 80% **Men** 20% **Minority** 31% **International** 3% **Part-time** 18%

Graduate Enrollment 60 **Women** 94% **Men** 6% **Minority** 9% **Part-time** 12%

Nursing Student Activities Sigma Theta Tau, Student Nurses' Association.

Nursing Student Resources Academic advising; academic or career counseling; assistance for students with disabilities; bookstore; campus computer network; career placement assistance; computer lab; computer-assisted instruction; daycare for children of students; e-mail services; interactive nursing skills videos; Internet; learning resource lab; library services; nursing audiovisuals; placement services for program completers; remedial services; resume preparation assistance; skills, simulation, or other laboratory; tutoring.

Library Facilities 23,000 volumes in health, 150 volumes in nursing; 780 periodical subscriptions health-care related.

BACCALAUREATE PROGRAMS

Degree BS

Available Programs Generic Baccalaureate; RN Baccalaureate.

Study Options Full-time and part-time.

Program Entrance Requirements Minimum overall college GPA of 2.7, transcript of college record, CPR certification, written essay, immunizations, 3 letters of recommendation, minimum GPA in nursing prerequisites of 2.7, professional liability insurance/malpractice insurance, prerequisite course work. Transfer students are accepted.

Advanced Placement Credit given for nursing courses completed elsewhere dependent upon specific evaluations.

Contact *Telephone:* 907-786-4550. *Fax:* 907-786-4558.

GRADUATE PROGRAMS

Contact *Telephone:* 907-786-4570. *Fax:* 907-786-4559.

MASTER'S DEGREE PROGRAM

Degree MS

Available Programs Master's.

Concentrations Available Health-care administration; nursing education. *Clinical nurse specialist programs in:* community health, psychiatric/mental health. *Nurse practitioner programs in:* family health, psychiatric/mental health.

Study Options Full-time and part-time.

Program Entrance Requirements Clinical experience, minimum overall college GPA of 3.0, transcript of college record, written essay, 3 letters of recommendation, nursing research course, prerequisite course work, statistics course, GRE or MAT.

Advanced Placement Credit given for nursing courses completed elsewhere dependent upon specific evaluations.

Degree Requirements 50 total credit hours, thesis or project.

ARIZONA

Arizona State University at the Downtown Phoenix Campus

College of Nursing
Phoenix, Arizona

http://nursing.asu.edu
Founded in 2006

DEGREES • BSN • DNP • MS • MS/MPH

Nursing Program Faculty 119 (44% with doctorates).

Baccalaureate Enrollment 1,625 **Women** 89% **Men** 11% **Minority** 29% **International** 1% **Part-time** 18%

Graduate Enrollment 179 **Women** 91% **Men** 9% **Minority** 7% **Part-time** 46%

Distance Learning Courses Available.

Nursing Student Activities Nursing Honor Society, Sigma Theta Tau, Student Nurses' Association, nursing club.

Nursing Student Resources Academic advising; academic or career counseling; assistance for students with disabilities; bookstore; campus computer network; career placement assistance; computer lab; computer-assisted instruction; daycare for children of students; e-mail services; employment services for current students; housing assistance; interactive nursing skills videos; Internet; learning resource lab; library services; nursing audiovisuals; paid internships; placement services for program completers; remedial services; resume preparation assistance; skills, simulation, or other laboratory; tutoring; unpaid internships.

Library Facilities 77,814 volumes in health, 7,501 volumes in nursing; 755 periodical subscriptions health-care related.

BACCALAUREATE PROGRAMS

Degree BSN

Available Programs Accelerated Baccalaureate for Second Degree; Accelerated RN Baccalaureate; Baccalaureate for Second Degree; Generic Baccalaureate; RN Baccalaureate.

Site Options Scottsdale, AZ; Phoenix, AZ.

Study Options Full-time.

Program Entrance Requirements Minimum overall college GPA of 2.75, transcript of college record, CPR certification, health exam, high school biology, high school chemistry, high school foreign language, 4 years high school math, 3 years high school science, high school transcript, immunizations, minimum high school GPA of 3.0, minimum high school rank 25%, minimum GPA in nursing prerequisites of 3.25, prerequisite course work. *Application deadline:* 5/1 (fall), 9/1 (spring), 2/1 (summer).

Financial Aid 70% of baccalaureate students in nursing programs received some form of financial aid in 2008-09.

Contact Ms. Maurine Lee, Senior Student Support Specialist, College of Nursing, Arizona State University at the Downtown Phoenix Campus, 500 North 3rd Street, Phoenix, AZ 85004. *Telephone:* 602-496-0888. *Fax:* 602-496-0705. *E-mail:* maurine.lee@asu.edu.

GRADUATE PROGRAMS

Financial Aid 75% of graduate students in nursing programs received some form of financial aid in 2008-09.

Contact Ms. Eula Bradley, Academic Success Coordinator, College of Nursing, Arizona State University at the Downtown Phoenix Campus, 550 North 3rd Street, Phoenix, AZ 85004. *Telephone:* 602-496-0703. *E-mail:* eula.bradley@asu.edu.

MASTER'S DEGREE PROGRAM

Degrees MS; MS/MPH

Available Programs Master's.

Concentrations Available *Clinical nurse specialist programs in:* acute care, adult health, community health, pediatric, psychiatric/mental health. *Nurse practitioner programs in:* acute care, adult health, family health, neonatal health, pediatric, psychiatric/mental health, women's health.

Site Options Phoenix, AZ.

Study Options Full-time and part-time.

Program Entrance Requirements Clinical experience, minimum overall college GPA of 3.0, transcript of college record, immunizations, interview, 3 letters of recommendation, physical assessment course, prerequisite course work, resume, statistics course, GRE.

Advanced Placement Credit given for nursing courses completed elsewhere dependent upon specific evaluations.
Degree Requirements 40 total credit hours, thesis or project.

POST-MASTER'S PROGRAM

Areas of Study *Clinical nurse specialist programs in:* acute care, adult health, community health, pediatric, psychiatric/mental health. *Nurse practitioner programs in:* acute care, adult health, family health, neonatal health, pediatric, psychiatric/mental health, women's health.

DOCTORAL DEGREE PROGRAM

Degree DNP
Available Programs Doctorate.
Areas of Study Advanced practice nursing.
Site Options Phoenix, AZ.

CONTINUING EDUCATION PROGRAM

Contact Daniel Weberg, Faculty Associate, College of Nursing, Arizona State University at the Downtown Phoenix Campus, 550 North 3rd Stret, Phoenix, AZ 85004. *Telephone:* 602-496-0878. *E-mail:* Daniel.Weberg@asu.edu.

Chamberlain College of Nursing

Chamberlain College of Nursing
Phoenix, Arizona

DEGREES • BSN • MSN

Distance Learning Courses Available.

BACCALAUREATE PROGRAMS

Degree BSN
Available Programs Accelerated Baccalaureate; Accelerated Baccalaureate for Second Degree; RN Baccalaureate.
Contact Admissions, Chamberlain College of Nursing, 2149 West Dunlap Avenue, Phoenix, AZ 85021. *Telephone:* 888-556-8226.

GRADUATE PROGRAMS

Contact Admissions, Chamberlain College of Nursing, 2149 West Dunlap Avenue, Phoenix, AZ 85021. *Telephone:* 888-556-8226.

MASTER'S DEGREE PROGRAM

Degree MSN
Available Programs Master's.

Grand Canyon University

College of Nursing and Health Sciences
Phoenix, Arizona

Founded in 1949

DEGREES • BSN • MS • MSN/MBA

Nursing Program Faculty 122 (3% with doctorates).
Baccalaureate Enrollment 1,067 **Women** 90% **Men** 10% **International** .01% **Part-time** 58%
Graduate Enrollment 297 **Women** 93% **Men** 7% **Part-time** 89%
Distance Learning Courses Available.
Nursing Student Activities Sigma Theta Tau, Student Nurses' Association.
Nursing Student Resources Academic advising; academic or career counseling; assistance for students with disabilities; bookstore; campus computer network; career placement assistance; computer lab; computer-assisted instruction; e-mail services; employment services for current students; housing assistance; Internet; learning resource lab; library services; nursing audiovisuals; other; paid internships; remedial services; resume preparation assistance; skills, simulation, or other laboratory; tutoring; unpaid internships.
Library Facilities 9,663 volumes in health; 177 periodical subscriptions health-care related.

BACCALAUREATE PROGRAMS

Degree BSN
Available Programs ADN to Baccalaureate; RN Baccalaureate.
Site Options Phoenix, AZ; Tucson, AZ; Albuquerque, NM.
Study Options Full-time.
Online Degree Options Yes.
Program Entrance Requirements Minimum overall college GPA of 3.0, transcript of college record, CPR certification, health exam, health insurance, high school transcript, immunizations, minimum GPA in nursing prerequisites of 3.0, prerequisite course work. Transfer students are accepted. *Application deadline:* 5/15 (fall), 9/15 (spring), 1/15 (summer).
Advanced Placement Credit by examination available. Credit given for nursing courses completed elsewhere dependent upon specific evaluations.
Expenses (2010-11) *Tuition:* full-time $16,500; part-time $688 per credit. *Room and board:* $3600 per academic year. *Required fees:* full-time $800.
Financial Aid 91% of baccalaureate students in nursing programs received some form of financial aid in 2009-10.
Contact Andrea Wolochuk, Manager Traditional Enrollment, College of Nursing and Health Sciences, Grand Canyon University, 3300 West Camelback Road, Phoenix, AZ 85017. *Telephone:* 602-639-6429. *E-mail:* andrea.wolochuk@gcu.edu.

GRADUATE PROGRAMS

Expenses (2010-11) *Tuition:* full-time $8960; part-time $560 per credit. *International tuition:* $8960 full-time.
Contact Mr. Christopher Landauer, Assistant Director of Enrollment CONHS, College of Nursing and Health Sciences, Grand Canyon University, 3300 West Camelback Road, Phoenix, AZ 85017. *Telephone:* 602-639-7982. *E-mail:* christopher.landauer@gcu.edu.

MASTER'S DEGREE PROGRAM

Degrees MS; MSN/MBA
Available Programs Master's.
Concentrations Available Nursing administration; nursing education. *Clinical nurse specialist programs in:* adult health. *Nurse practitioner programs in:* acute care, family health.
Site Options Phoenix, AZ; Tucson, AZ.
Study Options Full-time and part-time.
Online Degree Options Yes.
Program Entrance Requirements Clinical experience, computer literacy, minimum overall college GPA of 3.0, transcript of college record, CPR certification, written essay, immunizations, interview, nursing research course, physical assessment course, professional liability insurance/malpractice insurance, prerequisite course work, resume, statistics course. *Application deadline:* Applications may be processed on a rolling basis for some programs.
Advanced Placement Credit given for nursing courses completed elsewhere dependent upon specific evaluations.
Degree Requirements 52 total credit hours, thesis or project.

POST-MASTER'S PROGRAM

Areas of Study Nursing education. *Clinical nurse specialist programs in:* adult health. *Nurse practitioner programs in:* acute care, family health.

CONTINUING EDUCATION PROGRAM

Contact Mr. Christopher Landauer, Assistant Director of Enrollment CONHS, College of Nursing and Health Sciences, Grand Canyon University, 3300 West Camelback Road, Phoenix, AZ 85017. *Telephone:* 602-639-7982. *Fax:* 602-639-7982. *E-mail:* christopher.landauer@gcu.edu.

Northern Arizona University

School of Nursing
Flagstaff , Arizona

http://www.nau.edu/hp/dept/nurse
Founded in 1899

DEGREES • BSN • MS

Nursing Program Faculty 60 (25% with doctorates).
Baccalaureate Enrollment 450 **Women** 88% **Men** 12% **Minority** 20% **International** 1%
Graduate Enrollment 110 **Women** 96% **Men** 4% **Minority** 20% **Part-time** 65%
Distance Learning Courses Available.
Nursing Student Activities Nursing Honor Society, Sigma Theta Tau, Student Nurses' Association.

Nursing Student Resources Academic advising; academic or career counseling; bookstore; campus computer network; computer lab; computer-assisted instruction; e-mail services; externships; interactive nursing skills videos; Internet; learning resource lab; library services; nursing audiovisuals; paid internships; remedial services; skills, simulation, or other laboratory; tutoring.

Library Facilities 1.1 million volumes; 44,867 periodical subscriptions.

BACCALAUREATE PROGRAMS

Degree BSN

Available Programs Accelerated Baccalaureate for Second Degree; Generic Baccalaureate; RN Baccalaureate.

Site Options St. Michaels/Window Rock, AZ; Tucson, AZ; Yuma, AZ.

Study Options Full-time.

Online Degree Options Yes (online only).

Program Entrance Requirements Transcript of college record, CPR certification, health exam, health insurance, high school transcript, immunizations, 2 letters of recommendation, minimum GPA in nursing prerequisites of 2.75, professional liability insurance/malpractice insurance, prerequisite course work. Transfer students are accepted. *Application deadline:* 3/15 (fall), 9/15 (spring).

Advanced Placement Credit given for nursing courses completed elsewhere dependent upon specific evaluations.

Expenses (2010-11) *Tuition, state resident:* full-time $8000; part-time $380 per credit hour. *Tuition, nonresident:* full-time $18,000; part-time $1000 per credit hour. *Room and board:* room only: $4500 per academic year. *Required fees:* full-time $1200.

Financial Aid 75% of baccalaureate students in nursing programs received some form of financial aid in 2009-10.

Contact Mr. Gregg Schneider, Senior Academic Advisor, School of Nursing, Northern Arizona University, Box 15035, Flagstaff, AZ 86011. *Telephone:* 928-523-6717. *Fax:* 928-523-7171. *E-mail:* gregg.schneider@nau.edu.

GRADUATE PROGRAMS

Expenses (2010-11) *Tuition, state resident:* full-time $7000; part-time $375 per credit hour. *Tuition, nonresident:* full-time $18,000; part-time $1050 per credit hour. *International tuition:* $18,000 full-time.

Financial Aid 75% of graduate students in nursing programs received some form of financial aid in 2009-10. 4 teaching assistantships with partial tuition reimbursements available were awarded; career-related internships or fieldwork, Federal Work-Study, traineeships, tuition waivers, and unspecified assistantships also available. Aid available to part-time students. *Financial aid application deadline:* 3/30.

Contact Dr. Ilene Decker, Graduate Program Coordinator, School of Nursing, Northern Arizona University, Box 15035, Flagstaff, AZ 86011. *Telephone:* 928-523-2159. *Fax:* 928-523-7171. *E-mail:* ilene.decker@nau.edu.

MASTER'S DEGREE PROGRAM

Degree MS

Available Programs Master's.

Concentrations Available Nursing education. *Nurse practitioner programs in:* family health.

Site Options St. Michaels/Window Rock, AZ; Tucson, AZ; Yuma, AZ.

Study Options Full-time and part-time.

Online Degree Options Yes (online only).

Program Entrance Requirements Clinical experience, minimum overall college GPA of 3.0, transcript of college record, CPR certification, written essay, immunizations, interview, 3 letters of recommendation, nursing research course, physical assessment course, professional liability insurance/malpractice insurance, prerequisite course work, resume, statistics course, GRE General Test or minimum GPA of 3.0. *Application deadline:* 10/15 (fall), 1/15 (spring), 7/15 (summer).

Degree Requirements 40 total credit hours, thesis or project.

POST-MASTER'S PROGRAM

Areas of Study *Nurse practitioner programs in:* family health.

The University of Arizona
College of Nursing
Tucson, Arizona

http://www.nursing.arizona.edu/
Founded in 1885

DEGREES • BSN • MS • PHD

Nursing Program Faculty 64 (58% with doctorates).
Baccalaureate Enrollment 315 **Women** 88.9% **Men** 11.1% **Minority** 24.1% **International** 1.3% **Part-time** 1.3%
Graduate Enrollment 169 **Women** 89.9% **Men** 10.1% **Minority** 30% **International** 1.2% **Part-time** 36.1%
Distance Learning Courses Available.
Nursing Student Activities Nursing Honor Society, Sigma Theta Tau, Student Nurses' Association, nursing club.
Nursing Student Resources Academic advising; academic or career counseling; assistance for students with disabilities; bookstore; campus computer network; career placement assistance; computer lab; computer-assisted instruction; e-mail services; externships; housing assistance; interactive nursing skills videos; Internet; learning resource lab; library services; nursing audiovisuals; other; placement services for program completers; skills, simulation, or other laboratory; tutoring.
Library Facilities 112,500 volumes in health, 5,400 volumes in nursing; 10,785 periodical subscriptions health-care related.

BACCALAUREATE PROGRAMS

Degree BSN
Available Programs Generic Baccalaureate.
Site Options Yuma, AZ.
Study Options Full-time.
Program Entrance Requirements Minimum overall college GPA of 3.0, transcript of college record, CPR certification, written essay, health insurance, immunizations, interview, minimum GPA in nursing prerequisites of 3.0, prerequisite course work. Transfer students are accepted. *Application deadline:* 2/1 (fall), 9/1 (spring).
Advanced Placement Credit given for nursing courses completed elsewhere dependent upon specific evaluations.
Expenses (2010-11) *Tuition, state resident:* full-time $9614. *Tuition, nonresident:* full-time $25,972. *Room and board:* $9024; room only: $6530 per academic year. *Required fees:* full-time $636.
Financial Aid 75% of baccalaureate students in nursing programs received some form of financial aid in 2009-10.
Contact Ms. Vickie Radoye, Assistant Dean for Student Affairs, College of Nursing, The University of Arizona, 1305 North Martin, PO Box 210203, Tucson, AZ 85721-0203. *Telephone:* 520-626-3808. *Fax:* 520-626-6424. *E-mail:* vradoye@nursing.arizona.edu.

GRADUATE PROGRAMS

Expenses (2010-11) *Tuition, state resident:* full-time $13,640; part-time $974 per credit. *Tuition, nonresident:* full-time $29,466; part-time $2104 per credit. *International tuition:* $29,466 full-time. *Room and board:* $12,020; room only: $9028 per academic year. *Required fees:* full-time $636; part-time $318 per term.
Financial Aid 55% of graduate students in nursing programs received some form of financial aid in 2009-10. 6 research assistantships with full tuition reimbursements available (averaging $15,552 per year) were awarded; teaching assistantships, career-related internships or fieldwork, institutionally sponsored loans, scholarships, traineeships, tuition waivers (full), and unspecified assistantships also available. *Financial aid application deadline:* 6/1.
Contact Sue Rawley, Senior Academic Advisor, College of Nursing, The University of Arizona, 1305 North Martin, PO Box 210203, Tucson, AZ 85721-0203. *Telephone:* 520-626-3808. *Fax:* 520-626-6424. *E-mail:* srawley@nursing.arizona.edu.

MASTER'S DEGREE PROGRAM

Degree MS
Available Programs Accelerated Master's for Non-Nursing College Graduates; Accelerated RN to Master's; Master's.
Study Options Full-time and part-time.
Program Entrance Requirements Minimum overall college GPA of 3.0, transcript of college record, CPR certification, written essay, immunizations, interview, prerequisite course work, statistics course. *Application deadline:* 1/15 (fall). *Application fee:* $75.
Advanced Placement Credit given for nursing courses completed elsewhere dependent upon specific evaluations.
Degree Requirements 56 total credit hours.

POST-MASTER'S PROGRAM
Areas of Study *Nurse practitioner programs in:* acute care, family health, pediatric.

DOCTORAL DEGREE PROGRAM
Degree PhD
Available Programs Doctorate; Post-Baccalaureate Doctorate.
Areas of Study Aging, bio-behavioral research, biology of health and illness, gerontology, health policy, health promotion/disease prevention, illness and transition, information systems, nursing research, nursing science.
Online Degree Options Yes (online only).
Program Entrance Requirements Minimum overall college GPA of 3.0, interview by faculty committee, interview, 3 letters of recommendation, statistics course, vita. Application deadline: 12/15 (fall). Application fee: $75.
Degree Requirements 64 total credit hours, dissertation, oral exam, written exam, residency.

POSTDOCTORAL PROGRAM
Postdoctoral Program Contact Ms. Vickie Radoye, Assistant Dean for Student Affairs, College of Nursing, The University of Arizona, 1305 North Martin, PO Box 210203, Tucson, AZ 85721-0203. *Telephone:* 520-626-3808. *Fax:* 520-626-6424. *E-mail:* vradoye@nursing.arizona.edu.

University of Phoenix
Online Campus
Phoenix, Arizona

Founded in 1989

DEGREES • BSN • MSN • MSN/MBA • MSN/MHA • PHD
Nursing Program Faculty 444 (29% with doctorates).
Baccalaureate Enrollment 5,644 **Women** 92.2% **Men** 7.8% **Minority** 18.1%
Graduate Enrollment 5,878 **Women** 92.5% **Men** 7.5% **Minority** 23%
Distance Learning Courses Available.
Nursing Student Activities Sigma Theta Tau.
Nursing Student Resources Academic advising; academic or career counseling; assistance for students with disabilities; bookstore; campus computer network; computer lab; computer-assisted instruction; e-mail services; interactive nursing skills videos; Internet; learning resource lab; library services; nursing audiovisuals; remedial services; skills, simulation, or other laboratory; tutoring.
Library Facilities 16,781 periodical subscriptions (1,300 health-care related).

BACCALAUREATE PROGRAMS
Degree BSN
Available Programs Accelerated Baccalaureate.
Study Options Full-time.
Online Degree Options Yes.
Program Entrance Requirements Transcript of college record, CPR certification, immunizations, 1 letter of recommendation, RN licensure. Transfer students are accepted. *Application deadline:* Applications may be processed on a rolling basis for some programs.
Advanced Placement Credit by examination available. Credit given for nursing courses completed elsewhere dependent upon specific evaluations.
Expenses (2009-10) *Tuition:* full-time $10,800. *International tuition:* $10,800 full-time. *Required fees:* full-time $600.
Contact Program Chair, Healthcare, Online Campus, University of Phoenix, CF-A101, 3157 East Elwood Street, Phoenix, AZ 85034-7209. *Telephone:* 602-387-7000.

GRADUATE PROGRAMS
Expenses (2009-10) *Tuition:* full-time $13,200. *International tuition:* $13,200 full-time. *Required fees:* full-time $760.
Contact Program Chair, Healthcare, Online Campus, University of Phoenix, Phoenix, AZ 85034-7209. *Telephone:* 602-387-7000.

MASTER'S DEGREE PROGRAM
Degrees MSN; MSN/MBA; MSN/MHA
Available Programs Master's; Master's for Nurses with Non-Nursing Degrees.
Concentrations Available Health-care administration; nursing administration; nursing education. *Nurse practitioner programs in:* family health.
Study Options Full-time.
Online Degree Options Yes.
Program Entrance Requirements Clinical experience, computer literacy, minimum overall college GPA of 3.0, transcript of college record, CPR certification. *Application deadline:* Applications may be processed on a rolling basis for some programs.
Advanced Placement Credit given for nursing courses completed elsewhere dependent upon specific evaluations.
Degree Requirements 39 total credit hours, thesis or project.

POST-MASTER'S PROGRAM
Areas of Study *Nurse practitioner programs in:* family health.

DOCTORAL DEGREE PROGRAM
Degree PhD
Available Programs Doctorate.
Areas of Study Nursing administration, nursing education.
Online Degree Options Yes (online only).
Program Entrance Requirements Minimum overall college GPA of 3.0, MSN or equivalent. Application deadline: Applications may be processed on a rolling basis for some programs. Application fee: $45.
Degree Requirements 62 total credit hours, dissertation, residency.

CONTINUING EDUCATION PROGRAM
Contact Program Chair, Healthcare, Online Campus, University of Phoenix, Phoenix, AZ 85034. *Telephone:* 602-387-7000.

University of Phoenix–Phoenix Campus
College of Nursing
Phoenix, Arizona

Founded in 1976

DEGREES • BSN • MSN • MSN/MBA • MSN/MHA
Nursing Program Faculty 38 (32% with doctorates).
Baccalaureate Enrollment 239 **Women** 89.5% **Men** 10.5% **Minority** 23.4%
Graduate Enrollment 148 **Women** 91.9% **Men** 8.1% **Minority** 14.86%
Nursing Student Activities Sigma Theta Tau.
Nursing Student Resources Academic advising; academic or career counseling; assistance for students with disabilities; bookstore; campus computer network; computer lab; computer-assisted instruction; interactive nursing skills videos; Internet; learning resource lab; library services; nursing audiovisuals; skills, simulation, or other laboratory; tutoring.
Library Facilities 16,781 periodical subscriptions (1,300 health-care related).

BACCALAUREATE PROGRAMS
Degree BSN
Available Programs Accelerated Baccalaureate; LPN to Baccalaureate.
Site Options Scottsdale, AZ; Mesa, AZ; Chandler, AZ.
Study Options Full-time.
Online Degree Options Yes.
Program Entrance Requirements Transcript of college record, CPR certification, immunizations, 1 letter of recommendation, RN licensure. Transfer students are accepted. *Application deadline:* Applications may be processed on a rolling basis for some programs.
Advanced Placement Credit by examination available. Credit given for nursing courses completed elsewhere dependent upon specific evaluations.
Expenses (2009-10) *Tuition:* full-time $9300. *Required fees:* full-time $600.
Contact Campus College Chair, Nursing, College of Nursing, University of Phoenix–Phoenix Campus, 4635 East Elwood Street, Phoenix, AZ 85040-1958. *Telephone:* 480-804-7600.

GRADUATE PROGRAMS
Expenses (2009-10) *Tuition:* full-time $10,560. *Required fees:* full-time $760.
Financial Aid Institutionally sponsored loans and scholarships available.

Contact Campus College Chair, Nursing, College of Nursing, University of Phoenix–Phoenix Campus, 4635 East Elwood Street, Phoenix, AZ 85040-1958. *Telephone:* 480-804-7600.

MASTER'S DEGREE PROGRAM

Degrees MSN; MSN/MBA; MSN/MHA
Available Programs Master's.
Concentrations Available Health-care administration; nursing administration; nursing education. *Nurse practitioner programs in:* family health.
Site Options Scottsdale, AZ; Mesa, AZ; Chandler, AZ.
Study Options Full-time.
Online Degree Options Yes.
Program Entrance Requirements Clinical experience, computer literacy, minimum overall college GPA of 2.5, transcript of college record. *Application deadline:* Applications may be processed on a rolling basis for some programs. *Application fee:* $45.
Advanced Placement Credit given for nursing courses completed elsewhere dependent upon specific evaluations.
Degree Requirements 39 total credit hours, thesis or project.

POST-MASTER'S PROGRAM

Areas of Study *Nurse practitioner programs in:* family health.

CONTINUING EDUCATION PROGRAM

Contact Campus College Chair, Nursing, College of Nursing, University of Phoenix–Phoenix Campus, Mail Stop CJ A101, 4635 East Elwood Street, Phoenix, AZ 85040-1958. *Telephone:* 480-557-2279. *Fax:* 480-557-2338.

University of Phoenix–Southern Arizona Campus

College of Social Sciences
Tucson, Arizona

Founded in 1979

DEGREES • BSN • MSN

Nursing Program Faculty 19 (32% with doctorates).
Baccalaureate Enrollment 67 **Women** 85.1% **Men** 14.9% **Minority** 33.8%
Graduate Enrollment 97 **Women** 80.4% **Men** 19.6% **Minority** 18.56%
Nursing Student Activities Sigma Theta Tau.
Nursing Student Resources Academic advising; academic or career counseling; assistance for students with disabilities; bookstore; campus computer network; computer lab; computer-assisted instruction; e-mail services; interactive nursing skills videos; Internet; learning resource lab; library services; nursing audiovisuals; remedial services; skills, simulation, or other laboratory; tutoring.
Library Facilities 16,781 periodical subscriptions (1,300 health-care related).

BACCALAUREATE PROGRAMS

Degree BSN
Available Programs Accelerated Baccalaureate; LPN to Baccalaureate.
Site Options Sierra Vista, AZ; Yuma, AZ; Nogales, AZ.
Study Options Full-time.
Online Degree Options Yes.
Program Entrance Requirements Transcript of college record, CPR certification, immunizations, 1 letter of recommendation, RN licensure. Transfer students are accepted. *Application deadline:* Applications may be processed on a rolling basis for some programs.
Advanced Placement Credit by examination available. Credit given for nursing courses completed elsewhere dependent upon specific evaluations.
Expenses (2009-10) *Tuition:* full-time $9300. *Required fees:* full-time $600.
Contact Campus College Chair, Nursing, College of Social Sciences, University of Phoenix–Southern Arizona Campus, 300 South Craycroft Road, Tucson, AZ 85711-4574. *Telephone:* 520-881-6512.

GRADUATE PROGRAMS

Expenses (2009-10) *Tuition:* full-time $10,560. *Required fees:* full-time $760.
Financial Aid Institutionally sponsored loans and scholarships available.
Contact Campus College Chair, Nursing, College of Social Sciences, University of Phoenix–Southern Arizona Campus, 300 South Craycroft Road, Tucson, AZ 85711-4574. *Telephone:* 520-881-6512.

MASTER'S DEGREE PROGRAM

Degree MSN
Available Programs Master's.
Concentrations Available Health-care administration; nursing administration; nursing education. *Nurse practitioner programs in:* family health.
Site Options Sierra Vista, AZ; Yuma, AZ; Nogales, AZ.
Study Options Full-time.
Online Degree Options Yes.
Program Entrance Requirements Clinical experience, computer literacy, minimum overall college GPA of 2.5, transcript of college record. *Application deadline:* Applications may be processed on a rolling basis for some programs. *Application fee:* $45.
Advanced Placement Credit given for nursing courses completed elsewhere dependent upon specific evaluations.
Degree Requirements 39 total credit hours, thesis or project.

POST-MASTER'S PROGRAM

Areas of Study *Nurse practitioner programs in:* family health.

CONTINUING EDUCATION PROGRAM

Contact Campus College Chair, Nursing, College of Social Sciences, University of Phoenix–Southern Arizona Campus, 300 South Craycroft Road, Tucson, AZ 85711-4574. *Telephone:* 520-881-6512.

ARKANSAS

Arkansas State University - Jonesboro

Department of Nursing
Jonesboro, State University, Arkansas

http://www.conhp.astate.edu/Nursing/
Founded in 1909

DEGREES • BSN • MSN

Nursing Program Faculty 35 (20% with doctorates).
Baccalaureate Enrollment 245
Graduate Enrollment 91
Nursing Student Activities Nursing Honor Society, Sigma Theta Tau.
Library Facilities 631,161 volumes; 3,595 periodical subscriptions.

BACCALAUREATE PROGRAMS

Degree BSN
Available Programs Generic Baccalaureate; LPN to Baccalaureate; RN Baccalaureate.
Site Options Mountain Home, AR; Melbourne, AR; Beebe, AR.
Study Options Full-time.
Program Entrance Requirements Minimum overall college GPA of 2.5, transcript of college record, CPR certification, health exam, immunizations, minimum GPA in nursing prerequisites of 3.5, prerequisite course work. Transfer students are accepted.
Advanced Placement Credit given for nursing courses completed elsewhere dependent upon specific evaluations.
Contact *Telephone:* 870-972-3074. *Fax:* 870-972-2954.

GRADUATE PROGRAMS

Contact *Telephone:* 870-972-3074. *Fax:* 870-972-2954.

MASTER'S DEGREE PROGRAM

Degree MSN
Available Programs Master's.
Concentrations Available Nurse anesthesia; nursing education. *Clinical nurse specialist programs in:* adult health. *Nurse practitioner programs in:* primary care.
Site Options Mountain Home, AR; Melbourne, AR; Beebe, AR.
Study Options Full-time and part-time.
Program Entrance Requirements Clinical experience, minimum overall college GPA of 2.75, transcript of college record, CPR certifi-

cation, written essay, immunizations, interview, letters of recommendation, physical assessment course, professional liability insurance/malpractice insurance, statistics course.
Degree Requirements 39 total credit hours, thesis or project, comprehensive exam.

Arkansas Tech University
Program in Nursing
Russellville, Arkansas

http://nursing.atu.edu/
Founded in 1909

DEGREES • BSN • MSN

Nursing Program Faculty 26 (20% with doctorates).
Baccalaureate Enrollment 205 **Women** 84% **Men** 16% **Minority** 11% **Part-time** 14%
Graduate Enrollment 8 **Women** 87% **Men** 13% **Part-time** 13%
Distance Learning Courses Available.
Nursing Student Activities Nursing Honor Society, Sigma Theta Tau, Student Nurses' Association.
Nursing Student Resources Academic advising; academic or career counseling; assistance for students with disabilities; bookstore; campus computer network; career placement assistance; computer lab; computer-assisted instruction; e-mail services; employment services for current students; housing assistance; interactive nursing skills videos; Internet; learning resource lab; library services; nursing audiovisuals; other; paid internships; placement services for program completers; remedial services; resume preparation assistance; skills, simulation, or other laboratory; tutoring.
Library Facilities 289,158 volumes (16,900 in health, 2,100 in nursing); 829 periodical subscriptions (130 health-care related).

BACCALAUREATE PROGRAMS

Degree BSN
Available Programs ADN to Baccalaureate; Generic Baccalaureate; LPN to Baccalaureate; RN Baccalaureate.
Site Options Russellville, AR.
Study Options Full-time and part-time.
Online Degree Options Yes.
Program Entrance Requirements Transcript of college record, CPR certification, health exam, immunizations, minimum GPA in nursing prerequisites of 3.00, professional liability insurance/malpractice insurance, prerequisite course work. Transfer students are accepted. *Application deadline:* 3/1 (fall), 10/1 (spring).
Advanced Placement Credit by examination available. Credit given for nursing courses completed elsewhere dependent upon specific evaluations.
Expenses (2010-11) *Tuition, state resident:* full-time $5100; part-time $170 per credit hour. *Tuition, nonresident:* full-time $10,200; part-time $350 per credit hour. *Room and board:* $5444; room only: $3340 per academic year. *Required fees:* full-time $808; part-time $14 per credit; part-time $388 per term.
Financial Aid 80% of baccalaureate students in nursing programs received some form of financial aid in 2009-10.
Contact Dr. Rebecca F. Burris, Professor and Department Chair, Program in Nursing, Arkansas Tech University, 402 West O Street, Russellville, AR 72801. *Telephone:* 479-968-0383. *Fax:* 479-968-0219. *E-mail:* rburris@atu.edu.

GRADUATE PROGRAMS

Financial Aid 75% of graduate students in nursing programs received some form of financial aid in 2009-10.
Contact Dr. Mary Gunter, Dean of Graduate College, Program in Nursing, Arkansas Tech University, Tomlinson Graduate College, Russellville, AR 72801. *Telephone:* 479-968-0398. *E-mail:* mgunter@atu.edu.

MASTER'S DEGREE PROGRAM

Degree MSN
Available Programs Master's; Master's for Nurses with Non-Nursing Degrees; RN to Master's.
Concentrations Available Nursing administration.
Site Options Russellville, AR.
Study Options Full-time and part-time.
Program Entrance Requirements Clinical experience, computer literacy, minimum overall college GPA of 3.0, transcript of college record, statistics course. *Application deadline:* 3/1 (fall).
Advanced Placement Credit given for nursing courses completed elsewhere dependent upon specific evaluations.
Degree Requirements 39 total credit hours, thesis or project.

Harding University
College of Nursing
Searcy, Arkansas

http://www.harding.edu/nursing
Founded in 1924

DEGREE • BSN

Nursing Program Faculty 19 (25% with doctorates).
Baccalaureate Enrollment 89 **Women** 83% **Men** 17% **Minority** 1% **International** 1% **Part-time** 1%
Nursing Student Activities Nursing Honor Society, Sigma Theta Tau, Student Nurses' Association.
Nursing Student Resources Academic advising; academic or career counseling; assistance for students with disabilities; bookstore; campus computer network; career placement assistance; computer lab; computer-assisted instruction; e-mail services; employment services for current students; externships; housing assistance; interactive nursing skills videos; Internet; learning resource lab; library services; nursing audiovisuals; placement services for program completers; remedial services; resume preparation assistance; skills, simulation, or other laboratory; tutoring.
Library Facilities 253,771 volumes (5,000 in health, 1,729 in nursing); 24,513 periodical subscriptions (120 health-care related).

BACCALAUREATE PROGRAMS

Degree BSN
Available Programs ADN to Baccalaureate; Generic Baccalaureate; LPN to Baccalaureate; LPN to RN Baccalaureate; RN Baccalaureate.
Site Options Searcy, AR.
Study Options Full-time and part-time.
Program Entrance Requirements Minimum overall college GPA of 2.0, transcript of college record, CPR certification, health exam, high school transcript, immunizations, 3 letters of recommendation, minimum GPA in nursing prerequisites of 2.5, prerequisite course work. Transfer students are accepted. *Application deadline:* 3/1 (fall), 10/1 (spring).
Advanced Placement Credit by examination available. Credit given for nursing courses completed elsewhere dependent upon specific evaluations.
Expenses (2009-10) *Tuition:* full-time $6352; part-time $4600 per semester. *International tuition:* $6352 full-time. *Room and board:* $3051; room only: $1412 per academic year.
Financial Aid 95% of baccalaureate students in nursing programs received some form of financial aid in 2008-09. *Gift aid (need-based):* Federal Pell, FSEOG, state, private, college/university gift aid from institutional funds. *Loans:* Federal Nursing Student Loans, Perkins, state, college/university. *Work-study:* Federal Work-Study, part-time campus jobs. *Financial aid application deadline (priority):* 4/15.
Contact Ms. Jeanne L. Castleberry, Assistant to the Dean, College of Nursing, Harding University, Box 12265, 914 East Market Avenue, Searcy, AR 72149-2265. *Telephone:* 501-279-4682. *Fax:* 501-305-8902. *E-mail:* nursing@harding.edu.

CONTINUING EDUCATION PROGRAM

Contact Dr. Cathleen M. Shultz, Dean and Professor, College of Nursing, Harding University, Box 12265, Searcy, AR 72149-2265. *Telephone:* 501-279-4476. *Fax:* 501-279-4669. *E-mail:* nursing@harding.edu.

Henderson State University
Department of Nursing
Arkadelphia, Arkansas

http://www.hsu.edu/dept/nsg/index.html
Founded in 1890

DEGREE • BSN

Nursing Program Faculty 7 (29% with doctorates).

Baccalaureate Enrollment 50 **Women** 64% **Men** 36% **Minority** 35% **International** 2%
Distance Learning Courses Available.
Nursing Student Activities Student Nurses' Association, nursing club.
Nursing Student Resources Academic advising; academic or career counseling; assistance for students with disabilities; bookstore; campus computer network; career placement assistance; computer lab; computer-assisted instruction; e-mail services; interactive nursing skills videos; Internet; learning resource lab; library services; nursing audiovisuals; remedial services; resume preparation assistance; skills, simulation, or other laboratory; tutoring.
Library Facilities 264,367 volumes (1,000 in health, 200 in nursing); 216,738 periodical subscriptions (40 health-care related).

BACCALAUREATE PROGRAMS

Degree BSN
Available Programs ADN to Baccalaureate; Generic Baccalaureate; LPN to Baccalaureate.
Study Options Full-time.
Program Entrance Requirements Minimum overall college GPA of 2.5, transcript of college record, CPR certification, immunizations, minimum GPA in nursing prerequisites of 2.50, prerequisite course work. Transfer students are accepted. *Application deadline:* 2/15 (fall). *Application fee:* $57.
Advanced Placement Credit given for nursing courses completed elsewhere dependent upon specific evaluations.
Expenses (2010-11) *Tuition, state resident:* full-time $4272; part-time $178 per credit hour. *Tuition, nonresident:* full-time $8544; part-time $356 per credit hour. *Room and board:* $2983; room only: $1683 per academic year. *Required fees:* full-time $1021.
Financial Aid 80% of baccalaureate students in nursing programs received some form of financial aid in 2009-10. *Gift aid (need-based):* Federal Pell, FSEOG, state, private, college/university gift aid from institutional funds. *Loans:* Perkins. *Work-study:* Federal Work-Study, part-time campus jobs. *Financial aid application deadline (priority):* 6/1.
Contact Dr. Barbara J. Landrum, Professor and Department Chair, Department of Nursing, Henderson State University, Box 7803, 1100 Henderson Street, Arkadelphia, AR 71999-0001. *Telephone:* 870-230-5508. *Fax:* 870-230-5390. *E-mail:* landrub@hsu.edu.

Southern Arkansas University–Magnolia
Department of Nursing
Magnolia, Arkansas

http://www.saumag.edu/academics/science_and_technology/nursing/
Founded in 1909

DEGREE • BSN

Nursing Program Faculty 13 (23% with doctorates).
Baccalaureate Enrollment 51 **Women** 90% **Men** 10% **Minority** 15% **Part-time** 58%
Distance Learning Courses Available.
Nursing Student Activities Student Nurses' Association.
Nursing Student Resources Academic advising; academic or career counseling; assistance for students with disabilities; bookstore; campus computer network; career placement assistance; computer lab; computer-assisted instruction; e-mail services; employment services for current students; housing assistance; interactive nursing skills videos; Internet; learning resource lab; library services; nursing audiovisuals; remedial services; resume preparation assistance; skills, simulation, or other laboratory; tutoring.
Library Facilities 151,166 volumes (800 in health, 200 in nursing); 1,065 periodical subscriptions (2,000 health-care related).

BACCALAUREATE PROGRAMS

Degree BSN
Available Programs ADN to Baccalaureate; Generic Baccalaureate; RN Baccalaureate.
Study Options Full-time.
Online Degree Options Yes.
Program Entrance Requirements Minimum overall college GPA of 2.5, transcript of college record, CPR certification, high school chemistry, immunizations, minimum GPA in nursing prerequisites of 2.5, prerequisite course work. Transfer students are accepted. *Application deadline:* 2/28 (fall). Applications may be processed on a rolling basis for some programs.
Advanced Placement Credit given for nursing courses completed elsewhere dependent upon specific evaluations.
Expenses (2010-11) *Tuition, state resident:* full-time $5340; part-time $178 per credit hour. *Tuition, nonresident:* full-time $8100; part-time $270 per credit hour. *Room and board:* $2290; room only: $1145 per academic year. *Required fees:* full-time $250; part-time $125 per term.
Financial Aid 40% of baccalaureate students in nursing programs received some form of financial aid in 2009-10. *Gift aid (need-based):* Federal Pell, FSEOG, state, private, college/university gift aid from institutional funds. *Loans:* Perkins. *Work-study:* Federal Work-Study, part-time campus jobs. *Financial aid application deadline (priority):* 7/1.
Contact Dr. Shari Kist, BSN Program Director, Department of Nursing, Southern Arkansas University–Magnolia, 100 East University, Magnolia, AR 71753-5000. *Telephone:* 870-235-4331. *Fax:* 870-235-5058. *E-mail:* sharikist@saumag.edu.

University of Arkansas
Eleanor Mann School of Nursing
Fayetteville, Arkansas

http://www.uark.edu/coehp
Founded in 1871

DEGREES • BSN • MSN

Nursing Program Faculty 25 (26% with doctorates).
Baccalaureate Enrollment 220 **Women** 95% **Men** 5% **Minority** 7%
Graduate Enrollment 20
Nursing Student Activities Sigma Theta Tau, Student Nurses' Association.
Nursing Student Resources Academic advising; academic or career counseling; assistance for students with disabilities; bookstore; campus computer network; career placement assistance; computer lab; computer-assisted instruction; e-mail services; employment services for current students; housing assistance; interactive nursing skills videos; Internet; learning resource lab; library services; nursing audiovisuals; other; placement services for program completers; remedial services; resume preparation assistance; skills, simulation, or other laboratory; tutoring.
Library Facilities 1.8 million volumes (60,000 in health, 20,000 in nursing); 18,576 periodical subscriptions (130,000 health-care related).

BACCALAUREATE PROGRAMS

Degree BSN
Available Programs Generic Baccalaureate; LPN to Baccalaureate; LPN to RN Baccalaureate; RN Baccalaureate.
Study Options Full-time and part-time.
Program Entrance Requirements Minimum overall college GPA of 2.75, transcript of college record, CPR certification, health insurance, immunizations, minimum GPA in nursing prerequisites of 2.75, professional liability insurance/malpractice insurance, prerequisite course work. Transfer students are accepted.
Advanced Placement Credit by examination available. Credit given for nursing courses completed elsewhere dependent upon specific evaluations.
Contact ***Telephone:*** 479-575-3907. *Fax:* 479-575-3218.

GRADUATE PROGRAMS

Contact ***Telephone:*** 479-575-3907. *Fax:* 479-575-3218.

MASTER'S DEGREE PROGRAM

Degree MSN
Available Programs Master's.
Concentrations Available Nursing education. *Clinical nurse specialist programs in:* acute care, medical-surgical.
Study Options Full-time and part-time.
Online Degree Options Yes.
Program Entrance Requirements Computer literacy, minimum overall college GPA of 3.0, transcript of college record, CPR certification, immunizations, nursing research course, physical assessment course, statistics course.
Degree Requirements 42 total credit hours, thesis or project, comprehensive exam.

CONTINUING EDUCATION PROGRAM

Contact *Telephone:* 479-575-3907. *Fax:* 479-575-3218.

University of Arkansas at Fort Smith

Carol McKelvey Moore School of Nursing
Fort Smith, Arkansas

Founded in 1928

DEGREE • BSN

Nursing Program Faculty 18
Baccalaureate Enrollment 20 **Women** 60% **Men** 40% **Minority** 5%
Distance Learning Courses Available.
Nursing Student Activities Student Nurses' Association.
Nursing Student Resources Academic advising; academic or career counseling; assistance for students with disabilities; bookstore; campus computer network; career placement assistance; computer lab; computer-assisted instruction; e-mail services; housing assistance; interactive nursing skills videos; Internet; learning resource lab; library services; nursing audiovisuals; remedial services; resume preparation assistance; skills, simulation, or other laboratory; tutoring.
Library Facilities 85,898 volumes (2,231 in health, 1,183 in nursing); 2,196 periodical subscriptions (5,350 health-care related).

BACCALAUREATE PROGRAMS

Degree BSN
Available Programs ADN to Baccalaureate; Generic Baccalaureate.
Study Options Full-time.
Online Degree Options Yes (online only).
Program Entrance Requirements Minimum overall college GPA of 2.5, transcript of college record, CPR certification, health exam, health insurance, immunizations, interview, minimum GPA in nursing prerequisites of 2.5, prerequisite course work. Transfer students are accepted.
Advanced Placement Credit given for nursing courses completed elsewhere dependent upon specific evaluations.
Contact *Telephone:* 479-788-7840. *Fax:* 479-788-7869.

University of Arkansas at Little Rock

BSN Programs
Little Rock, Arkansas

Founded in 1927

DEGREE • BSN

Library Facilities 3,998 periodical subscriptions.

BACCALAUREATE PROGRAMS

Degree BSN
Available Programs RN Baccalaureate.
Contact Ann Schlumberger, Chairperson/Professor, BSN Programs, University of Arkansas at Little Rock, Little Rock, AR 72204. *Telephone:* 501-569-8081. *E-mail:* abschlumberg@ualr.edu.

University of Arkansas at Monticello

School of Nursing
Monticello, Arkansas

http://www.uamont.edu/Nursing/
Founded in 1909

DEGREE • BSN

Nursing Program Faculty 11 (11% with doctorates).
Baccalaureate Enrollment 58 **Women** 84% **Men** 16% **Minority** 9% **International** 2%
Distance Learning Courses Available.
Nursing Student Activities Student Nurses' Association.
Nursing Student Resources Academic advising; academic or career counseling; assistance for students with disabilities; bookstore; campus computer network; computer lab; computer-assisted instruction; e-mail services; interactive nursing skills videos; Internet; learning resource lab; library services; nursing audiovisuals; skills, simulation, or other laboratory; tutoring.
Library Facilities 241,822 volumes (3,888 in health, 539 in nursing); 956 periodical subscriptions (5,015 health-care related).

BACCALAUREATE PROGRAMS

Degree BSN
Available Programs ADN to Baccalaureate; Generic Baccalaureate; LPN to Baccalaureate; RN Baccalaureate.
Study Options Full-time.
Program Entrance Requirements Transcript of college record, immunizations, minimum GPA in nursing prerequisites of 2.5, professional liability insurance/malpractice insurance, prerequisite course work. Transfer students are accepted. *Application deadline:* 3/1 (spring).
Advanced Placement Credit by examination available. Credit given for nursing courses completed elsewhere dependent upon specific evaluations.
Expenses (2010-11) *Tuition, state resident:* full-time $3600; part-time $120 per credit hour. *Tuition, nonresident:* full-time $8250; part-time $275 per credit hour. *Room and board:* $3850 per academic year. *Required fees:* full-time $1390; part-time $46 per credit; part-time $5 per term.
Financial Aid 83% of baccalaureate students in nursing programs received some form of financial aid in 2009-10.
Contact Ms. Pamela D. Gouner, Dean, School of Nursing, University of Arkansas at Monticello, PO Box 3606, Monticello, AR 71656. *Telephone:* 870-460-1069. *Fax:* 870-460-1969. *E-mail:* gouner@uamont.edu.

University of Arkansas at Pine Bluff

Department of Nursing
Pine Bluff, Arkansas

http://www.uapb.com/
Founded in 1873

DEGREE • BSN

Nursing Program Faculty 5 (40% with doctorates).
Baccalaureate Enrollment 20 **Women** 95% **Men** 5% **Minority** 100% **International** 20%
Nursing Student Activities Student Nurses' Association.
Nursing Student Resources Academic advising; academic or career counseling; assistance for students with disabilities; bookstore; campus computer network; career placement assistance; computer lab; computer-assisted instruction; e-mail services; housing assistance; interactive nursing skills videos; Internet; learning resource lab; library services; nursing audiovisuals; remedial services; resume preparation assistance; skills, simulation, or other laboratory; tutoring.
Library Facilities 287,857 volumes (2,600 in health, 1,550 in nursing); 3,041 periodical subscriptions (60 health-care related).

BACCALAUREATE PROGRAMS

Degree BSN
Available Programs Generic Baccalaureate.
Study Options Full-time and part-time.
Program Entrance Requirements Minimum overall college GPA of 2.5, transcript of college record, CPR certification, written essay, health exam, immunizations, 3 letters of recommendation, minimum GPA in nursing prerequisites of 2.5, professional liability insurance/malpractice insurance, prerequisite course work. Transfer students are accepted.
Advanced Placement Credit by examination available. Credit given for nursing courses completed elsewhere dependent upon specific evaluations.
Financial Aid 88% of baccalaureate students in nursing programs received some form of financial aid in 2009-10.
Contact Dr. Irene T. Henderson, Interim Chairperson, Department of Nursing, University of Arkansas at Pine Bluff, 1200 University Drive, Mail Slot 4973, Pine Bluff, AR 71601. *Telephone:* 870-575-8220. *Fax:* 870-575-8229. *E-mail:* henderson_i@uapb.edu.

University of Arkansas for Medical Sciences

College of Nursing
Little Rock, Arkansas

http://www.nursing.uams.edu/
Founded in 1879

DEGREES • BSN • MN SC • PHD

Nursing Program Faculty 85 (38% with doctorates).
Baccalaureate Enrollment 299
Graduate Enrollment 217
Distance Learning Courses Available.
Nursing Student Activities Nursing Honor Society, Sigma Theta Tau, Student Nurses' Association.
Nursing Student Resources Academic advising; academic or career counseling; assistance for students with disabilities; bookstore; campus computer network; computer lab; computer-assisted instruction; e-mail services; externships; interactive nursing skills videos; Internet; learning resource lab; library services; nursing audiovisuals; remedial services; skills, simulation, or other laboratory; tutoring.
Library Facilities 183,975 volumes (183,975 in health); 1,567 periodical subscriptions (1,567 health-care related).

BACCALAUREATE PROGRAMS

Degree BSN
Available Programs ADN to Baccalaureate; Accelerated RN Baccalaureate; Baccalaureate for Second Degree; Generic Baccalaureate; LPN to Baccalaureate; RN Baccalaureate.
Site Options Hope, AR; Fayetteville, AR; El Dorado, AR; Texarkana, Helena, Jonesboro, AR.
Study Options Full-time.
Online Degree Options Yes.
Program Entrance Requirements Minimum overall college GPA of 2.5, transcript of college record, CPR certification, health insurance, immunizations, minimum GPA in nursing prerequisites of 2.5, prerequisite course work. Transfer students are accepted. *Application deadline:* 2/1 (summer). *Application fee:* $58.
Advanced Placement Credit by examination available. Credit given for nursing courses completed elsewhere dependent upon specific evaluations.
Expenses (2010-11) *Tuition, area resident:* full-time $8043; part-time $208 per credit hour. *Tuition, nonresident:* full-time $6540; part-time $545 per credit hour. *Required fees:* full-time $580.
Financial Aid 90% of baccalaureate students in nursing programs received some form of financial aid in 2009-10.
Contact Dr. Donna Middaugh, Associate Dean for Service, College of Nursing, University of Arkansas for Medical Sciences, 4301 West Markham, #529, Little Rock, AR 72205-7199. *Telephone:* 501-686-5374. *Fax:* 501-686-8350. *E-mail:* middaughdonnaj@uams.edu.

GRADUATE PROGRAMS

Expenses (2010-11) *Tuition, area resident:* full-time $2844; part-time $928 per credit hour. *Tuition, nonresident:* full-time $6102; part-time $678 per credit hour.
Financial Aid 90% of graduate students in nursing programs received some form of financial aid in 2009-10. Career-related internships or fieldwork and traineeships available. Aid available to part-time students.
Contact Dr. Donna Middaugh, Associate Dean for Service, College of Nursing, University of Arkansas for Medical Sciences, 4301 West Markham, #529, Little Rock, AR 72205-7199. *Telephone:* 501-686-8349. *Fax:* 501-686-8350. *E-mail:* middaughdonnaj@uams.edu.

MASTER'S DEGREE PROGRAM

Degree MN Sc
Available Programs Master's; Master's for Nurses with Non-Nursing Degrees; RN to Master's.
Concentrations Available Nursing administration; nursing education. *Clinical nurse specialist programs in:* acute care, adult health, pediatric. *Nurse practitioner programs in:* acute care, family health, gerontology, pediatric, psychiatric/mental health, women's health.
Site Options Fayetteville, AR; El Dorado, AR; Texarkana, Helena, Jonesboro, AR.
Study Options Full-time and part-time.
Program Entrance Requirements Clinical experience, minimum overall college GPA of 2.85, transcript of college record, CPR certification, immunizations, physical assessment course, professional liability insurance/malpractice insurance, statistics course. *Application deadline:* 4/1 (fall), 9/1 (spring). *Application fee:* $58.
Advanced Placement Credit given for nursing courses completed elsewhere dependent upon specific evaluations.
Degree Requirements 39 total credit hours, thesis or project, comprehensive exam.

DOCTORAL DEGREE PROGRAM

Degree PhD
Available Programs Doctorate; Doctorate for Nurses with Non-Nursing Degrees; Post-Baccalaureate Doctorate.
Areas of Study Advanced practice nursing, clinical practice, gerontology, health-care systems, nursing administration, nursing education, nursing research, nursing science, oncology, women's health.
Program Entrance Requirements Minimum overall college GPA of 3.65, interview by faculty committee, interview, 4 letters of recommendation, MSN or equivalent, scholarly papers, statistics course, writing sample, GRE. Application deadline: 1/2 (spring).
Degree Requirements 60 total credit hours, dissertation, oral exam, written exam.

POSTDOCTORAL PROGRAM

Areas of Study Aging, cancer care, gerontology, nursing research, nursing science.
Postdoctoral Program Contact Postdoctoral Contact, College of Nursing, University of Arkansas for Medical Sciences, 4301 West Markham, #529, Little Rock, AR 72205-7199. *Telephone:* 501-686-5374. *Fax:* 501-686-8350.

CONTINUING EDUCATION PROGRAM

Contact Dr. Claudia P. Barone, Dean and Professor, College of Nursing, University of Arkansas for Medical Sciences, 4301 West Markham, #529, Little Rock, AR 72205-7199. *Telephone:* 501-686-5374. *Fax:* 501-686-8350. *E-mail:* baroneclaudiap@uams.edu.

University of Central Arkansas

Department of Nursing
Conway, Arkansas

http://www.uca.edu/divisions/academic/nursing/
Founded in 1907

DEGREES • BSN • MSN

Nursing Program Faculty 32 (28% with doctorates).
Baccalaureate Enrollment 245 **Women** 84.9% **Men** 15.1% **Minority** 12.65% **International** 2.04% **Part-time** 23.67%
Graduate Enrollment 136 **Women** 95.59% **Men** 4.41% **Minority** 11.76% **International** .74% **Part-time** 95.59%
Distance Learning Courses Available.
Nursing Student Activities Sigma Theta Tau, Student Nurses' Association.
Nursing Student Resources Academic advising; academic or career counseling; assistance for students with disabilities; bookstore; campus computer network; career placement assistance; computer lab; computer-assisted instruction; e-mail services; employment services for current students; externships; housing assistance; interactive nursing skills videos; Internet; learning resource lab; library services; nursing audiovisuals; paid internships; placement services for program completers; remedial services; resume preparation assistance; skills, simulation, or other laboratory; tutoring; unpaid internships.
Library Facilities 600,084 volumes; 804 periodical subscriptions.

BACCALAUREATE PROGRAMS

Degree BSN
Available Programs ADN to Baccalaureate; Generic Baccalaureate; LPN to Baccalaureate; LPN to RN Baccalaureate; RN Baccalaureate.
Study Options Full-time and part-time.
Program Entrance Requirements Minimum overall college GPA of 2.5, transcript of college record, health exam, health insurance, immunizations, minimum GPA in nursing prerequisites, prerequisite course work. Transfer students are accepted. *Application deadline:* 3/1 (fall). *Application fee:* $50.
Advanced Placement Credit given for nursing courses completed elsewhere dependent upon specific evaluations.
Expenses (2009-10) *Tuition, area resident:* full-time $12,578; part-time $6289 per semester. *Room and board:* $4880 per academic year.

Contact Ms. Ann Mattison, Education Counselor, Department of Nursing, University of Central Arkansas, Doyne Health Science Center, 201 South Donaghey Avenue, Conway, AR 72035. *Telephone:* 501-450-5526. *Fax:* 501-450-5560. *E-mail:* annm@uca.edu.

GRADUATE PROGRAMS

Financial Aid Federal Work-Study, traineeships, and unspecified assistantships available.
Contact Ms. Rose Schlosser, Education Counselor, Department of Nursing, University of Central Arkansas, Doyne Health Science Center, 201 South Donaghey Avenue, Conway, AR 72035. *Telephone:* 501-450-5532. *Fax:* 501-450-5560. *E-mail:* RSchlosser@uca.edu.

MASTER'S DEGREE PROGRAM

Degree MSN
Available Programs Master's; RN to Master's.
Concentrations Available Nursing education. *Clinical nurse specialist programs in:* medical-surgical. *Nurse practitioner programs in:* adult health, family health.
Site Options Russelville, AR; Pine Bluff, AR; Fort Smith, AR.
Study Options Full-time and part-time.
Online Degree Options Yes (online only).
Program Entrance Requirements Clinical experience, minimum overall college GPA of 2.7, transcript of college record, CPR certification, immunizations, professional liability insurance/malpractice insurance, prerequisite course work, resume, statistics course, GRE General Test. *Application deadline:* 4/1 (fall), 8/1 (spring). *Application fee:* $50.
Degree Requirements 39 total credit hours, comprehensive exam.

POST-MASTER'S PROGRAM

Areas of Study Nursing education. *Clinical nurse specialist programs in:* medical-surgical. *Nurse practitioner programs in:* adult health, family health.

CALIFORNIA

Azusa Pacific University

School of Nursing
Azusa, California

http://www.apu.edu/nursing/grad
Founded in 1899

DEGREES • BSN • MSN • PHD

Nursing Program Faculty 77 (22% with doctorates).
Baccalaureate Enrollment 236 **Women** 90% **Men** 10% **Minority** 44% **International** 11% **Part-time** 2%
Graduate Enrollment 110 **Women** 89% **Men** 11% **Minority** 37%
Nursing Student Activities Sigma Theta Tau, Student Nurses' Association, nursing club.
Nursing Student Resources Academic advising; academic or career counseling; bookstore; campus computer network; career placement assistance; computer lab; computer-assisted instruction; e-mail services; employment services for current students; housing assistance; interactive nursing skills videos; Internet; learning resource lab; library services; nursing audiovisuals; remedial services; resume preparation assistance; skills, simulation, or other laboratory; tutoring.
Library Facilities 14,206 volumes in health, 4,712 volumes in nursing; 432 periodical subscriptions health-care related.

BACCALAUREATE PROGRAMS

Degree BSN
Available Programs ADN to Baccalaureate; Accelerated Baccalaureate; Accelerated RN Baccalaureate; Generic Baccalaureate.
Study Options Full-time and part-time.
Program Entrance Requirements Minimum overall college GPA of 3.0, transcript of college record, CPR certification, written essay, health exam, high school biology, high school chemistry, 2 years high school math, high school transcript, immunizations, 3 letters of recommendation, minimum high school GPA of 3.0, minimum GPA in nursing prerequisites of 3.0. Transfer students are accepted.
Advanced Placement Credit by examination available. Credit given for nursing courses completed elsewhere dependent upon specific evaluations.
Contact *Telephone:* 626-815-6000 Ext. 5501. *Fax:* 626-815-5414.

GRADUATE PROGRAMS

Contact *Telephone:* 626-815-5386. *Fax:* 626-815-5414.

MASTER'S DEGREE PROGRAM

Degree MSN
Available Programs Accelerated Master's for Non-Nursing College Graduates; Accelerated Master's for Nurses with Non-Nursing Degrees; Master's.
Concentrations Available Nursing administration; nursing education. *Clinical nurse specialist programs in:* adult health, medical-surgical, parent-child, pediatric, school health. *Nurse practitioner programs in:* adult health, family health, pediatric, primary care.
Study Options Full-time and part-time.
Program Entrance Requirements Clinical experience, computer literacy, minimum overall college GPA of 3.0, transcript of college record, CPR certification, written essay, immunizations, 3 letters of recommendation, nursing research course, physical assessment course, professional liability insurance/malpractice insurance, prerequisite course work, resume, statistics course.
Advanced Placement Credit by examination available. Credit given for nursing courses completed elsewhere dependent upon specific evaluations.
Degree Requirements 42 total credit hours, thesis or project, comprehensive exam.

POST-MASTER'S PROGRAM

Areas of Study Nursing administration; nursing education. *Clinical nurse specialist programs in:* adult health, medical-surgical, parent-child, pediatric, school health. *Nurse practitioner programs in:* adult health, family health, pediatric, primary care.

DOCTORAL DEGREE PROGRAM

Degree PhD
Available Programs Doctorate.
Areas of Study Community health, family health, nursing education.
Program Entrance Requirements Clinical experience, minimum overall college GPA of 3.5, interview by faculty committee, interview, 3 letters of recommendation, MSN or equivalent, scholarly papers, statistics course, vita, writing sample.
Degree Requirements 64 total credit hours, dissertation, oral exam, written exam.

CONTINUING EDUCATION PROGRAM

Contact *Telephone:* 626-815-5385. *Fax:* 626-815-5414.

Biola University

Department of Nursing
La Mirada, California

http://www.biola.edu/
Founded in 1908

DEGREE • BSN

Nursing Program Faculty 16 (19% with doctorates).
Baccalaureate Enrollment 106 **Women** 91% **Men** 9% **Minority** 25%
Nursing Student Activities Student Nurses' Association.
Nursing Student Resources Academic advising; academic or career counseling; assistance for students with disabilities; bookstore; campus computer network; career placement assistance; computer lab; computer-assisted instruction; e-mail services; employment services for current students; housing assistance; Internet; learning resource lab; library services; nursing audiovisuals; placement services for program completers; remedial services; resume preparation assistance; skills, simulation, or other laboratory; tutoring.
Library Facilities 20,000 volumes in health, 10,000 volumes in nursing; 750 periodical subscriptions health-care related.

BACCALAUREATE PROGRAMS

Degree BSN
Available Programs ADN to Baccalaureate; Generic Baccalaureate; LPN to Baccalaureate; RN Baccalaureate.

Study Options Full-time.
Program Entrance Requirements Minimum overall college GPA of 3.0, transcript of college record, CPR certification, written essay, health exam, health insurance, high school biology, high school chemistry, high school foreign language, 2 years high school math, high school transcript, immunizations, interview, 2 letters of recommendation, minimum high school GPA of 3.5, minimum GPA in nursing prerequisites of 3.0, professional liability insurance/malpractice insurance, prerequisite course work. Transfer students are accepted. *Application fee:* $50.
Advanced Placement Credit given for nursing courses completed elsewhere dependent upon specific evaluations.
Expenses (2010-11) *Tuition:* full-time $28,852. *Room and board:* $8038; room only: $4544 per academic year. *Required fees:* full-time $1500.
Financial Aid 95% of baccalaureate students in nursing programs received some form of financial aid in 2009-10. *Gift aid (need-based):* Federal Pell, FSEOG, state, private, college/university gift aid from institutional funds. *Loans:* Federal Nursing Student Loans, Federal Direct (Subsidized and Unsubsidized Stafford PLUS), Perkins, college/university, alternative loans. *Work-study:* Federal Work-Study, part-time campus jobs. *Financial aid application deadline:* Continuous.
Contact Dr. Anne L. Gewe, Associate Chair/Associate Professor, Department of Nursing, Biola University, 13800 Biola Avenue, La Mirada, CA 90639. *Telephone:* 562-903-4850. *Fax:* 562-903-4803. *E-mail:* anne.gewe@biola.edu.

California Baptist University
School of Nursing
Riverside, California

http://www.calbaptist.edu/nursing
Founded in 1950

DEGREES • BSN • MSN
Nursing Program Faculty 26 (4% with doctorates).
Baccalaureate Enrollment 180 **Women** 87.78% **Men** 12.22% **Minority** 33.89% **International** 1.67%
Graduate Enrollment 16 **Women** 87.5% **Men** 12.5% **Minority** 56.25%
Nursing Student Activities Student Nurses' Association.
Nursing Student Resources Academic advising; academic or career counseling; bookstore; campus computer network; career placement assistance; computer lab; e-mail services; employment services for current students; interactive nursing skills videos; Internet; learning resource lab; library services; nursing audiovisuals; resume preparation assistance; skills, simulation, or other laboratory; tutoring.
Library Facilities 203,175 volumes (335 in health, 236 in nursing); 17,037 periodical subscriptions (286 health-care related).

BACCALAUREATE PROGRAMS

Degree BSN
Available Programs ADN to Baccalaureate; Generic Baccalaureate; RN Baccalaureate.
Site Options Corona, CA; San Bernardino, CA; Fullerton, CA.
Study Options Full-time.
Program Entrance Requirements Minimum overall college GPA of 2.7, transcript of college record, CPR certification, written essay, health exam, health insurance, immunizations, 2 letters of recommendation, minimum GPA in nursing prerequisites of 2.7, professional liability insurance/malpractice insurance, prerequisite course work. Transfer students are accepted. *Application deadline:* 3/11 (fall), 8/31 (spring). *Application fee:* $50.
Expenses (2010-11) *Tuition:* full-time $11,427. *Room and board:* $6950; room only: $4160 per academic year. *Required fees:* full-time $4091.
Financial Aid 90% of baccalaureate students in nursing programs received some form of financial aid in 2009-10. *Gift aid (need-based):* Federal Pell, FSEOG, state, private, college/university gift aid from institutional funds. *Loans:* Perkins, alternative loans. *Work-study:* Federal Work-Study. *Financial aid application deadline (priority):* 3/2.
Contact Beth Wagner, Program Specialist, School of Nursing, California Baptist University, 8432 Magnolia Avenue, Riverside, CA 92504. *Telephone:* 951-343-4336. *E-mail:* bwagner@calbaptist.edu.

GRADUATE PROGRAMS

Expenses (2010-11) *Tuition:* full-time $24,024. *Room and board:* $6164; room only: $2080 per academic year.
Financial Aid 93% of graduate students in nursing programs received some form of financial aid in 2009-10.
Contact Beth Wagner, Program Specialist, School of Nursing, California Baptist University, 8432 Magnolia Avenue, Riverside, CA 92504. *Telephone:* 951-343-4336. *Fax:* 951-343-4703. *E-mail:* bwagner@calbaptist.edu.

MASTER'S DEGREE PROGRAM

Degree MSN
Available Programs Accelerated Master's for Non-Nursing College Graduates; Master's.
Concentrations Available Clinical nurse leader; nursing education. *Clinical nurse specialist programs in:* adult health.
Study Options Part-time.
Program Entrance Requirements Computer literacy, minimum overall college GPA of 3.25, transcript of college record, CPR certification, written essay, immunizations, interview, 3 letters of recommendation, professional liability insurance/malpractice insurance, prerequisite course work, resume, statistics course. *Application deadline:* Applications may be processed on a rolling basis for some programs. *Application fee:* $45.
Degree Requirements 42 total credit hours, thesis or project, comprehensive exam.

California State University, Bakersfield
Program in Nursing
Bakersfield, California

http://www.csub.edu/nursing
Founded in 1970

DEGREE • BSN
Nursing Program Faculty 24 (15% with doctorates).
Baccalaureate Enrollment 208 **Women** 86% **Men** 14% **Minority** 60% **International** 4% **Part-time** 6%
Distance Learning Courses Available.
Nursing Student Activities Nursing Honor Society, Sigma Theta Tau, Student Nurses' Association, nursing club.
Nursing Student Resources Academic advising; academic or career counseling; assistance for students with disabilities; bookstore; campus computer network; career placement assistance; computer lab; computer-assisted instruction; daycare for children of students; e-mail services; employment services for current students; externships; housing assistance; interactive nursing skills videos; Internet; learning resource lab; library services; nursing audiovisuals; paid internships; placement services for program completers; remedial services; resume preparation assistance; skills, simulation, or other laboratory; tutoring; unpaid internships.
Library Facilities 20,000 volumes in health, 1,850 volumes in nursing; 255 periodical subscriptions health-care related.

BACCALAUREATE PROGRAMS

Degree BSN
Available Programs ADN to Baccalaureate; Generic Baccalaureate.
Site Options Visalia, CA; Lancaster, CA.
Study Options Full-time.
Program Entrance Requirements Minimum overall college GPA of 2.0, transcript of college record, CPR certification, health exam, health insurance, high school transcript, immunizations, interview, minimum GPA in nursing prerequisites of 2.8, professional liability insurance/malpractice insurance, prerequisite course work. Transfer students are accepted. *Application deadline:* 4/30 (fall), 12/31 (spring). *Application fee:* $25.
Advanced Placement Credit by examination available. Credit given for nursing courses completed elsewhere dependent upon specific evaluations.
Financial Aid 78% of baccalaureate students in nursing programs received some form of financial aid in 2009-10.
Contact Mrs. Kathy Lewis, Pre-Nursing Advisor, Program in Nursing, California State University, Bakersfield, 9001 Stockdale Highway, Romberg Nursing Education Center, Bakersfield, CA 93311-1022. *Telephone:* 661-654-2508. *Fax:* 661-654-6347. *E-mail:* klewis3@csub.edu.

CONTINUING EDUCATION PROGRAM

Contact Dr. Craig Kelsey, Dean, Extended University, Program in Nursing, California State University, Bakersfield, 9001 Stockdale

Highway, Bakersfield, CA 93311-1099. *Telephone:* 661-654-2446. *Fax:* 661-664-2447. *E-mail:* ckelsey@csub.edu.

California State University Channel Islands

Nursing Program
Camarillo, California

Founded in 2002

DEGREE • BSN

Nursing Program Faculty 13 (20% with doctorates).
Baccalaureate Enrollment 120
Nursing Student Activities Student Nurses' Association.
Nursing Student Resources Academic advising; academic or career counseling; assistance for students with disabilities; bookstore; campus computer network; career placement assistance; computer lab; e-mail services; housing assistance; interactive nursing skills videos; Internet; learning resource lab; library services; nursing audiovisuals; remedial services; skills, simulation, or other laboratory; tutoring.

BACCALAUREATE PROGRAMS

Degree BSN
Available Programs Generic Baccalaureate; RN Baccalaureate.
Contact Nursing Program, Nursing Program, California State University Channel Islands, One University Drive, Camarillo, CA 93012. *Telephone:* 805-437-3307. *E-mail:* nursing@csuci.edu.

California State University, Chico

School of Nursing
Chico, California

http://www.csuchico.edu/nurs/nurs.html
Founded in 1887

DEGREES • BSN • MSN

Nursing Program Faculty 36 (25% with doctorates).
Baccalaureate Enrollment 279 **Women** 86% **Men** 14% **Minority** 35% **Part-time** 30%
Graduate Enrollment 30 **Women** 90% **Men** 10% **Minority** 23% **Part-time** 100%
Distance Learning Courses Available.
Nursing Student Activities Sigma Theta Tau, Student Nurses' Association, nursing club.
Nursing Student Resources Academic advising; academic or career counseling; assistance for students with disabilities; bookstore; campus computer network; career placement assistance; computer lab; computer-assisted instruction; daycare for children of students; e-mail services; employment services for current students; externships; housing assistance; interactive nursing skills videos; Internet; learning resource lab; library services; nursing audiovisuals; paid internships; placement services for program completers; remedial services; resume preparation assistance; skills, simulation, or other laboratory; tutoring; unpaid internships.
Library Facilities 951,276 volumes (17,727 in health, 1,467 in nursing); 22,000 periodical subscriptions (133 health-care related).

BACCALAUREATE PROGRAMS

Degree BSN
Available Programs ADN to Baccalaureate; Baccalaureate for Second Degree; Generic Baccalaureate; LPN to RN Baccalaureate; RN Baccalaureate.
Study Options Full-time.
Program Entrance Requirements Minimum overall college GPA of 3.0, transcript of college record, CPR certification, health exam, health insurance, immunizations, minimum GPA in nursing prerequisites of 3.0, professional liability insurance/malpractice insurance, prerequisite course work. Transfer students are accepted. *Application deadline:* 11/30 (fall), 8/30 (spring). *Application fee:* $55.
Advanced Placement Credit given for nursing courses completed elsewhere dependent upon specific evaluations.
Expenses (2010-11) *Tuition, state resident:* full-time $4230; part-time $1289 per semester. *Tuition, nonresident:* full-time $16,496; part-time $4214 per semester. *Room and board:* $9961; room only: $6861 per academic year. *Required fees:* full-time $1344; part-time $693 per term.
Financial Aid 75% of baccalaureate students in nursing programs received some form of financial aid in 2009-10.
Contact Dr. Carol L. Huston, Director, School of Nursing, California State University, Chico, Holt Hall 369, Chico, CA 95929-0200. *Telephone:* 530-898-5891. *Fax:* 530-898-4363. *E-mail:* chuston@csuchico.edu.

GRADUATE PROGRAMS

Expenses (2010-11) *Tuition, state resident:* full-time $4564; part-time $2282 per semester. *Tuition, nonresident:* full-time $6800; part-time $6796 per semester. *Room and board:* $9961; room only: $6861 per academic year. *Required fees:* full-time $2640; part-time $220 per credit.
Financial Aid 25% of graduate students in nursing programs received some form of financial aid in 2009-10. Career-related internships or fieldwork available.
Contact Irene Morgan, Graduate Coordinator, School of Nursing, California State University, Chico, 400 West 1st Street, Chico, CA 95929-0200. *Telephone:* 530-898-5891. *Fax:* 530-898-6709. *E-mail:* imorgan@csuchico.edu.

MASTER'S DEGREE PROGRAM

Degree MSN
Available Programs Master's.
Concentrations Available Nursing education. *Clinical nurse specialist programs in:* adult health.
Study Options Part-time.
Online Degree Options Yes (online only).
Program Entrance Requirements Clinical experience, minimum overall college GPA of 3.0, transcript of college record, CPR certification, written essay, immunizations, physical assessment course, professional liability insurance/malpractice insurance, statistics course, GRE. *Application deadline:* 11/30 (fall), 8/30 (spring). *Application fee:* $55.
Advanced Placement Credit given for nursing courses completed elsewhere dependent upon specific evaluations.
Degree Requirements 30 total credit hours, thesis or project.

POST-MASTER'S PROGRAM

Areas of Study Nursing education.

CONTINUING EDUCATION PROGRAM

Contact Ms. Elaina McReynolds, Program Director, School of Nursing, California State University, Chico, 400 West 1st Street, Chico, CA 95929-0250. *Telephone:* 530-898-6105. *E-mail:* rce@csuchico.edu.

California State University, Dominguez Hills

Program in Nursing
Carson, California

http://www.csudh.edu/cps/son
Founded in 1960

DEGREES • BSN • MSN

Nursing Program Faculty 79 (80% with doctorates).
Baccalaureate Enrollment 1,265 **Women** 90.5% **Men** 9.5% **Minority** 55.2% **Part-time** 91.3%
Graduate Enrollment 681 **Women** 90.1% **Men** 9.9% **Minority** 53.9% **Part-time** 76.7%
Distance Learning Courses Available.
Nursing Student Activities Nursing Honor Society, Sigma Theta Tau, Student Nurses' Association, nursing club.
Nursing Student Resources Academic advising; academic or career counseling; assistance for students with disabilities; bookstore; campus computer network; career placement assistance; computer lab; computer-assisted instruction; daycare for children of students; e-mail services; externships; housing assistance; interactive nursing skills videos; Internet; learning resource lab; library services; nursing audiovisuals; remedial services; skills, simulation, or other laboratory; tutoring.
Library Facilities 442,893 volumes (10,000 in nursing); 723 periodical subscriptions (215 health-care related).

BACCALAUREATE PROGRAMS

Degree BSN

Available Programs Baccalaureate for Second Degree; RN Baccalaureate.
Site Options Fullerton, CA; Whittier, CA; Ventura, CA.
Online Degree Options Yes.
Program Entrance Requirements Minimum overall college GPA of 2.0, transcript of college record, minimum GPA in nursing prerequisites of 2.0, prerequisite course work, RN licensure. Transfer students are accepted. *Application fee:* $55.
Expenses (2010-11) *Tuition, area resident:* full-time $4440; part-time $1287 per semester. *Tuition, nonresident:* part-time $372 per unit. *Required fees:* part-time $312 per term.
Contact Dr. Kathleen T. Chai, BSN Coordinator, Program in Nursing, California State University, Dominguez Hills, 1000 East Victoria Street, WH 335, Carson, CA 90747. *Telephone:* 310-243-2005. *Fax:* 310-516-3542. *E-mail:* kchai@csudh.edu.

GRADUATE PROGRAMS

Expenses (2010-11) *Tuition, area resident:* full-time $5472; part-time $1587 per semester. *Tuition, nonresident:* part-time $372 per unit. *Required fees:* part-time $312 per term.
Contact Dr. Cynthia Johnson, MSN Coordinator, Program in Nursing, California State University, Dominguez Hills, 1000 East Victoria Street, WH A320, Carson, CA 90747. *Telephone:* 310-243-2522. *Fax:* 310-516-3542. *E-mail:* cjohnson@csudh.edu.

MASTER'S DEGREE PROGRAM

Degree MSN
Available Programs Master's; Master's for Non-Nursing College Graduates; Master's for Nurses with Non-Nursing Degrees.
Concentrations Available Clinical nurse leader; nursing administration; nursing education. *Clinical nurse specialist programs in:* gerontology, parent-child. *Nurse practitioner programs in:* family health.
Site Options Fullerton, CA; Whittier, CA.
Study Options Full-time.
Program Entrance Requirements Minimum overall college GPA of 3.0, transcript of college record, written essay, nursing research course, physical assessment course, prerequisite course work, resume, statistics course. *Application deadline:* 4/1 (fall), 11/1 (spring). Applications may be processed on a rolling basis for some programs. *Application fee:* $55.
Advanced Placement Credit given for nursing courses completed elsewhere dependent upon specific evaluations.
Degree Requirements 45 total credit hours, comprehensive exam.

POST-MASTER'S PROGRAM

Areas of Study Nursing administration; nursing education. *Clinical nurse specialist programs in:* gerontology, parent-child. *Nurse practitioner programs in:* family health.

CONTINUING EDUCATION PROGRAM

Contact Cristina Prado, School of Nursing Staff, Program in Nursing, California State University, Dominguez Hills, 1000 East Victoria Street, Carson, CA 90747. *Telephone:* 310-243-1050. *Fax:* 310-516-3542. *E-mail:* cprado@csudh.edu.

California State University, East Bay

Department of Nursing and Health Sciences
Hayward, California

http://www.sci.csueastbay.edu/nursing/
Founded in 1957

DEGREE • BS

Nursing Program Faculty 39 (30% with doctorates).
Baccalaureate Enrollment 378 **Women** 80% **Men** 20% **Minority** 40% **International** 5% **Part-time** 1%
Distance Learning Courses Available.
Nursing Student Activities Sigma Theta Tau, Student Nurses' Association.
Nursing Student Resources Academic advising; academic or career counseling; assistance for students with disabilities; campus computer network; career placement assistance; computer lab; computer-assisted instruction; daycare for children of students; e-mail services; employment services for current students; externships; interactive nursing skills videos; Internet; learning resource lab; library services; nursing audiovisuals; other; paid internships; placement services for program completers; remedial services; resume preparation assistance; skills, simulation, or other laboratory; tutoring; unpaid internships.

BACCALAUREATE PROGRAMS

Degree BS
Available Programs ADN to Baccalaureate; Accelerated Baccalaureate; Generic Baccalaureate.
Site Options Concord, CA.
Study Options Full-time and part-time.
Program Entrance Requirements Minimum overall college GPA of 3.0, transcript of college record, health exam, minimum GPA in nursing prerequisites of 3.0, prerequisite course work. Transfer students are accepted. *Application deadline:* 11/30 (fall).
Advanced Placement Credit given for nursing courses completed elsewhere dependent upon specific evaluations.
Financial Aid *Gift aid (need-based):* Federal Pell, FSEOG, state, private, college/university gift aid from institutional funds. *Loans:* Federal Direct (Subsidized and Unsubsidized Stafford PLUS), Perkins, college/university. *Work-study:* Federal Work-Study. *Financial aid application deadline (priority):* 3/2.
Contact Lara Dungan, Preadmission Student Advisor, Department of Nursing and Health Sciences, California State University, East Bay, 25800 Carlos Bee Boulevard, Hayward, CA 94542. *Telephone:* 510-885-3481. *Fax:* 510-885-2156. *E-mail:* lara.dungan@csueastbay.edu.

California State University, Fresno

Department of Nursing
Fresno, California

http://www.csufresno.edu/nursing/
Founded in 1911

DEGREES • BSN • MSN

Nursing Program Faculty 56 (20% with doctorates).
Baccalaureate Enrollment 450 **Women** 80% **Men** 20% **Minority** 49% **Part-time** 5%
Graduate Enrollment 114 **Women** 84% **Men** 16% **Minority** 53% **International** 4% **Part-time** 36%
Distance Learning Courses Available.
Nursing Student Activities Sigma Theta Tau, Student Nurses' Association.
Nursing Student Resources Academic advising; academic or career counseling; assistance for students with disabilities; bookstore; campus computer network; career placement assistance; computer lab; computer-assisted instruction; daycare for children of students; e-mail services; externships; housing assistance; interactive nursing skills videos; Internet; learning resource lab; library services; nursing audiovisuals; paid internships; placement services for program completers; remedial services; skills, simulation, or other laboratory; tutoring.
Library Facilities 1.9 million volumes (23,961 in health, 1,287 in nursing); 28,249 periodical subscriptions (1,260 health-care related).

BACCALAUREATE PROGRAMS

Degree BSN
Available Programs ADN to Baccalaureate; Generic Baccalaureate.
Study Options Full-time.
Program Entrance Requirements Transcript of college record, CPR certification, health exam, immunizations, minimum GPA in nursing prerequisites of 3.0, professional liability insurance/malpractice insurance, prerequisite course work. Transfer students are accepted. *Application deadline:* 3/31 (fall), 8/31 (spring).
Advanced Placement Credit by examination available. Credit given for nursing courses completed elsewhere dependent upon specific evaluations.
Expenses (2009-10) *Tuition, state resident:* full-time $4672; part-time $1490 per semester. *Tuition, nonresident:* full-time $11,160. *International tuition:* $11,160 full-time. *Room and board:* $8495; room only: $4200 per academic year. *Required fees:* full-time $80.
Financial Aid 65% of baccalaureate students in nursing programs received some form of financial aid in 2008-09. *Gift aid (need-based):* Federal Pell, FSEOG, state, private, college/university gift aid from institutional funds. *Loans:* Federal Nursing Student Loans, Perkins, college/university, alternative loans. *Work-study:* Federal Work-Study. *Financial aid application deadline (priority):* 3/2.

Contact Dr. Michael F. Russler, Chair, Department of Nursing, California State University, Fresno, 2345 East San Ramon Avenue, MH25, Fresno, CA 93740-8031. *Telephone:* 559-278-2429. *Fax:* 559-278-6360. *E-mail:* michaelr@csufresno.edu.

GRADUATE PROGRAMS

Expenses (2009-10) *Tuition, state resident:* full-time $5608; part-time $2804 per semester. *Tuition, nonresident:* full-time $11,160; part-time $5580 per semester. *International tuition:* $11,160 full-time. *Room and board:* $8495; room only: $4200 per academic year. *Required fees:* full-time $40.
Financial Aid 30% of graduate students in nursing programs received some form of financial aid in 2008-09. 2 teaching assistantships were awarded; career-related internships or fieldwork, Federal Work-Study, scholarships, and traineeships also available. Aid available to part-time students. *Financial aid application deadline:* 3/1.
Contact Dr. Robert Fire, Graduate Coordinator, Department of Nursing, California State University, Fresno, 2345 East San Ramon Avenue, MH25, Fresno, CA 93740-8031. *Telephone:* 559-278-8852. *Fax:* 559-278-6360. *E-mail:* rfire@csufresno.edu.

MASTER'S DEGREE PROGRAM

Degree MSN
Available Programs Accelerated Master's; Master's; Master's for Nurses with Non-Nursing Degrees.
Concentrations Available Nursing education. *Clinical nurse specialist programs in:* acute care, community health, critical care, pediatric, psychiatric/mental health, public health. *Nurse practitioner programs in:* family health, pediatric.
Study Options Full-time and part-time.
Program Entrance Requirements Computer literacy, minimum overall college GPA of 3.0, transcript of college record, CPR certification, written essay, 3 letters of recommendation, nursing research course, physical assessment course, professional liability insurance/malpractice insurance, prerequisite course work, resume, statistics course, GRE General Test. *Application deadline:* 4/1 (fall).
Advanced Placement Credit given for nursing courses completed elsewhere dependent upon specific evaluations.
Degree Requirements 38 total credit hours, thesis or project, comprehensive exam.

POST-MASTER'S PROGRAM

Areas of Study *Nurse practitioner programs in:* family health, pediatric.

CONTINUING EDUCATION PROGRAM

Contact Dr. Berta Gonzalez, Associate Vice President, Department of Nursing, California State University, Fresno, 5005 North Maple Avenue, ED76, Fresno, CA 93740-0076. *Telephone:* 559-278-0333. *Fax:* 559-278-0395. *E-mail:* bertag@csufresno.edu.

California State University, Fullerton

Department of Nursing
Fullerton, California

http://nursing.fullerton.edu/
Founded in 1957

DEGREES • BSN • MSN
Nursing Program Faculty 71 (28% with doctorates).
Baccalaureate Enrollment 464 **Women** 83.2% **Men** 16.8% **Minority** 60.8% **International** 4.3% **Part-time** 69%
Graduate Enrollment 372 **Women** 84.9% **Men** 15.1% **Minority** 44.9% **International** 1.1% **Part-time** 46.5%
Distance Learning Courses Available.
Nursing Student Activities Nursing Honor Society, Sigma Theta Tau, Student Nurses' Association.
Nursing Student Resources Academic advising; academic or career counseling; assistance for students with disabilities; bookstore; campus computer network; computer lab; computer-assisted instruction; daycare for children of students; e-mail services; housing assistance; Internet; learning resource lab; library services; resume preparation assistance; skills, simulation, or other laboratory; tutoring.
Library Facilities 1.3 million volumes (17,340 in health, 837 in nursing); 10,902 periodical subscriptions (8,145 health-care related).

BACCALAUREATE PROGRAMS

Degree BSN
Available Programs ADN to Baccalaureate; Baccalaureate for Second Degree; Generic Baccalaureate.
Site Options Riverside, CA; Los Angeles, CA; Mission Viejo, CA.
Study Options Full-time and part-time.
Program Entrance Requirements Minimum overall college GPA of 2.5, transcript of college record, 2 letters of recommendation, prerequisite course work, RN licensure. Transfer students are accepted. *Application deadline:* 3/1 (fall), 10/1 (spring). Applications may be processed on a rolling basis for some programs. *Application fee:* $55.
Advanced Placement Credit given for nursing courses completed elsewhere dependent upon specific evaluations.
Financial Aid ***Gift aid (need-based):*** Federal Pell, FSEOG, state, private, college/university gift aid from institutional funds, Federal Nursing. *Loans:* Federal Direct (Subsidized and Unsubsidized Stafford PLUS), Perkins, college/university, private alternative loans. *Work-study:* Federal Work-Study. *Financial aid application deadline (priority):* 3/2.
Contact Nursing Advisor, Department of Nursing, California State University, Fullerton, EC-182, PO Box 6868, Fullerton, CA 92834-6868. *Telephone:* 657-278-3217. *Fax:* 657-278-2096. *E-mail:* nursingadvising@fullerton.edu.

GRADUATE PROGRAMS

Expenses (2010-11) *Room and board:* $9632; room only: $4866 per academic year.
Financial Aid 44% of graduate students in nursing programs received some form of financial aid in 2009-10.
Contact Ms. Mary Lehn-Mooney, Advisor, Department of Nursing, California State University, Fullerton, EC 190, 800 North State College Boulevard, Fullerton, CA 92834-6868. *Telephone:* 714-278-3217. *Fax:* 714-278-2096. *E-mail:* mlehn-mooney@fullerton.edu.

MASTER'S DEGREE PROGRAM

Degree MSN
Available Programs Accelerated AD/RN to Master's; Accelerated Master's for Non-Nursing College Graduates; Master's; Master's for Non-Nursing College Graduates.
Concentrations Available Nurse anesthesia; nurse-midwifery; nursing administration; nursing education. *Clinical nurse specialist programs in:* school health. *Nurse practitioner programs in:* women's health.
Study Options Full-time and part-time.
Online Degree Options Yes.
Program Entrance Requirements Clinical experience, minimum overall college GPA of 3.0, transcript of college record, CPR certification, written essay, immunizations, interview, 3 letters of recommendation, nursing research course, professional liability insurance/malpractice insurance, prerequisite course work, statistics course. *Application deadline:* 11/30 (fall). Applications may be processed on a rolling basis for some programs. *Application fee:* $55.
Advanced Placement Credit given for nursing courses completed elsewhere dependent upon specific evaluations.
Degree Requirements 71 total credit hours, thesis or project, comprehensive exam.

CONTINUING EDUCATION PROGRAM

Contact Ms. Rosabel Hernandez, Nursing Advisement Receptionist, Department of Nursing, California State University, Fullerton, Nursing Department, EC 190, 800 North State College Boulevard, Fullerton, CA 92834-9480. *Telephone:* 657-278-3217. *Fax:* 657-278-2096. *E-mail:* nursingadvising@fullerton.edu.

California State University, Long Beach

Department of Nursing
Long Beach, California

http://www.csulb.edu/depts/nursing/
Founded in 1949

DEGREES • BSN • MSN • MSN/MHEA
Nursing Program Faculty 82 (25% with doctorates).
Baccalaureate Enrollment 559 **Women** 81.22% **Men** 18.78% **Minority** 72.27% **International** .01%

Graduate Enrollment 323 **Women** 87.38% **Men** 12.62% **Minority** 70.73% **International** .01% **Part-time** 50%

Nursing Student Activities Nursing Honor Society, Sigma Theta Tau, Student Nurses' Association.

Nursing Student Resources Academic advising; Internet; library services; skills, simulation, or other laboratory; tutoring.

Library Facilities 35,860 periodical subscriptions.

BACCALAUREATE PROGRAMS

Degree BSN

Available Programs ADN to Baccalaureate; Accelerated Baccalaureate; Baccalaureate for Second Degree; Generic Baccalaureate; LPN to Baccalaureate.

Site Options Long Beach, CA; Huntington Beach, CA.

Study Options Full-time.

Program Entrance Requirements Transcript of college record, CPR certification, health exam, health insurance, immunizations, interview, minimum GPA in nursing prerequisites of 3.0, professional liability insurance/malpractice insurance, prerequisite course work. Transfer students are accepted. *Application deadline:* 2/15 (fall), 9/15 (spring).

Advanced Placement Credit given for nursing courses completed elsewhere dependent upon specific evaluations.

Expenses (2010-11) *Tuition, area resident:* full-time $4800; part-time $3050 per term. *International tuition:* $14,000 full-time. *Room and board:* $10,500; room only: $10,000 per academic year. *Required fees:* full-time $3000.

Financial Aid 75% of baccalaureate students in nursing programs received some form of financial aid in 2009-10. *Gift aid (need-based):* Federal Pell, FSEOG, state, private, college/university gift aid from institutional funds. *Loans:* Federal Direct (Subsidized and Unsubsidized Stafford PLUS), Perkins. *Work-study:* Federal Work-Study. *Financial aid application deadline (priority):* 3/2.

Contact Dr. Beth R. Keely, Assistant Director, Undergraduate Nursing Programs, Department of Nursing, California State University, Long Beach, 1250 Bellflower Boulevard, Long Beach, CA 90840. *Telephone:* 562-985-4478. *Fax:* 562-985-2382. *E-mail:* bkeely@csulb.edu.

GRADUATE PROGRAMS

Expenses (2010-11) *Tuition, area resident:* full-time $5800; part-time $3600 per semester. *Tuition, state resident:* full-time $18,000; part-time $8000 per semester. *Tuition, nonresident:* full-time $18,000; part-time $8000 per semester. *Room and board:* $10,500; room only: $10,000 per academic year. *Required fees:* full-time $3000.

Financial Aid 25% of graduate students in nursing programs received some form of financial aid in 2009-10. Federal Work-Study, institutionally sponsored loans, and scholarships available. *Financial aid application deadline:* 3/2.

Contact Alison Kliachko-Trafas, Administrative Assistant, Department of Nursing, California State University, Long Beach, 1250 Bellflower Boulevard, Long Beach, CA 90840. *Telephone:* 562-985-4473. *Fax:* 562-985-2382. *E-mail:* akliachk@csulb.edu.

MASTER'S DEGREE PROGRAM

Degrees MSN; MSN/MHeA

Available Programs Accelerated Master's; Master's; Master's for Non-Nursing College Graduates.

Concentrations Available Health-care administration; nursing education. *Clinical nurse specialist programs in:* adult health, public health. *Nurse practitioner programs in:* adult health, family health, gerontology, pediatric, psychiatric/mental health, women's health.

Study Options Full-time and part-time.

Program Entrance Requirements Clinical experience, minimum overall college GPA of 2.75, transcript of college record, written essay, 3 letters of recommendation, physical assessment course, prerequisite course work, resume, statistics course. *Application deadline:* 3/15 (fall), 10/15 (spring).

Advanced Placement Credit given for nursing courses completed elsewhere dependent upon specific evaluations.

Degree Requirements 37 total credit hours, thesis or project, comprehensive exam.

POST-MASTER'S PROGRAM

Areas of Study *Clinical nurse specialist programs in:* adult health. *Nurse practitioner programs in:* adult health, family health, gerontology, pediatric, psychiatric/mental health, women's health.

California State University, Los Angeles

School of Nursing
Los Angeles, California

http://www.calstatela.edu/dept/nursing/
Founded in 1947

DEGREES • BSN • MSN

Nursing Program Faculty 31 (39% with doctorates).

Baccalaureate Enrollment 300

Graduate Enrollment 100

Nursing Student Resources Academic advising.

Library Facilities 1.3 million volumes; 26,104 periodical subscriptions.

BACCALAUREATE PROGRAMS

Degree BSN

Available Programs Generic Baccalaureate; LPN to RN Baccalaureate; RN Baccalaureate.

Study Options Full-time.

Program Entrance Requirements Minimum overall college GPA of 2.75, CPR certification, health exam, health insurance, high school biology, immunizations, minimum GPA in nursing prerequisites of 2.75, professional liability insurance/malpractice insurance, prerequisite course work. Transfer students are accepted. *Application deadline:* 12/1 (fall).

Advanced Placement Credit given for nursing courses completed elsewhere dependent upon specific evaluations.

Contact *Telephone:* 323-343-4700. *Fax:* 323-343-6454.

GRADUATE PROGRAMS

Contact *Telephone:* 323-343-4700. *Fax:* 323-343-6454.

MASTER'S DEGREE PROGRAM

Degree MSN

Available Programs Accelerated Master's for Nurses with Non-Nursing Degrees; Accelerated RN to Master's; Master's; Master's for Non-Nursing College Graduates.

Concentrations Available Nursing administration; nursing education. *Clinical nurse specialist programs in:* psychiatric/mental health. *Nurse practitioner programs in:* acute care, adult health, family health, pediatric, primary care, psychiatric/mental health.

Study Options Full-time and part-time.

Program Entrance Requirements Clinical experience, minimum overall college GPA of 3.0, transcript of college record, written essay, immunizations, letters of recommendation, nursing research course, physical assessment course, professional liability insurance/malpractice insurance, resume, statistics course. *Application deadline:* 11/15 (fall), 5/15 (spring).

Advanced Placement Credit given for nursing courses completed elsewhere dependent upon specific evaluations.

Degree Requirements 45 total credit hours, comprehensive exam.

POST-MASTER'S PROGRAM

Areas of Study *Nurse practitioner programs in:* acute care, adult health, family health, pediatric, primary care.

California State University, Northridge

Nursing Program
Northridge, California

http://www.csun.edu/~nursing/
Founded in 1958

DEGREE • BSN

Nursing Program Faculty 15 (27% with doctorates).

Baccalaureate Enrollment 106 **Women** 92% **Men** 8% **Minority** 60% **International** 12% **Part-time** 66%

Nursing Student Activities Sigma Theta Tau, Student Nurses' Association.

Nursing Student Resources Academic advising; academic or career counseling; assistance for students with disabilities; bookstore; campus computer network; career placement assistance; computer lab; computer-assisted instruction; daycare for children of students; e-mail services;

housing assistance; interactive nursing skills videos; Internet; learning resource lab; library services; nursing audiovisuals; remedial services; resume preparation assistance; skills, simulation, or other laboratory; tutoring.

Library Facilities 61,848 volumes in health, 1,401 volumes in nursing; 303 periodical subscriptions health-care related.

BACCALAUREATE PROGRAMS

Degree BSN
Available Programs ADN to Baccalaureate; Accelerated Baccalaureate.
Study Options Full-time.
Program Entrance Requirements Minimum overall college GPA of 3.0, transcript of college record, CPR certification, written essay, health exam, health insurance, immunizations, interview, 3 letters of recommendation, minimum GPA in nursing prerequisites of 3.0, professional liability insurance/malpractice insurance, prerequisite course work, RN licensure. Transfer students are accepted. *Application deadline:* 12/4 (fall), 12/4 (summer). *Application fee:* $55.
Advanced Placement Credit by examination available. Credit given for nursing courses completed elsewhere dependent upon specific evaluations.
Contact *Telephone:* 818-677-3101. *Fax:* 818-677-2045.

California State University, Sacramento

Division of Nursing
Sacramento, California

http://www.hhs.csus.edu/nrs
Founded in 1947

DEGREES • BSN • MS

Nursing Program Faculty 64 (50% with doctorates).
Baccalaureate Enrollment 286 **Women** 89% **Men** 11%
Graduate Enrollment 180 **Women** 95% **Men** 5% **Part-time** 100%
Distance Learning Courses Available.
Nursing Student Activities Sigma Theta Tau, Student Nurses' Association.
Nursing Student Resources Academic advising; academic or career counseling; assistance for students with disabilities; bookstore; campus computer network; computer lab; computer-assisted instruction; daycare for children of students; e-mail services; externships; housing assistance; interactive nursing skills videos; Internet; learning resource lab; library services; nursing audiovisuals; paid internships; placement services for program completers; remedial services; resume preparation assistance; skills, simulation, or other laboratory; tutoring.
Library Facilities 33,000 volumes in health; 327 periodical subscriptions health-care related.

BACCALAUREATE PROGRAMS

Degree BSN
Available Programs ADN to Baccalaureate; Baccalaureate for Second Degree; Generic Baccalaureate; LPN to RN Baccalaureate.
Study Options Full-time.
Program Entrance Requirements Transcript of college record, CPR certification, health exam, health insurance, high school biology, high school math, immunizations, minimum GPA in nursing prerequisites of 3.3, professional liability insurance/malpractice insurance, prerequisite course work. Transfer students are accepted. *Application deadline:* 3/1 (fall), 10/1 (spring).
Advanced Placement Credit by examination available. Credit given for nursing courses completed elsewhere dependent upon specific evaluations.
Expenses (2010-11) *Tuition, area resident:* full-time $2013; part-time $1167 per semester. *Room and board:* $4776 per academic year. *Required fees:* full-time $437; part-time $437 per term.
Financial Aid 60% of baccalaureate students in nursing programs received some form of financial aid in 2009-10.
Contact Nancy Beers, Administrative Support Coordinator, Division of Nursing, California State University, Sacramento, 6000 J Street, Sacramento, CA 95819-6096. *Telephone:* 916-278-6525. *E-mail:* beersnj@csus.edu.

GRADUATE PROGRAMS

Expenses (2010-11) *Tuition, area resident:* full-time $2481; part-time $1440 per semester. *Required fees:* full-time $437; part-time $437 per credit.
Financial Aid 10% of graduate students in nursing programs received some form of financial aid in 2009-10. Research assistantships, teaching assistantships, career-related internships or fieldwork and Federal Work-Study available. Aid available to part-time students. *Financial aid application deadline:* 3/1.
Contact Dr. Alexa Curtis, Graduate Coordinator, Division of Nursing, California State University, Sacramento, 6000 J Street, Sacramento, CA 95819-6096. *Fax:* 916-278-6311. *E-mail:* curtisa@csus.edu.

MASTER'S DEGREE PROGRAM

Degree MS
Available Programs Master's.
Concentrations Available Nursing administration; nursing education. *Nurse practitioner programs in:* family health, primary care.
Study Options Part-time.
Program Entrance Requirements Clinical experience, computer literacy, minimum overall college GPA of 3.0, transcript of college record, CPR certification, immunizations, nursing research course, professional liability insurance/malpractice insurance, prerequisite course work, statistics course, GRE. *Application deadline:* 11/30 (fall).
Advanced Placement Credit given for nursing courses completed elsewhere dependent upon specific evaluations.
Degree Requirements 33 total credit hours, comprehensive exam.

California State University, San Bernardino

Department of Nursing
San Bernardino, California

http://nursing.csusb.edu
Founded in 1965

DEGREES • BSN • MSN

Nursing Program Faculty 42 (19% with doctorates).
Baccalaureate Enrollment 457 **Women** 81% **Men** 19% **Minority** 59%
Graduate Enrollment 19 **Women** 89% **Men** 11% **Minority** 47%
Distance Learning Courses Available.
Nursing Student Activities Sigma Theta Tau, Student Nurses' Association.
Nursing Student Resources Academic advising; academic or career counseling; assistance for students with disabilities; bookstore; campus computer network; computer lab; computer-assisted instruction; daycare for children of students; e-mail services; Internet; learning resource lab; library services; nursing audiovisuals; remedial services; skills, simulation, or other laboratory.
Library Facilities 731,259 volumes (1,500 in health, 1,000 in nursing); 2,028 periodical subscriptions (5,000 health-care related).

BACCALAUREATE PROGRAMS

Degree BSN
Available Programs Generic Baccalaureate; LPN to Baccalaureate; RN Baccalaureate.
Site Options Palm Desert, CA.
Study Options Full-time.
Program Entrance Requirements Minimum overall college GPA of 2.5, transcript of college record, 3 letters of recommendation, minimum GPA in nursing prerequisites of 2.5, prerequisite course work. Transfer students are accepted. *Application deadline:* 3/1 (fall), 10/1 (winter).
Advanced Placement Credit given for nursing courses completed elsewhere dependent upon specific evaluations.
Financial Aid 80% of baccalaureate students in nursing programs received some form of financial aid in 2008-09. *Gift aid (need-based):* Federal Pell, FSEOG, state, private, college/university gift aid from institutional funds, Academic Competitiveness Grants, National SMART Grants. *Loans:* Federal Direct (Subsidized and Unsubsidized Stafford PLUS), Perkins. *Work-study:* Federal Work-Study. *Financial aid application deadline (priority):* 3/2.
Contact Dr. Jean Nix, BSN Coordinator, Department of Nursing, California State University, San Bernardino, 5500 University Parkway, HP 231 Nursing, San Bernardino, CA 92407. *Telephone:* 909-537-5381. *E-mail:* pjnix@csusb.edu.

GRADUATE PROGRAMS

Financial Aid 60% of graduate students in nursing programs received some form of financial aid in 2008-09.
Contact Dr. Mary Molle, MSN Coordinator and Professor, Department of Nursing, California State University, San Bernardino, 5500 University Parkway, San Bernardino, CA 92407. *Telephone:* 909-537-7241. *E-mail:* mmolle@csusb.edu.

MASTER'S DEGREE PROGRAM

Degree MSN
Available Programs Master's.
Concentrations Available Nursing administration; nursing education. *Clinical nurse specialist programs in:* community health.
Study Options Full-time and part-time.
Program Entrance Requirements Clinical experience, minimum overall college GPA of 3.0, transcript of college record, letters of recommendation, prerequisite course work, resume, statistics course. *Application deadline:* 6/10 (fall).
Advanced Placement Credit given for nursing courses completed elsewhere dependent upon specific evaluations.
Degree Requirements 65 total credit hours, thesis or project, comprehensive exam.

California State University, San Marcos

School of Nursing
San Marcos, California

Founded in 1990

DEGREE • BSN

Nursing Student Activities Student Nurses' Association.
Library Facilities 326,393 volumes; 3,747 periodical subscriptions.

BACCALAUREATE PROGRAMS

Degree BSN
Available Programs Accelerated Baccalaureate; Generic Baccalaureate.
Contact Baccalaureate programs, School of Nursing, California State University, San Marcos, 333 South Twin Oaks Valley Road, San Marcos, CA 92096-0001. *Telephone:* 706-750-7550. *Fax:* 706-750-3646.

California State University, Stanislaus

Department of Nursing
Turlock, California

http://www.csustan.edu/Nursing/index.htm
Founded in 1957

DEGREE • BSN

Nursing Program Faculty 17 (24% with doctorates).
Baccalaureate Enrollment 164 **Women** 88% **Men** 12% **Minority** 42% **Part-time** 30%
Nursing Student Activities Sigma Theta Tau, Student Nurses' Association.
Nursing Student Resources Academic advising; academic or career counseling; assistance for students with disabilities; bookstore; campus computer network; career placement assistance; computer lab; computer-assisted instruction; daycare for children of students; e-mail services; employment services for current students; externships; interactive nursing skills videos; Internet; learning resource lab; library services; nursing audiovisuals; resume preparation assistance; skills, simulation, or other laboratory; tutoring.
Library Facilities 375,662 volumes (12,642 in health, 1,338 in nursing); 31,813 periodical subscriptions (93 health-care related).

BACCALAUREATE PROGRAMS

Degree BSN
Available Programs ADN to Baccalaureate; Generic Baccalaureate; LPN to Baccalaureate.
Study Options Full-time.
Program Entrance Requirements Minimum overall college GPA of 3.0, transcript of college record, CPR certification, health exam, immunizations, minimum GPA in nursing prerequisites of 3.0, professional liability insurance/malpractice insurance, prerequisite course work. Transfer students are accepted.
Advanced Placement Credit given for nursing courses completed elsewhere dependent upon specific evaluations.
Contact *Telephone:* 209-667-3141. *Fax:* 209-667-3690.

Concordia University

Bachelor of Science in Nursing Program
Irvine, California

Founded in 1972

DEGREE • BSN

Library Facilities 77,783 volumes; 24,480 periodical subscriptions.

BACCALAUREATE PROGRAMS

Degree BSN
Available Programs Accelerated Baccalaureate for Second Degree; RN Baccalaureate.
Program Entrance Requirements Transcript of college record, prerequisite course work, RN licensure.
Contact Nursing Program. *Telephone:* 949-854-8002 Ext. 1144.

Dominican University of California

Program in Nursing
San Rafael, California

http://www.dominican.edu/
Founded in 1890

DEGREES • BSN • MSN

Nursing Program Faculty 51 (24% with doctorates).
Baccalaureate Enrollment 507 **Women** 87% **Men** 13% **Minority** 61% **International** 1% **Part-time** 15%
Graduate Enrollment 27 **Women** 78% **Men** 22% **Minority** 48% **Part-time** 22%
Nursing Student Activities Sigma Theta Tau, Student Nurses' Association, nursing club.
Nursing Student Resources Academic advising; academic or career counseling; assistance for students with disabilities; bookstore; campus computer network; career placement assistance; computer lab; computer-assisted instruction; e-mail services; employment services for current students; housing assistance; interactive nursing skills videos; Internet; learning resource lab; library services; nursing audiovisuals; remedial services; resume preparation assistance; skills, simulation, or other laboratory; tutoring; unpaid internships.
Library Facilities 120,646 volumes (1,200 in health, 1,000 in nursing); 61,257 periodical subscriptions (1,300 health-care related).

BACCALAUREATE PROGRAMS

Degree BSN
Available Programs Baccalaureate for Second Degree; Generic Baccalaureate; RN Baccalaureate.
Study Options Full-time and part-time.
Program Entrance Requirements Minimum overall college GPA of 3.0, transcript of college record, CPR certification, written essay, health exam, health insurance, high school biology, high school chemistry, 2 years high school math, high school transcript, immunizations, 1 letter of recommendation, minimum high school GPA of 3.0, minimum GPA in nursing prerequisites of 3.0, prerequisite course work. Transfer students are accepted. *Application deadline:* 2/1 (fall), 9/1 (spring). Applications may be processed on a rolling basis for some programs. *Application fee:* $40.
Advanced Placement Credit given for nursing courses completed elsewhere dependent upon specific evaluations.
Expenses (2010-11) *Tuition:* full-time $35,220; part-time $1470 per unit. *Room and board:* $13,020; room only: $7720 per academic year. *Required fees:* full-time $330.
Financial Aid 91% of baccalaureate students in nursing programs received some form of financial aid in 2009-10.
Contact Rebecca Finn Kenney, Assistant Vice President of Undergraduate Admissions, Program in Nursing, Dominican University of Cal-

ifornia, 50 Acacia Avenue, San Rafael, CA 94901-2298. *Telephone:* 415-485-3204. *Fax:* 415-485-3214. *E-mail:* rebecca.finnkenney@dominican.edu.

GRADUATE PROGRAMS

Expenses (2010-11) *Tuition:* full-time $15,570; part-time $865 per unit. *International tuition:* $15,570 full-time. *Required fees:* full-time $200; part-time $100 per term.
Financial Aid 33% of graduate students in nursing programs received some form of financial aid in 2009-10. 10 fellowships (averaging $3,200 per year) were awarded; scholarships also available. Aid available to part-time students.
Contact Dr. Barbara Ganley, Director of Graduate Nursing, Program in Nursing, Dominican University of California, 50 Acacia Avenue, San Rafael, CA 94901-2298. *Telephone:* 415-482-1829. *Fax:* 415-482-1829. *E-mail:* bganley@dominican.edu.

MASTER'S DEGREE PROGRAM

Degree MSN
Available Programs Master's; Master's for Nurses with Non-Nursing Degrees; RN to Master's.
Concentrations Available Clinical nurse leader.
Study Options Full-time and part-time.
Program Entrance Requirements Clinical experience, minimum overall college GPA of 3.0, transcript of college record, CPR certification, written essay, interview, 2 letters of recommendation, nursing research course, prerequisite course work, resume, statistics course. *Application deadline:* 6/15 (fall), 11/15 (spring). Applications may be processed on a rolling basis for some programs. *Application fee:* $40.
Advanced Placement Credit given for nursing courses completed elsewhere dependent upon specific evaluations.
Degree Requirements 32 total credit hours, thesis or project.

Fresno Pacific University

RN to BSN Program
Fresno, California

Founded in 1944

DEGREE • BSN

Library Facilities 196,000 volumes; 16,000 periodical subscriptions.

BACCALAUREATE PROGRAMS

Degree BSN
Available Programs RN Baccalaureate.
Contact RN to BSN Program, RN to BSN Program, Fresno Pacific University, 1717 South Chestnut Avenue, Fresno, CA 93702-4709. *Telephone:* 559-453-2000.

Holy Names University

Department of Nursing
Oakland, California

http://www.hnu.edu/academics/adultBaccalaureateDegreePrograms/registeredNurse.html

Founded in 1868

DEGREES • BSN • MSN • MSN/MBA

Nursing Program Faculty 44 (8% with doctorates).
Baccalaureate Enrollment 68 **Women** 90% **Men** 10% **Minority** 52% **International** 1% **Part-time** 100%
Graduate Enrollment 70 **Women** 85% **Men** 15% **Minority** 60% **International** 2% **Part-time** 10%
Distance Learning Courses Available.
Nursing Student Activities Nursing Honor Society, Sigma Theta Tau, nursing club.
Nursing Student Resources Academic advising; academic or career counseling; assistance for students with disabilities; bookstore; campus computer network; career placement assistance; computer lab; computer-assisted instruction; e-mail services; employment services for current students; externships; housing assistance; interactive nursing skills videos; Internet; learning resource lab; library services; nursing audiovisuals; placement services for program completers; remedial services; resume preparation assistance; skills, simulation, or other laboratory; tutoring.
Library Facilities 117,760 volumes (500 in health, 200 in nursing); 8,003 periodical subscriptions (200 health-care related).

BACCALAUREATE PROGRAMS

Degree BSN
Available Programs LPN to RN Baccalaureate; RN Baccalaureate.
Site Options Stanford, CA; CHW hospitals, CA.
Study Options Full-time and part-time.
Program Entrance Requirements Minimum overall college GPA of 2.7, transcript of college record, written essay, prerequisite course work, RN licensure. Transfer students are accepted. *Application deadline:* Applications may be processed on a rolling basis for some programs. *Application fee:* $50.
Advanced Placement Credit given for nursing courses completed elsewhere dependent upon specific evaluations.
Expenses (2010-11) *Tuition:* full-time $19,000. *Required fees:* full-time $200.
Financial Aid 95% of baccalaureate students in nursing programs received some form of financial aid in 2009-10.
Contact Ms. Lisa Marie Gibson, Admission Counselor, Department of Nursing, Holy Names University, 3500 Mountain Boulevard, Oakland, CA 94619-1699. *Telephone:* 510-436-1317. *Fax:* 510-436-1376. *E-mail:* lgibson@hnu.edu.

GRADUATE PROGRAMS

Expenses (2010-11) *Tuition:* full-time $27,000. *Required fees:* full-time $200.
Financial Aid 95% of graduate students in nursing programs received some form of financial aid in 2009-10. Scholarships available. Aid available to part-time students. *Financial aid application deadline:* 3/2.
Contact Ms. Lisa Marie Gibson, Admission Counselor, Department of Nursing, Holy Names University, 3500 Mountain Boulevard, Oakland, CA 94619-1699. *Telephone:* 510-436-1317. *Fax:* 510-436-1376. *E-mail:* lgibson@hnu.edu.

MASTER'S DEGREE PROGRAM

Degrees MSN; MSN/MBA
Available Programs Master's; Master's for Nurses with Non-Nursing Degrees.
Concentrations Available Nursing administration; nursing education. *Nurse practitioner programs in:* family health.
Site Options CHW hospitals, CA.
Study Options Full-time and part-time.
Program Entrance Requirements Minimum overall college GPA of 2.8, transcript of college record, written essay, 2 letters of recommendation, resume. *Application deadline:* Applications may be processed on a rolling basis for some programs. *Application fee:* $65.
Degree Requirements 45 total credit hours, thesis or project.

POST-MASTER'S PROGRAM

Areas of Study Nursing administration; nursing education. *Nurse practitioner programs in:* family health.

Humboldt State University

Department of Nursing
Arcata, California

http://www.humboldt.edu/~nurs

Founded in 1913

DEGREE • BSN

Nursing Program Faculty 21 (14% with doctorates).
Baccalaureate Enrollment 150 **Women** 85% **Men** 15% **Minority** 21%
Distance Learning Courses Available.
Nursing Student Activities Nursing Honor Society, Sigma Theta Tau, Student Nurses' Association.
Nursing Student Resources Academic advising; academic or career counseling; assistance for students with disabilities; bookstore; campus computer network; career placement assistance; computer lab; computer-assisted instruction; daycare for children of students; e-mail services; employment services for current students; housing assistance; interactive nursing skills videos; Internet; learning resource lab; library services; nursing audiovisuals; placement services for program completers; remedial services; resume preparation assistance; skills, simulation, or other laboratory; tutoring.
Library Facilities 2 million volumes (16,000 in health, 750 in nursing); 864 periodical subscriptions (152 health-care related).

BACCALAUREATE PROGRAMS

Degree BSN
Available Programs ADN to Baccalaureate; Baccalaureate for Second Degree; Generic Baccalaureate; RN Baccalaureate.
Site Options Fortuna, CA; Eureka, CA; Arcata, CA.
Study Options Full-time.
Program Entrance Requirements Minimum overall college GPA of 2.5, transcript of college record, CPR certification, health exam, high school foreign language, 2 years high school math, 1 year of high school science, high school transcript, immunizations, minimum GPA in nursing prerequisites of 2.5, prerequisite course work. Transfer students are accepted. *Application deadline:* 2/1 (fall), 10/1 (spring).
Advanced Placement Credit given for nursing courses completed elsewhere dependent upon specific evaluations.
Expenses (2009-10) *Tuition, state resident:* full-time $4496; part-time $1437 per term. *Tuition, nonresident:* full-time $12,632. *Room and board:* $9510; room only: $9088 per academic year. *Required fees:* full-time $868; part-time $36 per credit; part-time $434 per term.
Financial Aid 75% of baccalaureate students in nursing programs received some form of financial aid in 2008-09. *Gift aid (need-based):* Federal Pell, FSEOG, state, private, college/university gift aid from institutional funds. *Loans:* Federal Direct (Subsidized and Unsubsidized Stafford PLUS), Perkins. *Work-study:* Federal Work-Study. *Financial aid application deadline (priority):* 3/2.
Contact Miss Marcie Evans, Administrative Support Assistant, Department of Nursing, Humboldt State University, 1 Harpst Street, Arcata, CA 95521-8299. *Telephone:* 707-826-3839. *Fax:* 707-826-5141. *E-mail:* naac@humboldt.edu.

Loma Linda University
School of Nursing
Loma Linda, California

http://www.llu.edu/nursing
Founded in 1905

DEGREES • BS • MS • PHD
Nursing Program Faculty 47 (55% with doctorates).
Baccalaureate Enrollment 496 **Women** 81% **Men** 19% **Minority** 62% **International** 19% **Part-time** 22%
Graduate Enrollment 128 **Women** 98% **Men** 2% **Minority** 40% **International** 8% **Part-time** 73%
Nursing Student Activities Nursing Honor Society, Sigma Theta Tau, Student Nurses' Association, nursing club.
Nursing Student Resources Academic advising; academic or career counseling; assistance for students with disabilities; bookstore; campus computer network; computer lab; computer-assisted instruction; e-mail services; employment services for current students; externships; housing assistance; interactive nursing skills videos; Internet; learning resource lab; library services; nursing audiovisuals; paid internships; remedial services; resume preparation assistance; skills, simulation, or other laboratory; tutoring.
Library Facilities 338,418 volumes (73,702 in health, 4,965 in nursing); 1,671 periodical subscriptions (6,516 health-care related).

BACCALAUREATE PROGRAMS

Degree BS
Available Programs ADN to Baccalaureate; Accelerated Baccalaureate for Second Degree; Accelerated RN Baccalaureate; Generic Baccalaureate; LPN to Baccalaureate; RN Baccalaureate.
Study Options Full-time and part-time.
Program Entrance Requirements Minimum overall college GPA of 3.0, transcript of college record, CPR certification, written essay, health exam, high school transcript, immunizations, interview, 3 letters of recommendation, minimum GPA in nursing prerequisites of 3.0, prerequisite course work. Transfer students are accepted. *Application deadline:* 3/31 (fall), 8/15 (winter), 11/1 (spring). Applications may be processed on a rolling basis for some programs. *Application fee:* $120.
Advanced Placement Credit by examination available. Credit given for nursing courses completed elsewhere dependent upon specific evaluations.
Expenses (2010-11) *Tuition:* full-time $25,000; part-time $535 per quarter hour. *Room and board:* room only: $2520 per academic year. *Required fees:* full-time $1770; part-time $590 per term.
Financial Aid 95% of baccalaureate students in nursing programs received some form of financial aid in 2009-10.
Contact Mrs. Heather Krause, Director of Admissions, Marketing and Recruitment, School of Nursing, Loma Linda University, 11262 Campus Street, Loma Linda, CA 92350. *Telephone:* 909-558-4923. *Fax:* 909-558-0175. *E-mail:* hkrause@llu.edu.

GRADUATE PROGRAMS

Expenses (2010-11) *Tuition:* part-time $634 per quarter hour. *Room and board:* room only: $2520 per academic year. *Required fees:* full-time $1770; part-time $590 per term.
Financial Aid 26% of graduate students in nursing programs received some form of financial aid in 2009-10.
Contact Mrs. Michelle Mohr, Assistant Director of Admissions, Marketing and Recruitment, School of Nursing, Loma Linda University, 11262 Campus Street, Loma Linda, CA 92350. *Telephone:* 909-558-1000 Ext. 83113. *Fax:* 909-558-4134. *E-mail:* graduatenursing@llu.edu.

MASTER'S DEGREE PROGRAM

Degree MS
Available Programs Master's; RN to Master's.
Concentrations Available Health-care administration; nurse anesthesia; nursing administration; nursing education. *Clinical nurse specialist programs in:* adult health, family health, maternity-newborn, medical-surgical, parent-child, pediatric. *Nurse practitioner programs in:* adult health, family health, pediatric, primary care, psychiatric/mental health.
Study Options Full-time and part-time.
Program Entrance Requirements Clinical experience, minimum overall college GPA of 3.0, transcript of college record, written essay, immunizations, interview, 3 letters of recommendation, nursing research course, prerequisite course work, statistics course.*Application fee:* $60.
Advanced Placement Credit given for nursing courses completed elsewhere dependent upon specific evaluations.
Degree Requirements Comprehensive exam.

POST-MASTER'S PROGRAM

Areas of Study *Clinical nurse specialist programs in:* adult health, family health, maternity-newborn, medical-surgical, parent-child, pediatric. *Nurse practitioner programs in:* adult health, family health, pediatric, primary care, psychiatric/mental health.

DOCTORAL DEGREE PROGRAM

Degree PhD
Available Programs Doctorate.
Areas of Study Ethics, faculty preparation, gerontology, health policy, health promotion/disease prevention, human health and illness, nursing education, nursing research.
Program Entrance Requirements Clinical experience, minimum overall college GPA of 3.5, interview by faculty committee, interview, 3 letters of recommendation, MSN or equivalent, scholarly papers, statistics course, vita, writing sample. Application deadline: 3/1 (summer). Application fee: $60.
Degree Requirements 90 total credit hours, dissertation, oral exam, written exam, residency.

Mount St. Mary's College
Department of Nursing
Los Angeles, California

http://www.msmc.la.edu/nursing/
Founded in 1925

DEGREES • BSN • BSC PN • MSN
Nursing Program Faculty 112 (10% with doctorates).
Baccalaureate Enrollment 326 **Women** 87% **Men** 13% **Minority** 80%
Graduate Enrollment 51 **Women** 91% **Men** 9% **Minority** 54%
Distance Learning Courses Available.
Nursing Student Activities Nursing Honor Society, Student Nurses' Association, nursing club.
Nursing Student Resources Academic advising; academic or career counseling; assistance for students with disabilities; bookstore; campus computer network; career placement assistance; computer lab; computer-assisted instruction; daycare for children of students; e-mail services; employment services for current students; housing assistance; interactive nursing skills videos; Internet; learning resource lab; library services; nursing audiovisuals; remedial services; resume preparation assistance; skills, simulation, or other laboratory; tutoring.

Library Facilities 140,000 volumes (4,000 in health, 1,000 in nursing); 26,000 periodical subscriptions (150 health-care related).

BACCALAUREATE PROGRAMS

Degrees BSN; BSc PN
Available Programs ADN to Baccalaureate; Accelerated Baccalaureate; Generic Baccalaureate.
Study Options Full-time.
Program Entrance Requirements Minimum overall college GPA of 2.7, transcript of college record, CPR certification, written essay, health exam, high school chemistry, high school transcript, immunizations, 1 letter of recommendation, minimum GPA in nursing prerequisites of 2.5, professional liability insurance/malpractice insurance, prerequisite course work. Transfer students are accepted. *Application deadline:* 2/1 (fall). *Application fee:* $20.
Advanced Placement Credit by examination available. Credit given for nursing courses completed elsewhere dependent upon specific evaluations.
Expenses (2009-10) *Tuition:* full-time $27,840. *Room and board:* $8810 per academic year. *Required fees:* full-time $705.
Financial Aid 95% of baccalaureate students in nursing programs received some form of financial aid in 2008-09. *Gift aid (need-based):* Federal Pell, FSEOG, state, private, college/university gift aid from institutional funds. *Loans:* Federal Nursing Student Loans, Federal Direct (Subsidized and Unsubsidized Stafford PLUS), college/university. *Work-study:* Federal Work-Study, part-time campus jobs. *Financial aid application deadline (priority):* 2/15.
Contact Anne Tumbarello, Director, Department of Nursing, Mount St. Mary's College, 12001 Chalon Road, Los Angeles, CA 90049-1599. *Telephone:* 310-954-4279. *Fax:* 310-954-4229. *E-mail:* atumbarello@msmc.la.edu.

GRADUATE PROGRAMS

Expenses (2009-10) *Tuition:* part-time $708 per unit.
Financial Aid 95% of graduate students in nursing programs received some form of financial aid in 2008-09.
Contact Dr. Marsha Sato, Program Director, Department of Nursing, Mount St. Mary's College, 10 Chester Place, Los Angeles, CA 90007. *Telephone:* 213-477-2980. *Fax:* 213-477-2639. *E-mail:* msato@msmc.la.edu.

MASTER'S DEGREE PROGRAM

Degree MSN
Available Programs Master's; RN to Master's.
Concentrations Available Nursing administration; nursing education. *Clinical nurse specialist programs in:* adult health, community health.
Study Options Full-time and part-time.
Program Entrance Requirements Minimum overall college GPA of 3.0, transcript of college record, CPR certification, written essay, immunizations, interview, professional liability insurance/malpractice insurance, statistics course. *Application deadline:* Applications may be processed on a rolling basis for some programs. *Application fee:* $50.
Advanced Placement Credit given for nursing courses completed elsewhere dependent upon specific evaluations.
Degree Requirements 39 total credit hours, thesis or project.

National University

Department of Nursing
La Jolla, California

http://www.nu.edu/Academics/Schools/SOHHS/nursing.html
Founded in 1971

DEGREE • BSN

Nursing Program Faculty 65 (9% with doctorates).
Baccalaureate Enrollment 188 **Women** 88% **Men** 12% **Minority** 27% **International** 2%
Distance Learning Courses Available.
Nursing Student Activities Student Nurses' Association.
Nursing Student Resources Academic advising; academic or career counseling; assistance for students with disabilities; bookstore; campus computer network; computer lab; Internet; library services; nursing audiovisuals; other; remedial services; resume preparation assistance; tutoring.
Library Facilities 303,000 volumes (14,446 in health, 1,167 in nursing); 22,700 periodical subscriptions (2,047 health-care related).

BACCALAUREATE PROGRAMS

Degree BSN
Available Programs Accelerated Baccalaureate; Generic Baccalaureate; LPN to Baccalaureate; RN Baccalaureate.
Study Options Full-time.
Program Entrance Requirements Minimum overall college GPA of 2.0, transcript of college record, CPR certification, written essay, health exam, health insurance, immunizations, minimum GPA in nursing prerequisites of 2.75, professional liability insurance/malpractice insurance, prerequisite course work. Transfer students are accepted.
Advanced Placement Credit given for nursing courses completed elsewhere dependent upon specific evaluations.
Contact *Telephone:* 800-628-8648 Ext. 8211. *Fax:* 858-642-8709.

Pacific Union College

Department of Nursing
Angwin, California

http://www.puc.edu/PUC/academics/Academic_Departments/Nursing_Dept/
Founded in 1882

DEGREE • BSN

Nursing Program Faculty 16 (14% with doctorates).
Baccalaureate Enrollment 56 **Women** 77% **Men** 23% **Minority** 39% **Part-time** 59%
Nursing Student Activities Student Nurses' Association.
Nursing Student Resources Academic advising; academic or career counseling; assistance for students with disabilities; bookstore; campus computer network; career placement assistance; computer lab; daycare for children of students; e-mail services; employment services for current students; externships; housing assistance; Internet; learning resource lab; library services; nursing audiovisuals; skills, simulation, or other laboratory; tutoring.
Library Facilities 125 volumes in health, 75 volumes in nursing; 109 periodical subscriptions health-care related.

BACCALAUREATE PROGRAMS

Degree BSN
Available Programs ADN to Baccalaureate.
Site Options Napa, CA.
Study Options Full-time and part-time.
Program Entrance Requirements Transcript of college record, CPR certification, health exam, health insurance, immunizations, interview, 2 letters of recommendation, minimum GPA in nursing prerequisites of 2.0, professional liability insurance/malpractice insurance, prerequisite course work, RN licensure. Transfer students are accepted.
Advanced Placement Credit given for nursing courses completed elsewhere dependent upon specific evaluations.
Expenses (2009-10) *Tuition:* full-time $23,844; part-time $695 per quarter hour. *Room and board:* $6750; room only: $3975 per academic year. *Required fees:* part-time $7948 per term.
Financial Aid 93% of baccalaureate students in nursing programs received some form of financial aid in 2008-09. *Gift aid (need-based):* Federal Pell, FSEOG, state, private, college/university gift aid from institutional funds. *Loans:* Federal Direct (Subsidized and Unsubsidized Stafford PLUS), Perkins, college/university. *Work-study:* Federal Work-Study. *Financial aid application deadline (priority):* 3/2.
Contact Mrs. Nancy Tucker, PhD, Coordinator, BSN Program, Department of Nursing, Pacific Union College, One Angwin Avenue, Angwin, CA 94508. *Telephone:* 707-965-7618. *Fax:* 707-965-6499. *E-mail:* ntucker@puc.edu.

CONTINUING EDUCATION PROGRAM

Contact Dr. Shana L. Ruggenberg, Chair, Department of Nursing, Pacific Union College, One Angwin Avenue, Angwin, CA 94508. *Telephone:* 707-965-7262. *Fax:* 707-965-6499. *E-mail:* sruggenberg@puc.edu.

Point Loma Nazarene University

School of Nursing
San Diego, California

http://www.ptloma.edu/nursing
Founded in 1902

DEGREES • BSN • MSN

Nursing Program Faculty 28 (40% with doctorates).
Baccalaureate Enrollment 170 **Women** 90% **Men** 10% **Minority** 23% **International** 1% **Part-time** 2%
Graduate Enrollment 43 **Women** 92% **Men** 8% **Minority** 45% **Part-time** 5%
Nursing Student Activities Sigma Theta Tau, Student Nurses' Association.
Nursing Student Resources Academic advising; academic or career counseling; bookstore; campus computer network; computer lab; computer-assisted instruction; daycare for children of students; e-mail services; employment services for current students; externships; housing assistance; interactive nursing skills videos; Internet; learning resource lab; library services; nursing audiovisuals; paid internships; resume preparation assistance; skills, simulation, or other laboratory; tutoring; unpaid internships.

BACCALAUREATE PROGRAMS

Degree BSN
Available Programs ADN to Baccalaureate; Generic Baccalaureate; LPN to RN Baccalaureate; RN Baccalaureate.
Site Options San Diego, CA.
Study Options Full-time.
Program Entrance Requirements Minimum overall college GPA of 2.7, transcript of college record, CPR certification, written essay, health exam, health insurance, 2 years high school math, immunizations, 1 letter of recommendation, minimum GPA in nursing prerequisites of 2.7, prerequisite course work. Transfer students are accepted. *Application deadline:* 2/1 (fall), 2/1 (winter).
Advanced Placement Credit by examination available. Credit given for nursing courses completed elsewhere dependent upon specific evaluations.
Expenses (2009-10) *Tuition:* full-time $30,000. *Room and board:* $12,000 per academic year. *Required fees:* full-time $700.
Financial Aid 90% of baccalaureate students in nursing programs received some form of financial aid in 2008-09. *Gift aid (need-based):* Federal Pell, FSEOG, state, private, college/university gift aid from institutional funds, Federal Nursing. *Loans:* Federal Nursing Student Loans, Perkins, college/university. *Work-study:* Federal Work-Study. *Financial aid application deadline (priority):* 3/2.
Contact Ms. Marsha Reece, Program Assistant, School of Nursing, Point Loma Nazarene University, 3900 Lomaland Drive, San Diego, CA 92106-2899. *Telephone:* 619-849-7055. *Fax:* 619-849-2672. *E-mail:* mreece@pointloma.edu.

GRADUATE PROGRAMS

Expenses (2009-10) *Tuition:* full-time $15,000.
Financial Aid 80% of graduate students in nursing programs received some form of financial aid in 2008-09.
Contact Prof. Larry Rankin, PhD, MSN Director/Associate Dean, School of Nursing, Point Loma Nazarene University, 4007 Camino Del Rio South, San Diego, CA 92108. *Telephone:* 619-849-2863. *Fax:* 619-849-2672. *E-mail:* lrankin@pointloma.edu.

MASTER'S DEGREE PROGRAM

Degree MSN
Available Programs Master's; RN to Master's.
Concentrations Available Nursing education. *Clinical nurse specialist programs in:* family health, gerontology, medical-surgical, psychiatric/mental health.
Site Options San Diego, CA.
Study Options Full-time and part-time.
Program Entrance Requirements Clinical experience, computer literacy, minimum overall college GPA of 3.0, transcript of college record, CPR certification, written essay, immunizations, interview, 3 letters of recommendation, professional liability insurance/malpractice insurance, resume. *Application deadline:* 8/1 (fall), 12/1 (winter), 8/1 (summer). *Application fee:* $40.
Degree Requirements 43 total credit hours, thesis or project.

POST-MASTER'S PROGRAM

Areas of Study Nursing education. *Clinical nurse specialist programs in:* family health, gerontology, medical-surgical, psychiatric/mental health.

CONTINUING EDUCATION PROGRAM

Contact Ms. Marsha Reece, Program Assistant, School of Nursing, Point Loma Nazarene University, 3900 Lomaland Drive, San Diego, CA 92106-2899. *Telephone:* 619-849-7055. *Fax:* 619-849-2672. *E-mail:* mreece@pointloma.edu.

Samuel Merritt University

School of Nursing
Oakland, California

http://www.samuelmerritt.edu/nursing
Founded in 1909

DEGREES • BSN • MSN

Nursing Program Faculty 171 (23% with doctorates).
Baccalaureate Enrollment 510 **Women** 86% **Men** 14% **Minority** 63% **Part-time** 2%
Graduate Enrollment 356 **Women** 80% **Men** 20% **Minority** 65% **Part-time** 28%
Distance Learning Courses Available.
Nursing Student Activities Sigma Theta Tau, Student Nurses' Association.
Nursing Student Resources Academic advising; academic or career counseling; assistance for students with disabilities; bookstore; campus computer network; computer lab; computer-assisted instruction; e-mail services; housing assistance; interactive nursing skills videos; Internet; learning resource lab; library services; nursing audiovisuals; remedial services; skills, simulation, or other laboratory; tutoring; unpaid internships.
Library Facilities 45,040 volumes (11,328 in health, 4,067 in nursing); 8,392 periodical subscriptions (10,947 health-care related).

BACCALAUREATE PROGRAMS

Degree BSN
Available Programs Accelerated Baccalaureate; Generic Baccalaureate.
Site Options San Mateo, CA; Sacramento, CA; San Francisco, CA.
Study Options Full-time and part-time.
Program Entrance Requirements Minimum overall college GPA of 3.0, transcript of college record, health exam, high school biology, high school chemistry, high school foreign language, 2 years high school math, 3 years high school science, high school transcript, immunizations, 1 letter of recommendation, minimum high school GPA of 2.5, minimum GPA in nursing prerequisites of 3.0, prerequisite course work. Transfer students are accepted. *Application deadline:* 3/1 (fall), 9/1 (spring). *Application fee:* $50.
Advanced Placement Credit by examination available. Credit given for nursing courses completed elsewhere dependent upon specific evaluations.
Expenses (2010-11) *Tuition:* full-time $35,686; part-time $1504 per unit. *Required fees:* full-time $1335.
Financial Aid 83% of baccalaureate students in nursing programs received some form of financial aid in 2009-10. *Gift aid (need-based):* Federal Pell, FSEOG, state, private, college/university gift aid from institutional funds, Federal Nursing. *Loans:* Federal Nursing Student Loans, Perkins, college/university. *Work-study:* Federal Work-Study, part-time campus jobs. *Financial aid application deadline (priority):* 3/2.
Contact Ms. Anne E. Seed, Director of Admissions, School of Nursing, Samuel Merritt University, 3100 Telegraph Avenue, Office of Admissions, Oakland, CA 94609. *Telephone:* 510-869-6610. *Fax:* 510-869-6525. *E-mail:* admission@samuelmerritt.edu.

GRADUATE PROGRAMS

Expenses (2010-11) *Tuition:* full-time $34,584; part-time $1011 per unit. *Required fees:* full-time $569.
Financial Aid 90% of graduate students in nursing programs received some form of financial aid in 2009-10. Career-related internships or fieldwork, Federal Work-Study, scholarships, and traineeships available. Aid available to part-time students. *Financial aid application deadline:* 3/2.
Contact Ms. Anne E. Seed, Director of Admissions, School of Nursing, Samuel Merritt University, 3100 Telegraph Avenue, Office of Admis-

sions, Oakland, CA 94609. *Telephone:* 510-869-6610. *Fax:* 510-869-6525. *E-mail:* aseed@samuelmerritt.edu.

MASTER'S DEGREE PROGRAM

Degree MSN
Available Programs Master's; Master's for Non-Nursing College Graduates; Master's for Nurses with Non-Nursing Degrees.
Concentrations Available Nurse anesthesia; nurse case management. *Nurse practitioner programs in:* family health.
Site Options Sacramento, CA.
Study Options Full-time and part-time.
Online Degree Options Yes.
Program Entrance Requirements Clinical experience, computer literacy, minimum overall college GPA of 3.0, transcript of college record, CPR certification, written essay, immunizations, interview, 2 letters of recommendation, prerequisite course work, statistics course. *Application deadline:* 1/15 (fall), 7/1 (spring). *Application fee:* $50.
Advanced Placement Credit by examination available. Credit given for nursing courses completed elsewhere dependent upon specific evaluations.
Degree Requirements 49 total credit hours, thesis or project, comprehensive exam.

POST-MASTER'S PROGRAM

Areas of Study Nurse anesthesia; nurse case management. *Nurse practitioner programs in:* family health.

San Diego State University

School of Nursing
San Diego, California

http://nursing.sdsu.edu/
Founded in 1897

DEGREES • BSN • MSN

Nursing Program Faculty 70 (30% with doctorates).
Baccalaureate Enrollment 540 **Women** 95% **Men** 5% **Minority** 60% **International** 1%
Graduate Enrollment 79 **Women** 95% **Men** 5% **Minority** 5% **Part-time** 75%
Distance Learning Courses Available.
Nursing Student Activities Sigma Theta Tau, Student Nurses' Association.
Nursing Student Resources Academic advising; academic or career counseling; assistance for students with disabilities; bookstore; campus computer network; career placement assistance; computer lab; daycare for children of students; e-mail services; housing assistance; Internet; learning resource lab; library services; nursing audiovisuals; paid internships; placement services for program completers; remedial services; resume preparation assistance; skills, simulation, or other laboratory; unpaid internships.
Library Facilities 1.3 million volumes (36,000 in health, 14,000 in nursing); 8,245 periodical subscriptions (335 health-care related).

BACCALAUREATE PROGRAMS

Degree BSN
Available Programs ADN to Baccalaureate; Generic Baccalaureate; RN Baccalaureate.
Study Options Full-time.
Online Degree Options Yes.
Program Entrance Requirements Minimum overall college GPA of 2.5, transcript of college record, CPR certification, health exam, health insurance, high school biology, high school chemistry, high school foreign language, 3 years high school math, 2 years high school science, high school transcript, immunizations, minimum high school GPA of 2.5, minimum GPA in nursing prerequisites of 2.5, professional liability insurance/malpractice insurance, prerequisite course work. Transfer students are accepted. *Application deadline:* 11/30 (fall), 4/5 (spring). Applications may be processed on a rolling basis for some programs. *Application fee:* $55.
Advanced Placement Credit by examination available. Credit given for nursing courses completed elsewhere dependent upon specific evaluations.
Financial Aid 75% of baccalaureate students in nursing programs received some form of financial aid in 2009-10. *Gift aid (need-based):* Federal Pell, FSEOG, state, private, college/university gift aid from institutional funds, Federal Nursing. *Loans:* Federal Direct (Subsidized and Unsubsidized Stafford PLUS), Perkins, college/university. *Work-study:* Federal Work-Study. *Financial aid application deadline:* 3/2.
Contact Nursing Contact, School of Nursing, San Diego State University, 5500 Campanile Drive, San Diego, CA 92182-0254. *Telephone:* 619-594-2540. *Fax:* 619-594-2765. *E-mail:* nursing@mail.sdsu.edu.

GRADUATE PROGRAMS

Financial Aid 90% of graduate students in nursing programs received some form of financial aid in 2009-10. Career-related internships or fieldwork, scholarships, traineeships, and unspecified assistantships available.
Contact Prof. Janet Wessels, Graduate Adviser, School of Nursing, San Diego State University, 5500 Campanile Drive, San Diego, CA 92182-0254. *Telephone:* 619-594-2763. *Fax:* 619-594-2765. *E-mail:* jwessels@mail.sdsu.edu.

MASTER'S DEGREE PROGRAM

Degree MSN
Available Programs Master's.
Concentrations Available Nurse-midwifery; nursing administration; nursing education. *Clinical nurse specialist programs in:* adult health, community health, critical care, gerontology, maternity-newborn, school health, women's health. *Nurse practitioner programs in:* acute care, adult health, gerontology, women's health.
Site Options La Jolla, CA.
Study Options Full-time and part-time.
Program Entrance Requirements Clinical experience, minimum overall college GPA of 3.0, transcript of college record, written essay, 3 letters of recommendation, nursing research course, physical assessment course, professional liability insurance/malpractice insurance, resume, statistics course, GRE General Test. *Application deadline:* 2/1 (fall), 2/1 (spring). Applications may be processed on a rolling basis for some programs. *Application fee:* $45.
Advanced Placement Credit by examination available. Credit given for nursing courses completed elsewhere dependent upon specific evaluations.
Degree Requirements 39 total credit hours, thesis or project, comprehensive exam.

POST-MASTER'S PROGRAM

Areas of Study Nurse-midwifery.

CONTINUING EDUCATION PROGRAM

Contact Prof. Janet Wessels, Graduate Advisor, School of Nursing, San Diego State University, 5500 Campanile Drive, San Diego, CA 92182-0254. *Telephone:* 619-594-2763. *Fax:* 619-594-2765. *E-mail:* jwessels@mail.sdsu.edu.

San Francisco State University

School of Nursing
San Francisco, California

Founded in 1899

DEGREES • BSN • MSN

Nursing Program Faculty 40 (50% with doctorates).
Baccalaureate Enrollment 250 **Women** 88% **Men** 12% **Minority** 53% **International** 2% **Part-time** 5%
Graduate Enrollment 180 **Women** 80% **Men** 20% **Minority** 80% **International** 10% **Part-time** 20%
Nursing Student Activities Sigma Theta Tau, Student Nurses' Association.
Nursing Student Resources Academic advising; academic or career counseling; assistance for students with disabilities; bookstore; campus computer network; career placement assistance; computer lab; computer-assisted instruction; daycare for children of students; e-mail services; employment services for current students; externships; housing assistance; interactive nursing skills videos; Internet; learning resource lab; library services; nursing audiovisuals; other; placement services for program completers; remedial services; resume preparation assistance; skills, simulation, or other laboratory; tutoring.
Library Facilities 1.1 million volumes (11,000 in health, 1,500 in nursing); 40,184 periodical subscriptions (200 health-care related).

BACCALAUREATE PROGRAMS

Degree BSN

Available Programs ADN to Baccalaureate; Accelerated LPN to Baccalaureate; Generic Baccalaureate; RN Baccalaureate.
Study Options Full-time.
Program Entrance Requirements Minimum overall college GPA of 2.5, transcript of college record, CPR certification, health exam, health insurance, immunizations, minimum GPA in nursing prerequisites of 2.5, professional liability insurance/malpractice insurance, prerequisite course work. Transfer students are accepted.
Advanced Placement Credit by examination available. Credit given for nursing courses completed elsewhere dependent upon specific evaluations.
Contact ***Telephone:*** 415-338-2315 Ext. 1. *Fax:* 415-338-0555.

GRADUATE PROGRAMS

Contact ***Telephone:*** 415-338-1802. *Fax:* 415-338-0555.

MASTER'S DEGREE PROGRAM

Degree MSN
Available Programs Accelerated Master's for Non-Nursing College Graduates; Accelerated Master's for Nurses with Non-Nursing Degrees; Master's; Master's for Non-Nursing College Graduates; Master's for Nurses with Non-Nursing Degrees.
Concentrations Available Nurse case management; nursing administration. *Clinical nurse specialist programs in:* adult health, perinatal, public health. *Nurse practitioner programs in:* family health.
Study Options Full-time and part-time.
Program Entrance Requirements Minimum overall college GPA of 3.0, transcript of college record, CPR certification, written essay, immunizations, 3 letters of recommendation, nursing research course, professional liability insurance/malpractice insurance, resume, statistics course.
Advanced Placement Credit by examination available. Credit given for nursing courses completed elsewhere dependent upon specific evaluations.
Degree Requirements 36 total credit hours, thesis or project.

POST-MASTER'S PROGRAM

Areas of Study Nursing administration. *Nurse practitioner programs in:* family health.

CONTINUING EDUCATION PROGRAM

Contact ***Telephone:*** 415-405-3660. *Fax:* 415-338-0555.

San Jose State University

The Valley Foundation School of Nursing
San Jose, California

Founded in 1857

DEGREES • BS • MS

Nursing Program Faculty 55 (52% with doctorates).
Baccalaureate Enrollment 550 **Women** 92% **Men** 8% **Minority** 76% **Part-time** 20%
Graduate Enrollment 101 **Women** 92% **Men** 8% **Minority** 46% **Part-time** 83%
Nursing Student Activities Sigma Theta Tau, Student Nurses' Association, nursing club.
Nursing Student Resources Academic advising; academic or career counseling; assistance for students with disabilities; bookstore; career placement assistance; computer lab; computer-assisted instruction; housing assistance; interactive nursing skills videos; Internet; learning resource lab; library services; nursing audiovisuals; skills, simulation, or other laboratory; tutoring.
Library Facilities 280 volumes in health, 250 volumes in nursing; 80 periodical subscriptions health-care related.

BACCALAUREATE PROGRAMS

Degree BS
Available Programs Generic Baccalaureate; RPN to Baccalaureate.
Site Options Salinas, CA; Gilroy, CA.
Study Options Full-time and part-time.
Program Entrance Requirements Transcript of college record, health insurance, 3 years high school math, minimum high school GPA of 2.0, minimum GPA in nursing prerequisites of 2.0, professional liability insurance/malpractice insurance, prerequisite course work. Transfer students are accepted.
Advanced Placement Credit by examination available. Credit given for nursing courses completed elsewhere dependent upon specific evaluations.
Contact ***Telephone:*** 408-924-3131. *Fax:* 408-924-3135.

GRADUATE PROGRAMS

Contact ***Telephone:*** 408-924-3144. *Fax:* 408-924-3135.

MASTER'S DEGREE PROGRAM

Degree MS
Available Programs Master's.
Concentrations Available Nursing administration; nursing education. *Clinical nurse specialist programs in:* gerontology, school health. *Nurse practitioner programs in:* family health.
Study Options Full-time and part-time.
Program Entrance Requirements Minimum overall college GPA of 3.0, transcript of college record, CPR certification, written essay, immunizations, 3 letters of recommendation, nursing research course, physical assessment course, professional liability insurance/malpractice insurance, resume, statistics course.
Degree Requirements 36 total credit hours, thesis or project.

Sonoma State University

Department of Nursing
Rohnert Park, California

http://www.sonoma.edu/nursing
Founded in 1960

DEGREES • BSN • MSN

Nursing Program Faculty 37 (22% with doctorates).
Baccalaureate Enrollment 134 **Women** 84% **Men** 16% **Minority** 25% **Part-time** 27%
Graduate Enrollment 176 **Women** 91% **Men** 9% **Minority** 29% **Part-time** 59%
Distance Learning Courses Available.
Nursing Student Activities Sigma Theta Tau, Student Nurses' Association, nursing club.
Nursing Student Resources Academic advising; academic or career counseling; assistance for students with disabilities; bookstore; campus computer network; career placement assistance; computer lab; computer-assisted instruction; daycare for children of students; e-mail services; employment services for current students; housing assistance; interactive nursing skills videos; Internet; learning resource lab; library services; nursing audiovisuals; remedial services; resume preparation assistance; skills, simulation, or other laboratory; tutoring; unpaid internships.
Library Facilities 678,474 volumes (26,700 in health, 1,400 in nursing); 21,117 periodical subscriptions (64 health-care related).

BACCALAUREATE PROGRAMS

Degree BSN
Available Programs ADN to Baccalaureate; Baccalaureate for Second Degree; Generic Baccalaureate; RN Baccalaureate.
Study Options Full-time.
Program Entrance Requirements Minimum overall college GPA of 3.5, transcript of college record, CPR certification, written essay, health exam, high school biology, high school chemistry, high school foreign language, 3 years high school math, 2 years high school science, high school transcript, immunizations, minimum high school GPA of 3.0, minimum GPA in nursing prerequisites of 3.5, prerequisite course work. Transfer students are accepted. *Application deadline:* 2/28 (fall). *Application fee:* $25.
Advanced Placement Credit given for nursing courses completed elsewhere dependent upon specific evaluations.
Financial Aid 53% of baccalaureate students in nursing programs received some form of financial aid in 2009-10. *Gift aid (need-based):* Federal Pell, FSEOG, state, private, college/university gift aid from institutional funds, Academic Competitiveness Grants, National SMART Grants. *Loans:* Federal Direct (Subsidized and Unsubsidized Stafford PLUS), Perkins. *Work-study:* Federal Work-Study, part-time campus jobs. *Financial aid application deadline (priority):* 1/31.
Contact Ms. Eileen P. O'Brien, Administrative Coordinator, Department of Nursing, Sonoma State University, 1801 East Cotati Avenue, Rohnert Park, CA 94928. *Telephone:* 707-664-2465. *Fax:* 707-664-2653. *E-mail:* nursing@sonoma.edu.

GRADUATE PROGRAMS

Financial Aid 70% of graduate students in nursing programs received some form of financial aid in 2009-10.
Contact Ms. Eileen P. O'Brien, Administrative Coordinator, Department of Nursing, Sonoma State University, 1801 East Cotati Avenue, Rohnert Park, CA 94928. *Telephone:* 707-664-2465. *Fax:* 707-664-2653. *E-mail:* nursing@sonoma.edu.

MASTER'S DEGREE PROGRAM

Degree MSN
Available Programs Accelerated Master's for Non-Nursing College Graduates; Master's.
Concentrations Available Nursing administration; nursing education. *Nurse practitioner programs in:* family health.
Site Options Turlock, CA; Chico, CA.
Study Options Full-time and part-time.
Program Entrance Requirements Clinical experience, computer literacy, minimum overall college GPA of 3.0, transcript of college record, CPR certification, written essay, immunizations, 3 letters of recommendation, physical assessment course, prerequisite course work, statistics course. *Application deadline:* 3/31 (fall). *Application fee:* $25.
Advanced Placement Credit by examination available. Credit given for nursing courses completed elsewhere dependent upon specific evaluations.
Degree Requirements 32 total credit hours, thesis or project, comprehensive exam.

POST-MASTER'S PROGRAM

Areas of Study *Nurse practitioner programs in:* family health.

University of California, Irvine

Program in Nursing Science
Irvine, California

http://www.cohs.uci.edu/nursing
Founded in 1965

DEGREES • BS • MS

Nursing Program Faculty 36 (27% with doctorates).
Baccalaureate Enrollment 162 **Women** 89% **Men** 11% **Minority** 72%
Graduate Enrollment 26 **Women** 88% **Men** 12% **Minority** 54% **Part-time** 35%
Nursing Student Activities Student Nurses' Association.
Nursing Student Resources Academic advising; academic or career counseling; assistance for students with disabilities; bookstore; campus computer network; computer lab; computer-assisted instruction; daycare for children of students; e-mail services; employment services for current students; housing assistance; interactive nursing skills videos; Internet; learning resource lab; library services; nursing audiovisuals; skills, simulation, or other laboratory; tutoring.
Library Facilities 3 million volumes (365,965 in health, 6,047 in nursing); 51,623 periodical subscriptions.

BACCALAUREATE PROGRAMS

Degree BS
Available Programs Generic Baccalaureate.
Study Options Full-time.
Program Entrance Requirements Written essay, high school biology, high school chemistry, 2 years high school science, 3 letters of recommendation. Transfer students are accepted. *Application deadline:* 11/30 (fall). *Application fee:* $60.
Expenses (2010-11) *Tuition, state resident:* full-time $10,302. *Tuition, nonresident:* full-time $22,879. *Required fees:* full-time $1625.
Financial Aid ***Gift aid (need-based):*** Federal Pell, FSEOG, state, private, college/university gift aid from institutional funds. *Loans:* Federal Direct (Subsidized and Unsubsidized Stafford PLUS), Perkins, college/university, private loans. *Work-study:* Federal Work-Study. *Financial aid application deadline:* 5/1(priority: 3/2).
Contact Baccalaureate Program, Program in Nursing Science, University of California, Irvine, 31 Irvine Hall, Irvine, CA 92697-3959. *Telephone:* 949-824-3580. *Fax:* 949-824-0470.

GRADUATE PROGRAMS

Expenses (2010-11) *Tuition, state resident:* full-time $10,212. *Tuition, nonresident:* full-time $12,245. *Required fees:* full-time $7980.
Contact Master's Program, Program in Nursing Science, University of California, Irvine, Program in Nursing Science, 244A Irvine Hall, Irvine, CA 92697-3959. *Telephone:* 949-824-3580. *Fax:* 949-824-0470. *E-mail:* gsnao@uci.edu.

MASTER'S DEGREE PROGRAM

Degree MS
Available Programs Master's.
Concentrations Available *Nurse practitioner programs in:* adult health, family health, gerontology.
Study Options Full-time and part-time.
Program Entrance Requirements Clinical experience, transcript of college record, 3 letters of recommendation, statistics course. *Application deadline:* 3/1 (winter). *Application fee:* $70.
Degree Requirements 72 total credit hours, comprehensive exam.

POST-MASTER'S PROGRAM

Areas of Study *Nurse practitioner programs in:* adult health, family health, gerontology.

University of California, Los Angeles

School of Nursing
Los Angeles, California

http://www.nursing.ucla.edu/
Founded in 1919

DEGREES • BS • MSN • MSN/MBA • PHD

Nursing Program Faculty 87 (54% with doctorates).
Baccalaureate Enrollment 242 **Women** 88% **Men** 12% **Minority** 65%
Graduate Enrollment 348 **Women** 89% **Men** 11% **Minority** 51%
International 1%
Nursing Student Activities Nursing Honor Society, Sigma Theta Tau, Student Nurses' Association, nursing club.
Nursing Student Resources Academic advising; academic or career counseling; assistance for students with disabilities; bookstore; campus computer network; computer lab; daycare for children of students; e-mail services; housing assistance; Internet; library services; nursing audiovisuals; skills, simulation, or other laboratory.
Library Facilities 9 million volumes (760,000 in health, 8,000 in nursing); 38,975 periodical subscriptions (600,000 health-care related).

BACCALAUREATE PROGRAMS

Degree BS
Available Programs Generic Baccalaureate.
Study Options Full-time.
Program Entrance Requirements Transcript of college record, written essay, high school transcript, 2 letters of recommendation, minimum high school GPA, prerequisite course work. Transfer students are accepted. *Application deadline:* 11/30 (fall). *Application fee:* $60.
Expenses (2010-11) *Tuition, nonresident:* full-time $34,747. *Room and board:* $13,734 per academic year. *Required fees:* full-time $11,868; part-time $3956 per term.
Financial Aid 71% of baccalaureate students in nursing programs received some form of financial aid in 2009-10. *Gift aid (need-based):* Federal Pell, FSEOG, state, private, college/university gift aid from institutional funds, United Negro College Fund, Federal Nursing. *Loans:* Federal Nursing Student Loans, Perkins, state, college/university. *Work-study:* Federal Work-Study, part-time campus jobs. *Financial aid application deadline:* Continuous.
Contact Ms. Rhonda Flenoy-Younger, Director of Recruitment, Outreach and Admissions, School of Nursing, University of California, Los Angeles, Box 951702, Los Angeles, CA 90095-1702. *Telephone:* 310-825-9193. *Fax:* 310-206-7433. *E-mail:* rflenoy@sonnet.ucla.edu.

GRADUATE PROGRAMS

Expenses (2010-11) *Tuition, nonresident:* full-time $29,601. *Room and board:* $15,600 per academic year. *Required fees:* full-time $17,356; part-time $5785 per term.
Financial Aid 88% of graduate students in nursing programs received some form of financial aid in 2009-10. 185 fellowships with full and partial tuition reimbursements available, 10 research assistantships with full and partial tuition reimbursements available, 34 teaching assistantships with full and partial tuition reimbursements available were awarded; Federal Work-Study, institutionally sponsored loans, scholar-

ships, tuition waivers (full and partial), and unspecified assistantships also available. *Financial aid application deadline:* 3/1.

Contact Ms. Rhonda Flenoy-Younger, Director of Recruitment, Outreach and Admissions, School of Nursing, University of California, Los Angeles, Box 951702, Los Angeles, CA 90095-1702. *Telephone:* 310-825-9193. *Fax:* 310-267-0330. *E-mail:* rflenoy@sonnet.ucla.edu.

MASTER'S DEGREE PROGRAM

Degrees MSN; MSN/MBA

Available Programs Master's; Master's for Non-Nursing College Graduates.

Concentrations Available Clinical nurse leader; nursing administration. *Clinical nurse specialist programs in:* acute care, adult health, gerontology, oncology, pediatric. *Nurse practitioner programs in:* acute care, adult health, family health, gerontology, occupational health, oncology, pediatric.

Study Options Full-time.

Program Entrance Requirements Minimum overall college GPA of 3.0, transcript of college record, written essay, 3 letters of recommendation, nursing research course, physical assessment course, prerequisite course work, statistics course. *Application deadline:* 11/1 (fall). *Application fee:* $70.

Degree Requirements 72 total credit hours, comprehensive exam.

POST-MASTER'S PROGRAM

Areas of Study Nursing administration. *Nurse practitioner programs in:* acute care, adult health, family health, gerontology, oncology, pediatric.

DOCTORAL DEGREE PROGRAM

Degree PhD

Available Programs Doctorate; Post-Baccalaureate Doctorate.

Areas of Study Addiction/substance abuse, advanced practice nursing, aging, bio-behavioral research, biology of health and illness, clinical practice, community health, critical care, family health, gerontology, health policy, health promotion/disease prevention, health-care systems, human health and illness, illness and transition, neuro-behavior, nursing administration, nursing research, nursing science, oncology, women's health.

Program Entrance Requirements Minimum overall college GPA of 3.5, 4 letters of recommendation, scholarly papers, statistics course, vita, writing sample, GRE General Test. Application deadline: 12/1 (fall). Application fee: $70.

Degree Requirements 127 total credit hours, dissertation, oral exam, written exam, residency.

POSTDOCTORAL PROGRAM

Areas of Study Addiction/substance abuse, adolescent health, aging, cancer care, gerontology, health promotion/disease prevention, nursing research, vulnerable population, women's health.

Postdoctoral Program Contact Dr. Peggy Compton, Associate Dean for Academic Affairs, School of Nursing, University of California, Los Angeles, Box 951702, Los Angeles, CA 90095-1702. *Telephone:* 310-206-2825. *Fax:* 310-206-7433. *E-mail:* pcompton@sonnet.ucla.edu.

CONTINUING EDUCATION PROGRAM

Contact Ms. Salpy Akaragian, Education Specialist, School of Nursing, University of California, Los Angeles, Box 951701, Los Angeles, CA 90095-1701. *Telephone:* 310-206-9581. *E-mail:* nssa@mednet.ucla.edu.

University of California, San Francisco

School of Nursing
San Francisco, California

http://www.nurseweb.ucsf.edu

Founded in 1864

DEGREES • MS • PHD

Nursing Program Faculty 151 (72% with doctorates).

Graduate Enrollment 721 **Women** 87% **Men** 13% **Minority** 30% **International** 10% **Part-time** 1%

Distance Learning Courses Available.

Nursing Student Activities Nursing Honor Society, Sigma Theta Tau, Student Nurses' Association, nursing club.

Nursing Student Resources Academic advising; academic or career counseling; assistance for students with disabilities; bookstore; campus computer network; career placement assistance; computer lab; computer-assisted instruction; daycare for children of students; e-mail services; employment services for current students; housing assistance; interactive nursing skills videos; Internet; learning resource lab; library services; nursing audiovisuals; other; paid internships; placement services for program completers; remedial services; resume preparation assistance; skills, simulation, or other laboratory; tutoring; unpaid internships.

Library Facilities 856,169 volumes in health, 131,046 volumes in nursing; 3,270 periodical subscriptions health-care related.

GRADUATE PROGRAMS

Expenses (2009-10) *Tuition, state resident:* full-time $14,695. *Tuition, nonresident:* full-time $26,940. *International tuition:* $26,940 full-time.

Financial Aid 59% of graduate students in nursing programs received some form of financial aid in 2008-09. Fellowships, career-related internships or fieldwork and Federal Work-Study available. Aid available to part-time students.

Contact Mr. Terry Linton, Admissions and Progression Officer, School of Nursing, University of California, San Francisco, Room N319X, 2 Koret Way, San Francisco, CA 94143-0602. *Telephone:* 415-476-1435. *Fax:* 415-476-9707. *E-mail:* terry.linton@nursing.ucsf.edu.

MASTER'S DEGREE PROGRAM

Degree MS

Available Programs Master's; Master's for Non-Nursing College Graduates; Master's for Nurses with Non-Nursing Degrees.

Concentrations Available Nurse-midwifery; nursing administration. *Clinical nurse specialist programs in:* cardiovascular, community health, critical care, gerontology, occupational health, oncology, pediatric, perinatal, psychiatric/mental health. *Nurse practitioner programs in:* acute care, adult health, family health, gerontology, neonatal health, occupational health, pediatric, psychiatric/mental health.

Study Options Full-time.

Program Entrance Requirements Clinical experience, computer literacy, minimum overall college GPA of 3.0, transcript of college record, written essay, immunizations, 4 letters of recommendation, statistics course, GRE General Test. *Application deadline:* 2/1 (fall). *Application fee:* $60.

Advanced Placement Credit given for nursing courses completed elsewhere dependent upon specific evaluations.

Degree Requirements 44 total credit hours, comprehensive exam.

POST-MASTER'S PROGRAM

Areas of Study *Clinical nurse specialist programs in:* cardiovascular, community health, critical care, gerontology, occupational health, oncology, pediatric, perinatal, psychiatric/mental health. *Nurse practitioner programs in:* acute care, adult health, family health, gerontology, neonatal health, occupational health, pediatric, psychiatric/mental health.

DOCTORAL DEGREE PROGRAM

Degree PhD

Available Programs Doctorate; Post-Baccalaureate Doctorate.

Areas of Study Addiction/substance abuse, aging, bio-behavioral research, biology of health and illness, community health, critical care, ethics, family health, gerontology, health policy, health promotion/disease prevention, health-care systems, human health and illness, illness and transition, individualized study, information systems, maternity-newborn, nursing administration, nursing policy, nursing research, nursing science, oncology, urban health, women's health.

Program Entrance Requirements Minimum overall college GPA of 3.0, 4 letters of recommendation, statistics course, writing sample, GRE General Test. Application deadline: 12/15 (fall). Application fee: $60.

Degree Requirements Dissertation, oral exam, written exam, residency.

POSTDOCTORAL PROGRAM

Areas of Study Individualized study.

Postdoctoral Program Contact Mr. Jeff Kilmer, Director, Office of Student and Curricular Affairs, School of Nursing, University of California, San Francisco, Room N319X, 2 Koret Way, San Francisco, CA 94143-0602. *Telephone:* 415-476-1435. *Fax:* 415-476-9707. *E-mail:* jeff.kilmer@nursing.ucsf.edu.

University of Phoenix–Bay Area Campus
College of Health and Human Services
Pleasanton, California

DEGREES • BSN • MSN • MSN/MBA • MSN/MHA
Nursing Program Faculty 12 (58% with doctorates).
Baccalaureate Enrollment 39 **Women** 92.3% **Men** 7.7% **Minority** 35.9%
Graduate Enrollment 22 **Women** 86.4% **Men** 13.6% **Minority** 40.91%
Nursing Student Activities Sigma Theta Tau.
Nursing Student Resources Academic advising; academic or career counseling; assistance for students with disabilities; bookstore; campus computer network; computer lab; computer-assisted instruction; e-mail services; interactive nursing skills videos; Internet; learning resource lab; library services; nursing audiovisuals; remedial services; skills, simulation, or other laboratory; tutoring.
Library Facilities 16,781 periodical subscriptions (1,300 health-care related).

BACCALAUREATE PROGRAMS

Degree BSN
Available Programs Accelerated Baccalaureate.
Site Options Oakland, CA; San Francisco, CA; Novato, CA.
Study Options Full-time.
Program Entrance Requirements Transcript of college record, CPR certification, immunizations, 1 letter of recommendation, RN licensure. Transfer students are accepted. *Application deadline:* Applications may be processed on a rolling basis for some programs.
Advanced Placement Credit by examination available. Credit given for nursing courses completed elsewhere dependent upon specific evaluations.
Expenses (2009-10) *Tuition:* full-time $9300. *Required fees:* full-time $600.
Contact Campus College Chair, Nursing, College of Health and Human Services, University of Phoenix–Bay Area Campus, 7901 Stoneridge Drive, Suite #130, Pleasanton, CA 94588-3677. *Telephone:* 877-416-4100.

GRADUATE PROGRAMS

Expenses (2009-10) *Tuition:* full-time $10,560. *Required fees:* full-time $760.
Financial Aid Institutionally sponsored loans and scholarships available.
Contact Campus College Chair, Nursing, College of Health and Human Services, University of Phoenix–Bay Area Campus, 7901 Stoneridge Drive, Suite #130, Pleasanton, CA 94588-3677. *Telephone:* 877-416-4100.

MASTER'S DEGREE PROGRAM

Degrees MSN; MSN/MBA; MSN/MHA
Available Programs Master's.
Concentrations Available Health-care administration; nursing administration; nursing education.
Site Options Oakland, CA; San Francisco, CA; Novato, CA.
Study Options Full-time.
Program Entrance Requirements Clinical experience, computer literacy, minimum overall college GPA of 2.5, transcript of college record. *Application deadline:* Applications may be processed on a rolling basis for some programs. *Application fee:* $45.
Advanced Placement Credit given for nursing courses completed elsewhere dependent upon specific evaluations.
Degree Requirements 39 total credit hours, thesis or project.

University of Phoenix–Central Valley Campus
College of Health and Human Services
Fresno, California

Founded in 2004
DEGREE • BSN
Nursing Program Faculty 8 (13% with doctorates).
Baccalaureate Enrollment 53 **Women** 94.3% **Men** 5.7% **Minority** 30.2%
Nursing Student Activities Sigma Theta Tau.
Nursing Student Resources Academic advising; academic or career counseling; bookstore; campus computer network; computer lab; computer-assisted instruction; e-mail services; interactive nursing skills videos; Internet; learning resource lab; library services; nursing audiovisuals; remedial services; skills, simulation, or other laboratory; tutoring.
Library Facilities 1,300 periodical subscriptions health-care related.

BACCALAUREATE PROGRAMS

Degree BSN
Available Programs RN Baccalaureate.
Site Options Fresno, CA; Visalia, CA; Bakersfield, CA.
Study Options Full-time.
Program Entrance Requirements Transcript of college record, CPR certification, immunizations, 1 letter of recommendation, RN licensure. Transfer students are accepted.
Advanced Placement Credit by examination available. Credit given for nursing courses completed elsewhere dependent upon specific evaluations.
Contact Campus College Chair, Nursing, College of Health and Human Services, University of Phoenix–Central Valley Campus, 4900 California Avenue, Tower A, Suite 300, Bakersfield, CA 93309-7018. *Telephone:* 661-663-0300. *Fax:* 661-633-2711.

University of Phoenix–Sacramento Valley Campus
College of Nursing
Sacramento, California

Founded in 1993
DEGREES • BSN • MSN • MSN/MHA
Nursing Program Faculty 29 (28% with doctorates).
Baccalaureate Enrollment 250 **Women** 88.8% **Men** 11.2% **Minority** 32%
Graduate Enrollment 53 **Women** 90.6% **Men** 9.4% **Minority** 15.09%
Nursing Student Activities Sigma Theta Tau.
Nursing Student Resources Academic advising; academic or career counseling; assistance for students with disabilities; bookstore; campus computer network; computer lab; computer-assisted instruction; e-mail services; interactive nursing skills videos; Internet; learning resource lab; library services; nursing audiovisuals; skills, simulation, or other laboratory; tutoring.
Library Facilities 16,781 periodical subscriptions (1,300 health-care related).

BACCALAUREATE PROGRAMS

Degree BSN
Available Programs Accelerated Baccalaureate; LPN to Baccalaureate.
Site Options Lathrop, CA; Modesto, CA; Fairfield, CA.
Study Options Full-time.
Online Degree Options Yes.
Program Entrance Requirements Transcript of college record, CPR certification, immunizations, 1 letter of recommendation, RN licensure. Transfer students are accepted. *Application deadline:* Applications may be processed on a rolling basis for some programs.
Advanced Placement Credit by examination available. Credit given for nursing courses completed elsewhere dependent upon specific evaluations.
Expenses (2009-10) *Tuition:* full-time $11,100. *Required fees:* full-time $600.
Contact Campus College Chair, Nursing, College of Nursing, University of Phoenix–Sacramento Valley Campus, 1760 Creekside Oaks Drive, #100, Sacramento, CA 95833-3632. *Telephone:* 800-266-2107.

GRADUATE PROGRAMS

Expenses (2009-10) *Tuition:* full-time $13,200. *Required fees:* full-time $760.
Financial Aid Institutionally sponsored loans and scholarships available.
Contact Campus College Chair, Nursing, College of Nursing, University of Phoenix–Sacramento Valley Campus, 1760 Creekside Oaks Drive, #100, Sacramento, CA 95833-3632. *Telephone:* 800-266-2107.

MASTER'S DEGREE PROGRAM

Degrees MSN; MSN/MHA
Available Programs Accelerated Master's.

Concentrations Available Health-care administration; nursing administration; nursing education. *Nurse practitioner programs in:* family health.
Site Options Lathrop, CA; Modesto, CA; Fairfield, CA.
Study Options Full-time and part-time.
Program Entrance Requirements Clinical experience, computer literacy, minimum overall college GPA of 2.5, transcript of college record. *Application deadline:* Applications may be processed on a rolling basis for some programs. *Application fee:* $45.
Advanced Placement Credit given for nursing courses completed elsewhere dependent upon specific evaluations.
Degree Requirements 39 total credit hours, thesis or project.

POST-MASTER'S PROGRAM

Areas of Study *Nurse practitioner programs in:* family health.

CONTINUING EDUCATION PROGRAM

Contact Campus College Chair, College of Nursing, University of Phoenix–Sacramento Valley Campus, 1760 Creekside Oaks Drive, #100, Scaramento, CA 95833-3632. *Telephone:* 800-266-2107.

University of Phoenix–San Diego Campus

College of Nursing
San Diego, California

Founded in 1988

DEGREES • BSN • MSN • MSN/ED D
Nursing Program Faculty 30 (37% with doctorates).
Baccalaureate Enrollment 103 **Women** 81.6% **Men** 18.4% **Minority** 29.1%
Graduate Enrollment 46 **Women** 89.1% **Men** 10.9% **Minority** 58.7%
Nursing Student Activities Sigma Theta Tau.
Nursing Student Resources Academic advising; academic or career counseling; assistance for students with disabilities; bookstore; campus computer network; computer lab; computer-assisted instruction; e-mail services; interactive nursing skills videos; Internet; learning resource lab; library services; nursing audiovisuals; skills, simulation, or other laboratory; tutoring.
Library Facilities 16,781 periodical subscriptions (1,300 health-care related).

BACCALAUREATE PROGRAMS

Degree BSN
Available Programs Accelerated Baccalaureate.
Site Options Chula Vista, CA; Imperial, CA; Palm Desert, CA.
Study Options Full-time.
Program Entrance Requirements Transcript of college record, CPR certification, immunizations, 1 letter of recommendation, RN licensure. Transfer students are accepted. *Application deadline:* Applications may be processed on a rolling basis for some programs.
Advanced Placement Credit by examination available. Credit given for nursing courses completed elsewhere dependent upon specific evaluations.
Expenses (2009-10) *Tuition:* full-time $10,560. *Required fees:* full-time $600.
Contact Campus College Chair, Nursing, College of Nursing, University of Phoenix–San Diego Campus, 3870 Murphy Canyon Road, #100, San Diego, CA 92123-4403. *Telephone:* 888-867-4636.

GRADUATE PROGRAMS

Expenses (2009-10) *Tuition:* full-time $13,200. *Required fees:* full-time $760.
Financial Aid Institutionally sponsored loans and scholarships available.
Contact Campus College Chair, Nursing, College of Nursing, University of Phoenix–San Diego Campus, 3870 Murphy Canyon Road, #100, San Diego, CA 92123-4403. *Telephone:* 888-867-4636.

MASTER'S DEGREE PROGRAM

Degrees MSN; MSN/Ed D
Available Programs Master's.
Concentrations Available Health-care administration; nursing administration; nursing education.
Site Options Chula Vista, CA; Imperial, CA; Palm Desert, CA.
Study Options Full-time.
Program Entrance Requirements Clinical experience, computer literacy, minimum overall college GPA of 2.5, transcript of college record. *Application deadline:* Applications may be processed on a rolling basis for some programs. *Application fee:* $45.
Advanced Placement Credit given for nursing courses completed elsewhere dependent upon specific evaluations.
Degree Requirements 39 total credit hours, thesis or project.

University of Phoenix–Southern California Campus

College of Nursing
Costa Mesa, California

Founded in 1980

DEGREES • BSN • MSN • MSN/MBA • MSN/MHA
Nursing Program Faculty 109 (23% with doctorates).
Baccalaureate Enrollment 563 **Women** 89.2% **Men** 10.8% **Minority** 36.8%
Graduate Enrollment 379 **Women** 90.2% **Men** 9.8% **Minority** 40.9%
Nursing Student Activities Sigma Theta Tau.
Nursing Student Resources Academic advising; academic or career counseling; assistance for students with disabilities; bookstore; campus computer network; computer lab; computer-assisted instruction; e-mail services; interactive nursing skills videos; Internet; learning resource lab; library services; nursing audiovisuals; remedial services; skills, simulation, or other laboratory; tutoring.
Library Facilities 16,781 periodical subscriptions (1,300 health-care related).

BACCALAUREATE PROGRAMS

Degree BSN
Available Programs Accelerated Baccalaureate.
Site Options Diamond Bar, CA; La Marada, CA; Lancaster, CA.
Study Options Full-time.
Program Entrance Requirements Transcript of college record, CPR certification, immunizations, 1 letter of recommendation, RN licensure. Transfer students are accepted. *Application deadline:* Applications may be processed on a rolling basis for some programs.
Advanced Placement Credit by examination available. Credit given for nursing courses completed elsewhere dependent upon specific evaluations.
Expenses (2009-10) *Tuition:* full-time $11,400. *Required fees:* full-time $600.
Contact Campus College Chair, Nursing, College of Nursing, University of Phoenix–Southern California Campus, 10540 Talbert Avenue, West Tower, Suite 120, Fountain Valley, CA 92708-6027. *Telephone:* 800-697-8223.

GRADUATE PROGRAMS

Expenses (2009-10) *Tuition:* full-time $15,120. *Required fees:* full-time $760.
Financial Aid Institutionally sponsored loans and scholarships available.
Contact Campus College Chair, Nursing, College of Nursing, University of Phoenix–Southern California Campus, 10540 Talbert Avenue, West Tower, Suite 120, Fountain Valley, CA 92708-6027. *Telephone:* 800-697-8223.

MASTER'S DEGREE PROGRAM

Degrees MSN; MSN/MBA; MSN/MHA
Available Programs Master's.
Concentrations Available Health-care administration; nursing administration; nursing education. *Nurse practitioner programs in:* family health.
Site Options Diamond Bar, CA; La Marada, CA; Lancaster, CA.
Study Options Full-time.
Program Entrance Requirements Clinical experience, computer literacy, minimum overall college GPA of 2.5, transcript of college record, 1 letter of recommendation. *Application deadline:* Applications may be processed on a rolling basis for some programs. *Application fee:* $45.
Advanced Placement Credit given for nursing courses completed elsewhere dependent upon specific evaluations.
Degree Requirements 39 total credit hours, thesis or project.

POST-MASTER'S PROGRAM

Areas of Study *Nurse practitioner programs in:* family health.

CONTINUING EDUCATION PROGRAM

Contact Campus College Chair, College of Nursing, University of Phoenix–Southern California Campus, 3100 Bristol Street, Costa Mesa, CA 92626-3099. *Telephone:* 714-338-1720.

University of San Diego

Hahn School of Nursing and Health Science
San Diego, California

http://www.sandiego.edu/academics/nursing

Founded in 1949

DEGREES • DNP • MSN • PHD

Nursing Program Faculty 44 (75% with doctorates).

Graduate Enrollment 324 **Women** 87% **Men** 13% **Minority** 36% **International** 1% **Part-time** 35%

Nursing Student Activities Nursing Honor Society, Sigma Theta Tau, Student Nurses' Association.

Nursing Student Resources Academic advising; academic or career counseling; assistance for students with disabilities; bookstore; campus computer network; career placement assistance; computer lab; computer-assisted instruction; daycare for children of students; e-mail services; employment services for current students; externships; interactive nursing skills videos; Internet; learning resource lab; library services; nursing audiovisuals; resume preparation assistance; skills, simulation, or other laboratory; tutoring.

Library Facilities 704,887 volumes (47,500 in health, 24,600 in nursing); 38,488 periodical subscriptions (2,200 health-care related).

GRADUATE PROGRAMS

Expenses (2010-11) *Tuition:* full-time $29,160; part-time $1215 per credit. *Room and board:* $14,000 per academic year. *Required fees:* full-time $525; part-time $200 per term.

Financial Aid 90% of graduate students in nursing programs received some form of financial aid in 2009-10. Scholarships and traineeships available. Aid available to part-time students. *Financial aid application deadline:* 4/1.

Contact Ms. Cathleen Mumper, Director of Student Services and Admissions Officer, Hahn School of Nursing and Health Science, University of San Diego, 5998 Alcala Park, San Diego, CA 92110-2492. *Telephone:* 619-260-4548. *Fax:* 619-260-6814. *E-mail:* cmm@sandiego.edu.

MASTER'S DEGREE PROGRAM

Degree MSN

Available Programs Accelerated Master's for Non-Nursing College Graduates; Master's; Master's for Nurses with Non-Nursing Degrees.

Concentrations Available Clinical nurse leader; nursing administration; nursing education. *Clinical nurse specialist programs in:* acute care, adult health, medical-surgical. *Nurse practitioner programs in:* adult health, family health, pediatric, psychiatric/mental health.

Study Options Full-time and part-time.

Program Entrance Requirements Clinical experience, computer literacy, minimum overall college GPA of 3.0, transcript of college record, CPR certification, written essay, immunizations, interview, 3 letters of recommendation, prerequisite course work, resume, statistics course, GRE General Test (entry-level nursing). *Application deadline:* 3/1 (fall), 11/1 (spring). *Application fee:* $45.

Advanced Placement Credit by examination available. Credit given for nursing courses completed elsewhere dependent upon specific evaluations.

Degree Requirements 30–53 total units, depending on specialty.

DOCTORAL DEGREE PROGRAM

Degree DNP

Available Programs Doctorate; Post-Baccalaureate Doctorate.

Areas of Study Advanced practice nursing; family, dual pediatric/family, or dual adult/family nurse practitioner, in psychiatric-mental health as a nurse practitioner or dual preparation as a nurse practitioner/clinical nurse specialist, and preparation in adult-gerontology as a clinical nurse specialist.

Program Entrance Requirements Vary by program, contact school for more details. *Application deadline*: 3/1 (fall).

Degree Requirements 78-91 semester credits (post-baccalaureate).

Degree PhD

Available Programs Doctorate.

Areas of Study Addiction/substance abuse, advanced practice nursing, aging, bio-behavioral research, clinical practice, community health, critical care, ethics, faculty preparation, family health, gerontology,

health policy, health promotion/disease prevention, health-care systems, human health and illness, illness and transition, individualized study, information systems, maternity-newborn, nurse case management, nursing administration, nursing education, nursing policy, nursing research, nursing science, oncology, urban health, women's health.
Program Entrance Requirements Clinical experience, minimum overall college GPA of 3.5, interview by faculty committee, interview, 3 letters of recommendation, MSN or equivalent, statistics course, vita, writing sample. Application deadline: 3/1 (fall). Application fee: $45.
Degree Requirements 48 total credit hours, dissertation, residency.

See full description on page 498.

University of San Francisco

School of Nursing
San Francisco, California

http://www.usfca.edu/nursing/
Founded in 1855

DEGREES • BSN • DNP • MSN
Nursing Program Faculty 75 (80% with doctorates).
Baccalaureate Enrollment 658 **Women** 86% **Men** 14% **Minority** 57% **International** 1% **Part-time** 1%
Graduate Enrollment 388 **Women** 84% **Men** 16% **Minority** 40% **Part-time** 1%
Distance Learning Courses Available.
Nursing Student Activities Nursing Honor Society, Sigma Theta Tau, Student Nurses' Association, nursing club.
Nursing Student Resources Academic advising; academic or career counseling; assistance for students with disabilities; bookstore; campus computer network; career placement assistance; computer lab; computer-assisted instruction; e-mail services; employment services for current students; housing assistance; interactive nursing skills videos; Internet; learning resource lab; library services; nursing audiovisuals; placement services for program completers; remedial services; resume preparation assistance; skills, simulation, or other laboratory; tutoring; unpaid internships.
Library Facilities 1.1 million volumes; 5,560 periodical subscriptions (200 health-care related).

BACCALAUREATE PROGRAMS

Degree BSN
Available Programs Baccalaureate for Second Degree; Generic Baccalaureate.
Study Options Full-time.
Program Entrance Requirements Minimum overall college GPA of 3.0, transcript of college record, written essay, health insurance, high school biology, high school chemistry, 3 years high school math, 2 years high school science, high school transcript, immunizations, 2 letters of recommendation, minimum high school GPA of 3.0, prerequisite course work. Transfer students are accepted.
Advanced Placement Credit given for nursing courses completed elsewhere dependent upon specific evaluations.
Expenses (2010-11) *Tuition:* full-time $37,040; part-time $1315 per unit. *Room and board:* $12,250; room only: $8240 per academic year. *Required fees:* full-time $664.
Financial Aid 95% of baccalaureate students in nursing programs received some form of financial aid in 2009-10.
Contact Office of Undergraduate Admissions, School of Nursing, University of San Francisco, 2130 Fulton Street, San Francisco, CA 94117. *Telephone:* 800-422-6563. *Fax:* 415-422-6877. *E-mail:* admission@usfca.edu.

GRADUATE PROGRAMS

Expenses (2010-11) *Tuition:* part-time $1085 per unit. *Required fees:* full-time $525.
Financial Aid 95% of graduate students in nursing programs received some form of financial aid in 2009-10. Institutionally sponsored loans available. *Financial aid application deadline:* 3/2.
Contact Ms. Megan McDrew, Graduate Programs Outreach, School of Nursing, University of San Francisco, 2130 Fulton Street, Cowell Hall, San Francisco, CA 94117-1080. *Telephone:* 415-422-6681. *Fax:* 415-422-6877. *E-mail:* msmcdrew@usfca.edu.

MASTER'S DEGREE PROGRAM

Degree MSN
Available Programs Accelerated AD/RN to Master's; Accelerated Master's for Non-Nursing College Graduates; Master's for Nurses with Non-Nursing Degrees; RN to Master's.
Concentrations Available Clinical nurse leader.
Site Options Cupertino, CA; San Ramon, CA; Santa Rosa, CA.
Study Options Full-time.
Program Entrance Requirements Clinical experience, minimum overall college GPA of 3.5, transcript of college record, written essay, 2 letters of recommendation, prerequisite course work, resume, statistics course.
Advanced Placement Credit given for nursing courses completed elsewhere dependent upon specific evaluations.
Degree Requirements 36 total credit hours, thesis or project, comprehensive exam.

DOCTORAL DEGREE PROGRAM

Degree DNP
Available Programs Doctorate.
Areas of Study Advanced practice nursing, family health, health-care systems, nursing administration.
Program Entrance Requirements Clinical experience, minimum overall college GPA of 3.0, 3 letters of recommendation, statistics course, vita, writing sample.
Degree Requirements 48 total credit hours, dissertation, oral exam, residency.

Vanguard University of Southern California

Nursing Program
Costa Mesa, California

Founded in 1920

DEGREE • BSN
Baccalaureate Enrollment 75
Library Facilities 164,333 volumes; 17,342 periodical subscriptions.

BACCALAUREATE PROGRAMS

Degree BSN
Available Programs RN Baccalaureate.
Contact Kristi Starkey, Director of Recruitment, School for Professional Studies, Nursing Program, Vanguard University of Southern California, 55 Fair Drive, Costa Mesa, CA 92626. *Telephone:* 714-668-6130 Ext. 3902. *Fax:* 714-668-6194. *E-mail:* kstarkey@vanguard.edu.

West Coast University

Nursing Programs
North Hollywood, California

Founded in 1909

DEGREE • BSN

BACCALAUREATE PROGRAMS

Degree BSN
Available Programs Accelerated RN Baccalaureate; RN Baccalaureate.
Contact Nursing Program, Nursing Programs, West Coast University, 4021 Rosewood Avenue, Los Angeles, CA 90004. *Telephone:* 866-508-2684.

Western University of Health Sciences

College of Graduate Nursing
Pomona, California

http://www.westernu.edu/cogn.html
Founded in 1977

DEGREES • DNP • MSN
Nursing Program Faculty 25 (65% with doctorates).

Graduate Enrollment 285 **Women** 85% **Men** 15% **Minority** 54% **International** 1% **Part-time** 5%
Distance Learning Courses Available.
Nursing Student Activities Nursing Honor Society, Sigma Theta Tau, Student Nurses' Association, nursing club.
Nursing Student Resources Academic advising; academic or career counseling; assistance for students with disabilities; bookstore; campus computer network; career placement assistance; computer lab; computer-assisted instruction; e-mail services; interactive nursing skills videos; Internet; learning resource lab; library services; nursing audiovisuals; other; remedial services; resume preparation assistance; skills, simulation, or other laboratory; tutoring.
Library Facilities 17,171 volumes in health, 322 volumes in nursing; 5,000 periodical subscriptions health-care related.

GRADUATE PROGRAMS

Expenses (2009-10) *Tuition:* full-time $20,000; part-time $673 per unit. *International tuition:* $20,000 full-time. *Required fees:* full-time $1800; part-time $600 per term.
Financial Aid 80% of graduate students in nursing programs received some form of financial aid in 2008-09. Institutionally sponsored loans, scholarships, and veterans educational benefits available. *Financial aid application deadline:* 3/2.
Contact Ms. Mitzi McKay, Assistant Dean of Student Affairs, College of Graduate Nursing, Western University of Health Sciences, 309 East Second Street, Pomona, CA 91766-1854. *Telephone:* 909-469-5255. *Fax:* 909-469-5521. *E-mail:* mmckay@westernu.edu.

MASTER'S DEGREE PROGRAM

Degree MSN
Available Programs Accelerated AD/RN to Master's; Accelerated Master's; Accelerated Master's for Non-Nursing College Graduates; Master's.
Concentrations Available Clinical nurse leader; nursing administration. *Nurse practitioner programs in:* family health.
Study Options Full-time and part-time.
Online Degree Options Yes (online only).
Program Entrance Requirements Computer literacy, minimum overall college GPA of 3.0, transcript of college record, CPR certification, written essay, immunizations, interview, 3 letters of recommendation, prerequisite course work, resume, statistics course, GRE General Test. *Application deadline:* 3/1 (fall). Applications may be processed on a rolling basis for some programs. *Application fee:* $60.
Advanced Placement Credit given for nursing courses completed elsewhere dependent upon specific evaluations.
Degree Requirements 50 total credit hours, thesis or project.

POST-MASTER'S PROGRAM

Areas of Study *Nurse practitioner programs in:* family health.

DOCTORAL DEGREE PROGRAM

Degree DNP
Available Programs Doctorate.
Online Degree Options Yes (online only).
Program Entrance Requirements Minimum overall college GPA of 3.0, 3 letters of recommendation, MSN or equivalent, scholarly papers, statistics course, vita, writing sample. Application deadline: 3/1 (fall). Applications may be processed on a rolling basis for some programs. Application fee: $60.
Degree Requirements 30 total credit hours, dissertation.

COLORADO

Adams State College

Nursing Program
Alamosa, Colorado

Founded in 1921

DEGREE • BSN

Nursing Program Faculty 10 (10% with doctorates).
Baccalaureate Enrollment 67 **Women** 89% **Men** 11% **Minority** 48% **International** 1% **Part-time** 39%
Nursing Student Activities Nursing Honor Society, Sigma Theta Tau, Student Nurses' Association.
Nursing Student Resources Academic advising; academic or career counseling; assistance for students with disabilities; bookstore; campus computer network; computer lab; computer-assisted instruction; daycare for children of students; e-mail services; employment services for current students; housing assistance; interactive nursing skills videos; Internet; learning resource lab; library services; nursing audiovisuals; remedial services; resume preparation assistance; skills, simulation, or other laboratory; tutoring; unpaid internships.
Library Facilities 125,288 volumes (565 in health, 565 in nursing); 16,724 periodical subscriptions (200 health-care related).

BACCALAUREATE PROGRAMS

Degree BSN
Available Programs Generic Baccalaureate; RN Baccalaureate.
Site Options Salida, CO; Trinidad, CO.
Study Options Full-time.
Program Entrance Requirements Minimum overall college GPA of 3.0, transcript of college record, written essay, immunizations, interview, 2 letters of recommendation, minimum GPA in nursing prerequisites of 3.0, prerequisite course work. Transfer students are accepted. *Application deadline:* 8/1 (fall).
Advanced Placement Credit by examination available. Credit given for nursing courses completed elsewhere dependent upon specific evaluations.
Expenses (2010-11) *Tuition, area resident:* full-time $2952; part-time $123 per credit hour. *Tuition, nonresident:* full-time $12,912; part-time $538 per credit hour. *Room and board:* $3980; room only: $2100 per academic year. *Required fees:* full-time $2016; part-time $84 per credit; part-time $1008 per term.
Financial Aid 90% of baccalaureate students in nursing programs received some form of financial aid in 2009-10.
Contact Amanda Jojola, Director of Nursing, Nursing Program, Adams State College, 208 Edgemont Boulevard, Alamosa, CO 81102. *Telephone:* 719-587-8134. *Fax:* 719-587-7522. *E-mail:* aidasahud@adams.edu.

American Sentinel University

RN to Bachelor of Science Nursing
Aurora, Colorado

Founded in 1988

DEGREES • BSN • MSN

Distance Learning Courses Available.

BACCALAUREATE PROGRAMS

Degree BSN
Available Programs RN Baccalaureate.
Program Entrance Requirements Transcript of college record, RN licensure.
Expenses (2010-11) *Tuition:* part-time $370 per credit hour. *Required fees:* part-time $55 per term.
Contact Dr. Catherine Garner, Provost and Dean of Health Sciences and Nursing. *Telephone:* 866-922-5690.

GRADUATE PROGRAMS

Expenses (2010-11) *Tuition:* part-time $450 per credit hour. *Required fees:* part-time $55 per term.
Contact Dr. Catherine Garner, Provost and Dean of Health Sciences and Nursing. *Telephone:* 866-922-5690.

MASTER'S DEGREE PROGRAM

Degree MSN
Available Programs Master's.
Concentrations Available Nurse case management; nursing administration; nursing education; nursing informatics.
Program Entrance Requirements Transcript of college record.
Degree Requirements 36 total credit hours.

Colorado State University–Pueblo

Department of Nursing
Pueblo, Colorado

Founded in 1933

DEGREES • BSN • MS

Nursing Program Faculty 30 (10% with doctorates).

Baccalaureate Enrollment 134 **Women** 90% **Men** 10% **Minority** 42% **International** 1% **Part-time** 2%

Graduate Enrollment 26 **Women** 73% **Men** 27% **Minority** 50% **Part-time** 92%

Nursing Student Activities Sigma Theta Tau, Student Nurses' Association.

Nursing Student Resources Academic advising; academic or career counseling; assistance for students with disabilities; bookstore; campus computer network; computer lab; computer-assisted instruction; daycare for children of students; e-mail services; employment services for current students; housing assistance; Internet; learning resource lab; library services; nursing audiovisuals; remedial services; resume preparation assistance; skills, simulation, or other laboratory; tutoring.

Library Facilities 274,890 volumes (2,891 in health, 1,168 in nursing); 14,672 periodical subscriptions (101 health-care related).

BACCALAUREATE PROGRAMS

Degree BSN

Available Programs ADN to Baccalaureate; Accelerated Baccalaureate for Second Degree; Accelerated RN Baccalaureate; Baccalaureate for Second Degree; Generic Baccalaureate; LPN to Baccalaureate; LPN to RN Baccalaureate; RN Baccalaureate.

Study Options Full-time.

Program Entrance Requirements Minimum overall college GPA of 2.75, transcript of college record, CPR certification, health exam, immunizations, minimum GPA in nursing prerequisites of 2.75, professional liability insurance/malpractice insurance, prerequisite course work. Transfer students are accepted. *Application deadline:* 5/25 (fall), 10/1 (summer). *Application fee:* $25.

Advanced Placement Credit by examination available. Credit given for nursing courses completed elsewhere dependent upon specific evaluations.

Contact ***Telephone:*** 719-549-2422. *Fax:* 719-549-2113.

GRADUATE PROGRAMS

Contact ***Telephone:*** 719-549-2502. *Fax:* 719-549-2949.

MASTER'S DEGREE PROGRAM

Degree MS

Available Programs Master's.

Concentrations Available Nursing education. *Clinical nurse specialist programs in:* acute care, psychiatric/mental health. *Nurse practitioner programs in:* acute care, family health, pediatric.

Study Options Full-time and part-time.

Program Entrance Requirements Clinical experience, computer literacy, minimum overall college GPA of 3.0, transcript of college record, CPR certification, written essay, immunizations, 3 letters of recommendation, nursing research course, professional liability insurance/malpractice insurance, prerequisite course work, resume, statistics course. *Application deadline:* 5/25 (fall). *Application fee:* $35.

Advanced Placement Credit given for nursing courses completed elsewhere dependent upon specific evaluations.

Degree Requirements 46 total credit hours, thesis or project, comprehensive exam.

POST-MASTER'S PROGRAM

Areas of Study Nursing education. *Clinical nurse specialist programs in:* acute care, psychiatric/mental health. *Nurse practitioner programs in:* acute care; family health, pediatric.

Denver College of Nursing

Denver College of Nursing
Denver, Colorado

DEGREE • BSN

Nursing Program Faculty 47 (11% with doctorates).

Baccalaureate Enrollment 185 **Women** 82% **Men** 18% **Minority** 23% **International** 1% **Part-time** 2%

Nursing Student Activities Student Nurses' Association.

Nursing Student Resources Academic advising; academic or career counseling; assistance for students with disabilities; bookstore; campus computer network; career placement assistance; computer lab; computer-assisted instruction; e-mail services; employment services for current students; externships; interactive nursing skills videos; Internet; learning resource lab; library services; nursing audiovisuals; placement services for program completers; remedial services; resume preparation assistance; skills, simulation, or other laboratory; tutoring.

Library Facilities 1,000 volumes in health, 1,000 volumes in nursing; 10,000 periodical subscriptions health-care related.

BACCALAUREATE PROGRAMS

Degree BSN

Available Programs Generic Baccalaureate; RN Baccalaureate.

Site Options Denver, CO.

Contact Dr. Deb Banik, Dean of Nursing Education Programs, Denver College of Nursing, 1401 19th Street, Denver, CO 80202. *Telephone:* 888-479-5550. *Fax:* 720-974-0290. *E-mail:* d.banik@denverschoolof-nursing.org.

Mesa State College

Department of Nursing and Radiologic Sciences
Grand Junction, Colorado

http://www.mesastate.edu/schools/sbps/nars/index.htm

Founded in 1925

DEGREE • BSN

Nursing Program Faculty 40 (7% with doctorates).

Baccalaureate Enrollment 190 **Women** 88% **Men** 12% **Minority** 11% **International** 4% **Part-time** 8%

Distance Learning Courses Available.

Nursing Student Activities Sigma Theta Tau, Student Nurses' Association.

Nursing Student Resources Academic advising; academic or career counseling; assistance for students with disabilities; bookstore; campus computer network; career placement assistance; computer lab; computer-assisted instruction; daycare for children of students; e-mail services; employment services for current students; housing assistance; interactive nursing skills videos; Internet; learning resource lab; library services; nursing audiovisuals; placement services for program completers; resume preparation assistance; skills, simulation, or other laboratory; tutoring; unpaid internships.

Library Facilities 260,784 volumes (7,500 in health, 6,576 in nursing); 31,992 periodical subscriptions (100 health-care related).

BACCALAUREATE PROGRAMS

Degree BSN

Available Programs ADN to Baccalaureate; Generic Baccalaureate; LPN to Baccalaureate; LPN to RN Baccalaureate; RN Baccalaureate.

Study Options Full-time and part-time.

Online Degree Options Yes.

Program Entrance Requirements Minimum overall college GPA of 2.0, transcript of college record, CPR certification, health exam, immunizations, minimum GPA in nursing prerequisites of 2.0, professional liability insurance/malpractice insurance, prerequisite course work. Transfer students are accepted. *Application deadline:* 3/1 (fall), 10/1 (spring).

Advanced Placement Credit by examination available. Credit given for nursing courses completed elsewhere dependent upon specific evaluations.

Expenses (2009-10) *Tuition, state resident:* full-time $5509; part-time $230 per credit hour. *Tuition, nonresident:* full-time $11,707; part-time $488 per credit hour. *Room and board:* $8515 per academic year. *Required fees:* full-time $591; part-time $25 per credit.

Financial Aid 90% of baccalaureate students in nursing programs received some form of financial aid in 2008-09. *Gift aid (need-based):* Federal Pell, FSEOG, state, private, college/university gift aid from institutional funds. *Loans:* Federal Direct (Subsidized and Unsubsidized Stafford PLUS), Perkins. *Work-study:* Federal Work-Study, part-time campus jobs. *Financial aid application deadline:* Continuous.

Contact Dr. Alma Jackson, Program Director, Department of Nursing and Radiologic Sciences, Mesa State College, 1100 North Avenue, Grand

Junction, CO 81501. *Telephone:* 970-248-1840. *Fax:* 970-248-1133. *E-mail:* ajackson@mesastate.edu.

Metropolitan State College of Denver
Department of Health Professions
Denver, Colorado

http://www.mscd.edu/~nursing
Founded in 1963

DEGREE • BS

Nursing Program Faculty 10 (10% with doctorates).
Baccalaureate Enrollment 124 **Women** 89% **Men** 11% **Minority** 17% **International** 2% **Part-time** 63%
Distance Learning Courses Available.
Nursing Student Activities Nursing club.
Nursing Student Resources Academic advising; academic or career counseling; assistance for students with disabilities; bookstore; campus computer network; computer lab; computer-assisted instruction; daycare for children of students; e-mail services; interactive nursing skills videos; Internet; library services; nursing audiovisuals; remedial services; resume preparation assistance; skills, simulation, or other laboratory.
Library Facilities 607,971 volumes (21,503 in health); 2,380 periodical subscriptions (204 health-care related).

BACCALAUREATE PROGRAMS

Degree BS
Available Programs ADN to Baccalaureate; RN Baccalaureate.
Study Options Full-time and part-time.
Program Entrance Requirements Transcript of college record, CPR certification, written essay, immunizations, minimum GPA in nursing prerequisites of 2.5, professional liability insurance/malpractice insurance, prerequisite course work, RN licensure. Transfer students are accepted.
Advanced Placement Credit given for nursing courses completed elsewhere dependent upon specific evaluations.
Contact ***Telephone:*** 303-556-4391. *Fax:* 303-556-5165.

Platt College
School of Nursing
Aurora, Colorado

Founded in 1986

DEGREE • BSN

Nursing Program Faculty 8 (2% with doctorates).
Baccalaureate Enrollment 134 **Women** 90% **Men** 10% **Minority** 2.5%
Nursing Student Activities Student Nurses' Association.
Nursing Student Resources Academic advising; academic or career counseling; assistance for students with disabilities; campus computer network; career placement assistance; housing assistance; Internet; learning resource lab; library services; nursing audiovisuals; resume preparation assistance; skills, simulation, or other laboratory; tutoring; unpaid internships.
Library Facilities 1,000 volumes in health, 888 volumes in nursing; 12 periodical subscriptions health-care related.

BACCALAUREATE PROGRAMS

Degree BSN
Available Programs Accelerated Baccalaureate.
Study Options Full-time.
Program Entrance Requirements Transcript of college record, CPR certification, written essay, health exam, health insurance, high school transcript, interview, letters of recommendation, minimum GPA in nursing prerequisites. Transfer students are accepted. *Application deadline:* 7/15 (fall), 11/15 (winter), 2/15 (spring), 5/15 (summer). Applications may be processed on a rolling basis for some programs. *Application fee:* $50.
Advanced Placement Credit by examination available. Credit given for nursing courses completed elsewhere dependent upon specific evaluations.
Expenses (2009-10) *Tuition:* full-time $15,500; part-time $338 per quarter hour.
Financial Aid 98% of baccalaureate students in nursing programs received some form of financial aid in 2008-09. *Gift aid (need-based):* Federal Pell, FSEOG. *Loans:* Perkins. *Financial aid application deadline:* Continuous.
Contact Ms. Barb Jones, BSN Coordinator, School of Nursing, Platt College, 3100 South Parker Road, Aurora, CO 80014. *Telephone:* 303-369-5151. *E-mail:* BarbJones@plattcolorado.edu.

Regis University
School of Nursing
Denver, Colorado

Founded in 1877

DEGREES • BSN • MS

Nursing Program Faculty 18 (55% with doctorates).
Distance Learning Courses Available.
Nursing Student Activities Nursing Honor Society, Sigma Theta Tau, Student Nurses' Association.
Nursing Student Resources Academic advising; academic or career counseling; assistance for students with disabilities; bookstore; campus computer network; computer lab; computer-assisted instruction; e-mail services; interactive nursing skills videos; Internet; learning resource lab; library services; nursing audiovisuals; resume preparation assistance; skills, simulation, or other laboratory; tutoring; unpaid internships.
Library Facilities 350,000 volumes; 20,800 periodical subscriptions.

BACCALAUREATE PROGRAMS

Degree BSN
Available Programs Accelerated Baccalaureate; Generic Baccalaureate; RN Baccalaureate.
Site Options Cheyenne, WY.
Study Options Full-time.
Program Entrance Requirements Minimum overall college GPA of 2.5, transcript of college record, written essay, 2 letters of recommendation, prerequisite course work. Transfer students are accepted.
Advanced Placement Credit by examination available.
Contact ***Telephone:*** 303-964-5178. *Fax:* 303-964-5400.

GRADUATE PROGRAMS

Contact ***Telephone:*** 303-458-3534. *Fax:* 303-964-5400.

MASTER'S DEGREE PROGRAM

Degree MS
Available Programs Master's; RN to Master's.
Concentrations Available Health-care administration; nursing administration; nursing education. *Nurse practitioner programs in:* family health, neonatal health.
Study Options Full-time and part-time.
Online Degree Options Yes.
Program Entrance Requirements Minimum overall college GPA of 2.75, transcript of college record, written essay, 3 letters of recommendation, prerequisite course work, statistics course.
Advanced Placement Credit by examination available.
Degree Requirements 42 total credit hours, thesis or project.

University of Colorado at Colorado Springs
Beth-El College of Nursing and Health Sciences
Colorado Springs, Colorado

http://www.uccs.edu/~bethel/
Founded in 1965

DEGREES • BSN • DNP • MSN

Nursing Program Faculty 43 (32% with doctorates).
Baccalaureate Enrollment 332 **Women** 92% **Men** 8% **Minority** 6.5% **Part-time** 5%
Graduate Enrollment 155 **Women** 94% **Men** 6% **Minority** 8% **Part-time** 38%
Distance Learning Courses Available.
Nursing Student Activities Nursing Honor Society, Sigma Theta Tau, Student Nurses' Association, nursing club.

Nursing Student Resources Academic advising; academic or career counseling; assistance for students with disabilities; bookstore; campus computer network; career placement assistance; computer lab; computer-assisted instruction; daycare for children of students; e-mail services; employment services for current students; externships; housing assistance; interactive nursing skills videos; Internet; learning resource lab; library services; nursing audiovisuals; resume preparation assistance; skills, simulation, or other laboratory; tutoring; unpaid internships.
Library Facilities 391,638 volumes (10,454 in health, 1,040 in nursing); 2,201 periodical subscriptions (331 health-care related).

BACCALAUREATE PROGRAMS

Degree BSN
Available Programs Accelerated Baccalaureate for Second Degree; Generic Baccalaureate; RN Baccalaureate.
Study Options Full-time.
Online Degree Options Yes.
Program Entrance Requirements Minimum overall college GPA of 3.3, transcript of college record, CPR certification, health insurance, high school biology, high school chemistry, high school foreign language, 3 years high school math, 1 year of high school science, high school transcript, immunizations, minimum high school GPA of 3.3, minimum GPA in nursing prerequisites of 3.0. Transfer students are accepted. *Application deadline:* Applications may be processed on a rolling basis for some programs. *Application fee:* $50.
Advanced Placement Credit given for nursing courses completed elsewhere dependent upon specific evaluations.
Expenses (2009-10) *Tuition, area resident:* full-time $6312; part-time $263 per credit hour. *Tuition, nonresident:* full-time $7800; part-time $780 per credit hour. *Room and board:* $4330; room only: $3745 per academic year. *Required fees:* full-time $1004; part-time $501 per term.
Financial Aid 68% of baccalaureate students in nursing programs received some form of financial aid in 2008-09. *Gift aid (need-based):* Federal Pell, FSEOG, state, private, college/university gift aid from institutional funds. *Loans:* Perkins. *Work-study:* Federal Work-Study, part-time campus jobs. *Financial aid application deadline (priority):* 3/1.
Contact Linda Goodwin, Advisor, Baccalaureate Nursing and Health Sciences, Beth-El College of Nursing and Health Sciences, University of Colorado at Colorado Springs, 1420 Austin Bluffs Parkway, Colorado Springs, CO 80918. *Telephone:* 719-255-3867. *Fax:* 719-255-3645. *E-mail:* lgoodwin@uccs.edu.

GRADUATE PROGRAMS

Expenses (2009-10) *Tuition, area resident:* full-time $5883; part-time $684 per credit hour. *Tuition, nonresident:* full-time $9686; part-time $1154 per credit hour. *Required fees:* full-time $2019.
Financial Aid 27% of graduate students in nursing programs received some form of financial aid in 2008-09.
Contact Diane Busch, Program Assistant, Nursing Department, Beth-El College of Nursing and Health Sciences, University of Colorado at Colorado Springs, 1420 Austin Bluffs Parkway, Colorado Springs, CO 80918. *Telephone:* 719-255-4424. *Fax:* 719-255-4496. *E-mail:* dbusch@uccs.edu.

MASTER'S DEGREE PROGRAM

Degree MSN
Available Programs Master's.
Concentrations Available *Clinical nurse specialist programs in:* adult health. *Nurse practitioner programs in:* adult health, family health.
Study Options Full-time and part-time.
Online Degree Options Yes (online only).
Program Entrance Requirements Clinical experience, computer literacy, minimum overall college GPA of 3.0, transcript of college record, CPR certification, immunizations, 4 letters of recommendation, nursing research course, physical assessment course, professional liability insurance/malpractice insurance, prerequisite course work, resume, statistics course. *Application deadline:* 7/1 (fall), 11/1 (spring). *Application fee:* $60.
Advanced Placement Credit given for nursing courses completed elsewhere dependent upon specific evaluations.
Degree Requirements 47 total credit hours, thesis or project, comprehensive exam.

POST-MASTER'S PROGRAM

Areas of Study Nursing education. *Clinical nurse specialist programs in:* adult health. *Nurse practitioner programs in:* adult health, family health.

DOCTORAL DEGREE PROGRAM

Degree DNP
Available Programs Doctorate.
Areas of Study Forensic nursing, gerontology, individualized study.
Online Degree Options Yes (online only).
Program Entrance Requirements Clinical experience, minimum overall college GPA of 3.3, interview, 3 letters of recommendation, MSN or equivalent, statistics course, vita. Application deadline: 3/1 (summer). Application fee: $60.
Degree Requirements 36 total credit hours, written exam, residency.

CONTINUING EDUCATION PROGRAM

Contact Dr. William Crouch, Director, Extended Studies, Beth-El College of Nursing and Health Sciences, University of Colorado at Colorado Springs, 1420 Austin Bluffs Parkway, Colorado Springs, CO 80918. *Telephone:* 719-255-4651. *Fax:* 719-255-4284. *E-mail:* wcrouch@uccs.edu.

University of Colorado Denver
College of Nursing
Denver, Colorado

http://www.nursing.ucdenver.edu/
Founded in 1912

DEGREES • BS • MS • PHD

Nursing Program Faculty 82 (63% with doctorates).
Baccalaureate Enrollment 416 **Women** 92% **Men** 8% **Minority** 16% **Part-time** 9%
Graduate Enrollment 230 **Women** 93% **Men** 7% **Minority** 13% **International** 1% **Part-time** 18%
Distance Learning Courses Available.
Nursing Student Activities Sigma Theta Tau, Student Nurses' Association, nursing club.
Nursing Student Resources Academic advising; academic or career counseling; assistance for students with disabilities; bookstore; campus computer network; computer lab; computer-assisted instruction; e-mail services; externships; interactive nursing skills videos; Internet; learning resource lab; library services; nursing audiovisuals; paid internships; remedial services; skills, simulation, or other laboratory; tutoring; unpaid internships.
Library Facilities 1,000 volumes in health, 40 volumes in nursing; 200 periodical subscriptions health-care related.

BACCALAUREATE PROGRAMS

Degree BS
Available Programs Generic Baccalaureate; RN Baccalaureate.
Site Options Aurora, CO.
Study Options Full-time and part-time.
Online Degree Options Yes.
Program Entrance Requirements Minimum overall college GPA of 3.0, transcript of college record, written essay, health exam, health insurance, immunizations, minimum GPA in nursing prerequisites of 3.0, prerequisite course work. Transfer students are accepted. *Application deadline:* 6/15 (spring), 9/15 (summer). *Application fee:* $65.
Advanced Placement Credit given for nursing courses completed elsewhere dependent upon specific evaluations.
Expenses (2010-11) *Tuition, state resident:* full-time $21,120. *Tuition, nonresident:* full-time $54,054. *Required fees:* full-time $7632; part-time $3816 per term.
Financial Aid 60% of baccalaureate students in nursing programs received some form of financial aid in 2009-10.
Contact Ms. Julie Aguilar, Admissions Manager, College of Nursing, University of Colorado Denver, 13120 East 19th Avenue, Box C288-6, Aurora, CO 80045. *Telephone:* 303-724-1484. *Fax:* 303-724-1710. *E-mail:* julie.aguilar@ucdenver.edu.

GRADUATE PROGRAMS

Expenses (2010-11) *Tuition, state resident:* full-time $460; part-time $460 per credit. *Tuition, nonresident:* full-time $979; part-time $979 per credit. *International tuition:* $979 full-time. *Required fees:* full-time $4626.
Financial Aid 40% of graduate students in nursing programs received some form of financial aid in 2009-10. Fellowships, research assistantships, teaching assistantships, career-related internships or fieldwork,

Federal Work-Study, and institutionally sponsored loans available. Aid available to part-time students. *Financial aid application deadline:* 3/15.
Contact Ms. Julie Aguilar, Admissions Manager, College of Nursing, University of Colorado Denver, 13120 East 19th Avenue, Box C288-6, Aurora, CO 80045. *Telephone:* 303-724-1484. *Fax:* 303-724-1710. *E-mail:* julie.aguilar@ucdenver.edu.

MASTER'S DEGREE PROGRAM

Degree MS
Available Programs Master's; RN to Master's.
Concentrations Available Nurse-midwifery; nursing administration; nursing informatics. *Clinical nurse specialist programs in:* acute care, adult health, palliative care. *Nurse practitioner programs in:* adult health, family health, pediatric, psychiatric/mental health, women's health.
Site Options Aurora, CO.
Study Options Full-time and part-time.
Online Degree Options Yes.
Program Entrance Requirements Computer literacy, minimum overall college GPA of 3.0, transcript of college record, written essay, immunizations, 4 letters of recommendation, nursing research course, resume, statistics course. *Application deadline:* 9/1 (fall), 4/1 (spring). *Application fee:* $65.
Advanced Placement Credit given for nursing courses completed elsewhere dependent upon specific evaluations.
Degree Requirements 35 total credit hours, comprehensive exam.

POST-MASTER'S PROGRAM

Areas of Study Nurse-midwifery; nursing administration; nursing informatics. *Clinical nurse specialist programs in:* acute care, adult health, palliative care. *Nurse practitioner programs in:* adult health, family health, pediatric, psychiatric/mental health, women's health.

DOCTORAL DEGREE PROGRAM

Degree PhD
Available Programs Doctorate; Post-Baccalaureate Doctorate.
Areas of Study Bio-behavioral research, health-care systems, human health and illness, illness and transition, individualized study, nursing research, nursing science.
Site Options Aurora, CO.
Program Entrance Requirements Minimum overall college GPA of 3.5, interview by faculty committee, interview, 4 letters of recommendation, MSN or equivalent, statistics course, vita, writing sample. Application deadline: 4/15 (spring). Application fee: $65.
Degree Requirements 75 total credit hours, dissertation, oral exam, written exam.

POSTDOCTORAL PROGRAM

Areas of Study Adolescent health, cancer care, community health, gerontology, individualized study, information systems, nursing informatics, nursing interventions, nursing research, nursing science, outcomes, vulnerable population.
Postdoctoral Program Contact Ms. Julie Aguilar, Admissions Manager, College of Nursing, University of Colorado Denver, 13120 East 19th Avenue, Box C288-6, Aurora, CO 80045. *Telephone:* 303-724-1484. *Fax:* 303-724-1450. *E-mail:* julie.aguilar@ucdenver.edu.

CONTINUING EDUCATION PROGRAM

Contact Ms. Jennifer Disabato, Manager, Extended Studies, College of Nursing, University of Colorado Denver, 13120 East 19th Avenue, Box C288-6, Aurora, CO 80045. *Telephone:* 303-724-1529. *Fax:* 303-724-1372. *E-mail:* jennifer.disabato@ucdenver.edu.

University of Northern Colorado

School of Nursing
Greeley, Colorado

http://www.unco.edu/nursing
Founded in 1890

DEGREES • BS • MS • PHD

Nursing Program Faculty 52 (60% with doctorates).
Baccalaureate Enrollment 216 **Women** 94% **Men** 6% **Minority** 18%
Graduate Enrollment 57 **Women** 98% **Men** 2% **Minority** 10% **Part-time** 60%
Distance Learning Courses Available.
Nursing Student Activities Sigma Theta Tau, Student Nurses' Association.
Nursing Student Resources Academic advising; academic or career counseling; assistance for students with disabilities; bookstore; campus computer network; career placement assistance; computer lab; computer-assisted instruction; e-mail services; employment services for current students; housing assistance; interactive nursing skills videos; Internet; learning resource lab; library services; nursing audiovisuals; paid internships; placement services for program completers; resume preparation assistance; skills, simulation, or other laboratory; tutoring.
Library Facilities 1 million volumes (43,602 in health, 25,700 in nursing); 3,417 periodical subscriptions (140 health-care related).

BACCALAUREATE PROGRAMS

Degree BS
Available Programs Accelerated Baccalaureate; Generic Baccalaureate; RN Baccalaureate.
Site Options Greeley, CO.
Study Options Full-time.
Program Entrance Requirements Minimum overall college GPA of 3.0, transcript of college record, CPR certification, health exam, immunizations, 2 letters of recommendation, minimum GPA in nursing prerequisites of 3.0, professional liability insurance/malpractice insurance, prerequisite course work. Transfer students are accepted.
Advanced Placement Credit given for nursing courses completed elsewhere dependent upon specific evaluations.
Financial Aid 70% of baccalaureate students in nursing programs received some form of financial aid in 2008-09.
Contact Dr. Audrey Bopp, Assistant Director, School of Nursing, University of Northern Colorado, Gunter Hall, Box 125, Greeley, CO 80639. *Telephone:* 970-351-2293. *Fax:* 970-351-1707. *E-mail:* Audrey.Bopp@unco.edu.

GRADUATE PROGRAMS

Financial Aid 80% of graduate students in nursing programs received some form of financial aid in 2008-09. 7 research assistantships (averaging $6,183 per year), 1 teaching assistantship (averaging $2,849 per year) were awarded; fellowships, unspecified assistantships also available. *Financial aid application deadline:* 3/1.
Contact Dr. Janice Hayes, Graduate Program Assistant Director and Professor, School of Nursing, University of Northern Colorado, Gunter Hall, Box 125, Greeley, CO 80639. *Telephone:* 970-351-2293. *Fax:* 970-351-1707. *E-mail:* janice.hayes@unco.edu.

MASTER'S DEGREE PROGRAM

Degree MS
Available Programs Master's.
Concentrations Available Nursing education. *Clinical nurse specialist programs in:* family health. *Nurse practitioner programs in:* family health.
Site Options Greeley, CO.
Study Options Full-time and part-time.
Online Degree Options Yes (online only).
Program Entrance Requirements Clinical experience, minimum overall college GPA of 3.0, transcript of college record, CPR certification, immunizations, 2 letters of recommendation, GRE General Test.
Advanced Placement Credit given for nursing courses completed elsewhere dependent upon specific evaluations.
Degree Requirements 45 total credit hours, thesis or project, comprehensive exam.

POST-MASTER'S PROGRAM

Areas of Study Nursing education. *Nurse practitioner programs in:* family health.

DOCTORAL DEGREE PROGRAM

Degree PhD
Available Programs Doctorate.
Areas of Study Nursing education.
Site Options Greeley, CO.
Online Degree Options Yes (online only).
Program Entrance Requirements Clinical experience, minimum overall college GPA of 3.0, 2 letters of recommendation, MSN or equivalent, vita, writing sample, GRE General Test.
Degree Requirements 60 total credit hours, dissertation.

University of Phoenix–Denver Campus
College of Nursing
Lone Tree, Colorado

DEGREES • BSN • MSN • MSN/ED D • MSN/MHA
Nursing Program Faculty 19 (5% with doctorates).
Baccalaureate Enrollment 330 **Women** 86.7% **Men** 13.3% **Minority** 23.3%
Graduate Enrollment 19 **Women** 78.9% **Men** 21.1% **Minority** 21.05%
Nursing Student Activities Sigma Theta Tau.
Nursing Student Resources Academic advising; academic or career counseling; assistance for students with disabilities; bookstore; campus computer network; computer lab; computer-assisted instruction; e-mail services; interactive nursing skills videos; Internet; learning resource lab; library services; nursing audiovisuals; remedial services; skills, simulation, or other laboratory; tutoring.
Library Facilities 16,781 periodical subscriptions (1,300 health-care related).

BACCALAUREATE PROGRAMS
Degree BSN
Available Programs Accelerated Baccalaureate; LPN to Baccalaureate.
Site Options Westminister, CO; Aurora, CO; Ft. Collins, CO.
Study Options Full-time.
Program Entrance Requirements Transcript of college record, CPR certification, immunizations, 1 letter of recommendation, RN licensure. Transfer students are accepted. *Application deadline:* Applications may be processed on a rolling basis for some programs.
Advanced Placement Credit by examination available. Credit given for nursing courses completed elsewhere dependent upon specific evaluations.
Expenses (2009-10) *Tuition:* full-time $8820. *Required fees:* full-time $600.
Contact Campus College Chair, Nursing, College of Nursing, University of Phoenix–Denver Campus, 10004 Park Meadow Drive, Lone Tree, CO 80124-5453. *Telephone:* 303-694-9093.

GRADUATE PROGRAMS
Expenses (2009-10) *Tuition:* full-time $12,480. *Required fees:* full-time $760.
Financial Aid Institutionally sponsored loans and scholarships available.
Contact Campus College Chair, Nursing, College of Nursing, University of Phoenix–Denver Campus, 10004 Park Meadow Drive, Lone Tree, CO 80124-5453. *Telephone:* 303-694-9003.

MASTER'S DEGREE PROGRAM
Degrees MSN; MSN/Ed D; MSN/MHA
Available Programs Master's.
Concentrations Available Nursing administration; nursing education.
Site Options Westminister, CO; Aurora, CO.
Study Options Full-time.
Program Entrance Requirements Clinical experience, computer literacy, minimum overall college GPA of 2.5, transcript of college record. *Application deadline:* Applications may be processed on a rolling basis for some programs. *Application fee:* $45.
Advanced Placement Credit given for nursing courses completed elsewhere dependent upon specific evaluations.
Degree Requirements 39 total credit hours, thesis or project.

University of Phoenix–Southern Colorado Campus
College of Nursing
Colorado Springs, Colorado

Founded in 1999
Nursing Program Faculty 2
Nursing Student Activities Sigma Theta Tau.
Nursing Student Resources Academic advising; academic or career counseling; assistance for students with disabilities; bookstore; campus computer network; computer lab; computer-assisted instruction; e-mail services; interactive nursing skills videos; Internet; learning resource lab; library services; nursing audiovisuals; remedial services; skills, simulation, or other laboratory; tutoring.
Library Facilities 16,781 periodical subscriptions (1,300 health-care related).

CONNECTICUT

Central Connecticut State University
Department of Nursing
New Britain, Connecticut

Founded in 1849
DEGREE • BSN
Nursing Program Faculty 4 (100% with doctorates).
Nursing Student Activities Sigma Theta Tau, nursing club.
Nursing Student Resources Academic advising; academic or career counseling; assistance for students with disabilities; bookstore; campus computer network; career placement assistance; computer lab; computer-assisted instruction; e-mail services; employment services for current students; externships; Internet; learning resource lab; library services; nursing audiovisuals; resume preparation assistance; skills, simulation, or other laboratory; tutoring.
Library Facilities 725,978 volumes; 40,128 periodical subscriptions.

BACCALAUREATE PROGRAMS
Degree BSN
Available Programs Generic Baccalaureate; RN Baccalaureate.
Site Options New Britain, CT.
Study Options Full-time and part-time.
Program Entrance Requirements Minimum overall college GPA of 2.7, CPR certification, health exam, high school transcript, immunizations, minimum GPA in nursing prerequisites of 2.7, prerequisite course work. Transfer students are accepted.
Advanced Placement Credit given for nursing courses completed elsewhere dependent upon specific evaluations.
Contact ***Telephone:*** 860-832-2147. *Fax:* 860-832-2188.

Fairfield University
School of Nursing
Fairfield, Connecticut

http://www.fairfield.edu/son/
Founded in 1942
DEGREES • BS • DNP • MSN
Nursing Program Faculty 51 (85% with doctorates).
Baccalaureate Enrollment 422 **Women** 93% **Men** 7% **Minority** 18% **International** 1% **Part-time** 21%
Graduate Enrollment 164 **Women** 89% **Men** 11% **Minority** 15% **International** 1% **Part-time** 98%
Nursing Student Activities Nursing Honor Society, Sigma Theta Tau, Student Nurses' Association.
Nursing Student Resources Academic advising; academic or career counseling; assistance for students with disabilities; bookstore; campus computer network; career placement assistance; computer lab; computer-assisted instruction; daycare for children of students; e-mail services; interactive nursing skills videos; Internet; learning resource lab; library services; nursing audiovisuals; placement services for program completers; resume preparation assistance; skills, simulation, or other laboratory; tutoring; unpaid internships.
Library Facilities 394,600 volumes (5,643 in health, 4,282 in nursing); 34,400 periodical subscriptions (270 health-care related).

BACCALAUREATE PROGRAMS
Degree BS
Available Programs Accelerated Baccalaureate for Second Degree; Generic Baccalaureate; RN Baccalaureate.
Site Options West Haven, CT.
Study Options Full-time.

Program Entrance Requirements Written essay, health exam, health insurance, high school biology, high school chemistry, high school foreign language, 3 years high school math, 3 years high school science, high school transcript, immunizations, 1 letter of recommendation, minimum high school GPA of 3.0. Transfer students are accepted. *Application deadline:* 1/15 (fall). *Application fee:* $60.

Advanced Placement Credit given for nursing courses completed elsewhere dependent upon specific evaluations.

Expenses (2010-11) *Tuition:* full-time $19,225; part-time $525 per credit hour. *Room and board:* $11,740; room only: $7010 per academic year. *Required fees:* full-time $590.

Financial Aid 70% of baccalaureate students in nursing programs received some form of financial aid in 2009-10. *Gift aid (need-based):* Federal Pell, FSEOG, state, private, college/university gift aid from institutional funds, United Negro College Fund, Federal Nursing, ACG and SMART Grants and Teach Grants. *Loans:* Federal Nursing Student Loans, Federal Direct (Subsidized and Unsubsidized Stafford PLUS), Perkins, alternative loans. *Work-study:* Federal Work-Study. *Financial aid application deadline:* 2/15.

Contact Ms. Karen Pellegrino, Director of Admission, School of Nursing, Fairfield University, 1073 North Benson Road, Kelley Center, Fairfield, CT 06824-5195. *Telephone:* 203-254-4100. *Fax:* 203-254-4199. *E-mail:* admis@fairfield.edu.

GRADUATE PROGRAMS

Expenses (2010-11) *Tuition:* part-time $575 per hour. *Required fees:* part-time $25 per term.

Financial Aid 11% of graduate students in nursing programs received some form of financial aid in 2009-10. Traineeships, unspecified assistantships, and Traineeships is a federally funded grant program available.

Contact Ms. Marianne Gumpper, Director of Graduate and Continuing Studies Admission, School of Nursing, Fairfield University, 1073 North Benson Road, Kelley Center, Fairfield, CT 06824-5195. *Telephone:* 203-254-4184. *Fax:* 203-254-4073. *E-mail:* gradadmis@fairfield.edu.

MASTER'S DEGREE PROGRAM

Degree MSN

Available Programs Master's; Master's for Nurses with Non-Nursing Degrees.

Concentrations Available Clinical nurse leader; health-care administration; nurse anesthesia. *Nurse practitioner programs in:* family health, psychiatric/mental health.

Study Options Full-time and part-time.

Program Entrance Requirements Computer literacy, minimum overall college GPA of 3.0, transcript of college record, written essay, immunizations, interview, 2 letters of recommendation, resume, statistics course, GRE (nurse anesthesia applicants only). *Application deadline:* Applications may be processed on a rolling basis for some programs. *Application fee:* $60.

Advanced Placement Credit given for nursing courses completed elsewhere dependent upon specific evaluations.

Degree Requirements 39 total credit hours.

POST-MASTER'S PROGRAM

Areas of Study *Nurse practitioner programs in:* family health, psychiatric/mental health.

DOCTORAL DEGREE PROGRAM

Degree DNP

Available Programs Doctorate.

Areas of Study Advanced practice nursing.

Program Entrance Requirements Clinical experience, minimum overall college GPA of 3.2, interview by faculty committee, interview, 2 letters of recommendation, vita, writing sample. Application deadline: Applications may be processed on a rolling basis for some programs. Application fee: $60.

CONTINUING EDUCATION PROGRAM

Contact Carol A. Pomarico, Adult Program Director, School of Nursing, Fairfield University, 1073 North Benson Road, Fairfield, CT 06824. *Telephone:* 203-254-4000 Ext. 2711. *Fax:* 203-254-4126. *E-mail:* capomarico@fairfield.edu.

Quinnipiac University

Department of Nursing
Hamden, Connecticut

http://www.quinnipiac.edu/x740.xml

Founded in 1929

DEGREES • BSN • MSN

Nursing Program Faculty 50 (90% with doctorates).

Baccalaureate Enrollment 540 **Women** 97% **Men** 3% **Minority** 7% **International** 2%

Graduate Enrollment 98 **Women** 98% **Men** 2% **Minority** 6% **International** 1% **Part-time** 60%

Nursing Student Activities Sigma Theta Tau, Student Nurses' Association.

Nursing Student Resources Academic advising; academic or career counseling; bookstore; campus computer network; career placement assistance; computer lab; computer-assisted instruction; e-mail services; employment services for current students; externships; housing assistance; interactive nursing skills videos; Internet; learning resource lab; library services; nursing audiovisuals; paid internships; placement services for program completers; resume preparation assistance; skills, simulation, or other laboratory; tutoring; unpaid internships.

Library Facilities 285,000 volumes (1,700 in nursing); 5,500 periodical subscriptions.

BACCALAUREATE PROGRAMS

Degree BSN

Available Programs Accelerated Baccalaureate for Second Degree; Generic Baccalaureate.

Site Options North Haven, CT.

Study Options Full-time.

Program Entrance Requirements Minimum overall college GPA of 3.0, transcript of college record, written essay, health exam, high school biology, high school chemistry, 4 years high school math, 4 years high school science, high school transcript, immunizations, 1 letter of recommendation, minimum high school GPA of 3.0, minimum high school rank 50%, minimum GPA in nursing prerequisites of 3.0. Transfer students are accepted. *Application deadline:* 11/1 (fall), 12/1 (spring). Applications may be processed on a rolling basis for some programs. *Application fee:* $45.

Advanced Placement Credit given for nursing courses completed elsewhere dependent upon specific evaluations.

Expenses (2010-11) *Tuition:* full-time $32,850; part-time $790 per credit. *Room and board:* $12,730; room only: $10,600 per academic year. *Required fees:* full-time $1400; part-time $35 per credit.

Financial Aid 72% of baccalaureate students in nursing programs received some form of financial aid in 2009-10. *Gift aid (need-based):* Federal Pell, FSEOG, state, private, college/university gift aid from institutional funds. *Loans:* Federal Nursing Student Loans, Federal Direct (Subsidized and Unsubsidized Stafford PLUS), Perkins. *Work-study:* Federal Work-Study, part-time campus jobs. *Financial aid application deadline (priority):* 3/1.

Contact Ms. Carla Knowlton, Director of Undergraduate Admissions, Department of Nursing, Quinnipiac University, 275 Mount Carmel Avenue, Hamden, CT 06518. *Telephone:* 203-582-8600. *Fax:* 203-582-8906. *E-mail:* admissions@quinnipiac.edu.

GRADUATE PROGRAMS

Expenses (2010-11) *Tuition:* full-time $16,830; part-time $810 per credit. *Required fees:* full-time $630; part-time $35 per credit.

Financial Aid 30% of graduate students in nursing programs received some form of financial aid in 2009-10.

Contact Kristin Parent, Associate Director of Graduate Admissions, Department of Nursing, Quinnipiac University, 275 Mount Carmel Avenue, Hamden, CT 06518. *Telephone:* 203-582-8672. *Fax:* 203-582-3443. *E-mail:* graduate@quinnipiac.edu.

MASTER'S DEGREE PROGRAM

Degree MSN

Available Programs Master's.

Concentrations Available Health-care administration. *Nurse practitioner programs in:* adult health, family health.

Site Options North Haven, CT.

Study Options Full-time and part-time.

Program Entrance Requirements Clinical experience, minimum overall college GPA of 3.0, transcript of college record, CPR certification, written essay, immunizations, interview, 3 letters of recommendation, prerequisite course work, resume. *Application deadline:* 6/1 (fall), 12/15 (spring). Applications may be processed on a rolling basis for some programs. *Application fee:* $45.
Advanced Placement Credit given for nursing courses completed elsewhere dependent upon specific evaluations.
Degree Requirements 47 total credit hours, thesis or project.

CONTINUING EDUCATION PROGRAM

Contact Ms. Mary Wargo, Director of Transfer and Part-Time Admissions, Department of Nursing, Quinnipiac University, 275 Mount Carmel Avenue, Hamden, CT 06518. *Telephone:* 203-582-8612. *Fax:* 203-582-8906. *E-mail:* mary.wargo@quinnipiac.edu.

See full description on page 490.

Sacred Heart University
Program in Nursing
Fairfield, Connecticut

http://www.sacredheart.edu/nursing.cfm
Founded in 1963

DEGREES • BS • DNP • MSN

Nursing Program Faculty 43 (27% with doctorates).
Baccalaureate Enrollment 262 **Women** 96% **Men** 4% **Minority** 12% **International** 1% **Part-time** 31%
Graduate Enrollment 227 **Women** 95% **Men** 5% **Minority** 24% **International** 1% **Part-time** 84%
Distance Learning Courses Available.
Nursing Student Activities Nursing Honor Society, Sigma Theta Tau, Student Nurses' Association.
Nursing Student Resources Academic advising; academic or career counseling; assistance for students with disabilities; bookstore; campus computer network; career placement assistance; computer lab; computer-assisted instruction; e-mail services; employment services for current students; externships; housing assistance; interactive nursing skills videos; Internet; learning resource lab; library services; nursing audiovisuals; paid internships; placement services for program completers; remedial services; resume preparation assistance; skills, simulation, or other laboratory; tutoring; unpaid internships.
Library Facilities 148,803 volumes (5,000 in health, 649 in nursing); 1,770 periodical subscriptions (328 health-care related).

BACCALAUREATE PROGRAMS

Degree BS
Available Programs ADN to Baccalaureate; Generic Baccalaureate; RN Baccalaureate.
Study Options Full-time and part-time.
Program Entrance Requirements Minimum overall college GPA of 2.8, transcript of college record, written essay, high school biology, high school chemistry, high school foreign language, 3 years high school math, 3 years high school science, high school transcript, interview, 1 letter of recommendation, minimum high school GPA of 3.2, minimum high school rank 30%, minimum GPA in nursing prerequisites of 3.0, prerequisite course work. Transfer students are accepted. *Application deadline:* 2/1 (fall), 12/1 (spring). Applications may be processed on a rolling basis for some programs. *Application fee:* $50.
Advanced Placement Credit given for nursing courses completed elsewhere dependent upon specific evaluations.
Expenses (2010-11) *Tuition:* full-time $31,224; part-time $475 per credit. *Room and board:* $8840 per academic year. *Required fees:* full-time $1130; part-time $50 per credit; part-time $85 per term.
Financial Aid 85% of baccalaureate students in nursing programs received some form of financial aid in 2009-10. *Gift aid (need-based):* Federal Pell, FSEOG, state, private, college/university gift aid from institutional funds. *Loans:* Federal Direct (Subsidized and Unsubsidized Stafford PLUS), Perkins, state. *Work-study:* Federal Work-Study, part-time campus jobs. *Financial aid application deadline (priority):* 2/15.
Contact Ms. Karen N. Guastelle, Dean of Undergraduate Admissions, Program in Nursing, Sacred Heart University, 5151 Park Avenue, Fairfield, CT 06825-1000. *Telephone:* 203-371-7880. *E-mail:* enroll@sacredheart.edu.

GRADUATE PROGRAMS

Expenses (2010-11) *Tuition:* part-time $565 per credit. *Required fees:* part-time $131 per term.
Contact Ms. Kathy Dilks, Associate Dean of Graduate Admissions, Program in Nursing, Sacred Heart University, 5151 Park Avenue, Fairfield, CT 06825-1000. *Telephone:* 203-396-8259. *E-mail:* dilksk@sacredheart.edu.

MASTER'S DEGREE PROGRAM

Degree MSN
Available Programs Master's; RN to Master's.
Concentrations Available Clinical nurse leader; nursing administration. *Nurse practitioner programs in:* family health.
Study Options Full-time and part-time.
Online Degree Options Yes.
Program Entrance Requirements Clinical experience, minimum overall college GPA of 3.0, transcript of college record, written essay, interview, 2 letters of recommendation, prerequisite course work, statistics course. *Application deadline:* Applications may be processed on a rolling basis for some programs. *Application fee:* $50.
Advanced Placement Credit given for nursing courses completed elsewhere dependent upon specific evaluations.
Degree Requirements 38 total credit hours, thesis or project.

POST-MASTER'S PROGRAM

Areas of Study *Nurse practitioner programs in:* family health.

DOCTORAL DEGREE PROGRAM

Degree DNP
Available Programs Doctorate.
Areas of Study Clinical practice, nursing administration.
Program Entrance Requirements Minimum overall college GPA of 3.2, interview by faculty committee, 2 letters of recommendation, MSN or equivalent, statistics course, writing sample. Application deadline: 4/1 (fall). Application fee: $50.
Degree Requirements 39 total credit hours, dissertation.

Saint Joseph College

Department of Nursing
West Hartford, Connecticut

http://www.sjc.edu/
Founded in 1932

DEGREES • BS • MS

Nursing Program Faculty 23 (44% with doctorates).
Baccalaureate Enrollment 250 **Women** 98% **Men** 2% **Minority** 21% **International** 2% **Part-time** 38%
Graduate Enrollment 125 **Women** 98% **Men** 2% **Minority** 25% **International** 1% **Part-time** 66%
Distance Learning Courses Available.
Nursing Student Activities Sigma Theta Tau, Student Nurses' Association, nursing club.
Nursing Student Resources Academic advising; academic or career counseling; assistance for students with disabilities; bookstore; campus computer network; career placement assistance; computer lab; computer-assisted instruction; daycare for children of students; e-mail services; employment services for current students; externships; housing assistance; interactive nursing skills videos; Internet; learning resource lab; library services; nursing audiovisuals; paid internships; placement services for program completers; remedial services; resume preparation assistance; skills, simulation, or other laboratory; tutoring; unpaid internships.
Library Facilities 7,058 volumes in health, 1,949 volumes in nursing; 1,495 periodical subscriptions health-care related.

BACCALAUREATE PROGRAMS

Degree BS
Available Programs Baccalaureate for Second Degree; Generic Baccalaureate; RN Baccalaureate.
Site Options Middletown, CT.
Study Options Full-time.
Program Entrance Requirements Minimum overall college GPA of 2.8, transcript of college record, CPR certification, written essay, health exam, health insurance, high school biology, high school chemistry, high school transcript, immunizations, minimum high school GPA, minimum GPA in nursing prerequisites of 2.8, prerequisite course work. Transfer students are accepted. *Application deadline:* 4/1 (fall), 12/1 (spring). Applications may be processed on a rolling basis for some programs. *Application fee:* $50.
Advanced Placement Credit given for nursing courses completed elsewhere dependent upon specific evaluations.
Financial Aid 85% of baccalaureate students in nursing programs received some form of financial aid in 2009-10. *Gift aid (need-based):* Federal Pell, FSEOG, state, private, college/university gift aid from institutional funds. *Loans:* Federal Direct (Subsidized and Unsubsidized Stafford PLUS), Perkins, state, private bank loans. *Work-study:* Federal Work-Study, part-time campus jobs. *Financial aid application deadline (priority):* 2/15.
Contact Dr. Joyce Fontana, Chairperson, Department of Nursing, Saint Joseph College, 1678 Asylum Avenue, West Hartford, CT 06117-2700. *Telephone:* 860-231-5304. *E-mail:* jfontana@sjc.edu.

GRADUATE PROGRAMS

Financial Aid 75% of graduate students in nursing programs received some form of financial aid in 2009-10.
Contact Dr. Pam Aselton, Director, Department of Nursing, Saint Joseph College, 1678 Asylum Avenue, West Hartford, CT 06117-2700. *Telephone:* 860-231-5211. *Fax:* 860-231-8396. *E-mail:* paselton@sjc.edu.

MASTER'S DEGREE PROGRAM

Degree MS
Available Programs Master's; Master's for Nurses with Non-Nursing Degrees.
Concentrations Available Nursing education. *Clinical nurse specialist programs in:* family health, psychiatric/mental health. *Nurse practitioner programs in:* family health.
Site Options Middletown, CT.
Study Options Full-time and part-time.
Program Entrance Requirements Clinical experience, minimum overall college GPA of 3.0, transcript of college record, CPR certification, written essay, immunizations, interview, 2 letters of recommendation, nursing research course, physical assessment course, professional liability insurance/malpractice insurance, resume, statistics course. *Application deadline:* Applications may be processed on a rolling basis for some programs. *Application fee:* $50.
Degree Requirements 47 total credit hours, thesis or project.

POST-MASTER'S PROGRAM

Areas of Study Nursing education. *Clinical nurse specialist programs in:* family health, psychiatric/mental health. *Nurse practitioner programs in:* family health.

Southern Connecticut State University

Department of Nursing
New Haven, Connecticut

http://www.southernct.edu/nursing/
Founded in 1893

DEGREES • BS • MSN

Nursing Program Faculty 42 (65% with doctorates).
Baccalaureate Enrollment 220 **Women** 85% **Men** 15% **Minority** 20% **Part-time** 5%
Graduate Enrollment 40 **Women** 97% **Men** 3% **Part-time** 97%
Distance Learning Courses Available.
Nursing Student Activities Nursing Honor Society, Sigma Theta Tau, Student Nurses' Association.
Nursing Student Resources Academic advising; academic or career counseling; assistance for students with disabilities; bookstore; campus computer network; career placement assistance; computer lab; daycare for children of students; e-mail services; employment services for current students; housing assistance; Internet; learning resource lab; library services; nursing audiovisuals; resume preparation assistance; skills, simulation, or other laboratory; tutoring.
Library Facilities 495,660 volumes (35,540 in health, 2,279 in nursing); 3,549 periodical subscriptions (318 health-care related).

BACCALAUREATE PROGRAMS

Degree BS
Available Programs ADN to Baccalaureate; Accelerated Baccalaureate; Generic Baccalaureate; RN Baccalaureate.

Study Options Full-time and part-time.
Program Entrance Requirements Minimum overall college GPA of 2.8, transcript of college record, CPR certification, health exam, high school transcript, minimum GPA in nursing prerequisites, prerequisite course work. Transfer students are accepted. *Application deadline:* 2/1 (spring).
Advanced Placement Credit given for nursing courses completed elsewhere dependent upon specific evaluations.
Financial Aid ***Gift aid (need-based):*** Federal Pell, FSEOG, state, private, college/university gift aid from institutional funds. *Loans:* Federal Direct (Subsidized and Unsubsidized Stafford PLUS). *Work-study:* Federal Work-Study. *Financial aid application deadline:* 3/9(priority: 3/5).
Contact Dr. Barbara Aronson, Coordinator, BSN Program in Nursing, Department of Nursing, Southern Connecticut State University, 501 Crescent Street, New Haven, CT 06515-1355. *Telephone:* 203-392-6496. *Fax:* 203-392-6493. *E-mail:* aronsonb1@southernct.edu.

GRADUATE PROGRAMS

Contact Dr. Leslie Neal Boylan, Coordinator, Graduate Programs in Nursing, Department of Nursing, Southern Connecticut State University, 501 Crescent Street, New Haven, CT 06515. *Telephone:* 203-392-6480. *Fax:* 203-392-6493. *E-mail:* nealboylanl1@southernct.edu.

MASTER'S DEGREE PROGRAM

Degree MSN
Available Programs Master's; RN to Master's.
Concentrations Available Clinical nurse leader; nursing education. *Nurse practitioner programs in:* family health.
Study Options Full-time and part-time.
Program Entrance Requirements Clinical experience, minimum overall college GPA of 3.0, transcript of college record, CPR certification, immunizations, interview, 2 letters of recommendation, nursing research course, physical assessment course, professional liability insurance/malpractice insurance, prerequisite course work, resume, statistics course, GRE, MAT. *Application deadline:* Applications may be processed on a rolling basis for some programs.
Advanced Placement Credit given for nursing courses completed elsewhere dependent upon specific evaluations.
Degree Requirements 42 total credit hours, thesis or project.

POST-MASTER'S PROGRAM

Areas of Study Nursing education. *Nurse practitioner programs in:* family health.

University of Connecticut

School of Nursing
Storrs, Connecticut

http://www.nursing.uconn.edu/
Founded in 1881

DEGREES • BS • MS • MS/MBA • PHD

Nursing Program Faculty 84 (85% with doctorates).
Baccalaureate Enrollment 551 **Women** 88% **Men** 12% **Minority** 19% **International** .3% **Part-time** .2%
Graduate Enrollment 188 **Women** 88% **Men** 12% **Minority** 16% **International** .5% **Part-time** 59%
Distance Learning Courses Available.
Nursing Student Activities Nursing Honor Society, Sigma Theta Tau, Student Nurses' Association.
Nursing Student Resources Academic advising; academic or career counseling; assistance for students with disabilities; bookstore; campus computer network; career placement assistance; computer lab; e-mail services; externships; housing assistance; interactive nursing skills videos; Internet; learning resource lab; library services; nursing audiovisuals; remedial services; resume preparation assistance; skills, simulation, or other laboratory; tutoring; unpaid internships.
Library Facilities 3 million volumes (46,250 in health, 1,170 in nursing); 17,378 periodical subscriptions (6,131 health-care related).

BACCALAUREATE PROGRAMS

Degree BS
Available Programs Generic Baccalaureate.
Site Options West Hartford, CT; Avery Point, Waterbury, Stamford, CT.
Study Options Full-time and part-time.
Program Entrance Requirements Minimum overall college GPA of 3.0, transcript of college record, written essay, health exam, health insurance, high school chemistry, high school foreign language, 3 years high school math, 2 years high school science, high school transcript, immunizations, minimum high school GPA of 3.0, minimum GPA in nursing prerequisites of 2.0, prerequisite course work. Transfer students are accepted. *Application deadline:* 2/1 (fall). *Application fee:* $70.
Advanced Placement Credit by examination available. Credit given for nursing courses completed elsewhere dependent upon specific evaluations.
Expenses (2010-11) *Tuition, state resident:* full-time $8064; part-time $336 per credit. *Tuition, nonresident:* full-time $24,528; part-time $1022 per credit. *Room and board:* $10,308; room only: $5774 per academic year. *Required fees:* full-time $4838.
Financial Aid 77% of baccalaureate students in nursing programs received some form of financial aid in 2009-10. *Gift aid (need-based):* Federal Pell, FSEOG, state, private, college/university gift aid from institutional funds. *Loans:* Federal Nursing Student Loans, Federal Direct (Subsidized and Unsubsidized Stafford PLUS), Perkins, state. *Work-study:* Federal Work-Study, part-time campus jobs. *Financial aid application deadline (priority):* 3/1.
Contact Ms. Ann Salina, Admissions and Recruitment Coordinator, School of Nursing, University of Connecticut, 231 Glenbrook Road, Unit 2026, Storrs, CT 06269-2026. *Telephone:* 860-486-1937. *Fax:* 860-486-0906. *E-mail:* ann.salina@uconn.edu.

GRADUATE PROGRAMS

Expenses (2010-11) *Tuition, state resident:* full-time $9972; part-time $554 per credit. *Tuition, nonresident:* full-time $25,884; part-time $1438 per credit. *Room and board:* $11,810; room only: $6802 per academic year. *Required fees:* full-time $1856; part-time $928 per term.
Financial Aid 24% of graduate students in nursing programs received some form of financial aid in 2009-10. 9 research assistantships with full tuition reimbursements available, 12 teaching assistantships with full tuition reimbursements available were awarded; fellowships, Federal Work-Study, scholarships, and unspecified assistantships also available. *Financial aid application deadline:* 2/1.
Contact Ms. Ann Salina, Admission and Recruitment Coordinator, School of Nursing, University of Connecticut, 231 Glenbrook Road, Unit 2026, Storrs, CT 06269-2026. *Telephone:* 860-486-1937. *Fax:* 860-486-0906. *E-mail:* ann.salina@uconn.edu.

MASTER'S DEGREE PROGRAM

Degrees MS; MS/MBA
Available Programs Accelerated Master's for Nurses with Non-Nursing Degrees; Master's; RN to Master's.
Concentrations Available Clinical nurse leader. *Clinical nurse specialist programs in:* acute care, maternity-newborn. *Nurse practitioner programs in:* acute care, neonatal health, primary care.
Site Options Farmington, CT.
Study Options Full-time and part-time.
Program Entrance Requirements Clinical experience, computer literacy, minimum overall college GPA of 3.0, transcript of college record, CPR certification, immunizations, interview, 3 letters of recommendation, nursing research course, physical assessment course, professional liability insurance/malpractice insurance, resume, statistics course. *Application deadline:* 2/1 (fall). *Application fee:* $55.
Advanced Placement Credit given for nursing courses completed elsewhere dependent upon specific evaluations.
Degree Requirements 24 total credit hours, comprehensive exam.

POST-MASTER'S PROGRAM

Areas of Study *Nurse practitioner programs in:* acute care, neonatal health, primary care.

DOCTORAL DEGREE PROGRAM

Degree PhD
Available Programs Doctorate; Post-Baccalaureate Doctorate.
Areas of Study Nursing research, nursing science.
Program Entrance Requirements Minimum overall college GPA of 3.25, interview by faculty committee, interview, 3 letters of recommendation, MSN or equivalent, statistics course, vita, writing sample. Application deadline: 2/1 (fall). Application fee: $55.
Degree Requirements 60 total credit hours, dissertation, oral exam, written exam.

CONTINUING EDUCATION PROGRAM

Contact Ms. Ann Salina, Admission and Recruitment Coordinator, School of Nursing, University of Connecticut, 231 Glenbrook Road, Unit

2026, Storrs, CT 06269-2026. *Telephone:* 860-486-1937. *Fax:* 860-486-0906. *E-mail:* ann.salina@uconn.edu.

University of Hartford

College of Education, Nursing, and Health Professions
West Hartford, Connecticut

http://www.hartford.edu/enhp
Founded in 1877

DEGREES • BSN • MSN • MSN/MSOB
Nursing Program Faculty 9 (60% with doctorates).
Baccalaureate Enrollment 88 **Women** 97% **Men** 3% **Minority** 32% **Part-time** 100%
Graduate Enrollment 140 **Women** 97% **Men** 3% **Minority** 25% **Part-time** 100%
Distance Learning Courses Available.
Nursing Student Activities Sigma Theta Tau.
Nursing Student Resources Academic advising; academic or career counseling; assistance for students with disabilities; bookstore; computer lab; e-mail services; Internet; library services; resume preparation assistance; tutoring.
Library Facilities 481,685 volumes; 2,424 periodical subscriptions.

BACCALAUREATE PROGRAMS

Degree BSN
Available Programs ADN to Baccalaureate; RN Baccalaureate.
Study Options Part-time.
Program Entrance Requirements Transcript of college record, professional liability insurance/malpractice insurance, prerequisite course work, RN licensure. Transfer students are accepted. *Application deadline:* Applications may be processed on a rolling basis for some programs. *Application fee:* $45.
Advanced Placement Credit by examination available. Credit given for nursing courses completed elsewhere dependent upon specific evaluations.
Expenses (2010-11) *Tuition:* part-time $420 per credit hour. *Required fees:* part-time $105 per term.
Financial Aid 50% of baccalaureate students in nursing programs received some form of financial aid in 2009-10. *Gift aid (need-based):* Federal Pell, FSEOG, state, private, college/university gift aid from institutional funds. *Loans:* Perkins. *Work-study:* Federal Work-Study, part-time campus jobs. *Financial aid application deadline (priority):* 2/1.
Contact Dr. Mary Jane Williams, Chair, Department of Nursing, College of Education, Nursing, and Health Professions, University of Hartford, 200 Bloomfield Avenue, West Hartford, CT 06117-1599. *Telephone:* 860-768-4213. *Fax:* 860-768-5346. *E-mail:* mjwilliam@hartford.edu.

GRADUATE PROGRAMS

Expenses (2010-11) *Tuition:* part-time $430 per credit. *Required fees:* part-time $105 per term.
Financial Aid 50% of graduate students in nursing programs received some form of financial aid in 2009-10. 4 research assistantships (averaging $4,500 per year) were awarded; teaching assistantships, institutionally sponsored loans and unspecified assistantships also available. *Financial aid application deadline:* 6/1.
Contact Ms. Marlene J. Hall, Director of Communication and Recruitment, ENHP, College of Education, Nursing, and Health Professions, University of Hartford, 200 Bloomfield Avenue, West Hartford, CT 06117-1599. *Telephone:* 860-768-5116. *Fax:* 860-768-5346. *E-mail:* mhall@hartford.edu.

MASTER'S DEGREE PROGRAM

Degrees MSN; MSN/MSOB
Available Programs Master's; Master's for Nurses with Non-Nursing Degrees.
Concentrations Available Nursing administration; nursing education. *Clinical nurse specialist programs in:* public health.
Study Options Part-time.
Program Entrance Requirements Clinical experience, minimum overall college GPA of 3.0, transcript of college record, written essay, immunizations, 2 letters of recommendation, nursing research course, physical assessment course, professional liability insurance/malpractice insurance, resume. *Application deadline:* 4/15 (fall), 11/15 (spring). *Application fee:* $45.
Advanced Placement Credit given for nursing courses completed elsewhere dependent upon specific evaluations.
Degree Requirements 34 total credit hours, thesis or project.

POST-MASTER'S PROGRAM

Areas of Study Nursing education.

DOCTORAL DEGREE PROGRAM

Program Entrance Requirements MAT.

CONTINUING EDUCATION PROGRAM

Contact Dr. Susan H. Diehl, Interim Chair, Department of Nursing, College of Education, Nursing, and Health Professions, University of Hartford, Department of Nursing, ENHP, West Hartford, CT 06117-1599. *Telephone:* 860-768-4214. *Fax:* 860-768-5346. *E-mail:* diehl@hartford.edu.

Western Connecticut State University

Department of Nursing
Danbury, Connecticut

http://www.wcsu.edu/
Founded in 1903

DEGREES • BS • MS
Nursing Program Faculty 18 (50% with doctorates).
Baccalaureate Enrollment 160 **Women** 95% **Men** 5% **Minority** 20%
Graduate Enrollment 35 **Women** 100% **Minority** 2% **Part-time** 100%
Distance Learning Courses Available.
Nursing Student Activities Sigma Theta Tau, Student Nurses' Association.
Nursing Student Resources Academic advising; academic or career counseling; assistance for students with disabilities; bookstore; campus computer network; career placement assistance; computer lab; computer-assisted instruction; daycare for children of students; e-mail services; employment services for current students; externships; housing assistance; interactive nursing skills videos; Internet; learning resource lab; library services; nursing audiovisuals; paid internships; remedial services; resume preparation assistance; skills, simulation, or other laboratory; tutoring.

BACCALAUREATE PROGRAMS

Degree BS
Available Programs Generic Baccalaureate; RN Baccalaureate.
Site Options Waterbury, CT.
Study Options Full-time.
Program Entrance Requirements Minimum overall college GPA of 2.5, transcript of college record, CPR certification, health exam, health insurance, high school biology, high school chemistry, high school foreign language, 3 years high school math, 2 years high school science, high school transcript, immunizations, minimum GPA in nursing prerequisites of 2.5, prerequisite course work. Transfer students are accepted. *Application deadline:* Applications may be processed on a rolling basis for some programs. *Application fee:* $60.
Advanced Placement Credit by examination available. Credit given for nursing courses completed elsewhere dependent upon specific evaluations.
Expenses (2010-11) *Tuition, state resident:* full-time $4250; part-time $380 per credit hour. *Tuition, nonresident:* full-time $13,250; part-time $425 per credit hour. *Room and board:* $11,250; room only: $5750 per academic year. *Required fees:* full-time $6000; part-time $75 per credit.
Financial Aid 50% of baccalaureate students in nursing programs received some form of financial aid in 2009-10.
Contact Dr. Karen Crouse, Chair, Department of Nursing, Western Connecticut State University, 181 White Street, Danbury, CT 06810. *Telephone:* 203-837-8556. *Fax:* 203-837-8550. *E-mail:* crousek@wcsu.edu.

GRADUATE PROGRAMS

Expenses (2010-11) *Tuition, state resident:* part-time $425 per credit hour. *Tuition, nonresident:* part-time $450 per credit hour. *Required fees:* full-time $2500.
Financial Aid 10% of graduate students in nursing programs received some form of financial aid in 2009-10.

Contact Dr. Karen Daley, Graduate Program Coordinator, Department of Nursing, Western Connecticut State University, 181 White Street, Danbury, CT 06810. *Telephone:* 203-837-8556. *Fax:* 203-837-8550. *E-mail:* daleyk@wcsu.edu.

MASTER'S DEGREE PROGRAM

Degree MS
Available Programs Master's.
Concentrations Available *Clinical nurse specialist programs in:* adult health. *Nurse practitioner programs in:* adult health.
Study Options Part-time.
Program Entrance Requirements Clinical experience, computer literacy, minimum overall college GPA of 3.0, transcript of college record, CPR certification, immunizations, interview, 2 letters of recommendation, nursing research course, physical assessment course, professional liability insurance/malpractice insurance, prerequisite course work, resume, statistics course. *Application deadline:* Applications may be processed on a rolling basis for some programs. *Application fee:* $60.
Advanced Placement Credit by examination available. Credit given for nursing courses completed elsewhere dependent upon specific evaluations.
Degree Requirements 36 total credit hours, thesis or project.

POST-MASTER'S PROGRAM

Areas of Study *Clinical nurse specialist programs in:* adult health. *Nurse practitioner programs in:* adult health.

Yale University

School of Nursing
New Haven, Connecticut

http://www.nursing.yale.edu/
Founded in 1701

DEGREES • MSN • MSN/MDIV • MSN/MPH • PHD

Nursing Program Faculty 149 (50% with doctorates).
Graduate Enrollment 340 **Women** 94% **Men** 6% **Minority** 17% **International** 5% **Part-time** 12%
Distance Learning Courses Available.
Nursing Student Activities Nursing Honor Society, Sigma Theta Tau.
Nursing Student Resources Academic advising; academic or career counseling; assistance for students with disabilities; bookstore; campus computer network; career placement assistance; computer lab; computer-assisted instruction; daycare for children of students; e-mail services; employment services for current students; housing assistance; interactive nursing skills videos; Internet; learning resource lab; library services; nursing audiovisuals; placement services for program completers; remedial services; resume preparation assistance; skills, simulation, or other laboratory; tutoring; unpaid internships.
Library Facilities 12.5 million volumes (400,000 in health); 85,000 periodical subscriptions (2,900 health-care related).

GRADUATE PROGRAMS

Expenses (2009-10) *Tuition:* full-time $30,185. *International tuition:* $30,185 full-time. *Required fees:* full-time $325.
Financial Aid 90% of graduate students in nursing programs received some form of financial aid in 2008-09. 239 fellowships (averaging $5,905 per year), 13 research assistantships with tuition reimbursements available (averaging $28,450 per year) were awarded; Federal Work-Study, scholarships, and traineeships also available. Aid available to part-time students. *Financial aid application deadline:* 2/1.
Contact Dr. Frank A. Grosso, Assistant Dean for Student Affairs, School of Nursing, Yale University, PO Box 9740, New Haven, CT 06536-0740. *Telephone:* 203-737-2257. *Fax:* 203-737-5409. *E-mail:* frank.grosso@yale.edu.

MASTER'S DEGREE PROGRAM

Degrees MSN; MSN/MDIV; MSN/MPH
Available Programs Master's; Master's for Non-Nursing College Graduates; Master's for Nurses with Non-Nursing Degrees.
Concentrations Available Nurse-midwifery; nursing administration. *Clinical nurse specialist programs in:* cardiovascular, critical care, oncology, psychiatric/mental health. *Nurse practitioner programs in:* acute care, adult health, family health, gerontology, oncology, pediatric, primary care, psychiatric/mental health, women's health.
Study Options Full-time.
Online Degree Options Yes.
Program Entrance Requirements Minimum overall college GPA of 3.0, transcript of college record, CPR certification, written essay, immunizations, interview, 3 letters of recommendation, resume, GRE General Test. *Application deadline:* 11/1 (fall). *Application fee:* $65.
Advanced Placement Credit by examination available. Credit given for nursing courses completed elsewhere dependent upon specific evaluations.
Degree Requirements 40 total credit hours, thesis or project.

POST-MASTER'S PROGRAM

Areas of Study *Clinical nurse specialist programs in:* psychiatric/mental health. *Nurse practitioner programs in:* acute care, adult health, gerontology, oncology, pediatric.

DOCTORAL DEGREE PROGRAM

Degree PhD
Available Programs Doctorate.
Areas of Study Aging, critical care, family health, gerontology, health policy, health promotion/disease prevention, health-care systems, human health and illness, maternity-newborn, neuro-behavior, nursing policy, nursing research, oncology.
Program Entrance Requirements Minimum overall college GPA of 3.0, interview by faculty committee, interview, 3 letters of recommendation, MSN or equivalent, statistics course, vita, writing sample, GRE General Test. Application deadline: 1/2 (fall). Application fee: $90.
Degree Requirements 60 total credit hours, dissertation, oral exam, written exam.

POSTDOCTORAL PROGRAM

Areas of Study Adolescent health, chronic illness.
Postdoctoral Program Contact Ms. Sarah Zaino, Assistant Director, Research Activities, School of Nursing, Yale University, PO Box 9740, New Haven, CT 06536-0740. *Telephone:* 203-737-2420. *Fax:* 203-737-4480. *E-mail:* sarah.zaino@yale.edu.

DELAWARE

Delaware State University

Department of Nursing
Dover, Delaware

http://www.dsc.edu/schools/professional_studies/nursing
Founded in 1891

DEGREE • BSN

Nursing Program Faculty 11
Nursing Student Activities Sigma Theta Tau, Student Nurses' Association.
Library Facilities 187,045 volumes; 74,881 periodical subscriptions.

BACCALAUREATE PROGRAMS

Degree BSN
Available Programs Generic Baccalaureate; LPN to Baccalaureate.
Study Options Full-time and part-time.
Program Entrance Requirements High school biology, high school chemistry, high school transcript, minimum high school GPA of 2.0, prerequisite course work. Transfer students are accepted.
Advanced Placement Credit by examination available. Credit given for nursing courses completed elsewhere dependent upon specific evaluations.
Contact *Telephone:* 302-857-6750. *Fax:* 302-857-6755.

University of Delaware

School of Nursing
Newark, Delaware

http://www.udel.edu/nursing/udnursing.html
Founded in 1743

DEGREES • BSN • MSN

Nursing Program Faculty 58 (48% with doctorates).

Baccalaureate Enrollment 674 **Women** 90% **Men** 10% **Minority** 17% **International** 1% **Part-time** 18%
Graduate Enrollment 121 **Women** 92% **Men** 8% **Minority** 21% **Part-time** 93%
Distance Learning Courses Available.
Nursing Student Activities Sigma Theta Tau, Student Nurses' Association.
Nursing Student Resources Academic advising; academic or career counseling; assistance for students with disabilities; bookstore; campus computer network; career placement assistance; computer lab; computer-assisted instruction; e-mail services; employment services for current students; housing assistance; interactive nursing skills videos; Internet; learning resource lab; library services; nursing audiovisuals; resume preparation assistance; skills, simulation, or other laboratory; tutoring.
Library Facilities 2.7 million volumes in health, 40,000 volumes in nursing; 240 periodical subscriptions health-care related.

BACCALAUREATE PROGRAMS

Degree BSN
Available Programs Accelerated Baccalaureate for Second Degree; Generic Baccalaureate; RN Baccalaureate.
Study Options Full-time.
Program Entrance Requirements CPR certification, written essay, high school biology, high school chemistry, high school foreign language, 3 years high school math, 4 years high school science, high school transcript, immunizations, 1 letter of recommendation, minimum high school GPA of 3.0. Transfer students are accepted.
Advanced Placement Credit given for nursing courses completed elsewhere dependent upon specific evaluations.
Contact ***Telephone:*** 302-831-1117. *Fax:* 302-831-2382.

GRADUATE PROGRAMS

Contact ***Telephone:*** 302-831-8386. *Fax:* 302-831-2382.

MASTER'S DEGREE PROGRAM

Degree MSN
Available Programs Master's; Master's for Nurses with Non-Nursing Degrees; RN to Master's.
Concentrations Available Health-care administration. *Clinical nurse specialist programs in:* adult health, pediatric, psychiatric/mental health, school health. *Nurse practitioner programs in:* adult health, family health.
Study Options Full-time and part-time.
Program Entrance Requirements Clinical experience, minimum overall college GPA of 3.0, transcript of college record, CPR certification, written essay, immunizations, interview, 3 letters of recommendation, professional liability insurance/malpractice insurance, resume.
Advanced Placement Credit given for nursing courses completed elsewhere dependent upon specific evaluations.
Degree Requirements 34 total credit hours.

POST-MASTER'S PROGRAM

Areas of Study Health-care administration. *Clinical nurse specialist programs in:* adult health, pediatric, psychiatric/mental health. *Nurse practitioner programs in:* adult health, family health.

Wesley College

Nursing Program
Dover, Delaware

http://www.wesley.edu/
Founded in 1873

DEGREES • BSN • MSN
Nursing Program Faculty 10 (80% with doctorates).
Baccalaureate Enrollment 210 **Women** 85% **Men** 15% **Minority** 35% **International** 1% **Part-time** 2%
Graduate Enrollment 87 **Women** 90% **Men** 10% **Minority** 25% **Part-time** 10%
Nursing Student Activities Sigma Theta Tau, Student Nurses' Association.
Nursing Student Resources Academic advising; academic or career counseling; assistance for students with disabilities; bookstore; campus computer network; career placement assistance; computer lab; computer-assisted instruction; e-mail services; employment services for current students; externships; housing assistance; interactive nursing skills videos; Internet; learning resource lab; library services; nursing audiovisuals; placement services for program completers; remedial services; resume preparation assistance; skills, simulation, or other laboratory; tutoring; unpaid internships.
Library Facilities 104,636 volumes (15,000 in health, 1,500 in nursing); 252 periodical subscriptions (40 health-care related).

BACCALAUREATE PROGRAMS

Degree BSN
Available Programs Generic Baccalaureate; International Nurse to Baccalaureate; LPN to Baccalaureate.
Study Options Full-time and part-time.
Program Entrance Requirements Minimum overall college GPA of 2.75, transcript of college record, CPR certification, written essay, health exam, health insurance, high school biology, high school chemistry, 2 years high school math, 2 years high school science, high school transcript, immunizations, minimum high school GPA of 2.75, minimum GPA in nursing prerequisites of 2.0, professional liability insurance/malpractice insurance. Transfer students are accepted. *Application deadline:* Applications may be processed on a rolling basis for some programs. *Application fee:* $40.
Advanced Placement Credit by examination available. Credit given for nursing courses completed elsewhere dependent upon specific evaluations.
Expenses (2010-11) *Tuition:* full-time $19,700; part-time $835 per credit. *Room and board:* $9550; room only: $4750 per academic year. *Required fees:* full-time $880; part-time $550 per term.
Financial Aid 90% of baccalaureate students in nursing programs received some form of financial aid in 2009-10.
Contact Dr. Karen Panunto, Program Director, Nursing Program, Wesley College, 120 North State Street, Dulany Hall, Dover, DE 19901. *Telephone:* 302-736-2511. *Fax:* 302-736-2548. *E-mail:* panuntka@wesley.edu.

GRADUATE PROGRAMS

Expenses (2010-11) *Tuition:* full-time $6100; part-time $435 per credit hour. *Required fees:* full-time $350; part-time $175 per term.
Financial Aid 100% of graduate students in nursing programs received some form of financial aid in 2009-10. Traineeships available.
Contact Dr. Lucille C. Gambardella, Chairperson, Nursing Program, Wesley College, 120 North State Street, Dover, DE 19901. *Telephone:* 302-736-2512. *Fax:* 302-736-2548. *E-mail:* gambarlu@wesley.edu.

MASTER'S DEGREE PROGRAM

Degree MSN
Available Programs Accelerated AD/RN to Master's; Accelerated RN to Master's; Master's; RN to Master's.
Concentrations Available *Clinical nurse specialist programs in:* community health, women's health. *Nurse practitioner programs in:* women's health.
Site Options New Castle, DE.
Study Options Full-time and part-time.
Program Entrance Requirements Clinical experience, computer literacy, minimum overall college GPA of 3.0, transcript of college record, written essay, interview, 2 letters of recommendation, professional liability insurance/malpractice insurance, resume, statistics course, GRE or MAT. *Application deadline:* Applications may be processed on a rolling basis for some programs. *Application fee:* $35.
Advanced Placement Credit by examination available. Credit given for nursing courses completed elsewhere dependent upon specific evaluations.
Degree Requirements 39 total credit hours, thesis or project.

POST-MASTER'S PROGRAM

Areas of Study Nursing education. *Clinical nurse specialist programs in:* palliative care, women's health.

CONTINUING EDUCATION PROGRAM

Contact Dr. Lucille C. Gambardella, Chair, Department of Nursing/Director, Graduate Programs, Nursing Program, Wesley College, 120 North State Street, Dover, DE 19901. *Telephone:* 302-736-2512. *Fax:* 302-736-2548. *E-mail:* gambarlu@wesley.edu.

Wilmington University

College of Health Professions
New Castle, Delaware

http://www.wilmu.edu/nursing/index.aspx
Founded in 1967

DEGREES • BSN • MSN • MSN/MBA • MSN/MS

Nursing Program Faculty 10 (60% with doctorates).
Baccalaureate Enrollment 474 **Women** 93% **Men** 7% **Minority** 8% **Part-time** 90%
Graduate Enrollment 263 **Women** 92% **Men** 8% **Minority** 17% **International** 5% **Part-time** 50%
Distance Learning Courses Available.
Nursing Student Activities Sigma Theta Tau.
Nursing Student Resources Academic advising; academic or career counseling; assistance for students with disabilities; bookstore; campus computer network; career placement assistance; computer lab; computer-assisted instruction; e-mail services; employment services for current students; housing assistance; interactive nursing skills videos; learning resource lab; library services; nursing audiovisuals; remedial services; resume preparation assistance; skills, simulation, or other laboratory; tutoring.
Library Facilities 98,713 volumes (6,000 in health, 3,500 in nursing); 425 periodical subscriptions (60 health-care related).

BACCALAUREATE PROGRAMS

Degree BSN
Available Programs Accelerated RN Baccalaureate; International Nurse to Baccalaureate; RN Baccalaureate.
Site Options Dover, DE; Georgetown, DE.
Study Options Full-time and part-time.
Online Degree Options Yes.
Program Entrance Requirements Transcript of college record, CPR certification, written essay, health exam, immunizations, prerequisite course work, RN licensure. Transfer students are accepted. *Application deadline:* 8/31 (fall), 1/1 (spring), 5/1 (summer). Applications may be processed on a rolling basis for some programs. *Application fee:* $35.
Advanced Placement Credit by examination available. Credit given for nursing courses completed elsewhere dependent upon specific evaluations.
Expenses (2010-11) *Tuition:* full-time $3396; part-time $308 per credit hour.
Financial Aid 60% of baccalaureate students in nursing programs received some form of financial aid in 2009-10.
Contact Ms. Denise Westbrook, BSN Program Coordinator, College of Health Professions, Wilmington University, 320 DuPont Highway, New Castle, DE 19720. *Telephone:* 302-856-5780. *Fax:* 302-322-7081. *E-mail:* denise.z.westbrook@wilmu.edu.

GRADUATE PROGRAMS

Expenses (2010-11) *Tuition:* part-time $395 per credit hour.
Financial Aid 65% of graduate students in nursing programs received some form of financial aid in 2009-10. 28 fellowships with tuition reimbursements available (averaging $2,200 per year) were awarded; traineeships also available.
Contact Ms. Misty Williams, Admissions Associate, College of Health Professions, Wilmington University, Wilson Graduate Center, 31 Read's Way, New Castle, DE 19720. *Telephone:* 302-295-1121. *E-mail:* kimberly.a.christensen@wilmu.edu.

MASTER'S DEGREE PROGRAM

Degrees MSN; MSN/MBA; MSN/MS
Available Programs Accelerated AD/RN to Master's; Master's.
Concentrations Available Legal nurse consultant; nursing administration; nursing education. *Nurse practitioner programs in:* adult health, family health, gerontology.
Site Options New Castle, DE; Georgetown, DE.
Study Options Full-time and part-time.
Program Entrance Requirements Clinical experience, computer literacy, minimum overall college GPA of 3.0, transcript of college record, CPR certification, written essay, immunizations, interview, 2 letters of recommendation, nursing research course, physical assessment course, professional liability insurance/malpractice insurance, prerequisite course work, resume, statistics course. *Application deadline:* 5/15 (fall). *Application fee:* $35.
Advanced Placement Credit given for nursing courses completed elsewhere dependent upon specific evaluations.
Degree Requirements 42 total credit hours, thesis or project.

POST-MASTER'S PROGRAM

Areas of Study Legal nurse consultant; nursing administration; nursing education. *Nurse practitioner programs in:* adult health, family health, gerontology.

DISTRICT OF COLUMBIA

The Catholic University of America

School of Nursing
Washington, District of Columbia

http://nursing.cua.edu/
Founded in 1887

DEGREES • BSN • DNP • MA/MSM • MSN • PHD

Nursing Program Faculty 47 (43% with doctorates).
Baccalaureate Enrollment 286 **Women** 94% **Men** 6% **Minority** 16% **International** 1% **Part-time** 1%
Graduate Enrollment 102 **Women** 96% **Men** 4% **Minority** 35% **International** 1% **Part-time** 69%
Distance Learning Courses Available.
Nursing Student Activities Nursing Honor Society, Sigma Theta Tau, Student Nurses' Association, nursing club.
Nursing Student Resources Academic advising; academic or career counseling; assistance for students with disabilities; bookstore; computer lab; computer-assisted instruction; e-mail services; interactive nursing skills videos; Internet; learning resource lab; library services; nursing audiovisuals; skills, simulation, or other laboratory.
Library Facilities 1.6 million volumes (39,000 in health, 17,500 in nursing); 10,047 periodical subscriptions (250 health-care related).

BACCALAUREATE PROGRAMS

Degree BSN
Available Programs Accelerated Baccalaureate; Accelerated Baccalaureate for Second Degree; Generic Baccalaureate.
Study Options Full-time and part-time.
Program Entrance Requirements Minimum overall college GPA of 3.0, transcript of college record, written essay, health exam, health insurance, high school chemistry, 3 years high school math, high school transcript, immunizations, 1 letter of recommendation, minimum high school GPA of 3.0, minimum GPA in nursing prerequisites of 2.75, prerequisite course work. Transfer students are accepted. *Application deadline:* 7/15 (fall), 11/15 (spring), 2/28 (summer). *Application fee:* $55.
Expenses (2010-11) *Tuition:* full-time $33,580; part-time $1315 per credit hour. *Room and board:* $11,800; room only: $7000 per academic year. *Required fees:* full-time $470; part-time $50 per credit; part-time $100 per term.
Financial Aid 50% of baccalaureate students in nursing programs received some form of financial aid in 2009-10. *Gift aid (need-based):* Federal Pell, FSEOG, state, private, college/university gift aid from institutional funds. *Loans:* Federal Direct (Subsidized and Unsubsidized Stafford PLUS), commercial loans. *Work-study:* Federal Work-Study. *Financial aid application deadline:* 4/10(priority: 2/15).
Contact Ms. Lynn Doyle, Administrative Assistant, School of Nursing, The Catholic University of America, 124 Gowan Hall, 620 Michigan Avenue NE, Washington, DC 20064. *Telephone:* 202-319-6457. *Fax:* 202-319-6485. *E-mail:* doyle@cua.edu.

GRADUATE PROGRAMS

Expenses (2010-11) *Tuition:* full-time $33,580; part-time $1315 per credit hour. *Room and board:* $12,000; room only: $7000 per academic year. *Required fees:* full-time $80; part-time $80 per term.
Financial Aid 80% of graduate students in nursing programs received some form of financial aid in 2009-10. Fellowships, research assistantships, teaching assistantships, Federal Work-Study, scholarships, tuition waivers (full and partial), and unspecified assistantships available. *Financial aid application deadline:* 2/1.

Contact Jacqueline Tintle, Administrative Assistant, School of Nursing, The Catholic University of America, 118 Gowan Hall, Washington, DC 20064. *Telephone:* 202-319-5403. *Fax:* 202-319-5403. *E-mail:* tintlej@cua.edu.

MASTER'S DEGREE PROGRAM

Degrees MA/MSM; MSN
Available Programs Master's.
Concentrations Available *Clinical nurse specialist programs in:* adult health, community health, pediatric. *Nurse practitioner programs in:* acute care, adult health, family health, gerontology, pediatric.
Site Options Washington, DC.
Study Options Full-time and part-time.
Program Entrance Requirements Clinical experience, minimum overall college GPA of 3.0, transcript of college record, written essay, immunizations, 3 letters of recommendation, professional liability insurance/malpractice insurance, prerequisite course work, statistics course. *Application deadline:* 8/1 (fall), 12/1 (spring). Applications may be processed on a rolling basis for some programs. *Application fee:* $55.
Advanced Placement Credit given for nursing courses completed elsewhere dependent upon specific evaluations.
Degree Requirements 44 total credit hours, comprehensive exam.

POST-MASTER'S PROGRAM

Areas of Study *Clinical nurse specialist programs in:* adult health, community health, pediatric. *Nurse practitioner programs in:* acute care, adult health, family health, gerontology, pediatric.

DOCTORAL DEGREE PROGRAM

Degree DNP
Available Programs Doctorate.
Online Degree Options Two-week residency requirement at the start of each semester, then the balance of the semester is online.
Program Entrance Requirements Clinical experience, minimum overall college GPA of 3.5, interview by faculty committee, interview, 3 letters of recommendation, MSN or equivalent, scholarly papers, writing sample; graduate level courses in health policy, bioethics, health promotion, and statistics; advanced practice certification or willingness to obtain post-master's certification in an area of advanced practice. Applications are processed on a rolling basis.
Degree Requirements 34-37 total credits for post-master's, which may include 6 graduate transfer credits.

Degree PhD
Available Programs Doctorate; Post-Baccalaureate Doctorate.
Areas of Study Advanced practice nursing, clinical practice, ethics, gerontology, human health and illness, nursing research, nursing science, women's health.
Online Degree Options Yes.
Program Entrance Requirements Clinical experience, minimum overall college GPA of 3.5, interview by faculty committee, interview, 3 letters of recommendation, MSN or equivalent, scholarly papers, statistics course, writing sample, GRE General Test. Application deadline: 8/1 (fall), 12/1 (spring). Applications may be processed on a rolling basis for some programs. Application fee: $55.
Degree Requirements 70 total credit hours, dissertation, oral exam, written exam, residency.

Georgetown University

School of Nursing and Health Studies
Washington, District of Columbia

http://nhs.georgetown.edu/
Founded in 1789

DEGREES • BSN • MS

Nursing Program Faculty 77 (35% with doctorates).
Baccalaureate Enrollment 480 **Women** 85% **Men** 15% **Minority** 26% **International** 1% **Part-time** 2%
Graduate Enrollment 235 **Women** 73% **Men** 27% **Minority** 24% **International** 1% **Part-time** 20%
Nursing Student Activities Nursing Honor Society, Sigma Theta Tau, Student Nurses' Association.
Nursing Student Resources Academic advising; academic or career counseling; assistance for students with disabilities; bookstore; campus computer network; career placement assistance; computer lab; computer-assisted instruction; e-mail services; employment services for current students; housing assistance; interactive nursing skills videos; Internet; learning resource lab; library services; nursing audiovisuals; placement services for program completers; resume preparation assistance; skills, simulation, or other laboratory; tutoring; unpaid internships.
Library Facilities 36,000 volumes in health, 20,000 volumes in nursing; 92 periodical subscriptions health-care related.

BACCALAUREATE PROGRAMS

Degree BSN
Available Programs Accelerated Baccalaureate for Second Degree; Generic Baccalaureate.
Study Options Full-time.
Program Entrance Requirements CPR certification, written essay, health exam, health insurance, 3 years high school math, 4 years high school science, high school transcript, immunizations, interview, 2 letters of recommendation. Transfer students are accepted. *Application deadline:* 1/10 (fall). *Application fee:* $65.
Expenses (2010-11) *Tuition:* full-time $39,768. *Room and board:* $12,758 per academic year. *Required fees:* full-time $760.
Financial Aid 70% of baccalaureate students in nursing programs received some form of financial aid in 2009-10. *Gift aid (need-based):* Federal Pell, FSEOG, state, private, college/university gift aid from institutional funds. *Loans:* Federal Nursing Student Loans, Perkins, alternative loans. *Work-study:* Federal Work-Study. *Financial aid application deadline:* 2/1.
Contact Office of Undergraduate Admissions, School of Nursing and Health Studies, Georgetown University, 37th and O Street NW, Washington, DC 20057. *Telephone:* 202-687-3600.

GRADUATE PROGRAMS

Expenses (2010-11) *Tuition:* full-time $39,768; part-time $1577 per credit. *Required fees:* full-time $400.
Financial Aid 70% of graduate students in nursing programs received some form of financial aid in 2009-10. Scholarships and traineeships available.
Contact Office of Graduate Admissions, School of Nursing and Health Studies, Georgetown University, 37th and O Street NW, Washington, DC 20057. *Telephone:* 202-687-5568.

MASTER'S DEGREE PROGRAM

Degree MS
Available Programs Master's; Master's for Non-Nursing College Graduates.
Concentrations Available Health-care administration; nurse anesthesia; nurse-midwifery; nursing education. *Clinical nurse specialist programs in:* acute care, critical care. *Nurse practitioner programs in:* acute care, family health, women's health.
Study Options Full-time and part-time.
Program Entrance Requirements Clinical experience, minimum overall college GPA of 3.0, transcript of college record, CPR certification, written essay, immunizations, interview, 3 letters of recommendation, resume, statistics course, GRE General Test or MAT. *Application deadline:* 1/15 (fall). Applications may be processed on a rolling basis for some programs. *Application fee:* $75.
Advanced Placement Credit given for nursing courses completed elsewhere dependent upon specific evaluations.
Degree Requirements 40 total credit hours, thesis or project.

POST-MASTER'S PROGRAM

Areas of Study Nurse-midwifery; nursing education. *Clinical nurse specialist programs in:* acute care, critical care. *Nurse practitioner programs in:* acute care, family health, women's health.

The George Washington University

Department of Nursing Education
Washington, District of Columbia

Founded in 1821

DEGREES • BSN • DNP • MSN

Distance Learning Courses Available.
Nursing Student Activities Sigma Theta Tau.
Nursing Student Resources Academic advising; academic or career counseling; bookstore; campus computer network; computer lab; computer-assisted instruction; e-mail services; interactive nursing skills

videos; Internet; learning resource lab; library services; nursing audiovisuals; skills, simulation, or other laboratory.

BACCALAUREATE PROGRAMS

Degree BSN
Available Programs Accelerated Baccalaureate for Second Degree.
Study Options Full-time.
Program Entrance Requirements Minimum overall college GPA of 2.8, transcript of college record, CPR certification, written essay, health exam, health insurance, immunizations, 2 letters of recommendation, minimum GPA in nursing prerequisites of 3.0, prerequisite course work. *Application deadline:* 6/15 (fall). *Application fee:* $60.
Contact Leigh Ellen Baca, Executive Coordinator, Department of Nursing Education, The George Washington University, 900 23rd Street NW, Suite 6167, Washington, DC 20037. *Telephone:* 202-994-7901. *Fax:* 202-994-2777. *E-mail:* hspleb@gwumc.edu.

GRADUATE PROGRAMS

Contact Joe Velez, Nursing Education Department, Department of Nursing Education, The George Washington University, 900 23rd Street NW, Suite 6167, Washington, DC 20037. *Telephone:* 202-994-7901. *Fax:* 202-994-2777. *E-mail:* nursing@gwumc.edu.

MASTER'S DEGREE PROGRAM

Degree MSN
Available Programs Master's.
Concentrations Available Clinical nurse leader; health-care administration; nursing administration. *Nurse practitioner programs in:* adult health, family health.

POST-MASTER'S PROGRAM

Areas of Study *Nurse practitioner programs in:* adult health, family health.

DOCTORAL DEGREE PROGRAM

Degree DNP
Available Programs Doctorate.

Howard University

Division of Nursing
Washington, District of Columbia

http://www.howard.edu
Founded in 1867

DEGREES • BSN • MSN

Nursing Program Faculty 32 (25% with doctorates).
Graduate Enrollment 22 **Women** 90% **Men** 10% **Minority** 55% **International** 45% **Part-time** 75%
Nursing Student Activities Sigma Theta Tau, Student Nurses' Association.
Nursing Student Resources Academic advising; academic or career counseling; assistance for students with disabilities; bookstore; campus computer network; career placement assistance; computer lab; computer-assisted instruction; e-mail services; externships; housing assistance; interactive nursing skills videos; Internet; learning resource lab; library services; nursing audiovisuals; paid internships; placement services for program completers; remedial services; resume preparation assistance; skills, simulation, or other laboratory.
Library Facilities 2.5 million volumes (219,448 in health, 4,500 in nursing); 26,382 periodical subscriptions (5,247 health-care related).

BACCALAUREATE PROGRAMS

Degree BSN
Available Programs Accelerated Baccalaureate for Second Degree; Baccalaureate for Second Degree; Generic Baccalaureate; LPN to Baccalaureate; RN Baccalaureate.
Study Options Full-time and part-time.
Program Entrance Requirements Minimum overall college GPA of 2.8, transcript of college record, CPR certification, written essay, health exam, high school biology, high school chemistry, 2 years high school math, 2 years high school science, high school transcript, immunizations, 2 letters of recommendation, minimum high school GPA of 2.8, minimum high school rank 50%, minimum GPA in nursing prerequisites of 2.5. Transfer students are accepted. *Application deadline:* 2/15 (fall), 4/1 (summer). *Application fee:* $45.
Advanced Placement Credit by examination available. Credit given for nursing courses completed elsewhere dependent upon specific evaluations.
Contact *Telephone:* 202-806-7854. *Fax:* 202-806-5958.

GRADUATE PROGRAMS

Contact *Telephone:* 202-806-7460. *Fax:* 202-806-5978.

MASTER'S DEGREE PROGRAM

Degree MSN
Available Programs Master's.
Concentrations Available *Nurse practitioner programs in:* family health.
Study Options Full-time and part-time.
Program Entrance Requirements Minimum overall college GPA of 3.0, transcript of college record, CPR certification, written essay, immunizations, interview, 3 letters of recommendation, physical assessment course, professional liability insurance/malpractice insurance, statistics course. *Application deadline:* Applications may be processed on a rolling basis for some programs. *Application fee:* $45.
Advanced Placement Credit given for nursing courses completed elsewhere dependent upon specific evaluations.
Degree Requirements 46 total credit hours, comprehensive exam.

POST-MASTER'S PROGRAM

Areas of Study *Nurse practitioner programs in:* family health.

Trinity (Washington) University

Nursing Program
Washington, District of Columbia

Founded in 1897

DEGREE • BSN

Nursing Program Faculty 9 (4% with doctorates).
Baccalaureate Enrollment 80
Nursing Student Activities Sigma Theta Tau, Student Nurses' Association.
Nursing Student Resources Academic advising; academic or career counseling; assistance for students with disabilities; bookstore; campus computer network; career placement assistance; computer lab; computer-assisted instruction; e-mail services; employment services for current students; housing assistance; Internet; learning resource lab; library services; nursing audiovisuals; paid internships; remedial services; resume preparation assistance; skills, simulation, or other laboratory; tutoring; unpaid internships.
Library Facilities 207,000 volumes (1,200 in health, 200 in nursing); 498 periodical subscriptions (40 health-care related).

BACCALAUREATE PROGRAMS

Degree BSN
Available Programs Generic Baccalaureate; RN Baccalaureate.
Study Options Full-time and part-time.
Program Entrance Requirements Transcript of college record, CPR certification, written essay, health exam, health insurance, high school transcript, immunizations, interview, 1 letter of recommendation, minimum GPA in nursing prerequisites of 2.0, professional liability insurance/malpractice insurance, prerequisite course work, RN licensure. Transfer students are accepted. *Application deadline:* Applications may be processed on a rolling basis for some programs.
Advanced Placement Credit by examination available. Credit given for nursing courses completed elsewhere dependent upon specific evaluations.
Contact *Telephone:* 202-884-9245. *Fax:* 202-884-9308.

University of the District of Columbia

Nursing Education Program
Washington, District of Columbia

Founded in 1976

DEGREE • BSN

Nursing Program Faculty 6 (3% with doctorates).

Baccalaureate Enrollment 40 **Women** 97% **Men** 3% **Minority** 98% **International** 50% **Part-time** 50%

Nursing Student Activities Student Nurses' Association.

Nursing Student Resources Academic advising; academic or career counseling; assistance for students with disabilities; bookstore; campus computer network; career placement assistance; computer lab; computer-assisted instruction; daycare for children of students; e-mail services; employment services for current students; Internet; learning resource lab; library services; nursing audiovisuals; remedial services; resume preparation assistance; skills, simulation, or other laboratory; tutoring.

Library Facilities 544,412 volumes (500 in health, 250 in nursing); 594 periodical subscriptions (75 health-care related).

BACCALAUREATE PROGRAMS

Degree BSN

Available Programs RN Baccalaureate.

Site Options Washington, DC.

Study Options Full-time and part-time.

Program Entrance Requirements Minimum overall college GPA of 2.7, transcript of college record, CPR certification, written essay, health exam, health insurance, immunizations, 2 letters of recommendation, minimum GPA in nursing prerequisites of 2.7, professional liability insurance/malpractice insurance, prerequisite course work, RN licensure. Transfer students are accepted. *Application deadline:* 6/15 (fall), 11/15 (spring), 4/15 (summer).

Advanced Placement Credit by examination available. Credit given for nursing courses completed elsewhere dependent upon specific evaluations.

Expenses (2010-11) *Tuition, area resident:* full-time $7000; part-time $266 per credit. *Tuition, state resident:* full-time $8000; part-time $308 per credit. *Tuition, nonresident:* full-time $14,000; part-time $558 per credit. *Required fees:* full-time $690; part-time $30 per credit.

Financial Aid 30% of baccalaureate students in nursing programs received some form of financial aid in 2009-10. *Gift aid (need-based):* Federal Pell, FSEOG, state, college/university gift aid from institutional funds. *Loans:* Perkins, college/university. *Work-study:* Federal Work-Study, part-time campus jobs. *Financial aid application deadline (priority):* 3/31.

Contact Dr. Pier Angeli Broadnax, Director, Nursing Program, Nursing Education Program, University of the District of Columbia, Building 44, Room 104A, 4200 Connecticut Avenue NW, Washington, DC 20008-1175. *Telephone:* 202-274-5916. *Fax:* 202-274-5952. *E-mail:* pbroadnax@udc.edu.

FLORIDA

Barry University

School of Nursing
Miami Shores, Florida

http://www.barry.edu/nursing
Founded in 1940

DEGREES • BSN • MSN • MSN/MBA • PHD

Nursing Program Faculty 30 (50% with doctorates).

Baccalaureate Enrollment 431 **Women** 87% **Men** 13% **Minority** 51% **International** 2% **Part-time** 20%

Graduate Enrollment 161 **Women** 93% **Men** 7% **Minority** 51% **International** 1% **Part-time** 99%

Nursing Student Activities Sigma Theta Tau, Student Nurses' Association.

Nursing Student Resources Academic advising; academic or career counseling; assistance for students with disabilities; bookstore; campus computer network; career placement assistance; computer lab; computer-assisted instruction; e-mail services; employment services for current students; housing assistance; interactive nursing skills videos; Internet; learning resource lab; library services; nursing audiovisuals; paid internships; remedial services; resume preparation assistance; skills, simulation, or other laboratory; tutoring.

Library Facilities 316,517 volumes (15,000 in health, 8,500 in nursing); 2,880 periodical subscriptions (400 health-care related).

BACCALAUREATE PROGRAMS

Degree BSN

Available Programs ADN to Baccalaureate; Accelerated Baccalaureate; Accelerated Baccalaureate for Second Degree; Baccalaureate for Second Degree; Generic Baccalaureate; LPN to Baccalaureate; LPN to RN Baccalaureate; RN Baccalaureate.

Site Options Davie, FL; Kendall, FL.

Study Options Full-time and part-time.

Program Entrance Requirements Minimum overall college GPA of 3.0, transcript of college record, CPR certification, health exam, health insurance, high school biology, high school chemistry, high school math, high school science, high school transcript, immunizations, 2 letters of recommendation, minimum high school GPA of 3.0, minimum GPA in nursing prerequisites of 3.0, professional liability insurance/malpractice insurance. Transfer students are accepted. *Application deadline:* Applications may be processed on a rolling basis for some programs.

Advanced Placement Credit given for nursing courses completed elsewhere dependent upon specific evaluations.

Expenses (2009-10) *Tuition:* full-time $26,400; part-time $790 per credit.

Financial Aid 90% of baccalaureate students in nursing programs received some form of financial aid in 2008-09.

Contact Ms. Rosanne Sonshine, Recruiter and Clinical Coordinator, School of Nursing, Barry University, 11300 NE Second Avenue, Miami Shores, FL 33161-6695. *Telephone:* 305-899-3813. *Fax:* 305-899-3831. *E-mail:* rsonshine@mail.barry.edu.

GRADUATE PROGRAMS

Expenses (2009-10) *Tuition:* part-time $845 per credit.

Financial Aid 90% of graduate students in nursing programs received some form of financial aid in 2008-09. 3 research assistantships (averaging $5,000 per year), 3 teaching assistantships (averaging $5,000 per year) were awarded; scholarships and tuition waivers (full) also available. *Financial aid application deadline:* 5/1.

Contact Rosanne Sonshine, Recruiter and Clinical Coordinator, School of Nursing, Barry University, 11300 NE Second Avenue, Miami Shores, FL 33161-6695. *Telephone:* 305-899-3813. *Fax:* 305-899-3831. *E-mail:* rsonshine@mail.barry.edu.

MASTER'S DEGREE PROGRAM

Degrees MSN; MSN/MBA

Available Programs Master's.

Concentrations Available Nursing administration; nursing education. *Nurse practitioner programs in:* acute care, family health.

Study Options Part-time.

Program Entrance Requirements Clinical experience, computer literacy, minimum overall college GPA of 3.0, transcript of college record, written essay, 2 letters of recommendation, nursing research course, professional liability insurance/malpractice insurance, statistics course, GRE General Test or MAT. *Application deadline:* Applications may be processed on a rolling basis for some programs.

Advanced Placement Credit given for nursing courses completed elsewhere dependent upon specific evaluations.

Degree Requirements 45 total credit hours.

POST-MASTER'S PROGRAM

Areas of Study Nursing administration; nursing education. *Nurse practitioner programs in:* acute care, family health.

DOCTORAL DEGREE PROGRAM

Degree PhD

Available Programs Doctorate.

Areas of Study Nursing research, nursing science.

Program Entrance Requirements Clinical experience, minimum overall college GPA of 3.0, interview, 2 letters of recommendation, MSN or equivalent, statistics course, writing sample, GRE General Test or MAT. Application deadline: Applications may be processed on a rolling basis for some programs.

Degree Requirements 45 total credit hours, dissertation, written exam, residency.

Bethune-Cookman University

School of Nursing
Daytona Beach, Florida

http://www.cookman.edu/Nursing
Founded in 1904

DEGREE • BSN
Nursing Program Faculty 11 (2% with doctorates).
Baccalaureate Enrollment 137 **Women** 93% **Men** 7% **Minority** 95% **International** 2%
Nursing Student Activities Nursing Honor Society, Student Nurses' Association.
Nursing Student Resources Academic advising; bookstore; campus computer network; computer lab; computer-assisted instruction; e-mail services; interactive nursing skills videos; Internet; learning resource lab; library services; nursing audiovisuals; resume preparation assistance; skills, simulation, or other laboratory; tutoring; unpaid internships.
Library Facilities 164,874 volumes; 800 periodical subscriptions.

BACCALAUREATE PROGRAMS
Degree BSN
Available Programs Generic Baccalaureate; RN Baccalaureate.
Study Options Full-time.
Program Entrance Requirements Minimum overall college GPA of 2.8, transcript of college record, CPR certification, written essay, health exam, high school transcript, immunizations, interview, 2 letters of recommendation, minimum GPA in nursing prerequisites of 2.8, prerequisite course work. Transfer students are accepted.
Advanced Placement Credit by examination available. Credit given for nursing courses completed elsewhere dependent upon specific evaluations.
Contact ***Telephone:*** 386-481-2000.

Florida Agricultural and Mechanical University

School of Nursing
Tallahassee, Florida

http://www.famu.edu/acad/colleges/son
Founded in 1887

DEGREES • BSN • MSN • PHD
Nursing Program Faculty 28 (18% with doctorates).
Baccalaureate Enrollment 161 **Women** 90% **Men** 10% **Minority** 98%
Graduate Enrollment 17 **Women** 83% **Men** 17% **Minority** 76% **Part-time** 12%
Nursing Student Activities Sigma Theta Tau, Student Nurses' Association.
Nursing Student Resources Academic advising; academic or career counseling; bookstore; campus computer network; career placement assistance; computer lab; computer-assisted instruction; daycare for children of students; e-mail services; employment services for current students; externships; interactive nursing skills videos; Internet; library services; nursing audiovisuals; placement services for program completers; remedial services; resume preparation assistance; skills, simulation, or other laboratory; tutoring.
Library Facilities 889,272 volumes (5,000 in health, 4,091 in nursing); 59,695 periodical subscriptions (385 health-care related).

BACCALAUREATE PROGRAMS
Degree BSN
Available Programs Generic Baccalaureate.
Study Options Part-time.
Program Entrance Requirements CPR certification, health exam, immunizations, 3 letters of recommendation, minimum high school GPA of 2.5, prerequisite course work. Transfer students are accepted.
Contact ***Telephone:*** 850-599-3458. *Fax:* 850-599-3508.

GRADUATE PROGRAMS
Contact ***Telephone:*** 850-599-3017. *Fax:* 850-599-3508.

MASTER'S DEGREE PROGRAM
Degree MSN
Available Programs Master's.
Concentrations Available *Nurse practitioner programs in:* adult health, gerontology, women's health.
Study Options Full-time and part-time.
Program Entrance Requirements Clinical experience, minimum overall college GPA of 3.0, CPR certification, immunizations, interview, nursing research course, physical assessment course, professional liability insurance/malpractice insurance, statistics course.
Degree Requirements 42 total credit hours, thesis or project.

POST-MASTER'S PROGRAM
Areas of Study *Nurse practitioner programs in:* adult health, gerontology, women's health.

DOCTORAL DEGREE PROGRAM
Degree PhD
Program Entrance Requirements Minimum overall college GPA of 3.5, 3 letters of recommendation, MSN or equivalent.
Degree Requirements 90 total credit hours, dissertation, oral exam, written exam.

CONTINUING EDUCATION PROGRAM
Contact ***Telephone:*** 850-599-3017. *Fax:* 850-599-3508.

Florida Atlantic University

Christine E. Lynn College of Nursing
Boca Raton, Florida

http://www.fau.edu/nursing
Founded in 1961

DEGREES • BS • MS • MSN/MBA • PHD
Nursing Program Faculty 73 (49% with doctorates).
Baccalaureate Enrollment 528 **Women** 85% **Men** 15% **Minority** 40% **International** 5% **Part-time** 40%
Graduate Enrollment 515 **Women** 89% **Men** 11% **Minority** 39% **International** 2% **Part-time** 85%
Distance Learning Courses Available.
Nursing Student Activities Sigma Theta Tau, Student Nurses' Association.
Nursing Student Resources Academic advising; academic or career counseling; assistance for students with disabilities; bookstore; campus computer network; computer lab; computer-assisted instruction; e-mail services; housing assistance; interactive nursing skills videos; Internet; learning resource lab; library services; nursing audiovisuals; remedial services; skills, simulation, or other laboratory; tutoring.
Library Facilities 1.3 million volumes (17,825 in health, 4,889 in nursing); 12,811 periodical subscriptions (333 health-care related).

BACCALAUREATE PROGRAMS
Degree BS
Available Programs Accelerated Baccalaureate for Second Degree; Generic Baccalaureate; RN Baccalaureate.
Site Options Port St. Lucie, FL; Davie, FL.
Study Options Full-time.
Program Entrance Requirements Minimum overall college GPA of 3.0, transcript of college record, CPR certification, health exam, health insurance, high school transcript, immunizations, minimum GPA in nursing prerequisites of 2.0, professional liability insurance/malpractice insurance, prerequisite course work. Transfer students are accepted. *Application deadline:* 11/30 (fall). *Application fee:* $30.
Advanced Placement Credit by examination available. Credit given for nursing courses completed elsewhere dependent upon specific evaluations.
Expenses (2009-10) *Tuition, state resident:* full-time $1680; part-time $840 per semester. *Tuition, nonresident:* full-time $7008; part-time $3500 per semester. *International tuition:* $7008 full-time. *Room and board:* $9500; room only: $5000 per academic year. *Required fees:* full-time $300; part-time $100 per term.
Financial Aid 75% of baccalaureate students in nursing programs received some form of financial aid in 2008-09. *Gift aid (need-based):* Federal Pell, FSEOG, state, private, college/university gift aid from institutional funds, Federal Nursing. *Loans:* Perkins, college/university. *Work-study:* Federal Work-Study, part-time campus jobs. *Financial aid application deadline (priority):* 3/1.
Contact Ms. Mary Ellen Wright, Interim Director, Undergraduate Programs, Christine E. Lynn College of Nursing, Florida Atlantic University,

777 Glades Road, Boca Raton, FL 33431. *Telephone:* 561-297-2535. *Fax:* 561-297-3652. *E-mail:* mehodges@fau.edu.

GRADUATE PROGRAMS

Expenses (2009-10) *Tuition, state resident:* full-time $7055; part-time $294 per credit hour. *Tuition, nonresident:* full-time $22,095; part-time $921 per credit hour. *International tuition:* $22,095 full-time. *Room and board:* $9500; room only: $5000 per academic year. *Required fees:* full-time $1500; part-time $500 per term.
Financial Aid 15% of graduate students in nursing programs received some form of financial aid in 2008-09. Research assistantships with partial tuition reimbursements available, teaching assistantships with partial tuition reimbursements available, career-related internships or fieldwork, Federal Work-Study, institutionally sponsored loans, scholarships, and traineeships available. Aid available to part-time students.
Contact Dr. Shirley Gordon, Masters Program Director, Christine E. Lynn College of Nursing, Florida Atlantic University, 777 Glades Road, Boca Raton, FL 33431. *Telephone:* 561-297-3389. *Fax:* 561-297-3652. *E-mail:* sgordon@fau.edu.

MASTER'S DEGREE PROGRAM

Degrees MS; MSN/MBA
Available Programs Master's; Master's for Nurses with Non-Nursing Degrees; RN to Master's.
Concentrations Available Clinical nurse leader; nursing administration; nursing education. *Nurse practitioner programs in:* adult health, family health, gerontology.
Site Options Port St. Lucie, FL; Davie, FL.
Online Degree Options Yes.
Program Entrance Requirements Minimum overall college GPA of 3.0, transcript of college record, CPR certification, written essay, immunizations, interview, 2 letters of recommendation, nursing research course, physical assessment course, professional liability insurance/malpractice insurance, prerequisite course work, resume, statistics course, GRE General Test. *Application deadline:* 6/1 (fall), 10/1 (spring), 2/1 (summer). *Application fee:* $30.
Degree Requirements 30 total credit hours.

POST-MASTER'S PROGRAM

Areas of Study Clinical nurse leader; nursing administration; nursing education. *Nurse practitioner programs in:* adult health, family health, gerontology.

DOCTORAL DEGREE PROGRAM

Degree PhD
Available Programs Doctorate; Post-Baccalaureate Doctorate.
Areas of Study Aging, bio-behavioral research, gerontology, human health and illness, individualized study, nursing administration, nursing research, nursing science.
Program Entrance Requirements Minimum overall college GPA of 3.5, interview by faculty committee, interview, 3 letters of recommendation, MSN or equivalent, scholarly papers, statistics course, vita, writing sample, GRE General Test. Application deadline: 2/28 (fall). Application fee: $30.
Degree Requirements 62 total credit hours, dissertation, oral exam, written exam, residency.

CONTINUING EDUCATION PROGRAM

Contact Dr. Beth King, Director, Christine E. Lynn College of Nursing, Florida Atlantic University, 777 Glades Road, Boca Raton, FL 33431. *Telephone:* 561-297-3887. *Fax:* 561-297-3652. *E-mail:* bking@fau.edu.

Florida Gulf Coast University
School of Nursing
Fort Myers, Florida

http://www.fgcu.edu/chp/nursing/
Founded in 1991

DEGREES • BSN • MSN

Nursing Program Faculty 17 (57% with doctorates).
Baccalaureate Enrollment 160 **Women** 96.5% **Men** 3.5% **Minority** 29.5% **International** 7%
Graduate Enrollment 48 **Women** 86% **Men** 14% **Minority** 20% **Part-time** 10%
Nursing Student Activities Sigma Theta Tau, Student Nurses' Association.
Nursing Student Resources Academic advising; academic or career counseling; assistance for students with disabilities; bookstore; campus computer network; career placement assistance; computer lab; computer-assisted instruction; e-mail services; employment services for current students; Internet; learning resource lab; library services; nursing audiovisuals; skills, simulation, or other laboratory; tutoring.
Library Facilities 387,860 volumes (13,943 in health, 6,742 in nursing); 12,374 periodical subscriptions (471 health-care related).

BACCALAUREATE PROGRAMS

Degree BSN
Available Programs ADN to Baccalaureate; Generic Baccalaureate.
Study Options Full-time.
Program Entrance Requirements Minimum overall college GPA of 3.0, transcript of college record, CPR certification, health insurance, high school foreign language, immunizations, professional liability insurance/malpractice insurance, prerequisite course work. Transfer students are accepted.
Advanced Placement Credit by examination available. Credit given for nursing courses completed elsewhere dependent upon specific evaluations.
Contact School of Nursing Advising, School of Nursing, Florida Gulf Coast University, 10501 FGCU Boulevard South, Fort Myers, FL 33965-6565. *Telephone:* 239-590-7485. *Fax:* 239-590-7474. *E-mail:* ayoung@fgcu.edu.

GRADUATE PROGRAMS

Financial Aid 45% of graduate students in nursing programs received some form of financial aid in 2009-10.
Contact Dr. Marydelle Polk, Program Director, School of Nursing, Florida Gulf Coast University, 10501 FGCU Boulevard South, Fort Myers, FL 33965-6565. *Telephone:* 239-590-7518. *Fax:* 239-590-7474. *E-mail:* mpolk@fgcu.edu.

MASTER'S DEGREE PROGRAM

Degree MSN
Available Programs Master's.
Concentrations Available Nurse anesthesia; nursing education. *Nurse practitioner programs in:* acute care, adult health, family health.
Study Options Full-time and part-time.
Program Entrance Requirements Minimum overall college GPA of 3.0, physical assessment course, resume, statistics course.
Advanced Placement Credit given for nursing courses completed elsewhere dependent upon specific evaluations.

POST-MASTER'S PROGRAM

Areas of Study *Nurse practitioner programs in:* family health.

CONTINUING EDUCATION PROGRAM

Contact Dr. Anne Nolan, Associate Professor, School of Nursing, Florida Gulf Coast University, 10501 FGCU Boulevard South, Fort Myers, FL 33931. *Telephone:* 239-590-7513. *Fax:* 239-590-7474. *E-mail:* anolan@fgcu.edu.

Florida Hospital College of Health Sciences
Department of Nursing
Orlando, Florida

http://www.fhchs.edu/
Founded in 1913

DEGREE • BS

Nursing Program Faculty 12 (16% with doctorates).
Nursing Student Resources Campus computer network; computer lab; computer-assisted instruction; Internet; learning resource lab; library services; nursing audiovisuals; skills, simulation, or other laboratory.
Library Facilities 74,581 volumes; 158 periodical subscriptions.

BACCALAUREATE PROGRAMS

Degree BS
Available Programs Generic Baccalaureate; RN Baccalaureate.
Study Options Full-time and part-time.

Program Entrance Requirements Minimum overall college GPA of 2.5, transcript of college record, health exam, 1 letter of recommendation, prerequisite course work, RN licensure. Transfer students are accepted.
Advanced Placement Credit by examination available. Credit given for nursing courses completed elsewhere dependent upon specific evaluations.
Contact *Telephone:* 407-303-9798. *Fax:* 407-303-9408.

Florida International University
Nursing Program
Miami, Florida

http://www.fiu.edu
Founded in 1965

DEGREES • BSN • MSN • PHD

Nursing Program Faculty 77 (29% with doctorates).
Baccalaureate Enrollment 474 **Women** 73% **Men** 27% **Minority** 88% **International** 1% **Part-time** 25%
Graduate Enrollment 395 **Women** 82% **Men** 18% **Minority** 74% **International** 1% **Part-time** 60%
Distance Learning Courses Available.
Nursing Student Activities Sigma Theta Tau, Student Nurses' Association.
Nursing Student Resources Academic advising; academic or career counseling; assistance for students with disabilities; bookstore; campus computer network; career placement assistance; computer lab; computer-assisted instruction; daycare for children of students; e-mail services; externships; housing assistance; interactive nursing skills videos; Internet; learning resource lab; library services; nursing audiovisuals; paid internships; remedial services; resume preparation assistance; skills, simulation, or other laboratory; tutoring.
Library Facilities 2.1 million volumes (25,000 in health, 3,300 in nursing); 48,143 periodical subscriptions (1,500 health-care related).

BACCALAUREATE PROGRAMS

Degree BSN
Available Programs Accelerated Baccalaureate for Second Degree; Generic Baccalaureate; RN Baccalaureate.
Site Options St. Petersburg, FL; North Miami, FL.
Study Options Full-time.
Online Degree Options Yes.
Program Entrance Requirements Minimum overall college GPA of 3.0, transcript of college record, CPR certification, written essay, health exam, health insurance, high school foreign language, high school transcript, immunizations, minimum GPA in nursing prerequisites of 3.0, prerequisite course work. Transfer students are accepted. *Application deadline:* 5/15 (fall), 2/15 (summer). *Application fee:* $30.
Advanced Placement Credit by examination available. Credit given for nursing courses completed elsewhere dependent upon specific evaluations.
Expenses (2009-10) *Tuition, state resident:* full-time $4004; part-time $128 per credit. *Tuition, nonresident:* full-time $16,782; part-time $542 per credit. *International tuition:* $16,782 full-time. *Room and board:* $16,000; room only: $10,000 per academic year. *Required fees:* full-time $1500; part-time $62 per credit; part-time $500 per term.
Financial Aid 75% of baccalaureate students in nursing programs received some form of financial aid in 2008-09.
Contact Diane M. Loffredo, Director for Admissions and Student Services, Nursing Program, Florida International University, 11200 SW 8th Street, Modesto A. Maidique Campus, HLS 2, RM 482, Miami, FL 33199. *Telephone:* 305-348-7717. *Fax:* 305-348-7764. *E-mail:* dloffred@fiu.edu.

GRADUATE PROGRAMS

Expenses (2009-10) *Tuition, state resident:* full-time $9174; part-time $341 per credit. *Tuition, nonresident:* full-time $22,822; part-time $845 per credit. *International tuition:* $22,822 full-time. *Room and board:* $16,000; room only: $10,000 per academic year. *Required fees:* full-time $1600; part-time $65 per credit; part-time $600 per term.
Financial Aid 60% of graduate students in nursing programs received some form of financial aid in 2008-09. Institutionally sponsored loans and scholarships available. *Financial aid application deadline:* 3/1.
Contact Diane M. Loffredo, Director for Admissions and Student Services, Nursing Program, Florida International University, 11200 SW 8th Street, Modesto A. Maidique Campus, HLS 2, RM 482, Miami, FL 33199. *Telephone:* 305-348-7717. *Fax:* 305-348-7764. *E-mail:* dloffred@fiu.edu.

MASTER'S DEGREE PROGRAM

Degree MSN
Available Programs Accelerated AD/RN to Master's; Master's; Master's for Nurses with Non-Nursing Degrees.
Concentrations Available Nurse anesthesia; nursing administration; nursing education. *Nurse practitioner programs in:* adult health, family health, pediatric.
Study Options Full-time and part-time.
Program Entrance Requirements Clinical experience, computer literacy, minimum overall college GPA of 3.0, transcript of college record, CPR certification, written essay, immunizations, interview, 3 letters of recommendation, nursing research course, physical assessment course, professional liability insurance/malpractice insurance, prerequisite course work, resume, statistics course. *Application deadline:* 6/1 (fall), 10/1 (spring), 3/1 (summer). *Application fee:* $30.
Advanced Placement Credit given for nursing courses completed elsewhere dependent upon specific evaluations.
Degree Requirements 43 total credit hours.

POST-MASTER'S PROGRAM

Areas of Study Nursing administration; nursing education. *Nurse practitioner programs in:* adult health, family health, pediatric.

DOCTORAL DEGREE PROGRAM

Degree PhD
Available Programs Doctorate.
Areas of Study Faculty preparation, health policy, health-care systems, individualized study, nursing administration, nursing education, nursing policy, nursing research, nursing science.
Program Entrance Requirements Clinical experience, minimum overall college GPA of 3.0, interview by faculty committee, 3 letters of recommendation, MSN or equivalent, statistics course, writing sample, GRE. Application deadline: Applications may be processed on a rolling basis for some programs. Application fee: $30.
Degree Requirements 84 total credit hours, dissertation, oral exam, written exam.

Florida Southern College
Department of Nursing
Lakeland, Florida

http://www.flsouthern.edu/academics/nursing/
Founded in 1885

DEGREES • BSN • MSN • MSN/MBA

Nursing Program Faculty 12 (75% with doctorates).
Baccalaureate Enrollment 149
Graduate Enrollment 89
Nursing Student Activities Nursing Honor Society, Sigma Theta Tau, Student Nurses' Association.
Nursing Student Resources Academic advising; academic or career counseling; assistance for students with disabilities; bookstore; campus computer network; career placement assistance; computer lab; computer-assisted instruction; e-mail services; externships; interactive nursing skills videos; Internet; learning resource lab; library services; nursing audiovisuals; paid internships; placement services for program completers; remedial services; resume preparation assistance; skills, simulation, or other laboratory; tutoring.
Library Facilities 175,213 volumes (4,000 in health, 3,500 in nursing); 50,328 periodical subscriptions (40 health-care related).

BACCALAUREATE PROGRAMS

Degree BSN
Available Programs ADN to Baccalaureate; Generic Baccalaureate.
Study Options Full-time.
Program Entrance Requirements Minimum overall college GPA of 3.2, transcript of college record, CPR certification, written essay, health exam, immunizations, minimum high school GPA of 3.2, minimum GPA in nursing prerequisites of 3.0, prerequisite course work. Transfer students are accepted. *Application deadline:* 3/1 (fall).
Advanced Placement Credit given for nursing courses completed elsewhere dependent upon specific evaluations.
Contact Dr. John Welton, Dean, Department of Nursing, Florida Southern College, 111 Lake Hollingsworth Drive, Blanton School of

Nursing, Lakeland, FL 33801. *Telephone:* 863-680-3951. *Fax:* 863-680-3860. *E-mail:* jwelton@flsouthern.edu.

GRADUATE PROGRAMS

Contact Dr. Beverley Brown, Graduate Program Director, Department of Nursing, Florida Southern College, 111 Lake Hollingsworth Drive, Blanton School of Nursing, Lakeland, FL 33801. *Telephone:* 863-680-3951. *Fax:* 863-680-3860. *E-mail:* bbrown@flsouthern.edu.

MASTER'S DEGREE PROGRAM

Degrees MSN; MSN/MBA
Available Programs Accelerated AD/RN to Master's; Master's; Master's for Nurses with Non-Nursing Degrees; RN to Master's.
Concentrations Available Nursing administration; nursing education. *Clinical nurse specialist programs in:* adult health, family health, gerontology. *Nurse practitioner programs in:* primary care.
Study Options Full-time and part-time.
Program Entrance Requirements Clinical experience, computer literacy, minimum overall college GPA of 3.0, transcript of college record, written essay, immunizations, 3 letters of recommendation, nursing research course, physical assessment course, professional liability insurance/malpractice insurance, resume, statistics course. *Application deadline:* 6/1 (fall), 11/1 (spring). *Application fee:* $30.
Advanced Placement Credit given for nursing courses completed elsewhere dependent upon specific evaluations.
Degree Requirements 39 total credit hours, thesis or project.

POST-MASTER'S PROGRAM

Areas of Study Nursing administration; nursing education. *Clinical nurse specialist programs in:* adult health, family health, gerontology. *Nurse practitioner programs in:* primary care.

Florida State College at Jacksonville

Nursing Department
Jacksonville, Florida

Founded in 1963

DEGREE • BSN

Nursing Program Faculty 6 (50% with doctorates).
Baccalaureate Enrollment 52
Distance Learning Courses Available.
Nursing Student Resources Academic advising; academic or career counseling; assistance for students with disabilities; bookstore; campus computer network; computer lab; computer-assisted instruction; daycare for children of students; e-mail services; employment services for current students; interactive nursing skills videos; Internet; learning resource lab; library services; nursing audiovisuals; skills, simulation, or other laboratory; tutoring.
Library Facilities 302,146 volumes; 3,326 periodical subscriptions.

BACCALAUREATE PROGRAMS

Degree BSN
Available Programs RN Baccalaureate.
Program Entrance Requirements Transcript of college record, CPR certification, health exam, immunizations, 1 letter of recommendation, minimum GPA in nursing prerequisites of 2.0, professional liability insurance/malpractice insurance, prerequisite course work, RN licensure. Transfer students are accepted.
Contact Dr. Mary Kathleen Ebener, Associate Dean of Nursing for BSN Program, Nursing Department, Florida State College at Jacksonville, North campus, 4501 Capper Road, Jacksonville, FL 32218. *Telephone:* 904-713-6015. *Fax:* 904-713-4850. *E-mail:* mebener@fscj.edu.

Florida State University

College of Nursing
Tallahassee, Florida

http://nursing.fsu.edu/
Founded in 1851

DEGREES • BSN • DNP • MSN

Nursing Program Faculty 46 (39% with doctorates).
Baccalaureate Enrollment 226 **Women** 89% **Men** 11% **Minority** 29% **International** 1% **Part-time** 10%
Graduate Enrollment 81 **Women** 98% **Men** 2% **Minority** 5% **Part-time** 55%
Distance Learning Courses Available.
Nursing Student Activities Sigma Theta Tau, Student Nurses' Association.
Nursing Student Resources Academic advising; academic or career counseling; assistance for students with disabilities; bookstore; campus computer network; career placement assistance; computer lab; computer-assisted instruction; e-mail services; housing assistance; interactive nursing skills videos; Internet; learning resource lab; library services; nursing audiovisuals; resume preparation assistance; skills, simulation, or other laboratory; tutoring; unpaid internships.
Library Facilities 3 million volumes; 78,300 periodical subscriptions.

BACCALAUREATE PROGRAMS

Degree BSN
Available Programs Accelerated Baccalaureate; Generic Baccalaureate; RN Baccalaureate.
Site Options Panama City, FL.
Study Options Full-time.
Online Degree Options Yes.
Program Entrance Requirements Minimum overall college GPA of 3.0, transcript of college record, CPR certification, health exam, health insurance, high school foreign language, immunizations, minimum GPA in nursing prerequisites of 3.0, professional liability insurance/malpractice insurance, prerequisite course work. Transfer students are accepted. *Application deadline:* 2/1 (fall).
Advanced Placement Credit given for nursing courses completed elsewhere dependent upon specific evaluations.
Expenses (2010-11) *Tuition, state resident:* full-time $4840; part-time $151 per credit hour. *Tuition, nonresident:* full-time $20,952; part-time $655 per credit hour. *Room and board:* $8390; room only: $4950 per academic year. *Required fees:* full-time $1240; part-time $100 per credit; part-time $20 per term.
Financial Aid 96% of baccalaureate students in nursing programs received some form of financial aid in 2009-10. *Gift aid (need-based):* Federal Pell, FSEOG, state, private, college/university gift aid from institutional funds, Academic Competitiveness Grants, National SMART Grants. *Loans:* Federal Direct (Subsidized and Unsubsidized Stafford PLUS), Perkins, college/university. *Work-study:* Federal Work-Study, part-time campus jobs. *Financial aid application deadline:* Continuous.
Contact Ms. Brenda Pereira, Director of Student Services, College of Nursing, Florida State University, 98 Varsity Way, 103 SCN, Tallahassee, FL 32306-4310. *Telephone:* 850-644-5638. *Fax:* 850-645-7249. *E-mail:* bpereira@fsu.edu.

GRADUATE PROGRAMS

Expenses (2010-11) *Tuition, state resident:* full-time $8908; part-time $371 per credit hour. *Tuition, nonresident:* full-time $24,060; part-time $1003 per credit hour. *Room and board:* $8390; room only: $4950 per academic year. *Required fees:* full-time $40; part-time $20 per term.
Financial Aid 91% of graduate students in nursing programs received some form of financial aid in 2009-10. Fellowships with partial tuition reimbursements available (averaging $6,300 per year), research assistantships with partial tuition reimbursements available (averaging $3,000 per year), 3 teaching assistantships with partial tuition reimbursements available (averaging $3,000 per year) were awarded; career-related internships or fieldwork, Federal Work-Study, institutionally sponsored loans, scholarships, traineeships, and tuition waivers (partial) also available. *Financial aid application deadline:* 4/15.
Contact Ms. Brenda Pereira, Director of Student Services, College of Nursing, Florida State University, 98 Varsity Way, 103 SCN, Tallahassee, FL 32306-4310. *Telephone:* 850-644-5638. *Fax:* 850-645-7249. *E-mail:* bpereira@fsu.edu.

MASTER'S DEGREE PROGRAM

Degree MSN
Available Programs Master's.
Concentrations Available Nursing education. *Nurse practitioner programs in:* family health.
Study Options Full-time and part-time.
Online Degree Options Yes (online only).
Program Entrance Requirements Minimum overall college GPA of 3.0, transcript of college record, CPR certification, immunizations, 2 letters of recommendation, professional liability insurance/malpractice insurance, GRE General Test, MAT. *Application deadline:* 7/1 (fall).

Advanced Placement Credit given for nursing courses completed elsewhere dependent upon specific evaluations.
Degree Requirements 38 total credit hours.

POST-MASTER'S PROGRAM
Areas of Study Nursing education.

DOCTORAL DEGREE PROGRAM
Degree DNP
Available Programs Doctorate.
Areas of Study Family health, health-care systems.
Site Options Panama City, FL; Sarasota, FL.
Program Entrance Requirements Minimum overall college GPA of 3.0, 2 letters of recommendation, GRE General Test, MAT. Application deadline: 4/15 (fall).
Degree Requirements 90 total credit hours, residency.

Indian River State College
Bachelor of Science in Nursing Program
Fort Pierce, Florida

Founded in 1960

DEGREE • BSN
Library Facilities 88,397 volumes; 198 periodical subscriptions.

BACCALAUREATE PROGRAMS
Degree BSN
Available Programs RN Baccalaureate.
Contact Nursing Program, Bachelor of Science in Nursing Program, Indian River State College, 3209 Virginia Avenue, Fort Pierce, FL 34981-5596. *Telephone:* 772-462-7415.

Jacksonville University
School of Nursing
Jacksonville, Florida

http://ju.edu/depts/nursing/default.aspx
Founded in 1934

DEGREES • BSN • MSN • MSN/MBA
Nursing Program Faculty 31 (52% with doctorates).
Baccalaureate Enrollment 700 **Women** 90% **Men** 10% **Minority** 40% **International** .5% **Part-time** 15%
Graduate Enrollment 90 **Women** 87% **Men** 13% **Minority** 37%
Distance Learning Courses Available.
Nursing Student Activities Nursing Honor Society, Sigma Theta Tau, Student Nurses' Association, nursing club.
Nursing Student Resources Academic advising; academic or career counseling; assistance for students with disabilities; bookstore; campus computer network; career placement assistance; computer lab; computer-assisted instruction; e-mail services; employment services for current students; externships; interactive nursing skills videos; Internet; learning resource lab; library services; nursing audiovisuals; placement services for program completers; remedial services; resume preparation assistance; skills, simulation, or other laboratory; tutoring; unpaid internships.

BACCALAUREATE PROGRAMS
Degree BSN
Available Programs ADN to Baccalaureate; Accelerated Baccalaureate; Accelerated Baccalaureate for Second Degree; Baccalaureate for Second Degree; Generic Baccalaureate.
Site Options Jacksonville, FL.
Study Options Full-time.
Online Degree Options Yes.
Program Entrance Requirements Minimum overall college GPA of 2.5, transcript of college record, CPR certification, written essay, health exam, health insurance, immunizations, interview, 3 letters of recommendation, minimum GPA in nursing prerequisites of 2.0, prerequisite course work. Transfer students are accepted. *Application deadline:* 4/1 (fall), 12/1 (summer). *Application fee:* $15.
Advanced Placement Credit given for nursing courses completed elsewhere dependent upon specific evaluations.
Expenses (2010-11) *Tuition:* full-time $26,600; part-time $883 per credit hour. *Room and board:* $4660; room only: $2780 per academic year.
Financial Aid 92% of baccalaureate students in nursing programs received some form of financial aid in 2009-10. *Gift aid (need-based):* Federal Pell, FSEOG, state, private, college/university gift aid from institutional funds, Academic Competitiveness Grants, National SMART Grants. *Loans:* Perkins, college/university, private loans. *Work-study:* Federal Work-Study. *Financial aid application deadline (priority):* 3/1.
Contact Mr. Chris Rillstone, Director of Enrollment and Program Development, School of Nursing, Jacksonville University, 2800 University Boulevard North, Jacksonville, FL 32211. *Telephone:* 904-256-7286. *Fax:* 904-256-7287. *E-mail:* crillst@ju.edu.

GRADUATE PROGRAMS
Expenses (2010-11) *Tuition:* full-time $5340; part-time $445 per credit hour.
Financial Aid 59% of graduate students in nursing programs received some form of financial aid in 2009-10.
Contact Ms. Laura Winn, Graduate Program Advisor, School of Nursing, Jacksonville University, 2800 University Boulevard North, Jacksonville, FL 32211. *Telephone:* 904-256-7034. *Fax:* 904-256-7287. *E-mail:* lwinn@ju.edu.

MASTER'S DEGREE PROGRAM
Degrees MSN; MSN/MBA
Available Programs Master's.
Concentrations Available Nursing administration; nursing education. *Nurse practitioner programs in:* family health.
Site Options Jacksonville, FL.
Study Options Full-time and part-time.
Online Degree Options Yes.
Program Entrance Requirements Clinical experience, minimum overall college GPA of 3.0, transcript of college record, CPR certification, written essay, immunizations, interview, 3 letters of recommendation, prerequisite course work, resume. *Application deadline:* 4/30 (fall). Applications may be processed on a rolling basis for some programs. *Application fee:* $30.
Advanced Placement Credit given for nursing courses completed elsewhere dependent upon specific evaluations.
Degree Requirements 46 total credit hours, thesis or project, comprehensive exam.

POST-MASTER'S PROGRAM
Areas of Study *Nurse practitioner programs in:* family health.

Kaplan University Online
The School of Nursing Online
Fort Lauderdale, Florida

DEGREES • BSN • MSN

BACCALAUREATE PROGRAMS
Degree BSN
Available Programs Generic Baccalaureate.
Contact Sheila Burke, Dean, School of Nursing. *Telephone:* 866-527-5268.

GRADUATE PROGRAMS
Contact Sheila Burke, Dean, School of Nursing. *Telephone:* 866-527-5268.

MASTER'S DEGREE PROGRAM
Degree MSN
Available Programs Master's; RN to Master's.
Concentrations Available Health-care administration; nursing education; nursing informatics. *Nurse practitioner programs in:* adult health, family health.

Miami Dade College
School of Nursing
Miami, Florida

Founded in 1960

DEGREE • BSN

Library Facilities 363,432 volumes; 3,824 periodical subscriptions.

BACCALAUREATE PROGRAMS

Degree BSN
Available Programs Accelerated Baccalaureate; Generic Baccalaureate; RN Baccalaureate.
Contact Gloria McWhirter, Chairperson. *Telephone:* 305-237-4047. *E-mail:* gmcwhirt@mdc.edu.

Northwest Florida State College
RN to BSN Degree Program
Niceville, Florida

http://www.nwfsc.edu/RNtoBSN/
Founded in 1963

DEGREE • BSN

Nursing Program Faculty 3 (2% with doctorates).
Baccalaureate Enrollment 83
Distance Learning Courses Available.
Nursing Student Activities Student Nurses' Association, nursing club.
Nursing Student Resources Academic advising; academic or career counseling; assistance for students with disabilities; bookstore; campus computer network; career placement assistance; computer lab; computer-assisted instruction; daycare for children of students; employment services for current students; interactive nursing skills videos; Internet; learning resource lab; library services; nursing audiovisuals; placement services for program completers; remedial services; resume preparation assistance; skills, simulation, or other laboratory; tutoring; unpaid internships.
Library Facilities 106,383 volumes (1,880 in health, 1,048 in nursing); 480 periodical subscriptions (70 health-care related).

BACCALAUREATE PROGRAMS

Degree BSN
Available Programs ADN to Baccalaureate; Accelerated RN Baccalaureate; RN Baccalaureate.
Program Entrance Requirements Transcript of college record, CPR certification, health exam, immunizations, RN licensure. Transfer students are accepted. *Application deadline:* 8/10 (fall), 1/3 (spring), 5/1 (summer). Applications may be processed on a rolling basis for some programs.
Advanced Placement Credit given for nursing courses completed elsewhere dependent upon specific evaluations.
Expenses (2010-11) *Tuition, area resident:* full-time $2360; part-time $98 per credit. *Tuition, state resident:* full-time $2384; part-time $99 per credit. *Tuition, nonresident:* full-time $9354; part-time $390 per credit. *Required fees:* full-time $200; part-time $100 per credit.
Contact Dr. Beth C. Norton, Division Director, Allied Health and BSN Programs, RN to BSN Degree Program, Northwest Florida State College, 100 College Boulevard, Niceville, FL 32578. *Telephone:* 850-729-6473. *Fax:* 850-729-6484. *E-mail:* nortonb@nwfsc.edu.

Nova Southeastern University
College of Allied Health and Nursing
Fort Lauderdale, Florida

Founded in 1964

DEGREES • BSN • MSN • MSN/MBA

Library Facilities 850,095 volumes; 50,033 periodical subscriptions.

BACCALAUREATE PROGRAMS

Degree BSN
Available Programs Generic Baccalaureate; RN Baccalaureate.
Study Options Full-time.
Program Entrance Requirements Minimum overall college GPA of 2.75, transcript of college record, written essay, health exam, immunizations, 2 letters of recommendation, prerequisite course work.
Contact *Telephone:* 800-356-0026 Ext. 1983. *Fax:* 954-262-1036.

GRADUATE PROGRAMS

Contact *Telephone:* 954-262-1956. *Fax:* 954-262-1036.

MASTER'S DEGREE PROGRAM

Degrees MSN; MSN/MBA
Available Programs Master's.
Concentrations Available Nursing administration; nursing education.
Study Options Full-time and part-time.
Program Entrance Requirements Minimum overall college GPA of 3.0, transcript of college record, 3 letters of recommendation, GRE General Test.
Degree Requirements 42 total credit hours, thesis or project.

DOCTORAL DEGREE PROGRAM

Program Entrance Requirements GRE General Test.

Palm Beach Atlantic University
School of Nursing
West Palm Beach, Florida

Founded in 1968

DEGREE • BSN

Nursing Student Activities Student Nurses' Association.
Library Facilities 160,714 volumes; 317 periodical subscriptions.

BACCALAUREATE PROGRAMS

Degree BSN
Available Programs RN Baccalaureate.
Program Entrance Requirements RN licensure.
Contact *Telephone:* 561-803-2825. *Fax:* 561-803-2828.

Remington College of Nursing
Remington College of Nursing
Lake Mary, Florida

DEGREE • BSN

BACCALAUREATE PROGRAMS

Degree BSN
Available Programs Accelerated RN Baccalaureate.
Study Options Full-time.
Contact Kathi Rinker, Admissions Coordinator, Remington College of Nursing, 660 Century Point, Suite 1050, Lake Mary, FL 32746. *Telephone:* 800-294-4434. *E-mail:* nursing.info@remingtoncollege.edu.

St. Petersburg College
Department of Nursing
St. Petersburg, Florida

http://www.spcollege.edu/
Founded in 1927

DEGREE • BSN

Nursing Program Faculty 23 (60% with doctorates).
Baccalaureate Enrollment 628 **Women** 87% **Men** 13% **Minority** 29% **International** 1%
Distance Learning Courses Available.
Nursing Student Activities Sigma Theta Tau, Student Nurses' Association, nursing club.
Nursing Student Resources Academic advising; academic or career counseling; assistance for students with disabilities; bookstore; campus computer network; computer lab; computer-assisted instruction; e-mail services; employment services for current students; interactive nursing skills videos; Internet; learning resource lab; library services; nursing audiovisuals; paid internships; remedial services; resume preparation

assistance; skills, simulation, or other laboratory; tutoring; unpaid internships.
Library Facilities 334,769 volumes (10,000 in health, 1,000 in nursing); 1,134 periodical subscriptions (385 health-care related).

BACCALAUREATE PROGRAMS

Degree BSN
Available Programs ADN to Baccalaureate; RN Baccalaureate.
Site Options Pinellas Park, FL.
Study Options Full-time.
Online Degree Options Yes.
Program Entrance Requirements Minimum overall college GPA of 2.0, transcript of college record, high school transcript, RN licensure. Transfer students are accepted. *Application deadline:* Applications may be processed on a rolling basis for some programs. *Application fee:* $40.
Advanced Placement Credit given for nursing courses completed elsewhere dependent upon specific evaluations.
Expenses (2010-11) *Tuition, area resident:* full-time $2140; part-time $102 per credit hour. *Tuition, nonresident:* full-time $8232. *Required fees:* full-time $148.
Financial Aid 80% of baccalaureate students in nursing programs received some form of financial aid in 2009-10. *Gift aid (need-based):* Federal Pell, FSEOG, state, private, college/university gift aid from institutional funds. *Loans:* college/university. *Work-study:* Federal Work-Study. *Financial aid application deadline (priority):* 4/15.
Contact Dr. Jean M. Wortock, Dean, Department of Nursing, St. Petersburg College, PO Box 13489, St. Petersburg, FL 33733. *Telephone:* 727-341-3640. *Fax:* 727-341-3646. *E-mail:* wortock.jean@spcollege.edu.

CONTINUING EDUCATION PROGRAM

Contact Denise Kerwin, Program Director, Department of Nursing, St. Petersburg College, PO Box 13489, St. Petersburg, FL 33733. *Telephone:* 727-341-3374. *Fax:* 727-341-4197. *E-mail:* kerwin.denise@spcollege.edu.

South University
Nursing Program
Royal Palm Beach, Florida

http://www.southuniversity.edu/campus/campus_programs.asp?plid=4&id=2
Founded in 1899

DEGREES • BSN • MSN

Nursing Program Faculty 89 (50% with doctorates).
Baccalaureate Enrollment 1,150 **Women** 93% **Men** 7% **Minority** 40%
Graduate Enrollment 212 **Women** 93% **Men** 7% **Minority** 40%
Distance Learning Courses Available.
Nursing Student Activities Nursing Honor Society, Student Nurses' Association.
Nursing Student Resources Academic advising; academic or career counseling; assistance for students with disabilities; bookstore; campus computer network; career placement assistance; computer lab; computer-assisted instruction; e-mail services; externships; interactive nursing skills videos; Internet; learning resource lab; library services; nursing audiovisuals; placement services for program completers; remedial services; resume preparation assistance; skills, simulation, or other laboratory; tutoring.
Library Facilities 6,000 volumes in health, 2,000 volumes in nursing; 50 periodical subscriptions health-care related.

BACCALAUREATE PROGRAMS

Degree BSN
Available Programs Generic Baccalaureate; RN Baccalaureate.
Site Options Tampa, FL; West Palm Beach, FL; Columbia, SC.
Study Options Full-time.
Online Degree Options Yes.
Program Entrance Requirements Minimum overall college GPA of 2.5, transcript of college record, health exam, high school transcript, immunizations, minimum GPA in nursing prerequisites of 2.5, prerequisite course work. Transfer students are accepted.
Financial Aid 95% of baccalaureate students in nursing programs received some form of financial aid in 2008-09.
Contact Admissions, Nursing Program, South University, 709 Mall Boulevard, Savannah, GA 31406. *Telephone:* 800-688-0932.

GRADUATE PROGRAMS

Contact Admissions, Nursing Program, South University, 709 Mall Boulevard, Savannah, GA 31406-4805. *Telephone:* 888-444-3404.

MASTER'S DEGREE PROGRAM

Degree MSN
Available Programs Master's; RN to Master's.
Concentrations Available Nursing education.
Site Options West Palm Beach, FL.
Study Options Full-time and part-time.
Online Degree Options Yes.
Program Entrance Requirements Minimum overall college GPA of 2.7, transcript of college record, written essay, 3 letters of recommendation, nursing research course, prerequisite course work, resume, statistics course. *Application deadline:* Applications may be processed on a rolling basis for some programs.
Advanced Placement Credit given for nursing courses completed elsewhere dependent upon specific evaluations.
Degree Requirements 48 total credit hours, thesis or project.

South University
College of Nursing
Tampa, Florida

DEGREES • BSN • MS

BACCALAUREATE PROGRAMS

Degree BSN
Available Programs RN Baccalaureate.
Online Degree Options Yes.
Program Entrance Requirements Minimum overall college GPA of 2.5, RN licensure.
Contact Nursing Program, College of Nursing, South University, 4401 North Himes Avenue, Tampa, FL 33614-7095. *Telephone:* 800-846-1472. *Fax:* 813-393-3814.

GRADUATE PROGRAMS

Contact Nursing Program, College of Nursing, South University, 4401 North Himes Avenue, Tampa, FL 33614-7095. *Telephone:* 800-846-1472. *Fax:* 813-393-3814.

MASTER'S DEGREE PROGRAM

Degree MS
Available Programs Master's.
Program Entrance Requirements 3 Letters of recommendation, resume.

University of Central Florida
College of Nursing
Orlando, Florida

http://www.cohpa.ucf.edu/nursing
Founded in 1963

DEGREES • BSN • MSN • PHD

Nursing Program Faculty 56 (43% with doctorates).
Baccalaureate Enrollment 379 **Women** 91% **Men** 9% **Minority** 25% **Part-time** 32%
Graduate Enrollment 136 **Women** 87% **Men** 13% **Minority** 10% **Part-time** 75%
Nursing Student Activities Sigma Theta Tau, Student Nurses' Association.
Nursing Student Resources Academic advising; academic or career counseling; assistance for students with disabilities; bookstore; campus computer network; computer lab; computer-assisted instruction; daycare for children of students; e-mail services; employment services for current students; externships; housing assistance; interactive nursing skills videos; Internet; learning resource lab; library services; nursing audiovisuals; skills, simulation, or other laboratory; tutoring.
Library Facilities 1.9 million volumes (38,944 in health, 2,848 in nursing); 32,009 periodical subscriptions (360 health-care related).

BACCALAUREATE PROGRAMS

Degree BSN
Available Programs Accelerated Baccalaureate for Second Degree; Generic Baccalaureate; RN Baccalaureate.
Study Options Full-time and part-time.
Program Entrance Requirements Minimum overall college GPA of 2.5, transcript of college record, CPR certification, health exam, health insurance, high school foreign language, high school math, high school transcript, immunizations, minimum high school GPA of 2.5, prerequisite course work. Transfer students are accepted.
Advanced Placement Credit given for nursing courses completed elsewhere dependent upon specific evaluations.
Contact ***Telephone:*** 407-823-2744. *Fax:* 407-823-5675.

GRADUATE PROGRAMS

Contact ***Telephone:*** 407-823-2744. *Fax:* 407-823-5675.

MASTER'S DEGREE PROGRAM

Degree MSN
Available Programs Master's; RN to Master's.
Concentrations Available Nurse case management; nursing administration; nursing education. *Clinical nurse specialist programs in:* acute care, critical care. *Nurse practitioner programs in:* adult health, family health, pediatric.
Study Options Full-time and part-time.
Program Entrance Requirements Clinical experience, minimum overall college GPA of 3.0, transcript of college record, CPR certification, written essay, immunizations, 3 letters of recommendation, physical assessment course, resume, statistics course.
Advanced Placement Credit given for nursing courses completed elsewhere dependent upon specific evaluations.
Degree Requirements 47 total credit hours, thesis or project.

POST-MASTER'S PROGRAM

Areas of Study *Nurse practitioner programs in:* adult health, family health, pediatric.

DOCTORAL DEGREE PROGRAM

Degree PhD
Available Programs Doctorate.
Areas of Study Health policy, health-care systems, individualized study, information systems, nursing research.
Program Entrance Requirements Minimum overall college GPA of 3.5, interview by faculty committee, 3 letters of recommendation, MSN or equivalent, statistics course, vita.
Degree Requirements 57 total credit hours, dissertation.

University of Florida

College of Nursing
Gainesville, Florida

http://www.nursing.ufl.edu
Founded in 1853

DEGREES • BSN • MSN • MSN/PHD • PHD

Nursing Program Faculty 62 (50% with doctorates).
Baccalaureate Enrollment 374 **Women** 94% **Men** 6% **Minority** 23% **International** 1%
Graduate Enrollment 364 **Women** 97% **Men** 3% **Minority** 17% **International** 1% **Part-time** 56%
Distance Learning Courses Available.
Nursing Student Activities Nursing Honor Society, Sigma Theta Tau, Student Nurses' Association.
Nursing Student Resources Academic advising; academic or career counseling; assistance for students with disabilities; bookstore; campus computer network; career placement assistance; computer lab; computer-assisted instruction; daycare for children of students; e-mail services; employment services for current students; housing assistance; interactive nursing skills videos; Internet; learning resource lab; library services; nursing audiovisuals; placement services for program completers; remedial services; resume preparation assistance; skills, simulation, or other laboratory; tutoring.
Library Facilities 5.6 million volumes (260,000 in health, 3,000 in nursing); 89,741 periodical subscriptions (200 health-care related).

BACCALAUREATE PROGRAMS

Degree BSN
Available Programs Accelerated Baccalaureate for Second Degree; Generic Baccalaureate.
Study Options Full-time.
Program Entrance Requirements Minimum overall college GPA of 2.8, transcript of college record, CPR certification, written essay, health exam, health insurance, high school biology, high school chemistry, high school foreign language, high school transcript, immunizations, 2 letters of recommendation, minimum GPA in nursing prerequisites of 2.8, prerequisite course work. Transfer students are accepted. *Application deadline:* 3/15 (fall), 1/15 (summer). *Application fee:* $30.
Advanced Placement Credit by examination available. Credit given for nursing courses completed elsewhere dependent upon specific evaluations.
Expenses (2009-10) *Tuition, state resident:* part-time $146 per credit hour. *Tuition, nonresident:* part-time $791 per credit hour. *Room and board:* $8330; room only: $7020 per academic year.
Financial Aid 90% of baccalaureate students in nursing programs received some form of financial aid in 2008-09.
Contact Mr. Kenneth H. Foote, Coordinator, Admissions and Registration, College of Nursing, University of Florida, PO Box 100197, HPNP Complex, Gainesville, FL 32610-0197. *Telephone:* 352-273-6383. *Fax:* 352-273-6440. *E-mail:* kfoote@ufl.edu.

GRADUATE PROGRAMS

Expenses (2009-10) *Tuition, state resident:* part-time $395 per credit hour. *Tuition, nonresident:* part-time $1120 per credit hour.
Financial Aid 59% of graduate students in nursing programs received some form of financial aid in 2008-09. 1 research assistantship with partial tuition reimbursement available (averaging $14,942 per year), 1 teaching assistantship with partial tuition reimbursement available (averaging $14,942 per year) were awarded; fellowships with partial tuition reimbursements available, career-related internships or fieldwork and Federal Work-Study also available. Aid available to part-time students.
Contact Ms. Cecile Kiley, Coordinator, Academic Support Services, College of Nursing, University of Florida, PO Box 100197, HPNP Complex, Gainesville, FL 32610-0197. *Telephone:* 352-273-6331. *Fax:* 352-273-6440. *E-mail:* ckiley@ufl.edu.

MASTER'S DEGREE PROGRAM

Degrees MSN; MSN/PhD
Available Programs Master's.
Concentrations Available Clinical nurse leader; nurse-midwifery. *Clinical nurse specialist programs in:* psychiatric/mental health, public health. *Nurse practitioner programs in:* acute care, adult health, family health, neonatal health, pediatric, psychiatric/mental health.
Site Options Jacksonville, FL.
Study Options Full-time and part-time.
Online Degree Options Yes.
Program Entrance Requirements Minimum overall college GPA of 3.0, transcript of college record, CPR certification, written essay, immunizations, 2 letters of recommendation, resume, GRE General Test. *Application deadline:* 3/15 (fall). Applications may be processed on a rolling basis for some programs. *Application fee:* $30.
Advanced Placement Credit given for nursing courses completed elsewhere dependent upon specific evaluations.
Degree Requirements 46 total credit hours, comprehensive exam.

POST-MASTER'S PROGRAM

Areas of Study Clinical nurse leader; nurse-midwifery. *Clinical nurse specialist programs in:* psychiatric/mental health, public health. *Nurse practitioner programs in:* acute care, adult health, family health, neonatal health, pediatric, psychiatric/mental health.

DOCTORAL DEGREE PROGRAM

Degree PhD
Available Programs Doctorate; Post-Baccalaureate Doctorate.
Areas of Study Aging, bio-behavioral research, health policy, nursing policy, nursing science, oncology, women's health.
Site Options Jacksonville, FL.
Online Degree Options Yes.
Program Entrance Requirements Minimum overall college GPA of 3.5, 3 letters of recommendation, MSN or equivalent, vita, writing sample, GRE General Test. Application deadline: 3/15 (fall). Applications may be processed on a rolling basis for some programs. Application fee: $30.
Degree Requirements 62 total credit hours, dissertation.

University of Miami
School of Nursing and Health Studies
Coral Gables, Florida

http://www6.miami.edu/sonhs/
Founded in 1925

DEGREES • BSN • MSN • PHD

Nursing Program Faculty 46 (37% with doctorates).
Baccalaureate Enrollment 405 **Women** 86.55% **Men** 13.45% **Minority** 55.86% **International** 4.14% **Part-time** 3.45%
Graduate Enrollment 85 **Women** 72% **Men** 28% **Minority** 53% **International** 1% **Part-time** 26.5%
Distance Learning Courses Available.
Nursing Student Activities Sigma Theta Tau, Student Nurses' Association.
Nursing Student Resources Academic advising; academic or career counseling; assistance for students with disabilities; bookstore; campus computer network; career placement assistance; computer lab; computer-assisted instruction; daycare for children of students; e-mail services; employment services for current students; externships; housing assistance; interactive nursing skills videos; Internet; learning resource lab; library services; nursing audiovisuals; placement services for program completers; remedial services; resume preparation assistance; skills, simulation, or other laboratory; tutoring; unpaid internships.
Library Facilities 3.3 million volumes (2,000 in nursing); 76,869 periodical subscriptions (89 health-care related).

BACCALAUREATE PROGRAMS

Degree BSN
Available Programs Accelerated Baccalaureate for Second Degree; Baccalaureate for Second Degree; Generic Baccalaureate; RN Baccalaureate.
Study Options Full-time.
Program Entrance Requirements Minimum overall college GPA of 3.5, transcript of college record, written essay, health exam, health insurance, immunizations, 2 letters of recommendation, minimum GPA in nursing prerequisites of 3.3, professional liability insurance/malpractice insurance, prerequisite course work. Transfer students are accepted. *Application deadline:* 11/1 (fall), 3/1 (spring). Applications may be processed on a rolling basis for some programs. *Application fee:* $65.
Expenses (2010-11) *Tuition:* full-time $36,962; part-time $1538 per credit. *Room and board:* $10,800; room only: $6322 per academic year. *Required fees:* full-time $1040; part-time $520 per credit; part-time $520 per term.
Financial Aid ***Gift aid (need-based):*** Federal Pell, FSEOG, state, private, college/university gift aid from institutional funds, Federal Nursing, Academic Competitiveness Grants, National SMART Grants. *Loans:* Federal Nursing Student Loans, Perkins, college/university, private alternative loans. *Work-study:* Federal Work-Study, part-time campus jobs. *Financial aid application deadline (priority):* 2/1.
Contact Ms. Deborah Paris, Assistant Dean for the Office of Student Services, School of Nursing and Health Studies, University of Miami, 5030 Brunson Drive, Coral Gables, FL 33143. *Telephone:* 305-284-4325. *Fax:* 305-284-4827. *E-mail:* dparis@miami.edu.

GRADUATE PROGRAMS

Expenses (2010-11) *Tuition:* part-time $1538 per credit. *Room and board:* $10,800; room only: $6322 per academic year. *Required fees:* full-time $770; part-time $500 per credit; part-time $170 per term.
Financial Aid 95% of graduate students in nursing programs received some form of financial aid in 2009-10. 1 fellowship (averaging $36,000 per year), 6 research assistantships with tuition reimbursements available (averaging $36,000 per year), 4 teaching assistantships with tuition reimbursements available (averaging $36,000 per year) were awarded; Federal Work-Study, institutionally sponsored loans, scholarships, and unspecified assistantships also available. Aid available to part-time students. *Financial aid application deadline:* 3/1.
Contact Ms. Deborah Paris, Assistant Dean for the Office of Student Services, School of Nursing and Health Studies, University of Miami, PO Box 248153, M. Christine Schwartz Center, Coral Gables, FL 33124-3850. *Telephone:* 305-284-4199. *Fax:* 305-284-4827. *E-mail:* dparis@miami.edu.

MASTER'S DEGREE PROGRAM

Degree MSN
Available Programs Master's; Master's for Non-Nursing College Graduates.
Concentrations Available Nurse anesthesia; nurse-midwifery; nursing education. *Nurse practitioner programs in:* acute care, adult health, family health.
Study Options Full-time and part-time.
Program Entrance Requirements Clinical experience, minimum overall college GPA of 3.0, transcript of college record, CPR certification, written essay, immunizations, interview, 3 letters of recommendation, professional liability insurance/malpractice insurance, resume, statistics course, GRE General Test. *Application deadline:* 4/1 (fall), 11/1 (spring). Applications may be processed on a rolling basis for some programs.
Degree Requirements 30 total credit hours, comprehensive exam.

POST-MASTER'S PROGRAM

Areas of Study Nurse-midwifery. *Nurse practitioner programs in:* acute care, adult health, family health.

DOCTORAL DEGREE PROGRAM

Degree PhD
Available Programs Doctorate; Post-Baccalaureate Doctorate.
Areas of Study Addiction/substance abuse, health policy, health promotion/disease prevention, maternity-newborn, nursing policy, nursing research.
Program Entrance Requirements Minimum overall college GPA of 3.0, interview, 3 letters of recommendation, MSN or equivalent, statistics course, vita, writing sample, GRE General Test. Application deadline: 6/1 (fall), 3/1 (summer). Applications may be processed on a rolling basis for some programs. Application fee: $65.
Degree Requirements Dissertation, oral exam, written exam, residency.

CONTINUING EDUCATION PROGRAM

Contact Ms. Deborah Paris, Assistant Dean, School of Nursing and Health Studies, University of Miami, PO Box 248153, M. Christine Schwartz Center, Room 152, Coral Gables, FL 33124-3850. *Telephone:* 305-284-4325. *Fax:* 305-284-4827. *E-mail:* dparis@miami.edu.

University of North Florida
School of Nursing
Jacksonville, Florida

http://www.unf.edu/coh/cohnursi.htm
Founded in 1965

DEGREES • BSN • MSN

Nursing Program Faculty 19 (50% with doctorates).
Baccalaureate Enrollment 279 **Women** 85% **Men** 15% **Minority** 20% **International** 1% **Part-time** 27%
Graduate Enrollment 35 **Women** 86% **Men** 14% **Minority** 6% **Part-time** 70%
Nursing Student Activities Sigma Theta Tau, Student Nurses' Association.
Nursing Student Resources Academic advising; academic or career counseling; assistance for students with disabilities; bookstore; campus computer network; career placement assistance; computer lab; computer-assisted instruction; e-mail services; interactive nursing skills videos; Internet; learning resource lab; library services; nursing audiovisuals; resume preparation assistance; skills, simulation, or other laboratory.
Library Facilities 957,625 volumes (30,466 in health, 3,000 in nursing); 3,979 periodical subscriptions (200 health-care related).

BACCALAUREATE PROGRAMS

Degree BSN
Available Programs Accelerated Baccalaureate for Second Degree; Generic Baccalaureate; RN Baccalaureate.
Study Options Full-time.
Program Entrance Requirements Minimum overall college GPA of 2.7, CPR certification, written essay, health exam, immunizations, interview, minimum high school GPA, minimum GPA in nursing prerequisites of 3.0, professional liability insurance/malpractice insurance, prerequisite course work. Transfer students are accepted.
Advanced Placement Credit given for nursing courses completed elsewhere dependent upon specific evaluations.
Contact ***Telephone:*** 904-620-2418.

GRADUATE PROGRAMS

Contact ***Telephone:*** 904-620-2684. *Fax:* 904-620-2848.

MASTER'S DEGREE PROGRAM

Degree MSN
Available Programs Master's; RN to Master's.
Concentrations Available *Clinical nurse specialist programs in:* adult health, cardiovascular, community health, critical care, gerontology, maternity-newborn, medical-surgical, pediatric, psychiatric/mental health, women's health. *Nurse practitioner programs in:* family health, primary care.
Study Options Full-time and part-time.
Program Entrance Requirements Clinical experience, computer literacy, minimum overall college GPA of 3.0, transcript of college record, CPR certification, written essay, immunizations, 2 letters of recommendation, nursing research course, physical assessment course, professional liability insurance/malpractice insurance, resume, statistics course.
Advanced Placement Credit given for nursing courses completed elsewhere dependent upon specific evaluations.
Degree Requirements 43 total credit hours, thesis or project.

POST-MASTER'S PROGRAM

Areas of Study *Nurse practitioner programs in:* family health, primary care.

University of Phoenix–Central Florida Campus

College of Nursing
Maitland, Florida

Founded in 1996

DEGREES • BSN • MSN • MSN/ED D

Nursing Program Faculty 10 (60% with doctorates).
Baccalaureate Enrollment 35 **Women** 88.6% **Men** 11.4% **Minority** 45.7%
Graduate Enrollment 18 **Women** 94.4% **Men** 5.6% **Minority** 50%
Nursing Student Activities Sigma Theta Tau.
Nursing Student Resources Academic advising; academic or career counseling; assistance for students with disabilities; bookstore; campus computer network; computer lab; computer-assisted instruction; e-mail services; interactive nursing skills videos; Internet; learning resource lab; library services; nursing audiovisuals; remedial services; skills, simulation, or other laboratory; tutoring.
Library Facilities 16,781 periodical subscriptions (1,300 health-care related).

BACCALAUREATE PROGRAMS

Degree BSN
Available Programs Accelerated Baccalaureate.
Site Options Orlando, FL; Daytona Beach, FL.
Study Options Full-time.
Program Entrance Requirements Transcript of college record, CPR certification, immunizations, 1 letter of recommendation, RN licensure. Transfer students are accepted. *Application deadline:* Applications may be processed on a rolling basis for some programs.
Advanced Placement Credit by examination available. Credit given for nursing courses completed elsewhere dependent upon specific evaluations.
Expenses (2009-10) *Tuition:* full-time $9300. *Required fees:* full-time $600.
Contact Campus College Chair, Nursing, College of Nursing, University of Phoenix–Central Florida Campus, 2290 Lucien Way, Suite 400, Maitland, FL 32751-7057. *Telephone:* 407-667-0555.

GRADUATE PROGRAMS

Expenses (2009-10) *Tuition:* full-time $11,640. *Required fees:* full-time $760.
Financial Aid Institutionally sponsored loans and scholarships available.
Contact Campus College Chair, Nursing, College of Nursing, University of Phoenix–Central Florida Campus, 2290 Lucien Way, Suite 400, Maitland, FL 32751-7057. *Telephone:* 407-667-0555.

MASTER'S DEGREE PROGRAM

Degrees MSN; MSN/Ed D
Available Programs Master's.
Concentrations Available Nursing administration; nursing education.
Site Options Orlando, FL; Daytona Beach, FL.
Study Options Full-time.
Program Entrance Requirements Clinical experience, computer literacy, minimum overall college GPA of 2.5, transcript of college record. *Application deadline:* Applications may be processed on a rolling basis for some programs. *Application fee:* $45.
Advanced Placement Credit given for nursing courses completed elsewhere dependent upon specific evaluations.
Degree Requirements 39 total credit hours, thesis or project.

University of Phoenix–North Florida Campus

College of Nursing
Jacksonville, Florida

Founded in 1976

DEGREES • BSN • MSN • MSN/ED D • MSN/MHA

Nursing Program Faculty 7 (29% with doctorates).
Baccalaureate Enrollment 13 **Women** 92.3% **Men** 7.7% **Minority** 38.5%
Graduate Enrollment 10 **Women** 100% **Minority** 20%
Nursing Student Activities Sigma Theta Tau.
Nursing Student Resources Academic advising; academic or career counseling; assistance for students with disabilities; bookstore; campus computer network; computer lab; computer-assisted instruction; e-mail services; interactive nursing skills videos; Internet; learning resource lab; library services; nursing audiovisuals; remedial services; skills, simulation, or other laboratory; tutoring.
Library Facilities 1,300 periodical subscriptions health-care related.

BACCALAUREATE PROGRAMS

Degree BSN
Available Programs Accelerated Baccalaureate.
Site Options Orange Park, FL.
Study Options Full-time.
Program Entrance Requirements Transcript of college record, CPR certification, immunizations, 1 letter of recommendation, RN licensure. Transfer students are accepted. *Application deadline:* Applications may be processed on a rolling basis for some programs.
Advanced Placement Credit by examination available. Credit given for nursing courses completed elsewhere dependent upon specific evaluations.
Expenses (2009-10) *Tuition:* full-time $9300. *Required fees:* full-time $600.
Contact Campus College Chair, Nursing, College of Nursing, University of Phoenix–North Florida Campus, 4500 Salisbury Road, Suite 200, Jacksonville, FL 32216-0959. *Telephone:* 904-636-6645.

GRADUATE PROGRAMS

Expenses (2009-10) *Tuition:* full-time $11,640. *Required fees:* full-time $760.
Financial Aid Institutionally sponsored loans and scholarships available.
Contact Campus College Chair, Nursing, College of Nursing, University of Phoenix–North Florida Campus, 4500 Salisbury Road, Suite 200, Jacksonville, FL 32216-0959. *Telephone:* 904-636-6645.

MASTER'S DEGREE PROGRAM

Degrees MSN; MSN/Ed D; MSN/MHA
Available Programs Master's.
Concentrations Available Health-care administration; nursing administration; nursing education.
Site Options Orange Park, FL.
Study Options Full-time.
Program Entrance Requirements Clinical experience, computer literacy, minimum overall college GPA of 2.5, transcript of college record. *Application deadline:* Applications may be processed on a rolling basis for some programs. *Application fee:* $45.
Advanced Placement Credit given for nursing courses completed elsewhere dependent upon specific evaluations.
Degree Requirements 39 total credit hours, thesis or project.

University of Phoenix–South Florida Campus

College of Nursing
Fort Lauderdale, Florida

DEGREES • BSN • MSN • MSN/MBA • MSN/MHA

Nursing Program Faculty 24 (21% with doctorates).
Baccalaureate Enrollment 135 **Women** 96.3% **Men** 3.7% **Minority** 38.5%
Graduate Enrollment 102 **Women** 91.2% **Men** 8.8% **Minority** 41.18%
Nursing Student Activities Sigma Theta Tau.
Nursing Student Resources Academic advising; academic or career counseling; assistance for students with disabilities; bookstore; campus computer network; computer lab; computer-assisted instruction; e-mail services; interactive nursing skills videos; Internet; learning resource lab; library services; nursing audiovisuals; skills, simulation, or other laboratory; tutoring.
Library Facilities 16,781 periodical subscriptions (1,300 health-care related).

BACCALAUREATE PROGRAMS

Degree BSN
Available Programs RN Baccalaureate.
Site Options Palm Beach Gardens, FL; Ft. Lauderdale, FL; Miramar, FL.
Study Options Full-time.
Online Degree Options Yes.
Program Entrance Requirements Transcript of college record, CPR certification, immunizations, 1 letter of recommendation, RN licensure. Transfer students are accepted. *Application deadline:* Applications may be processed on a rolling basis for some programs.
Advanced Placement Credit by examination available. Credit given for nursing courses completed elsewhere dependent upon specific evaluations.
Expenses (2009-10) *Tuition:* full-time $9420. *Required fees:* full-time $600.
Contact Campus College Chair, Nursing, College of Nursing, University of Phoenix–South Florida Campus, 600 North Pine Island Road, Suite #500, Plantation, FL 33324-1393. *Telephone:* 954-382-5303.

GRADUATE PROGRAMS

Expenses (2009-10) *Tuition:* full-time $11,640.
Financial Aid Institutionally sponsored loans and scholarships available.
Contact Campus College Chair, Nursing, College of Nursing, University of Phoenix–South Florida Campus, 600 North Pine Island Road, Suite #500, Plantation, FL 33324-1393. *Telephone:* 954-382-5303.

MASTER'S DEGREE PROGRAM

Degrees MSN; MSN/MBA; MSN/MHA
Available Programs Master's.
Concentrations Available Health-care administration; nursing administration; nursing education.
Site Options Palm Beach Gardens, FL; Ft. Lauderdale, FL; Miramar, FL.
Study Options Full-time.
Online Degree Options Yes.
Program Entrance Requirements Clinical experience, computer literacy, minimum overall college GPA of 2.5, transcript of college record. *Application deadline:* Applications may be processed on a rolling basis for some programs. *Application fee:* $45.
Advanced Placement Credit given for nursing courses completed elsewhere dependent upon specific evaluations.
Degree Requirements 39 total credit hours, thesis or project.

University of Phoenix–West Florida Campus

College of Nursing
Temple Terrace, Florida

DEGREE • BSN

Nursing Program Faculty 5 (60% with doctorates).
Baccalaureate Enrollment 8 **Women** 87.5% **Men** 12.5% **Minority** 12.5%
Nursing Student Activities Sigma Theta Tau.
Nursing Student Resources Academic advising; academic or career counseling; assistance for students with disabilities; bookstore; campus computer network; computer lab; computer-assisted instruction; e-mail services; interactive nursing skills videos; Internet; learning resource lab; library services; nursing audiovisuals; remedial services; skills, simulation, or other laboratory; tutoring.
Library Facilities 16,781 periodical subscriptions (1,300 health-care related).

BACCALAUREATE PROGRAMS

Degree BSN
Available Programs Accelerated Baccalaureate.
Site Options Tampa, FL; Clearwater, FL; Sarasota, FL.
Study Options Full-time.
Online Degree Options Yes.
Program Entrance Requirements Transcript of college record, CPR certification, immunizations, 1 letter of recommendation, RN licensure. Transfer students are accepted. *Application deadline:* Applications may be processed on a rolling basis for some programs.
Advanced Placement Credit by examination available. Credit given for nursing courses completed elsewhere dependent upon specific evaluations.
Expenses (2009-10) *Tuition:* full-time $9300. *Required fees:* full-time $600.
Contact Campus College Chair, Nursing, College of Nursing, University of Phoenix–West Florida Campus, 100 Tampa Oaks Boulevard, Suite #200, Temple Terrace, FL 33637-1920. *Telephone:* 813-626-7911.

University of South Florida

College of Nursing
Tampa, Florida

http://hsc.usf.edu/nursing
Founded in 1956

DEGREES • BS • MS • MS/MPH • PHD

Nursing Program Faculty 75 (45% with doctorates).
Baccalaureate Enrollment 597 **Women** 86% **Men** 14% **Minority** 32% **International** 2% **Part-time** 38%
Graduate Enrollment 711 **Women** 88% **Men** 12% **Minority** 27% **International** 1% **Part-time** 83%
Distance Learning Courses Available.
Nursing Student Activities Nursing Honor Society, Sigma Theta Tau, Student Nurses' Association.
Nursing Student Resources Academic advising; academic or career counseling; assistance for students with disabilities; bookstore; campus computer network; career placement assistance; computer lab; computer-assisted instruction; daycare for children of students; e-mail services; employment services for current students; housing assistance; Internet; learning resource lab; library services; nursing audiovisuals; remedial services; resume preparation assistance; skills, simulation, or other laboratory; tutoring.
Library Facilities 2.3 million volumes (106,028 in health, 3,898 in nursing); 81,762 periodical subscriptions (1,581 health-care related).

BACCALAUREATE PROGRAMS

Degree BS
Available Programs ADN to Baccalaureate; Accelerated Baccalaureate for Second Degree; Generic Baccalaureate.
Study Options Full-time.
Program Entrance Requirements Minimum overall college GPA of 3.2, transcript of college record, CPR certification, health insurance, immunizations, prerequisite course work. Transfer students are accepted. *Application deadline:* 6/15 (fall), 3/15 (summer). *Application fee:* $30.
Expenses (2010-11) *Tuition, state resident:* part-time $2562 per semester. *Tuition, nonresident:* part-time $7967 per semester. *International tuition:* $7967 full-time. *Room and board:* room only: $4500 per academic year. *Required fees:* part-time $42 per term.
Financial Aid 60% of baccalaureate students in nursing programs received some form of financial aid in 2009-10.
Contact Ms. McKenzie McDonald, Coordinator, Baccalaureate Admissions, College of Nursing, University of South Florida, 12901 Bruce B. Downs Boulevard, MDC Box 22, Tampa, FL 33612-4766. *Telephone:* 813-974-2191. *Fax:* 813-974-3118. *E-mail:* nurstudent@health.usf.edu.

GRADUATE PROGRAMS

Expenses (2010-11) *Tuition, state resident:* part-time $3291 per semester. *Tuition, nonresident:* part-time $6981 per semester. *International tuition:* $6981 full-time.
Financial Aid 30% of graduate students in nursing programs received some form of financial aid in 2009-10. Teaching assistantships (averaging $24,202 per year); tuition waivers (partial) and unspecified assistantships also available. *Financial aid application deadline:* 2/1.
Contact Ms. Melinda Kretschmer, Admissions Recruiter Advisor, College of Nursing, University of South Florida, 12901 Bruce B. Downs Boulevard, MDC Box 22, Tampa, FL 33612-4766. *Telephone:* 813-974-2952. *Fax:* 813-974-5418. *E-mail:* nurstudent@health.usf.edu.

MASTER'S DEGREE PROGRAM

Degrees MS; MS/MPH
Available Programs Master's; Master's for Nurses with Non-Nursing Degrees; RN to Master's.
Concentrations Available Clinical nurse leader; nurse anesthesia; nursing education. *Nurse practitioner programs in:* adult health, family health, occupational health, oncology, pediatric.
Study Options Full-time and part-time.
Program Entrance Requirements Computer literacy, minimum overall college GPA of 3.0, transcript of college record, CPR certification, immunizations, interview, 3 letters of recommendation, resume, GRE General Test. *Application deadline:* 2/15 (fall), 10/15 (spring), 2/15 (summer). *Application fee:* $30.
Advanced Placement Credit given for nursing courses completed elsewhere dependent upon specific evaluations.
Degree Requirements 41 total credit hours, thesis or project, comprehensive exam.

POST-MASTER'S PROGRAM

Areas of Study Clinical nurse leader; nursing education. *Nurse practitioner programs in:* adult health, family health, occupational health, oncology, pediatric.

DOCTORAL DEGREE PROGRAM

Degree PhD
Available Programs Doctorate.
Areas of Study Bio-behavioral research, clinical practice, critical care, ethics, faculty preparation, family health, gerontology, health promotion/disease prevention, human health and illness, illness and transition, maternity-newborn, nursing education, nursing research, nursing science, oncology, women's health.
Program Entrance Requirements Minimum overall college GPA of 3.0, interview by faculty committee, interview, 3 letters of recommendation, MSN or equivalent, vita, writing sample, GRE General Test. Application deadline: 2/1 (fall). Application fee: $30.
Degree Requirements 63 total credit hours, dissertation.

CONTINUING EDUCATION PROGRAM

Contact Dr. Patricia Gorzka, Coordinator of Continuing Medical Education, College of Nursing, University of South Florida, 12901 Bruce B. Downs Boulevard, MDC Box 22, Tampa, FL 33612-4766. *Telephone:* 813-974-4392. *Fax:* 813-974-5418. *E-mail:* pgorzka@hsc.usf.edu.

The University of Tampa
Department of Nursing
Tampa, Florida

http://www.ut.edu/nursing
Founded in 1931

DEGREES • BSN • MSN
Nursing Program Faculty 25 (45% with doctorates).
Baccalaureate Enrollment 133 **Women** 94% **Men** 6% **Minority** 20% **International** 6% **Part-time** 5%
Graduate Enrollment 135 **Women** 95% **Men** 5% **Minority** 21% **International** 3% **Part-time** 66%
Nursing Student Activities Sigma Theta Tau, Student Nurses' Association.
Nursing Student Resources Academic advising; academic or career counseling; assistance for students with disabilities; bookstore; campus computer network; career placement assistance; computer lab; computer-assisted instruction; e-mail services; employment services for current students; externships; housing assistance; interactive nursing skills videos; Internet; learning resource lab; library services; nursing audiovisuals; paid internships; placement services for program completers; remedial services; resume preparation assistance; skills, simulation, or other laboratory; tutoring; unpaid internships.
Library Facilities 292,202 volumes (252,147 in health, 3,000 in nursing); 42,916 periodical subscriptions (10,854 health-care related).

BACCALAUREATE PROGRAMS

Degree BSN
Available Programs ADN to Baccalaureate; Generic Baccalaureate; RN Baccalaureate.
Study Options Full-time.
Program Entrance Requirements Minimum overall college GPA of 3.25, transcript of college record, CPR certification, written essay, health exam, health insurance, high school transcript, immunizations, 1 letter of recommendation, minimum GPA in nursing prerequisites, professional liability insurance/malpractice insurance, prerequisite course work. Transfer students are accepted. *Application deadline:* 10/15 (spring).
Expenses (2010-11) *Tuition:* full-time $22,116; part-time $470 per credit. *Room and board:* $8590 per academic year. *Required fees:* full-time $1102; part-time $184 per term.
Financial Aid 85% of baccalaureate students in nursing programs received some form of financial aid in 2009-10. *Gift aid (need-based):* Federal Pell, FSEOG, state, private, college/university gift aid from institutional funds. *Loans:* Federal Direct (Subsidized and Unsubsidized Stafford PLUS), Perkins, state, college/university. *Work-study:* Federal Work-Study, part-time campus jobs. *Financial aid application deadline:* Continuous.
Contact Admissions Office, Department of Nursing, The University of Tampa, 401 West Kennedy Boulevard, Box F, Tampa, FL 33606. *Telephone:* 813-253-6211. *Fax:* 813-258-7398. *E-mail:* admissions@ut.edu.

GRADUATE PROGRAMS

Expenses (2010-11) *Tuition:* part-time $504 per credit. *Room and board:* $8590 per academic year. *Required fees:* full-time $375.
Financial Aid 80% of graduate students in nursing programs received some form of financial aid in 2009-10.
Contact Graduate Studies Office, Department of Nursing, The University of Tampa, 401 West Kennedy Boulevard, Tampa, FL 33606. *Telephone:* 813-258-7409. *E-mail:* utgrad@ut.edu.

MASTER'S DEGREE PROGRAM

Degree MSN
Available Programs Master's; RN to Master's.
Concentrations Available *Nurse practitioner programs in:* adult health, family health.
Study Options Full-time and part-time.
Program Entrance Requirements Computer literacy, minimum overall college GPA of 3.0, transcript of college record, CPR certification, written essay, immunizations, interview, 2 letters of recommendation, physical assessment course, professional liability insurance/malpractice insurance, prerequisite course work, resume, statistics course. *Application deadline:* Applications may be processed on a rolling basis for some programs.
Advanced Placement Credit given for nursing courses completed elsewhere dependent upon specific evaluations.
Degree Requirements 48 total credit hours, comprehensive exam.

POST-MASTER'S PROGRAM

Areas of Study *Nurse practitioner programs in:* adult health, family health.

CONTINUING EDUCATION PROGRAM

Contact Dr. Kim Curry, Assistant Professor/Associate Director, Department of Nursing, The University of Tampa, 401 West Kennedy Boulevard, Box 10-F, Tampa, FL 33606-1490. *Telephone:* 813-257-3633. *Fax:* 813-258-7214. *E-mail:* kcurry@ut.edu.

University of West Florida
Department of Nursing
Pensacola, Florida

http://uwf.edu/nursing
Founded in 1963

DEGREE • BSN
Nursing Program Faculty 14 (1% with doctorates).

Baccalaureate Enrollment 134 **Women** 87% **Men** 13% **Minority** 14% **Part-time** 31%

Distance Learning Courses Available.

Nursing Student Activities Sigma Theta Tau, Student Nurses' Association.

Nursing Student Resources Academic advising; academic or career counseling; assistance for students with disabilities; bookstore; campus computer network; career placement assistance; computer lab; computer-assisted instruction; daycare for children of students; e-mail services; employment services for current students; housing assistance; interactive nursing skills videos; Internet; learning resource lab; library services; nursing audiovisuals; remedial services; resume preparation assistance; skills, simulation, or other laboratory; tutoring.

Library Facilities 1 million volumes (3,500 in health, 1,950 in nursing); 4,619 periodical subscriptions (54 health-care related).

BACCALAUREATE PROGRAMS

Degree BSN

Available Programs ADN to Baccalaureate; Generic Baccalaureate.

Study Options Full-time.

Online Degree Options Yes.

Program Entrance Requirements Minimum overall college GPA of 2.75, transcript of college record, CPR certification, health exam, health insurance, immunizations, minimum GPA in nursing prerequisites of 2.75, professional liability insurance/malpractice insurance, prerequisite course work. Transfer students are accepted. *Application deadline:* 3/1 (fall).

Advanced Placement Credit by examination available. Credit given for nursing courses completed elsewhere dependent upon specific evaluations.

Expenses (2009-10) *Tuition, state resident:* full-time $3649; part-time $140 per credit hour. *Tuition, nonresident:* full-time $14,813; part-time $570 per credit hour. *International tuition:* $14,813 full-time. *Room and board:* $7576 per academic year. *Required fees:* full-time $102.

Financial Aid 70% of baccalaureate students in nursing programs received some form of financial aid in 2008-09. *Gift aid (need-based):* Federal Pell, FSEOG, state, private, college/university gift aid from institutional funds. *Loans:* Federal Direct (Subsidized and Unsubsidized Stafford PLUS), Perkins, college/university. *Work-study:* Federal Work-Study, part-time campus jobs. *Financial aid application deadline:* Continuous.

Contact Ms. Carol K. Hatcher, Nursing Advisor, Department of Nursing, University of West Florida, 11000 University Parkway, Pensacola, FL 32514. *Telephone:* 850-473-7757. *Fax:* 850-473-7769. *E-mail:* chatcher@uwf.edu.

GEORGIA

Albany State University

College of Sciences and Health Professions
Albany, Georgia

http://asuweb.asurams.edu/

Founded in 1903

DEGREES • BSN • MSN

Nursing Program Faculty 17 (41% with doctorates).

Baccalaureate Enrollment 314 **Women** 93% **Men** 7% **Minority** 94% **International** 1% **Part-time** 26%

Graduate Enrollment 78 **Women** 91% **Men** 9% **Minority** 49% **International** 3% **Part-time** 51%

Distance Learning Courses Available.

Nursing Student Activities Nursing Honor Society, Student Nurses' Association, nursing club.

Nursing Student Resources Academic advising; academic or career counseling; assistance for students with disabilities; bookstore; campus computer network; career placement assistance; computer lab; computer-assisted instruction; e-mail services; interactive nursing skills videos; Internet; learning resource lab; library services; nursing audiovisuals; paid internships; placement services for program completers; remedial services; resume preparation assistance; skills, simulation, or other laboratory; tutoring; unpaid internships.

Library Facilities 196,411 volumes (15,075 in health, 7,032 in nursing); 791,635 periodical subscriptions (75 health-care related).

BACCALAUREATE PROGRAMS

Degree BSN

Available Programs ADN to Baccalaureate; Accelerated Baccalaureate for Second Degree; Accelerated RN Baccalaureate; Baccalaureate for Second Degree; Generic Baccalaureate; RN Baccalaureate.

Study Options Full-time.

Online Degree Options Yes.

Program Entrance Requirements Minimum overall college GPA of 2.75, transcript of college record, CPR certification, written essay, health exam, health insurance, high school biology, high school foreign language, 4 years high school math, 3 years high school science, high school transcript, immunizations, interview, minimum GPA in nursing prerequisites of 2.75, professional liability insurance/malpractice insurance, prerequisite course work. Transfer students are accepted. *Application deadline:* 7/1 (fall), 11/15 (spring), 4/1 (summer). Applications may be processed on a rolling basis for some programs. *Application fee:* $20.

Advanced Placement Credit given for nursing courses completed elsewhere dependent upon specific evaluations.

Expenses (2010-11) *Tuition, state resident:* full-time $4258; part-time $354 per credit hour. *Tuition, nonresident:* full-time $13,880; part-time $764 per credit hour. *Room and board:* $8724; room only: $5875 per academic year. *Required fees:* full-time $1160; part-time $580 per term.

Financial Aid 92% of baccalaureate students in nursing programs received some form of financial aid in 2009-10.

Contact Dr. Linda P. Grimsley, Chair, Department of Nursing, College of Sciences and Health Professions, Albany State University, 504 College Drive, Albany, GA 31705. *Telephone:* 229-430-4724. *Fax:* 229-430-3937. *E-mail:* linda.grimsley@asurams.edu.

GRADUATE PROGRAMS

Expenses (2010-11) *Tuition, state resident:* full-time $3951; part-time $439 per credit hour. *Tuition, nonresident:* full-time $3951; part-time $439 per credit hour. *Required fees:* full-time $1609; part-time $179 per credit; part-time $179 per term.

Financial Aid 70% of graduate students in nursing programs received some form of financial aid in 2009-10. Scholarships and traineeships available. *Financial aid application deadline:* 6/30.

Contact Dr. Linda P. Grimsley, Chair, Department of Nursing, College of Sciences and Health Professions, Albany State University, 504 College Drive, Albany, GA 31705. *Telephone:* 229-430-4724. *Fax:* 229-430-3937. *E-mail:* linda.grimsley@asurams.edu.

MASTER'S DEGREE PROGRAM

Degree MSN

Available Programs Accelerated AD/RN to Master's; Accelerated Master's; Master's; RN to Master's.

Concentrations Available Health-care administration; nursing education. *Nurse practitioner programs in:* family health.

Study Options Full-time and part-time.

Online Degree Options Yes (online only).

Program Entrance Requirements Clinical experience, computer literacy, minimum overall college GPA of 3.0, transcript of college record, CPR certification, immunizations, 2 letters of recommendation, nursing research course, physical assessment course, professional liability insurance/malpractice insurance, prerequisite course work, resume, statistics course, GRE General Test or MAT. *Application deadline:* 7/1 (fall), 11/15 (spring), 4/1 (summer). Applications may be processed on a rolling basis for some programs. *Application fee:* $20.

Advanced Placement Credit given for nursing courses completed elsewhere dependent upon specific evaluations.

Degree Requirements 36 total credit hours, thesis or project, comprehensive exam.

POST-MASTER'S PROGRAM

Areas of Study Health-care administration; nursing education. *Nurse practitioner programs in:* family health.

Armstrong Atlantic State University

Program in Nursing
Savannah, Georgia

http://www.nursing.armstrong.edu/
Founded in 1935

DEGREES • BSN • MS/MHSA • MSN

Nursing Program Faculty 40 (40% with doctorates).
Baccalaureate Enrollment 380 **Women** 85% **Men** 15% **Minority** 30% **International** 2% **Part-time** 10%
Graduate Enrollment 39 **Women** 93% **Men** 7% **Minority** 38% **Part-time** 70%
Distance Learning Courses Available.
Nursing Student Activities Nursing Honor Society, Sigma Theta Tau, Student Nurses' Association.
Nursing Student Resources Academic advising; academic or career counseling; assistance for students with disabilities; bookstore; campus computer network; career placement assistance; computer lab; computer-assisted instruction; e-mail services; employment services for current students; housing assistance; interactive nursing skills videos; Internet; learning resource lab; library services; nursing audiovisuals; placement services for program completers; remedial services; resume preparation assistance; skills, simulation, or other laboratory; tutoring.
Library Facilities 231,500 volumes (8,200 in nursing); 925 periodical subscriptions (171 health-care related).

BACCALAUREATE PROGRAMS

Degree BSN
Available Programs ADN to Baccalaureate; Baccalaureate for Second Degree; Generic Baccalaureate; LPN to Baccalaureate; RN Baccalaureate.
Study Options Full-time and part-time.
Program Entrance Requirements Transcript of college record, CPR certification, health exam, health insurance, immunizations, minimum GPA in nursing prerequisites of 2.7, professional liability insurance/malpractice insurance, prerequisite course work. Transfer students are accepted. *Application deadline:* 2/15 (fall), 10/15 (spring). *Application fee:* $200.
Advanced Placement Credit by examination available.
Expenses (2010-11) *Tuition, state resident:* full-time $3432; part-time $143 per credit. *Tuition, nonresident:* full-time $12,720; part-time $530 per credit. *Room and board:* $4200; room only: $3034 per academic year. *Required fees:* full-time $1078; part-time $539 per term.
Financial Aid 90% of baccalaureate students in nursing programs received some form of financial aid in 2009-10.
Contact Dr. Helen Taggart, Undergraduate Coordinator, Program in Nursing, Armstrong Atlantic State University, 11935 Abercorn Street, Savannah, GA 31419-1997. *Telephone:* 912-344-2667. *Fax:* 912-344-3481. *E-mail:* helen.taggart@armstrong.edu.

GRADUATE PROGRAMS

Financial Aid 85% of graduate students in nursing programs received some form of financial aid in 2009-10. Research assistantships with partial tuition reimbursements available (averaging $2,500 per year); Federal Work-Study, scholarships, and unspecified assistantships also available. Aid available to part-time students.
Contact Dr. Anita Nivens, Graduate Program Coordinator, Program in Nursing, Armstrong Atlantic State University, 11935 Abercorn Street, Savannah, GA 31419-1997. *Telephone:* 912-344-2724. *Fax:* 912-344-3481. *E-mail:* anita.nivens@armstrong.edu.

MASTER'S DEGREE PROGRAM

Degrees MS/MHSA; MSN
Available Programs Master's; RN to Master's.
Concentrations Available Nursing administration. *Clinical nurse specialist programs in:* adult health. *Nurse practitioner programs in:* adult health.
Study Options Full-time and part-time.
Program Entrance Requirements Clinical experience, minimum overall college GPA of 3.0, transcript of college record, CPR certification, written essay, immunizations, interview, 3 letters of recommendation, nursing research course, physical assessment course, professional liability insurance/malpractice insurance, prerequisite course work, statistics course, GRE General Test or MAT. *Application deadline:* 5/15 (fall), 11/15 (spring).
Advanced Placement Credit by examination available.
Degree Requirements 36 total credit hours, thesis or project.

POST-MASTER'S PROGRAM

Areas of Study Nursing administration. *Clinical nurse specialist programs in:* adult health. *Nurse practitioner programs in:* adult health.

CONTINUING EDUCATION PROGRAM

Contact Mrs. Linda Tuck, Assistant Professor, Program in Nursing, Armstrong Atlantic State University, 11935 Abercorn Street, Savannah, GA 31419-1997. *Telephone:* 912-344-2886. *Fax:* 912-920-6579. *E-mail:* linda.tuck@armstrong.edu.

Augusta State University

Department of Nursing
Augusta, Georgia

Founded in 1925

DEGREE • BSN

BACCALAUREATE PROGRAMS

Degree BSN
Available Programs Generic Baccalaureate; LPN to Baccalaureate; RN Baccalaureate.
Contact Nursing Department, Department of Nursing, Augusta State University, 2500 Walton Way, Augusta, GA 30904. *Telephone:* 706-737-1725. *Fax:* 706-737-1726.

Brenau University

School of Health and Science
Gainesville, Georgia

Founded in 1878

DEGREES • BSN • MSN

Nursing Program Faculty 14 (65% with doctorates).
Baccalaureate Enrollment 300 **Women** 95% **Men** 5% **Minority** 40% **International** 10% **Part-time** 50%
Graduate Enrollment 55 **Women** 95% **Men** 5% **Minority** 20% **Part-time** 100%
Distance Learning Courses Available.
Nursing Student Activities Sigma Theta Tau, Student Nurses' Association.
Nursing Student Resources Academic advising; academic or career counseling; assistance for students with disabilities; bookstore; campus computer network; career placement assistance; computer lab; computer-assisted instruction; e-mail services; housing assistance; interactive nursing skills videos; Internet; learning resource lab; library services; nursing audiovisuals; remedial services; skills, simulation, or other laboratory; tutoring.
Library Facilities 89,016 volumes (6,000 in health, 5,000 in nursing); 17,512 periodical subscriptions (275 health-care related).

BACCALAUREATE PROGRAMS

Degree BSN
Available Programs ADN to Baccalaureate; Generic Baccalaureate; RN Baccalaureate.
Study Options Full-time and part-time.
Online Degree Options Yes.
Program Entrance Requirements Minimum overall college GPA of 2.5, transcript of college record, health exam, high school biology, high school chemistry, high school foreign language, 2 years high school math, 1 year of high school science, high school transcript, immunizations, minimum high school GPA of 2.5, minimum GPA in nursing prerequisites of 2.5, professional liability insurance/malpractice insurance, prerequisite course work. Transfer students are accepted. *Application deadline:* 7/15 (spring), 11/15 (summer). *Application fee:* $35.
Advanced Placement Credit by examination available. Credit given for nursing courses completed elsewhere dependent upon specific evaluations.
Financial Aid 75% of baccalaureate students in nursing programs received some form of financial aid in 2009-10. *Gift aid (need-based):* Federal Pell, FSEOG, state, private, college/university gift aid from institutional funds, Academic Competitiveness Grants, National SMART

Grants. *Loans:* Federal Direct (Subsidized and Unsubsidized Stafford PLUS), Perkins, state. *Work-study:* Federal Work-Study. *Financial aid application deadline (priority):* 3/15.
Contact Ms. Christina White, Undergraduate Admissions Coordinator for Women's College, School of Health and Science, Brenau University, 500 Washington Street SE, Gainesville, GA 30501. *Telephone:* 770-534-6100. *Fax:* 770-538-4306. *E-mail:* cwhite@brenau.edu.

GRADUATE PROGRAMS

Financial Aid 90% of graduate students in nursing programs received some form of financial aid in 2009-10. Scholarships and traineeships available. Aid available to part-time students. *Financial aid application deadline:* 7/15.
Contact Dr. Cathy Dyches, Coordinator of Graduate Nursing Programs, School of Health and Science, Brenau University, 500 Washington Street SE, Gainesville, GA 30501. *Telephone:* 770-534-6125. *Fax:* 770-534-4666. *E-mail:* cdyches@brenau.edu.

MASTER'S DEGREE PROGRAM

Degree MSN
Available Programs Accelerated AD/RN to Master's; Accelerated RN to Master's; Master's; RN to Master's.
Concentrations Available Clinical nurse leader; nursing education. *Nurse practitioner programs in:* family health.
Site Options Atlanta, GA.
Study Options Part-time.
Program Entrance Requirements Clinical experience, minimum overall college GPA of 3.0, transcript of college record, CPR certification, written essay, immunizations, 3 letters of recommendation, nursing research course, physical assessment course, prerequisite course work, statistics course, GRE General Test or MAT (for some programs). *Application deadline:* Applications may be processed on a rolling basis for some programs.
Degree Requirements Thesis or project.

POST-MASTER'S PROGRAM

Areas of Study *Nurse practitioner programs in:* family health.

CONTINUING EDUCATION PROGRAM

Contact Dr. Keeta Wilborn, Chair, Department of Nursing, School of Health and Science, Brenau University, 500 Washington Street SE, Gainesville, GA 30501. *Telephone:* 770-534-6206. *Fax:* 770-538-4666. *E-mail:* kwilborn@brenau.edu.

Clayton State University

Department of Nursing
Morrow, Georgia

http://nursing.clayton.edu/default.htm
Founded in 1969

DEGREES • BSN • MSN

Nursing Program Faculty 38 (56% with doctorates).
Baccalaureate Enrollment 195 **Women** 83.33% **Men** 16.67% **Minority** 65.79% **International** 2.19% **Part-time** 17.98%
Graduate Enrollment 7 **Women** 94.44% **Men** 5.56% **Minority** 72.22% **Part-time** 66.67%
Distance Learning Courses Available.
Nursing Student Activities Nursing Honor Society, Sigma Theta Tau, Student Nurses' Association.
Nursing Student Resources Academic advising; academic or career counseling; assistance for students with disabilities; bookstore; campus computer network; career placement assistance; computer lab; computer-assisted instruction; e-mail services; employment services for current students; externships; housing assistance; interactive nursing skills videos; Internet; learning resource lab; library services; nursing audiovisuals; paid internships; placement services for program completers; remedial services; resume preparation assistance; skills, simulation, or other laboratory; tutoring.
Library Facilities 77,043 volumes (3,450 in health, 1,800 in nursing); 4,250 periodical subscriptions (151 health-care related).

BACCALAUREATE PROGRAMS

Degree BSN
Available Programs Generic Baccalaureate; RN Baccalaureate.
Study Options Full-time.
Online Degree Options Yes.
Program Entrance Requirements Minimum overall college GPA of 2.5, transcript of college record, CPR certification, health exam, health insurance, immunizations, interview, minimum GPA in nursing prerequisites of 2.5, professional liability insurance/malpractice insurance, prerequisite course work. Transfer students are accepted. *Application deadline:* 3/15 (fall), 9/15 (spring). *Application fee:* $25.
Expenses (2010-11) *Tuition, state resident:* full-time $4274; part-time $143 per credit hour. *Tuition, nonresident:* full-time $15,888; part-time $530 per credit hour. *Room and board:* $8352; room only: $5254 per academic year. *Required fees:* part-time $12 per credit; part-time $567 per term.
Financial Aid 61% of baccalaureate students in nursing programs received some form of financial aid in 2009-10.
Contact Dr. Sue E. Odom, Director of the Undergraduate Nursing PRogram, Department of Nursing, Clayton State University, 2000 Clayton State Boulevard, Morrow, GA 30260. *Telephone:* 678-466-4959. *Fax:* 678-466-4999. *E-mail:* sueodom@clayton.edu.

GRADUATE PROGRAMS

Expenses (2010-11) *Tuition, area resident:* full-time $5094; part-time $220 per credit hour. *Tuition, nonresident:* full-time $16,974; part-time $880 per credit hour. *Required fees:* full-time $1134.
Financial Aid 86% of graduate students in nursing programs received some form of financial aid in 2009-10.
Contact Dr. Katherine Willock, Director of the MSN Program, Department of Nursing, Clayton State University, 2000 Clayton State Boulevard, Morrow, GA 30260. *Telephone:* 678-466-4987. *Fax:* 678-466-4999. *E-mail:* katherinewillock@clayton.edu.

MASTER'S DEGREE PROGRAM

Degree MSN
Available Programs Master's; RN to Master's.
Concentrations Available Nursing administration; nursing education.
Study Options Full-time and part-time.
Online Degree Options Yes (online only).
Program Entrance Requirements Computer literacy, minimum overall college GPA of 3.0, transcript of college record, CPR certification, written essay, immunizations, interview, 3 letters of recommendation, professional liability insurance/malpractice insurance. *Application deadline:* 7/1 (fall), 11/1 (spring), 3/1 (summer). Applications may be processed on a rolling basis for some programs. *Application fee:* $25.
Advanced Placement Credit given for nursing courses completed elsewhere dependent upon specific evaluations.
Degree Requirements 36 total credit hours, thesis or project.

College of Coastal Georgia

Department of Nursing and Health Sciences
Brunswick, Georgia

Founded in 1961

DEGREE • BS

Library Facilities 535 periodical subscriptions.

BACCALAUREATE PROGRAMS

Degree BS
Available Programs Generic Baccalaureate; RN Baccalaureate.
Program Entrance Requirements Transcript of college record.
Contact Kay Hampton, Interim Chair for Nursing and Health Sciences. *Telephone:* 912-279-5705. *E-mail:* khampton@ccga.edu.

Columbus State University

Nursing Program
Columbus, Georgia

http://nursing.ColumbusState.edu/
Founded in 1958

DEGREE • BSN

Nursing Program Faculty 31 (12% with doctorates).
Baccalaureate Enrollment 187 **Women** 91% **Men** 9% **Minority** 42% **International** 6% **Part-time** 3%
Distance Learning Courses Available.

Nursing Student Activities Sigma Theta Tau, Student Nurses' Association.

Nursing Student Resources Academic advising; academic or career counseling; assistance for students with disabilities; bookstore; campus computer network; career placement assistance; computer lab; computer-assisted instruction; e-mail services; housing assistance; interactive nursing skills videos; Internet; learning resource lab; library services; nursing audiovisuals; remedial services; resume preparation assistance; skills, simulation, or other laboratory; tutoring.

Library Facilities 368,486 volumes (284 in health, 260 in nursing); 1,508 periodical subscriptions (81 health-care related).

BACCALAUREATE PROGRAMS

Degree BSN

Available Programs Generic Baccalaureate; RN Baccalaureate.

Study Options Full-time.

Online Degree Options Yes.

Program Entrance Requirements Minimum overall college GPA of 2.75, transcript of college record, CPR certification, health exam, health insurance, immunizations, 3 letters of recommendation, minimum GPA in nursing prerequisites of 2.75, professional liability insurance/malpractice insurance, prerequisite course work. *Application deadline:* 2/28 (fall).

Advanced Placement Credit given for nursing courses completed elsewhere dependent upon specific evaluations.

Expenses (2010-11) *Tuition, state resident:* full-time $4596; part-time $154 per credit hour. *Tuition, nonresident:* full-time $16,572; part-time $553 per credit hour. *Room and board:* $3125; room only: $2050 per academic year. *Required fees:* full-time $3806; part-time $65 per credit; part-time $650 per term.

Financial Aid 95% of baccalaureate students in nursing programs received some form of financial aid in 2009-10. *Gift aid (need-based):* Federal Pell, FSEOG, state, private, college/university gift aid from institutional funds. *Loans:* Federal Nursing Student Loans, Federal Direct (Subsidized and Unsubsidized Stafford PLUS), Perkins, state, college/university. *Work-study:* Federal Work-Study. *Financial aid application deadline (priority):* 5/1.

Contact Dr. June S. Goyne, Director, School of Nursing, Nursing Program, Columbus State University, 4225 University Avenue, Columbus, GA 31907. *Telephone:* 706-568-5050. *Fax:* 706-569-3101. *E-mail:* goyne_june@colstate.edu.

Emory University
Nell Hodgson Woodruff School of Nursing
Atlanta, Georgia

http://www.nursing.emory.edu/

Founded in 1836

DEGREES • BSN • MSN • MSN/MPH • PHD

Nursing Program Faculty 62 (56% with doctorates).

Baccalaureate Enrollment 256 **Women** 93% **Men** 7% **Minority** 46% **International** 1% **Part-time** 1%

Graduate Enrollment 200 **Women** 92% **Men** 8% **Minority** 46% **International** 2% **Part-time** 23%

Nursing Student Activities Sigma Theta Tau, Student Nurses' Association.

Nursing Student Resources Academic advising; academic or career counseling; assistance for students with disabilities; bookstore; campus computer network; career placement assistance; computer lab; computer-assisted instruction; daycare for children of students; e-mail services; employment services for current students; externships; housing assistance; interactive nursing skills videos; Internet; learning resource lab; library services; nursing audiovisuals; other; resume preparation assistance; skills, simulation, or other laboratory; tutoring; unpaid internships.

Library Facilities 3.5 million volumes (250,000 in health); 83,514 periodical subscriptions (1,800 health-care related).

BACCALAUREATE PROGRAMS

Degree BSN

Available Programs Accelerated Baccalaureate; Baccalaureate for Second Degree; Generic Baccalaureate.

Study Options Full-time.

Program Entrance Requirements Minimum overall college GPA of 3.0, transcript of college record, written essay, 3 letters of recommendation, minimum GPA in nursing prerequisites of 3.0, prerequisite course work. Transfer students are accepted. *Application deadline:* 1/15 (fall), 12/1 (summer). *Application fee:* $50.

Advanced Placement Credit given for nursing courses completed elsewhere dependent upon specific evaluations.

Expenses (2010-11) *Tuition:* full-time $34,800; part-time $1450 per credit hour. *Required fees:* full-time $329.

Financial Aid 94% of baccalaureate students in nursing programs received some form of financial aid in 2009-10. *Gift aid (need-based):* Federal Pell, FSEOG, state, private, college/university gift aid from institutional funds. *Loans:* Federal Nursing Student Loans, Perkins, state, college/university. *Work-study:* Federal Work-Study, part-time campus jobs. *Financial aid application deadline:* 3/1(priority: 2/15).

Contact Office of Admission and Student Services, Nell Hodgson Woodruff School of Nursing, Emory University, 1520 Clifton Road NE, Atlanta, GA 30322. *Telephone:* 404-727-7980. *Fax:* 404-727-8509. *E-mail:* admit@nursing.emory.edu.

GRADUATE PROGRAMS

Expenses (2010-11) *Tuition:* full-time $34,800; part-time $1450 per credit hour. *Required fees:* full-time $296.

Financial Aid 89% of graduate students in nursing programs received some form of financial aid in 2009-10. 14 fellowships (averaging $28,000 per year) were awarded; career-related internships or fieldwork, Federal Work-Study, institutionally sponsored loans, and scholarships also available. Aid available to part-time students. *Financial aid application deadline:* 3/1.

Contact Office of Admission and Student Services, Nell Hodgson Woodruff School of Nursing, Emory University, 1520 Clifton Road NE, Atlanta, GA 30322. *Telephone:* 404-727-7980. *Fax:* 404-727-8509. *E-mail:* admit@nursing.emory.edu.

MASTER'S DEGREE PROGRAM

Degrees MSN; MSN/MPH

Available Programs Master's; RN to Master's.

Concentrations Available Nurse-midwifery. *Clinical nurse specialist programs in:* public health. *Nurse practitioner programs in:* acute care, adult health, family health, gerontology, pediatric, primary care, women's health.

Study Options Full-time and part-time.

Program Entrance Requirements Clinical experience, minimum overall college GPA of 3.0, transcript of college record, written essay, interview, 3 letters of recommendation, physical assessment course, prerequisite course work, resume, statistics course, GRE General Test or MAT. *Application deadline:* 1/15 (fall), 10/1 (spring), 1/15 (summer). Applications may be processed on a rolling basis for some programs. *Application fee:* $50.

Advanced Placement Credit given for nursing courses completed elsewhere dependent upon specific evaluations.

Degree Requirements 41 total credit hours.

POST-MASTER'S PROGRAM

Areas of Study Nurse-midwifery; nursing education. *Clinical nurse specialist programs in:* public health. *Nurse practitioner programs in:* acute care, adult health, family health, gerontology, pediatric, primary care, women's health.

DOCTORAL DEGREE PROGRAM

Degree PhD

Available Programs Doctorate; Post-Baccalaureate Doctorate.

Areas of Study Aging, biology of health and illness, ethics, faculty preparation, gerontology, health policy, human health and illness, illness and transition, individualized study, neuro-behavior, nursing policy, nursing research, nursing science, women's health.

Program Entrance Requirements Minimum overall college GPA of 3.0, interview by faculty committee, 3 letters of recommendation, MSN or equivalent, statistics course, vita, writing sample. Application deadline: 1/3 (fall). Applications may be processed on a rolling basis for some programs.

Degree Requirements 50 total credit hours, dissertation, oral exam, written exam, residency.

POSTDOCTORAL PROGRAM

Postdoctoral Program Contact Ms. Teresa Fosque, Senior Business Manager, Nell Hodgson Woodruff School of Nursing, Emory University, 1520 Clifton Road NE, Atlanta, GA 30322. *E-mail:* tfosque@emory.edu.

Georgia Baptist College of Nursing of Mercer University
Department of Nursing
Atlanta, Georgia

http://www.mercer.edu/nursing
Founded in 1988

DEGREES • BSN • MSN • PHD
Nursing Program Faculty 31 (45% with doctorates).
Baccalaureate Enrollment 391 **Women** 99% **Men** 1% **Minority** 42% **International** 1% **Part-time** 13%
Graduate Enrollment 13 **Women** 99% **Men** 1% **Minority** 72% **International** 12% **Part-time** 54%
Nursing Student Activities Nursing Honor Society, Sigma Theta Tau, Student Nurses' Association, nursing club.
Nursing Student Resources Academic advising; academic or career counseling; assistance for students with disabilities; bookstore; campus computer network; career placement assistance; computer lab; computer-assisted instruction; e-mail services; employment services for current students; housing assistance; interactive nursing skills videos; Internet; learning resource lab; library services; nursing audiovisuals; placement services for program completers; remedial services; resume preparation assistance; skills, simulation, or other laboratory; tutoring.
Library Facilities 12,836 volumes (4,072 in health, 2,805 in nursing); 182 periodical subscriptions (218 health-care related).

BACCALAUREATE PROGRAMS

Degree BSN
Available Programs Generic Baccalaureate; RN Baccalaureate.
Study Options Full-time and part-time.
Program Entrance Requirements Transcript of college record, written essay, health exam, health insurance, high school biology, high school foreign language, 3 years high school math, 3 years high school science, high school transcript, immunizations, prerequisite course work. Transfer students are accepted. *Application deadline:* 5/15 (fall). *Application fee:* $50.
Advanced Placement Credit by examination available. Credit given for nursing courses completed elsewhere dependent upon specific evaluations.
Expenses (2010-11) *Tuition:* full-time $19,888; part-time $829 per credit hour. *Room and board:* $3875; room only: $3875 per academic year. *Required fees:* full-time $1004.
Financial Aid 80% of baccalaureate students in nursing programs received some form of financial aid in 2009-10.
Contact Mrs. Lynn Vines, Director of Admissions, Department of Nursing, Georgia Baptist College of Nursing of Mercer University, 3001 Mercer University Drive, Atlanta, GA 30341. *Telephone:* 678-547-6700. *Fax:* 678-547-6794. *E-mail:* vines_ml@mercer.edu.

GRADUATE PROGRAMS

Expenses (2010-11) *Tuition:* full-time $17,646; part-time $981 per credit hour. *Room and board:* room only: $3875 per academic year. *Required fees:* full-time $400.
Financial Aid 90% of graduate students in nursing programs received some form of financial aid in 2009-10.
Contact Dr. Linda A. Streit, Associate Dean for the Graduate Program, Department of Nursing, Georgia Baptist College of Nursing of Mercer University, 3001 Mercer University Drive, Atlanta, GA 30341. *Telephone:* 678-547-6774. *Fax:* 678-547-6777. *E-mail:* streit_la@mercer.edu.

MASTER'S DEGREE PROGRAM
Degree MSN
Available Programs Master's.
Concentrations Available Nursing education. *Clinical nurse specialist programs in:* acute care, critical care.
Study Options Full-time and part-time.
Program Entrance Requirements Clinical experience, computer literacy, minimum overall college GPA of 3.0, transcript of college record, CPR certification, written essay, immunizations, interview, 3 letters of recommendation, nursing research course, physical assessment course, statistics course. *Application deadline:* 5/15 (fall), 11/1 (spring). *Application fee:* $50.
Advanced Placement Credit given for nursing courses completed elsewhere dependent upon specific evaluations.
Degree Requirements 36 total credit hours, thesis or project.

POST-MASTER'S PROGRAM
Areas of Study Nursing education.

DOCTORAL DEGREE PROGRAM
Degree PhD
Available Programs Doctorate.
Areas of Study Clinical practice, ethics, nursing education.
Program Entrance Requirements Minimum overall college GPA of 3.2, interview, 3 letters of recommendation, MSN or equivalent, scholarly papers, statistics course, vita, writing sample. Application deadline: 2/28 (fall). Applications may be processed on a rolling basis for some programs. Application fee: $50.
Degree Requirements 52 total credit hours, dissertation, oral exam, written exam, residency.

Georgia College & State University
College of Health Sciences
Milledgeville, Georgia

http://www.gcsu.edu/acad_affairs/school_healthsci/healthsci
Founded in 1889

DEGREES • BSN • MSN • MSN/MBA
Nursing Program Faculty 36 (25% with doctorates).
Baccalaureate Enrollment 267 **Women** 85% **Men** 15% **Minority** 12% **International** 1% **Part-time** 30%
Graduate Enrollment 70 **Women** 80% **Men** 20% **Minority** 16% **International** 1% **Part-time** 100%
Nursing Student Activities Sigma Theta Tau, Student Nurses' Association.
Nursing Student Resources Academic advising; academic or career counseling; assistance for students with disabilities; bookstore; campus computer network; career placement assistance; computer lab; computer-assisted instruction; e-mail services; employment services for current students; housing assistance; interactive nursing skills videos; Internet; learning resource lab; library services; nursing audiovisuals; remedial services; resume preparation assistance; skills, simulation, or other laboratory; tutoring; unpaid internships.
Library Facilities 199,506 volumes (3,095 in health, 1,465 in nursing); 5,625 periodical subscriptions (315 health-care related).

BACCALAUREATE PROGRAMS

Degree BSN
Available Programs Generic Baccalaureate; RN Baccalaureate.
Site Options Macon, GA.
Study Options Full-time and part-time.
Program Entrance Requirements Minimum overall college GPA of 2.5, transcript of college record, CPR certification, health exam, health insurance, high school biology, high school foreign language, 4 years high school math, 3 years high school science, high school transcript, immunizations, minimum GPA in nursing prerequisites of 2.5, professional liability insurance/malpractice insurance, prerequisite course work. Transfer students are accepted.
Advanced Placement Credit by examination available. Credit given for nursing courses completed elsewhere dependent upon specific evaluations.
Contact ***Telephone:*** 478-445-4004. *Fax:* 478-445-1913.

GRADUATE PROGRAMS

Contact ***Telephone:*** 478-445-1795. *Fax:* 478-445-1913.

MASTER'S DEGREE PROGRAM
Degrees MSN; MSN/MBA
Available Programs Master's; RN to Master's.
Concentrations Available Nursing administration; nursing education; nursing informatics. *Clinical nurse specialist programs in:* adult health. *Nurse practitioner programs in:* family health.
Site Options Macon, GA.
Study Options Part-time.
Program Entrance Requirements Clinical experience, computer literacy, minimum overall college GPA of 2.75, transcript of college record, CPR certification, immunizations, interview, nursing research course, professional liability insurance/malpractice insurance, resume, statistics course, GRE, GMAT or MAT.

Advanced Placement Credit given for nursing courses completed elsewhere dependent upon specific evaluations.
Degree Requirements 36 total credit hours, thesis or project, comprehensive exam.

POST-MASTER'S PROGRAM
Areas of Study Nursing education; nursing informatics. *Nurse practitioner programs in:* family health.

Georgia Health Sciences University
School of Nursing
Augusta, Georgia

http://www.mcg.edu/son
Founded in 1828

DEGREES • BSN • MSN • PHD
Nursing Program Faculty 73 (40% with doctorates).
Baccalaureate Enrollment 289 **Women** 94% **Men** 6% **Minority** 14.5% **Part-time** 1%
Graduate Enrollment 298 **Women** 89.6% **Men** 10.4% **Minority** 21.14% **Part-time** 27.85%
Distance Learning Courses Available.
Nursing Student Activities Nursing Honor Society, Sigma Theta Tau, Student Nurses' Association, nursing club.
Nursing Student Resources Academic advising; academic or career counseling; assistance for students with disabilities; bookstore; campus computer network; career placement assistance; computer lab; computer-assisted instruction; daycare for children of students; e-mail services; employment services for current students; externships; housing assistance; interactive nursing skills videos; Internet; learning resource lab; library services; nursing audiovisuals; paid internships; remedial services; skills, simulation, or other laboratory; tutoring.
Library Facilities 165,901 volumes (178,650 in health, 14,650 in nursing); 4,674 periodical subscriptions (1,307 health-care related).

BACCALAUREATE PROGRAMS
Degree BSN
Available Programs Generic Baccalaureate.
Site Options Columbus, GA; Athens, GA.
Study Options Full-time.
Program Entrance Requirements Minimum overall college GPA of 2.8, transcript of college record, CPR certification, written essay, health insurance, immunizations, 2 letters of recommendation, prerequisite course work. Transfer students are accepted. *Application deadline:* 12/1 (fall). *Application fee:* $30.
Expenses (2009-10) *Tuition, area resident:* full-time $9105; part-time $203 per credit hour. *Tuition, nonresident:* full-time $36,420; part-time $810 per credit hour. *Room and board:* room only: $1500 per academic year. *Required fees:* full-time $842.
Financial Aid 80% of baccalaureate students in nursing programs received some form of financial aid in 2008-09. *Gift aid (need-based):* Federal Pell, FSEOG, state, private, college/university gift aid from institutional funds, Federal Nursing. *Loans:* Federal Nursing Student Loans, Federal Direct (Subsidized and Unsubsidized Stafford PLUS), Perkins, state, college/university. *Work-study:* Federal Work-Study. *Financial aid application deadline:* Continuous.
Contact Office of Academic Admissions, School of Nursing, Georgia Health Sciences University, AA-170 Kelly Building, Augusta, GA 30912. *Telephone:* 706-721-2725. *Fax:* 706-721-0186. *E-mail:* underadm@mail.mcg.edu.

GRADUATE PROGRAMS
Expenses (2009-10) *Tuition, area resident:* full-time $11,469; part-time $319 per credit hour. *Tuition, nonresident:* full-time $31,881; part-time $886 per credit hour. *Room and board:* room only: $1500 per academic year. *Required fees:* full-time $607.
Financial Aid 75% of graduate students in nursing programs received some form of financial aid in 2008-09.
Contact Director, Academic Admissions, School of Nursing, Georgia Health Sciences University, AA-170 Kelly Building, Augusta, GA 30912. *Telephone:* 706-721-2725. *Fax:* 706-721-0186. *E-mail:* gradadm@mail.mcg.edu.

MASTER'S DEGREE PROGRAM
Degree MSN
Available Programs Accelerated Master's; Accelerated Master's for Non-Nursing College Graduates; Master's; RN to Master's.
Concentrations Available Clinical nurse leader; nurse anesthesia. *Nurse practitioner programs in:* family health, pediatric.
Site Options Columbus, GA; Athens, GA.
Study Options Full-time and part-time.
Online Degree Options Yes.
Program Entrance Requirements Clinical experience, computer literacy, minimum overall college GPA of 3.0, transcript of college record, CPR certification, written essay, immunizations, interview, 3 letters of recommendation, professional liability insurance/malpractice insurance, prerequisite course work, resume, statistics course.*Application fee:* $30.
Degree Requirements 46 total credit hours, thesis or project.

POST-MASTER'S PROGRAM
Areas of Study Nurse anesthesia. *Nurse practitioner programs in:* family health, pediatric.

DOCTORAL DEGREE PROGRAM
Degree PhD
Available Programs Doctorate; Post-Baccalaureate Doctorate.
Areas of Study Bio-behavioral research, nursing research.
Site Options Columbus, GA; Athens, GA.
Program Entrance Requirements Clinical experience, minimum overall college GPA of 3.2, interview by faculty committee, interview, 3 letters of recommendation, MSN or equivalent, scholarly papers, statistics course, vita, writing sample. Application fee: $30.
Degree Requirements 60 total credit hours, dissertation, oral exam, written exam.

Georgia Southern University
School of Nursing
Statesboro, Georgia

http://chhs.georgiasouthern.edu/nursing/
Founded in 1906

DEGREES • BSN • DNP • MSN
Nursing Program Faculty 36 (35% with doctorates).
Baccalaureate Enrollment 267 **Women** 86.5% **Men** 13.5% **Minority** 15.3% **International** .4% **Part-time** 24.7%
Graduate Enrollment 66 **Women** 94% **Men** 6% **Minority** 27% **Part-time** 1.5%
Distance Learning Courses Available.
Nursing Student Activities Sigma Theta Tau, Student Nurses' Association.
Nursing Student Resources Academic advising; academic or career counseling; assistance for students with disabilities; bookstore; campus computer network; career placement assistance; computer lab; computer-assisted instruction; daycare for children of students; e-mail services; employment services for current students; housing assistance; interactive nursing skills videos; Internet; learning resource lab; library services; nursing audiovisuals; placement services for program completers; resume preparation assistance; skills, simulation, or other laboratory; tutoring.
Library Facilities 607,542 volumes (25,000 in health, 12,000 in nursing); 49,100 periodical subscriptions (20,000 health-care related).

BACCALAUREATE PROGRAMS
Degree BSN
Available Programs ADN to Baccalaureate; Generic Baccalaureate; LPN to RN Baccalaureate.
Study Options Full-time.
Online Degree Options Yes.
Program Entrance Requirements Minimum overall college GPA of 3.0, transcript of college record, CPR certification, written essay, health exam, health insurance, high school biology, high school chemistry, high school foreign language, 2 years high school math, 4 years high school science, high school transcript, immunizations, minimum GPA in nursing prerequisites of 3.0, professional liability insurance/malpractice insurance, prerequisite course work. Transfer students are accepted. *Application deadline:* 2/4 (fall), 8/5 (spring).
Advanced Placement Credit by examination available. Credit given for nursing courses completed elsewhere dependent upon specific evaluations.

Expenses (2010-11) *Tuition, state resident:* full-time $3196; part-time $134 per credit hour. *Tuition, nonresident:* full-time $12,778; part-time $533 per credit hour. *Room and board:* $9050; room only: $6000 per academic year. *Required fees:* full-time $1644; part-time $822 per term.
Financial Aid 94% of baccalaureate students in nursing programs received some form of financial aid in 2009-10.
Contact Dr. Melissa Garno, BSN Program Director, School of Nursing, Georgia Southern University, PO Box 8158, Statesboro, GA 30460-8158. *Telephone:* 912-478-5454. *Fax:* 912-478-1159. *E-mail:* mel@georgiasouthern.edu.

GRADUATE PROGRAMS

Expenses (2010-11) *Tuition, state resident:* full-time $6000; part-time $250 per credit hour. *Tuition, nonresident:* full-time $23,976; part-time $999 per credit hour. *Room and board:* $9050; room only: $6000 per academic year. *Required fees:* full-time $1644; part-time $822 per term.
Financial Aid 39% of graduate students in nursing programs received some form of financial aid in 2009-10. Research assistantships with partial tuition reimbursements available (averaging $7,200 per year), teaching assistantships with partial tuition reimbursements available (averaging $7,200 per year) were awarded; career-related internships or fieldwork, Federal Work-Study, scholarships, traineeships, tuition waivers (partial), and unspecified assistantships also available. Aid available to part-time students. *Financial aid application deadline:* 4/15.
Contact Dr. Deborah Allen, Director, Graduate Program, School of Nursing, Georgia Southern University, PO Box 8158, Statesboro, GA 30460-8158. *Telephone:* 912-478-0017. *Fax:* 912-478-1679. *E-mail:* debbieallen@georgiasouthern.edu.

MASTER'S DEGREE PROGRAM
Degree MSN
Available Programs Master's; RN to Master's.
Concentrations Available *Clinical nurse specialist programs in:* community health. *Nurse practitioner programs in:* family health.
Study Options Full-time and part-time.
Program Entrance Requirements Clinical experience, computer literacy, minimum overall college GPA of 3.0, transcript of college record, CPR certification, immunizations, interview, 3 letters of recommendation, professional liability insurance/malpractice insurance, prerequisite course work, statistics course, GRE General Test or MAT. *Application deadline:* 3/15 (fall).
Advanced Placement Credit given for nursing courses completed elsewhere dependent upon specific evaluations.
Degree Requirements 48 total credit hours, comprehensive exam.

POST-MASTER'S PROGRAM
Areas of Study *Clinical nurse specialist programs in:* community health. *Nurse practitioner programs in:* family health.

DOCTORAL DEGREE PROGRAM
Degree DNP
Available Programs Doctorate.
Areas of Study Nursing science.
Online Degree Options Yes (online only).
Program Entrance Requirements Minimum overall college GPA of 3.0, interview by faculty committee, 3 letters of recommendation, MSN or equivalent, vita, writing sample, GRE, MAT. Application deadline: 3/1 (fall).
Degree Requirements 40 total credit hours, oral exam, written exam.

Georgia Southwestern State University
School of Nursing
Americus, Georgia

http://www.gsw.edu/
Founded in 1906

DEGREE • BSN
Nursing Program Faculty 13 (32% with doctorates).
Baccalaureate Enrollment 331 **Women** 88% **Men** 12% **Minority** 30% **International** 8% **Part-time** 35%
Distance Learning Courses Available.
Nursing Student Activities Sigma Theta Tau, Student Nurses' Association.
Nursing Student Resources Academic advising; academic or career counseling; assistance for students with disabilities; bookstore; campus computer network; career placement assistance; computer lab; computer-assisted instruction; e-mail services; employment services for current students; interactive nursing skills videos; Internet; learning resource lab; library services; nursing audiovisuals; placement services for program completers; remedial services; resume preparation assistance; skills, simulation, or other laboratory; tutoring.
Library Facilities 627 volumes in health, 528 volumes in nursing; 141 periodical subscriptions health-care related.

BACCALAUREATE PROGRAMS
Degree BSN
Available Programs Accelerated Baccalaureate for Second Degree; Baccalaureate for Second Degree; Generic Baccalaureate; LPN to RN Baccalaureate; RN Baccalaureate.
Study Options Full-time and part-time.
Online Degree Options Yes (online only).
Program Entrance Requirements Minimum overall college GPA of 2.8, transcript of college record, CPR certification, written essay, health exam, health insurance, high school foreign language, 4 years high school math, 4 years high school science, high school transcript, immunizations, 2 letters of recommendation, minimum high school GPA of 2.8, minimum GPA in nursing prerequisites of 2.8, professional liability insurance/malpractice insurance, prerequisite course work, RN licensure. Transfer students are accepted. *Application deadline:* 2/15 (fall), 8/15 (spring).
Advanced Placement Credit given for nursing courses completed elsewhere dependent upon specific evaluations.
Expenses (2010-11) *Tuition, state resident:* full-time $4274; part-time $143 per credit hour. *Tuition, nonresident:* full-time $15,888; part-time $530 per credit hour. *Room and board:* $6200; room only: $3400 per academic year. *Required fees:* full-time $858; part-time $400 per term.
Financial Aid 91% of baccalaureate students in nursing programs received some form of financial aid in 2009-10. *Gift aid (need-based):* Federal Pell, FSEOG, state, private, college/university gift aid from institutional funds. *Loans:* Perkins, state, college/university. *Work-study:* Federal Work-Study, part-time campus jobs. *Financial aid application deadline (priority):* 4/1.
Contact Dr. Sandra Daniel, Dean and Professor, School of Nursing, Georgia Southwestern State University, 800 Georgia Southwestern State University Drive, Americus, GA 31709. *Telephone:* 229-931-2280. *Fax:* 229-931-2288. *E-mail:* sdd@canes.gsw.edu.

Georgia State University
Byrdine F. Lewis School of Nursing
Atlanta, Georgia

http://chhs.gsu.edu/nursing/
Founded in 1913

DEGREES • BS • MSN • PHD
Nursing Program Faculty 60 (40% with doctorates).
Baccalaureate Enrollment 269 **Women** 82% **Men** 18% **Minority** 35% **International** 5% **Part-time** 5%
Graduate Enrollment 200 **Women** 90% **Men** 10% **Minority** 33% **Part-time** 90%
Distance Learning Courses Available.
Nursing Student Activities Sigma Theta Tau, Student Nurses' Association.
Nursing Student Resources Academic advising; academic or career counseling; assistance for students with disabilities; bookstore; campus computer network; career placement assistance; computer lab; computer-assisted instruction; e-mail services; interactive nursing skills videos; Internet; learning resource lab; library services; nursing audiovisuals; remedial services; resume preparation assistance; skills, simulation, or other laboratory; tutoring.
Library Facilities 1.8 million volumes (52,835 in health, 20,856 in nursing); 11,994 periodical subscriptions (725 health-care related).

BACCALAUREATE PROGRAMS
Degree BS
Available Programs Generic Baccalaureate.
Study Options Full-time and part-time.
Program Entrance Requirements Minimum overall college GPA of 3.0, transcript of college record, CPR certification, written essay, health exam, immunizations, 2 letters of recommendation, minimum GPA in

nursing prerequisites of 3.0, professional liability insurance/malpractice insurance, prerequisite course work. Transfer students are accepted. *Application deadline:* 3/1 (fall), 10/1 (spring).

Advanced Placement Credit given for nursing courses completed elsewhere dependent upon specific evaluations.

Expenses (2009-10) *Tuition, state resident:* full-time $6000; part-time $203 per credit hour. *Tuition, nonresident:* full-time $24,200; part-time $810 per credit hour. *International tuition:* $24,200 full-time. *Room and board:* room only: $3000 per academic year. *Required fees:* full-time $1500; part-time $203 per credit.

Financial Aid 90% of baccalaureate students in nursing programs received some form of financial aid in 2008-09. *Gift aid (need-based):* Federal Pell, FSEOG, state, private, college/university gift aid from institutional funds. *Loans:* Federal Direct (Subsidized and Unsubsidized Stafford PLUS), Perkins, state. *Work-study:* Federal Work-Study. *Financial aid application deadline:* 11/1(priority: 4/1).

Contact Ms. Denisa Hightower, Admissions Counselor, Byrdine F. Lewis School of Nursing, Georgia State University, College of Health and Human Sciences, Office of Academic Assistance, Atlanta, GA 30303-3083. *Telephone:* 404-413-1000. *Fax:* 404-413-1001. *E-mail:* dhightower@gsu.edu.

GRADUATE PROGRAMS

Expenses (2009-10) *Tuition, state resident:* full-time $26,000; part-time $221 per credit hour. *Room and board:* $12,000; room only: $4000 per academic year. *Required fees:* full-time $2500.

Financial Aid 50% of graduate students in nursing programs received some form of financial aid in 2008-09. Research assistantships with full and partial tuition reimbursements available (averaging $3,108 per year); fellowships with full tuition reimbursements available, teaching assistantships, Federal Work-Study, institutionally sponsored loans, scholarships, traineeships, tuition waivers (partial), and unspecified assistantships also available. Aid available to part-time students. *Financial aid application deadline:* 4/1.

Contact Ms. Barbara Smith, Admissions Counselor, Byrdine F. Lewis School of Nursing, Georgia State University, College of Health and Human Sciences, PO Box 3995, Atlanta, GA 30302-3995. *Telephone:* 404-413-1007. *Fax:* 404-413-1001. *E-mail:* alhbbs@langate.gsu.edu.

MASTER'S DEGREE PROGRAM

Degree MSN

Available Programs Master's; RN to Master's.

Concentrations Available Nursing informatics. *Clinical nurse specialist programs in:* adult health, pediatric, perinatal, psychiatric/mental health, women's health. *Nurse practitioner programs in:* adult health, family health, pediatric, psychiatric/mental health, women's health.

Site Options Alpharetta, GA.

Study Options Full-time and part-time.

Program Entrance Requirements Clinical experience, computer literacy, minimum overall college GPA of 3.0, transcript of college record, CPR certification, written essay, interview, 2 letters of recommendation, professional liability insurance/malpractice insurance, MAT (preferred) or GRE. *Application deadline:* 3/1 (fall), 10/15 (spring), 3/1 (summer). *Application fee:* $50.

Advanced Placement Credit given for nursing courses completed elsewhere dependent upon specific evaluations.

Degree Requirements 48 total credit hours.

POST-MASTER'S PROGRAM

Areas of Study *Clinical nurse specialist programs in:* adult health, pediatric, perinatal, psychiatric/mental health, women's health. *Nurse practitioner programs in:* adult health, family health, pediatric, psychiatric/mental health, women's health.

DOCTORAL DEGREE PROGRAM

Degree PhD

Available Programs Doctorate; Post-Baccalaureate Doctorate.

Areas of Study Bio-behavioral research, health promotion/disease prevention, individualized study, nursing research, nursing science.

Site Options Alpharetta, GA.

Program Entrance Requirements Minimum overall college GPA of 3.0, interview by faculty committee, interview, 3 letters of recommendation, MSN or equivalent, vita, GRE General Test. Application deadline: 3/1 (fall). Application fee: $50.

Degree Requirements 60 total credit hours, dissertation, written exam, residency.

Gordon College

Division of Nursing and Health Sciences
Barnesville, Georgia

http://www.gdn.edu/

Founded in 1852

DEGREE • BSN

Nursing Program Faculty 2 (50% with doctorates).

Baccalaureate Enrollment 26

Nursing Student Activities Student Nurses' Association.

Nursing Student Resources Academic advising; academic or career counseling; assistance for students with disabilities; bookstore; campus computer network; computer lab; computer-assisted instruction; e-mail services; employment services for current students; externships; interactive nursing skills videos; Internet; learning resource lab; library services; nursing audiovisuals; remedial services; skills, simulation, or other laboratory; tutoring.

Library Facilities 15 volumes in nursing.

BACCALAUREATE PROGRAMS

Degree BSN

Available Programs RN Baccalaureate.

Program Entrance Requirements Transcript of college record.

Contact Dr. Joan S. Cranford, Program Director. *Telephone:* 678-359-5085. *Fax:* 678-359-5064. *E-mail:* j_cranford@gdn.edu.

Kennesaw State University

School of Nursing
Kennesaw, Georgia

http://www.kennesaw.edu/chhs/schoolofnursing

Founded in 1963

DEGREES • BSN • MSN

Distance Learning Courses Available.

Nursing Student Activities Sigma Theta Tau, Student Nurses' Association.

Nursing Student Resources Academic advising; academic or career counseling; assistance for students with disabilities; bookstore; campus computer network; career placement assistance; computer lab; computer-assisted instruction; e-mail services; employment services for current students; externships; housing assistance; interactive nursing skills videos; Internet; learning resource lab; library services; nursing audiovisuals; paid internships; placement services for program completers; remedial services; resume preparation assistance; skills, simulation, or other laboratory; tutoring.

Library Facilities 556,325 volumes (20,000 in health, 10,000 in nursing); 42,000 periodical subscriptions (503 health-care related).

BACCALAUREATE PROGRAMS

Degree BSN

Available Programs ADN to Baccalaureate; Accelerated Baccalaureate; Accelerated Baccalaureate for Second Degree; Baccalaureate for Second Degree; Generic Baccalaureate; RN Baccalaureate.

Site Options Rome, GA; Jasper, GA.

Study Options Full-time and part-time.

Program Entrance Requirements Minimum overall college GPA of 2.7, transcript of college record, CPR certification, health exam, health insurance, 2 years high school math, 2 years high school science, high school transcript, immunizations, interview, 1 letter of recommendation, minimum high school GPA of 2.5, minimum GPA in nursing prerequisites of 2.7, professional liability insurance/malpractice insurance, prerequisite course work. Transfer students are accepted.

Advanced Placement Credit by examination available. Credit given for nursing courses completed elsewhere dependent upon specific evaluations.

Contact ***Telephone:*** 770-499-3211. *Fax:* 770-423-6627.

GRADUATE PROGRAMS

Contact ***Telephone:*** 770-423-6061. *Fax:* 770-423-6627.

MASTER'S DEGREE PROGRAM

Degree MSN

Available Programs Master's.

Concentrations Available *Clinical nurse specialist programs in:* adult health. *Nurse practitioner programs in:* adult health, family health, primary care.
Study Options Full-time.
Program Entrance Requirements Clinical experience, minimum overall college GPA of 3.0, transcript of college record, CPR certification, written essay, immunizations, 2 letters of recommendation, nursing research course, physical assessment course, professional liability insurance/malpractice insurance, prerequisite course work, resume.
Advanced Placement Credit given for nursing courses completed elsewhere dependent upon specific evaluations.
Degree Requirements 40 total credit hours, thesis or project.

CONTINUING EDUCATION PROGRAM

Contact *Telephone:* 770-423-6064. *Fax:* 770-423-6627.

LaGrange College
Department of Nursing
LaGrange, Georgia

http://www.lagrange.edu/
Founded in 1831

DEGREE • BSN
Nursing Program Faculty 6 (20% with doctorates).
Baccalaureate Enrollment 65 **Women** 85% **Men** 15% **Minority** 20%
Nursing Student Activities Nursing Honor Society, Student Nurses' Association.
Nursing Student Resources Academic advising; academic or career counseling; assistance for students with disabilities; bookstore; campus computer network; career placement assistance; computer lab; computer-assisted instruction; e-mail services; employment services for current students; externships; interactive nursing skills videos; Internet; learning resource lab; library services; nursing audiovisuals; paid internships; placement services for program completers; remedial services; resume preparation assistance; skills, simulation, or other laboratory; tutoring; unpaid internships.
Library Facilities 116,300 volumes (19,000 in health, 10,000 in nursing); 374 periodical subscriptions (100 health-care related).

BACCALAUREATE PROGRAMS

Degree BSN
Available Programs Generic Baccalaureate; RN Baccalaureate.
Study Options Full-time.
Program Entrance Requirements Minimum overall college GPA of 2.5, transcript of college record, CPR certification, written essay, health exam, health insurance, immunizations, interview, 2 letters of recommendation, minimum GPA in nursing prerequisites of 2.5, professional liability insurance/malpractice insurance, prerequisite course work. Transfer students are accepted. *Application deadline:* 4/15 (fall).
Advanced Placement Credit given for nursing courses completed elsewhere dependent upon specific evaluations.
Expenses (2010-11) *Tuition:* full-time $29,000; part-time $912 per credit hour. *Room and board:* $4503; room only: $2631 per academic year. *Required fees:* full-time $375.
Financial Aid 95% of baccalaureate students in nursing programs received some form of financial aid in 2009-10. *Gift aid (need-based):* Federal Pell, FSEOG, state, private, college/university gift aid from institutional funds. *Loans:* Perkins, state. *Work-study:* Federal Work-Study, part-time campus jobs. *Financial aid application deadline (priority):* 3/1.
Contact Dr. Celia G. Hay, Chair, Department of Nursing, LaGrange College, 601 Broad Street, LaGrange, GA 30240-2999. *Telephone:* 706-880-8220. *Fdx:* 706-880-8029. *E-mail:* chay@lagrange.edu.

Macon State College
School of Nursing and Health Sciences
Macon, Georgia

http://www.maconstate.edu/nursing/nursing_introduction.aspx
Founded in 1968

DEGREE • BSN
Nursing Program Faculty 30 (7% with doctorates).
Baccalaureate Enrollment 104 **Women** 88% **Men** 12% **Minority** 21% **International** 2%
Nursing Student Activities Student Nurses' Association.
Nursing Student Resources Academic advising; academic or career counseling; assistance for students with disabilities; bookstore; campus computer network; career placement assistance; computer lab; computer-assisted instruction; e-mail services; interactive nursing skills videos; Internet; learning resource lab; library services; nursing audiovisuals; remedial services; resume preparation assistance; skills, simulation, or other laboratory; tutoring.
Library Facilities 80,000 volumes (4,000 in health, 920 in nursing); 513 periodical subscriptions (90 health-care related).

BACCALAUREATE PROGRAMS

Degree BSN
Available Programs ADN to Baccalaureate; Generic Baccalaureate.
Study Options Full-time and part-time.
Program Entrance Requirements Minimum overall college GPA of 2.0, transcript of college record, CPR certification, health exam, health insurance, immunizations, minimum GPA in nursing prerequisites of 2.5, professional liability insurance/malpractice insurance, prerequisite course work. Transfer students are accepted. *Application deadline:* 2/15 (fall).
Financial Aid 67% of baccalaureate students in nursing programs received some form of financial aid in 2009-10.
Contact Ms. Christine Elliot, Admissions Coordinator, School of Nursing and Health Sciences, Macon State College, 100 College Station Drive, Macon, GA 31206-5145.. *Telephone:* 478-471-2761. *Fax:* 478-471-2983. *E-mail:* christine.elliot@maconstate.edu.

North Georgia College & State University
Department of Nursing
Dahlonega, Georgia

http://www.ngcsu.edu
Founded in 1873

DEGREES • BSN • MS
Nursing Program Faculty 42 (17% with doctorates).
Baccalaureate Enrollment 70 **Women** 90% **Men** 10% **Minority** 12% **International** 4% **Part-time** 40%
Graduate Enrollment 50 **Women** 90% **Men** 10% **Minority** 10% **International** 2% **Part-time** 5%
Distance Learning Courses Available.
Nursing Student Activities Nursing Honor Society, Sigma Theta Tau, Student Nurses' Association.
Nursing Student Resources Academic advising; academic or career counseling; assistance for students with disabilities; bookstore; campus computer network; career placement assistance; computer lab; computer-assisted instruction; e-mail services; externships; interactive nursing skills videos; Internet; learning resource lab; library services; nursing audiovisuals; remedial services; resume preparation assistance; skills, simulation, or other laboratory; tutoring.
Library Facilities 173,074 volumes (6,875 in health, 619 in nursing); 4,633 periodical subscriptions (2,377 health-care related).

BACCALAUREATE PROGRAMS

Degree BSN
Available Programs ADN to Baccalaureate.
Study Options Full-time and part-time.
Online Degree Options Yes (online only).
Program Entrance Requirements Minimum overall college GPA of 2.75, transcript of college record, CPR certification, health exam, health insurance, high school biology, high school chemistry, high school foreign language, 3 years high school math, 2 years high school science, high school transcript, immunizations, 2 letters of recommendation, professional liability insurance/malpractice insurance, prerequisite course work, RN licensure. Transfer students are accepted. *Application deadline:* 2/1 (fall). *Application fee:* $25.
Financial Aid 75% of baccalaureate students in nursing programs received some form of financial aid in 2008-09.
Contact Mrs. Nancy Stahl, RN, Coordinator, BSN Program, Department of Nursing, North Georgia College & State University, 82 College Circle, Dahlonega, GA 30597. *Telephone:* 706-864-1937. *Fax:* 706-864-1845. *E-mail:* nstahl@ngcsu.edu.

GRADUATE PROGRAMS

Financial Aid 100% of graduate students in nursing programs received some form of financial aid in 2008-09.
Contact Dr. Grace Newsome, Coordinator, MS Program, Department of Nursing, North Georgia College & State University, 82 College Circle, Dahlonega, GA 30597. *Telephone:* 706-864-1489. *Fax:* 706-864-1845. *E-mail:* gnewsome@ngsu.edu.

MASTER'S DEGREE PROGRAM

Degree MS
Available Programs Master's.
Concentrations Available Nursing education. *Nurse practitioner programs in:* family health.
Study Options Full-time and part-time.
Program Entrance Requirements Clinical experience, computer literacy, minimum overall college GPA of 2.75, transcript of college record, CPR certification, written essay, immunizations, 3 letters of recommendation, nursing research course, physical assessment course, professional liability insurance/malpractice insurance, prerequisite course work. *Application deadline:* 2/28 (spring). *Application fee:* $25.
Degree Requirements 46 total credit hours, thesis or project, comprehensive exam.

POST-MASTER'S PROGRAM

Areas of Study Nursing education. *Nurse practitioner programs in:* family health.

Piedmont College

School of Nursing
Demorest, Georgia

http://www.piedmont.edu/schools/index.html#nursing
Founded in 1897

DEGREE • BSN
Nursing Program Faculty 8 (25% with doctorates).
Baccalaureate Enrollment 60 **Women** 99% **Men** 1% **Minority** 10% **International** 1% **Part-time** 20%
Distance Learning Courses Available.
Nursing Student Activities Nursing Honor Society, Student Nurses' Association.
Nursing Student Resources Academic advising; academic or career counseling; assistance for students with disabilities; bookstore; campus computer network; career placement assistance; computer lab; computer-assisted instruction; e-mail services; externships; housing assistance; interactive nursing skills videos; Internet; learning resource lab; library services; nursing audiovisuals; other; paid internships; resume preparation assistance; skills, simulation, or other laboratory; tutoring.
Library Facilities 115,400 volumes (3,000 in health, 500 in nursing); 365 periodical subscriptions (75 health-care related).

BACCALAUREATE PROGRAMS

Degree BSN
Available Programs Generic Baccalaureate; LPN to Baccalaureate; RN Baccalaureate.
Study Options Full-time.
Program Entrance Requirements Transcript of college record, CPR certification, health exam, health insurance, high school foreign language, 2 years high school math, 3 years high school science, high school transcript, immunizations, minimum GPA in nursing prerequisites of 3.0, professional liability insurance/malpractice insurance, prerequisite course work. Transfer students are accepted. *Application deadline:* 10/15 (fall).
Advanced Placement Credit given for nursing courses completed elsewhere dependent upon specific evaluations.
Expenses (2009-10) *Tuition:* full-time $18,000; part-time $9000 per semester. *International tuition:* $18,000 full-time. *Room and board:* $6000 per academic year.
Financial Aid 50% of baccalaureate students in nursing programs received some form of financial aid in 2008-09. *Gift aid (need-based):* Federal Pell, FSEOG, state, private, college/university gift aid from institutional funds. *Loans:* Federal Direct (Subsidized and Unsubsidized Stafford PLUS). *Work-study:* Federal Work-Study, part-time campus jobs. *Financial aid application deadline (priority):* 3/1.
Contact Dr. Linda Scott, Dean, School of Nursing, Piedmont College, 165 Central Avenue, Demorest, GA 30535. *Telephone:* 706-776-0116. *Fax:* 706-778-0701. *E-mail:* lscott@piedmont.edu.

Thomas University

Division of Nursing
Thomasville, Georgia

http://www.thomasu.edu/nursing.htm
Founded in 1950

DEGREES • BSN • MSN • MSN/MBA
Nursing Program Faculty 12 (40% with doctorates).
Baccalaureate Enrollment 85 **Women** 85% **Men** 15% **Minority** 30%
Graduate Enrollment 35 **Women** 90% **Men** 10% **Minority** 30% **Part-time** 40%
Distance Learning Courses Available.
Nursing Student Activities Nursing Honor Society, Sigma Theta Tau.
Nursing Student Resources Academic advising; academic or career counseling; assistance for students with disabilities; bookstore; campus computer network; career placement assistance; computer lab; computer-assisted instruction; e-mail services; housing assistance; interactive nursing skills videos; Internet; learning resource lab; library services; nursing audiovisuals; remedial services; resume preparation assistance; skills, simulation, or other laboratory; tutoring.
Library Facilities 41,467 volumes (1,200 in health, 400 in nursing); 451 periodical subscriptions (150 health-care related).

BACCALAUREATE PROGRAMS

Degree BSN
Available Programs ADN to Baccalaureate; Accelerated RN Baccalaureate; RN Baccalaureate.
Site Options Tallahassee, FL; Moultrie, GA.
Study Options Full-time and part-time.
Program Entrance Requirements Minimum overall college GPA of 2.5, transcript of college record, CPR certification, health exam, health insurance, immunizations, minimum GPA in nursing prerequisites of 2.5, professional liability insurance/malpractice insurance, prerequisite course work, RN licensure. Transfer students are accepted. *Application deadline:* 8/1 (fall), 12/1 (spring), 4/15 (summer). Applications may be processed on a rolling basis for some programs. *Application fee:* $35.
Advanced Placement Credit by examination available. Credit given for nursing courses completed elsewhere dependent upon specific evaluations.
Financial Aid 90% of baccalaureate students in nursing programs received some form of financial aid in 2009-10. *Gift aid (need-based):* Federal Pell, FSEOG, state, private, college/university gift aid from institutional funds. *Loans:* state, alternative loans. *Work-study:* Federal Work-Study. *Financial aid application deadline:* Continuous.
Contact Deryl Ouzts, Associate Director of Enrollment Management, Division of Nursing, Thomas University, 1501 Millpond Road, Thomasville, GA 31792. *Telephone:* 229-227-6884. *Fax:* 229-226-1653. *E-mail:* douzts@thomasu.edu.

GRADUATE PROGRAMS

Financial Aid 50% of graduate students in nursing programs received some form of financial aid in 2009-10.
Contact Deryl Ouzts, Associate Director of Enrollment Management, Division of Nursing, Thomas University, 1501 Millpond Road, Thomasville, GA 31792. *Telephone:* 229-227-6884. *Fax:* 229-226-1653. *E-mail:* douzts@thomasu.edu.

MASTER'S DEGREE PROGRAM

Degrees MSN; MSN/MBA
Available Programs Accelerated Master's; Master's; Master's for Nurses with Non-Nursing Degrees.
Concentrations Available Health-care administration; nursing administration; nursing education.
Study Options Full-time and part-time.
Program Entrance Requirements Computer literacy, minimum overall college GPA of 3.0, transcript of college record, CPR certification, written essay, immunizations, 3 letters of recommendation, professional liability insurance/malpractice insurance, resume, statistics course. *Application deadline:* 8/1 (fall), 12/1 (spring), 4/15 (summer). Applications may be processed on a rolling basis for some programs. *Application fee:* $50.
Advanced Placement Credit given for nursing courses completed elsewhere dependent upon specific evaluations.
Degree Requirements 36 total credit hours, thesis or project.

POST-MASTER'S PROGRAM

Areas of Study Health-care administration; nursing administration; nursing education.

University of Phoenix–Atlanta Campus

College of Health and Human Services
Sandy Springs, Georgia

Nursing Student Activities Sigma Theta Tau.
Nursing Student Resources Academic advising; academic or career counseling; assistance for students with disabilities; bookstore; campus computer network; computer lab; computer-assisted instruction; e-mail services; interactive nursing skills videos; Internet; learning resource lab; library services; nursing audiovisuals; remedial services; skills, simulation, or other laboratory; tutoring.
Library Facilities 16,781 periodical subscriptions (1,300 health-care related).

University of West Georgia

School of Nursing
Carrollton, Georgia

http://www.westga.edu/~nurs/
Founded in 1933

DEGREES • BSN • MSN
Nursing Program Faculty 31 (32% with doctorates).
Baccalaureate Enrollment 394 **Women** 87.5% **Men** 12.5% **Minority** 35% **International** 2% **Part-time** 69.5%
Graduate Enrollment 17 **Women** 100% **Minority** 12% **Part-time** 18%
Distance Learning Courses Available.
Nursing Student Activities Sigma Theta Tau, Student Nurses' Association.
Nursing Student Resources Academic advising; academic or career counseling; assistance for students with disabilities; bookstore; campus computer network; career placement assistance; computer lab; computer-assisted instruction; e-mail services; employment services for current students; externships; housing assistance; interactive nursing skills videos; Internet; learning resource lab; library services; nursing audiovisuals; remedial services; resume preparation assistance; skills, simulation, or other laboratory; tutoring.
Library Facilities 541,488 volumes (1,795 in health, 1,308 in nursing); 17,000 periodical subscriptions (81 health-care related).

BACCALAUREATE PROGRAMS

Degree BSN
Available Programs Generic Baccalaureate; RN Baccalaureate.
Site Options Dalton, GA; Newnan, GA; Rome, GA.
Study Options Full-time and part-time.
Program Entrance Requirements Minimum overall college GPA of 2.75, transcript of college record, CPR certification, health exam, health insurance, immunizations, minimum GPA in nursing prerequisites of 2.75, professional liability insurance/malpractice insurance, prerequisite course work. Transfer students are accepted. *Application deadline:* 1/15 (spring).
Advanced Placement Credit given for nursing courses completed elsewhere dependent upon specific evaluations.
Expenses (2010-11) *Tuition, state resident:* full-time $4558; part-time $154 per credit hour. *Tuition, nonresident:* full-time $16,796; part-time $533 per credit hour. *Room and board:* $7003; room only: $4560 per academic year. *Required fees:* full-time $2768; part-time $772 per credit.
Financial Aid 77% of baccalaureate students in nursing programs received some form of financial aid in 2009-10. *Gift aid (need-based):* Federal Pell, FSEOG, state, private, college/university gift aid from institutional funds, United Negro College Fund. *Loans:* Federal Direct (Subsidized and Unsubsidized Stafford PLUS), Perkins, state, college/university. *Work-study:* Federal Work-Study, part-time campus jobs. *Financial aid application deadline:* 7/1(priority: 4/1).
Contact Dr. Cynthia D. Epps, Associate Dean and Undergraduate Program Coordinator, School of Nursing, University of West Georgia, 1601 Maple Street, Carrollton, GA 30118. *Telephone:* 678-839-6552. *Fax:* 678-839-6553. *E-mail:* cepps@westga.edu.

GRADUATE PROGRAMS

Expenses (2010-11) *Tuition, state resident:* full-time $3460; part-time $173 per credit hour. *Tuition, nonresident:* full-time $13,780; part-time $689 per credit hour. *Room and board:* $5344; room only: $3700 per academic year. *Required fees:* full-time $1646; part-time $410 per credit.
Financial Aid 52% of graduate students in nursing programs received some form of financial aid in 2009-10.
Contact Dr. Laurie Jowers Ware, Assistant Dean and Director of Graduate Program, School of Nursing, University of West Georgia, 1601 Maple Street, Carrollton, GA 30118. *Telephone:* 678-839-6552. *Fax:* 678-839-6553. *E-mail:* lware@westga.edu.

MASTER'S DEGREE PROGRAM

Degree MSN
Available Programs Master's.
Concentrations Available Clinical nurse leader; nursing administration; nursing education.
Study Options Full-time and part-time.
Program Entrance Requirements Clinical experience, computer literacy, minimum overall college GPA of 3.0, transcript of college record, CPR certification, immunizations, 3 letters of recommendation, nursing research course, professional liability insurance/malpractice insurance, prerequisite course work, resume, statistics course. *Application deadline:* 7/1 (summer).
Degree Requirements 36 total credit hours, thesis or project, comprehensive exam.

POST-MASTER'S PROGRAM

Areas of Study Clinical nurse leader; nursing administration; nursing education.

Valdosta State University

College of Nursing
Valdosta, Georgia

http://www.valdosta.edu/nursing/
Founded in 1906

DEGREES • BSN • MSN
Nursing Program Faculty 23 (52% with doctorates).
Baccalaureate Enrollment 183 **Women** 87% **Men** 13% **Minority** 21% **International** 1% **Part-time** 7%
Graduate Enrollment 25 **Women** 99% **Men** 1% **Minority** 15% **International** 1% **Part-time** 49%
Nursing Student Activities Sigma Theta Tau, Student Nurses' Association.
Nursing Student Resources Academic advising; academic or career counseling; assistance for students with disabilities; bookstore; campus computer network; career placement assistance; computer lab; computer-assisted instruction; e-mail services; employment services for current students; externships; housing assistance; Internet; learning resource lab; library services; nursing audiovisuals; placement services for program completers; resume preparation assistance; skills, simulation, or other laboratory; tutoring; unpaid internships.
Library Facilities 636,608 volumes (21,688 in health); 2,732 periodical subscriptions (75 health-care related).

BACCALAUREATE PROGRAMS

Degree BSN
Available Programs Generic Baccalaureate; RN Baccalaureate.
Study Options Full-time.
Program Entrance Requirements Minimum overall college GPA of 2.8, transcript of college record, CPR certification, health exam, health insurance, immunizations, minimum GPA in nursing prerequisites of 2.8, professional liability insurance/malpractice insurance, prerequisite course work. Transfer students are accepted.
Advanced Placement Credit given for nursing courses completed elsewhere dependent upon specific evaluations.
Contact *Telephone:* 229-333-5959. *Fax:* 229-333-7300.

GRADUATE PROGRAMS

Contact *Telephone:* 229-333-5959. *Fax:* 229-333-7300.

MASTER'S DEGREE PROGRAM

Degree MSN
Available Programs Master's; RN to Master's.

Concentrations Available Nurse case management; nursing administration; nursing education. *Clinical nurse specialist programs in:* adult health, family health, psychiatric/mental health.
Study Options Full-time and part-time.
Program Entrance Requirements Minimum overall college GPA of 2.8, transcript of college record, CPR certification, immunizations, 3 letters of recommendation, physical assessment course, professional liability insurance/malpractice insurance, statistics course, GRE General Test.
Advanced Placement Credit given for nursing courses completed elsewhere dependent upon specific evaluations.
Degree Requirements 36 total credit hours, thesis or project, comprehensive exam.

CONTINUING EDUCATION PROGRAM

Contact *Telephone:* 229-333-5960.

GUAM

University of Guam
School of Nursing and Health Sciences
Mangilao, Guam

http://www.uog.edu/cnhs/index.html
Founded in 1952

DEGREE • BSN
Nursing Program Faculty 10 (30% with doctorates).
Baccalaureate Enrollment 175 **Women** 97% **Men** 3% **International** 2%
Nursing Student Activities Student Nurses' Association.
Nursing Student Resources Academic advising; academic or career counseling; assistance for students with disabilities; bookstore; campus computer network; career placement assistance; computer lab; daycare for children of students; e-mail services; employment services for current students; interactive nursing skills videos; Internet; learning resource lab; library services; nursing audiovisuals; remedial services; skills, simulation, or other laboratory; tutoring.
Library Facilities 309,528 volumes (5,246 in health, 982 in nursing); 28,845 periodical subscriptions (53 health-care related).

BACCALAUREATE PROGRAMS

Degree BSN
Available Programs ADN to Baccalaureate; Generic Baccalaureate; RN Baccalaureate.
Study Options Full-time and part-time.
Program Entrance Requirements Transcript of college record, CPR certification, written essay, health exam, high school biology, high school chemistry, 1 year of high school math, 1 year of high school science, high school transcript, immunizations, interview, minimum high school GPA of 2.5, minimum GPA in nursing prerequisites of 2.7, prerequisite course work. Transfer students are accepted.
Advanced Placement Credit by examination available. Credit given for nursing courses completed elsewhere dependent upon specific evaluations.
Contact *Telephone:* 671-735-2210. *Fax:* 671-734-4245.

HAWAII

Hawai`i Pacific University
College of Nursing and Health Sciences
Honolulu, Hawaii

http://www.hpu.edu/
Founded in 1965

DEGREES • BSN • MSN • MSN/MBA
Nursing Program Faculty 100 (16% with doctorates).
Baccalaureate Enrollment 1,388 **Women** 84% **Men** 16% **Minority** 73% **International** 2% **Part-time** 32%
Graduate Enrollment 56 **Women** 84% **Men** 16% **Minority** 36% **International** 20% **Part-time** 27%

Distance Learning Courses Available.
Nursing Student Activities Nursing Honor Society, Sigma Theta Tau, Student Nurses' Association.
Nursing Student Resources Academic advising; academic or career counseling; assistance for students with disabilities; bookstore; campus computer network; career placement assistance; computer lab; computer-assisted instruction; e-mail services; employment services for current students; externships; housing assistance; Internet; learning resource lab; library services; paid internships; placement services for program completers; resume preparation assistance; skills, simulation, or other laboratory; tutoring.
Library Facilities 160,800 volumes (4,825 in health, 1,170 in nursing); 38,050 periodical subscriptions (7,954 health-care related).

BACCALAUREATE PROGRAMS

Degree BSN
Available Programs Generic Baccalaureate; International Nurse to Baccalaureate; LPN to Baccalaureate; RN Baccalaureate.
Site Options Kailua, Kaneohe, Honolulu, HI; Aiea, Kahuku, Wahiawa, HI.
Study Options Full-time and part-time.
Program Entrance Requirements Minimum overall college GPA of 2.75, transcript of college record, CPR certification, health exam, health insurance, immunizations, minimum GPA in nursing prerequisites of 2.75, prerequisite course work. Transfer students are accepted. *Application deadline:* Applications may be processed on a rolling basis for some programs. *Application fee:* $50.
Advanced Placement Credit given for nursing courses completed elsewhere dependent upon specific evaluations.
Expenses (2010-11) *Tuition:* full-time $22,920; part-time $955 per credit. *Room and board:* $11,648 per academic year. *Required fees:* full-time $100.
Financial Aid 81% of baccalaureate students in nursing programs received some form of financial aid in 2009-10. *Gift aid (need-based):* Federal Pell, FSEOG, state, private, college/university gift aid from institutional funds, Federal Nursing. *Loans:* Federal Nursing Student Loans, Perkins. *Work-study:* Federal Work-Study. *Financial aid application deadline (priority):* 3/1.
Contact Miss Sara Sato, Director of Admissions, College of Nursing and Health Sciences, Hawai`i Pacific University, 1164 Bishop Street, Honolulu, HI 96813. *Telephone:* 808-544-0238. *Fax:* 808-544-1136. *E-mail:* ssato@hpu.edu.

GRADUATE PROGRAMS

Expenses (2010-11) *Tuition:* full-time $12,600; part-time $700 per credit. *Required fees:* full-time $100.
Financial Aid 52% of graduate students in nursing programs received some form of financial aid in 2009-10. Career-related internships or fieldwork, Federal Work-Study, scholarships, and traineeships available. Aid available to part-time students. *Financial aid application deadline:* 3/1.
Contact Dr. Patricia Burrell, Chair, Department of Graduate and Post-Baccalaureate Nursing Programs, College of Nursing and Health Sciences, Hawai`i Pacific University, 45-045 Kamehameha Highway, Kaneohe, HI 96744-5297. *Telephone:* 808-236-5813. *Fax:* 808-236-3524. *E-mail:* pburrell@hpu.edu.

MASTER'S DEGREE PROGRAM

Degrees MSN; MSN/MBA
Available Programs Master's; RN to Master's.
Concentrations Available Nursing education. *Clinical nurse specialist programs in:* community health. *Nurse practitioner programs in:* family health.
Study Options Full-time and part-time.
Program Entrance Requirements Clinical experience, minimum overall college GPA of 3.0, transcript of college record, written essay, 2 letters of recommendation, nursing research course, prerequisite course work, statistics course. *Application deadline:* Applications may be processed on a rolling basis for some programs. *Application fee:* $50.
Advanced Placement Credit given for nursing courses completed elsewhere dependent upon specific evaluations.
Degree Requirements 48 total credit hours, thesis or project.

POST-MASTER'S PROGRAM

Areas of Study Nursing education. *Nurse practitioner programs in:* family health.

See full description on page 476

University of Hawaii at Hilo

Department in Nursing
Hilo, Hawaii

http://www.uhh.hawaii.edu/
Founded in 1970

DEGREE • BSN
Nursing Program Faculty 11 (36% with doctorates).
Baccalaureate Enrollment 77 **Women** 77% **Men** 23% **Minority** 74% **Part-time** 17%
Distance Learning Courses Available.
Nursing Student Activities Nursing Honor Society, Sigma Theta Tau, Student Nurses' Association.
Nursing Student Resources Academic advising; academic or career counseling; assistance for students with disabilities; bookstore; campus computer network; career placement assistance; computer lab; computer-assisted instruction; e-mail services; employment services for current students; externships; housing assistance; interactive nursing skills videos; Internet; learning resource lab; library services; nursing audiovisuals; paid internships; remedial services; resume preparation assistance; skills, simulation, or other laboratory; tutoring.
Library Facilities 250,000 volumes (680 in health, 284 in nursing); 2,500 periodical subscriptions (15,000 health-care related).

BACCALAUREATE PROGRAMS

Degree BSN
Available Programs ADN to Baccalaureate; Generic Baccalaureate; RN Baccalaureate.
Site Options Kahalui, HI; Kona, HI; Lihue, HI.
Study Options Full-time.
Program Entrance Requirements Minimum overall college GPA of 2.7, transcript of college record, CPR certification, written essay, health exam, health insurance, high school biology, high school chemistry, high school foreign language, 1 year of high school math, 3 years high school science, high school transcript, immunizations, 2 letters of recommendation, minimum high school GPA of 3.0, minimum GPA in nursing prerequisites of 2.7, professional liability insurance/malpractice insurance, prerequisite course work. *Application deadline:* 1/15 (fall).
Expenses (2010-11) *Tuition, state resident:* full-time $6112; part-time $213 per credit hour. *Tuition, nonresident:* full-time $16,600; part-time $650 per credit hour. *Room and board:* $7736; room only: $3916 per academic year. *Required fees:* full-time $1152; part-time $652 per term.
Financial Aid 88% of baccalaureate students in nursing programs received some form of financial aid in 2009-10. *Gift aid (need-based):* Federal Pell, FSEOG, state, private, college/university gift aid from institutional funds. *Loans:* Federal Direct (Subsidized and Unsubsidized Stafford PLUS), Perkins, state. *Work-study:* Federal Work-Study, part-time campus jobs. *Financial aid application deadline (priority):* 3/1.
Contact Dr. Katharyn Daub, Chair and Program Director, Department in Nursing, University of Hawaii at Hilo, 200 West Kawili Street, UCB 235, Hilo, HI 96720. *Telephone:* 808-974-7760. *Fax:* 808-974-7665. *E-mail:* katharyn@hawaii.edu.

University of Hawaii at Manoa

School of Nursing and Dental Hygiene
Honolulu, Hawaii

http://www.nursing.hawaii.edu
Founded in 1907

DEGREES • BSN • MS • MSN/MBA • PHD
Nursing Program Faculty 97 (35% with doctorates).
Baccalaureate Enrollment 336 **Women** 77% **Men** 23% **Minority** 83% **International** 3% **Part-time** 56%
Graduate Enrollment 170 **Women** 88% **Men** 12% **Minority** 60% **International** 2% **Part-time** 66%
Distance Learning Courses Available.
Nursing Student Activities Nursing Honor Society, Sigma Theta Tau, Student Nurses' Association, nursing club.
Nursing Student Resources Academic advising; academic or career counseling; assistance for students with disabilities; bookstore; computer lab; computer-assisted instruction; e-mail services; employment services for current students; housing assistance; Internet; learning resource lab; library services; nursing audiovisuals; resume preparation assistance; skills, simulation, or other laboratory.

Library Facilities 3.4 million volumes; 51,928 periodical subscriptions.

BACCALAUREATE PROGRAMS

Degree BSN
Available Programs ADN to Baccalaureate; Generic Baccalaureate; RN Baccalaureate.
Study Options Full-time and part-time.
Program Entrance Requirements Minimum overall college GPA of 2.5, transcript of college record, CPR certification, health exam, health insurance, immunizations, minimum GPA in nursing prerequisites of 2.5, prerequisite course work. Transfer students are accepted. *Application deadline:* 3/1 (fall), 10/1 (spring). *Application fee:* $50.
Advanced Placement Credit by examination available. Credit given for nursing courses completed elsewhere dependent upon specific evaluations.
Contact ***Telephone:*** 808-956-8939. *Fax:* 808-956-5977.

GRADUATE PROGRAMS

Contact ***Telephone:*** 808-956-3519. *Fax:* 808-956-5977.

MASTER'S DEGREE PROGRAM

Degrees MS; MSN/MBA
Available Programs Accelerated Master's; Master's; Master's for Non-Nursing College Graduates; RN to Master's.
Concentrations Available Nursing administration; nursing education. *Clinical nurse specialist programs in:* psychiatric/mental health. *Nurse practitioner programs in:* adult health, community health, family health, gerontology, pediatric.
Site Options Kahului, HI; Lihue, HI; Kailua Kona, HI.
Study Options Full-time and part-time.
Online Degree Options Yes.
Program Entrance Requirements Minimum overall college GPA of 3.0, transcript of college record, CPR certification, written essay, immunizations, interview, 2 letters of recommendation, resume, statistics course. *Application deadline:* 3/1 (fall). *Application fee:* $60.
Advanced Placement Credit given for nursing courses completed elsewhere dependent upon specific evaluations.
Degree Requirements 52 total credit hours.

POST-MASTER'S PROGRAM

Areas of Study Nursing administration; nursing education. *Clinical nurse specialist programs in:* psychiatric/mental health. *Nurse practitioner programs in:* adult health, community health, family health, gerontology, pediatric.

DOCTORAL DEGREE PROGRAM

Degree PhD
Available Programs Doctorate.
Areas of Study Faculty preparation, nursing education, nursing research, nursing science.
Site Options Kahului, HI; Lihue, HI; Kailua Kona, HI.
Online Degree Options Yes (online only).
Program Entrance Requirements Clinical experience, minimum overall college GPA of 3.0, interview by faculty committee, interview, 3 letters of recommendation, MSN or equivalent, scholarly papers, statistics course, vita, writing sample. Application deadline: 2/1 (fall).
Degree Requirements 46 total credit hours, dissertation, oral exam, residency.

University of Phoenix–Hawaii Campus

College of Nursing
Honolulu, Hawaii

DEGREES • BSN • MSN • MSN/ED D

Nursing Program Faculty 26 (15% with doctorates).
Baccalaureate Enrollment 70 **Women** 90% **Men** 10% **Minority** 40%
Graduate Enrollment 14 **Women** 71.4% **Men** 28.6% **Minority** 57.14%
Nursing Student Activities Sigma Theta Tau.
Nursing Student Resources Academic advising; academic or career counseling; assistance for students with disabilities; bookstore; campus computer network; computer lab; computer-assisted instruction; e-mail services; interactive nursing skills videos; Internet; learning resource lab; library services; nursing audiovisuals; remedial services; skills, simulation, or other laboratory; tutoring.
Library Facilities 16,781 periodical subscriptions (1,300 health-care related).

BACCALAUREATE PROGRAMS

Degree BSN
Available Programs Accelerated Baccalaureate; LPN to Baccalaureate.
Site Options Kaneohe, HI; Mililani, HI; Kapolei, HI.
Study Options Full-time.
Program Entrance Requirements Transcript of college record, CPR certification, immunizations, 1 letter of recommendation, RN licensure. Transfer students are accepted. *Application deadline:* Applications may be processed on a rolling basis for some programs.
Advanced Placement Credit by examination available. Credit given for nursing courses completed elsewhere dependent upon specific evaluations.
Expenses (2009-10) *Tuition:* full-time $10,560. *Required fees:* full-time $600.
Contact Campus College Chair, Nursing, College of Nursing, University of Phoenix–Hawaii Campus, 827 Fort Street, Hololulu, HI 96813-4317. *Telephone:* 808-536-2686.

GRADUATE PROGRAMS

Expenses (2009-10) *Tuition:* full-time $13,200. *Required fees:* full-time $760.
Financial Aid Institutionally sponsored loans and scholarships available.
Contact Campus College Chair, Nursing, College of Nursing, University of Phoenix–Hawaii Campus, 827 Fort Street, Hololulu, HI 96813-4317. *Telephone:* 808-536-2686.

MASTER'S DEGREE PROGRAM

Degrees MSN; MSN/Ed D
Available Programs Master's.
Concentrations Available Health-care administration; nursing administration; nursing education. *Nurse practitioner programs in:* family health.
Site Options Kaneohe, HI; Mililani, HI; Kapolei, HI.
Study Options Full-time.
Program Entrance Requirements Clinical experience, computer literacy, minimum overall college GPA of 2.5, transcript of college record. *Application deadline:* Applications may be processed on a rolling basis for some programs. *Application fee:* $45.
Advanced Placement Credit given for nursing courses completed elsewhere dependent upon specific evaluations.
Degree Requirements 39 total credit hours, thesis or project.

IDAHO

Boise State University

Department of Nursing
Boise, Idaho

http://nursing.boisestate.edu/
Founded in 1932

DEGREES • BS • MSN • MSN/MS

Nursing Program Faculty 55 (25% with doctorates).
Baccalaureate Enrollment 540 **Women** 75% **Men** 25% **Minority** 1% **International** 1%
Graduate Enrollment 12
Distance Learning Courses Available.
Nursing Student Activities Nursing Honor Society, Sigma Theta Tau, Student Nurses' Association.
Nursing Student Resources Academic advising; academic or career counseling; assistance for students with disabilities; bookstore; campus computer network; career placement assistance; computer lab; computer-assisted instruction; daycare for children of students; e-mail services; employment services for current students; housing assistance; interactive nursing skills videos; Internet; learning resource lab; library services; nursing audiovisuals; placement services for program completers; remedial services; resume preparation assistance; skills, simulation, or other laboratory; tutoring.
Library Facilities 838,932 volumes (27,919 in health, 2,617 in nursing); 5,575 periodical subscriptions (158 health-care related).

BACCALAUREATE PROGRAMS

Degree BS
Available Programs Accelerated RN Baccalaureate; Generic Baccalaureate; LPN to Baccalaureate; RN Baccalaureate.
Site Options Nampa, ID.
Study Options Full-time.
Online Degree Options Yes.
Program Entrance Requirements Transcript of college record, immunizations, minimum GPA in nursing prerequisites of 3.0, professional liability insurance/malpractice insurance, prerequisite course work. Transfer students are accepted. *Application deadline:* 3/1 (fall), 10/1 (spring). *Application fee:* $20.
Advanced Placement Credit by examination available. Credit given for nursing courses completed elsewhere dependent upon specific evaluations.
Contact ***Telephone:*** 208-426-4143. *Fax:* 208-426-1370.

GRADUATE PROGRAMS

Contact ***Telephone:*** 208-426-4143.

MASTER'S DEGREE PROGRAM

Degrees MSN; MSN/MS
Available Programs Master's.
Concentrations Available Clinical nurse leader; health-care administration; nurse case management; nursing administration; nursing education.
Study Options Part-time.
Program Entrance Requirements Minimum overall college GPA of 3.0, transcript of college record, CPR certification, written essay, letters of recommendation, nursing research course, professional liability insurance/malpractice insurance, prerequisite course work, resume, statistics course. *Application deadline:* 3/31 (spring).
Degree Requirements 39 total credit hours, thesis or project.

Brigham Young University–Idaho

Department of Nursing
Rexburg, Idaho

Founded in 1888

DEGREE • BSN

BACCALAUREATE PROGRAMS

Degree BSN
Available Programs RN Baccalaureate.
Program Entrance Requirements RN licensure. Transfer students are accepted. *Application deadline:* 6/1 (fall), 10/1 (winter), 2/1 (spring).
Expenses (2010-11) *Tuition:* part-time $280 per credit. *Required fees:* part-time $42 per term.
Contact Susan Dicus, Department Chair. *Telephone:* 208-496-4555. *Fax:* 208-496-4553. *E-mail:* dicuss@byui.edu.

Idaho State University

Department of Nursing
Pocatello, Idaho

Founded in 1901

DEGREES • BSN • MS

Nursing Program Faculty 22 (36% with doctorates).
Baccalaureate Enrollment 195 **Women** 76% **Men** 24% **Minority** 14%
Graduate Enrollment 124 **Women** 85% **Men** 15% **Minority** 6% **Part-time** 58%
Distance Learning Courses Available.
Nursing Student Activities Sigma Theta Tau, Student Nurses' Association.
Nursing Student Resources Academic advising; academic or career counseling; assistance for students with disabilities; bookstore; campus computer network; computer lab; computer-assisted instruction; daycare for children of students; e-mail services; employment services for current students; housing assistance; interactive nursing skills videos; Internet; learning resource lab; library services; nursing audiovisuals; resume preparation assistance; skills, simulation, or other laboratory; tutoring.
Library Facilities 2.2 million volumes (35,948 in health, 1,775 in nursing); 5,124 periodical subscriptions (5,312 health-care related).

BACCALAUREATE PROGRAMS

Degree BSN
Available Programs ADN to Baccalaureate; Accelerated Baccalaureate for Second Degree; Generic Baccalaureate; LPN to Baccalaureate.
Site Options Boise, ID; Idaho Falls, ID; Twin Falls, ID.
Study Options Full-time.
Program Entrance Requirements Minimum overall college GPA, transcript of college record, CPR certification, written essay, health exam, health insurance, high school transcript, immunizations, 3 letters of recommendation, minimum high school GPA of 2.0, minimum GPA in nursing prerequisites of 3.0, professional liability insurance/malpractice insurance, prerequisite course work. Transfer students are accepted. *Application deadline:* 9/15 (spring). *Application fee:* $50.
Advanced Placement Credit given for nursing courses completed elsewhere dependent upon specific evaluations.
Expenses (2009-10) *Tuition, state resident:* full-time $4968; part-time $253 per credit. *Tuition, nonresident:* full-time $7385; part-time $393 per credit. *International tuition:* $14,770 full-time. *Room and board:* $4293; room only: $2943 per academic year. *Required fees:* full-time $1200; part-time $600 per term.
Contact Dr. Carol A. Ashton, Associate Dean and Director, School of Nursing, Department of Nursing, Idaho State University, 921 South 8th Avenue, Stop 8101, Pocatello, ID 83209-8101. *Telephone:* 208-282-2443. *Fax:* 208-236-4476. *E-mail:* ashtcaro@isu.edu.

GRADUATE PROGRAMS

Expenses (2009-10) *Tuition, state resident:* full-time $5848; part-time $297 per credit. *Tuition, nonresident:* full-time $7825; part-time $437 per credit. *International tuition:* $15,650 full-time. *Room and board:* $4075; room only: $3375 per academic year. *Required fees:* full-time $1540; part-time $770 per term.
Financial Aid 1 research assistantship (averaging $9,401 per year), 4 teaching assistantships (averaging $10,841 per year) were awarded; career-related internships or fieldwork, Federal Work-Study, institutionally sponsored loans, scholarships, tuition waivers (full and partial), and unspecified assistantships also available.
Contact Dr. Carol A. Ashton, Associate Dean and Director, School of Nursing, Department of Nursing, Idaho State University, 921 South 8th Avenue, Stop 8101, Pocatello, ID 83209-8101. *Telephone:* 208-282-2443. *Fax:* 208-282-4476. *E-mail:* ashtcaro@isu.edu.

MASTER'S DEGREE PROGRAM

Degree MS
Available Programs Accelerated AD/RN to Master's; Master's.
Concentrations Available Clinical nurse leader; nursing administration; nursing education. *Clinical nurse specialist programs in:* adult health. *Nurse practitioner programs in:* family health.
Study Options Full-time and part-time.
Online Degree Options Yes (online only).
Program Entrance Requirements Minimum overall college GPA of 3.0, transcript of college record, CPR certification, immunizations, interview, 3 letters of recommendation, professional liability insurance/malpractice insurance, prerequisite course work, statistics course, GRE General Test. *Application deadline:* 2/2 (fall). *Application fee:* $50.
Advanced Placement Credit given for nursing courses completed elsewhere dependent upon specific evaluations.
Degree Requirements 46 total credit hours, comprehensive exam.

POST-MASTER'S PROGRAM

Areas of Study Nursing administration; nursing education. *Clinical nurse specialist programs in:* adult health. *Nurse practitioner programs in:* family health.

Lewis-Clark State College

Division of Nursing and Health Sciences
Lewiston, Idaho

http://www.lcsc.edu/Nurdiv/
Founded in 1893

DEGREE • BSN

Nursing Program Faculty 22 (23% with doctorates).
Baccalaureate Enrollment 155 **Women** 85% **Men** 15% **Minority** 10% **International** 5% **Part-time** 20%
Distance Learning Courses Available.
Nursing Student Activities Student Nurses' Association.

Nursing Student Resources Academic advising; academic or career counseling; assistance for students with disabilities; bookstore; campus computer network; career placement assistance; computer lab; computer-assisted instruction; daycare for children of students; e-mail services; housing assistance; interactive nursing skills videos; Internet; learning resource lab; library services; nursing audiovisuals; remedial services; resume preparation assistance; skills, simulation, or other laboratory; tutoring; unpaid internships.
Library Facilities 19,920 volumes in health, 5,101 volumes in nursing; 12,058 periodical subscriptions health-care related.

BACCALAUREATE PROGRAMS

Degree BSN
Available Programs ADN to Baccalaureate; Generic Baccalaureate; LPN to Baccalaureate.
Site Options Coeur d'Alene, ID.
Study Options Full-time.
Program Entrance Requirements Minimum overall college GPA of 2.5, transcript of college record, CPR certification, health insurance, immunizations, minimum GPA in nursing prerequisites of 2.5, prerequisite course work. Transfer students are accepted. *Application deadline:* 1/15 (fall), 9/15 (spring). *Application fee:* $35.
Advanced Placement Credit given for nursing courses completed elsewhere dependent upon specific evaluations.
Expenses (2010-11) *Tuition, state resident:* full-time $4998; part-time $255 per credit. *Tuition, nonresident:* full-time $13,906. *Room and board:* $6400; room only: $3600 per academic year. *Required fees:* full-time $400.
Financial Aid 80% of baccalaureate students in nursing programs received some form of financial aid in 2009-10.
Contact Advising Center, Division of Nursing and Health Sciences, Lewis-Clark State College, 500 8th Avenue, Lewiston, ID 83501. *Telephone:* 208-792-2688. *Fax:* 208-792-2062. *E-mail:* nhs@lcsc.edu.

Northwest Nazarene University
School of Health and Science
Nampa, Idaho

http://www.nnu.edu/
Founded in 1913

DEGREES • BSN • MSN
Nursing Program Faculty 26 (27% with doctorates).
Baccalaureate Enrollment 98 **Women** 92% **Men** 8% **Minority** 12% **International** 3% **Part-time** 1%
Graduate Enrollment 17 **Women** 100%
Distance Learning Courses Available.
Nursing Student Activities Student Nurses' Association.
Nursing Student Resources Academic advising; academic or career counseling; assistance for students with disabilities; bookstore; campus computer network; career placement assistance; computer lab; computer-assisted instruction; e-mail services; housing assistance; interactive nursing skills videos; Internet; learning resource lab; library services; nursing audiovisuals; remedial services; resume preparation assistance; skills, simulation, or other laboratory; tutoring; unpaid internships.
Library Facilities 127,036 volumes (1,500 in health, 950 in nursing); 144,043 periodical subscriptions (218 health-care related).

BACCALAUREATE PROGRAMS

Degree BSN
Available Programs Generic Baccalaureate.
Study Options Full-time.
Program Entrance Requirements Transcript of college record, CPR certification, health exam, health insurance, high school chemistry, immunizations, minimum GPA in nursing prerequisites of 2.75, professional liability insurance/malpractice insurance, prerequisite course work. Transfer students are accepted. *Application deadline:* 4/15 (fall), 4/15 (spring).
Advanced Placement Credit given for nursing courses completed elsewhere dependent upon specific evaluations.
Expenses (2010-11) *Tuition:* full-time $22,810; part-time $988 per credit. *Room and board:* $6020; room only: $3420 per academic year. *Required fees:* full-time $697; part-time $349 per term.
Financial Aid 90% of baccalaureate students in nursing programs received some form of financial aid in 2009-10.
Contact Dr. Patricia D. Kissell, Dean, School of Nursing and Health Sciences, School of Health and Science, Northwest Nazarene University, 623 South University Boulevard, Nampa, ID 83686. *Telephone:* 208-467-8650. *Fax:* 208-467-8651. *E-mail:* nursing@nnu.edu.

GRADUATE PROGRAMS

Expenses (2010-11) *Tuition:* full-time $10,350; part-time $575 per credit. *Required fees:* full-time $150.
Financial Aid 90% of graduate students in nursing programs received some form of financial aid in 2009-10.
Contact Mrs. Kathy L. Hanson, Program Administrator, School of Health and Science, Northwest Nazarene University, 623 South University Boulevard, Nampa, ID 83686. *Telephone:* 208-467-8642. *Fax:* 208-467-8651. *E-mail:* klhanson@nnu.edu.

MASTER'S DEGREE PROGRAM

Degree MSN
Available Programs Master's; RN to Master's.
Concentrations Available Nursing education.
Study Options Full-time.
Online Degree Options Yes (online only).
Program Entrance Requirements Computer literacy, minimum overall college GPA of 3.0, transcript of college record, nursing research course, prerequisite course work, resume, statistics course. *Application deadline:* 7/31 (fall). Applications may be processed on a rolling basis for some programs. *Application fee:* $50.
Degree Requirements 36 total credit hours, thesis or project.

ILLINOIS

Aurora University
School of Nursing
Aurora, Illinois

http://www.aurora.edu/
Founded in 1893

DEGREES • BSN • MSN
Nursing Program Faculty 17 (27% with doctorates).
Baccalaureate Enrollment 223 **Women** 94% **Men** 6% **Minority** 28% **Part-time** 43%
Graduate Enrollment 11 **Women** 82% **Men** 18% **Minority** 18% **Part-time** 100%
Nursing Student Activities Sigma Theta Tau, Student Nurses' Association, nursing club.
Nursing Student Resources Academic advising; academic or career counseling; assistance for students with disabilities; bookstore; campus computer network; career placement assistance; computer lab; computer-assisted instruction; e-mail services; externships; interactive nursing skills videos; Internet; learning resource lab; library services; nursing audiovisuals; remedial services; resume preparation assistance; skills, simulation, or other laboratory; tutoring.
Library Facilities 95,869 volumes (3,791 in health, 620 in nursing); 30,124 periodical subscriptions (1,700 health-care related).

BACCALAUREATE PROGRAMS

Degree BSN
Available Programs Generic Baccalaureate; RN Baccalaureate.
Site Options Williams Bay, WI; Aurora, IL; Winfield, IL.
Study Options Full-time.
Program Entrance Requirements Minimum overall college GPA of 2.75, transcript of college record, CPR certification, written essay, health exam, health insurance, immunizations, interview, minimum GPA in nursing prerequisites of 2.75, prerequisite course work. Transfer students are accepted. *Application deadline:* 1/15 (fall). *Application fee:* $25.
Advanced Placement Credit given for nursing courses completed elsewhere dependent upon specific evaluations.
Expenses (2010-11) *Tuition:* full-time $18,600; part-time $550 per credit hour. *Room and board:* $8170 per academic year. *Required fees:* full-time $200; part-time $100 per term.
Financial Aid 85% of baccalaureate students in nursing programs received some form of financial aid in 2009-10. *Gift aid (need-based):* Federal Pell, FSEOG, state, private, college/university gift aid from institutional funds. *Loans:* Perkins, college/university. *Work-study:* Federal

Work-Study, part-time campus jobs. *Financial aid application deadline (priority):* 4/15.
Contact Dr. Carmella M. Moran, Director and Associate Professor of Nursing, School of Nursing, Aurora University, 347 South Gladstone Avenue, Aurora, IL 60506-4892. *Telephone:* 630-844-5130. *Fax:* 630-844-7822. *E-mail:* cmoran@aurora.edu.

GRADUATE PROGRAMS

Expenses (2010-11) *Tuition:* part-time $615 per credit hour.
Financial Aid 75% of graduate students in nursing programs received some form of financial aid in 2009-10.
Contact Dr. Barbara Lockwood, Coordinator, MSN Program, School of Nursing, Aurora University, 347 South Gladstone Avenue, Aurora, IL 60506-4892. *Telephone:* 630-844-5139. *Fax:* 630-844-7822. *E-mail:* lockwood@aurora.edu.

MASTER'S DEGREE PROGRAM

Degree MSN
Available Programs Master's.
Concentrations Available Nursing administration; nursing education.
Site Options Aurora, IL.
Study Options Part-time.
Program Entrance Requirements Computer literacy, minimum overall college GPA of 2.75, transcript of college record, CPR certification, written essay, immunizations, interview, 3 letters of recommendation, nursing research course, physical assessment course, professional liability insurance/malpractice insurance, resume, statistics course. *Application deadline:* Applications may be processed on a rolling basis for some programs. *Application fee:* $25.
Degree Requirements 36 total credit hours, thesis or project.

Benedictine University

Department of Nursing
Lisle, Illinois

http://www.ben.edu/nursing
Founded in 1887

DEGREES • BSN • MSN
Nursing Program Faculty 27 (70% with doctorates).
Baccalaureate Enrollment 100 **Women** 95% **Men** 5% **Minority** 25% **International** 1%
Graduate Enrollment 231 **Women** 96% **Men** 4% **Minority** 37%
Distance Learning Courses Available.
Nursing Student Activities Nursing Honor Society, Sigma Theta Tau.
Nursing Student Resources Academic advising; academic or career counseling; assistance for students with disabilities; bookstore; campus computer network; career placement assistance; computer lab; computer-assisted instruction; e-mail services; interactive nursing skills videos; Internet; learning resource lab; library services; nursing audiovisuals; placement services for program completers; remedial services; resume preparation assistance; skills, simulation, or other laboratory; tutoring.
Library Facilities 126,358 volumes (1,350 in health, 850 in nursing); 25,851 periodical subscriptions (291 health-care related).

BACCALAUREATE PROGRAMS

Degree BSN
Available Programs Accelerated RN Baccalaureate.
Site Options River Grove, IL; Springfield, IL; Glen Ellyn, IL.
Study Options Full-time.
Program Entrance Requirements Minimum overall college GPA of 2.50, transcript of college record, 1 letter of recommendation, RN licensure. Transfer students are accepted. *Application deadline:* 7/1 (fall), 11/1 (winter), 2/1 (spring), 5/1 (summer). Applications may be processed on a rolling basis for some programs.
Advanced Placement Credit given for nursing courses completed elsewhere dependent upon specific evaluations.
Financial Aid 50% of baccalaureate students in nursing programs received some form of financial aid in 2009-10. *Gift aid (need-based):* Federal Pell, FSEOG, state, private, college/university gift aid from institutional funds. *Loans:* Federal Direct (Subsidized and Unsubsidized Stafford PLUS), Perkins, alternative loans. *Work-study:* Federal Work-Study. *Financial aid application deadline:* Continuous.
Contact Crystal Pace, Office Assistant, Department of Nursing, Benedictine University, 5700 College Road, Kindlon Hall 249, Lisle, IL 60532-0900. *Telephone:* 630-829-1152. *Fax:* 630-829-1154. *E-mail:* cpace@ben.edu.

GRADUATE PROGRAMS

Financial Aid 90% of graduate students in nursing programs received some form of financial aid in 2009-10.
Contact Pamela Bush, Associate Director, Department of Nursing, Benedictine University, 851 Trafalgar Court, Suite 420, Matland, FL 32751. *Telephone:* 866-295-3104 Ext. 5349. *Fax:* 866-789-5608. *E-mail:* pbush@ben.edu.

MASTER'S DEGREE PROGRAM

Degree MSN
Available Programs Accelerated Master's; Master's.
Study Options Full-time and part-time.
Online Degree Options Yes (online only).
Program Entrance Requirements Minimum overall college GPA of 3.00, transcript of college record, written essay, 1 letter of recommendation, resume. *Application deadline:* Applications may be processed on a rolling basis for some programs.
Advanced Placement Credit given for nursing courses completed elsewhere dependent upon specific evaluations.
Degree Requirements 36 total credit hours, thesis or project.

Blessing–Rieman College of Nursing

Blessing–Rieman College of Nursing
Quincy, Illinois

http://www.brcn.edu/

DEGREES • BSN • MSN
Nursing Program Faculty 23 (21% with doctorates).
Baccalaureate Enrollment 300 **Women** 90% **Men** 10% **Minority** 5% **International** 1% **Part-time** 8%
Graduate Enrollment 8 **Women** 100% **Part-time** 100%
Distance Learning Courses Available.
Nursing Student Activities Nursing Honor Society, Sigma Theta Tau, Student Nurses' Association.
Nursing Student Resources Academic advising; academic or career counseling; bookstore; campus computer network; computer lab; computer-assisted instruction; daycare for children of students; e-mail services; employment services for current students; externships; interactive nursing skills videos; Internet; learning resource lab; library services; nursing audiovisuals; paid internships; resume preparation assistance; skills, simulation, or other laboratory; tutoring.
Library Facilities 3,752 volumes in health, 3,752 volumes in nursing; 125 periodical subscriptions health-care related.

BACCALAUREATE PROGRAMS

Degree BSN
Available Programs ADN to Baccalaureate; Accelerated Baccalaureate for Second Degree; Generic Baccalaureate; RN Baccalaureate.
Study Options Full-time and part-time.
Online Degree Options Yes.
Program Entrance Requirements Minimum overall college GPA of 2.5, transcript of college record, CPR certification, health insurance, high school biology, high school chemistry, 2 years high school math, 2 years high school science, high school transcript, immunizations, minimum high school GPA of 3.0, minimum GPA in nursing prerequisites of 2.5, prerequisite course work. Transfer students are accepted. *Application deadline:* Applications may be processed on a rolling basis for some programs.
Advanced Placement Credit by examination available. Credit given for nursing courses completed elsewhere dependent upon specific evaluations.
Expenses (2010-11) *Tuition:* full-time $17,088; part-time $450 per credit hour. *Room and board:* room only: $2840 per academic year. *Required fees:* full-time $570.
Financial Aid 90% of baccalaureate students in nursing programs received some form of financial aid in 2009-10.
Contact Mrs. Heather Mutter, Admission Counselor, Blessing–Rieman College of Nursing, Broadway at 11th Street, PO Box 7005, Quincy, IL 62305-7005. *Telephone:* 217-228-5520 Ext. 6949. *Fax:* 217-223-4661. *E-mail:* admissions@brcn.edu.

GRADUATE PROGRAMS

Expenses (2010-11) *Tuition:* full-time $10,200; part-time $300 per credit hour.. *Required fees:* full-time $100.

Contact Mrs. Heather Mutter, Admissions Counselor, Blessing–Rieman College of Nursing, Broadway at 11th Street, PO Box 7005, Quincy, IL 62305-7005. *Telephone:* 217-228-5520 Ext. 6949. *Fax:* 217-223-4661. *E-mail:* admissions@brcn.edu.

MASTER'S DEGREE PROGRAM

Degree MSN
Available Programs Master's.
Concentrations Available Nursing administration; nursing education.
Study Options Part-time.
Program Entrance Requirements Clinical experience, computer literacy, minimum overall college GPA of 3.0, transcript of college record, CPR certification, written essay, immunizations, letters of recommendation, nursing research course, physical assessment course, professional liability insurance/malpractice insurance, resume, statistics course. *Application deadline:* 4/15 (spring). Applications may be processed on a rolling basis for some programs.
Advanced Placement Credit given for nursing courses completed elsewhere dependent upon specific evaluations.
Degree Requirements 40 total credit hours, thesis or project.

Bradley University

Department of Nursing
Peoria, Illinois

http://www.bradley.edu/academics/ehs/nur/nur_index.html
Founded in 1897

DEGREES • BSN • BSC PN • MSN

Nursing Program Faculty 36 (25% with doctorates).
Baccalaureate Enrollment 328 **Women** 92% **Men** 8% **Minority** 16% **Part-time** 2%
Graduate Enrollment 40 **Women** 68% **Men** 32% **Minority** 2% **Part-time** 80%
Nursing Student Activities Sigma Theta Tau, Student Nurses' Association.
Nursing Student Resources Academic advising; academic or career counseling; bookstore; campus computer network; career placement assistance; computer lab; computer-assisted instruction; e-mail services; externships; housing assistance; Internet; learning resource lab; library services; nursing audiovisuals; placement services for program completers; remedial services; resume preparation assistance; skills, simulation, or other laboratory; tutoring.
Library Facilities 511,000 volumes (11,159 in health, 2,214 in nursing); 41,689 periodical subscriptions (210 health-care related).

BACCALAUREATE PROGRAMS

Degrees BSN; BSc PN
Available Programs ADN to Baccalaureate; Accelerated Baccalaureate for Second Degree; Generic Baccalaureate; LPN to Baccalaureate; RN Baccalaureate.
Study Options Full-time and part-time.
Program Entrance Requirements Written essay, high school biology, high school chemistry, 3 years high school math, 3 years high school science, high school transcript, immunizations, 1 letter of recommendation, minimum high school GPA of 3.0. Transfer students are accepted. *Application deadline:* Applications may be processed on a rolling basis for some programs.
Expenses (2010-11) *Tuition:* full-time $25,150; part-time $680 per hour. *Room and board:* $7950 per academic year. *Required fees:* full-time $250.
Financial Aid 93% of baccalaureate students in nursing programs received some form of financial aid in 2009-10. *Gift aid (need-based):* Federal Pell, FSEOG, state, private, college/university gift aid from institutional funds. *Loans:* Federal Nursing Student Loans, Federal Direct (Subsidized and Unsubsidized Stafford PLUS), Perkins. *Work-study:* Federal Work-Study. *Financial aid application deadline (priority):* 3/1.
Contact Ms. Marilyn Miller-Luster, Student Records Coordinator, Department of Nursing, Bradley University, 1501 West Bradley Avenue, Peoria, IL 61625. *Telephone:* 309-677-2530. *Fax:* 309-677-2566. *E-mail:* mmiller@bradley.edu.

GRADUATE PROGRAMS

Expenses (2010-11) *Tuition:* part-time $680 per hour.
Financial Aid Research assistantships, scholarships, tuition waivers (partial), and unspecified assistantships available.
Contact Ms. Marilyn Miller-Luster, Student Records Coordinator, Department of Nursing, Bradley University, 1501 West Bradley Avenue, Peoria, IL 61625. *Telephone:* 309-677-2530. *Fax:* 309-677-2527. *E-mail:* mmiller@bradley.edu.

MASTER'S DEGREE PROGRAM

Degree MSN
Available Programs Accelerated Master's for Nurses with Non-Nursing Degrees; Master's; RN to Master's.
Concentrations Available Nurse anesthesia; nursing administration; nursing education.
Study Options Full-time and part-time.
Program Entrance Requirements Clinical experience, minimum overall college GPA of 3.0, transcript of college record, interview, 3 letters of recommendation, nursing research course, physical assessment course, resume, statistics course, GRE General Test or MAT. *Application deadline:* Applications may be processed on a rolling basis for some programs.
Advanced Placement Credit given for nursing courses completed elsewhere dependent upon specific evaluations.
Degree Requirements 36 total credit hours, thesis or project, comprehensive exam.

Chicago State University

Department of Nursing
Chicago, Illinois

http://www.csu.edu
Founded in 1867

DEGREE • BSN

Nursing Program Faculty 23 (60% with doctorates).
Baccalaureate Enrollment 372 **Women** 90% **Men** 10% **Minority** 97% **International** 15% **Part-time** 24%
Nursing Student Activities Nursing Honor Society, Student Nurses' Association.
Nursing Student Resources Academic advising; academic or career counseling; assistance for students with disabilities; bookstore; campus computer network; computer lab; computer-assisted instruction; daycare for children of students; e-mail services; employment services for current students; externships; interactive nursing skills videos; Internet; learning resource lab; library services; nursing audiovisuals; remedial services; resume preparation assistance; skills, simulation, or other laboratory; tutoring; unpaid internships.
Library Facilities 426,691 volumes; 1,654 periodical subscriptions.

BACCALAUREATE PROGRAMS

Degree BSN
Available Programs Generic Baccalaureate; LPN to Baccalaureate; RN Baccalaureate.
Study Options Full-time.
Program Entrance Requirements Minimum overall college GPA of 2.5, transcript of college record, written essay, health exam, health insurance, 3 years high school math, 3 years high school science, high school transcript, immunizations, interview, 3 letters of recommendation, minimum GPA in nursing prerequisites of 2.5, professional liability insurance/malpractice insurance, prerequisite course work. Transfer students are accepted.
Advanced Placement Credit by examination available.
Contact *Telephone:* 773-995-3992. *Fax:* 773-821-2438.

DePaul University

Department of Nursing
Chicago, Illinois

http://www.depaul.edu/~nursing
Founded in 1898

DEGREES • BS • MS

Nursing Program Faculty 19 (89% with doctorates).

Baccalaureate Enrollment 5
Graduate Enrollment 131 **Women** 87% **Men** 13% **Minority** 23% **Part-time** 35%
Nursing Student Activities Sigma Theta Tau, Student Nurses' Association.
Nursing Student Resources Academic advising; academic or career counseling; assistance for students with disabilities; bookstore; campus computer network; computer lab; computer-assisted instruction; e-mail services; employment services for current students; externships; housing assistance; interactive nursing skills videos; Internet; learning resource lab; library services; nursing audiovisuals; resume preparation assistance; skills, simulation, or other laboratory; tutoring.
Library Facilities 927,400 volumes; 42,321 periodical subscriptions (193 health-care related).

BACCALAUREATE PROGRAMS

Degree BS
Available Programs Accelerated RN Baccalaureate.
Study Options Full-time and part-time.
Program Entrance Requirements Minimum overall college GPA of 2.5, transcript of college record, CPR certification, health exam, immunizations, professional liability insurance/malpractice insurance, RN licensure. Transfer students are accepted.
Advanced Placement Credit given for nursing courses completed elsewhere dependent upon specific evaluations.
Contact *Telephone:* 773-325-7280. *Fax:* 773-325-7282.

GRADUATE PROGRAMS

Contact *Telephone:* 773-325-7280. *Fax:* 773-325-7282.

MASTER'S DEGREE PROGRAM

Degree MS
Available Programs Master's; Master's for Non-Nursing College Graduates; Master's for Nurses with Non-Nursing Degrees; RN to Master's.
Concentrations Available Nurse anesthesia; nurse case management; nursing administration; nursing education. *Clinical nurse specialist programs in:* community health, medical-surgical. *Nurse practitioner programs in:* adult health, community health, family health, pediatric, women's health.
Study Options Full-time and part-time.
Program Entrance Requirements Computer literacy, minimum overall college GPA of 2.75, transcript of college record, CPR certification, physical assessment course, professional liability insurance/malpractice insurance, prerequisite course work, statistics course, GRE (if bachelor's GPA less than 3.2).
Advanced Placement Credit given for nursing courses completed elsewhere dependent upon specific evaluations.
Degree Requirements 52 total credit hours, thesis or project.

POST-MASTER'S PROGRAM

Areas of Study Nurse anesthesia. *Nurse practitioner programs in:* adult health, community health, family health, pediatric, women's health.

Eastern Illinois University

Nursing Program
Charleston, Illinois

Founded in 1895

DEGREE • BSN

Nursing Program Faculty 3
Baccalaureate Enrollment 32 **Women** 65% **Men** 35% **Minority** 45% **Part-time** 100%
Distance Learning Courses Available.
Nursing Student Resources Academic advising; academic or career counseling; assistance for students with disabilities; bookstore; campus computer network; computer lab; computer-assisted instruction; e-mail services; interactive nursing skills videos; Internet; library services; nursing audiovisuals; remedial services; resume preparation assistance; skills, simulation, or other laboratory; tutoring.
Library Facilities 992,487 volumes (500 in nursing); 34,190 periodical subscriptions (50 health-care related).

BACCALAUREATE PROGRAMS

Degree BSN
Available Programs RN Baccalaureate.
Study Options Full-time and part-time.
Online Degree Options Yes (online only).
Program Entrance Requirements CPR certification, written essay, health exam, health insurance, immunizations, 2 letters of recommendation, professional liability insurance/malpractice insurance, prerequisite course work, RN licensure. *Application deadline:* 11/15 (fall), 7/15 (summer). *Application fee:* $30.
Expenses (2010-11) *Tuition, state resident:* part-time $294 per credit hour.
Contact RN to BS in Nursing Program, Nursing Program, Eastern Illinois University, 600 Lincoln Avenue, 2230 McAfee, Charleston, IL 61920. *Telephone:* 217-581-7049. *Fax:* 217-581-7050.

Elmhurst College

Deicke Center for Nursing Education
Elmhurst, Illinois

Founded in 1871

DEGREES • BS • MS • MSN/MBA

Nursing Program Faculty 13 (55% with doctorates).
Baccalaureate Enrollment 195
Graduate Enrollment 34
Nursing Student Activities Sigma Theta Tau, Student Nurses' Association.
Nursing Student Resources Academic advising; academic or career counseling; assistance for students with disabilities; bookstore; campus computer network; career placement assistance; computer lab; daycare for children of students; e-mail services; employment services for current students; housing assistance; Internet; learning resource lab; library services; nursing audiovisuals; remedial services; resume preparation assistance; skills, simulation, or other laboratory; tutoring.
Library Facilities 228,015 volumes (6,000 in health); 1,907 periodical subscriptions (80 health-care related).

BACCALAUREATE PROGRAMS

Degree BS
Available Programs Generic Baccalaureate; RN Baccalaureate.
Study Options Full-time.
Program Entrance Requirements Minimum overall college GPA of 2.75, transcript of college record, CPR certification, written essay, health insurance, immunizations, 2 letters of recommendation, minimum GPA in nursing prerequisites of 2.75, prerequisite course work. Transfer students are accepted. *Application deadline:* 6/1 (fall).
Advanced Placement Credit given for nursing courses completed elsewhere dependent upon specific evaluations.
Contact Dr. Jan Strom, Director, Deicke Center for Nursing Education, Elmhurst College, 190 Prospect Avenue, Elmhurst, IL 60126. *Telephone:* 630-617-3344. *Fax:* 630-617-3237. *E-mail:* janstrom@elmhurst.edu.

GRADUATE PROGRAMS

Contact Dr. Mary Oesterle, Director, Master of Science in Nursing, Deicke Center for Nursing Education, Elmhurst College, 190 Prospect Avenue, Elmhurst, IL 60126. *Fax:* 630-617-3514. *E-mail:* oesterle@elmhurst.edu.

MASTER'S DEGREE PROGRAM

Degrees MS; MSN/MBA
Available Programs Master's.
Concentrations Available Clinical nurse leader; nursing education.
Study Options Full-time.
Program Entrance Requirements Clinical experience, computer literacy, transcript of college record, CPR certification, written essay, immunizations, interview, 3 letters of recommendation, nursing research course, physical assessment course, prerequisite course work, resume, statistics course. *Application deadline:* Applications may be processed on a rolling basis for some programs.
Degree Requirements 33 total credit hours.

Governors State University
College of Health and Human Services
University Park, Illinois

http://www.govst.edu/nursing/index.html
Founded in 1969

DEGREES • BS • MS

Nursing Program Faculty 7 (85% with doctorates).
Baccalaureate Enrollment 31 **Women** 98% **Men** 2% **Minority** 92% **International** 1% **Part-time** 100%
Graduate Enrollment 72 **Women** 97% **Men** 3% **Minority** 89% **International** 6% **Part-time** 4%
Nursing Student Activities Sigma Theta Tau.
Nursing Student Resources Academic advising; assistance for students with disabilities; bookstore; campus computer network; computer lab; daycare for children of students; e-mail services; Internet; learning resource lab; library services; nursing audiovisuals; tutoring.
Library Facilities 462,924 volumes; 3,046 periodical subscriptions.

BACCALAUREATE PROGRAMS

Degree BS
Available Programs RN Baccalaureate.
Study Options Part-time.
Program Entrance Requirements Transcript of college record, CPR certification, health exam, health insurance, immunizations, minimum GPA in nursing prerequisites of 2.0, professional liability insurance/malpractice insurance, prerequisite course work, RN licensure. Transfer students are accepted.
Contact ***Telephone:*** 708-534-4053. *Fax:* 708-534-2197.

GRADUATE PROGRAMS

Contact ***Telephone:*** 708-534-4053. *Fax:* 708-534-2197.

MASTER'S DEGREE PROGRAM

Degree MS
Available Programs Master's.
Concentrations Available *Clinical nurse specialist programs in:* adult health.
Study Options Full-time and part-time.
Program Entrance Requirements Clinical experience, computer literacy, minimum overall college GPA of 3.0, transcript of college record, CPR certification, written essay, immunizations, nursing research course, physical assessment course, professional liability insurance/malpractice insurance, prerequisite course work, statistics course.
Degree Requirements 42 total credit hours, comprehensive exam.

POST-MASTER'S PROGRAM

Areas of Study Nursing education.

Illinois State University
Mennonite College of Nursing
Normal, Illinois

http://www.mcn.ilstu.edu/
Founded in 1857

DEGREES • BSN • MSN • PHD

Nursing Program Faculty 47 (34% with doctorates).
Baccalaureate Enrollment 232 **Women** 95% **Men** 5% **Minority** 10% **Part-time** 8%
Graduate Enrollment 123 **Women** 97% **Men** 3% **Minority** 11% **International** 1% **Part-time** 78%
Distance Learning Courses Available.
Nursing Student Activities Nursing Honor Society, Sigma Theta Tau, Student Nurses' Association.
Nursing Student Resources Academic advising; academic or career counseling; assistance for students with disabilities; bookstore; campus computer network; career placement assistance; computer lab; computer-assisted instruction; daycare for children of students; e-mail services; employment services for current students; externships; interactive nursing skills videos; Internet; learning resource lab; library services; nursing audiovisuals; placement services for program completers; resume preparation assistance; skills, simulation, or other laboratory; tutoring.
Library Facilities 1.6 million volumes (36,000 in health, 4,000 in nursing); 14,166 periodical subscriptions (700 health-care related).

BACCALAUREATE PROGRAMS

Degree BSN
Available Programs Accelerated Baccalaureate for Second Degree; Generic Baccalaureate; RN Baccalaureate.
Site Options Normal, IL.
Study Options Full-time.
Online Degree Options Yes.
Program Entrance Requirements Minimum overall college GPA of 2.7, transcript of college record, CPR certification, health exam, health insurance, immunizations, minimum GPA in nursing prerequisites of 2.0, prerequisite course work. Transfer students are accepted. *Application deadline:* 1/15 (fall), 1/15 (spring), 1/15 (summer). *Application fee:* $40.
Advanced Placement Credit given for nursing courses completed elsewhere dependent upon specific evaluations.
Expenses (2010-11) *Tuition, state resident:* full-time $6336; part-time $364 per credit. *Tuition, nonresident:* full-time $13,152; part-time $548 per credit. *Room and board:* $10,172; room only: $5862 per academic year. *Required fees:* full-time $240; part-time $68 per credit.
Financial Aid 74% of baccalaureate students in nursing programs received some form of financial aid in 2009-10. *Gift aid (need-based):* Federal Pell, FSEOG, state, private, college/university gift aid from institutional funds, Federal Nursing. *Loans:* Federal Nursing Student Loans, Federal Direct (Subsidized and Unsubsidized Stafford PLUS), Perkins. *Work-study:* Federal Work-Study, part-time campus jobs. *Financial aid application deadline (priority):* 3/1.
Contact Ms. Nancy Jakubczyk, Academic Advisor, Mennonite College of Nursing, Illinois State University, 5810 Edwards Hall, 100 North University, Normal, IL 61790-5810. *Telephone:* 309-438-7400. *Fax:* 309-438-2620. *E-mail:* njakub@ilstu.edu.

GRADUATE PROGRAMS

Expenses (2010-11) *Tuition, state resident:* full-time $6336; part-time $264 per credit. *Tuition, nonresident:* full-time $13,152; part-time $548 per credit. *Room and board:* $10,172; room only: $5862 per academic year. *Required fees:* full-time $240; part-time $68 per credit.
Financial Aid 100% of graduate students in nursing programs received some form of financial aid in 2009-10.
Contact Ms. Melissa K. Moody, Academic Advisor, Mennonite College of Nursing, Illinois State University, 5810 Edwards Hall, 100 North University, Normal, IL 61790-5810. *Telephone:* 309-438-7400. *Fax:* 309-438-2280. *E-mail:* mkmoody@ilstu.edu.

MASTER'S DEGREE PROGRAM

Degree MSN
Available Programs Master's.
Concentrations Available Clinical nurse leader; nursing administration. *Nurse practitioner programs in:* family health.
Site Options Normal, IL.
Study Options Full-time and part-time.
Program Entrance Requirements Minimum overall college GPA of 3.0, transcript of college record, CPR certification, written essay, immunizations, 3 letters of recommendation, nursing research course, physical assessment course, prerequisite course work, resume, statistics course. *Application deadline:* 2/1 (fall), 9/1 (spring), 2/1 (summer). Applications may be processed on a rolling basis for some programs. *Application fee:* $40.
Advanced Placement Credit given for nursing courses completed elsewhere dependent upon specific evaluations.
Degree Requirements 44 total credit hours, comprehensive exam.

POST-MASTER'S PROGRAM

Areas of Study Nursing education. *Nurse practitioner programs in:* family health.

DOCTORAL DEGREE PROGRAM

Degree PhD
Available Programs Doctorate.
Areas of Study Aging.
Site Options Normal, IL.
Program Entrance Requirements Minimum overall college GPA of 3.0, interview by faculty committee, interview, 3 letters of recommendation, MSN or equivalent, statistics course, vita. Application deadline: 2/1 (fall). Applications may be processed on a rolling basis for some programs. Application fee: $40.
Degree Requirements 66 total credit hours, dissertation, oral exam, written exam, residency.

Illinois Wesleyan University
School of Nursing
Bloomington, Illinois

http://www2.iwu.edu/nursing/
Founded in 1850

DEGREE • BSN

Nursing Program Faculty 24 (38% with doctorates).
Baccalaureate Enrollment 130 **Women** 93% **Men** 7% **Minority** 15%
Nursing Student Activities Nursing Honor Society, Sigma Theta Tau, Student Nurses' Association, nursing club.
Nursing Student Resources Academic advising; academic or career counseling; assistance for students with disabilities; bookstore; campus computer network; career placement assistance; computer lab; computer-assisted instruction; e-mail services; employment services for current students; externships; housing assistance; interactive nursing skills videos; Internet; learning resource lab; library services; nursing audiovisuals; paid internships; placement services for program completers; resume preparation assistance; skills, simulation, or other laboratory; tutoring; unpaid internships.
Library Facilities 5,500 volumes in health, 3,000 volumes in nursing; 200 periodical subscriptions health-care related.

BACCALAUREATE PROGRAMS

Degree BSN
Available Programs Generic Baccalaureate.
Study Options Full-time and part-time.
Program Entrance Requirements Minimum overall college GPA of 3.0, transcript of college record, written essay, health exam, health insurance, high school biology, high school chemistry, 2 years high school math, 2 years high school science, high school transcript, immunizations, interview, minimum high school GPA of 3.0, minimum high school rank 25%, minimum GPA in nursing prerequisites of 3.0. Transfer students are accepted. *Application deadline:* Applications may be processed on a rolling basis for some programs.
Expenses (2010-11) *Tuition:* full-time $35,076; part-time $4385 per course. *Room and board:* $8116; room only: $5040 per academic year. *Required fees:* full-time $180.
Financial Aid 91% of baccalaureate students in nursing programs received some form of financial aid in 2009-10. *Gift aid (need-based):* Federal Pell, FSEOG, state, private, college/university gift aid from institutional funds. *Loans:* Federal Nursing Student Loans, Federal Direct (Subsidized and Unsubsidized Stafford PLUS), Perkins, college/university. *Work-study:* Federal Work-Study, part-time campus jobs. *Financial aid application deadline:* 3/1.
Contact Dr. Victoria N. Folse, Director and Associate Professor, School of Nursing, Illinois Wesleyan University, PO Box 2900, Bloomington, IL 61702-2900. *Telephone:* 309-556-3051. *Fax:* 309-556-3043. *E-mail:* vfolse@iwu.edu.

Lakeview College of Nursing
Lakeview College of Nursing
Danville, Illinois

http://www.lakeviewcol.edu/
Founded in 1987

DEGREE • BSN

Nursing Program Faculty 24 (2% with doctorates).
Baccalaureate Enrollment 284 **Women** 87% **Men** 13% **Minority** 20% **Part-time** 8%
Nursing Student Activities Nursing Honor Society, Sigma Theta Tau, Student Nurses' Association.
Nursing Student Resources Academic advising; academic or career counseling; assistance for students with disabilities; bookstore; campus computer network; career placement assistance; computer lab; Internet; library services; nursing audiovisuals; resume preparation assistance; skills, simulation, or other laboratory; tutoring.
Library Facilities 2,000 volumes in health; 41 periodical subscriptions health-care related.

BACCALAUREATE PROGRAMS

Degree BSN
Available Programs Accelerated RN Baccalaureate; Generic Baccalaureate; RN Baccalaureate.
Site Options Charleston, IL.
Study Options Full-time and part-time.
Program Entrance Requirements Minimum overall college GPA of 2.5, transcript of college record, CPR certification, written essay, health exam, immunizations, 2 letters of recommendation, prerequisite course work. Transfer students are accepted. *Application deadline:* 4/1 (fall), 10/1 (spring). *Application fee:* $100.
Advanced Placement Credit given for nursing courses completed elsewhere dependent upon specific evaluations.
Expenses (2010-11) *Tuition:* part-time $370 per credit. *Required fees:* full-time $1800.
Financial Aid 52% of baccalaureate students in nursing programs received some form of financial aid in 2009-10. *Gift aid (need-based):* Federal Pell, state, private, college/university gift aid from institutional funds. *Loans:* Federal Direct (Subsidized and Unsubsidized Stafford PLUS). *Financial aid application deadline:* Continuous.
Contact Mrs. Connie Young, Director of Enrollment/Registrar, Lakeview College of Nursing, 903 North Logan Avenue, Danville, IL 61832. *Telephone:* 217-709-0931. *Fax:* 217-709-0953. *E-mail:* cyoung@lakeviewcol.edu.

Lewis University
Program in Nursing
Romeoville, Illinois

http://www.lewisu.edu/academics/nursing/index.htm
Founded in 1932

DEGREES • BSN • MSN • MSN/MBA

Nursing Program Faculty 30 (40% with doctorates).
Baccalaureate Enrollment 630 **Women** 90% **Men** 10% **Minority** 31% **International** 9% **Part-time** 69%
Graduate Enrollment 147 **Women** 91% **Men** 9% **Minority** 16% **International** 2%
Distance Learning Courses Available.
Nursing Student Activities Sigma Theta Tau, Student Nurses' Association.
Nursing Student Resources Academic advising; academic or career counseling; assistance for students with disabilities; bookstore; campus computer network; career placement assistance; computer lab; computer-assisted instruction; e-mail services; employment services for current students; externships; interactive nursing skills videos; Internet; learning resource lab; library services; nursing audiovisuals; other; placement services for program completers; remedial services; resume preparation assistance; skills, simulation, or other laboratory; tutoring.
Library Facilities 149,870 volumes (3,100 in health, 2,038 in nursing); 1,990 periodical subscriptions (90 health-care related).

BACCALAUREATE PROGRAMS

Degree BSN
Available Programs Accelerated Baccalaureate for Second Degree; Accelerated RN Baccalaureate; Generic Baccalaureate.
Site Options Hickory Hills, IL; Shorewood, IL; Oak Brook, IL; Tinley Park, IL.
Study Options Full-time.
Program Entrance Requirements Minimum overall college GPA of 2.75, transcript of college record, CPR certification, health exam, health insurance, high school biology, high school chemistry, 3 years high school math, high school transcript, immunizations, minimum high school GPA of 2.75, minimum GPA in nursing prerequisites of 2.75, prerequisite course work. Transfer students are accepted.
Advanced Placement Credit given for nursing courses completed elsewhere dependent upon specific evaluations.
Contact *Telephone:* 815-836-5245. *Fax:* 815-838-8306.

GRADUATE PROGRAMS

Contact *Telephone:* 815-836-5878 Ext. 815. *Fax:* 815-836-5806.

MASTER'S DEGREE PROGRAM

Degrees MSN; MSN/MBA
Available Programs Accelerated Master's; Accelerated Master's for Nurses with Non-Nursing Degrees; Accelerated RN to Master's; RN to Master's.
Concentrations Available Nurse case management; nursing administration; nursing education. *Nurse practitioner programs in:* adult health.
Site Options Hickory Hills, IL; Shorewood, IL; Oak Brook, IL; Tinley Park, IL.

Study Options Full-time and part-time.
Online Degree Options Yes (online only).
Program Entrance Requirements Clinical experience, computer literacy, minimum overall college GPA of 3.0, transcript of college record, CPR certification, immunizations, interview, 2 letters of recommendation, nursing research course, physical assessment course, professional liability insurance/malpractice insurance, prerequisite course work, resume, statistics course.
Advanced Placement Credit given for nursing courses completed elsewhere dependent upon specific evaluations.
Degree Requirements 45 total credit hours, thesis or project.

POST-MASTER'S PROGRAM
Areas of Study Nursing administration; nursing education. *Nurse practitioner programs in:* adult health.

CONTINUING EDUCATION PROGRAM
Contact ***Telephone:*** 815-836-5889. *Fax:* 815-838-8306.

Loyola University Chicago
Marcella Niehoff School of Nursing
Maywood, Illinois

http://www.luc.edu/schools/nursing/
Founded in 1870

DEGREES • BSN • MSN • MSN/MBA • MSN/MDIV • PHD
Nursing Program Faculty 40 (90% with doctorates).
Nursing Student Activities Nursing Honor Society, Sigma Theta Tau, Student Nurses' Association.
Library Facilities 1.7 million volumes (51,674 in health, 4,966 in nursing); 54,309 periodical subscriptions (2,630 health-care related).

BACCALAUREATE PROGRAMS
Degree BSN
Available Programs Accelerated Baccalaureate; Generic Baccalaureate; RN Baccalaureate.
Site Options Maywood, IL; Chicago, IL.
Study Options Full-time and part-time.
Program Entrance Requirements Transcript of college record, CPR certification, written essay, health exam, health insurance, high school biology, high school chemistry, 2 years high school math, high school transcript, immunizations, 2 letters of recommendation, minimum high school GPA of 3.0, minimum high school rank 25%, prerequisite course work. Transfer students are accepted.
Advanced Placement Credit given for nursing courses completed elsewhere dependent upon specific evaluations.
Contact ***Telephone:*** 773-508-3249. *Fax:* 773-508-3241.

GRADUATE PROGRAMS
Contact ***Telephone:*** 773-508-3249. *Fax:* 773-508-3241.

MASTER'S DEGREE PROGRAM
Degrees MSN; MSN/MBA; MSN/MDIV
Available Programs Master's; RN to Master's.
Concentrations Available Nurse-midwifery; nursing administration. *Clinical nurse specialist programs in:* acute care, cardiovascular, oncology. *Nurse practitioner programs in:* acute care, adult health, family health, pediatric, women's health.
Site Options Maywood, IL; Chicago, IL.
Study Options Full-time and part-time.
Program Entrance Requirements Clinical experience, minimum overall college GPA of 3.0, transcript of college record, CPR certification, written essay, immunizations, interview, 3 letters of recommendation, physical assessment course, professional liability insurance/malpractice insurance, statistics course.
Advanced Placement Credit given for nursing courses completed elsewhere dependent upon specific evaluations.
Degree Requirements 48 total credit hours, comprehensive exam.

DOCTORAL DEGREE PROGRAM
Degree PhD
Available Programs Post-Baccalaureate Doctorate.
Areas of Study Ethics, nursing education, nursing research, nursing science.
Site Options Maywood, IL; Chicago, IL.
Program Entrance Requirements interview by faculty committee, interview, 3 letters of recommendation, scholarly papers, statistics course, vita, writing sample, GRE General Test.
Degree Requirements 64 total credit hours, dissertation, oral exam, written exam.

MacMurray College
Department of Nursing
Jacksonville, Illinois

http://www.mac.edu/academics/nursing.html
Founded in 1846

DEGREE • BSN
Nursing Program Faculty 9 (25% with doctorates).
Baccalaureate Enrollment 102 **Women** 91% **Men** 9% **Minority** 6% **Part-time** 11%
Nursing Student Activities Sigma Theta Tau, nursing club.
Nursing Student Resources Academic advising; academic or career counseling; bookstore; campus computer network; career placement assistance; computer lab; computer-assisted instruction; e-mail services; interactive nursing skills videos; Internet; learning resource lab; library services; nursing audiovisuals; paid internships; resume preparation assistance; skills, simulation, or other laboratory; tutoring.
Library Facilities 1.8 million volumes (1,800 in health, 1,300 in nursing); 185 periodical subscriptions (50 health-care related).

BACCALAUREATE PROGRAMS
Degree BSN
Available Programs ADN to Baccalaureate; Baccalaureate for Second Degree; Generic Baccalaureate; LPN to RN Baccalaureate; RN Baccalaureate.
Study Options Full-time and part-time.
Program Entrance Requirements Minimum overall college GPA of 2.5, transcript of college record, CPR certification, health exam, health insurance, high school chemistry, high school transcript, immunizations, minimum high school GPA of 2.5, minimum GPA in nursing prerequisites of 2.5. Transfer students are accepted. *Application deadline:* 5/30 (fall). Applications may be processed on a rolling basis for some programs.
Expenses (2010-11) *Tuition:* full-time $18,838; part-time $625 per credit hour. *Room and board:* $6982; room only: $3602 per academic year. *Required fees:* full-time $750.
Financial Aid 98% of baccalaureate students in nursing programs received some form of financial aid in 2009-10. *Gift aid (need-based):* Federal Pell, FSEOG, state, private, college/university gift aid from institutional funds. *Loans:* Federal Direct (Subsidized and Unsubsidized Stafford PLUS), Perkins. *Work-study:* Federal Work-Study. *Financial aid application deadline (priority):* 5/1.
Contact Vice President for Enrollment, Department of Nursing, MacMurray College, 447 East College Avenue, Jacksonville, IL 62650. *Telephone:* 800-252-7485. *Fax:* 217-291-0702. *E-mail:* admissions@mac.edu.

McKendree University
Department of Nursing
Lebanon, Illinois

http://www.mckendree.edu/nursing
Founded in 1828

DEGREES • BSN • MSN
Nursing Program Faculty 26 (35% with doctorates).
Baccalaureate Enrollment 319 **Women** 91% **Men** 9% **Minority** 8% **Part-time** 76%
Graduate Enrollment 87 **Women** 94% **Men** 6% **Minority** 7% **International** 1% **Part-time** 82%
Distance Learning Courses Available.
Nursing Student Activities Nursing Honor Society.
Nursing Student Resources Academic advising; academic or career counseling; assistance for students with disabilities; bookstore; campus computer network; career placement assistance; computer lab; computer-assisted instruction; e-mail services; interactive nursing skills videos; Internet; learning resource lab; library services; nursing audiovisuals; resume preparation assistance; tutoring.

Library Facilities 109,000 volumes (4,450 in health, 2,880 in nursing); 450 periodical subscriptions (80 health-care related).

BACCALAUREATE PROGRAMS

Degree BSN
Available Programs ADN to Baccalaureate.
Site Options Marion, IL; Belleville, IL; Louisville, KY.
Study Options Full-time and part-time.
Program Entrance Requirements Minimum overall college GPA of 2.0, transcript of college record, CPR certification, health exam, high school transcript, immunizations, prerequisite course work, RN licensure. Transfer students are accepted. *Application deadline:* Applications may be processed on a rolling basis for some programs.
Advanced Placement Credit given for nursing courses completed elsewhere dependent upon specific evaluations.
Expenses (2010-11) *Tuition:* part-time $265 per credit hour.
Financial Aid 32% of baccalaureate students in nursing programs received some form of financial aid in 2009-10. *Gift aid (need-based):* Federal Pell, FSEOG, state, private, college/university gift aid from institutional funds. *Loans:* Federal Direct (Subsidized and Unsubsidized Stafford PLUS), Perkins. *Work-study:* Federal Work-Study, part-time campus jobs. *Financial aid application deadline (priority):* 5/31.
Contact Kim Eichelberger, Director of Nursing Admissions, Department of Nursing, McKendree University, 701 College Road, Lebanon, IL 62254. *Telephone:* 800-232-7228 Ext. 6411. *Fax:* 618-537-6259. *E-mail:* kaeichelberger@mckendree.edu.

GRADUATE PROGRAMS

Expenses (2010-11) *Tuition:* part-time $350 per credit hour.
Financial Aid 23% of graduate students in nursing programs received some form of financial aid in 2009-10.
Contact Kim Eichelberger, Director of Nursing Admissions, Department of Nursing, McKendree University, 701 College Road, Lebanon, IL 62254. *Telephone:* 618-537-6411. *Fax:* 618-537-6410. *E-mail:* kaeichelberger@mckendree.edu.

MASTER'S DEGREE PROGRAM

Degree MSN
Available Programs Master's; RN to Master's.
Concentrations Available Nursing administration; nursing education.
Site Options Marion, IL; Belleville, IL; Louisville, KY.
Study Options Full-time and part-time.
Online Degree Options Yes.
Program Entrance Requirements Minimum overall college GPA of 3.0, transcript of college record, CPR certification, written essay, immunizations, interview, resume. *Application deadline:* Applications may be processed on a rolling basis for some programs.
Advanced Placement Credit given for nursing courses completed elsewhere dependent upon specific evaluations.
Degree Requirements 38 total credit hours, thesis or project.

POST-MASTER'S PROGRAM

Areas of Study Nursing administration; nursing education.

Methodist College of Nursing

Methodist College of Nursing
Peoria, Illinois

DEGREE • BSN

Nursing Program Faculty 40 (20% with doctorates).
Baccalaureate Enrollment 468 **Women** 89.6% **Men** 10.4% **Minority** 13.6% **Part-time** 19.5%
Distance Learning Courses Available.
Nursing Student Activities Nursing Honor Society, Student Nurses' Association.
Nursing Student Resources Academic advising; academic or career counseling; assistance for students with disabilities; bookstore; campus computer network; career placement assistance; computer lab; computer-assisted instruction; daycare for children of students; e-mail services; housing assistance; interactive nursing skills videos; Internet; learning resource lab; library services; nursing audiovisuals; remedial services; resume preparation assistance; skills, simulation, or other laboratory; tutoring; unpaid internships.
Library Facilities 1,260 volumes in health, 480 volumes in nursing; 825 periodical subscriptions health-care related.

BACCALAUREATE PROGRAMS

Degree BSN
Available Programs Accelerated Baccalaureate for Second Degree; Baccalaureate for Second Degree; Generic Baccalaureate; RN Baccalaureate.
Study Options Full-time and part-time.
Online Degree Options Yes (online only).
Program Entrance Requirements Transcript of college record, CPR certification, health exam, high school transcript, immunizations, minimum high school GPA of 2.5, minimum GPA in nursing prerequisites of 3.0, professional liability insurance/malpractice insurance. Transfer students are accepted. *Application deadline:* 4/15 (fall), 9/15 (spring). *Application fee:* $35.
Advanced Placement Credit by examination available. Credit given for nursing courses completed elsewhere dependent upon specific evaluations.
Expenses (2010-11) *Tuition:* full-time $13,680; part-time $570 per credit hour. *Room and board:* $2300; room only: $1800 per academic year. *Required fees:* full-time $1080; part-time $540 per term.
Financial Aid 98% of baccalaureate students in nursing programs received some form of financial aid in 2009-10.
Contact Mary Jane Dowling, Recruitment Coordinator, Methodist College of Nursing, 415 St. Mark Court, Peoria, IL 60613. *Telephone:* 309-672-5513. *Fax:* 309-671-8303. *E-mail:* mjdowling@mcon.edu.

Millikin University

School of Nursing
Decatur, Illinois

http://www.millikin.edu/
Founded in 1901

DEGREES • BSN • MSN

Nursing Program Faculty 20 (60% with doctorates).
Baccalaureate Enrollment 218 **Women** 91% **Men** 9% **Minority** 12% **International** 1% **Part-time** 5%
Graduate Enrollment 19 **Women** 89% **Men** 11% **Minority** 11% **Part-time** 35%
Distance Learning Courses Available.
Nursing Student Activities Nursing Honor Society, Sigma Theta Tau, Student Nurses' Association.
Nursing Student Resources Academic advising; academic or career counseling; assistance for students with disabilities; bookstore; campus computer network; career placement assistance; computer lab; computer-assisted instruction; e-mail services; employment services for current students; housing assistance; interactive nursing skills videos; Internet; learning resource lab; library services; nursing audiovisuals; other; placement services for program completers; remedial services; resume preparation assistance; skills, simulation, or other laboratory; tutoring; unpaid internships.
Library Facilities 218,618 volumes (10,000 in health, 6,000 in nursing); 363 periodical subscriptions (64 health-care related).

BACCALAUREATE PROGRAMS

Degree BSN
Available Programs Generic Baccalaureate; RN Baccalaureate.
Study Options Full-time and part-time.
Program Entrance Requirements Minimum overall college GPA of 2.5, transcript of college record, CPR certification, written essay, health exam, high school biology, high school chemistry, 2 years high school math, 2 years high school science, high school transcript, immunizations, minimum high school GPA of 3.0, minimum high school rank 75%, minimum GPA in nursing prerequisites of 2.5. Transfer students are accepted. *Application deadline:* Applications may be processed on a rolling basis for some programs.
Advanced Placement Credit given for nursing courses completed elsewhere dependent upon specific evaluations.
Expenses (2010-11) *Tuition:* full-time $26,780; part-time $895 per credit hour. *Room and board:* $8291; room only: $4621 per academic year. *Required fees:* full-time $645; part-time $88 per term.
Financial Aid 98% of baccalaureate students in nursing programs received some form of financial aid in 2009-10. *Gift aid (need-based):* Federal Pell, FSEOG, state, private, college/university gift aid from institutional funds. *Loans:* Perkins, state. *Work-study:* Federal Work-Study, part-time campus jobs. *Financial aid application deadline (priority):* 3/15.
Contact Ms. Kim Wenthe, Administrative Assistant, School of Nursing, Millikin University, 1184 West Main Street, Decatur, IL 62522. *Tele-*

phone: 217-424-6348. *Fax:* 217-420-6731. *E-mail:* kwenthe@mail.millikin.edu.

GRADUATE PROGRAMS

Contact Ms. Marianne G. Taylor, Administrative Assistant II, School of Nursing, Millikin University, 1184 West Main Street, Decatur, IL 62522. *Telephone:* 800-373-7733 Ext. 5034. *Fax:* 217-424-5034. *E-mail:* mgtaylor@mail.millikin.edu.

MASTER'S DEGREE PROGRAM

Degree MSN
Available Programs Accelerated Master's for Non-Nursing College Graduates; Master's.
Concentrations Available Clinical nurse leader; nurse anesthesia; nursing education.
Study Options Full-time and part-time.
Program Entrance Requirements Clinical experience, minimum overall college GPA of 3.0, transcript of college record, CPR certification, written essay, immunizations, interview, 3 letters of recommendation, professional liability insurance/malpractice insurance, resume, statistics course. *Application deadline:* Applications may be processed on a rolling basis for some programs.
Advanced Placement Credit given for nursing courses completed elsewhere dependent upon specific evaluations.
Degree Requirements 36 total credit hours, thesis or project.

Northern Illinois University

School of Nursing and Health Studies
De Kalb, Illinois

http://www.nursing.niu.edu
Founded in 1895

DEGREES • BS • MS • MSN/MPH
Nursing Program Faculty 43 (44% with doctorates).
Baccalaureate Enrollment 469 **Women** 92% **Men** 8% **Minority** 20% **Part-time** 23%
Graduate Enrollment 164 **Women** 96% **Men** 4% **Minority** 23% **Part-time** 96%
Distance Learning Courses Available.
Nursing Student Activities Nursing Honor Society, Sigma Theta Tau, Student Nurses' Association, nursing club.
Nursing Student Resources Academic advising; academic or career counseling; assistance for students with disabilities; bookstore; campus computer network; career placement assistance; computer lab; computer-assisted instruction; daycare for children of students; e-mail services; employment services for current students; externships; housing assistance; interactive nursing skills videos; Internet; learning resource lab; library services; nursing audiovisuals; paid internships; placement services for program completers; remedial services; resume preparation assistance; skills, simulation, or other laboratory; tutoring; unpaid internships.
Library Facilities 3.1 million volumes (39,869 in health, 7,600 in nursing); 24,696 periodical subscriptions (676 health-care related).

BACCALAUREATE PROGRAMS

Degree BS
Available Programs ADN to Baccalaureate; Generic Baccalaureate; RN Baccalaureate.
Site Options Rockford, IL; Palatine, IL; Aurora, IL.
Study Options Full-time and part-time.
Program Entrance Requirements Transcript of college record, CPR certification, health exam, health insurance, high school transcript, immunizations, minimum high school GPA of 3.25, minimum high school rank 50%, minimum GPA in nursing prerequisites of 2.5, professional liability insurance/malpractice insurance. Transfer students are accepted.
Advanced Placement Credit given for nursing courses completed elsewhere dependent upon specific evaluations.
Contact ***Telephone:*** 815-753-0665. *Fax:* 815-753-0814.

GRADUATE PROGRAMS

Contact ***Telephone:*** 815-753-6551. *Fax:* 815-753-0814.

MASTER'S DEGREE PROGRAM

Degrees MS; MSN/MPH
Available Programs Master's.
Concentrations Available Nursing education. *Clinical nurse specialist programs in:* adult health, community health. *Nurse practitioner programs in:* adult health, family health.
Study Options Full-time and part-time.
Program Entrance Requirements Minimum overall college GPA of 3.0, transcript of college record, CPR certification, written essay, immunizations, 2 letters of recommendation, nursing research course, physical assessment course, professional liability insurance/malpractice insurance, statistics course.
Degree Requirements 48 total credit hours.

POST-MASTER'S PROGRAM

Areas of Study Nursing education. *Nurse practitioner programs in:* family health.

North Park University

School of Nursing
Chicago, Illinois

http://www.northpark.edu/nursing/
Founded in 1891

DEGREES • BS • MS • MSN/MA • MSN/MBA • MSN/MM
Nursing Program Faculty 35 (63% with doctorates).
Baccalaureate Enrollment 278 **Women** 88.4% **Men** 11.6% **Minority** 57% **International** 4% **Part-time** 36%
Graduate Enrollment 189 **Women** 95% **Men** 5% **Minority** 76% **International** 7% **Part-time** 80%
Nursing Student Activities Sigma Theta Tau, Student Nurses' Association.
Nursing Student Resources Academic advising; academic or career counseling; assistance for students with disabilities; bookstore; campus computer network; career placement assistance; computer lab; computer-assisted instruction; e-mail services; employment services for current students; interactive nursing skills videos; Internet; learning resource lab; library services; nursing audiovisuals; remedial services; skills, simulation, or other laboratory; tutoring.
Library Facilities 260,685 volumes (3,959 in health, 1,791 in nursing); 1,178 periodical subscriptions (239 health-care related).

BACCALAUREATE PROGRAMS

Degree BS
Available Programs Generic Baccalaureate; RN Baccalaureate.
Site Options Evanston, IL; Arlington Heights, IL; Grayslake, IL.
Study Options Full-time.
Program Entrance Requirements Minimum overall college GPA of 2.75, transcript of college record, CPR certification, health exam, health insurance, immunizations, 1 letter of recommendation, minimum GPA in nursing prerequisites of 2.75, prerequisite course work. Transfer students are accepted.
Financial Aid 92% of baccalaureate students in nursing programs received some form of financial aid in 2008-09.
Contact Mr. Robert Berki, Admissions Counselor, School of Nursing, North Park University, 3225 West Foster Avenue, Chicago, IL 60625. *Telephone:* 773-244-5516. *E-mail:* rberki@northpark.edu.

GRADUATE PROGRAMS

Financial Aid 95% of graduate students in nursing programs received some form of financial aid in 2008-09.
Contact Ms. Jennifer Hulting, Assistant Director of Admissions, School of Nursing, North Park University, 3225 West Foster Avenue, Chicago, IL 60625. *Telephone:* 773-244-5508. *Fax:* 773-279-7082. *E-mail:* jhulting@northpark.edu.

MASTER'S DEGREE PROGRAM

Degrees MS; MSN/MA; MSN/MBA; MSN/MM
Available Programs Master's; RN to Master's.
Concentrations Available Nursing administration. *Clinical nurse specialist programs in:* community health. *Nurse practitioner programs in:* adult health, family health.
Site Options Arlington Heights, IL; Grayslake, IL.
Study Options Full-time and part-time.
Program Entrance Requirements Clinical experience, minimum overall college GPA of 3.0, transcript of college record, CPR certification, immunizations, 2 letters of recommendation, nursing research

course, physical assessment course, professional liability insurance/malpractice insurance, prerequisite course work, resume, statistics course.
Degree Requirements 37 total credit hours.

POST-MASTER'S PROGRAM

Areas of Study *Nurse practitioner programs in:* adult health, family health.

Olivet Nazarene University

Division of Nursing
Bourbonnais, Illinois

http://web.olivet.edu/nursing/
Founded in 1907

DEGREES • BSN • MSN
Nursing Program Faculty 15 (44% with doctorates).
Baccalaureate Enrollment 344 **Women** 95% **Men** 5% **Minority** 34% **Part-time** 60%
Graduate Enrollment 108 **Women** 94% **Men** 6% **Minority** 27% **Part-time** 99%
Nursing Student Activities Sigma Theta Tau, Student Nurses' Association.
Nursing Student Resources Academic advising; academic or career counseling; assistance for students with disabilities; bookstore; campus computer network; career placement assistance; computer lab; computer-assisted instruction; e-mail services; employment services for current students; externships; housing assistance; interactive nursing skills videos; Internet; learning resource lab; library services; nursing audiovisuals; placement services for program completers; remedial services; resume preparation assistance; skills, simulation, or other laboratory; tutoring.
Library Facilities 160,039 volumes (2,989 in health, 2,129 in nursing); 925 periodical subscriptions (3,864 health-care related).

BACCALAUREATE PROGRAMS

Degree BSN
Available Programs Accelerated RN Baccalaureate; Generic Baccalaureate.
Site Options Chicago, IL.
Study Options Full-time.
Program Entrance Requirements Minimum overall college GPA of 2.75, transcript of college record, CPR certification, health exam, health insurance, high school biology, high school chemistry, 2 years high school science, high school transcript, immunizations, minimum GPA in nursing prerequisites of 2.75, prerequisite course work. Transfer students are accepted. *Application deadline:* Applications may be processed on a rolling basis for some programs.
Expenses (2010-11) *Tuition:* full-time $12,375; part-time $1032 per credit hour. *Room and board:* $3200 per academic year. *Required fees:* full-time $420.
Financial Aid 98% of baccalaureate students in nursing programs received some form of financial aid in 2009-10. *Gift aid (need-based):* Federal Pell, FSEOG, state, private, college/university gift aid from institutional funds. *Loans:* Federal Direct (Subsidized and Unsubsidized Stafford PLUS), Perkins, private loans. *Work-study:* Federal Work-Study, part-time campus jobs. *Financial aid application deadline (priority):* 3/1.
Contact Mrs. Susan Wolff, Director of Admissions, Division of Nursing, Olivet Nazarene University, One University Avenue, Bourbonnais, IL 60914-2345. *Telephone:* 815-939-5203. *Fax:* 815-935-4998. *E-mail:* swolff@olivet.edu.

GRADUATE PROGRAMS

Expenses (2010-11) *Tuition:* part-time $22,280 per degree program. *Required fees:* full-time $250.
Financial Aid 56% of graduate students in nursing programs received some form of financial aid in 2009-10.
Contact Holly Nelson, Division of Nursing, Olivet Nazarene University, One University Avenue, Bourbonnais, IL 60914-2345. *Telephone:* 815-939-5036. *Fax:* 815-935-4991. *E-mail:* hnelson@olivet.edu.

MASTER'S DEGREE PROGRAM

Degree MSN
Available Programs Master's.
Study Options Full-time.
Program Entrance Requirements Computer literacy, minimum overall college GPA of 2.75, transcript of college record, nursing research course, statistics course.
Degree Requirements 32 total credit hours, thesis or project.

CONTINUING EDUCATION PROGRAM

Contact Dr. Pamela Lee, Professor of Nursing, Division of Nursing, Olivet Nazarene University, One University Avenue, Bourbonnais, IL 60914. *Telephone:* 815-939-5316. *Fax:* 815-939-5383. *E-mail:* plee@olivet.edu.

Quincy University

Blessing–Rieman College of Nursing
Quincy, Illinois

http://www.quincy.edu/

See description of programs under
Blessing–Rieman College of Nursing (Quincy, Illinois).

Resurrection University

Resurrection University
Oak Park, Illinois

Founded in 1982

DEGREES • BSN • MSN
Nursing Program Faculty 20 (20% with doctorates).
Baccalaureate Enrollment 237 **Women** 82.7% **Men** 17.3% **Minority** 64.5% **Part-time** 21.5%
Graduate Enrollment 20 **Women** 98% **Men** 2% **Minority** 52% **Part-time** 100%
Distance Learning Courses Available.
Nursing Student Activities Student Nurses' Association.
Nursing Student Resources Academic advising; academic or career counseling; bookstore; campus computer network; career placement assistance; computer lab; computer-assisted instruction; e-mail services; employment services for current students; externships; Internet; learning resource lab; library services; nursing audiovisuals; resume preparation assistance; skills, simulation, or other laboratory; tutoring.
Library Facilities 2,400 volumes in health, 1,100 volumes in nursing; 300 periodical subscriptions health-care related.

BACCALAUREATE PROGRAMS

Degree BSN
Available Programs ADN to Baccalaureate; Accelerated Baccalaureate; Accelerated Baccalaureate for Second Degree; Accelerated RN Baccalaureate; Baccalaureate for Second Degree; RN Baccalaureate.
Study Options Full-time and part-time.
Program Entrance Requirements Minimum overall college GPA of 2.75, transcript of college record, CPR certification, written essay, health exam, health insurance, immunizations, 1 letter of recommendation, minimum GPA in nursing prerequisites of 2.75, prerequisite course work. Transfer students are accepted. *Application deadline:* 2/1 (fall), 9/15 (spring), 2/1 (summer). Applications may be processed on a rolling basis for some programs. *Application fee:* $30.
Advanced Placement Credit by examination available. Credit given for nursing courses completed elsewhere dependent upon specific evaluations.
Expenses (2009-10) *Tuition:* full-time $22,000; part-time $711 per credit. *Required fees:* full-time $250.
Financial Aid 90% of baccalaureate students in nursing programs received some form of financial aid in 2008-09. *Gift aid (need-based):* Federal Pell, FSEOG, state, college/university gift aid from institutional funds. *Loans:* Federal Direct (Subsidized and Unsubsidized Stafford PLUS). *Work-study:* Federal Work-Study.
Contact Mrs. Wilda Tutol-Ortiz, Senior Admissions Counselor, Resurrection University, 3 Erie Court, Oak Park, IL 60302. *Telephone:* 708-763-6532. *Fax:* 708-763-1531. *E-mail:* admissions@wscn.edu.

GRADUATE PROGRAMS

Expenses (2009-10) *Tuition:* part-time $550 per credit.

Financial Aid 80% of graduate students in nursing programs received some form of financial aid in 2008-09.
Contact Dr. Cindy Valdez, EdD, Director of Office of Enrollment Management, Resurrection University, 3 Erie Court, Oak Park, IL 60302. *Telephone:* 708-763-6532. *Fax:* 708-763-1531. *E-mail:* admissions@wscn.edu.

MASTER'S DEGREE PROGRAM

Degree MSN
Available Programs Accelerated Master's for Nurses with Non-Nursing Degrees; Master's; Master's for Nurses with Non-Nursing Degrees; RN to Master's.
Concentrations Available Clinical nurse leader; health-care administration; nursing administration; nursing education.
Study Options Part-time.
Program Entrance Requirements Computer literacy, minimum overall college GPA of 3.0, transcript of college record, CPR certification, written essay, immunizations, 3 letters of recommendation, resume. *Application deadline:* 7/1 (fall). Applications may be processed on a rolling basis for some programs. *Application fee:* $30.
Advanced Placement Credit given for nursing courses completed elsewhere dependent upon specific evaluations.
Degree Requirements 32 total credit hours, thesis or project.

POST-MASTER'S PROGRAM

Areas of Study Clinical nurse leader; health-care administration; nursing administration; nursing education.

Rockford College

Department of Nursing
Rockford, Illinois

http://www.rockford.edu/
Founded in 1847

DEGREE • BSN
Nursing Program Faculty 7
Baccalaureate Enrollment 101 **Women** 94% **Men** 6% **Minority** 22% **Part-time** 7%
Nursing Student Activities Student Nurses' Association.
Nursing Student Resources Academic advising; academic or career counseling; assistance for students with disabilities; bookstore; campus computer network; career placement assistance; computer lab; computer-assisted instruction; e-mail services; employment services for current students; externships; housing assistance; interactive nursing skills videos; Internet; learning resource lab; library services; nursing audiovisuals; paid internships; placement services for program completers; remedial services; resume preparation assistance; skills, simulation, or other laboratory; tutoring.
Library Facilities 140,000 volumes (655 in health, 600 in nursing); 831 periodical subscriptions (55 health-care related).

BACCALAUREATE PROGRAMS

Degree BSN
Available Programs ADN to Baccalaureate; Generic Baccalaureate; RN Baccalaureate.
Study Options Full-time.
Program Entrance Requirements Minimum overall college GPA of 2.75, transcript of college record, CPR certification, health exam, health insurance, high school biology, high school chemistry, 4 years high school math, 2 years high school science, high school transcript, immunizations, minimum high school GPA of 2.75, minimum high school rank 50%, minimum GPA in nursing prerequisites of 2.75, prerequisite course work. Transfer students are accepted. *Application deadline:* 3/1 (fall), 9/1 (spring).
Advanced Placement Credit given for nursing courses completed elsewhere dependent upon specific evaluations.
Expenses (2010-11) *Tuition:* full-time $24,750; part-time $675 per credit hour. *Room and board:* $6950; room only: $3000 per academic year. *Required fees:* full-time $300.
Financial Aid 98% of baccalaureate students in nursing programs received some form of financial aid in 2009-10. *Gift aid (need-based):* Federal Pell, FSEOG, state, private, college/university gift aid from institutional funds. *Loans:* Federal Direct (Subsidized and Unsubsidized Stafford PLUS), Perkins, college/university, alternative loans. *Work-study:* Federal Work-Study, part-time campus jobs. *Financial aid application deadline (priority):* 3/1.
Contact Ms. Jennifer Nordstrom, Associate Vice President for Undergraduate Admissions, Department of Nursing, Rockford College, 5050 East State Street, Rockford, IL 61108-2393. *Telephone:* 815-226-4050. *E-mail:* jnordstrom@rockford.edu.

Rush University

College of Nursing
Chicago, Illinois

http://www.rushu.rush.edu/nursing
Founded in 1969

DEGREES • DNP • MSN
Nursing Program Faculty 93 (66% with doctorates).
Graduate Enrollment 700 **Women** 91% **Men** 9% **Minority** 16% **Part-time** 68%
Distance Learning Courses Available.
Nursing Student Activities Nursing Honor Society, Sigma Theta Tau, Student Nurses' Association.
Nursing Student Resources Academic advising; academic or career counseling; assistance for students with disabilities; bookstore; campus computer network; computer lab; computer-assisted instruction; e-mail services; employment services for current students; housing assistance; interactive nursing skills videos; Internet; learning resource lab; library services; nursing audiovisuals; remedial services; resume preparation assistance; skills, simulation, or other laboratory; tutoring; unpaid internships.
Library Facilities 120,042 volumes; 1,100 periodical subscriptions (5,228 health-care related).

GRADUATE PROGRAMS

Expenses (2009-10) *Tuition:* full-time $30,696; part-time $674 per credit. *Room and board:* room only: $7848 per academic year.
Financial Aid 88% of graduate students in nursing programs received some form of financial aid in 2008-09. Fellowships, research assistantships with partial tuition reimbursements available, teaching assistantships with partial tuition reimbursements available, Federal Work-Study, institutionally sponsored loans, scholarships, and traineeships available. Aid available to part-time students. *Financial aid application deadline:* 4/15.
Contact Ms. Angela Mason-Johnson, Acting Director of Admissions, College of Nursing, Rush University, 600 South Paulina Street, Armour Academic Center, Room 440, Chicago, IL 60612. *Telephone:* 312-942-7100. *Fax:* 312-942-2219. *E-mail:* Rush_Admissions@rush.edu.

MASTER'S DEGREE PROGRAM

Degree MSN
Available Programs Master's; Master's for Non-Nursing College Graduates; Master's for Nurses with Non-Nursing Degrees; RN to Master's.
Concentrations Available Clinical nurse leader; nurse anesthesia. *Clinical nurse specialist programs in:* community health, critical care, gerontology, medical-surgical, pediatric, psychiatric/mental health, public health. *Nurse practitioner programs in:* acute care, adult health, family health, gerontology, neonatal health, pediatric, psychiatric/mental health.
Study Options Full-time and part-time.
Online Degree Options Yes.
Program Entrance Requirements Minimum overall college GPA of 3.0, transcript of college record, CPR certification, written essay, immunizations, interview, 3 letters of recommendation, resume, GRE General Test (waived if nursing GPA is greater than 3.0 or cumulative GPA is greater than 3.25). *Application deadline:* 4/1 (fall), 5/1 (winter), 10/1 (spring), 1/1 (summer). Applications may be processed on a rolling basis for some programs.
Advanced Placement Credit given for nursing courses completed elsewhere dependent upon specific evaluations.
Degree Requirements 55 total credit hours, thesis or project.

POST-MASTER'S PROGRAM

Areas of Study Nurse anesthesia. *Clinical nurse specialist programs in:* community health, critical care, gerontology, medical-surgical, pediatric, psychiatric/mental health, public health. *Nurse practitioner programs in:* acute care, adult health, family health, gerontology, neonatal health, pediatric, psychiatric/mental health.

DOCTORAL DEGREE PROGRAM

Degree DNP

Available Programs Doctorate; Post-Baccalaureate Doctorate.
Areas of Study Nursing administration.
Online Degree Options Yes (online only).
Program Entrance Requirements Clinical experience, minimum overall college GPA of 3.0, interview, 3 letters of recommendation, MSN or equivalent, statistics course, vita, writing sample, GRE General Test. Application deadline: 7/15 (winter), 1/15 (summer). Applications may be processed on a rolling basis for some programs. Application fee: $40.
Degree Requirements 41 total credit hours, dissertation, oral exam.

POSTDOCTORAL PROGRAM

Postdoctoral Program Contact Dr. Carol Farran, PhD Program Director, College of Nursing, Rush University, 600 South Paulina Street, 1064 AR, Chicago, IL 60612. *Telephone:* 312-942-6955. *Fax:* 312-942-3043. *E-mail:* Carol_J_Farran@rush.edu.

CONTINUING EDUCATION PROGRAM

Contact Dr. Marilyn Wideman, RN, Director of Faculty Practice, College of Nursing, Rush University, 600 South Paulina Street, Suite 1080, Chicago, IL 60612-3832. *Telephone:* 312-942-7013. *Fax:* 312-942-3043. *E-mail:* Marlyn_Wideman@rush.edu.

Saint Anthony College of Nursing

Saint Anthony College of Nursing
Rockford, Illinois

http://www.sacn.edu/
Founded in 1915

DEGREES • BSN • MSN

Nursing Program Faculty 17 (23% with doctorates).
Baccalaureate Enrollment 178 **Women** 93% **Men** 7% **Minority** 30% **Part-time** 24%
Graduate Enrollment 25 **Women** 96% **Men** 4% **Minority** 8% **Part-time** 100%

Nursing Student Activities Nursing Honor Society, Student Nurses' Association.
Nursing Student Resources Academic advising; academic or career counseling; campus computer network; computer lab; computer-assisted instruction; e-mail services; interactive nursing skills videos; Internet; learning resource lab; library services; nursing audiovisuals; skills, simulation, or other laboratory; tutoring.
Library Facilities 1,258 volumes (1,751 in health, 1,385 in nursing); 3,136 periodical subscriptions (60 health-care related).

BACCALAUREATE PROGRAMS

Degree BSN
Available Programs Baccalaureate for Second Degree; Generic Baccalaureate; RN Baccalaureate.
Site Options Freeport, IL.
Study Options Full-time and part-time.
Program Entrance Requirements Minimum overall college GPA of 2.5, transcript of college record, CPR certification, written essay, health exam, health insurance, immunizations, interview, 3 letters of recommendation, minimum GPA in nursing prerequisites of 2.7, prerequisite course work. Transfer students are accepted. *Application deadline:* 2/15 (fall), 9/15 (spring). *Application fee:* $50.
Advanced Placement Credit by examination available. Credit given for nursing courses completed elsewhere dependent upon specific evaluations.
Expenses (2010-11) *Tuition:* full-time $9443; part-time $590 per credit hour. *Required fees:* full-time $240; part-time $120 per term.
Financial Aid 91% of baccalaureate students in nursing programs received some form of financial aid in 2009-10.
Contact Ms. Cheryl Delgado, Supervisor for Enrollment Management, Saint Anthony College of Nursing, 5658 East State Street, Rockford, IL 61108-2468. *Telephone:* 815-227-2141. *Fax:* 815-227-2730. *E-mail:* cheryldelgado@sacn.edu.

GRADUATE PROGRAMS

Expenses (2010-11) *Tuition:* part-time $719 per credit hour. *Required fees:* full-time $60; part-time $30 per term.

Financial Aid 92% of graduate students in nursing programs received some form of financial aid in 2009-10.
Contact Ms. Melissa Wrolstad, Student Affairs Specialist, Graduate Affairs, Saint Anthony College of Nursing, 5658 East State Street, Rockford, IL 61108-2468. *Telephone:* 815-395-5476. *Fax:* 815-395-2275. *E-mail:* melissawrolstad@sacn.edu.

MASTER'S DEGREE PROGRAM

Degree MSN
Available Programs Master's.
Concentrations Available Clinical nurse leader; nursing education. *Clinical nurse specialist programs in:* adult health. *Nurse practitioner programs in:* family health.
Study Options Part-time.
Program Entrance Requirements Minimum overall college GPA of 2.7, transcript of college record, CPR certification, written essay, immunizations, interview, 3 letters of recommendation, professional liability insurance/malpractice insurance, prerequisite course work, resume, statistics course. *Application deadline:* 4/1 (fall). *Application fee:* $50.
Advanced Placement Credit given for nursing courses completed elsewhere dependent upon specific evaluations.
Degree Requirements 48 total credit hours, thesis or project.

POST-MASTER'S PROGRAM

Areas of Study Nursing education.

See full description on page 492.

Saint Francis Medical Center College of Nursing

Baccalaureate Nursing Program
Peoria, Illinois

http://www.sfmccon.edu/
Founded in 1986

DEGREES • BSN • DNP • MSN

Nursing Program Faculty 47 (19% with doctorates).
Baccalaureate Enrollment 339 **Women** 90% **Men** 10% **Minority** 13% **Part-time** 21%
Graduate Enrollment 151 **Women** 93% **Men** 7% **Minority** 6% **Part-time** 97%
Distance Learning Courses Available.
Nursing Student Activities Sigma Theta Tau, Student Nurses' Association.
Nursing Student Resources Academic advising; academic or career counseling; campus computer network; computer lab; computer-assisted instruction; e-mail services; housing assistance; interactive nursing skills videos; Internet; learning resource lab; library services; nursing audiovisuals; skills, simulation, or other laboratory; tutoring.
Library Facilities 6,790 volumes (2,045 in nursing); 139 periodical subscriptions (124 health-care related).

BACCALAUREATE PROGRAMS

Degree BSN
Available Programs Generic Baccalaureate; RN Baccalaureate.
Study Options Full-time and part-time.
Program Entrance Requirements Transcript of college record, CPR certification, written essay, health exam, high school transcript, immunizations, minimum GPA in nursing prerequisites of 2.5, professional liability insurance/malpractice insurance, prerequisite course work. Transfer students are accepted. *Application deadline:* 9/15 (fall), 2/15 (spring). *Application fee:* $50.
Advanced Placement Credit given for nursing courses completed elsewhere dependent upon specific evaluations.
Expenses (2010-11) *Tuition:* full-time $14,880; part-time $480 per credit hour. *Room and board:* room only: $2400 per academic year. *Required fees:* full-time $260; part-time $260 per credit.
Financial Aid 86% of baccalaureate students in nursing programs received some form of financial aid in 2009-10. *Gift aid (need-based):* Federal Pell, state, private, college/university gift aid from institutional funds. *Loans:* Federal Direct (Subsidized and Unsubsidized Stafford PLUS), college/university. *Financial aid application deadline (priority):* 3/1.
Contact Ms. Janice E. Farquharson, Director of Admissions/Registrar, Baccalaureate Nursing Program, Saint Francis Medical Center College of Nursing, 511 NE Greenleaf Street, Peoria, IL 61603. *Telephone:* 309-624-8980. *Fax:* 309-624-8973. *E-mail:* janice.farquharson@osfhealthcare.org.

GRADUATE PROGRAMS

Expenses (2010-11) *Tuition:* full-time $8640; part-time $480 per credit hour. *Room and board:* room only: $2800 per academic year. *Required fees:* full-time $260; part-time $130 per term.
Financial Aid 91% of graduate students in nursing programs received some form of financial aid in 2009-10.
Contact Dr. Janice F. Boundy, Associate Dean of Graduate Program, Baccalaureate Nursing Program, Saint Francis Medical Center College of Nursing, 511 NE Greenleaf Street, Peoria, IL 61603. *Telephone:* 309-655-2230. *Fax:* 309-655-3648. *E-mail:* janice.f.boundy@osfhealthcare.org.

MASTER'S DEGREE PROGRAM

Degree MSN
Available Programs Accelerated RN to Master's; Master's; Master's for Nurses with Non-Nursing Degrees.
Concentrations Available Clinical nurse leader; nursing education. *Clinical nurse specialist programs in:* medical-surgical. *Nurse practitioner programs in:* neonatal health.
Study Options Full-time and part-time.
Online Degree Options Yes (online only).
Program Entrance Requirements Clinical experience, computer literacy, minimum overall college GPA of 2.8, transcript of college record, CPR certification, written essay, immunizations, interview, 3 letters of recommendation, nursing research course, physical assessment course, professional liability insurance/malpractice insurance, prerequisite course work, resume, statistics course. *Application deadline:* Applications may be processed on a rolling basis for some programs. *Application fee:* $50.
Advanced Placement Credit given for nursing courses completed elsewhere dependent upon specific evaluations.
Degree Requirements 45 total credit hours, thesis or project.

DOCTORAL DEGREE PROGRAM

Degree DNP
Available Programs Doctorate.
Areas of Study Clinical practice.
Online Degree Options Yes (online only).
Program Entrance Requirements Clinical experience, minimum overall college GPA of 3.2, 3 letters of recommendation, scholarly papers, statistics course, vita, writing sample. Application deadline: Applications may be processed on a rolling basis for some programs. Application fee: $50.
Degree Requirements 39 total credit hours, oral exam, residency.

St. John's College

Department of Nursing
Springfield, Illinois

http://www.st-johns.org/collegeofnursing
Founded in 1886

DEGREE • BSN

Nursing Program Faculty 15 (13% with doctorates).
Baccalaureate Enrollment 81 **Women** 93% **Men** 7% **Minority** 4% **International** 1% **Part-time** 5%
Nursing Student Activities Student Nurses' Association.
Nursing Student Resources Academic advising; computer lab; daycare for children of students; interactive nursing skills videos; Internet; library services; resume preparation assistance; skills, simulation, or other laboratory.

BACCALAUREATE PROGRAMS

Degree BSN
Available Programs Generic Baccalaureate.
Study Options Full-time and part-time.
Program Entrance Requirements Transcript of college record, CPR certification, health exam, high school transcript, immunizations, 2 letters of recommendation, minimum GPA in nursing prerequisites of 2.4, professional liability insurance/malpractice insurance, prerequisite course work. Transfer students are accepted.
Advanced Placement Credit given for nursing courses completed elsewhere dependent upon specific evaluations.
Contact ***Telephone:*** 217-525-5628. *Fax:* 217-757-6870.

Saint Xavier University

School of Nursing
Chicago, Illinois

http://www.sxu.edu/son
Founded in 1847

DEGREES • BSN • MSN • MSN/MBA

Nursing Program Faculty 36 (61% with doctorates).
Baccalaureate Enrollment 685 **Women** 90% **Men** 10% **Minority** 39% **Part-time** 16%
Graduate Enrollment 193 **Women** 94% **Men** 6% **Minority** 34% **International** .03% **Part-time** 21%
Distance Learning Courses Available.
Nursing Student Activities Nursing Honor Society, Sigma Theta Tau, Student Nurses' Association.
Nursing Student Resources Academic advising; academic or career counseling; assistance for students with disabilities; bookstore; campus computer network; career placement assistance; computer lab; computer-assisted instruction; e-mail services; employment services for current students; externships; housing assistance; interactive nursing skills videos; Internet; learning resource lab; library services; nursing audiovisuals; other; placement services for program completers; remedial services; resume preparation assistance; skills, simulation, or other laboratory; tutoring; unpaid internships.
Library Facilities 170,753 volumes (4,720 in health, 2,800 in nursing); 717 periodical subscriptions (5,225 health-care related).

BACCALAUREATE PROGRAMS

Degree BSN
Available Programs Generic Baccalaureate; LPN to RN Baccalaureate.
Site Options Elk Grove Village, IL; Orland Park, IL; Chicago, IL.
Study Options Full-time and part-time.
Program Entrance Requirements Minimum overall college GPA of 2.75, transcript of college record, CPR certification, written essay, health exam, health insurance, high school biology, high school chemistry, high school foreign language, 3 years high school math, 4 years high school science, high school transcript, immunizations, minimum high school GPA of 2.75, minimum GPA in nursing prerequisites of 2.75, prerequisite course work. Transfer students are accepted. *Application deadline:* 5/1 (fall), 11/1 (spring). Applications may be processed on a rolling basis for some programs.
Advanced Placement Credit by examination available. Credit given for nursing courses completed elsewhere dependent upon specific evaluations.
Expenses (2010-11) *Tuition:* full-time $24,790; part-time $830 per credit hour. *Room and board:* $8692; room only: $5142 per academic year. *Required fees:* full-time $730; part-time $245 per term.
Financial Aid 94% of baccalaureate students in nursing programs received some form of financial aid in 2009-10. *Gift aid (need-based):* Federal Pell, FSEOG, state, private, college/university gift aid from institutional funds, United Negro College Fund, Federal Nursing. *Loans:* Perkins. *Work-study:* Federal Work-Study, part-time campus jobs. *Financial aid application deadline (priority):* 3/1.
Contact Mr. Brian Hotzfield, Director, Undergraduate Admission, School of Nursing, Saint Xavier University, 3700 West 103rd Street, Chicago, IL 60655. *Telephone:* 773-298-3050. *Fax:* 773-298-3076. *E-mail:* admission@sxu.edu.

GRADUATE PROGRAMS

Expenses (2010-11) *Tuition:* full-time $4458; part-time $743 per credit hour. *Required fees:* full-time $420; part-time $210 per term.
Financial Aid 42% of graduate students in nursing programs received some form of financial aid in 2009-10. Available to part-time students.
Contact Kelly Fox, Assistant Director, Graduate Admission, School of Nursing, Saint Xavier University, 3700 West 103rd Street, Chicago, IL 60655. *Telephone:* 773-298-3053. *Fax:* 773-298-3951. *E-mail:* graduateadmission@sxu.edu.

MASTER'S DEGREE PROGRAM

Degrees MSN; MSN/MBA
Available Programs Master's; Master's for Nurses with Non-Nursing Degrees.
Concentrations Available Clinical nurse leader; nursing administration. *Nurse practitioner programs in:* family health.
Site Options Elk Grove Village, IL; Chicago, IL.
Study Options Full-time and part-time.
Online Degree Options Yes.
Program Entrance Requirements Minimum overall college GPA of 3.0, transcript of college record, written essay, 2 letters of recommendation, prerequisite course work, GRE General Test or MAT. *Application deadline:* Applications may be processed on a rolling basis for some programs.
Advanced Placement Credit given for nursing courses completed elsewhere dependent upon specific evaluations.
Degree Requirements 36 total credit hours, thesis or project.

POST-MASTER'S PROGRAM

Areas of Study Nursing education. *Nurse practitioner programs in:* family health.

CONTINUING EDUCATION PROGRAM

Contact Darlene O'Callaghan, Assistant Dean, Special Initiatives, School of Nursing, Saint Xavier University, 3700 West 103rd Street, Chicago, IL 60655. *Telephone:* 773-298-3742. *Fax:* 773-298-3704. *E-mail:* ocallaghan@sxu.edu.

Southern Illinois University Edwardsville

School of Nursing
Edwardsville, Illinois

http://www.siue.edu/nursing
Founded in 1957

DEGREES • BS • DNP • MS

Nursing Program Faculty 75 (37% with doctorates).
Baccalaureate Enrollment 640 **Women** 86% **Men** 14% **Minority** 15% **International** 1% **Part-time** 23%
Graduate Enrollment 217 **Women** 83% **Men** 17% **Minority** 11% **International** 3% **Part-time** 60%
Distance Learning Courses Available.
Nursing Student Activities Sigma Theta Tau, Student Nurses' Association, nursing club.
Nursing Student Resources Academic advising; academic or career counseling; assistance for students with disabilities; bookstore; campus computer network; career placement assistance; computer lab; computer-assisted instruction; daycare for children of students; e-mail services; employment services for current students; externships; housing assistance; interactive nursing skills videos; Internet; learning resource lab; library services; nursing audiovisuals; placement services for program completers; remedial services; resume preparation assistance; skills, simulation, or other laboratory; tutoring.
Library Facilities 1.4 million volumes; 25,872 periodical subscriptions.

BACCALAUREATE PROGRAMS

Degree BS
Available Programs ADN to Baccalaureate; Accelerated Baccalaureate; Generic Baccalaureate.
Site Options Carbondale, IL.
Study Options Full-time.
Program Entrance Requirements Minimum overall college GPA of 2.5, transcript of college record, CPR certification, written essay, health exam, health insurance, immunizations, minimum GPA in nursing prerequisites of 2.7, prerequisite course work. Transfer students are accepted. *Application deadline:* 3/1 (fall).
Advanced Placement Credit given for nursing courses completed elsewhere dependent upon specific evaluations.
Expenses (2010-11) *Tuition, state resident:* full-time $6201; part-time $207 per credit hour. *Tuition, nonresident:* full-time $15,502; part-time $517 per credit hour. *Room and board:* $7790; room only: $4970 per academic year. *Required fees:* full-time $3171.
Financial Aid ***Gift aid (need-based):*** Federal Pell, FSEOG, state, private, college/university gift aid from institutional funds, Federal Nursing. *Loans:* Federal Nursing Student Loans, Federal Direct (Subsidized and Unsubsidized Stafford PLUS), Perkins, college/university, alternative loans. *Work-study:* Federal Work-Study, part-time campus jobs. *Financial aid application deadline (priority):* 3/1.
Contact Mrs. Karen Montgomery, Coordinator, Academic Advising, School of Nursing, Southern Illinois University Edwardsville, Box 1066, Edwardsville, IL 62026-1066. *Telephone:* 618-650-3956. *Fax:* 618-650-3854. *E-mail:* kmontgo@siue.edu.

GRADUATE PROGRAMS

Expenses (2010-11) *Tuition, state resident:* full-time $4500; part-time $251 per credit hour. *Tuition, nonresident:* full-time $11,272; part-time $626 per credit hour. *International tuition:* $11,272 full-time. *Room and board:* $7645; room only: $4825 per academic year. *Required fees:* full-time $1750.
Financial Aid 2 fellowships (averaging $8,370 per year), 1 teaching assistantship (averaging $8,064 per year) were awarded; research assistantships, career-related internships or fieldwork, Federal Work-Study, institutionally sponsored loans, scholarships, traineeships, and unspecified assistantships also available.
Contact Dr. Kathy Ketchum, Assistant Dean, Graduate Programs, School of Nursing, Southern Illinois University Edwardsville, Alumni Hall, Room 2107, Edwardsville, IL 62026-1066. *Telephone:* 618-650-3956. *Fax:* 618-650-3854. *E-mail:* kketchu@siue.edu.

MASTER'S DEGREE PROGRAM

Degree MS
Available Programs Master's.
Concentrations Available Health-care administration; nurse anesthesia; nursing education. *Nurse practitioner programs in:* family health.
Site Options Springfield, IL.
Study Options Full-time and part-time.
Program Entrance Requirements Clinical experience, minimum overall college GPA of 3.0, transcript of college record, CPR certification, written essay, immunizations, interview, 3 letters of recommendation, prerequisite course work, statistics course. *Application deadline:* 3/1 (fall), 6/1 (summer).
Advanced Placement Credit given for nursing courses completed elsewhere dependent upon specific evaluations.
Degree Requirements 35 total credit hours, thesis or project.

POST-MASTER'S PROGRAM

Areas of Study Health-care administration; nurse anesthesia; nursing education. *Nurse practitioner programs in:* family health.

DOCTORAL DEGREE PROGRAM

Degree DNP
Available Programs Doctorate.
Program Entrance Requirements Clinical experience, minimum overall college GPA of 3.0, interview by faculty committee, 3 letters of recommendation, MSN or equivalent, statistics course, writing sample. Application deadline: 3/1 (fall).
Degree Requirements Oral exam, residency.

CONTINUING EDUCATION PROGRAM

Contact Dr. Karen Kelly, Associate Professor and Coordinator, Continuing Education, School of Nursing, Southern Illinois University Edwardsville, Box 1066, Edwardsville, IL 62026-1066. *Telephone:* 618-650-3908. *Fax:* 618-650-3854. *E-mail:* kkelly@siue.edu.

Trinity Christian College

Department of Nursing
Palos Heights, Illinois

http://www.trnty/depts/nursing/
Founded in 1959

DEGREE • BSN

Nursing Program Faculty 8 (37% with doctorates).
Baccalaureate Enrollment 145 **Women** 94.5% **Men** 5.5% **Minority** 14% **International** 3%
Nursing Student Activities Student Nurses' Association.
Nursing Student Resources Academic advising; academic or career counseling; assistance for students with disabilities; bookstore; campus computer network; career placement assistance; computer lab; computer-assisted instruction; e-mail services; interactive nursing skills videos; Internet; learning resource lab; library services; nursing audiovisuals; resume preparation assistance; skills, simulation, or other laboratory; tutoring; unpaid internships.
Library Facilities 66,232 volumes (2,500 in health, 500 in nursing); 221 periodical subscriptions (100 health-care related).

BACCALAUREATE PROGRAMS

Degree BSN
Available Programs Generic Baccalaureate; RN Baccalaureate.
Study Options Full-time.
Program Entrance Requirements Minimum overall college GPA of 2.5, transcript of college record, CPR certification, health exam, health insurance, high school biology, 3 years high school math, 2 years high school science, high school transcript, immunizations, minimum high school GPA of 2.0, minimum GPA in nursing prerequisites of 2.5, prerequisite course work. Transfer students are accepted.
Advanced Placement Credit given for nursing courses completed elsewhere dependent upon specific evaluations.
Contact *Telephone:* 866-874-6463. *Fax:* 708-385-5665.

Trinity College of Nursing and Health Sciences

Trinity College of Nursing and Health Sciences
Rock Island, Illinois

http://www.trinityqc.com/college/default.htm
Founded in 1994

DEGREE • BSN

Nursing Program Faculty 16 (25% with doctorates).
Baccalaureate Enrollment 58 **Women** 94% **Men** 6% **Minority** 6% **Part-time** 87%
Distance Learning Courses Available.
Nursing Student Activities Nursing Honor Society.
Nursing Student Resources Academic advising; academic or career counseling; assistance for students with disabilities; bookstore; campus computer network; computer lab; computer-assisted instruction; daycare for children of students; e-mail services; interactive nursing skills videos; Internet; learning resource lab; library services; nursing audiovisuals; placement services for program completers; remedial services; skills, simulation, or other laboratory; tutoring.
Library Facilities 6,000 volumes in health, 3,400 volumes in nursing; 746 periodical subscriptions health-care related.

BACCALAUREATE PROGRAMS

Degree BSN
Available Programs ADN to Baccalaureate; Accelerated Baccalaureate for Second Degree; Generic Baccalaureate; RN Baccalaureate.
Study Options Full-time and part-time.
Program Entrance Requirements Minimum overall college GPA of 2.75, transcript of college record, letters of recommendation, prerequisite course work. Transfer students are accepted. *Application deadline:* Applications may be processed on a rolling basis for some programs. *Application fee:* $50.
Advanced Placement Credit given for nursing courses completed elsewhere dependent upon specific evaluations.
Expenses (2010-11) *Tuition:* part-time $567 per credit hour. *Required fees:* full-time $1572; part-time $786 per term.
Financial Aid 90% of baccalaureate students in nursing programs received some form of financial aid in 2009-10. *Gift aid (need-based):* Federal Pell, FSEOG, state, private, college/university gift aid from institutional funds. *Loans:* Federal Nursing Student Loans, Federal Direct (Subsidized and Unsubsidized Stafford PLUS). *Financial aid application deadline:* Continuous.
Contact Mrs. Tracy L. Poelvoorde, Dean of Nursing and Health Sciences, Trinity College of Nursing and Health Sciences, 2122 25th Avenue, Rock Island, IL 61201. *Telephone:* 309-779-7708. *Fax:* 309-779-7798. *E-mail:* poelvoordet@ihs.org.

University of Illinois at Chicago

College of Nursing
Chicago, Illinois

http://www.uic.edu/nursing
Founded in 1946

DEGREES • BSN • MS • MS/MBA • MS/MPH • PHD

Nursing Program Faculty 200 (75% with doctorates).
Baccalaureate Enrollment 300 **Women** 90% **Men** 10% **Minority** 23% **International** 3% **Part-time** 20%
Graduate Enrollment 600 **Women** 95% **Men** 5% **Minority** 10% **International** 6%
Distance Learning Courses Available.

Nursing Student Activities Sigma Theta Tau, Student Nurses' Association.
Nursing Student Resources Academic advising; academic or career counseling; assistance for students with disabilities; bookstore; campus computer network; computer lab; computer-assisted instruction; daycare for children of students; e-mail services; employment services for current students; externships; Internet; learning resource lab; library services; nursing audiovisuals; resume preparation assistance; skills, simulation, or other laboratory; tutoring.
Library Facilities 3.3 million volumes (500,000 in health); 66,350 periodical subscriptions (5,100 health-care related).

BACCALAUREATE PROGRAMS

Degree BSN
Available Programs ADN to Baccalaureate; Baccalaureate for Second Degree; Generic Baccalaureate; RN Baccalaureate.
Site Options Urbana, IL.
Study Options Full-time and part-time.
Online Degree Options Yes.
Program Entrance Requirements Minimum overall college GPA of 2.5, transcript of college record, written essay, immunizations, 2 letters of recommendation, minimum GPA in nursing prerequisites of 2.5, prerequisite course work. Transfer students are accepted.
Contact ***Telephone:*** 312-996-5786. *Fax:* 312-996-8066.

GRADUATE PROGRAMS

Contact ***Telephone:*** 312-996-5786. *Fax:* 312-996-8066.

MASTER'S DEGREE PROGRAM

Degrees MS; MS/MBA; MS/MPH
Available Programs Master's; Master's for Non-Nursing College Graduates; Master's for Nurses with Non-Nursing Degrees.
Concentrations Available Health-care administration; nurse-midwifery; nursing administration; nursing informatics. *Clinical nurse specialist programs in:* acute care, adult health, cardiovascular, community health, family health, gerontology, maternity-newborn, medical-surgical, occupational health, pediatric, perinatal, psychiatric/mental health, public health, school health, women's health. *Nurse practitioner programs in:* acute care, adult health, family health, gerontology, occupational health, pediatric, psychiatric/mental health, school health, women's health.
Site Options Urbana, IL; Rockford, IL; Peoria, IL.
Study Options Full-time and part-time.
Program Entrance Requirements Clinical experience, computer literacy, minimum overall college GPA of 3.0, transcript of college record, CPR certification, written essay, immunizations, interview, 3 letters of recommendation, nursing research course, physical assessment course, prerequisite course work, resume, statistics course, GRE General Test.
Advanced Placement Credit given for nursing courses completed elsewhere dependent upon specific evaluations.
Degree Requirements Thesis or project.

POST-MASTER'S PROGRAM

Areas of Study Health-care administration; nurse-midwifery; nursing administration; nursing education; nursing informatics. *Clinical nurse specialist programs in:* acute care, adult health, cardiovascular, family health, forensic nursing, gerontology, medical-surgical, occupational health, palliative care, pediatric, psychiatric/mental health, public health, school health, women's health. *Nurse practitioner programs in:* acute care, adult health, family health, gerontology, occupational health, pediatric, psychiatric/mental health, school health, women's health.

DOCTORAL DEGREE PROGRAM

Degree PhD
Available Programs Doctorate; Post-Baccalaureate Doctorate.
Areas of Study Advanced practice nursing, aging, bio-behavioral research, clinical practice, community health, faculty preparation, family health, forensic nursing, gerontology, health policy, health-care systems, individualized study, information systems, maternity-newborn, nursing administration, nursing policy, nursing research, nursing science, women's health.
Site Options Urbana, IL; Rockford, IL; Peoria, IL.
Program Entrance Requirements Minimum overall college GPA of 3.0, interview by faculty committee, interview, 3 letters of recommendation, MSN or equivalent, statistics course, vita, writing sample, GRE General Test.
Degree Requirements 96 total credit hours, dissertation.

POSTDOCTORAL PROGRAM

Areas of Study Individualized study, information systems, nursing informatics, nursing interventions, nursing research, nursing science, vulnerable population.
Postdoctoral Program Contact ***Telephone:*** 312-996-8431.

CONTINUING EDUCATION PROGRAM

Contact ***Telephone:*** 312-413-2978.

University of St. Francis
College of Nursing and Allied Health
Joliet, Illinois

https://www.stfrancis.edu/academics/college-of-nursing/
Founded in 1920

DEGREES • BSN • DNP • MSN
Nursing Program Faculty 46 (30% with doctorates).
Baccalaureate Enrollment 459 **Women** 92% **Men** 8% **Minority** 22% **International** 1% **Part-time** 29%
Graduate Enrollment 198 **Women** 92% **Men** 8% **Minority** 24% **International** 1% **Part-time** 91%
Distance Learning Courses Available.
Nursing Student Activities Sigma Theta Tau, Student Nurses' Association.
Nursing Student Resources Academic advising; academic or career counseling; assistance for students with disabilities; bookstore; campus computer network; career placement assistance; computer lab; computer-assisted instruction; e-mail services; employment services for current students; externships; housing assistance; interactive nursing skills videos; Internet; learning resource lab; library services; nursing audiovisuals; remedial services; resume preparation assistance; skills, simulation, or other laboratory; tutoring.
Library Facilities 134,400 volumes (723 in health, 624 in nursing); 15,002 periodical subscriptions (123 health-care related).

BACCALAUREATE PROGRAMS

Degree BSN
Available Programs Accelerated RN Baccalaureate; Generic Baccalaureate.
Study Options Full-time and part-time.
Online Degree Options Yes.
Program Entrance Requirements Minimum overall college GPA of 2.75, transcript of college record, CPR certification, health exam, high school biology, high school chemistry, 3 years high school math, 2 years high school science, high school transcript, immunizations, minimum high school GPA of 2.5, minimum high school rank 50%, minimum GPA in nursing prerequisites of 2.0, prerequisite course work. Transfer students are accepted. *Application deadline:* Applications may be processed on a rolling basis for some programs.
Advanced Placement Credit by examination available. Credit given for nursing courses completed elsewhere dependent upon specific evaluations.
Expenses (2010-11) *Tuition:* full-time $24,292; part-time $790 per credit hour. *Room and board:* $8176 per academic year. *Required fees:* full-time $450.
Financial Aid 85% of baccalaureate students in nursing programs received some form of financial aid in 2009-10. *Gift aid (need-based):* Federal Pell, FSEOG, state, private, college/university gift aid from institutional funds. *Loans:* Federal Direct (Subsidized and Unsubsidized Stafford PLUS), Perkins, alternative loans. *Work-study:* Federal Work-Study, part-time campus jobs. *Financial aid application deadline (priority):* 4/1.
Contact Julie Marlatt, Director, Undergraduate Admissions, College of Nursing and Allied Health, University of St. Francis, 500 Wilcox Street, Joliet, IL 60435. *Telephone:* 800-735-7500. *Fax:* 815-740-3431. *E-mail:* jmarlatt@stfrancis.edu.

GRADUATE PROGRAMS

Expenses (2010-11) *Tuition:* part-time $628 per credit hour.
Financial Aid 65% of graduate students in nursing programs received some form of financial aid in 2009-10.
Contact Ms. Sandee Sloka, Director, Graduate/Degree Completion Admissions, College of Nursing and Allied Health, University of St. Francis, 500 Wilcox Street, Joliet, IL 60435. *Telephone:* 800-735-7500. *Fax:* 815-740-3431. *E-mail:* ssloka@stfrancis.edu.

MASTER'S DEGREE PROGRAM

Degree MSN
Available Programs Master's; Master's for Nurses with Non-Nursing Degrees.
Concentrations Available Nursing education. *Clinical nurse specialist programs in:* adult health. *Nurse practitioner programs in:* adult health, family health.
Site Options Albuquerque, NM.
Study Options Part-time.
Online Degree Options Yes.
Program Entrance Requirements Clinical experience, computer literacy, minimum overall college GPA of 3.0, transcript of college record, CPR certification, written essay, immunizations, interview, 3 letters of recommendation, nursing research course, physical assessment course, professional liability insurance/malpractice insurance, prerequisite course work, resume, statistics course. *Application deadline:* Applications may be processed on a rolling basis for some programs. *Application fee:* $30.
Advanced Placement Credit given for nursing courses completed elsewhere dependent upon specific evaluations.
Degree Requirements 44 total credit hours, thesis or project.

POST-MASTER'S PROGRAM

Areas of Study *Clinical nurse specialist programs in:* adult health. *Nurse practitioner programs in:* adult health, family health.

DOCTORAL DEGREE PROGRAM

Degree DNP
Available Programs Doctorate.
Areas of Study Nursing education.
Online Degree Options Yes (online only).
Program Entrance Requirements Clinical experience, minimum overall college GPA of 3.0, interview by faculty committee, interview, letters of recommendation, MSN or equivalent, statistics course, vita. Application deadline: Applications may be processed on a rolling basis for some programs. Application fee: $50.
Degree Requirements 37 total credit hours, residency.

Western Illinois University

School of Nursing
Macomb, Illinois

http://www.wiu.edu/nursing
Founded in 1899

DEGREE • BSN
Nursing Program Faculty 9 (10% with doctorates).
Baccalaureate Enrollment 50 **Women** 86% **Men** 14% **Minority** 12% **International** 5%
Distance Learning Courses Available.
Nursing Student Activities Nursing Honor Society, Student Nurses' Association.
Nursing Student Resources Academic advising; academic or career counseling; assistance for students with disabilities; bookstore; campus computer network; career placement assistance; computer lab; computer-assisted instruction; daycare for children of students; e-mail services; housing assistance; interactive nursing skills videos; Internet; learning resource lab; library services; nursing audiovisuals; resume preparation assistance; skills, simulation, or other laboratory.
Library Facilities 998,041 volumes; 3,200 periodical subscriptions.

BACCALAUREATE PROGRAMS

Degree BSN
Available Programs Baccalaureate for Second Degree; Generic Baccalaureate; RN Baccalaureate.
Site Options Moline, IL.
Study Options Full-time.
Online Degree Options Yes.
Program Entrance Requirements Minimum overall college GPA of 3.0, transcript of college record, CPR certification, written essay, health exam, health insurance, immunizations, 2 letters of recommendation, minimum GPA in nursing prerequisites of 3.0, professional liability insurance/malpractice insurance, prerequisite course work. Transfer students are accepted. *Application deadline:* 3/1 (fall).
Expenses (2010-11) *Tuition, state resident:* full-time $3850; part-time $241 per contact hour. *Tuition, nonresident:* full-time $5776; part-time $361 per contact hour. *Room and board:* $4690; room only: $2479 per academic year. *Required fees:* full-time $1211; part-time $76 per credit.
Financial Aid 90% of baccalaureate students in nursing programs received some form of financial aid in 2009-10. *Gift aid (need-based):* Federal Pell, FSEOG, state, private, college/university gift aid from institutional funds. *Loans:* Perkins, college/university. *Work-study:* Federal Work-Study, part-time campus jobs. *Financial aid application deadline (priority):* 2/15.
Contact Mr. Theo E. Schultz, Academic Advisor, School of Nursing, Western Illinois University, 1 University Circle, Macomb, IL 61455. *Telephone:* 309-298-2571. *E-mail:* t-schultz@wiu.ecu.

INDIANA

Anderson University

School of Nursing
Anderson, Indiana

http://www.anderson.edu/academics/nurs/
Founded in 1917

DEGREES • BSN • MSN • MSN/MBA
Nursing Program Faculty 12 (17% with doctorates).
Baccalaureate Enrollment 96 **Women** 94% **Men** 6% **Minority** 10% **Part-time** 13%
Graduate Enrollment 32 **Women** 94% **Men** 6% **Minority** 28% **Part-time** 100%
Distance Learning Courses Available.
Nursing Student Activities Nursing Honor Society, Sigma Theta Tau, Student Nurses' Association.
Nursing Student Resources Academic advising; academic or career counseling; assistance for students with disabilities; bookstore; campus computer network; career placement assistance; computer lab; computer-assisted instruction; e-mail services; housing assistance; interactive nursing skills videos; Internet; learning resource lab; library services; nursing audiovisuals; placement services for program completers; remedial services; resume preparation assistance; skills, simulation, or other laboratory; tutoring.
Library Facilities 307,239 volumes (6,954 in health, 1,259 in nursing); 652 periodical subscriptions (818 health-care related).

BACCALAUREATE PROGRAMS

Degree BSN
Available Programs ADN to Baccalaureate; Generic Baccalaureate.
Study Options Full-time and part-time.
Program Entrance Requirements Minimum overall college GPA of 3.0, transcript of college record, CPR certification, health exam, high school biology, high school chemistry, 2 years high school math, 3 years high school science, high school transcript, immunizations, minimum high school GPA of 3.5, minimum high school rank 33%, minimum GPA in nursing prerequisites of 3.0, professional liability insurance/malpractice insurance, prerequisite course work. Transfer students are accepted. *Application deadline:* 5/31 (spring), 8/30 (summer).
Advanced Placement Credit given for nursing courses completed elsewhere dependent upon specific evaluations.
Expenses (2010-11) *Tuition:* full-time $23,940. *Room and board:* $8350 per academic year.
Contact Dr. Karen S. Williams, Dean, School of Nursing, School of Nursing, Anderson University, 1100 East 5th Street, Anderson, IN 46012-3495. *Telephone:* 765-641-4385. *Fax:* 765-641-3095. *E-mail:* kswilliams@anderson.edu.

GRADUATE PROGRAMS

Financial Aid 90% of graduate students in nursing programs received some form of financial aid in 2009-10.
Contact Mrs. Lynn Schmidt, Graduate Coordinator and Assistant Professor, School of Nursing, Anderson University, 1100 East 5th Street, Anderson, IN 46012-3495. *Telephone:* 765-641-4388. *Fax:* 765-641-3095. *E-mail:* lmschmidt@anderson.edu.

MASTER'S DEGREE PROGRAM

Degrees MSN; MSN/MBA
Available Programs Master's; RN to Master's.
Concentrations Available Nursing administration; nursing education.
Site Options Indianapolis, IN.

Study Options Full-time and part-time.
Program Entrance Requirements Clinical experience, minimum overall college GPA of 2.75, transcript of college record, CPR certification, written essay, immunizations, 3 letters of recommendation, professional liability insurance/malpractice insurance. *Application deadline:* Applications may be processed on a rolling basis for some programs. *Application fee:* $50.
Advanced Placement Credit given for nursing courses completed elsewhere dependent upon specific evaluations.
Degree Requirements 55 total credit hours, thesis or project.

POST-MASTER'S PROGRAM

Areas of Study Nursing administration; nursing education.

Ball State University

School of Nursing
Muncie, Indiana

http://www.bsu.edu/nursing
Founded in 1918

DEGREES • BS • DNP • MS

Nursing Program Faculty 55 (29% with doctorates).
Baccalaureate Enrollment 428 **Women** 86% **Men** 14% **Minority** 4% **International** .5% **Part-time** 6%
Graduate Enrollment 387 **Women** 92% **Men** 8% **Minority** 7% **International** 100%
Distance Learning Courses Available.
Nursing Student Activities Nursing Honor Society, Sigma Theta Tau, Student Nurses' Association.
Nursing Student Resources Academic advising; academic or career counseling; assistance for students with disabilities; bookstore; campus computer network; career placement assistance; computer lab; computer-assisted instruction; e-mail services; employment services for current students; housing assistance; interactive nursing skills videos; Internet; learning resource lab; library services; nursing audiovisuals; placement services for program completers; remedial services; resume preparation assistance; skills, simulation, or other laboratory; tutoring.
Library Facilities 1.1 million volumes (16,885 in health, 9,221 in nursing); 3,093 periodical subscriptions (3,713 health-care related).

BACCALAUREATE PROGRAMS

Degree BS
Available Programs Accelerated Baccalaureate for Second Degree; Baccalaureate for Second Degree; Generic Baccalaureate; LPN to Baccalaureate; RN Baccalaureate.
Study Options Full-time and part-time.
Online Degree Options Yes.
Program Entrance Requirements Minimum overall college GPA of 3.00, transcript of college record, CPR certification, health exam, immunizations, prerequisite course work. Transfer students are accepted. *Application deadline:* 8/28 (fall), 1/21 (spring).
Advanced Placement Credit given for nursing courses completed elsewhere dependent upon specific evaluations.
Expenses (2009-10) *Tuition, state resident:* full-time $7228; part-time $1070 per course. *Tuition, nonresident:* full-time $9898; part-time $2628 per course. *International tuition:* $9898 full-time. *Room and board:* $8438; room only: $7390 per academic year. *Required fees:* full-time $900.
Financial Aid 90% of baccalaureate students in nursing programs received some form of financial aid in 2008-09. *Gift aid (need-based):* Federal Pell, FSEOG, state, private, college/university gift aid from institutional funds. *Loans:* Federal Direct (Subsidized and Unsubsidized Stafford PLUS), Perkins. *Work-study:* Federal Work-Study, part-time campus jobs. *Financial aid application deadline (priority):* 3/10.
Contact Dr. Nancy Dillard, RN, Baccalaureate Program Director, School of Nursing, Ball State University, CN 418, Muncie, IN 47306. *Telephone:* 765-285-5589. *Fax:* 765-285-2169. *E-mail:* ndillard@bsu.edu.

GRADUATE PROGRAMS

Expenses (2009-10) *Tuition, state resident:* part-time $256 per credit hour. *Tuition, nonresident:* part-time $454 per credit hour. *Required fees:* part-time $400 per term.
Financial Aid 3 teaching assistantships (averaging $9,874 per year) were awarded; research assistantships, career-related internships or fieldwork also available.
Contact Dr. Marilyn Ryan, RN, Associate Director, Graduate Program, School of Nursing, Ball State University, Muncie, IN 47306. *Telephone:* 765-285-5764. *Fax:* 765-285-2169. *E-mail:* mryan@bsu.edu.

MASTER'S DEGREE PROGRAM

Degree MS
Available Programs Master's; RN to Master's.
Concentrations Available Nursing administration; nursing education. *Clinical nurse specialist programs in:* adult health. *Nurse practitioner programs in:* adult health, family health.
Study Options Part-time.
Online Degree Options Yes (online only).
Program Entrance Requirements Clinical experience, computer literacy, minimum overall college GPA of 2.8, transcript of college record, CPR certification, written essay, immunizations, interview, 1 letter of recommendation, nursing research course, physical assessment course, prerequisite course work, statistics course. *Application deadline:* Applications may be processed on a rolling basis for some programs. *Application fee:* $35.
Advanced Placement Credit given for nursing courses completed elsewhere dependent upon specific evaluations.

POST-MASTER'S PROGRAM

Areas of Study Nursing education. *Nurse practitioner programs in:* adult health, family health.

DOCTORAL DEGREE PROGRAM

Degree DNP
Available Programs Doctorate.
Areas of Study Advanced practice nursing.
Online Degree Options Yes (online only).
Program Entrance Requirements Clinical experience, minimum overall college GPA of 3.2, interview by faculty committee, letters of recommendation, MSN or equivalent, statistics course, writing sample. Application deadline: 4/5 (fall). Application fee: $35.
Degree Requirements 38 total credit hours, residency.

Bethel College

Department of Nursing
Mishawaka, Indiana

http://www.bethelcollege.edu/
Founded in 1947

DEGREES • BSN • MSN

Nursing Program Faculty 30 (17% with doctorates).
Baccalaureate Enrollment 153 **Part-time** 39%
Graduate Enrollment 18 **Part-time** 100%
Nursing Student Activities Sigma Theta Tau, Student Nurses' Association.
Nursing Student Resources Academic advising; academic or career counseling; assistance for students with disabilities; bookstore; campus computer network; career placement assistance; computer lab; computer-assisted instruction; e-mail services; employment services for current students; housing assistance; interactive nursing skills videos; Internet; learning resource lab; library services; nursing audiovisuals; placement services for program completers; remedial services; resume preparation assistance; skills, simulation, or other laboratory; tutoring.
Library Facilities 136,958 volumes (3,000 in health, 2,050 in nursing); 1,381 periodical subscriptions (175 health-care related).

BACCALAUREATE PROGRAMS

Degree BSN
Available Programs ADN to Baccalaureate; Generic Baccalaureate; RN Baccalaureate.
Site Options Mishawaka, IN; Winona Lake, IN; St. Joseph, MI.
Study Options Full-time and part-time.
Program Entrance Requirements Minimum overall college GPA of 2.5, transcript of college record, CPR certification, written essay, health exam, health insurance, high school chemistry, high school transcript, immunizations, 1 letter of recommendation, minimum high school GPA of 2.5, minimum high school rank 35%, minimum GPA in nursing prerequisites of 2.5. Transfer students are accepted. *Application deadline:* 8/28 (fall). *Application fee:* $25.
Advanced Placement Credit by examination available. Credit given for nursing courses completed elsewhere dependent upon specific evaluations.

Financial Aid 77% of baccalaureate students in nursing programs received some form of financial aid in 2009-10. *Gift aid (need-based):* Federal Pell, FSEOG, state, private, college/university gift aid from institutional funds, Federal Nursing. *Loans:* Federal Nursing Student Loans, Perkins, college/university, GATE Loans. *Work-study:* Federal Work-Study, part-time campus jobs. *Financial aid application deadline (priority):* 3/1.
Contact Dr. Carol Dorough, Dean of Nursing, Department of Nursing, Bethel College, 1001 Bethel Circle, Mishawaka, IN 46545. *Telephone:* 574-257-3382. *Fax:* 574-257-2683. *E-mail:* carol.dorough@bethelcollege.edu.

GRADUATE PROGRAMS

Financial Aid 95% of graduate students in nursing programs received some form of financial aid in 2009-10.
Contact Dr. Karon Schwartz, Graduate Nursing Program Director, Department of Nursing, Bethel College, 1001 Bethel Circle, Mishawaka, IN 46545. *Telephone:* 574-257-3382. *Fax:* 574-257-7616. *E-mail:* schwark@bethelcollege.edu.

MASTER'S DEGREE PROGRAM

Degree MSN
Available Programs Master's.
Concentrations Available Nursing administration; nursing education.
Site Options Mishawaka, IN.
Study Options Part-time.
Program Entrance Requirements Clinical experience, minimum overall college GPA of 3.0, transcript of college record, CPR certification, immunizations, 3 letters of recommendation, nursing research course, physical assessment course, statistics course. *Application deadline:* 8/28 (fall). Applications may be processed on a rolling basis for some programs. *Application fee:* $25.
Advanced Placement Credit given for nursing courses completed elsewhere dependent upon specific evaluations.
Degree Requirements 36 total credit hours, thesis or project.

POST-MASTER'S PROGRAM

Areas of Study Nursing administration; nursing education.

Goshen College

Department of Nursing
Goshen, Indiana

http://www.goshen.edu/
Founded in 1894

DEGREE • BSN

Nursing Program Faculty 11 (18% with doctorates).
Baccalaureate Enrollment 120 **Women** 90% **Men** 10% **Minority** 11% **International** 3%
Graduate Enrollment 34 **Women** 86% **Men** 14% **International** 1%
Nursing Student Activities Sigma Theta Tau, Student Nurses' Association.
Nursing Student Resources Academic advising; academic or career counseling; bookstore; campus computer network; career placement assistance; computer lab; e-mail services; employment services for current students; externships; library services; nursing audiovisuals; placement services for program completers; remedial services; resume preparation assistance.
Library Facilities 137,000 volumes (80 in health, 80 in nursing); 350 periodical subscriptions (68 health-care related).

BACCALAUREATE PROGRAMS

Degree BSN
Available Programs Generic Baccalaureate; RN Baccalaureate.
Site Options Elkhart, IN.
Study Options Full-time and part-time.
Program Entrance Requirements Minimum overall college GPA of 2.5, transcript of college record, CPR certification, health exam, health insurance, high school chemistry, high school foreign language, 2 years high school math, high school science, high school transcript, immunizations, 2 letters of recommendation, minimum high school GPA of 2.5, minimum high school rank 50%. Transfer students are accepted. *Application deadline:* 3/1 (spring).
Advanced Placement Credit by examination available. Credit given for nursing courses completed elsewhere dependent upon specific evaluations.
Expenses (2010-11) *Tuition:* full-time $24,500; part-time $1020 per credit hour. *Room and board:* $8300; room only: $4350 per academic year.
Financial Aid 98% of baccalaureate students in nursing programs received some form of financial aid in 2009-10. *Gift aid (need-based):* Federal Pell, FSEOG, state, private, college/university gift aid from institutional funds. *Loans:* Federal Nursing Student Loans, Federal Direct (Subsidized and Unsubsidized Stafford PLUS), Perkins. *Work-study:* Federal Work-Study, part-time campus jobs. *Financial aid application deadline (priority):* 3/15.
Contact Admissions, Department of Nursing, Goshen College, 1700 South Main Street, Goshen, IN 46526. *Telephone:* 574-535-7535. *Fax:* 574-535-7609. *E-mail:* admissions@goshen.edu.

GRADUATE PROGRAMS

Expenses (2010-11) *Tuition:* full-time $8480; part-time $530 per credit hour. *Room and board:* $8300; room only: $4350 per academic year.
Financial Aid 25% of graduate students in nursing programs received some form of financial aid in 2009-10.
Contact Dr. Brenda Srof, Director, Masters in Nursing, Department of Nursing, Goshen College, 1700 South Main Street, Goshen, IN 46526. *Telephone:* 574-535-7375. *Fax:* 575-535-7375. *E-mail:* brendajs@goshen.edu.

Huntington University

Department of Nursing
Huntington, Indiana

http://www.huntington.edu/nursing/
Founded in 1897

DEGREE • BSN

Nursing Program Faculty 7 (33% with doctorates).
Baccalaureate Enrollment 30 **Women** 85% **Men** 15% **Minority** 15% **International** 10%
Nursing Student Activities Nursing club.
Nursing Student Resources Academic advising; academic or career counseling; assistance for students with disabilities; bookstore; campus computer network; career placement assistance; computer lab; computer-assisted instruction; daycare for children of students; e-mail services; employment services for current students; housing assistance; interactive nursing skills videos; Internet; learning resource lab; library services; nursing audiovisuals; other; placement services for program completers; remedial services; resume preparation assistance; skills, simulation, or other laboratory; tutoring; unpaid internships.
Library Facilities 181,291 volumes (1,544 in health, 100 in nursing); 28,414 periodical subscriptions (114 health-care related).

BACCALAUREATE PROGRAMS

Degree BSN
Available Programs RN Baccalaureate.
Study Options Full-time.
Program Entrance Requirements Minimum overall college GPA of 2.75, transcript of college record, CPR certification, health exam, high school chemistry, 2 years high school math, 2 years high school science, high school transcript, immunizations, interview, minimum high school GPA of 2.3, minimum high school rank 33%, minimum GPA in nursing prerequisites of 2.5, professional liability insurance/malpractice insurance, prerequisite course work. Transfer students are accepted. *Application deadline:* 3/31 (fall).
Expenses (2010-11) *Tuition:* full-time $20,820. *Room and board:* $7180 per academic year. *Required fees:* full-time $470.
Financial Aid 95% of baccalaureate students in nursing programs received some form of financial aid in 2009-10. *Gift aid (need-based):* Federal Pell, FSEOG, state, private, college/university gift aid from institutional funds. *Loans:* Perkins. *Work-study:* Federal Work-Study. *Financial aid application deadline (priority):* 3/1.
Contact Dr. Margaret Winter, Director, Department of Nursing, Department of Nursing, Huntington University, 2303 College Avenue, Huntington, IN 46750. *Telephone:* 260-359-4360. *Fax:* 260-359-4133. *E-mail:* mwinter@huntington.edu.

Indiana State University
Department of Nursing
Terre Haute, Indiana

http://www.indstate.edu/nhhs
Founded in 1865

DEGREES • BS • DNP • MSN

Nursing Program Faculty 42 (47% with doctorates).
Baccalaureate Enrollment 578 **Women** 88% **Men** 12% **Minority** 14% **International** 1% **Part-time** 47%
Graduate Enrollment 345 **Women** 92% **Men** 8% **Minority** 18% **International** 1% **Part-time** 82%
Distance Learning Courses Available.
Nursing Student Activities Sigma Theta Tau, Student Nurses' Association.
Nursing Student Resources Academic advising; academic or career counseling; assistance for students with disabilities; bookstore; campus computer network; career placement assistance; computer lab; computer-assisted instruction; daycare for children of students; e-mail services; employment services for current students; externships; housing assistance; interactive nursing skills videos; Internet; learning resource lab; library services; nursing audiovisuals; paid internships; placement services for program completers; remedial services; resume preparation assistance; skills, simulation, or other laboratory; tutoring; unpaid internships.
Library Facilities 1.2 million volumes (54,890 in health, 33,560 in nursing); 53,422 periodical subscriptions (104 health-care related).

BACCALAUREATE PROGRAMS

Degree BS
Available Programs ADN to Baccalaureate; Generic Baccalaureate; LPN to Baccalaureate; LPN to RN Baccalaureate; RN Baccalaureate.
Site Options Terre Haute, IN.
Study Options Full-time and part-time.
Online Degree Options Yes.
Program Entrance Requirements Minimum overall college GPA of 2.25, transcript of college record, CPR certification, health exam, high school chemistry, high school foreign language, 3 years high school math, 3 years high school science, high school transcript, immunizations, minimum high school GPA of 2.5, minimum high school rank 40%, minimum GPA in nursing prerequisites of 2.5, prerequisite course work. Transfer students are accepted. *Application deadline:* 6/1 (fall), 11/1 (spring).
Advanced Placement Credit by examination available. Credit given for nursing courses completed elsewhere dependent upon specific evaluations.
Expenses (2010-11) *Tuition, state resident:* full-time $7514; part-time $272 per credit hour. *Tuition, nonresident:* full-time $16,426; part-time $580 per credit hour. *Room and board:* $7463 per academic year. *Required fees:* full-time $1200; part-time $300 per term.
Financial Aid 7.5% of baccalaureate students in nursing programs received some form of financial aid in 2009-10. *Gift aid (need-based):* Federal Pell, FSEOG, state, private, college/university gift aid from institutional funds. *Loans:* Federal Direct (Subsidized and Unsubsidized Stafford PLUS), Perkins, alternative loans. *Work-study:* Federal Work-Study, part-time campus jobs. *Financial aid application deadline (priority):* 3/1.
Contact Ms. Lynn C. Foster, Director of Student Affairs, Department of Nursing, Indiana State University, 749 Chestnut Street, Terre Haute, IN 47809. *Telephone:* 812-237-2316. *Fax:* 812-237-8022. *E-mail:* lfoster@indstate.edu.

GRADUATE PROGRAMS

Expenses (2010-11) *Tuition, state resident:* part-time $341 per credit hour. *Tuition, nonresident:* part-time $426 per credit hour. *Room and board:* $8262 per academic year. *Required fees:* part-time $50 per term.
Financial Aid 7.5% of graduate students in nursing programs received some form of financial aid in 2009-10. 5 research assistantships with partial tuition reimbursements available (averaging $7,500 per year) were awarded; teaching assistantships with partial tuition reimbursements available, career-related internships or fieldwork and Federal Work-Study also available. Aid available to part-time students. *Financial aid application deadline:* 3/1.
Contact Ms. Cherie Howk, Chairperson, Advanced Practice Nursing, Department of Nursing, Indiana State University, 749 Chestnut Street, Terre Haute, IN 47809. *Telephone:* 812-237-2591. *Fax:* 812-237-4300. *E-mail:* cherie.howk@indstate.edu.

MASTER'S DEGREE PROGRAM

Degree MSN
Available Programs Master's.
Concentrations Available Nursing administration; nursing education. *Nurse practitioner programs in:* family health.
Site Options Terre Haute, IN.
Study Options Full-time and part-time.
Online Degree Options Yes (online only).
Program Entrance Requirements Minimum overall college GPA of 3.0, transcript of college record, CPR certification, written essay, immunizations, 3 letters of recommendation, nursing research course, prerequisite course work. *Application deadline:* 3/1 (fall), 10/1 (spring).
Advanced Placement Credit given for nursing courses completed elsewhere dependent upon specific evaluations.
Degree Requirements 36 total credit hours, thesis or project.

POST-MASTER'S PROGRAM

Areas of Study Nursing education. *Nurse practitioner programs in:* family health.

DOCTORAL DEGREE PROGRAM

Degree DNP
Available Programs Doctorate.
Areas of Study Advanced practice nursing.
Site Options Terre Haute, IN.
Online Degree Options Yes (online only).
Program Entrance Requirements Clinical experience, 3 letters of recommendation, MSN or equivalent, statistics course. Application deadline: Applications may be processed on a rolling basis for some programs.
Degree Requirements 39 total credit hours, residency.

CONTINUING EDUCATION PROGRAM

Contact Ms. Deb Bartnick, Director of Continuing Education, Department of Nursing, Indiana State University, Landsbaum Center, LCHE 208, 1433 North 61/2 Street, Terre Haute, IN 47807. *Telephone:* 812-237-3695. *Fax:* 812-237-8248. *E-mail:* deborah.bartnick@indstate.edu.

Indiana University Bloomington
Department of Nursing–Bloomington Division
Bloomington, Indiana

Founded in 1820

DEGREE • BSN

Nursing Program Faculty 25 (3.5% with doctorates).
Baccalaureate Enrollment 187 **Women** 97% **Men** 3% **Minority** 1%
Distance Learning Courses Available.
Nursing Student Activities Nursing Honor Society, Sigma Theta Tau, Student Nurses' Association.
Nursing Student Resources Academic advising; academic or career counseling; assistance for students with disabilities; campus computer network; computer lab; computer-assisted instruction; e-mail services; employment services for current students; interactive nursing skills videos; Internet; learning resource lab; library services; nursing audiovisuals; remedial services; resume preparation assistance; skills, simulation, or other laboratory; tutoring.
Library Facilities 7.6 million volumes (8,500 in nursing); 1,000 periodical subscriptions health-care related.

BACCALAUREATE PROGRAMS

Degree BSN
Available Programs Baccalaureate for Second Degree; Generic Baccalaureate; RN Baccalaureate.
Site Options Columbus , IN; Bedford, IN; Bloomington , IN.
Study Options Full-time.
Program Entrance Requirements Minimum overall college GPA of 2.5, transcript of college record, CPR certification, written essay, health exam, health insurance, high school chemistry, 3 years high school math, high school transcript, immunizations, interview, minimum GPA in nursing prerequisites of 2.7, prerequisite course work. Transfer students are accepted. *Application deadline:* 3/15 (fall).
Advanced Placement Credit by examination available. Credit given for nursing courses completed elsewhere dependent upon specific evaluations.

Expenses (2010-11) *Tuition, state resident:* full-time $8124; part-time $254 per credit. *Tuition, nonresident:* full-time $26,784; part-time $837 per credit. *Room and board:* $5018 per academic year. *Required fees:* full-time $4259.

Financial Aid 50% of baccalaureate students in nursing programs received some form of financial aid in 2009-10.

Contact Mrs. Deborah Hrisomalos, Academic Advisor, Department of Nursing–Bloomington Division, Indiana University Bloomington, Sycamore Hall, Room 401, Bloomington, IN 47405. *Telephone:* 812-855-2592. *Fax:* 812-855-6986. *E-mail:* dhrisoma@indiana.edu.

Indiana University East

School of Nursing
Richmond, Indiana

http://www.indiana.edu/nursing
Founded in 1971

DEGREE • BSN

Nursing Program Faculty 15 (7% with doctorates).

Baccalaureate Enrollment 201 **Women** 92.5% **Men** 7.5% **Minority** 5% **International** 1%

Nursing Student Activities Sigma Theta Tau, Student Nurses' Association.

Nursing Student Resources Academic advising; academic or career counseling; assistance for students with disabilities; bookstore; campus computer network; career placement assistance; computer lab; computer-assisted instruction; daycare for children of students; e-mail services; externships; interactive nursing skills videos; Internet; learning resource lab; library services; nursing audiovisuals; placement services for program completers; remedial services; resume preparation assistance; skills, simulation, or other laboratory; tutoring; unpaid internships.

Library Facilities 67,036 volumes (5,039 in health, 3,418 in nursing); 435 periodical subscriptions (70 health-care related).

BACCALAUREATE PROGRAMS

Degree BSN

Available Programs ADN to Baccalaureate; Generic Baccalaureate; RN Baccalaureate.

Study Options Full-time.

Program Entrance Requirements Minimum overall college GPA of 2.7, transcript of college record, CPR certification, high school biology, high school chemistry, 3 years high school math, 3 years high school science, high school transcript, immunizations, minimum high school GPA of 2.0, minimum high school rank 50%, minimum GPA in nursing prerequisites of 2.0, prerequisite course work. Transfer students are accepted. *Application deadline:* 3/1 (fall).

Advanced Placement Credit by examination available. Credit given for nursing courses completed elsewhere dependent upon specific evaluations.

Contact ***Telephone:*** 765-973-8353. *Fax:* 765-973-8220.

Indiana University Kokomo

Indiana University School of Nursing
Kokomo, Indiana

Founded in 1945

DEGREE • BSN

Nursing Program Faculty 14 (43% with doctorates).

Baccalaureate Enrollment 235 **Women** 95% **Men** 5% **Minority** 1% **International** 1% **Part-time** 32%

Nursing Student Activities Sigma Theta Tau, Student Nurses' Association.

Nursing Student Resources Academic advising; academic or career counseling; assistance for students with disabilities; bookstore; campus computer network; career placement assistance; computer lab; computer-assisted instruction; daycare for children of students; e-mail services; employment services for current students; externships; interactive nursing skills videos; Internet; learning resource lab; library services; nursing audiovisuals; paid internships; remedial services; resume preparation assistance; skills, simulation, or other laboratory; tutoring.

Library Facilities 132,424 volumes (2,881 in health, 1,513 in nursing); 1,513 periodical subscriptions (75 health-care related).

BACCALAUREATE PROGRAMS

Degree BSN

Available Programs Accelerated RN Baccalaureate; Generic Baccalaureate.

Site Options Peru, IN; Marion, IN; Logansport, IN.

Study Options Full-time.

Program Entrance Requirements Minimum overall college GPA of 2.5, transcript of college record, CPR certification, high school biology, high school chemistry, 4 years high school math, high school transcript, immunizations, minimum high school GPA of 2.0, minimum high school rank 50%, minimum GPA in nursing prerequisites of 2.7, prerequisite course work. Transfer students are accepted.

Financial Aid 75% of baccalaureate students in nursing programs received some form of financial aid in 2008-09.

Contact Mr. Morris S. Starkey, Coordinator, Nursing Student Services, Indiana University School of Nursing, Indiana University Kokomo, 2300 South Washington Street, PO Box 9003, Kokomo, IN 46904-9003. *Telephone:* 765-455-9384. *Fax:* 765-455-9421. *E-mail:* mstarke@iuk.edu.

CONTINUING EDUCATION PROGRAM

Contact Mr. Morris S. Starkey, Advisor, Nursing/Allied Health, Indiana University School of Nursing, Indiana University Kokomo, 2300 South Washington Street, PO Box 9003, Kokomo, IN 46904-9003. *Telephone:* 765-455-9384. *Fax:* 765-455-9421. *E-mail:* mstarke@iuk.edu.

Indiana University Northwest

School of Nursing and Health Professions
Gary, Indiana

http://www.iun.edu/~nurse
Founded in 1959

DEGREE • BSN

Nursing Program Faculty 25 (15% with doctorates).

Baccalaureate Enrollment 178 **Women** 90% **Men** 10% **Minority** 30% **International** .6% **Part-time** 6%

Nursing Student Activities Sigma Theta Tau, Student Nurses' Association.

Nursing Student Resources Academic advising; academic or career counseling; assistance for students with disabilities; bookstore; campus computer network; career placement assistance; computer lab; computer-assisted instruction; daycare for children of students; e-mail services; externships; interactive nursing skills videos; Internet; learning resource lab; library services; nursing audiovisuals; placement services for program completers; skills, simulation, or other laboratory; tutoring.

Library Facilities 251,508 volumes (42,000 in health, 15,000 in nursing); 1,541 periodical subscriptions (200 health-care related).

BACCALAUREATE PROGRAMS

Degree BSN

Available Programs Baccalaureate for Second Degree; Generic Baccalaureate; RN Baccalaureate.

Study Options Full-time.

Program Entrance Requirements Minimum overall college GPA of 2.5, transcript of college record, CPR certification, health exam, health insurance, high school biology, high school chemistry, high school foreign language, 4 years high school science, high school transcript, immunizations, minimum high school rank 25%, minimum GPA in nursing prerequisites, prerequisite course work. Transfer students are accepted.

Advanced Placement Credit given for nursing courses completed elsewhere dependent upon specific evaluations.

Contact ***Telephone:*** 219-980-6611. *Fax:* 219-980-6578.

Indiana University–Purdue University Fort Wayne

Department of Nursing
Fort Wayne, Indiana

http://www.ipfw.edu/nursing
Founded in 1917

DEGREES • BS • MS

Nursing Program Faculty 48 (10% with doctorates).
Baccalaureate Enrollment 251 **Women** 90% **Men** 10% **Minority** 14% **International** 2% **Part-time** 23%
Graduate Enrollment 37 **Women** 95% **Men** 5% **Minority** 10% **Part-time** 89%
Distance Learning Courses Available.
Nursing Student Activities Sigma Theta Tau.
Nursing Student Resources Academic advising; academic or career counseling; assistance for students with disabilities; bookstore; campus computer network; career placement assistance; computer lab; computer-assisted instruction; daycare for children of students; e-mail services; employment services for current students; housing assistance; interactive nursing skills videos; Internet; learning resource lab; library services; nursing audiovisuals; placement services for program completers; remedial services; resume preparation assistance; skills, simulation, or other laboratory; tutoring.
Library Facilities 441,647 volumes (1,100 in health, 500 in nursing); 19,822 periodical subscriptions (120 health-care related).

BACCALAUREATE PROGRAMS

Degree BS
Available Programs Generic Baccalaureate; LPN to RN Baccalaureate; RN Baccalaureate.
Study Options Full-time and part-time.
Program Entrance Requirements Minimum overall college GPA, transcript of college record, CPR certification, health exam, high school transcript, immunizations, minimum GPA in nursing prerequisites, professional liability insurance/malpractice insurance, prerequisite course work, RN licensure. Transfer students are accepted. *Application deadline:* 5/1 (fall), 12/1 (spring).
Advanced Placement Credit by examination available. Credit given for nursing courses completed elsewhere dependent upon specific evaluations.
Expenses (2009-10) *Tuition, state resident:* full-time $6045; part-time $202 per credit hour. *Tuition, nonresident:* full-time $15,597; part-time $520 per credit hour. *International tuition:* $15,597 full-time. *Room and board:* room only: $4900 per academic year. *Required fees:* full-time $881; part-time $29 per credit.
Financial Aid 60% of baccalaureate students in nursing programs received some form of financial aid in 2008-09.
Contact Ms. Joanne Bauman, Nursing Advisor, Department of Nursing, Indiana University–Purdue University Fort Wayne, 2101 East Coliseum Boulevard, Fort Wayne, IN 46805. *Telephone:* 260-481-6282. *Fax:* 260-481-6482. *E-mail:* baumanj@ipfw.edu.

GRADUATE PROGRAMS

Expenses (2009-10) *Tuition, state resident:* full-time $7658; part-time $255 per credit hour. *Tuition, nonresident:* full-time $18,272; part-time $609 per credit hour. *International tuition:* $18,272 full-time. *Room and board:* room only: $4900 per academic year. *Required fees:* full-time $881; part-time $29 per credit.
Financial Aid 46% of graduate students in nursing programs received some form of financial aid in 2008-09.
Contact Dr. Susan Ahrens, Director of Graduate Programs and Associate Professor, Department of Nursing, Indiana University–Purdue University Fort Wayne, 2101 East Coliseum Boulevard, Fort Wayne, IN 46805. *Telephone:* 260-481-6278. *Fax:* 260-481-6482. *E-mail:* ahrenss@ipfw.edu.

MASTER'S DEGREE PROGRAM

Degree MS
Available Programs Master's.
Concentrations Available Nursing administration; nursing education. *Nurse practitioner programs in:* adult health, women's health.
Study Options Part-time.
Program Entrance Requirements Computer literacy, minimum overall college GPA of 3, transcript of college record, CPR certification, immunizations, 3 letters of recommendation, nursing research course, professional liability insurance/malpractice insurance, prerequisite course work, resume, statistics course. *Application deadline:* 7/15 (fall), 11/15 (spring), 4/1 (summer). *Application fee:* $40.
Advanced Placement Credit by examination available. Credit given for nursing courses completed elsewhere dependent upon specific evaluations.
Degree Requirements 43 total credit hours, thesis or project.

POST-MASTER'S PROGRAM

Areas of Study Nursing administration.

CONTINUING EDUCATION PROGRAM

Contact Mersiha Alic, Registrar, Continuing Studies, Department of Nursing, Indiana University–Purdue University Fort Wayne, 2101 East Coliseum Boulevard, Fort Wayne, IN 46805. *Telephone:* 260-481-6627. *E-mail:* alicm@ipfw.edu.

Indiana University–Purdue University Indianapolis

School of Nursing
Indianapolis, Indiana

http://www.nursing.iupui.edu
Founded in 1969

DEGREES • BSN • MSN • MSN/MPH • PHD

Nursing Program Faculty 182 (37% with doctorates).
Nursing Student Activities Sigma Theta Tau, Student Nurses' Association.
Nursing Student Resources Academic advising; academic or career counseling; assistance for students with disabilities; bookstore; campus computer network; career placement assistance; computer lab; computer-assisted instruction; e-mail services; employment services for current students; externships; housing assistance; interactive nursing skills videos; Internet; learning resource lab; library services; nursing audiovisuals; other; paid internships; remedial services; resume preparation assistance; skills, simulation, or other laboratory; tutoring; unpaid internships.
Library Facilities 1.5 million volumes (318,211 in health, 8,258 in nursing); 14,673 periodical subscriptions (1,951 health-care related).

BACCALAUREATE PROGRAMS

Degree BSN
Available Programs ADN to Baccalaureate; Accelerated Baccalaureate for Second Degree; Generic Baccalaureate; RN Baccalaureate.
Site Options Columbus, IN.
Study Options Full-time and part-time.
Program Entrance Requirements Minimum overall college GPA of 2.5, transcript of college record, CPR certification, health insurance, 2 years high school math, 1 year of high school science, high school transcript, immunizations, interview, minimum GPA in nursing prerequisites of 2.7, prerequisite course work. Transfer students are accepted.
Advanced Placement Credit by examination available. Credit given for nursing courses completed elsewhere dependent upon specific evaluations.
Contact *Telephone:* 317-274-2806. *Fax:* 317-274-2996.

GRADUATE PROGRAMS

Contact *Telephone:* 317-274-2806. *Fax:* 317-274-2996.

MASTER'S DEGREE PROGRAM

Degrees MSN; MSN/MPH
Available Programs Master's; RN to Master's.
Concentrations Available Nursing administration. *Clinical nurse specialist programs in:* acute care, adult health, community health, critical care, oncology, pediatric, psychiatric/mental health. *Nurse practitioner programs in:* acute care, adult health, family health, neonatal health, pediatric, women's health.
Study Options Full-time and part-time.
Program Entrance Requirements Clinical experience, computer literacy, minimum overall college GPA of 3.0, transcript of college record, written essay, immunizations, 3 letters of recommendation, physical assessment course, resume, statistics course.
Advanced Placement Credit given for nursing courses completed elsewhere dependent upon specific evaluations.
Degree Requirements 42 total credit hours, thesis or project.

POST-MASTER'S PROGRAM

Areas of Study Nursing administration. *Clinical nurse specialist programs in:* adult health, community health, pediatric, psychiatric/mental health. *Nurse practitioner programs in:* acute care, adult health, family health, neonatal health, pediatric, women's health.

DOCTORAL DEGREE PROGRAM

Degree PhD
Available Programs Doctorate; Post-Baccalaureate Doctorate.
Areas of Study Aging, bio-behavioral research, faculty preparation, family health, health policy, health promotion/disease prevention, health-care systems, human health and illness, information systems, nursing administration, nursing education, nursing policy, nursing research, nursing science, oncology.
Program Entrance Requirements Minimum overall college GPA of 3.0, interview by faculty committee, 3 letters of recommendation, scholarly papers, statistics course, vita, GRE General Test.
Degree Requirements 90 total credit hours, dissertation, oral exam, written exam, residency.

POSTDOCTORAL PROGRAM

Areas of Study Adolescent health, cancer care, chronic illness, family health, health promotion/disease prevention, individualized study, nursing informatics, nursing research, nursing science.
Postdoctoral Program Contact ***Telephone:*** 317-274-2806. *Fax:* 317-274-2996.

CONTINUING EDUCATION PROGRAM

Contact ***Telephone:*** 317-274-7779. *Fax:* 317-274-0012.

Indiana University South Bend

Division of Nursing and Health Professions
South Bend, Indiana

http://www.iusb.edu/~health/
Founded in 1922

DEGREES • BSN • MSN

Nursing Program Faculty 24 (25% with doctorates).
Baccalaureate Enrollment 170 **Women** 94% **Men** 6% **Minority** 11% **International** 1% **Part-time** 36%
Nursing Student Activities Sigma Theta Tau, Student Nurses' Association.
Nursing Student Resources Academic advising; academic or career counseling; assistance for students with disabilities; bookstore; campus computer network; career placement assistance; computer lab; computer-assisted instruction; daycare for children of students; e-mail services; employment services for current students; externships; interactive nursing skills videos; Internet; learning resource lab; library services; nursing audiovisuals; placement services for program completers; resume preparation assistance; skills, simulation, or other laboratory; tutoring.
Library Facilities 300,202 volumes (4,300 in health, 2,300 in nursing); 1,937 periodical subscriptions (145 health-care related).

BACCALAUREATE PROGRAMS

Degree BSN
Available Programs Accelerated Baccalaureate for Second Degree; Generic Baccalaureate; RN Baccalaureate.
Site Options Indianapolis, IN.
Study Options Full-time and part-time.
Program Entrance Requirements Minimum overall college GPA of 2.5, transcript of college record, CPR certification, written essay, health exam, health insurance, high school biology, high school chemistry, high school transcript, immunizations, minimum high school GPA of 2.0, minimum high school rank 50%, minimum GPA in nursing prerequisites of 2.5, prerequisite course work. Transfer students are accepted.
Advanced Placement Credit given for nursing courses completed elsewhere dependent upon specific evaluations.
Contact ***Telephone:*** 574-520-4571. *Fax:* 574-520-4461.

GRADUATE PROGRAMS

Contact ***Telephone:*** 574-520-4569. *Fax:* 574-520-4461.

MASTER'S DEGREE PROGRAM

Degree MSN
Available Programs Master's.
Concentrations Available *Nurse practitioner programs in:* family health.
Study Options Part-time.
Program Entrance Requirements Clinical experience, computer literacy, minimum overall college GPA of 3.0, transcript of college record, CPR certification, written essay, immunizations, 3 letters of recommendation, nursing research course, physical assessment course, statistics course.
Advanced Placement Credit given for nursing courses completed elsewhere dependent upon specific evaluations.
Degree Requirements 42 total credit hours, thesis or project.

Indiana University Southeast

Division of Nursing
New Albany, Indiana

http://www.ius.edu/Nursing/homepage1.htm
Founded in 1941

DEGREE • BSN

Nursing Program Faculty 23 (27% with doctorates).
Baccalaureate Enrollment 162 **Women** 92% **Men** 8% **Minority** 2% **International** 2%
Distance Learning Courses Available.
Nursing Student Activities Sigma Theta Tau, Student Nurses' Association.
Nursing Student Resources Academic advising; academic or career counseling; assistance for students with disabilities; bookstore; campus computer network; career placement assistance; computer lab; computer-assisted instruction; daycare for children of students; e-mail services; externships; housing assistance; interactive nursing skills videos; Internet; learning resource lab; library services; nursing audiovisuals; paid internships; remedial services; resume preparation assistance; skills, simulation, or other laboratory; tutoring.
Library Facilities 215,429 volumes (35 in health, 15 in nursing); 962 periodical subscriptions (35 health-care related).

BACCALAUREATE PROGRAMS

Degree BSN
Available Programs Generic Baccalaureate; RN Baccalaureate.
Study Options Full-time.
Program Entrance Requirements Transcript of college record, CPR certification, immunizations, minimum GPA in nursing prerequisites of 2.5, prerequisite course work. Transfer students are accepted.
Advanced Placement Credit given for nursing courses completed elsewhere dependent upon specific evaluations.
Contact ***Telephone:*** 812-941-2283. *Fax:* 812-941-2687.

Indiana Wesleyan University

School of Nursing
Marion, Indiana

http://www.indwes.edu/academics/Nursing
Founded in 1920

DEGREES • BSN • MSN

Nursing Program Faculty 210 (21% with doctorates).
Baccalaureate Enrollment 1,581 **Women** 93% **Men** 7% **Minority** 16% **Part-time** 9%
Graduate Enrollment 427 **Women** 95% **Men** 5% **Minority** 13% **Part-time** 10%
Distance Learning Courses Available.
Nursing Student Activities Nursing Honor Society, Sigma Theta Tau, Student Nurses' Association, nursing club.
Nursing Student Resources Academic advising; academic or career counseling; assistance for students with disabilities; bookstore; campus computer network; career placement assistance; computer lab; computer-assisted instruction; e-mail services; housing assistance; interactive nursing skills videos; Internet; learning resource lab; library services; nursing audiovisuals; remedial services; resume preparation assistance; skills, simulation, or other laboratory; tutoring.
Library Facilities 164,272 volumes (7,142 in health, 5,672 in nursing); 85,642 periodical subscriptions (160 health-care related).

BACCALAUREATE PROGRAMS

Degree BSN
Available Programs Accelerated Baccalaureate for Second Degree; Generic Baccalaureate; RN Baccalaureate.
Site Options Lexington, KY; Merrillville, IN; Louisville, KY.
Study Options Full-time and part-time.
Program Entrance Requirements Minimum overall college GPA of 2.75, transcript of college record, CPR certification, written essay, health exam, health insurance, high school biology, high school chemistry, high school foreign language, 3 years high school math, 3 years high school science, high school transcript, immunizations, minimum high school GPA of 2.8, minimum GPA in nursing prerequisites of 2.75, prerequisite course work. Transfer students are accepted. *Application deadline:* 5/30 (fall), 12/1 (spring).
Advanced Placement Credit given for nursing courses completed elsewhere dependent upon specific evaluations.
Expenses (2009-10) *Tuition:* full-time $20,496; part-time $436 per credit. *International tuition:* $20,496 full-time. *Room and board:* $6770; room only: $3260 per academic year. *Required fees:* full-time $750.
Financial Aid 92% of baccalaureate students in nursing programs received some form of financial aid in 2008-09.
Contact Teresa Weaver, Secretary, School of Nursing, Indiana Wesleyan University, 4201 South Washington Street, Marion, IN 46953. *Telephone:* 765-677-2268. *Fax:* 765-677-2284. *E-mail:* teresa.weaver@indwes.edu.

GRADUATE PROGRAMS

Expenses (2009-10) *Tuition:* full-time $9765; part-time $465 per credit. *International tuition:* $9765 full-time. *Required fees:* full-time $323.
Financial Aid 48% of graduate students in nursing programs received some form of financial aid in 2008-09. 15 fellowships were awarded; career-related internships or fieldwork, scholarships, and traineeships also available. Aid available to part-time students. *Financial aid application deadline:* 3/15.
Contact Mr. Steve Evans, Recruitment, School of Nursing, Indiana Wesleyan University, 1900 West 50th Street, Marion, IN 46953. *Telephone:* 765-677-2045. *Fax:* 765-677-2380. *E-mail:* steve.evans@indwes.edu.

MASTER'S DEGREE PROGRAM

Degree MSN
Available Programs Master's.
Concentrations Available Nursing administration; nursing education. *Nurse practitioner programs in:* family health.
Site Options Lexington, KY; Merrillville, IN; Louisville, KY.
Study Options Full-time and part-time.
Online Degree Options Yes.
Program Entrance Requirements Clinical experience, minimum overall college GPA of 3.0, transcript of college record, written essay, immunizations, interview, 3 letters of recommendation, nursing research course, physical assessment course, resume, statistics course.
Advanced Placement Credit given for nursing courses completed elsewhere dependent upon specific evaluations.
Degree Requirements 41 total credit hours, thesis or project.

POST-MASTER'S PROGRAM

Areas of Study Nursing administration; nursing education. *Nurse practitioner programs in:* family health.

Marian University

Department of Nursing and Nutritional Science
Indianapolis, Indiana

http://www.sonak.marian.edu/academ/nursing/index.html
Founded in 1851

DEGREE • BSN

Nursing Program Faculty 16
Baccalaureate Enrollment 225 **Women** 95% **Men** 5% **Minority** 15% **International** 2% **Part-time** 10%
Nursing Student Activities Nursing Honor Society, Sigma Theta Tau, Student Nurses' Association.
Nursing Student Resources Academic advising; academic or career counseling; assistance for students with disabilities; bookstore; campus computer network; career placement assistance; computer lab; computer-assisted instruction; e-mail services; employment services for current students; interactive nursing skills videos; Internet; learning resource lab; library services; nursing audiovisuals; resume preparation assistance; skills, simulation, or other laboratory; tutoring.
Library Facilities 102,237 volumes (3,250 in health, 2,000 in nursing); 337 periodical subscriptions (116 health-care related).

BACCALAUREATE PROGRAMS

Degree BSN
Available Programs Accelerated Baccalaureate for Second Degree; Generic Baccalaureate; LPN to Baccalaureate; RN Baccalaureate.
Study Options Full-time and part-time.
Program Entrance Requirements Minimum overall college GPA of 2.5, transcript of college record, CPR certification, high school biology, high school chemistry, high school transcript, immunizations, minimum high school GPA of 2.7, minimum GPA in nursing prerequisites of 2.67, prerequisite course work. Transfer students are accepted.
Advanced Placement Credit by examination available. Credit given for nursing courses completed elsewhere dependent upon specific evaluations.
Contact *Telephone:* 317-955-6157. *Fax:* 317-955-6135.

Purdue University

School of Nursing
West Lafayette, Indiana

http://www.nursing.purdue.edu
Founded in 1869

DEGREES • BS • DNP • MS

Nursing Program Faculty 60 (15% with doctorates).
Baccalaureate Enrollment 552 **Women** 94% **Men** 6% **Minority** 3% **International** .5% **Part-time** .06%
Graduate Enrollment 48 **Women** 96% **Men** 4% **Minority** 2% **Part-time** 50%
Nursing Student Activities Sigma Theta Tau, Student Nurses' Association.
Nursing Student Resources Academic advising; academic or career counseling; assistance for students with disabilities; bookstore; campus computer network; career placement assistance; computer lab; computer-assisted instruction; e-mail services; interactive nursing skills videos; Internet; learning resource lab; library services; nursing audiovisuals; remedial services; resume preparation assistance; skills, simulation, or other laboratory; tutoring.
Library Facilities 2.5 million volumes (200,000 in health, 10,000 in nursing); 48,283 periodical subscriptions (1,000 health-care related).

BACCALAUREATE PROGRAMS

Degree BS
Available Programs ADN to Baccalaureate; Accelerated Baccalaureate for Second Degree; Baccalaureate for Second Degree; Generic Baccalaureate; RN Baccalaureate.
Site Options Indianapolis, IN.
Study Options Full-time and part-time.
Program Entrance Requirements Transcript of college record, CPR certification, health exam, health insurance, high school biology, high school chemistry, high school foreign language, 3 years high school math, 3 years high school science, high school transcript, immunizations, letters of recommendation, minimum high school GPA of 3.0. Transfer students are accepted.
Advanced Placement Credit by examination available. Credit given for nursing courses completed elsewhere dependent upon specific evaluations.
Contact *Telephone:* 765-494-1776. *Fax:* 765-494-0544.

GRADUATE PROGRAMS

Contact *Telephone:* 765-494-4015. *Fax:* 765-496-1800.

MASTER'S DEGREE PROGRAM

Degree MS
Available Programs Master's.
Concentrations Available *Nurse practitioner programs in:* adult health, pediatric.
Study Options Full-time and part-time.
Program Entrance Requirements Clinical experience, computer literacy, minimum overall college GPA of 3.0, transcript of college record, CPR certification, written essay, interview, 3 letters of recommendation,

professional liability insurance/malpractice insurance, prerequisite course work, resume, statistics course.
Advanced Placement Credit given for nursing courses completed elsewhere dependent upon specific evaluations.
Degree Requirements 46 total credit hours, thesis or project.

POST-MASTER'S PROGRAM

Areas of Study *Nurse practitioner programs in:* adult health, pediatric.

DOCTORAL DEGREE PROGRAM

Degree DNP
Available Programs Doctorate.
Areas of Study Advanced practice nursing, aging, biology of health and illness, clinical practice, critical care, ethics, gerontology, health policy, health promotion/disease prevention, health-care systems, illness and transition, individualized study, information systems, nursing administration, nursing education, nursing policy, nursing research, nursing science, oncology, urban health, women's health.
Program Entrance Requirements Clinical experience, minimum overall college GPA of 3.0, interview by faculty committee, interview, letters of recommendation, MSN or equivalent, statistics course, vita, writing sample.
Degree Requirements 83 total credit hours, oral exam, residency.

CONTINUING EDUCATION PROGRAM

Contact ***Telephone:*** 765-494-4030. *Fax:* 765-494-6339.

Purdue University Calumet

School of Nursing
Hammond, Indiana

http://www.calumet.purdue.edu/nursing/
Founded in 1951

DEGREES • BS • MS

Nursing Program Faculty 29 (31% with doctorates).
Baccalaureate Enrollment 451 **Women** 89% **Men** 11% **Minority** 27% **Part-time** 37%
Graduate Enrollment 133 **Women** 95% **Men** 5% **Minority** 28% **International** 3% **Part-time** 93%
Distance Learning Courses Available.
Nursing Student Activities Sigma Theta Tau, Student Nurses' Association, nursing club.
Nursing Student Resources Academic advising; academic or career counseling; assistance for students with disabilities; bookstore; campus computer network; career placement assistance; computer lab; computer-assisted instruction; daycare for children of students; e-mail services; employment services for current students; externships; housing assistance; interactive nursing skills videos; Internet; learning resource lab; library services; nursing audiovisuals; other; paid internships; placement services for program completers; remedial services; resume preparation assistance; skills, simulation, or other laboratory; tutoring; unpaid internships.
Library Facilities 7,900 volumes in health, 1,140 volumes in nursing; 204 periodical subscriptions health-care related.

BACCALAUREATE PROGRAMS

Degree BS
Available Programs Accelerated Baccalaureate for Second Degree; Accelerated RN Baccalaureate; Generic Baccalaureate; LPN to Baccalaureate; RN Baccalaureate.
Study Options Full-time and part-time.
Online Degree Options Yes.
Program Entrance Requirements Minimum overall college GPA of 2.5, transcript of college record, CPR certification, health exam, high school biology, high school chemistry, 3 years high school math, 3 years high school science, high school transcript, immunizations, minimum high school rank 65%, minimum GPA in nursing prerequisites of 2.0, prerequisite course work. Transfer students are accepted. *Application deadline:* 2/1 (fall).
Advanced Placement Credit by examination available. Credit given for nursing courses completed elsewhere dependent upon specific evaluations.
Expenses (2010-11) *Tuition, area resident:* full-time $6474; part-time $202 per credit hour. *Tuition, nonresident:* full-time $15,368; part-time $480 per credit hour. *Room and board:* room only: $4900 per academic year. *Required fees:* full-time $1158; part-time $27 per credit; part-time $579 per term.
Financial Aid 35% of baccalaureate students in nursing programs received some form of financial aid in 2009-10.
Contact Prof. Kathleen Ann Nix, Undergraduate Program Coordinator, School of Nursing, Purdue University Calumet, 2200 169th Street, Hammond, IN 46323-2094. *Telephone:* 219-989-2859. *Fax:* 219-989-2848. *E-mail:* nix@calumet.purdue.edu.

GRADUATE PROGRAMS

Expenses (2010-11) *Tuition, state resident:* full-time $5757; part-time $256 per credit hour. *Tuition, nonresident:* full-time $12,591; part-time $560 per credit hour. *International tuition:* $12,591 full-time. *Room and board:* room only: $4900 per academic year. *Required fees:* full-time $382; part-time $17 per credit; part-time $34 per term.
Financial Aid 50% of graduate students in nursing programs received some form of financial aid in 2009-10.
Contact Dr. Jane Walker, Graduate Program Coordinator, School of Nursing, Purdue University Calumet, 2200 169th Street, Hammond, IN 46323-2094. *Telephone:* 219-989-2815. *Fax:* 219-989-2848. *E-mail:* walkerj@calumet.purdue.edu.

MASTER'S DEGREE PROGRAM

Degree MS
Available Programs Master's.
Concentrations Available Nursing administration. *Clinical nurse specialist programs in:* adult health, critical care. *Nurse practitioner programs in:* family health.
Study Options Full-time and part-time.
Online Degree Options Yes.
Program Entrance Requirements Minimum overall college GPA of 3.0, transcript of college record, written essay, 3 letters of recommendation, physical assessment course, resume, statistics course. *Application deadline:* 2/15 (fall), 9/15 (spring), 2/15 (summer). *Application fee:* $55.
Advanced Placement Credit given for nursing courses completed elsewhere dependent upon specific evaluations.
Degree Requirements 45 total credit hours.

POST-MASTER'S PROGRAM

Areas of Study Nursing education. *Clinical nurse specialist programs in:* adult health, critical care. *Nurse practitioner programs in:* family health.

Purdue University North Central

Department of Nursing
Westville, Indiana

Founded in 1967

DEGREE • BS

Nursing Program Faculty 27 (11% with doctorates).
Baccalaureate Enrollment 52 **Women** 98% **Men** 2% **Minority** 12% **Part-time** 87%
Nursing Student Activities Nursing Honor Society, Student Nurses' Association.
Nursing Student Resources Academic advising; academic or career counseling; assistance for students with disabilities; bookstore; campus computer network; career placement assistance; computer lab; computer-assisted instruction; daycare for children of students; e-mail services; interactive nursing skills videos; Internet; learning resource lab; library services; nursing audiovisuals; placement services for program completers; resume preparation assistance; skills, simulation, or other laboratory; tutoring.
Library Facilities 88,379 volumes (1,100 in health, 560 in nursing); 26,045 periodical subscriptions (229 health-care related).

BACCALAUREATE PROGRAMS

Degree BS
Available Programs ADN to Baccalaureate; RN Baccalaureate.
Site Options Valparaiso, IN.
Study Options Full-time and part-time.
Program Entrance Requirements Minimum overall college GPA of 2.5, transcript of college record, high school biology, high school chemistry, 3 years high school math, 3 years high school science, high school transcript, minimum high school GPA of 2.5, minimum high school rank

50%, minimum GPA in nursing prerequisites of 2.5. Transfer students are accepted. *Application deadline:* 1/16 (fall), 8/16 (spring).
Advanced Placement Credit given for nursing courses completed elsewhere dependent upon specific evaluations.
Expenses (2009-10) *Tuition, state resident:* part-time $195 per credit hour. *Tuition, nonresident:* part-time $484 per credit hour. *Required fees:* part-time $16 per credit.
Financial Aid 44% of baccalaureate students in nursing programs received some form of financial aid in 2008-09.
Contact Nursing Contact, Department of Nursing, Purdue University North Central, 1401 South U.S. 421, Westville, IN 46391. *Telephone:* 219-785-5226. *E-mail:* nursing@pnc.edu.

Saint Mary's College

Department of Nursing
Notre Dame, Indiana

http://www3.saintmarys.edu/nursing
Founded in 1844

DEGREE • BS

Nursing Program Faculty 15 (9% with doctorates).
Baccalaureate Enrollment 228 **Women** 100% **Minority** 4%
Distance Learning Courses Available.
Nursing Student Activities Nursing Honor Society, Sigma Theta Tau, Student Nurses' Association.
Nursing Student Resources Academic advising; academic or career counseling; assistance for students with disabilities; bookstore; campus computer network; career placement assistance; computer lab; computer-assisted instruction; daycare for children of students; e-mail services; employment services for current students; externships; interactive nursing skills videos; Internet; learning resource lab; library services; nursing audiovisuals; paid internships; placement services for program completers; remedial services; resume preparation assistance; skills, simulation, or other laboratory; tutoring; unpaid internships.
Library Facilities 271,161 volumes (9,787 in health, 5,149 in nursing); 20,780 periodical subscriptions (70 health-care related).

BACCALAUREATE PROGRAMS

Degree BS
Available Programs Accelerated Baccalaureate; Generic Baccalaureate.
Site Options South Bend, IN; Goshen, IN.
Study Options Full-time.
Program Entrance Requirements Minimum overall college GPA of 3.0, transcript of college record, CPR certification, written essay, health exam, high school foreign language, 3 years high school math, 2 years high school science, high school transcript, immunizations, 2 letters of recommendation, minimum GPA in nursing prerequisites of 2.75. Transfer students are accepted. *Application deadline:* Applications may be processed on a rolling basis for some programs. *Application fee:* $30.
Advanced Placement Credit given for nursing courses completed elsewhere dependent upon specific evaluations.
Expenses (2010-11) *Tuition:* full-time $29,400; part-time $1100 per credit hour. *Room and board:* $9209 per academic year. *Required fees:* full-time $200.
Financial Aid 75% of baccalaureate students in nursing programs received some form of financial aid in 2009-10. *Gift aid (need-based):* Federal Pell, FSEOG, state, private, college/university gift aid from institutional funds. *Loans:* Federal Direct (Subsidized and Unsubsidized Stafford PLUS), Perkins. *Work-study:* Federal Work-Study, part-time campus jobs. *Financial aid application deadline:* 3/1(priority: 3/1).
Contact Mrs. Mona Bowe, Vice President for Enrollment Management, Department of Nursing, Saint Mary's College, 124 LeMans, Notre Dame, IN 46556. *Telephone:* 574-284-4587. *Fax:* 574-284-4716. *E-mail:* mbowe@saintmarys.edu.

University of Evansville

Department of Nursing
Evansville, Indiana

http://nursing.evansville.edu/
Founded in 1854

DEGREE • BSN

Nursing Program Faculty 10 (20% with doctorates).
Baccalaureate Enrollment 188 **Women** 86% **Men** 14% **Minority** 4% **International** 1% **Part-time** 20%
Distance Learning Courses Available.
Nursing Student Activities Sigma Theta Tau, Student Nurses' Association.
Nursing Student Resources Academic advising; academic or career counseling; assistance for students with disabilities; bookstore; campus computer network; career placement assistance; computer lab; computer-assisted instruction; e-mail services; employment services for current students; externships; housing assistance; interactive nursing skills videos; Internet; learning resource lab; library services; nursing audiovisuals; paid internships; placement services for program completers; remedial services; resume preparation assistance; skills, simulation, or other laboratory; tutoring; unpaid internships.
Library Facilities 277,330 volumes (11,000 in nursing); 768 periodical subscriptions (155 health-care related).

BACCALAUREATE PROGRAMS

Degree BSN
Available Programs Accelerated RN Baccalaureate; Generic Baccalaureate; RN Baccalaureate.
Study Options Full-time and part-time.
Program Entrance Requirements CPR certification, health exam, health insurance, high school chemistry, 3 years high school math, 2 years high school science, high school transcript, immunizations, minimum high school rank 67%, professional liability insurance/malpractice insurance. Transfer students are accepted. *Application deadline:* Applications may be processed on a rolling basis for some programs. *Application fee:* $35.
Advanced Placement Credit given for nursing courses completed elsewhere dependent upon specific evaluations.
Expenses (2010-11) *Tuition:* full-time $28,076; part-time $760 per credit hour. *International tuition:* $40,886 full-time. *Room and board:* $9110 per academic year. *Required fees:* full-time $550.
Financial Aid 100% of baccalaureate students in nursing programs received some form of financial aid in 2009-10. *Gift aid (need-based):* Federal Pell, FSEOG, state, college/university gift aid from institutional funds. *Loans:* Federal Nursing Student Loans, Federal Direct (Subsidized and Unsubsidized Stafford PLUS), Perkins, college/university. *Work-study:* Federal Work-Study, part-time campus jobs. *Financial aid application deadline (priority):* 3/10.
Contact Dr. Amy M. Hall, Chair/Professor of Nursing, Department of Nursing, University of Evansville, 1800 Lincoln Avenue, Evansville, IN 47722. *Telephone:* 812-488-2414. *Fax:* 812-488-2717. *E-mail:* ah169@evansville.edu.

University of Indianapolis

School of Nursing
Indianapolis, Indiana

http://www.uindy.edu/
Founded in 1902

DEGREES • BSN • MSN • MSN/MBA

Nursing Program Faculty 29 (40% with doctorates).
Baccalaureate Enrollment 261 **Women** 97.4% **Men** 2.6% **Minority** 6.5% **Part-time** 40%
Graduate Enrollment 146 **Women** 93.2% **Men** 6.8% **Minority** 12% **International** 1% **Part-time** 90%
Distance Learning Courses Available.
Nursing Student Activities Nursing Honor Society, Sigma Theta Tau, Student Nurses' Association.
Nursing Student Resources Academic advising; academic or career counseling; assistance for students with disabilities; bookstore; campus computer network; career placement assistance; computer lab; computer-assisted instruction; e-mail services; employment services for current students; externships; housing assistance; interactive nursing skills videos; Internet; learning resource lab; library services; nursing audiovisuals; other; paid internships; placement services for program completers; remedial services; resume preparation assistance; skills, simulation, or other laboratory; tutoring; unpaid internships.
Library Facilities 173,363 volumes (15,600 in health, 1,000 in nursing); 1,015 periodical subscriptions (600 health-care related).

BACCALAUREATE PROGRAMS

Degree BSN

Available Programs ADN to Baccalaureate; Accelerated Baccalaureate for Second Degree; Generic Baccalaureate.

Site Options Indianapolis, IN.

Study Options Full-time.

Program Entrance Requirements Minimum overall college GPA of 2.82, transcript of college record, CPR certification, health exam, health insurance, high school biology, high school chemistry, 2 years high school math, 2 years high school science, high school transcript, immunizations, minimum GPA in nursing prerequisites of 2.0, prerequisite course work. Transfer students are accepted. *Application deadline:* 4/15 (fall), 10/15 (winter).

Advanced Placement Credit by examination available. Credit given for nursing courses completed elsewhere dependent upon specific evaluations.

Expenses (2010-11) *Tuition:* full-time $22,020; part-time $917 per credit. *Room and board:* $7990 per academic year. *Required fees:* full-time $300.

Financial Aid 88% of baccalaureate students in nursing programs received some form of financial aid in 2009-10.

Contact Dr. Cheryl M. Martin, Director, BSN Program, School of Nursing, University of Indianapolis, 1400 East Hanna Avenue, Indianapolis, IN 46227-3697. *Telephone:* 317-788-3324. *Fax:* 317-788-3542. *E-mail:* martincm@uindy.edu.

GRADUATE PROGRAMS

Expenses (2010-11) *Tuition:* part-time $590 per credit. *Required fees:* full-time $300.

Financial Aid 90% of graduate students in nursing programs received some form of financial aid in 2009-10.

Contact Dr. Anne Thomas, Director, Graduate Program, School of Nursing, University of Indianapolis, 1400 East Hanna Avenue, Indianapolis, IN 46227-3697. *Telephone:* 317-788-3206. *Fax:* 317-788-6208. *E-mail:* athomas@uindy.edu.

MASTER'S DEGREE PROGRAM

Degrees MSN; MSN/MBA

Available Programs Accelerated Master's for Non-Nursing College Graduates; Master's.

Concentrations Available Nurse-midwifery; nursing administration; nursing education. *Nurse practitioner programs in:* family health, gerontology, women's health.

Site Options Indianapolis, IN.

Study Options Full-time and part-time.

Online Degree Options Yes.

Program Entrance Requirements Clinical experience, minimum overall college GPA of 3.0, transcript of college record, CPR certification, written essay, immunizations, interview, 3 letters of recommendation, nursing research course, professional liability insurance/malpractice insurance, resume, statistics course. *Application deadline:* 4/15 (fall). Applications may be processed on a rolling basis for some programs. *Application fee:* $60.

Advanced Placement Credit given for nursing courses completed elsewhere dependent upon specific evaluations.

Degree Requirements 36 total credit hours, thesis or project, comprehensive exam.

POST-MASTER'S PROGRAM

Areas of Study Nurse-midwifery; nursing administration; nursing education. *Nurse practitioner programs in:* family health, gerontology, women's health.

University of Saint Francis

Department of Nursing
Fort Wayne, Indiana

http://www.sf.edu/

Founded in 1890

DEGREES • BSN • MSN

Nursing Program Faculty 77 (7% with doctorates).

Baccalaureate Enrollment 261 **Women** 93% **Men** 7% **Minority** 6.8% **Part-time** 3.4%

Graduate Enrollment 98 **Women** 96% **Men** 4% **Minority** 7% **Part-time** 75%

Distance Learning Courses Available.

Nursing Student Activities Sigma Theta Tau, Student Nurses' Association.

Nursing Student Resources Academic advising; academic or career counseling; assistance for students with disabilities; bookstore; campus computer network; career placement assistance; computer lab; computer-assisted instruction; e-mail services; employment services for current students; externships; housing assistance; interactive nursing skills videos; Internet; learning resource lab; library services; nursing audiovisuals; paid internships; remedial services; resume preparation assistance; skills, simulation, or other laboratory; tutoring; unpaid internships.

Library Facilities 95,991 volumes (8,549 in health, 1,825 in nursing); 567 periodical subscriptions (2,913 health-care related).

BACCALAUREATE PROGRAMS

Degree BSN

Available Programs Generic Baccalaureate; RN Baccalaureate.

Study Options Full-time and part-time.

Program Entrance Requirements Minimum overall college GPA of 2.7, transcript of college record, CPR certification, health exam, high school biology, high school chemistry, 1 year of high school math, high school transcript, immunizations, minimum high school GPA of 2.7, minimum GPA in nursing prerequisites of 2.7, prerequisite course work. Transfer students are accepted. *Application deadline:* 7/31 (fall), 11/19 (spring).

Advanced Placement Credit given for nursing courses completed elsewhere dependent upon specific evaluations.

Expenses (2010-11) *Tuition:* full-time $22,000; part-time $695 per credit hour. *Room and board:* $8338; room only: $7528 per academic year. *Required fees:* full-time $810; part-time $252 per credit; part-time $115 per term.

Financial Aid 96% of baccalaureate students in nursing programs received some form of financial aid in 2009-10. *Gift aid (need-based):* Federal Pell, FSEOG, state, private, college/university gift aid from institutional funds. *Loans:* Perkins. *Work-study:* Federal Work-Study, part-time campus jobs. *Financial aid application deadline:* 6/30(priority: 3/10).

Contact Mindy Yoder, BSN/MSN Program Director, Department of Nursing, University of Saint Francis, 2701 Spring Street, Fort Wayne, IN 46808. *Telephone:* 260-399-7700 Ext. 8510. *Fax:* 260-434-7404. *E-mail:* myoder@sf.edu.

GRADUATE PROGRAMS

Expenses (2010-11) *Tuition:* part-time $735 per credit hour. *Required fees:* full-time $660; part-time $115 per term.

Financial Aid 97% of graduate students in nursing programs received some form of financial aid in 2009-10. Federal Work-Study and unspecified assistantships available.

Contact Mindy Yoder, BSN/MSN Program Director, Department of Nursing, University of Saint Francis, 2701 Spring Street, Fort Wayne, IN 46808. *Telephone:* 260-399-7700 Ext. 8510. *Fax:* 260-434-7404. *E-mail:* myoder@sf.edu.

MASTER'S DEGREE PROGRAM

Degree MSN

Available Programs Master's; Master's for Nurses with Non-Nursing Degrees.

Concentrations Available *Nurse practitioner programs in:* community health, family health.

Study Options Full-time and part-time.

Program Entrance Requirements Computer literacy, minimum overall college GPA of 3.2, transcript of college record, CPR certification, written essay, immunizations, interview, 3 letters of recommendation, nursing research course, physical assessment course, resume, statistics course, GRE. *Application deadline:* 7/29 (fall), 4/15 (summer).

Advanced Placement Credit given for nursing courses completed elsewhere dependent upon specific evaluations.

Degree Requirements 48 total credit hours.

POST-MASTER'S PROGRAM

Areas of Study *Nurse practitioner programs in:* family health.

University of Southern Indiana

College of Nursing and Health Professions
Evansville, Indiana

http://health.usi.edu/
Founded in 1965

DEGREES • BSN • DNP • MSN

Nursing Program Faculty 30 (50% with doctorates).
Baccalaureate Enrollment 410 **Women** 90% **Men** 10% **Minority** 5% **International** 1% **Part-time** 26%
Graduate Enrollment 306 **Women** 93% **Men** 7% **Minority** 8% **Part-time** 72%
Distance Learning Courses Available.
Nursing Student Activities Sigma Theta Tau, Student Nurses' Association.
Nursing Student Resources Academic advising; academic or career counseling; assistance for students with disabilities; bookstore; campus computer network; career placement assistance; computer lab; computer-assisted instruction; daycare for children of students; e-mail services; employment services for current students; housing assistance; interactive nursing skills videos; Internet; learning resource lab; library services; nursing audiovisuals; placement services for program completers; remedial services; resume preparation assistance; skills, simulation, or other laboratory; tutoring; unpaid internships.
Library Facilities 328,129 volumes (9,200 in health, 1,500 in nursing); 22,046 periodical subscriptions (2,000 health-care related).

BACCALAUREATE PROGRAMS

Degree BSN
Available Programs Generic Baccalaureate; RN Baccalaureate.
Study Options Full-time.
Online Degree Options Yes.
Program Entrance Requirements Minimum overall college GPA of 3.0, transcript of college record, CPR certification, written essay, health exam, health insurance, high school transcript, immunizations, minimum GPA in nursing prerequisites of 2.0, professional liability insurance/malpractice insurance, prerequisite course work. Transfer students are accepted. *Application deadline:* 8/15 (fall).
Advanced Placement Credit given for nursing courses completed elsewhere dependent upon specific evaluations.
Expenses (2010-11) *Tuition, state resident:* full-time $6095; part-time $185 per credit hour. *Tuition, nonresident:* full-time $9140; part-time $277 per credit hour. *Room and board:* $6920; room only: $3560 per academic year. *Required fees:* full-time $500; part-time $15 per credit; part-time $250 per term.
Financial Aid 70% of baccalaureate students in nursing programs received some form of financial aid in 2009-10. *Gift aid (need-based):* Federal Pell, FSEOG, state, private, college/university gift aid from institutional funds, Federal Nursing. *Loans:* Federal Direct (Subsidized and Unsubsidized Stafford PLUS). *Work-study:* Federal Work-Study. *Financial aid application deadline:* 3/1.
Contact Dr. Ann H. White, Associate Dean, College of Nursing and Health Professions, University of Southern Indiana, 8600 University Boulevard, Evansville, IN 47712. *Telephone:* 812-465-1173. *Fax:* 812-465-7092. *E-mail:* awhite@usi.edu.

GRADUATE PROGRAMS

Expenses (2010-11) *Tuition, state resident:* full-time $6430; part-time $268 per credit hour. *Tuition, nonresident:* full-time $6430; part-time $268 per credit hour. *International tuition:* $12,720 full-time. *Room and board:* $6920; room only: $3560 per academic year. *Required fees:* full-time $500; part-time $15 per credit; part-time $250 per term.
Financial Aid 45% of graduate students in nursing programs received some form of financial aid in 2009-10. Federal Work-Study, scholarships, tuition waivers (full and partial), and unspecified assistantships available. *Financial aid application deadline:* 3/1.
Contact Dr. Ann H. White, Associate Dean, College of Nursing and Health Professions, University of Southern Indiana, 8600 University Boulevard, Evansville, IN 47712. *Telephone:* 812-465-1173. *Fax:* 812-465-7092. *E-mail:* awhite@usi.edu.

MASTER'S DEGREE PROGRAM

Degree MSN
Available Programs Master's; RN to Master's.
Concentrations Available Nursing administration; nursing education. *Nurse practitioner programs in:* acute care, family health.
Study Options Full-time and part-time.
Online Degree Options Yes (online only).
Program Entrance Requirements Computer literacy, minimum overall college GPA of 3.0, transcript of college record, CPR certification, written essay, immunizations, 2 letters of recommendation, professional liability insurance/malpractice insurance, resume, statistics course. *Application deadline:* 2/15 (fall), 10/1 (winter). *Application fee:* $25.
Advanced Placement Credit given for nursing courses completed elsewhere dependent upon specific evaluations.
Degree Requirements 42 total credit hours.

POST-MASTER'S PROGRAM

Areas of Study Nursing administration; nursing education. *Nurse practitioner programs in:* acute care, family health.

DOCTORAL DEGREE PROGRAM

Degree DNP
Available Programs Doctorate.
Areas of Study Clinical practice, nursing administration.
Program Entrance Requirements Clinical experience, minimum overall college GPA of 3.25, 3 letters of recommendation, MSN or equivalent, vita, writing sample. Application deadline: 1/15 (fall). Application fee: $25.
Degree Requirements 78 total credit hours.

CONTINUING EDUCATION PROGRAM

Contact Peggy Graul, Coordinator of Continuing Education for Nursing and Health Professions, College of Nursing and Health Professions, University of Southern Indiana, 8600 University Boulevard, Evansville, IN 47712. *Telephone:* 812-465-1161. *Fax:* 812-465-7092. *E-mail:* pgraul@usi.edu.

See full description on page 500.

Valparaiso University

College of Nursing
Valparaiso, Indiana

http://www.valpo.edu/nursing
Founded in 1859

DEGREES • BSN • MSN • MSN/MBA

Nursing Program Faculty 13 (38% with doctorates).
Baccalaureate Enrollment 310 **Women** 92% **Men** 8% **Minority** 12% **International** 2% **Part-time** 6%
Graduate Enrollment 34 **Women** 91% **Men** 9% **Minority** 12% **Part-time** 59%
Nursing Student Activities Sigma Theta Tau, Student Nurses' Association.
Nursing Student Resources Academic advising; academic or career counseling; assistance for students with disabilities; bookstore; campus computer network; career placement assistance; computer lab; computer-assisted instruction; e-mail services; employment services for current students; externships; housing assistance; interactive nursing skills videos; Internet; learning resource lab; library services; nursing audiovisuals; placement services for program completers; remedial services; resume preparation assistance; skills, simulation, or other laboratory; tutoring; unpaid internships.
Library Facilities 537,234 volumes (9,500 in health, 995 in nursing); 47,914 periodical subscriptions (1,000 health-care related).

BACCALAUREATE PROGRAMS

Degree BSN
Available Programs Accelerated Baccalaureate; Generic Baccalaureate; RN Baccalaureate.
Study Options Full-time and part-time.
Program Entrance Requirements Minimum overall college GPA of 3.0, transcript of college record, written essay, high school biology, high school chemistry, 2 years high school math, 4 years high school science, high school transcript, immunizations, minimum high school GPA of 2.0, minimum GPA in nursing prerequisites of 2.5. Transfer students are accepted.
Advanced Placement Credit by examination available. Credit given for nursing courses completed elsewhere dependent upon specific evaluations.
Contact *Telephone:* 219-464-5011. *Fax:* 219-464-6888.

GRADUATE PROGRAMS

Contact *Telephone:* 219-464-5289. *Fax:* 219-464-5425.

MASTER'S DEGREE PROGRAM

Degrees MSN; MSN/MBA
Available Programs Master's; RN to Master's.
Concentrations Available *Clinical nurse specialist programs in:* adult health, gerontology, women's health.
Study Options Full-time and part-time.
Program Entrance Requirements Minimum overall college GPA of 3.0, transcript of college record, CPR certification, written essay, immunizations, 2 letters of recommendation, nursing research course, physical assessment course, statistics course.
Advanced Placement Credit given for nursing courses completed elsewhere dependent upon specific evaluations.
Degree Requirements 36 total credit hours, thesis or project.

POST-MASTER'S PROGRAM

Areas of Study *Nurse practitioner programs in:* family health.

CONTINUING EDUCATION PROGRAM

Contact *Telephone:* 219-464-5291. *Fax:* 219-464-5425.

Vincennes University

Department of Nursing
Vincennes, Indiana

Founded in 1801

DEGREE • BSN

BACCALAUREATE PROGRAMS

Degree BSN
Available Programs RN Baccalaureate.
Contact Nursing Program, Department of Nursing, Vincennes University, 1002 North First Street, Vincennes, IN 47591. *Telephone:* 812-888-8888.

IOWA

Allen College

Program in Nursing
Waterloo, Iowa

http://www.allencollege.edu/
Founded in 1989

DEGREES • BSN • MSN

Nursing Program Faculty 32 (25% with doctorates).
Baccalaureate Enrollment 277 **Women** 94% **Men** 6% **Minority** 5% **Part-time** 21%
Graduate Enrollment 151 **Women** 97% **Men** 3% **Minority** 4% **Part-time** 80%
Distance Learning Courses Available.
Nursing Student Activities Sigma Theta Tau, Student Nurses' Association, nursing club.
Nursing Student Resources Academic advising; academic or career counseling; campus computer network; career placement assistance; computer lab; computer-assisted instruction; e-mail services; employment services for current students; externships; housing assistance; interactive nursing skills videos; Internet; library services; nursing audiovisuals; other; paid internships; placement services for program completers; resume preparation assistance; skills, simulation, or other laboratory; tutoring.
Library Facilities 3,300 volumes (3,340 in health, 3,340 in nursing); 214 periodical subscriptions (240 health-care related).

BACCALAUREATE PROGRAMS

Degree BSN
Available Programs ADN to Baccalaureate; Accelerated Baccalaureate; Accelerated Baccalaureate for Second Degree; Accelerated RN Baccalaureate; Baccalaureate for Second Degree; Generic Baccalaureate; LPN to Baccalaureate; RN Baccalaureate.
Study Options Full-time.
Program Entrance Requirements Minimum overall college GPA of 2.7, transcript of college record, CPR certification, health exam, immunizations, 1 letter of recommendation, prerequisite course work. Transfer students are accepted. *Application deadline:* Applications may be processed on a rolling basis for some programs. *Application fee:* $50.
Advanced Placement Credit given for nursing courses completed elsewhere dependent upon specific evaluations.
Expenses (2010-11) *Tuition:* full-time $13,458; part-time $500 per credit hour. *Room and board:* $7157; room only: $3579 per academic year. *Required fees:* part-time $68 per credit.
Financial Aid 90% of baccalaureate students in nursing programs received some form of financial aid in 2009-10.
Contact Dina Dowden, Student Services Education Secretary, Program in Nursing, Allen College, 1825 Logan Avenue, Waterloo, IA 50703. *Telephone:* 319-226-2000. *Fax:* 319-226-2051. *E-mail:* allencollegeadmissions@ihs.org.

GRADUATE PROGRAMS

Expenses (2010-11) *Tuition:* full-time $13,709; part-time $677 per credit hour. *Room and board:* $7157; room only: $3579 per academic year. *Required fees:* full-time $68; part-time $68 per credit.
Financial Aid 93% of graduate students in nursing programs received some form of financial aid in 2009-10. Teaching assistantships, institutionally sponsored loans, scholarships, and traineeships available. Aid available to part-time students. *Financial aid application deadline:* 8/15.
Contact Dina Dowden, Student Services Education Secretary, Program in Nursing, Allen College, 1825 Logan Avenue, Waterloo, IA 50703. *Telephone:* 319-226-2000. *Fax:* 319-226-2051. *E-mail:* allencollegeadmissions@ihs.org.

MASTER'S DEGREE PROGRAM

Degree MSN
Available Programs Master's; Master's for Nurses with Non-Nursing Degrees; RN to Master's.
Concentrations Available Nursing administration; nursing education. *Nurse practitioner programs in:* acute care, adult health, family health, gerontology, psychiatric/mental health.
Study Options Full-time and part-time.
Online Degree Options Yes.
Program Entrance Requirements Clinical experience, computer literacy, minimum overall college GPA of 3.0, transcript of college record, CPR certification, written essay, immunizations, interview, 3 letters of recommendation, nursing research course, professional liability insurance/malpractice insurance, prerequisite course work, resume, statistics course. *Application deadline:* Applications may be processed on a rolling basis for some programs. *Application fee:* $50.
Advanced Placement Credit given for nursing courses completed elsewhere dependent upon specific evaluations.
Degree Requirements 44 total credit hours, thesis or project.

POST-MASTER'S PROGRAM

Areas of Study Nursing administration; nursing education. *Nurse practitioner programs in:* acute care, adult health, family health, gerontology, psychiatric/mental health.

POSTDOCTORAL PROGRAM

Postdoctoral Program Contact Dr. Diane Young, Department Chair, MSN Program, Program in Nursing, Allen College, 1825 Logan Avenue, Waterloo, IA 50703. *Telephone:* 319-226-2047. *Fax:* 319-226-2070. *E-mail:* youngdm@ihs.org.

CONTINUING EDUCATION PROGRAM

Contact Mrs. Mary Kay Frost, Continuing Education Coordinator, Program in Nursing, Allen College, 1825 Logan Avenue, Waterloo, IA 50703. *Telephone:* 319-226-2028. *Fax:* 319-226-2051. *E-mail:* frostmk@ihs.org.

Briar Cliff University
Department of Nursing
Sioux City, Iowa

http://www.briarcliff.edu/nursing
Founded in 1930

DEGREES • BSN • MSN

Nursing Program Faculty 8 (38% with doctorates).
Baccalaureate Enrollment 125 **Women** 90% **Men** 10% **Minority** 5% **Part-time** 25%
Graduate Enrollment 50 **Women** 95% **Men** 5% **Minority** 5% **Part-time** 75%
Distance Learning Courses Available.
Nursing Student Activities Sigma Theta Tau, Student Nurses' Association, nursing club.
Nursing Student Resources Academic advising; academic or career counseling; assistance for students with disabilities; bookstore; campus computer network; career placement assistance; computer lab; computer-assisted instruction; e-mail services; employment services for current students; externships; interactive nursing skills videos; Internet; learning resource lab; library services; nursing audiovisuals; placement services for program completers; remedial services; resume preparation assistance; skills, simulation, or other laboratory; tutoring.
Library Facilities 81,794 volumes; 154 periodical subscriptions.

BACCALAUREATE PROGRAMS

Degree BSN
Available Programs ADN to Baccalaureate; Generic Baccalaureate; LPN to Baccalaureate; RN Baccalaureate.
Study Options Full-time and part-time.
Program Entrance Requirements Minimum overall college GPA of 2.75, transcript of college record, CPR certification, written essay, health exam, high school foreign language, high school transcript, immunizations, minimum GPA in nursing prerequisites of 2.75, prerequisite course work. Transfer students are accepted. *Application deadline:* 6/15 (fall), 7/1 (winter), 10/31 (spring), 4/1 (summer). Applications may be processed on a rolling basis for some programs. *Application fee:* $25.
Advanced Placement Credit given for nursing courses completed elsewhere dependent upon specific evaluations.
Expenses (2010-11) *Tuition:* full-time $22,719; part-time $759 per credit. *Room and board:* $6500; room only: $3489 per academic year. *Required fees:* full-time $699; part-time $23 per credit; part-time $233 per term.
Financial Aid 99% of baccalaureate students in nursing programs received some form of financial aid in 2009-10. *Gift aid (need-based):* Federal Pell, FSEOG, state, private, college/university gift aid from institutional funds. *Loans:* Federal Direct (Subsidized and Unsubsidized Stafford PLUS), Perkins, alternative loans, partnership loans, Minnesota SELF Loans. *Work-study:* Federal Work-Study, part-time campus jobs. *Financial aid application deadline:* 3/15.
Contact Dr. Richard A. Petersen, Department Chair and Associate Professor, Department of Nursing, Briar Cliff University, 3303 Rebecca Street, Sioux City, IA 51104. *Telephone:* 712-279-1662. *E-mail:* rick.petersen@briarcliff.edu.

GRADUATE PROGRAMS

Expenses (2010-11) *Tuition:* part-time $492 per credit. *Required fees:* part-time $23 per credit.
Financial Aid 60% of graduate students in nursing programs received some form of financial aid in 2009-10.
Contact Dr. Richard A. Petersen, Department Chair and Associate Professor, Department of Nursing, Briar Cliff University, 3303 Rebecca Street, Sioux City, IA 51104. *Telephone:* 712-279-1662. *E-mail:* rick.petersen@briarcliff.edu.

MASTER'S DEGREE PROGRAM

Degree MSN
Available Programs Master's.
Concentrations Available Nursing education. *Nurse practitioner programs in:* family health.
Study Options Part-time.
Program Entrance Requirements Clinical experience, computer literacy, minimum overall college GPA of 3.0, transcript of college record, CPR certification, written essay, immunizations, 2 letters of recommendation, nursing research course, physical assessment course, resume, statistics course. *Application deadline:* 4/15 (fall). Applications may be processed on a rolling basis for some programs. *Application fee:* $25.
Advanced Placement Credit given for nursing courses completed elsewhere dependent upon specific evaluations.
Degree Requirements 40 total credit hours, thesis or project, comprehensive exam.

CONTINUING EDUCATION PROGRAM

Contact Dr. Richard A. Petersen, Chair and Associate Professor, Department of Nursing, Briar Cliff University, 3303 Rebecca Street, Sioux City, IA 51104. *Telephone:* 712-279-1662. *Fax:* 712-279-5463. *E-mail:* rick.petersen@briarcliff.edu.

Clarke University
Department of Nursing and Health
Dubuque, Iowa

Founded in 1843

DEGREES • BS • MSN

Nursing Program Faculty 18 (3% with doctorates).
Baccalaureate Enrollment 104 **Women** 92% **Men** 8% **Minority** 1% **International** 1% **Part-time** 9%
Graduate Enrollment 52 **Women** 99% **Men** 1% **Part-time** 35%
Nursing Student Activities Nursing Honor Society, Sigma Theta Tau, Student Nurses' Association.
Nursing Student Resources Academic advising; academic or career counseling; assistance for students with disabilities; bookstore; campus computer network; career placement assistance; computer lab; computer-assisted instruction; e-mail services; employment services for current students; externships; housing assistance; interactive nursing skills videos; Internet; learning resource lab; library services; nursing audiovisuals; paid internships; placement services for program completers; remedial services; resume preparation assistance; skills, simulation, or other laboratory; tutoring; unpaid internships.
Library Facilities 110,000 volumes (7,000 in health, 2,856 in nursing); 28,000 periodical subscriptions (124 health-care related).

BACCALAUREATE PROGRAMS

Degree BS
Available Programs Baccalaureate for Second Degree; Generic Baccalaureate; RN Baccalaureate.
Site Options Dubuque, IA.
Study Options Full-time and part-time.
Program Entrance Requirements Minimum overall college GPA of 2.75, transcript of college record, CPR certification, written essay, health exam, health insurance, high school chemistry, high school foreign language, high school math, high school transcript, immunizations, interview, 2 letters of recommendation, minimum high school GPA of 2.0, minimum GPA in nursing prerequisites of 1.67, professional liability insurance/malpractice insurance, prerequisite course work. Transfer students are accepted. *Application deadline:* Applications may be processed on a rolling basis for some programs.
Advanced Placement Credit given for nursing courses completed elsewhere dependent upon specific evaluations.
Expenses (2009-10) *Tuition:* full-time $22,800; part-time $578 per credit. *Room and board:* $6840; room only: $3360 per academic year. *Required fees:* full-time $10,000.
Financial Aid 98% of baccalaureate students in nursing programs received some form of financial aid in 2008-09. *Gift aid (need-based):* Federal Pell, FSEOG, state, private, college/university gift aid from institutional funds. *Loans:* Federal Nursing Student Loans, Perkins, state, college/university, private loans. *Work-study:* Federal Work-Study, part-time campus jobs. *Financial aid application deadline (priority):* 4/15.
Contact Keith Tackett, Interim Chairperson, Department of Nursing and Health, Clarke University, 1550 Clarke Drive, Dubuque, IA 52001. *Telephone:* 563-588-8109. *Fax:* 563-588-8684. *E-mail:* keith.tackett@clarke.edu.

GRADUATE PROGRAMS

Expenses (2009-10) *Tuition:* part-time $602 per credit.
Financial Aid 30% of graduate students in nursing programs received some form of financial aid in 2008-09. Career-related internships or fieldwork available. Aid available to part-time students.
Contact Keith Tackett, Interim Chairperson, Department of Nursing and Health, Clarke University, 1550 Clarke Drive, Dubuque, IA 52001. *Telephone:* 563-588-8109. *Fax:* 563-588-8684. *E-mail:* keith.tackett@clarke.edu.

MASTER'S DEGREE PROGRAM

Degree MSN
Available Programs Master's.
Concentrations Available Nursing education. *Nurse practitioner programs in:* family health.
Study Options Full-time and part-time.
Program Entrance Requirements Computer literacy, minimum overall college GPA of 3.0, transcript of college record, CPR certification, written essay, immunizations, interview, 3 letters of recommendation, nursing research course, physical assessment course, prerequisite course work, resume, statistics course, GRE General Test or MAT. *Application deadline:* Applications may be processed on a rolling basis for some programs. *Application fee:* $35.
Advanced Placement Credit given for nursing courses completed elsewhere dependent upon specific evaluations.
Degree Requirements 37 total credit hours, thesis or project.

POST-MASTER'S PROGRAM

Areas of Study *Nurse practitioner programs in:* family health.

CONTINUING EDUCATION PROGRAM

Contact Scott Schneider, Director of Adult Education and Timesaver Programs, Department of Nursing and Health, Clarke University, 1550 Clarke Drive, Dubuque, IA 52001. *Telephone:* 563-588-6378. *Fax:* 563-588-8684. *E-mail:* scott.schneider@clarke.edu.

Coe College
Department of Nursing
Cedar Rapids, Iowa

Founded in 1851

DEGREE • BSN
Nursing Program Faculty 9 (33% with doctorates).
Baccalaureate Enrollment 45 **Women** 98% **Men** 2%
Nursing Student Activities Student Nurses' Association.
Nursing Student Resources Academic advising; academic or career counseling; assistance for students with disabilities; bookstore; campus computer network; career placement assistance; computer lab; e-mail services; employment services for current students; housing assistance; Internet; learning resource lab; library services; nursing audiovisuals; remedial services; resume preparation assistance; skills, simulation, or other laboratory; tutoring; unpaid internships.
Library Facilities 2,929 volumes in health, 492 volumes in nursing; 34 periodical subscriptions health-care related.

BACCALAUREATE PROGRAMS

Degree BSN
Available Programs Generic Baccalaureate; RN Baccalaureate.
Study Options Full-time and part-time.
Program Entrance Requirements Minimum overall college GPA of 2.7, transcript of college record, CPR certification, written essay, health exam, health insurance, high school chemistry, high school transcript, immunizations, minimum high school GPA of 2.0, minimum GPA in nursing prerequisites of 2.7, prerequisite course work. Transfer students are accepted.
Advanced Placement Credit given for nursing courses completed elsewhere dependent upon specific evaluations.
Contact *Telephone:* 319-399-8120. *Fax:* 319-399-8121.

Dordt College
Nursing Program
Sioux Center, Iowa

Founded in 1955

DEGREE • BSN
Nursing Program Faculty 3
Library Facilities 170,000 volumes; 6,597 periodical subscriptions.

BACCALAUREATE PROGRAMS

Degree BSN
Available Programs Generic Baccalaureate.
Contact *Telephone:* 712-722-6000.

Grand View University
Division of Nursing
Des Moines, Iowa

http://www.gvc.edu/academics/nursing/
Founded in 1896

DEGREES • BSN • MS
Nursing Program Faculty 18 (33% with doctorates).
Baccalaureate Enrollment 200 **Women** 90% **Men** 10% **Minority** 15% **Part-time** 5%
Graduate Enrollment 6 **Women** 83% **Men** 17% **Part-time** 100%
Distance Learning Courses Available.
Nursing Student Activities Sigma Theta Tau, Student Nurses' Association.
Nursing Student Resources Academic advising; academic or career counseling; assistance for students with disabilities; bookstore; campus computer network; career placement assistance; computer lab; computer-assisted instruction; e-mail services; employment services for current students; externships; housing assistance; interactive nursing skills videos; Internet; learning resource lab; library services; nursing audiovisuals; placement services for program completers; remedial services; resume preparation assistance; skills, simulation, or other laboratory; tutoring; unpaid internships.
Library Facilities 137,138 volumes (5,672 in health, 4,061 in nursing); 21,536 periodical subscriptions (370 health-care related).

BACCALAUREATE PROGRAMS

Degree BSN
Available Programs Generic Baccalaureate; RN Baccalaureate.
Study Options Full-time and part-time.
Program Entrance Requirements Minimum overall college GPA of 2.75, transcript of college record, CPR certification, health exam, health insurance, high school chemistry, high school transcript, immunizations, 3 letters of recommendation, minimum GPA in nursing prerequisites of 2.75, prerequisite course work. Transfer students are accepted. *Application deadline:* 2/1 (fall), 10/1 (spring). Applications may be processed on a rolling basis for some programs.
Advanced Placement Credit by examination available. Credit given for nursing courses completed elsewhere dependent upon specific evaluations.
Financial Aid ***Gift aid (need-based):*** Federal Pell, FSEOG, state, private, college/university gift aid from institutional funds, Academic Competitiveness Grants, National SMART Grants. *Loans:* Federal Nursing Student Loans, Federal Direct (Subsidized and Unsubsidized Stafford PLUS), Perkins. *Work-study:* Federal Work-Study, part-time campus jobs. *Financial aid application deadline (priority):* 3/1.
Contact Dr. Debra Franzen, Head, Division of Nursing, Grand View University, 1200 Grandview Avenue, Des Moines, IA 50316. *Telephone:* 515-263-2859. *Fax:* 515-263-6077. *E-mail:* dfranzen@grandview.edu.

GRADUATE PROGRAMS

Contact Dr. Debra Franzen, Division Head for Nursing, Division of Nursing, Grand View University, 1200 Grandview Avenue, Des Moines, IA 50316. *Telephone:* 515-263-2859. *Fax:* 515-263-6077. *E-mail:* dfranzen@grandview.edu.

MASTER'S DEGREE PROGRAM

Degree MS
Available Programs Master's.
Concentrations Available Clinical nurse leader.
Study Options Part-time.
Program Entrance Requirements Clinical experience, computer literacy, minimum overall college GPA of 3.0, transcript of college record, CPR certification, written essay, immunizations, interview, 3 letters of recommendation, nursing research course, physical assessment course, professional liability insurance/malpractice insurance, prerequisite course work, resume, statistics course. *Application deadline:* 7/1 (fall). Applications may be processed on a rolling basis for some programs.
Degree Requirements 40 total credit hours, thesis or project.

CONTINUING EDUCATION PROGRAM

Contact Dr. Beth Gaul, CE Provider Coordinator, Division of Nursing, Grand View University, 1200 Grandview Avenue, Des Moines, IA 50316-1599. *Telephone:* 515-263-2869. *Fax:* 515-263-6700. *E-mail:* bgaul@grandview.edu.

Iowa Wesleyan College
Division of Health and Natural Sciences
Mount Pleasant, Iowa

http://www.iwc.edu/
Founded in 1842

DEGREE • BSN

Nursing Program Faculty 6 (17% with doctorates).
Baccalaureate Enrollment 80 **Women** 93% **Men** 7% **Minority** 7% **Part-time** 2%
Distance Learning Courses Available.
Nursing Student Activities Student Nurses' Association.
Nursing Student Resources Academic advising; academic or career counseling; assistance for students with disabilities; bookstore; campus computer network; career placement assistance; computer lab; computer-assisted instruction; e-mail services; interactive nursing skills videos; Internet; learning resource lab; library services; nursing audiovisuals; remedial services; resume preparation assistance; skills, simulation, or other laboratory; tutoring; unpaid internships.
Library Facilities 102,869 volumes (500 in health, 300 in nursing); 9,452 periodical subscriptions (40 health-care related).

BACCALAUREATE PROGRAMS

Degree BSN
Available Programs ADN to Baccalaureate; Baccalaureate for Second Degree; Generic Baccalaureate; LPN to Baccalaureate; LPN to RN Baccalaureate; RN Baccalaureate.
Study Options Full-time and part-time.
Program Entrance Requirements Minimum overall college GPA of 2.25, transcript of college record, CPR certification, health exam, health insurance, high school transcript, immunizations, interview, minimum high school GPA of 2.25, minimum high school rank 50%, minimum GPA in nursing prerequisites of 2.0, professional liability insurance/malpractice insurance, prerequisite course work. Transfer students are accepted. *Application deadline:* 8/1 (fall).
Financial Aid 98% of baccalaureate students in nursing programs received some form of financial aid in 2009-10. *Gift aid (need-based):* Federal Pell, FSEOG, state, private, college/university gift aid from institutional funds. *Loans:* Federal Direct (Subsidized and Unsubsidized Stafford PLUS), Perkins, alternative loans. *Work-study:* Federal Work-Study.
Contact Mr. Mark Petty, Director, Enrollment Management, Division of Health and Natural Sciences, Iowa Wesleyan College, 601 North Main Street, Mount Pleasant, IA 52641. *Telephone:* 800-582-2383 Ext. 6231. *Fax:* 319-385-6296. *E-mail:* mpetty@iwc.edu.

Luther College
Department of Nursing
Decorah, Iowa

http://nursing.luther.edu/
Founded in 1861

DEGREE • BA

Nursing Program Faculty 12 (33% with doctorates).
Baccalaureate Enrollment 130 **Women** 96% **Men** 4% **Minority** 3% **International** 2%
Nursing Student Activities Nursing club.
Nursing Student Resources Academic advising; academic or career counseling; assistance for students with disabilities; bookstore; campus computer network; career placement assistance; computer lab; computer-assisted instruction; e-mail services; Internet; learning resource lab; library services; nursing audiovisuals; placement services for program completers; remedial services; resume preparation assistance; skills, simulation, or other laboratory; tutoring; unpaid internships.
Library Facilities 329,949 volumes (4,324 in health, 3,337 in nursing); 828 periodical subscriptions (35 health-care related).

BACCALAUREATE PROGRAMS

Degree BA
Available Programs ADN to Baccalaureate; Generic Baccalaureate.
Site Options Rochester, MN.
Study Options Full-time and part-time.
Program Entrance Requirements Minimum overall college GPA of 2.5, transcript of college record, CPR certification, written essay, health exam, health insurance, 3 years high school math, 2 years high school science, high school transcript, immunizations, minimum high school

rank 50%, minimum GPA in nursing prerequisites of 2.5, prerequisite course work. Transfer students are accepted.
Advanced Placement Credit given for nursing courses completed elsewhere dependent upon specific evaluations.
Expenses (2010-11) *Tuition:* full-time $33,330. *Room and board:* $5600 per academic year.
Financial Aid 98% of baccalaureate students in nursing programs received some form of financial aid in 2009-10. *Gift aid (need-based):* Federal Pell, FSEOG, state, private, college/university gift aid from institutional funds. *Loans:* Federal Direct (Subsidized and Unsubsidized Stafford PLUS), Perkins, college/university. *Work-study:* Federal Work-Study, part-time campus jobs. *Financial aid application deadline (priority):* 3/1.
Contact Ms. Ruth Green, Administrative Assistant, Department of Nursing, Luther College, 700 College Drive, Decorah, IA 52101. *Telephone:* 563-387-1057. *Fax:* 563-387-2149. *E-mail:* greenru@luther.edu.

CONTINUING EDUCATION PROGRAM

Contact Ms. Ruth Green, Administrative Assistant, Department of Nursing, Luther College, 700 College Drive, Decorah, IA 52101. *Telephone:* 563-387-1057. *Fax:* 563-387-2149. *E-mail:* greenru@luther.edu.

See full description on page 484.

Mercy College of Health Sciences
Division of Nursing
Des Moines, Iowa

http://www.mchs.edu/divnurs.html
Founded in 1995

DEGREE • BSN
Nursing Program Faculty 22 (2% with doctorates).
Baccalaureate Enrollment 76 **Women** 98% **Men** 2% **Minority** 1% **Part-time** 98%
Nursing Student Activities Sigma Theta Tau, Student Nurses' Association.
Nursing Student Resources Academic advising; academic or career counseling; assistance for students with disabilities; campus computer network; career placement assistance; computer lab; computer-assisted instruction; daycare for children of students; e-mail services; employment services for current students; interactive nursing skills videos; Internet; learning resource lab; library services; nursing audiovisuals; placement services for program completers; skills, simulation, or other laboratory.
Library Facilities 20,334 volumes; 5,281 periodical subscriptions.

BACCALAUREATE PROGRAMS

Degree BSN
Available Programs ADN to Baccalaureate.
Study Options Full-time and part-time.
Program Entrance Requirements Minimum overall college GPA of 2.7, transcript of college record, CPR certification, health exam, high school biology, high school chemistry, high school transcript, immunizations, minimum GPA in nursing prerequisites of 2.7, prerequisite course work, RN licensure. Transfer students are accepted. *Application deadline:* Applications may be processed on a rolling basis for some programs. *Application fee:* $25.
Advanced Placement Credit given for nursing courses completed elsewhere dependent upon specific evaluations.
Contact *Telephone:* 515-643-3180. *Fax:* 515-643-6698.

Morningside College
Department of Nursing Education
Sioux City, Iowa

http://webs.morningside.edu/nursing/
Founded in 1894

DEGREE • BSN
Nursing Program Faculty 11 (18% with doctorates).
Baccalaureate Enrollment 82 **Women** 90% **Men** 10% **Minority** 2% **Part-time** 7%
Nursing Student Activities Sigma Theta Tau, Student Nurses' Association.
Nursing Student Resources Academic advising; academic or career counseling; assistance for students with disabilities; bookstore; campus computer network; computer lab; computer-assisted instruction; e-mail services; employment services for current students; externships; housing assistance; interactive nursing skills videos; Internet; learning resource lab; library services; nursing audiovisuals; remedial services; resume preparation assistance; skills, simulation, or other laboratory; tutoring; unpaid internships.
Library Facilities 91,926 volumes (2,500 in health, 2,500 in nursing); 300 periodical subscriptions (125 health-care related).

BACCALAUREATE PROGRAMS

Degree BSN
Available Programs Baccalaureate for Second Degree; Generic Baccalaureate; International Nurse to Baccalaureate; LPN to Baccalaureate; RN Baccalaureate.
Study Options Full-time and part-time.
Program Entrance Requirements Minimum overall college GPA of 2.75, transcript of college record, CPR certification, high school transcript, immunizations, interview, minimum GPA in nursing prerequisites of 2.75, prerequisite course work. Transfer students are accepted. *Application deadline:* 8/15 (fall).
Advanced Placement Credit given for nursing courses completed elsewhere dependent upon specific evaluations.
Expenses (2010-11) *Tuition:* full-time $21,810; part-time $400 per credit hour. *Room and board:* $7040 per academic year. *Required fees:* full-time $1170; part-time $215 per term.
Financial Aid 99% of baccalaureate students in nursing programs received some form of financial aid in 2009-10. *Gift aid (need-based):* Federal Pell, FSEOG, state, private, college/university gift aid from institutional funds. *Loans:* Perkins, state, college/university, private loans. *Work-study:* Federal Work-Study, part-time campus jobs. *Financial aid application deadline (priority):* 3/1.
Contact Dr. Mary B. Kovarna, Professor and Chair, Department of Nursing Education, Morningside College, 1501 Morningside Avenue, Sioux City, IA 51106-1751. *Telephone:* 712-274-5156. *Fax:* 712-274-5101. *E-mail:* kovarna@morningside.edu.

Mount Mercy University
Department of Nursing
Cedar Rapids, Iowa

http://www.mtmercy.edu/
Founded in 1928

DEGREES • BSN • MSN
Nursing Program Faculty 43 (15% with doctorates).
Baccalaureate Enrollment 289 **Women** 97% **Men** 3% **Minority** 3% **Part-time** 30%
Graduate Enrollment 13
Nursing Student Activities Sigma Theta Tau, Student Nurses' Association.
Nursing Student Resources Academic advising; academic or career counseling; assistance for students with disabilities; bookstore; campus computer network; career placement assistance; computer lab; computer-assisted instruction; e-mail services; employment services for current students; externships; housing assistance; interactive nursing skills videos; Internet; learning resource lab; library services; nursing audiovisuals; paid internships; placement services for program completers; remedial services; resume preparation assistance; skills, simulation, or other laboratory; tutoring; unpaid internships.
Library Facilities 140,319 volumes (5,200 in health, 1,475 in nursing); 870 periodical subscriptions (130 health-care related).

BACCALAUREATE PROGRAMS

Degree BSN
Available Programs Accelerated RN Baccalaureate; Generic Baccalaureate.
Study Options Full-time and part-time.
Program Entrance Requirements Minimum overall college GPA of 2.7, transcript of college record, CPR certification, health exam, health insurance, high school chemistry, 2 years high school math, 2 years high school science, high school transcript, immunizations, minimum high school rank 75%, minimum GPA in nursing prerequisites of 2.7, prerequisite course work. Transfer students are accepted. *Application deadline:*

5/31 (fall), 10/1 (winter), 10/1 (spring), 4/1 (summer). *Application fee:* $25.
Advanced Placement Credit by examination available. Credit given for nursing courses completed elsewhere dependent upon specific evaluations.
Expenses (2010-11) *Tuition:* full-time $23,260; part-time $640 per credit hour. *Room and board:* $7260; room only: $4400 per academic year. *Required fees:* full-time $300; part-time $150 per term.
Financial Aid 90% of baccalaureate students in nursing programs received some form of financial aid in 2009-10. *Gift aid (need-based):* Federal Pell, FSEOG, state, private, college/university gift aid from institutional funds. *Loans:* Federal Direct (Subsidized and Unsubsidized Stafford PLUS), Perkins, state, college/university. *Work-study:* Federal Work-Study, part-time campus jobs. *Financial aid application deadline (priority):* 3/1.
Contact Dr. Mary P. Tarbox, Professor and Chair, Department of Nursing, Mount Mercy University, 1330 Elmhurst Drive NE, Cedar Rapids, IA 52402. *Telephone:* 800-248-4504 Ext. 6460. *Fax:* 319-368-6479. *E-mail:* mtarbox@mtmercy.edu.

GRADUATE PROGRAMS

Expenses (2010-11) *Tuition:* full-time $15,750; part-time $525 per credit hour. *International tuition:* $15,750 full-time. *Required fees:* full-time $100; part-time $50 per term.
Financial Aid 90% of graduate students in nursing programs received some form of financial aid in 2009-10.
Contact Dr. Mary P. Tarbox, Chair, Department of Nursing, Mount Mercy University, 1330 Elmhurst DR NE, Cedar Rapids, IA 52402. *Telephone:* 319-368-6471. *Fax:* 319-368-6479. *E-mail:* mtarbox@mtmercy.edu.

MASTER'S DEGREE PROGRAM

Degree MSN
Available Programs Master's.
Concentrations Available Nursing education. *Clinical nurse specialist programs in:* public health.
Study Options Full-time and part-time.
Program Entrance Requirements Clinical experience, transcript of college record, written essay, 2 letters of recommendation, statistics course. *Application deadline:* 7/15 (fall), 12/15 (spring). *Application fee:* $25.
Advanced Placement Credit given for nursing courses completed elsewhere dependent upon specific evaluations.
Degree Requirements 36 total credit hours.

CONTINUING EDUCATION PROGRAM

Contact Dr. Mary P. Tarbox, Professor and Chair, Department of Nursing, Mount Mercy University, 1330 Elmhurst Drive NE, Cedar Rapids, IA 52402. *Telephone:* 319-368-6471. *Fax:* 319-368-6479. *E-mail:* mtarbox@mtmercy.edu.

Northwestern College
Nursing Program
Orange City, Iowa

http://www.nwciowa.edu/nursing
Founded in 1882

DEGREE • BSN
Nursing Program Faculty 8 (12% with doctorates).
Baccalaureate Enrollment 58 **Women** 93% **Men** 7% **Part-time** 3%
Nursing Student Activities Nursing Honor Society, Sigma Theta Tau, Student Nurses' Association, nursing club.
Nursing Student Resources Academic advising; assistance for students with disabilities; bookstore; campus computer network; career placement assistance; computer lab; e-mail services; housing assistance; interactive nursing skills videos; Internet; learning resource lab; library services; nursing audiovisuals; placement services for program completers; remedial services; resume preparation assistance; skills, simulation, or other laboratory; tutoring.
Library Facilities 125,000 volumes; 615 periodical subscriptions.

BACCALAUREATE PROGRAMS

Degree BSN
Available Programs Generic Baccalaureate.
Study Options Full-time.
Program Entrance Requirements Transcript of college record, CPR certification, written essay, health exam, immunizations, minimum GPA in nursing prerequisites of 2.7, prerequisite course work. Transfer students are accepted. *Application deadline:* 4/10 (spring). *Application fee:* $550.
Advanced Placement Credit given for nursing courses completed elsewhere dependent upon specific evaluations.
Expenses (2010-11) *Tuition:* full-time $23,330. *Room and board:* $7090 per academic year. *Required fees:* full-time $200.
Financial Aid 100% of baccalaureate students in nursing programs received some form of financial aid in 2009-10.
Contact Dr. Ruth Daumer, Associate Professor of Nursing, Nursing Program, Northwestern College, 101 7th Street SW, Orange City, IA 51041. *Telephone:* 712-707-7086. *E-mail:* rdaumer@nwciowa.edu.

St. Ambrose University
Program in Nursing (BSN)
Davenport, Iowa

http://www.sau.edu/
Founded in 1882

DEGREES • BSN • MSN
Nursing Program Faculty 15 (27% with doctorates).
Baccalaureate Enrollment 170 **Women** 94% **Men** 6% **Minority** 5% **International** 1% **Part-time** 2%
Graduate Enrollment 14 **Women** 100% **Part-time** 100%
Nursing Student Activities Student Nurses' Association.
Nursing Student Resources Academic advising; academic or career counseling; assistance for students with disabilities; bookstore; campus computer network; career placement assistance; computer lab; e-mail services; employment services for current students; housing assistance; interactive nursing skills videos; Internet; learning resource lab; library services; nursing audiovisuals; resume preparation assistance; skills, simulation, or other laboratory; tutoring; unpaid internships.
Library Facilities 156,303 volumes (1,793 in health, 674 in nursing); 679 periodical subscriptions (157 health-care related).

BACCALAUREATE PROGRAMS

Degree BSN
Available Programs Generic Baccalaureate; RN Baccalaureate.
Study Options Full-time and part-time.
Program Entrance Requirements Minimum overall college GPA of 3.0, transcript of college record, CPR certification, health exam, health insurance, high school biology, high school chemistry, high school foreign language, 3 years high school math, high school transcript, immunizations, minimum GPA in nursing prerequisites of 3.0, prerequisite course work. Transfer students are accepted. *Application deadline:* 4/1 (fall), 10/25 (winter), 11/30 (spring), 4/15 (summer). Applications may be processed on a rolling basis for some programs. *Application fee:* $25.
Advanced Placement Credit by examination available. Credit given for nursing courses completed elsewhere dependent upon specific evaluations.
Expenses (2010-11) *Tuition:* full-time $23,670; part-time $735 per credit hour. *Room and board:* $6860; room only: $4060 per academic year. *Required fees:* full-time $400; part-time $200 per credit; part-time $200 per term.
Financial Aid 95% of baccalaureate students in nursing programs received some form of financial aid in 2009-10. *Gift aid (need-based):* Federal Pell, FSEOG, state, private, college/university gift aid from institutional funds. *Loans:* Federal Direct (Subsidized and Unsubsidized Stafford PLUS), Perkins, private loans. *Work-study:* Federal Work-Study, part-time campus jobs. *Financial aid application deadline (priority):* 3/15.
Contact Nursing Department, Program in Nursing (BSN), St. Ambrose University, 518 West Locust Street, Davenport, IA 52803. *Telephone:* 563-333-6076. *E-mail:* nursing@sau.edu.

GRADUATE PROGRAMS

Expenses (2010-11) *Tuition:* full-time $23,670; part-time $735 per credit hour. *International tuition:* $23,670 full-time. *Room and board:* $4060; room only: $2800 per academic year. *Required fees:* full-time $50; part-time $50 per credit; part-time $50 per term.
Financial Aid 100% of graduate students in nursing programs received some form of financial aid in 2009-10.

Contact Ms. Kathryn M. McKnight, Director of MSN Program, Program in Nursing (BSN), St. Ambrose University, 1320 West Lombard Street, Davenport, IA 52804-2029. *Telephone:* 563-333-6069. *Fax:* 563-333-6063. *E-mail:* mcknightkathrynm@sau.edu.

MASTER'S DEGREE PROGRAM

Degree MSN
Available Programs Master's.
Concentrations Available Nursing administration.
Study Options Part-time.
Program Entrance Requirements Clinical experience, minimum overall college GPA of 3.0, transcript of college record, CPR certification, immunizations, 3 letters of recommendation, physical assessment course, resume, statistics course. *Application deadline:* 4/15 (fall). Applications may be processed on a rolling basis for some programs. *Application fee:* $25.
Advanced Placement Credit given for nursing courses completed elsewhere dependent upon specific evaluations.
Degree Requirements 40 total credit hours, thesis or project.

CONTINUING EDUCATION PROGRAM

Contact Dr. Dolores A. Hilden, Chairperson, Program in Nursing (BSN), St. Ambrose University, 1320 West Lombard Street, Davenport, IA 52804-2029. *Telephone:* 563-333-6076. *Fax:* 563-333-6063. *E-mail:* hildendoloresa@sau.edu.

University of Dubuque
School of Professional Programs
Dubuque, Iowa

http://www.dbq.edu/academics/nursing
Founded in 1852

DEGREE • BSN

Nursing Program Faculty 8 (1% with doctorates).
Baccalaureate Enrollment 58 **Women** 86% **Men** 14% **Minority** 2%
Nursing Student Activities Student Nurses' Association.
Nursing Student Resources Academic advising; academic or career counseling; assistance for students with disabilities; bookstore; campus computer network; career placement assistance; computer lab; daycare for children of students; e-mail services; employment services for current students; interactive nursing skills videos; Internet; learning resource lab; library services; nursing audiovisuals; resume preparation assistance; skills, simulation, or other laboratory; tutoring; unpaid internships.
Library Facilities 184,728 volumes; 37,169 periodical subscriptions.

BACCALAUREATE PROGRAMS

Degree BSN
Available Programs RN Baccalaureate.
Study Options Full-time.
Program Entrance Requirements Transcript of college record, CPR certification, health exam, health insurance, immunizations, 2 letters of recommendation, minimum GPA in nursing prerequisites of 2.75, professional liability insurance/malpractice insurance, prerequisite course work. Transfer students are accepted.
Financial Aid ***Gift aid (need-based):*** Federal Pell, FSEOG, state, private, college/university gift aid from institutional funds. *Loans:* Federal Direct (Subsidized and Unsubsidized Stafford PLUS), Perkins, state, college/university. *Work-study:* Federal Work-Study, part-time campus jobs. *Financial aid application deadline:* Continuous.
Contact BSN Program, School of Professional Programs, University of Dubuque, 2000 University Avenue, Dubuque, IA 52001. *Telephone:* 563-589-3000.

The University of Iowa
College of Nursing
Iowa City, Iowa

http://www.nursing.uiowa.edu
Founded in 1847

DEGREES • BSN • MSN • MSN/MBA • MSN/MPH • PHD

Nursing Program Faculty 67 (63% with doctorates).
Baccalaureate Enrollment 618 **Women** 93% **Men** 7% **Minority** 6% **Part-time** 25%
Graduate Enrollment 258 **Women** 89% **Men** 11% **Minority** 4% **International** 7% **Part-time** 50%
Nursing Student Activities Sigma Theta Tau, Student Nurses' Association.
Nursing Student Resources Academic advising; academic or career counseling; assistance for students with disabilities; campus computer network; career placement assistance; computer lab; computer-assisted instruction; e-mail services; employment services for current students; Internet; learning resource lab; nursing audiovisuals; placement services for program completers; resume preparation assistance; skills, simulation, or other laboratory; tutoring.
Library Facilities 4.1 million volumes (273,469 in health); 49,279 periodical subscriptions (2,500 health-care related).

BACCALAUREATE PROGRAMS

Degree BSN
Available Programs Generic Baccalaureate; RN Baccalaureate.
Study Options Full-time and part-time.
Program Entrance Requirements Minimum overall college GPA of 2.7, transcript of college record, CPR certification, written essay, health exam, health insurance, high school biology, high school chemistry, high school foreign language, 3 years high school math, 3 years high school science, high school transcript, immunizations, minimum GPA in nursing prerequisites of 2.7, professional liability insurance/malpractice insurance, prerequisite course work. Transfer students are accepted.
Advanced Placement Credit given for nursing courses completed elsewhere dependent upon specific evaluations.
Contact ***Telephone:*** 319-335-7016. *Fax:* 319-384-4423.

GRADUATE PROGRAMS

Contact ***Telephone:*** 319-335-7021. *Fax:* 319-335-9990.

MASTER'S DEGREE PROGRAM

Degrees MSN; MSN/MBA; MSN/MPH
Available Programs Accelerated RN to Master's; Master's; Master's for Nurses with Non-Nursing Degrees.
Concentrations Available Nurse anesthesia; nursing administration; nursing education; nursing informatics. *Clinical nurse specialist programs in:* adult health, community health, gerontology, occupational health, psychiatric/mental health. *Nurse practitioner programs in:* adult health, family health, gerontology, neonatal health, pediatric, psychiatric/mental health.
Study Options Full-time and part-time.
Program Entrance Requirements Computer literacy, minimum overall college GPA of 3.0, transcript of college record, written essay, immunizations, 3 letters of recommendation, nursing research course, physical assessment course, professional liability insurance/malpractice insurance, prerequisite course work, resume, statistics course.
Advanced Placement Credit given for nursing courses completed elsewhere dependent upon specific evaluations.
Degree Requirements 33 total credit hours, thesis or project.

POST-MASTER'S PROGRAM

Areas of Study Nursing informatics. *Clinical nurse specialist programs in:* adult health, psychiatric/mental health. *Nurse practitioner programs in:* adult health, family health, gerontology, pediatric, psychiatric/mental health.

DOCTORAL DEGREE PROGRAM

Degree PhD
Available Programs Doctorate; Post-Baccalaureate Doctorate.
Areas of Study Aging, family health, gerontology, individualized study, information systems, nursing administration.
Program Entrance Requirements Minimum overall college GPA of 3.0, interview, 3 letters of recommendation, statistics course, vita, GRE General Test.
Degree Requirements 60 total credit hours, dissertation, oral exam, written exam, residency.

POSTDOCTORAL PROGRAM

Areas of Study Family health, nursing informatics, nursing interventions, outcomes.
Postdoctoral Program Contact ***Telephone:*** 319-335-7021. *Fax:* 319-335-9990.

CONTINUING EDUCATION PROGRAM

Contact ***Telephone:*** 319-335-7075. *Fax:* 319-335-9990.

Upper Iowa University
RN-BSN Nursing Program
Fayette, Iowa

Founded in 1857

DEGREE • BSN

Nursing Program Faculty 10
Library Facilities 73,237 volumes; 282 periodical subscriptions.

BACCALAUREATE PROGRAMS

Degree BSN
Available Programs RN Baccalaureate.
Site Options Cedar Rapids, IA; West Des Moines, IA.
Program Entrance Requirements Minimum overall college GPA of 2.5, transcript of college record, CPR certification, health exam, high school transcript, RN licensure. Transfer students are accepted.
Contact *Telephone:* 563-425-5357.

KANSAS

Baker University
School of Nursing
Topeka, Kansas

http://www.bakeru.edu/
Founded in 1858

DEGREE • BSN

Nursing Program Faculty 16 (24% with doctorates).
Baccalaureate Enrollment 171 **Women** 88% **Men** 12% **Minority** 15% **Part-time** .1%
Nursing Student Activities Sigma Theta Tau, Student Nurses' Association.
Nursing Student Resources Academic advising; assistance for students with disabilities; campus computer network; computer lab; computer-assisted instruction; e-mail services; Internet; learning resource lab; library services; nursing audiovisuals; resume preparation assistance; skills, simulation, or other laboratory; tutoring.
Library Facilities 103,243 volumes (5,000 in health, 2,716 in nursing); 567 periodical subscriptions (414 health-care related).

BACCALAUREATE PROGRAMS

Degree BSN
Available Programs Generic Baccalaureate; RN Baccalaureate.
Study Options Full-time and part-time.
Program Entrance Requirements Transcript of college record, CPR certification, written essay, health exam, health insurance, high school transcript, immunizations, interview, minimum GPA in nursing prerequisites of 2.7, prerequisite course work. Transfer students are accepted. *Application deadline:* 12/1 (fall), 8/1 (spring).
Advanced Placement Credit given for nursing courses completed elsewhere dependent upon specific evaluations.
Expenses (2010-11) *Tuition:* full-time $14,400; part-time $480 per credit hour. *Required fees:* full-time $500.
Financial Aid 89% of baccalaureate students in nursing programs received some form of financial aid in 2009-10.
Contact Ms. Janet Creager, Student Affairs Specialist, School of Nursing, Baker University, 1500 SW 10th Street, Topeka, KS 66604-1353. *Telephone:* 785-354-5850. *Fax:* 785-354-5832. *E-mail:* janet.creager@bakeru.edu.

Bethel College
Department of Nursing
North Newton, Kansas

http://www.bethelks.edu
Founded in 1887

DEGREE • BSN

Nursing Program Faculty 9
Baccalaureate Enrollment 100 **Women** 75% **Men** 25% **Minority** 30% **International** 25% **Part-time** 1%
Nursing Student Activities Nursing Honor Society, Sigma Theta Tau, Student Nurses' Association.
Nursing Student Resources Academic advising; academic or career counseling; assistance for students with disabilities; bookstore; computer lab; e-mail services; employment services for current students; housing assistance; Internet; learning resource lab; library services; nursing audiovisuals; resume preparation assistance; skills, simulation, or other laboratory; tutoring.
Library Facilities 1.1 million volumes (5,690 in health, 3,150 in nursing); 32,765 periodical subscriptions (445 health-care related).

BACCALAUREATE PROGRAMS

Degree BSN
Available Programs Generic Baccalaureate; LPN to Baccalaureate; RN Baccalaureate.
Study Options Full-time and part-time.
Program Entrance Requirements Minimum overall college GPA of 3.0, transcript of college record, CPR certification, written essay, health exam, health insurance, high school transcript, immunizations, interview, 2 letters of recommendation, minimum high school GPA of 3.0, minimum GPA in nursing prerequisites of 2.0, prerequisite course work. Transfer students are accepted.
Advanced Placement Credit given for nursing courses completed elsewhere dependent upon specific evaluations.
Contact *Telephone:* 316-283-2500 Ext. 377. *Fax:* 316-284-5286.

Emporia State University
Newman Division of Nursing
Emporia, Kansas

http://www.emporia.edu/ndn
Founded in 1863

DEGREE • BSN

Nursing Program Faculty 12 (25% with doctorates).
Baccalaureate Enrollment 124 **Women** 90% **Men** 10% **Minority** 16% **International** 2% **Part-time** 8%
Nursing Student Activities Student Nurses' Association.
Nursing Student Resources Academic advising; academic or career counseling; assistance for students with disabilities; bookstore; campus computer network; career placement assistance; computer lab; computer-assisted instruction; daycare for children of students; e-mail services; employment services for current students; housing assistance; interactive nursing skills videos; Internet; learning resource lab; library services; nursing audiovisuals; placement services for program completers; remedial services; resume preparation assistance; skills, simulation, or other laboratory; tutoring.
Library Facilities 2.5 million volumes (52,844 in health, 2,248 in nursing); 41,417 periodical subscriptions (144 health-care related).

BACCALAUREATE PROGRAMS

Degree BSN
Available Programs ADN to Baccalaureate; Generic Baccalaureate; LPN to Baccalaureate; RN Baccalaureate.
Study Options Full-time and part-time.
Program Entrance Requirements Transcript of college record, written essay, minimum GPA in nursing prerequisites of 2.5, prerequisite course work. Transfer students are accepted. *Application deadline:* 5/1 (fall). *Application fee:* $25.
Advanced Placement Credit given for nursing courses completed elsewhere dependent upon specific evaluations.
Expenses (2010-11) *Tuition, area resident:* full-time $3614; part-time $120 per credit hour. *Tuition, state resident:* full-time $5420; part-time $181 per credit hour. *Tuition, nonresident:* full-time $13,324; part-time $444 per credit hour. *Room and board:* $6230 per academic year. *Required fees:* full-time $1022; part-time $62 per credit.
Financial Aid 90% of baccalaureate students in nursing programs received some form of financial aid in 2009-10. *Gift aid (need-based):* Federal Pell, FSEOG, state, private, college/university gift aid from institutional funds, Jones Foundation Grants, grants from outside sources. *Loans:* Perkins, Alaska Loans, alternative loans. *Work-study:* Federal Work-Study, part-time campus jobs. *Financial aid application deadline (priority):* 3/15.
Contact Dr. Judith E. Calhoun, Division Chair, Newman Division of Nursing, Emporia State University, 1127 Chestnut Street, Emporia, KS

66801. *Telephone:* 620-343-6800 Ext. 5641. *Fax:* 620-341-7871. *E-mail:* jcalhoun@emporia.edu.

Fort Hays State University
Department of Nursing
Hays, Kansas

http://www.fhsu.edu/nursing/
Founded in 1902

DEGREES • BSN • MSN
Nursing Program Faculty 21 (19% with doctorates).
Baccalaureate Enrollment 115 **Women** 92% **Men** 8% **Minority** 3% **Part-time** 44%
Graduate Enrollment 78 **Women** 99% **Men** 1% **Minority** 1% **Part-time** 99%
Distance Learning Courses Available.
Nursing Student Activities Sigma Theta Tau, Student Nurses' Association, nursing club.
Nursing Student Resources Academic advising; academic or career counseling; assistance for students with disabilities; bookstore; campus computer network; career placement assistance; computer lab; computer-assisted instruction; daycare for children of students; e-mail services; employment services for current students; housing assistance; interactive nursing skills videos; Internet; learning resource lab; library services; nursing audiovisuals; paid internships; placement services for program completers; remedial services; resume preparation assistance; skills, simulation, or other laboratory; tutoring.
Library Facilities 11,390 volumes in health, 1,750 volumes in nursing; 205 periodical subscriptions health-care related.

BACCALAUREATE PROGRAMS
Degree BSN
Available Programs Generic Baccalaureate; RN Baccalaureate.
Study Options Full-time and part-time.
Online Degree Options Yes.
Program Entrance Requirements Minimum overall college GPA of 2.5, transcript of college record, CPR certification, written essay, health exam, health insurance, high school transcript, immunizations, 2 letters of recommendation, minimum GPA in nursing prerequisites of 2.0, professional liability insurance/malpractice insurance, prerequisite course work. Transfer students are accepted. *Application deadline:* 3/1 (fall), 10/1 (spring).
Advanced Placement Credit by examination available. Credit given for nursing courses completed elsewhere dependent upon specific evaluations.
Expenses (2009-10) *Tuition, area resident:* full-time $1881; part-time $125 per credit hour. *Tuition, state resident:* full-time $2618; part-time $175 per credit hour. *Tuition, nonresident:* full-time $5957; part-time $397 per credit hour. *International tuition:* $5957 full-time. *Room and board:* $6560; room only: $3335 per academic year.
Financial Aid 96% of baccalaureate students in nursing programs received some form of financial aid in 2008-09.
Contact Ms. Rebecca Sander, Coordinator of Quality and Advising, Department of Nursing, Fort Hays State University, 600 Park Street, Stroup Hall, Room 139, Hays, KS 67601-4099. *Telephone:* 785-628-5561. *Fax:* 785-628-4080. *E-mail:* rsander@fhsu.edu.

GRADUATE PROGRAMS
Expenses (2009-10) *Tuition, area resident:* full-time $2087; part-time $174 per credit hour. *Tuition, state resident:* full-time $2968; part-time $247 per credit hour. *Tuition, nonresident:* full-time $5545; part-time $462 per credit hour. *International tuition:* $462 full-time. *Room and board:* $6560; room only: $3335 per academic year.
Financial Aid 94% of graduate students in nursing programs received some form of financial aid in 2008-09. 1 teaching assistantship (averaging $5,000 per year) was awarded; research assistantships.
Contact Dr. Liane Connelly, Chair, Department of Nursing, Fort Hays State University, 600 Park Street, Stroup Hall, Room 127, Hays, KS 67601-4099. *Telephone:* 785-628-4511. *Fax:* 785-628-4080. *E-mail:* lconnell@fhsu.edu.

MASTER'S DEGREE PROGRAM
Degree MSN
Available Programs Master's.
Concentrations Available Nursing administration; nursing education. *Nurse practitioner programs in:* family health.
Study Options Full-time and part-time.
Online Degree Options Yes.
Program Entrance Requirements Clinical experience, computer literacy, minimum overall college GPA of 3.0, transcript of college record, CPR certification, written essay, immunizations, 2 letters of recommendation, physical assessment course, professional liability insurance/malpractice insurance, prerequisite course work, statistics course, GRE General Test or MAT. *Application deadline:* 2/1 (fall), 9/1 (spring), 2/1 (summer).
Advanced Placement Credit given for nursing courses completed elsewhere dependent upon specific evaluations.
Degree Requirements 34 total credit hours, thesis or project, comprehensive exam.

POST-MASTER'S PROGRAM
Areas of Study Nursing administration; nursing education. *Nurse practitioner programs in:* family health.

Kansas Wesleyan University
Department of Nursing Education
Salina, Kansas

http://www.kwu.edu/nursing
Founded in 1886

DEGREE • BSN
Nursing Program Faculty 8 (13% with doctorates).
Baccalaureate Enrollment 68 **Women** 91% **Men** 9% **Minority** 12% **International** 3% **Part-time** 2%
Nursing Student Activities Nursing club.
Nursing Student Resources Academic advising; academic or career counseling; assistance for students with disabilities; bookstore; campus computer network; career placement assistance; computer lab; computer-assisted instruction; e-mail services; employment services for current students; housing assistance; Internet; learning resource lab; library services; nursing audiovisuals; resume preparation assistance; skills, simulation, or other laboratory; tutoring.
Library Facilities 97,060 volumes (15,921 in health, 8,700 in nursing); 188 periodical subscriptions (1,123 health-care related).

BACCALAUREATE PROGRAMS
Degree BSN
Available Programs ADN to Baccalaureate; Generic Baccalaureate; RN Baccalaureate.
Study Options Full-time and part-time.
Program Entrance Requirements Minimum overall college GPA of 2.6, transcript of college record, health exam, high school transcript, immunizations, minimum GPA in nursing prerequisites of 2.6, prerequisite course work. Transfer students are accepted. *Application deadline:* Applications may be processed on a rolling basis for some programs.
Advanced Placement Credit by examination available. Credit given for nursing courses completed elsewhere dependent upon specific evaluations.
Financial Aid 100% of baccalaureate students in nursing programs received some form of financial aid in 2009-10.
Contact Dr. Linda M. Adams-Wendling, Chair/Director of Division/Department Nursing Education, Department of Nursing Education, Kansas Wesleyan University, 100 East Claflin Avenue, Campus Box 39, Salina, KS 67401-6196. *Telephone:* 785-827-5541 Ext. 2311. *Fax:* 785-827-0927. *E-mail:* linda.adams-wendling@kwu.edu.

MidAmerica Nazarene University
Division of Nursing
Olathe, Kansas

http://www.mnu.edu
Founded in 1966

DEGREE • BSN
Nursing Program Faculty 14 (36% with doctorates).
Baccalaureate Enrollment 63 **Women** 81% **Men** 19% **Minority** 16% **International** 17%
Nursing Student Activities Student Nurses' Association, nursing club.
Nursing Student Resources Academic advising; academic or career counseling; assistance for students with disabilities; bookstore; campus

computer network; career placement assistance; computer lab; computer-assisted instruction; e-mail services; employment services for current students; housing assistance; Internet; learning resource lab; library services; nursing audiovisuals; resume preparation assistance; skills, simulation, or other laboratory; tutoring; unpaid internships.
Library Facilities 133,140 volumes (1,903 in health, 547 in nursing); 1,260 periodical subscriptions (115 health-care related).

BACCALAUREATE PROGRAMS

Degree BSN
Available Programs ADN to Baccalaureate; Accelerated Baccalaureate; Accelerated Baccalaureate for Second Degree; Accelerated LPN to Baccalaureate; Accelerated RN Baccalaureate; Generic Baccalaureate; RN Baccalaureate.
Study Options Full-time.
Program Entrance Requirements Minimum overall college GPA of 2.6, transcript of college record, CPR certification, written essay, health exam, health insurance, high school transcript, immunizations, 2 letters of recommendation, minimum GPA in nursing prerequisites of 2.6, prerequisite course work. Transfer students are accepted.
Advanced Placement Credit by examination available. Credit given for nursing courses completed elsewhere dependent upon specific evaluations.
Contact ***Telephone:*** 913-971-3698. *Fax:* 913-971-3408.

CONTINUING EDUCATION PROGRAM

Contact ***Telephone:*** 913-971-3696. *Fax:* 913-971-3408.

Newman University

Division of Nursing
Wichita, Kansas

http://www.newmanu.edu/
Founded in 1933

DEGREE • BSN

Nursing Program Faculty 12 (25% with doctorates).
Baccalaureate Enrollment 116 **Women** 88% **Men** 12% **Minority** 8% **International** 1% **Part-time** 3%
Graduate Enrollment 41 **Women** 60% **Men** 40% **Minority** 7%
Nursing Student Activities Sigma Theta Tau, nursing club.
Nursing Student Resources Academic advising; academic or career counseling; assistance for students with disabilities; bookstore; campus computer network; computer lab; computer-assisted instruction; e-mail services; Internet; learning resource lab; library services; nursing audiovisuals; remedial services; resume preparation assistance; skills, simulation, or other laboratory; tutoring.
Library Facilities 110,167 volumes (2,940 in health, 763 in nursing); 122 periodical subscriptions (769 health-care related).

BACCALAUREATE PROGRAMS

Degree BSN
Available Programs Generic Baccalaureate; LPN to Baccalaureate; RN Baccalaureate.
Study Options Full-time and part-time.
Program Entrance Requirements Minimum overall college GPA of 2.75, transcript of college record, CPR certification, written essay, health exam, health insurance, immunizations, interview, 2 letters of recommendation, minimum GPA in nursing prerequisites of 2.75, professional liability insurance/malpractice insurance, prerequisite course work. Transfer students are accepted. *Application deadline:* Applications may be processed on a rolling basis for some programs.
Advanced Placement Credit given for nursing courses completed elsewhere dependent upon specific evaluations.
Expenses (2010-11) *Tuition:* full-time $19,872; part-time $662 per credit hour. *Room and board:* $3520 per academic year. *Required fees:* full-time $487; part-time $15 per credit.
Financial Aid 78% of baccalaureate students in nursing programs received some form of financial aid in 2009-10. *Gift aid (need-based):* Federal Pell, FSEOG, state, private, college/university gift aid from institutional funds. *Loans:* Federal Direct (Subsidized and Unsubsidized Stafford PLUS), Perkins. *Work-study:* Federal Work-Study, part-time campus jobs. *Financial aid application deadline (priority):* 3/1.
Contact Dr. Bernadette M. Fetterolf, Associate Dean, School of Nursing and Allied Health, Division of Nursing, Newman University, 3100 McCormick Avenue, Wichita, KS 67213-2097. *Telephone:* 316-942-4291 Ext. 2244. *Fax:* 316-942-4483. *E-mail:* fetterolfb@newmanu.edu.

GRADUATE PROGRAMS

Expenses (2010-11) *Tuition:* full-time $20,000. *Room and board:* $3520 per academic year. *Required fees:* full-time $350.
Financial Aid 100% of graduate students in nursing programs received some form of financial aid in 2009-10. *Application deadline:* 8/15.
Contact Ms. Sharon Niemann, Director, Master of Science in Nurse Anesthesia Program, Division of Nursing, Newman University, 3100 McCormick Avenue, Wichita, KS 67213-2097. *Telephone:* 316-942-4291 Ext. 2272. *Fax:* 316-942-4483. *E-mail:* niemanns@newmanu.edu.

MASTER'S DEGREE PROGRAM

Program Entrance Requirements MAT.

Pittsburg State University

Department of Nursing
Pittsburg, Kansas

http://www.pittstate.edu/nurs
Founded in 1903

DEGREES • BSN • MSN

Nursing Program Faculty 23 (25% with doctorates).
Baccalaureate Enrollment 142 **Women** 93% **Men** 7% **Minority** 100% **International** 1%
Graduate Enrollment 67 **Women** 90% **Men** 10% **Minority** 100% **International** 1%
Distance Learning Courses Available.
Nursing Student Activities Nursing Honor Society, Sigma Theta Tau, Student Nurses' Association.
Nursing Student Resources Academic advising; academic or career counseling; assistance for students with disabilities; bookstore; campus computer network; career placement assistance; computer lab; computer-assisted instruction; e-mail services; employment services for current students; externships; housing assistance; interactive nursing skills videos; Internet; learning resource lab; library services; nursing audiovisuals; placement services for program completers; resume preparation assistance; skills, simulation, or other laboratory; tutoring; unpaid internships.
Library Facilities 712,681 volumes (45,044 in nursing); 35,360 periodical subscriptions.

BACCALAUREATE PROGRAMS

Degree BSN
Available Programs Generic Baccalaureate; RN Baccalaureate.
Study Options Full-time and part-time.
Online Degree Options Yes.
Program Entrance Requirements Minimum overall college GPA of 2.5, transcript of college record, CPR certification, health exam, immunizations, 3 letters of recommendation, minimum GPA in nursing prerequisites of 2.5, professional liability insurance/malpractice insurance, prerequisite course work. Transfer students are accepted. *Application deadline:* 12/15 (fall). *Application fee:* $25.
Advanced Placement Credit by examination available. Credit given for nursing courses completed elsewhere dependent upon specific evaluations.
Expenses (2010-11) *Tuition, area resident:* full-time $2424; part-time $173 per credit hour. *Tuition, nonresident:* full-time $6794; part-time $464 per credit hour. *Room and board:* $2955 per academic year. *Required fees:* part-time $173 per credit.
Financial Aid 95% of baccalaureate students in nursing programs received some form of financial aid in 2009-10. *Gift aid (need-based):* Federal Pell, FSEOG, state, private, college/university gift aid from institutional funds. *Loans:* Federal Nursing Student Loans, Federal Direct (Subsidized and Unsubsidized Stafford PLUS), Perkins, college/university. *Work-study:* Federal Work-Study, part-time campus jobs. *Financial aid application deadline (priority):* 3/1.
Contact Dr. Barbara Ruth McClaskey, Coordinator of Bachelor of Science in Nursing Program, Department of Nursing, Pittsburg State University, 1701 South Broadway, Pittsburg, KS 66762. *Telephone:* 620-235-4437. *Fax:* 620-235-4449. *E-mail:* bmcclask@pittstate.edu.

GRADUATE PROGRAMS

Expenses (2010-11) *Tuition, area resident:* full-time $2720; part-time $230 per credit hour. *Tuition, nonresident:* full-time $6503; part-time

$545 per credit hour. *International tuition:* $6503 full-time. *Room and board:* $2955 per academic year. *Required fees:* part-time $230 per credit.

Financial Aid 90% of graduate students in nursing programs received some form of financial aid in 2009-10.

Contact Dr. Mary Carol Pomatto, Master of Science Coordinator, Department of Nursing, Pittsburg State University, 1701 South Broadway, Pittsburg, KS 66762. *Telephone:* 620-235-4431. *Fax:* 620-235-4449. *E-mail:* mpomatto@pittstate.edu.

MASTER'S DEGREE PROGRAM

Degree MSN

Available Programs Master's.

Concentrations Available Clinical nurse leader; nursing administration; nursing education. *Clinical nurse specialist programs in:* family health. *Nurse practitioner programs in:* family health.

Study Options Full-time and part-time.

Program Entrance Requirements Clinical experience, minimum overall college GPA of 3.0, transcript of college record, CPR certification, written essay, immunizations, 3 letters of recommendation, nursing research course, physical assessment course, professional liability insurance/malpractice insurance, prerequisite course work, statistics course, GRE General Test. *Application deadline:* 3/15 (fall). *Application fee:* $50.

Advanced Placement Credit given for nursing courses completed elsewhere dependent upon specific evaluations.

Degree Requirements 47 total credit hours, thesis or project, comprehensive exam.

POST-MASTER'S PROGRAM

Areas of Study Clinical nurse leader; nursing administration; nursing education. *Clinical nurse specialist programs in:* family health. *Nurse practitioner programs in:* family health.

CONTINUING EDUCATION PROGRAM

Contact Ms. Kristy L. Frisbee, Coordinator of Continuing Nursing Education, Department of Nursing, Pittsburg State University, 1701 South Broadway, McPherson Hall, RM 121, Pittsburg, KS 66762. *Telephone:* 620-235-4434. *Fax:* 620-235-4449. *E-mail:* kfrisbee@pittstate.edu.

Southwestern College

Nursing Program
Winfield, Kansas

Founded in 1885

DEGREE • BSN

Nursing Program Faculty 6 (33% with doctorates).

Baccalaureate Enrollment 79

Nursing Student Activities Nursing Honor Society, Sigma Theta Tau, Student Nurses' Association, nursing club.

Nursing Student Resources Academic advising; academic or career counseling; assistance for students with disabilities; bookstore; campus computer network; career placement assistance; computer lab; computer-assisted instruction; e-mail services; externships; housing assistance; interactive nursing skills videos; Internet; learning resource lab; library services; nursing audiovisuals; paid internships; placement services for program completers; remedial services; resume preparation assistance; skills, simulation, or other laboratory; tutoring; unpaid internships.

Library Facilities 56,237 volumes; 40,660 periodical subscriptions.

BACCALAUREATE PROGRAMS

Degree BSN

Available Programs Accelerated RN Baccalaureate; Generic Baccalaureate; LPN to Baccalaureate; RN Baccalaureate.

Site Options Wichita, KS.

Study Options Full-time and part-time.

Online Degree Options Yes.

Program Entrance Requirements Transcript of college record, CPR certification, written essay, health exam, health insurance, high school transcript, immunizations, interview, minimum high school GPA of 2.75, minimum GPA in nursing prerequisites of 2.75, professional liability insurance/malpractice insurance, prerequisite course work. Transfer students are accepted.

Advanced Placement Credit given for nursing courses completed elsewhere dependent upon specific evaluations.

Contact *Telephone:* 620-229-6207. *Fax:* 620-229-6152 Ext. 6152.

Tabor College

Department of Nursing
Hillsboro, Kansas

http://www.tabor.edu/adult-graduate

Founded in 1908

DEGREE • BSN

Nursing Program Faculty 12

Baccalaureate Enrollment 71 **Women** 90% **Men** 10% **Minority** 10% **Part-time** 100%

Distance Learning Courses Available.

Nursing Student Activities Sigma Theta Tau.

Nursing Student Resources Academic advising; academic or career counseling; bookstore; campus computer network; computer lab; e-mail services; Internet; learning resource lab; library services; nursing audiovisuals; remedial services; resume preparation assistance; skills, simulation, or other laboratory; tutoring.

Library Facilities 80,099 volumes (240 in health, 140 in nursing); 265 periodical subscriptions (600 health-care related).

BACCALAUREATE PROGRAMS

Degree BSN

Available Programs ADN to Baccalaureate; Accelerated RN Baccalaureate.

Site Options Wichita, KS; Colby, KS; Larned, KS.

Study Options Full-time and part-time.

Online Degree Options Yes (online only).

Program Entrance Requirements Minimum overall college GPA of 2.5, transcript of college record, RN licensure. Transfer students are accepted. *Application deadline:* 8/31 (fall), 12/31 (spring), 4/30 (summer). Applications may be processed on a rolling basis for some programs. *Application fee:* $30.

Advanced Placement Credit by examination available. Credit given for nursing courses completed elsewhere dependent upon specific evaluations.

Expenses (2009-10) *Tuition:* part-time $340 per credit hour.

Financial Aid 90% of baccalaureate students in nursing programs received some form of financial aid in 2008-09. *Gift aid (need-based):* Federal Pell, FSEOG, state, private, college/university gift aid from institutional funds. *Loans:* Federal Direct (Subsidized and Unsubsidized Stafford PLUS), Perkins. *Work-study:* Federal Work-Study, part-time campus jobs. *Financial aid application deadline:* 8/15(priority: 3/1).

Contact Ms. Tona L. Leiker, Dean, Nursing Department, Department of Nursing, Tabor College, 7348 West 21st Street, Suite 117, Wichita, KS 67205. *Telephone:* 316-729-6333 Ext. 206. *Fax:* 316-773-5436. *E-mail:* tonal@tabor.edu.

The University of Kansas

School of Nursing
Kansas City, Kansas

http://www2.kumc.edu/son

Founded in 1866

DEGREES • BSN • MS • MS/MHSA • MS/MPH • PHD

Nursing Program Faculty 74 (58% with doctorates).

Baccalaureate Enrollment 283 **Women** 88% **Men** 12% **Minority** 11% **International** 1% **Part-time** 10%

Graduate Enrollment 387 **Women** 93% **Men** 7% **Minority** 16% **International** 1% **Part-time** 93%

Distance Learning Courses Available.

Nursing Student Activities Nursing Honor Society, Sigma Theta Tau, Student Nurses' Association, nursing club.

Nursing Student Resources Academic advising; academic or career counseling; assistance for students with disabilities; bookstore; campus computer network; computer lab; computer-assisted instruction; e-mail services; employment services for current students; interactive nursing skills videos; Internet; learning resource lab; library services; nursing audiovisuals; remedial services; resume preparation assistance; skills, simulation, or other laboratory.

Library Facilities 5 million volumes (180,000 in health, 5,050 in nursing); 73,613 periodical subscriptions (6,500 health-care related).

BACCALAUREATE PROGRAMS

Degree BSN
Available Programs ADN to Baccalaureate; Generic Baccalaureate; RN Baccalaureate.
Study Options Full-time and part-time.
Program Entrance Requirements Minimum overall college GPA of 2.5, transcript of college record, CPR certification, written essay, health exam, health insurance, immunizations, 3 letters of recommendation, minimum GPA in nursing prerequisites of 2.5, prerequisite course work. Transfer students are accepted. *Application deadline:* 10/15 (fall). *Application fee:* $60.
Advanced Placement Credit given for nursing courses completed elsewhere dependent upon specific evaluations.
Expenses (2010-11) *Tuition, state resident:* part-time $234 per credit hour. *Tuition, nonresident:* part-time $289 per credit hour. *International tuition:* $289 full-time. *Required fees:* full-time $473.
Financial Aid 65% of baccalaureate students in nursing programs received some form of financial aid in 2009-10.
Contact Dr. Rita Clifford, Associate Dean of Student Affairs, School of Nursing, The University of Kansas, 3901 Rainbow Boulevard, Mail Stop 2029, Kansas City, KS 66160. *Telephone:* 913-588-1619. *Fax:* 913-588-1615. *E-mail:* soninfo@kumc.edu.

GRADUATE PROGRAMS

Expenses (2010-11) *Tuition, state resident:* part-time $615 per credit hour. *Tuition, nonresident:* part-time $692 per credit hour. *International tuition:* $692 full-time. *Required fees:* full-time $473.
Financial Aid 52% of graduate students in nursing programs received some form of financial aid in 2009-10. 7 research assistantships (averaging $24,000 per year), 23 teaching assistantships with full and partial tuition reimbursements available (averaging $24,000 per year) were awarded; traineeships also available. *Financial aid application deadline:* 2/14.
Contact Dr. Rita Clifford, Associate Dean, Student Affairs, School of Nursing, The University of Kansas, 3901 Rainbow Boulevard, Mail Stop 2029, Kansas City, KS 66160. *Telephone:* 913-588-1619. *Fax:* 913-588-1615. *E-mail:* soninfo@kumc.edu.

MASTER'S DEGREE PROGRAM

Degrees MS; MS/MHSA; MS/MPH
Available Programs Master's; RN to Master's.
Concentrations Available Health-care administration; nurse-midwifery; nursing administration; nursing informatics. *Clinical nurse specialist programs in:* adult health, gerontology. *Nurse practitioner programs in:* adult health, family health, gerontology, psychiatric/mental health.
Site Options Garden City, KS.
Study Options Full-time and part-time.
Online Degree Options Yes.
Program Entrance Requirements Clinical experience, minimum overall college GPA of 3.0, transcript of college record, CPR certification, immunizations, interview, 3 letters of recommendation, physical assessment course, resume, statistics course. *Application deadline:* 4/1 (fall), 9/1 (spring). *Application fee:* $60.
Degree Requirements 37 total credit hours, thesis or project, comprehensive exam.

POST-MASTER'S PROGRAM

Areas of Study Health-care administration; nurse-midwifery; nursing administration; nursing informatics. *Clinical nurse specialist programs in:* adult health, gerontology. *Nurse practitioner programs in:* adult health, family health, gerontology, psychiatric/mental health.

DOCTORAL DEGREE PROGRAM

Degree PhD
Available Programs Doctorate; Post-Baccalaureate Doctorate.
Areas of Study Advanced practice nursing, nursing administration, nursing research.
Online Degree Options Yes.
Program Entrance Requirements Clinical experience, minimum overall college GPA of 3.5, interview by faculty committee, interview, 3 letters of recommendation, statistics course, vita, writing sample, GRE General Test. Application deadline: 3/1 (fall), 9/1 (spring), 12/1 (summer). Application fee: $60.
Degree Requirements 65 total credit hours, dissertation, oral exam, written exam, residency.

POSTDOCTORAL PROGRAM

Areas of Study Gerontology, nursing research, outcomes, self-care.
Postdoctoral Program Contact Dr. Marjorie J. Bott, Associate Dean, Research, School of Nursing, The University of Kansas, 3901 Rainbow Boulevard, Mail Stop 4043, Kansas City, KS 66160. *Telephone:* 913-588-1692. *E-mail:* mbott@kumc.edu.

CONTINUING EDUCATION PROGRAM

Contact Dr. Mary Gambino, Assistant Dean, Community Affairs, School of Nursing, The University of Kansas, 3901 Rainbow Boulevard, Mail Stop 4001, Kansas City, KS 66160. *Telephone:* 913-588-4488. *Fax:* 913-588-4486. *E-mail:* ceinfo@kumc.edu.

University of Saint Mary

Bachelor of Science in Nursing Program
Leavenworth, Kansas

Founded in 1923

DEGREE • BSN

Nursing Program Faculty 22 (9% with doctorates).
Baccalaureate Enrollment 168 **Women** 93% **Men** 7% **Minority** 12.5% **International** 3.5% **Part-time** 39%
Distance Learning Courses Available.
Nursing Student Activities Student Nurses' Association.
Nursing Student Resources Academic advising; academic or career counseling; bookstore; campus computer network; e-mail services; employment services for current students; Internet; learning resource lab; library services; nursing audiovisuals; placement services for program completers; resume preparation assistance; skills, simulation, or other laboratory; tutoring.
Library Facilities 120,753 volumes; 157 periodical subscriptions.

BACCALAUREATE PROGRAMS

Degree BSN
Available Programs Generic Baccalaureate; RN Baccalaureate.
Site Options Overland Park, KS.
Study Options Full-time.
Online Degree Options Yes (online only).
Program Entrance Requirements Minimum overall college GPA of 2.5, transcript of college record, CPR certification, written essay, health exam, health insurance, immunizations, 2 letters of recommendation, minimum GPA in nursing prerequisites of 2.5, prerequisite course work. Transfer students are accepted. *Application deadline:* 3/1 (fall). Applications may be processed on a rolling basis for some programs.
Contact Michelle Johnson, Nursing Program Specialist, Bachelor of Science in Nursing Program, University of Saint Mary, 4100 South 4th Street, Leavenworth, KS 66007. *Telephone:* 913-758-4381. *Fax:* 913-758-4356. *E-mail:* johnsonm@stmary.edu.

Washburn University

School of Nursing
Topeka, Kansas

http://www.washburn.edu/sonu/index.html
Founded in 1865

DEGREES • BSN • MSN

Nursing Program Faculty 29 (24% with doctorates).
Baccalaureate Enrollment 315 **Women** 89% **Men** 11% **Minority** 10% **International** 1% **Part-time** 1%
Graduate Enrollment 51 **Women** 90% **Men** 10% **Minority** 1% **Part-time** 70%
Nursing Student Activities Sigma Theta Tau, Student Nurses' Association, nursing club.
Nursing Student Resources Academic advising; academic or career counseling; assistance for students with disabilities; bookstore; campus computer network; career placement assistance; computer lab; computer-assisted instruction; e-mail services; employment services for current students; interactive nursing skills videos; Internet; learning resource lab; library services; nursing audiovisuals; remedial services; resume preparation assistance; skills, simulation, or other laboratory; tutoring; unpaid internships.
Library Facilities 356,990 volumes (12,880 in health, 1,612 in nursing); 35,312 periodical subscriptions (84 health-care related).

BACCALAUREATE PROGRAMS

Degree BSN
Available Programs ADN to Baccalaureate; Baccalaureate for Second Degree; Generic Baccalaureate; LPN to Baccalaureate; RN Baccalaureate.
Study Options Full-time.
Program Entrance Requirements Minimum overall college GPA of 2.7, transcript of college record, CPR certification, written essay, health exam, health insurance, immunizations, interview, 2 letters of recommendation, minimum GPA in nursing prerequisites of 2.0, professional liability insurance/malpractice insurance, prerequisite course work. Transfer students are accepted.
Advanced Placement Credit by examination available. Credit given for nursing courses completed elsewhere dependent upon specific evaluations.
Contact *Telephone:* 785-231-1032 Ext. 1525. *Fax:* 785-231-1032.

GRADUATE PROGRAMS

Contact *Telephone:* 785-231-1010 Ext. 1533. *Fax:* 785-213-1032.

MASTER'S DEGREE PROGRAM

Degree MSN
Available Programs Master's.
Concentrations Available Nursing administration. *Nurse practitioner programs in:* adult health, family health.
Study Options Full-time and part-time.
Program Entrance Requirements Computer literacy, transcript of college record, CPR certification, written essay, immunizations, 2 letters of recommendation, nursing research course, physical assessment course, professional liability insurance/malpractice insurance, prerequisite course work, resume, statistics course. *Application deadline:* 3/15 (fall). *Application fee:* $35.
Degree Requirements 42 total credit hours, thesis or project.

POST-MASTER'S PROGRAM

Areas of Study Nursing education.

CONTINUING EDUCATION PROGRAM

Contact *Telephone:* 785-231-1010 Ext. 1526. *Fax:* 785-231-1032.

Wichita State University
School of Nursing
Wichita, Kansas

http://www.wichita.edu/nurs
Founded in 1895

DEGREES • BSN • DNP • MSN • MSN/MBA

Nursing Program Faculty 51 (25% with doctorates).
Baccalaureate Enrollment 251 **Women** 90% **Men** 10% **Minority** 21% **International** 4% **Part-time** 1%
Graduate Enrollment 150 **Women** 94% **Men** 6% **Minority** 6% **International** 1% **Part-time** 66%
Distance Learning Courses Available.
Nursing Student Activities Sigma Theta Tau, Student Nurses' Association.
Nursing Student Resources Academic advising; academic or career counseling; assistance for students with disabilities; bookstore; campus computer network; career placement assistance; computer lab; computer-assisted instruction; daycare for children of students; e-mail services; employment services for current students; housing assistance; interactive nursing skills videos; Internet; learning resource lab; library services; nursing audiovisuals; resume preparation assistance; skills, simulation, or other laboratory.
Library Facilities 1.8 million volumes (31,320 in health, 2,746 in nursing); 54,615 periodical subscriptions (406 health-care related).

BACCALAUREATE PROGRAMS

Degree BSN
Available Programs ADN to Baccalaureate; Accelerated Baccalaureate; Accelerated Baccalaureate for Second Degree; Generic Baccalaureate; LPN to RN Baccalaureate; RN Baccalaureate.
Site Options Derby, KS.
Study Options Full-time.
Online Degree Options Yes.
Program Entrance Requirements Minimum overall college GPA of 2.75, transcript of college record, CPR certification, written essay, health exam, health insurance, immunizations, interview, minimum GPA in nursing prerequisites of 2.0, professional liability insurance/malpractice insurance, prerequisite course work. Transfer students are accepted. *Application deadline:* 2/1 (fall), 9/1 (spring).
Advanced Placement Credit given for nursing courses completed elsewhere dependent upon specific evaluations.
Expenses (2009-10) *Tuition, area resident:* full-time $5325; part-time $178 per credit hour. *Tuition, nonresident:* full-time $13,359; part-time $445 per credit hour. *Room and board:* $6000; room only: $3350 per academic year. *Required fees:* full-time $212.
Financial Aid 80% of baccalaureate students in nursing programs received some form of financial aid in 2008-09. *Gift aid (need-based):* Federal Pell, FSEOG, state, private, college/university gift aid from institutional funds, Academic Competitiveness Grants, National SMART Grants. *Loans:* Perkins. *Work-study:* Federal Work-Study, part-time campus jobs. *Financial aid application deadline (priority):* 3/1.
Contact Ms. Courtney Fleetwood, Senior Academic Advisor, School of Nursing, Wichita State University, 1845 Fairmount Street, Wichita, KS 67260-0041. *Telephone:* 316-978-5732. *Fax:* 316-978-3094. *E-mail:* courtney.fleetwood@wichita.edu.

GRADUATE PROGRAMS

Expenses (2009-10) *Tuition, area resident:* full-time $4247; part-time $236 per credit hour. *Tuition, nonresident:* full-time $11,170; part-time $621 per credit hour. *Room and board:* $6400; room only: $3700 per academic year. *Required fees:* full-time $600.
Financial Aid 60% of graduate students in nursing programs received some form of financial aid in 2008-09.
Contact Dr. Alicia Huckstadt, Director, Graduate Program, School of Nursing, Wichita State University, 1845 Fairmount Street, Wichita, KS 67260-0041. *Telephone:* 316-978-3610. *Fax:* 316-978-3094. *E-mail:* alicia.huckstadt@wichita.edu.

MASTER'S DEGREE PROGRAM

Degrees MSN; MSN/MBA
Available Programs Master's; Master's for Nurses with Non-Nursing Degrees; RN to Master's.
Concentrations Available Nurse-midwifery. *Clinical nurse specialist programs in:* acute care. *Nurse practitioner programs in:* acute care, family health, pediatric, psychiatric/mental health.
Study Options Full-time and part-time.
Program Entrance Requirements Clinical experience, computer literacy, minimum overall college GPA of 3.0, transcript of college record, CPR certification, immunizations, physical assessment course, professional liability insurance/malpractice insurance, resume, statistics course. *Application deadline:* Applications may be processed on a rolling basis for some programs. *Application fee:* $35.
Advanced Placement Credit given for nursing courses completed elsewhere dependent upon specific evaluations.
Degree Requirements 49 total credit hours, comprehensive exam.

POST-MASTER'S PROGRAM

Areas of Study *Clinical nurse specialist programs in:* acute care. *Nurse practitioner programs in:* acute care, family health, pediatric, psychiatric/mental health.

DOCTORAL DEGREE PROGRAM

Degree DNP
Available Programs Doctorate; Post-Baccalaureate Doctorate.
Areas of Study Advanced practice nursing, clinical practice, critical care, faculty preparation, family health, health policy, health promotion/disease prevention, health-care systems, human health and illness, nursing administration, nursing education, nursing policy, nursing research, nursing science.
Program Entrance Requirements Clinical experience, minimum overall college GPA of 3.0, interview by faculty committee, interview, 2 letters of recommendation, statistics course, vita. Application deadline: 2/15 (fall), 10/15 (spring). Application fee: $35.
Degree Requirements 74 total credit hours, written exam, residency.

KENTUCKY

Bellarmine University

Donna and Allan Lansing School of Nursing and Health Sciences
Louisville, Kentucky

http://www.bellarmine.edu/
Founded in 1950

DEGREES • BSN • DNP • MSN • MSN/MBA
Nursing Program Faculty 64 (6.4% with doctorates).
Baccalaureate Enrollment 210 **Women** 90% **Men** 10% **Minority** 10% **International** 5% **Part-time** 20%
Graduate Enrollment 79 **Women** 95% **Men** 5% **Minority** 5% **Part-time** 100%
Nursing Student Activities Sigma Theta Tau, Student Nurses' Association.
Nursing Student Resources Academic advising; academic or career counseling; assistance for students with disabilities; bookstore; campus computer network; career placement assistance; computer lab; computer-assisted instruction; e-mail services; employment services for current students; externships; housing assistance; interactive nursing skills videos; Internet; learning resource lab; library services; nursing audiovisuals; paid internships; placement services for program completers; remedial services; resume preparation assistance; skills, simulation, or other laboratory; tutoring; unpaid internships.
Library Facilities 132,323 volumes (1,795 in health, 1,395 in nursing); 420 periodical subscriptions (93 health-care related).

BACCALAUREATE PROGRAMS

Degree BSN
Available Programs Accelerated Baccalaureate for Second Degree; Accelerated RN Baccalaureate; Baccalaureate for Second Degree; Generic Baccalaureate; RN Baccalaureate.
Study Options Full-time and part-time.
Program Entrance Requirements Minimum overall college GPA of 2.5, transcript of college record, CPR certification, written essay, health exam, health insurance, high school biology, high school chemistry, 2 years high school math, 2 years high school science, high school transcript, immunizations, interview, minimum high school GPA of 2.75, minimum GPA in nursing prerequisites of 2.75, prerequisite course work. Transfer students are accepted. *Application deadline:* 8/15 (fall), 1/3 (winter), 1/3 (spring), 5/3 (summer). Applications may be processed on a rolling basis for some programs. *Application fee:* $25.
Advanced Placement Credit by examination available. Credit given for nursing courses completed elsewhere dependent upon specific evaluations.
Expenses (2010-11) *Tuition:* full-time $30,310; part-time $590 per credit hour. *International tuition:* $40,000 full-time. *Room and board:* $7100; room only: $5700 per academic year.
Financial Aid 77% of baccalaureate students in nursing programs received some form of financial aid in 2009-10. *Gift aid (need-based):* Federal Pell, FSEOG, state, private, college/university gift aid from institutional funds. *Loans:* Perkins, college/university. *Work-study:* Federal Work-Study, part-time campus jobs. *Financial aid application deadline (priority):* 3/1.
Contact Dr. Beverley Holland, BSN Department Chairperson, Donna and Allan Lansing School of Nursing and Health Sciences, Bellarmine University, 2001 Newburg Road, Miles Hall, #202, Louisville, KY 40205-0671. *Telephone:* 502-452-8279. *Fax:* 502-452-8058. *E-mail:* bholland@bellarmine.edu.

GRADUATE PROGRAMS

Expenses (2010-11) *Tuition:* part-time $643 per credit hour.
Financial Aid 77% of graduate students in nursing programs received some form of financial aid in 2009-10. Career-related internships or fieldwork and scholarships available.
Contact Ms. Julie Armstrong-Binnix, Marketing/Recruiter, Donna and Allan Lansing School of Nursing and Health Sciences, Bellarmine University, 2001 Newburg Road, Miles Hall, #201, Louisville, KY 40205-0671. *Telephone:* 502-452-8364. *Fax:* 502-452-8058. *E-mail:* julieab@bellarmine.edu.

MASTER'S DEGREE PROGRAM

Degrees MSN; MSN/MBA
Available Programs Master's; Master's for Nurses with Non-Nursing Degrees; RN to Master's.
Concentrations Available Nursing administration; nursing education.
Study Options Part-time.
Program Entrance Requirements Minimum overall college GPA of 2.75, transcript of college record, professional liability insurance/malpractice insurance, GRE General Test. *Application deadline:* 8/20 (fall), 1/5 (winter), 1/5 (spring), 5/1 (summer). Applications may be processed on a rolling basis for some programs. *Application fee:* $25.
Advanced Placement Credit given for nursing courses completed elsewhere dependent upon specific evaluations.
Degree Requirements 38 total credit hours, thesis or project.

POST-MASTER'S PROGRAM

Areas of Study *Nurse practitioner programs in:* family health.

DOCTORAL DEGREE PROGRAM

Degree DNP
Available Programs Doctorate for Nurses with Non-Nursing Degrees.
Areas of Study Family health.
Program Entrance Requirements Minimum overall college GPA of 3.5, interview by faculty committee, 3 letters of recommendation, MSN or equivalent, vita, GRE General Test. Application deadline: 8/15 (fall), 1/5 (spring), 5/3 (summer).
Degree Requirements Residency.

CONTINUING EDUCATION PROGRAM

Contact Ms. Linda Bailey, Director, Continuing Education, Donna and Allan Lansing School of Nursing and Health Sciences, Bellarmine University, 2001 Newburg Road, Continuing Education Office, Louisville, KY 40205-0671. *Telephone:* 502-452-8161. *Fax:* 502-452-8203. *E-mail:* lbailey@bellarmine.edu.

Berea College

Department of Nursing
Berea, Kentucky

http://www.berea.edu/nursing
Founded in 1855

DEGREE • BSN
Nursing Program Faculty 9 (2% with doctorates).
Baccalaureate Enrollment 48 **Women** 90% **Men** 10% **Minority** 10% **International** 12.5%
Nursing Student Activities Student Nurses' Association.
Nursing Student Resources Academic advising; academic or career counseling; assistance for students with disabilities; bookstore; campus computer network; career placement assistance; computer lab; computer-assisted instruction; daycare for children of students; e-mail services; employment services for current students; externships; housing assistance; interactive nursing skills videos; Internet; learning resource lab; library services; nursing audiovisuals; paid internships; placement services for program completers; remedial services; resume preparation assistance; skills, simulation, or other laboratory; tutoring; unpaid internships.
Library Facilities 381,418 volumes; 1,879 periodical subscriptions.

BACCALAUREATE PROGRAMS

Degree BSN
Available Programs Generic Baccalaureate.
Study Options Full-time.
Program Entrance Requirements Minimum overall college GPA of 2.5, transcript of college record, CPR certification, written essay, high school transcript, immunizations, interview, 3 letters of recommendation, minimum high school GPA, minimum high school rank 15%, minimum GPA in nursing prerequisites of 2.5, prerequisite course work. Transfer students are accepted. *Application deadline:* Applications may be processed on a rolling basis for some programs.
Advanced Placement Credit given for nursing courses completed elsewhere dependent upon specific evaluations.
Financial Aid 100% of baccalaureate students in nursing programs received some form of financial aid in 2009-10. *Gift aid (need-based):* Federal Pell, FSEOG, state, private, college/university gift aid from institutional funds. *Loans:* Perkins, college/university. *Work-study:* Federal Work-Study, part-time campus jobs. *Financial aid application deadline (priority):* 3/15.

Contact Luke Hodson, Director of Admissions/Operations, Department of Nursing, Berea College, CPO 2220, Berea, KY 40404. *Telephone:* 859-985-3503. *E-mail:* luke_hodson@berea.edu.

Eastern Kentucky University

Department of Baccalaureate and Graduate Nursing
Richmond, Kentucky

http://www.bsn-gn.eku.edu
Founded in 1906

DEGREES • BSN • MSN

Nursing Program Faculty 42 (40% with doctorates).
Baccalaureate Enrollment 500
Graduate Enrollment 200
Distance Learning Courses Available.
Nursing Student Activities Sigma Theta Tau, Student Nurses' Association.
Nursing Student Resources Academic advising; academic or career counseling; assistance for students with disabilities; bookstore; campus computer network; computer lab; computer-assisted instruction; e-mail services; housing assistance; interactive nursing skills videos; Internet; learning resource lab; library services; nursing audiovisuals; skills, simulation, or other laboratory.
Library Facilities 799,496 volumes; 2,901 periodical subscriptions.

BACCALAUREATE PROGRAMS

Degree BSN
Available Programs Accelerated RN Baccalaureate; Baccalaureate for Second Degree; Generic Baccalaureate; RN Baccalaureate.
Site Options Hazard, KY; Corbin, KY; Danville, KY.
Study Options Full-time and part-time.
Program Entrance Requirements Minimum overall college GPA of 2.5, CPR certification, immunizations, professional liability insurance/malpractice insurance, prerequisite course work. Transfer students are accepted.
Advanced Placement Credit given for nursing courses completed elsewhere dependent upon specific evaluations.
Contact ***Telephone:*** 859-622-1827. *Fax:* 859-622-1972.

GRADUATE PROGRAMS

Contact ***Telephone:*** 859-622-1838. *Fax:* 859-622-1972.

MASTER'S DEGREE PROGRAM

Degree MSN
Available Programs Master's.
Concentrations Available Nursing education. *Clinical nurse specialist programs in:* public health. *Nurse practitioner programs in:* family health, psychiatric/mental health.
Site Options Hazard, KY; Corbin, KY; Danville, KY.
Study Options Full-time and part-time.
Program Entrance Requirements Minimum overall college GPA of 2.75, transcript of college record, written essay, 3 letters of recommendation, statistics course.
Advanced Placement Credit given for nursing courses completed elsewhere dependent upon specific evaluations.
Degree Requirements 48 total credit hours, thesis or project, comprehensive exam.

Frontier School of Midwifery and Family Nursing

Nursing Degree Programs
Hyden, Kentucky

Founded in 1939

DEGREES • DNP • MSN

GRADUATE PROGRAMS

Contact Doctorate and Master in Nursing Programs, Nursing Degree Programs, Frontier School of Midwifery and Family Nursing, PO Box 528, 195 School Street, Hyden, KY 41749. *Telephone:* 606-672-2312. *E-mail:* fsmfn@midwives.org.

MASTER'S DEGREE PROGRAM

Degree MSN
Available Programs Accelerated AD/RN to Master's.

DOCTORAL DEGREE PROGRAM

Degree DNP
Available Programs Doctorate.

Kentucky Christian University

School of Nursing
Grayson, Kentucky

Founded in 1919

DEGREE • BSN

Nursing Program Faculty 6 (20% with doctorates).
Baccalaureate Enrollment 63 **Women** 90% **Men** 10% **Minority** 1% **International** 1%
Nursing Student Activities Student Nurses' Association.
Nursing Student Resources Academic advising; assistance for students with disabilities; bookstore; campus computer network; computer lab; e-mail services; housing assistance;, interactive nursing skills videos; Internet; learning resource lab; library services; nursing audiovisuals; other; remedial services; skills, simulation, or other laboratory.
Library Facilities 103,323 volumes (400 in health, 300 in nursing); 395 periodical subscriptions (200 health-care related).

BACCALAUREATE PROGRAMS

Degree BSN
Available Programs Generic Baccalaureate.
Study Options Full-time.
Program Entrance Requirements Transcript of college record, written essay, health exam, health insurance, high school transcript, immunizations, minimum GPA in nursing prerequisites of 2.5, prerequisite course work. Transfer students are accepted.
Contact ***Telephone:*** 606-474-3255. *Fax:* 606-474-3342.

CONTINUING EDUCATION PROGRAM

Contact ***Telephone:*** 606-474-3271. *Fax:* 606-474-3342.

Kentucky State University

School of Nursing
Frankfort, Kentucky

Founded in 1886

DEGREE • BSN

Nursing Program Faculty 18 (11% with doctorates).
Baccalaureate Enrollment 25
Nursing Student Activities Student Nurses' Association.
Nursing Student Resources Academic advising; academic or career counseling; assistance for students with disabilities; bookstore; campus computer network; career placement assistance; computer lab; computer-assisted instruction; e-mail services; externships; housing assistance; interactive nursing skills videos; Internet; learning resource lab; library services; nursing audiovisuals; other; placement services for program completers; remedial services; resume preparation assistance; skills, simulation, or other laboratory; tutoring.
Library Facilities 333,642 volumes; 864 periodical subscriptions.

BACCALAUREATE PROGRAMS

Degree BSN
Available Programs ADN to Baccalaureate.
Program Entrance Requirements Transfer students are accepted.
Contact ***Telephone:*** 502-597-6963. *Fax:* 502-597-5818.

Midway College
Program in Nursing (Baccalaureate)
Midway, Kentucky

http://www.midway.edu/degreeprograms/nursing.html
Founded in 1847

DEGREE • BSN

Nursing Program Faculty 12 (25% with doctorates).
Baccalaureate Enrollment 20 **Women** 100% **Minority** 30% **Part-time** 10%
Distance Learning Courses Available.
Nursing Student Activities Student Nurses' Association, nursing club.
Nursing Student Resources Academic advising; academic or career counseling; assistance for students with disabilities; bookstore; campus computer network; career placement assistance; computer lab; computer-assisted instruction; e-mail services; externships; interactive nursing skills videos; Internet; learning resource lab; library services; nursing audiovisuals; placement services for program completers; remedial services; resume preparation assistance; skills, simulation, or other laboratory; tutoring; unpaid internships.
Library Facilities 96,236 volumes (1,200 in health, 800 in nursing); 250 periodical subscriptions (102 health-care related).

BACCALAUREATE PROGRAMS

Degree BSN
Available Programs ADN to Baccalaureate; Accelerated RN Baccalaureate; RN Baccalaureate.
Site Options Lexington, KY; Lexington, NT.
Study Options Full-time and part-time.
Program Entrance Requirements Minimum overall college GPA of 2.8, transcript of college record, CPR certification, health exam, health insurance, high school chemistry, 2 years high school math, high school transcript, immunizations, interview, 1 letter of recommendation, minimum high school GPA of 3.0, minimum GPA in nursing prerequisites of 3.0, professional liability insurance/malpractice insurance, prerequisite course work, RN licensure. Transfer students are accepted. *Application deadline:* Applications may be processed on a rolling basis for some programs. *Application fee:* $25.
Advanced Placement Credit given for nursing courses completed elsewhere dependent upon specific evaluations.
Expenses (2009-10) *Tuition:* full-time $12,360; part-time $515 per credit hour. *International tuition:* $12,360 full-time.
Financial Aid 95% of baccalaureate students in nursing programs received some form of financial aid in 2008-09.
Contact Dr. Barbara R. Kitchen, RN, Chair, Nursing and Science Programs, Program in Nursing (Baccalaureate), Midway College, 512 East Stephens Street, Midway, KY 40347. *Telephone:* 859-846-5335. *Fax:* 859-846-5876. *E-mail:* bkitchen@midway.edu.

CONTINUING EDUCATION PROGRAM

Contact Dr. Barbara R. Kitchen, RN, Chair, Nursing and Science Programs, Program in Nursing (Baccalaureate), Midway College, 512 East Stephens Street, Midway, KY 40347. *Telephone:* 859-846-5335. *Fax:* 859-846-5876. *E-mail:* bkitchen@midway.edu.

Morehead State University
Department of Nursing
Morehead, Kentucky

http://www.moreheadstate.edu/nursing
Founded in 1922

DEGREE • BSN

Nursing Program Faculty 42 (12% with doctorates).
Baccalaureate Enrollment 144 **Women** 81% **Men** 19% **Minority** 3% **Part-time** 22%
Distance Learning Courses Available.
Nursing Student Activities Student Nurses' Association.
Nursing Student Resources Academic advising; academic or career counseling; assistance for students with disabilities; bookstore; campus computer network; career placement assistance; computer lab; computer-assisted instruction; e-mail services; interactive nursing skills videos; Internet; learning resource lab; library services; nursing audiovisuals; remedial services; resume preparation assistance; skills, simulation, or other laboratory; tutoring.
Library Facilities 537,675 volumes (500,000 in health, 855 in nursing); 41,041 periodical subscriptions (286 health-care related).

BACCALAUREATE PROGRAMS

Degree BSN
Available Programs ADN to Baccalaureate; Generic Baccalaureate; RN Baccalaureate.
Site Options Ashland, KY; Prestonsburg, KY; Mt. Sterling, KY.
Study Options Full-time.
Online Degree Options Yes.
Program Entrance Requirements Minimum overall college GPA of 2.0, transcript of college record, CPR certification, immunizations, minimum GPA in nursing prerequisites of 2.5, prerequisite course work. Transfer students are accepted. *Application deadline:* 3/15 (fall).
Advanced Placement Credit by examination available. Credit given for nursing courses completed elsewhere dependent upon specific evaluations.
Expenses (2010-11) *Tuition, state resident:* full-time $6492; part-time $246 per credit hour. *Tuition, nonresident:* full-time $16,236; part-time $615 per credit hour. *Room and board:* $6582; room only: $3500 per academic year. *Required fees:* full-time $500.
Financial Aid 80% of baccalaureate students in nursing programs received some form of financial aid in 2009-10. *Gift aid (need-based):* Federal Pell, FSEOG, state, private, college/university gift aid from institutional funds. *Loans:* Federal Direct (Subsidized and Unsubsidized Stafford PLUS), Perkins, college/university. *Work-study:* Federal Work-Study, part-time campus jobs. *Financial aid application deadline (priority):* 3/15.
Contact Ms. Carla June Aagaard, Academic Counseling Coordinator, Department of Nursing, Morehead State University, CHER 201, 316 West 2nd Street, Suite 201, Morehead, KY 40351. *Telephone:* 606-783-2641. *Fax:* 606-783-9211. *E-mail:* c.aagaard@moreheadstate.edu.

Murray State University
Program in Nursing
Murray, Kentucky

http://www.murraystate.edu/
Founded in 1922

DEGREES • BSN • MSN

Nursing Program Faculty 16 (47% with doctorates).
Baccalaureate Enrollment 206 **Women** 94% **Men** 6% **Minority** 3%
Graduate Enrollment 48 **Women** 85% **Men** 15%
Distance Learning Courses Available.
Nursing Student Activities Sigma Theta Tau, Student Nurses' Association.
Nursing Student Resources Academic advising; academic or career counseling; assistance for students with disabilities; bookstore; campus computer network; career placement assistance; computer lab; computer-assisted instruction; daycare for children of students; e-mail services; employment services for current students; externships; housing assistance; interactive nursing skills videos; Internet; learning resource lab; library services; nursing audiovisuals; placement services for program completers; remedial services; resume preparation assistance; skills, simulation, or other laboratory; tutoring; unpaid internships.
Library Facilities 933,635 volumes (4,060 in health, 2,160 in nursing); 1,381 periodical subscriptions (124 health-care related).

BACCALAUREATE PROGRAMS

Degree BSN
Available Programs Generic Baccalaureate; RN Baccalaureate.
Site Options Hopkinsville, KY; Paducah, KY; Madisonville, KY.
Study Options Full-time.
Program Entrance Requirements Transcript of college record, CPR certification, immunizations, minimum GPA in nursing prerequisites of 2.5, professional liability insurance/malpractice insurance, prerequisite course work. Transfer students are accepted. *Application deadline:* 5/1 (fall), 11/22 (spring).
Advanced Placement Credit by examination available. Credit given for nursing courses completed elsewhere dependent upon specific evaluations.
Expenses (2009-10) *Tuition, state resident:* full-time $3200; part-time $300 per credit hour. *Tuition, nonresident:* full-time $7000; part-time $600 per credit hour. *Room and board:* $2400; room only: $1400 per academic year. *Required fees:* full-time $300.

Financial Aid 70% of baccalaureate students in nursing programs received some form of financial aid in 2008-09. *Gift aid (need-based):* Federal Pell, FSEOG, state, private, college/university gift aid from institutional funds. *Loans:* Federal Nursing Student Loans, Perkins, state, college/university. *Work-study:* Federal Work-Study, part-time campus jobs. *Financial aid application deadline (priority):* 4/1.

Contact Dr. Michael B. Perlow, Chair, Program in Nursing, Murray State University, 120 Mason Hall, Murray, KY 42071-0009. *Telephone:* 270-809-2193. *Fax:* 270-809-6662. *E-mail:* michael.perlow@murraystate.edu.

GRADUATE PROGRAMS

Expenses (2009-10) *Tuition, state resident:* full-time $4000; part-time $400 per credit hour. *Tuition, nonresident:* full-time $8000; part-time $800 per credit hour. *International tuition:* $4000 full-time. *Room and board:* $2000; room only: $900 per academic year. *Required fees:* full-time $400.

Financial Aid 70% of graduate students in nursing programs received some form of financial aid in 2008-09. Traineeships available. *Financial aid application deadline:* 4/1.

Contact Dr. Nancey E.M. France, RN, Graduate Coordinator, Program in Nursing, Murray State University, 120 Mason Hall, Murray, KY 42071-0009. *Telephone:* 270-809-6671. *Fax:* 270-809-6662. *E-mail:* nancey.france@murraystate.edu.

MASTER'S DEGREE PROGRAM

Degree MSN

Available Programs Master's.

Concentrations Available Nurse anesthesia. *Clinical nurse specialist programs in:* adult health, critical care, medical-surgical. *Nurse practitioner programs in:* family health.

Site Options Hopkinsville, KY; Paducah, KY; Madisonville, KY.

Study Options Full-time and part-time.

Program Entrance Requirements Clinical experience, minimum overall college GPA of 3.0, transcript of college record, CPR certification, immunizations, interview, 3 letters of recommendation, nursing research course, physical assessment course, professional liability insurance/malpractice insurance, prerequisite course work, statistics course, GRE General Test. *Application deadline:* 11/1 (fall).

Advanced Placement Credit given for nursing courses completed elsewhere dependent upon specific evaluations.

Degree Requirements 46 total credit hours.

POST-MASTER'S PROGRAM

Areas of Study Nurse anesthesia. *Clinical nurse specialist programs in:* adult health, critical care, medical-surgical. *Nurse practitioner programs in:* family health.

CONTINUING EDUCATION PROGRAM

Contact Michele Hack, Program in Nursing, Murray State University, 120 Mason Hall, Murray, KY 42071-0009. *Telephone:* 270-809-6674. *Fax:* 270-809-6662. *E-mail:* mhack@murraystate.edu.

Northern Kentucky University

Department of Nursing
Highland Heights, Kentucky

http://www.nku.edu/~nursing/

Founded in 1968

DEGREES • BSN • MSN

Nursing Program Faculty 75 (20% with doctorates).

Baccalaureate Enrollment 600 **Women** 93% **Men** 7% **Minority** 2% **International** 1% **Part-time** 50%

Graduate Enrollment 275 **Women** 95% **Men** 5% **Minority** 1% **Part-time** 90%

Distance Learning Courses Available.

Nursing Student Activities Sigma Theta Tau, Student Nurses' Association.

Nursing Student Resources Academic advising; academic or career counseling; assistance for students with disabilities; bookstore; campus computer network; career placement assistance; computer lab; computer-assisted instruction; daycare for children of students; e-mail services; employment services for current students; housing assistance; interactive nursing skills videos; Internet; learning resource lab; library services; nursing audiovisuals; resume preparation assistance; skills, simulation, or other laboratory; tutoring.

Library Facilities 871,092 volumes (6,380 in health, 3,500 in nursing); 1,001 periodical subscriptions (100 health-care related).

BACCALAUREATE PROGRAMS

Degree BSN

Available Programs Accelerated Baccalaureate for Second Degree; Generic Baccalaureate; RN Baccalaureate.

Study Options Full-time.

Program Entrance Requirements Minimum overall college GPA of 2.5, transcript of college record, CPR certification, health exam, health insurance, high school biology, high school chemistry, 3 years high school math, high school transcript, immunizations, minimum GPA in nursing prerequisites of 3.0, prerequisite course work. Transfer students are accepted. *Application deadline:* 1/15 (fall), 8/15 (spring).

Advanced Placement Credit by examination available. Credit given for nursing courses completed elsewhere dependent upon specific evaluations.

Expenses (2010-11) *Tuition, state resident:* full-time $3564; part-time $297 per credit hour. *Tuition, nonresident:* full-time $6948; part-time $579 per credit hour. *Room and board:* $7600; room only: $4200 per academic year. *Required fees:* full-time $250; part-time $125 per term.

Contact Dr. Carrie McCoy, Chair, Department of Nursing, Northern Kentucky University, Nunn Drive, AHC 303, Highland Heights, KY 41099. *Telephone:* 859-572-5248. *Fax:* 859-572-6098. *E-mail:* mccoy@nku.edu.

GRADUATE PROGRAMS

Expenses (2010-11) *Tuition, state resident:* part-time $403 per credit hour. *Tuition, nonresident:* part-time $694 per credit hour. *Room and board:* $7600; room only: $4200 per academic year. *Required fees:* part-time $45 per term.

Financial Aid 10% of graduate students in nursing programs received some form of financial aid in 2009-10.

Contact Dr. Marilyn Schleyer, Chair of Advanced Nursing Studies, Department of Nursing, Northern Kentucky University, HC 206, Highland Heights, KY 41099. *Telephone:* 859-572-5579. *Fax:* 859-572-1934. *E-mail:* schleyerm1@nku.edu.

MASTER'S DEGREE PROGRAM

Degree MSN

Available Programs Master's.

Concentrations Available Nursing administration; nursing education. *Nurse practitioner programs in:* acute care, adult health, family health, pediatric.

Study Options Full-time and part-time.

Online Degree Options Yes.

Program Entrance Requirements Clinical experience, minimum overall college GPA of 3.0, transcript of college record, CPR certification, immunizations, 1 letter of recommendation, nursing research course, physical assessment course, professional liability insurance/malpractice insurance, prerequisite course work, resume, statistics course. *Application deadline:* 2/15 (fall), 10/15 (spring).

Advanced Placement Credit by examination available. Credit given for nursing courses completed elsewhere dependent upon specific evaluations.

Degree Requirements 44 total credit hours, thesis or project.

POST-MASTER'S PROGRAM

Areas of Study Nursing administration; nursing education. *Nurse practitioner programs in:* acute care, adult health, family health, pediatric, psychiatric/mental health.

CONTINUING EDUCATION PROGRAM

Contact Mary Gers, Director of Simulation and Technology, Department of Nursing, Northern Kentucky University, NKU, HC 303, Highland Heights, KY 41099. *Telephone:* 859-572-6322. *Fax:* 859-572-1934. *E-mail:* gersm@nku.edu.

Spalding University
School of Nursing
Louisville, Kentucky

http://www.spalding.edu/nursing
Founded in 1814

DEGREES • BSN • MSN

Nursing Program Faculty 33 (18% with doctorates).
Baccalaureate Enrollment 170 **Women** 94% **Men** 6% **Minority** 10% **International** 6%
Graduate Enrollment 56 **Women** 99.5% **Men** .5% **Minority** 2% **International** 3.4% **Part-time** 50%
Nursing Student Activities Sigma Theta Tau, Student Nurses' Association.
Nursing Student Resources Academic advising; academic or career counseling; assistance for students with disabilities; bookstore; campus computer network; career placement assistance; computer lab; computer-assisted instruction; e-mail services; employment services for current students; externships; interactive nursing skills videos; Internet; learning resource lab; library services; nursing audiovisuals; remedial services; resume preparation assistance; skills, simulation, or other laboratory; tutoring; unpaid internships.
Library Facilities 109,292 volumes (2,875 in health, 1,125 in nursing); 200 periodical subscriptions (367 health-care related).

BACCALAUREATE PROGRAMS

Degree BSN
Available Programs Accelerated Baccalaureate for Second Degree; Accelerated RN Baccalaureate; Generic Baccalaureate.
Study Options Full-time and part-time.
Program Entrance Requirements Minimum overall college GPA of 2.5, transcript of college record, CPR certification, health exam, health insurance, high school transcript, immunizations, minimum GPA in nursing prerequisites of 2.5, professional liability insurance/malpractice insurance, prerequisite course work. Transfer students are accepted.
Advanced Placement Credit given for nursing courses completed elsewhere dependent upon specific evaluations.
Contact ***Telephone:*** 502-585-7125. *Fax:* 502-588-7175.

GRADUATE PROGRAMS

Contact ***Telephone:*** 502-585-9911 Ext. 2332. *Fax:* 502-588-7175.

MASTER'S DEGREE PROGRAM

Degree MSN
Available Programs Accelerated RN to Master's; Master's.
Concentrations Available Nursing administration; nursing education. *Nurse practitioner programs in:* adult health, family health, pediatric.
Study Options Full-time and part-time.
Program Entrance Requirements Computer literacy, minimum overall college GPA of 3.0, transcript of college record, CPR certification, written essay, immunizations, interview, 2 letters of recommendation, physical assessment course, professional liability insurance/malpractice insurance, prerequisite course work, resume, statistics course, GRE General Test.
Advanced Placement Credit by examination available. Credit given for nursing courses completed elsewhere dependent upon specific evaluations.
Degree Requirements 53 total credit hours, thesis or project.

POST-MASTER'S PROGRAM

Areas of Study Nursing administration; nursing education. *Nurse practitioner programs in:* adult health, family health, pediatric.

CONTINUING EDUCATION PROGRAM

Contact ***Telephone:*** 502-585-9911 Ext. 2332. *Fax:* 502-588-7175.

Thomas More College
Program in Nursing
Crestview Hills, Kentucky

http://www.thomasmore.edu/
Founded in 1921

DEGREE • BSN

Nursing Program Faculty 7 (29% with doctorates).
Baccalaureate Enrollment 101 **Women** 95% **Men** 5% **Minority** 1% **Part-time** 5%
Nursing Student Activities Student Nurses' Association.
Nursing Student Resources Academic advising; academic or career counseling; assistance for students with disabilities; bookstore; campus computer network; career placement assistance; computer lab; computer-assisted instruction; e-mail services; employment services for current students; externships; interactive nursing skills videos; Internet; learning resource lab; library services; nursing audiovisuals; other; placement services for program completers; remedial services; resume preparation assistance; skills, simulation, or other laboratory; tutoring.
Library Facilities 110,565 volumes (350 in health, 200 in nursing); 506 periodical subscriptions (50 health-care related).

BACCALAUREATE PROGRAMS

Degree BSN
Available Programs Generic Baccalaureate.
Study Options Full-time.
Program Entrance Requirements Transcript of college record, CPR certification, health exam, health insurance, high school transcript, immunizations, minimum GPA in nursing prerequisites of 2.75, professional liability insurance/malpractice insurance, prerequisite course work. Transfer students are accepted. *Application deadline:* 5/1 (fall). *Application fee:* $25.
Advanced Placement Credit given for nursing courses completed elsewhere dependent upon specific evaluations.
Expenses (2010-11) *Tuition:* full-time $12,000; part-time $545 per credit hour. *Required fees:* full-time $720.
Financial Aid 90% of baccalaureate students in nursing programs received some form of financial aid in 2009-10. *Gift aid (need-based):* Federal Pell, FSEOG, state, private, college/university gift aid from institutional funds, Federal Nursing. *Loans:* Federal Nursing Student Loans, Federal Direct (Subsidized and Unsubsidized Stafford PLUS), Perkins, college/university. *Work-study:* Federal Work-Study, part-time campus jobs. *Financial aid application deadline (priority):* 3/15.
Contact Dr. Lisa Spangler Torok, Chair, Program in Nursing, Thomas More College, 333 Thomas More Parkway, Crestview Hills, KY 41017. *Telephone:* 859-344-3413. *Fax:* 859-344-3537. *E-mail:* lisa.spangler-torok@thomasmore.edu.

University of Kentucky
Graduate School Programs in the College of Nursing
Lexington, Kentucky

http://www.mc.uky.edu/nursing
Founded in 1865

DEGREES • BSN • MSN • PHD

Nursing Program Faculty 65 (54% with doctorates).
Baccalaureate Enrollment 260 **Women** 97% **Men** 3% **Minority** 6% **Part-time** 14%
Graduate Enrollment 221 **Women** 92% **Men** 8% **Minority** 9% **International** 5% **Part-time** 35%
Nursing Student Activities Sigma Theta Tau, Student Nurses' Association.
Nursing Student Resources Academic advising; academic or career counseling; assistance for students with disabilities; bookstore; campus computer network; career placement assistance; computer lab; computer-assisted instruction; e-mail services; interactive nursing skills videos; Internet; learning resource lab; library services; nursing audiovisuals; skills, simulation, or other laboratory.
Library Facilities 105,793 volumes in health; 3,347 periodical subscriptions health-care related.

BACCALAUREATE PROGRAMS

Degree BSN
Available Programs Baccalaureate for Second Degree; Generic Baccalaureate; RN Baccalaureate.
Study Options Full-time and part-time.
Program Entrance Requirements Minimum overall college GPA of 2.5, transcript of college record, CPR certification, written essay, high school transcript, immunizations, minimum GPA in nursing prerequisites of 2.5, prerequisite course work. Transfer students are accepted.
Advanced Placement Credit by examination available. Credit given for nursing courses completed elsewhere dependent upon specific evaluations.

Contact ***Telephone:*** 859-323-5108. *Fax:* 859-323-1057.

GRADUATE PROGRAMS

Contact ***Telephone:*** 859-323-5108. *Fax:* 859-323-1057.

MASTER'S DEGREE PROGRAM

Degree MSN
Available Programs Master's; RN to Master's.
Concentrations Available Nurse case management; nursing administration. *Clinical nurse specialist programs in:* acute care, adult health, community health, critical care, gerontology, medical-surgical, oncology, parent-child, pediatric, perinatal, psychiatric/mental health, public health, women's health. *Nurse practitioner programs in:* acute care, adult health, family health, gerontology, pediatric, psychiatric/mental health.
Site Options Morehead, KY.
Study Options Full-time and part-time.
Program Entrance Requirements Clinical experience, minimum overall college GPA of 2.75, transcript of college record, written essay, interview, 3 letters of recommendation, physical assessment course, statistics course, GRE General Test.
Advanced Placement Credit given for nursing courses completed elsewhere dependent upon specific evaluations.
Degree Requirements 40 total credit hours, comprehensive exam.

POST-MASTER'S PROGRAM

Areas of Study Nurse case management. *Nurse practitioner programs in:* acute care, adult health, family health, gerontology, pediatric, psychiatric/mental health.

DOCTORAL DEGREE PROGRAM

Degree PhD
Available Programs Doctorate.
Areas of Study Nursing research.
Program Entrance Requirements Minimum overall college GPA of 3.3, interview, 3 letters of recommendation, MSN or equivalent, statistics course, writing sample, GRE General Test.
Degree Requirements 63 total credit hours, dissertation, oral exam, written exam, residency.

CONTINUING EDUCATION PROGRAM

Contact ***Telephone:*** 859-323-3851. *Fax:* 859-323-1057.

University of Louisville

School of Nursing
Louisville, Kentucky

http://www.louisville.edu/nursing
Founded in 1798

DEGREES • BSN • MSN • PHD

Nursing Program Faculty 65 (49% with doctorates).
Baccalaureate Enrollment 302 **Women** 88% **Men** 12% **Minority** 12% **International** 1% **Part-time** 1%
Graduate Enrollment 152 **Women** 99% **Men** 1% **Minority** 18% **International** 1% **Part-time** 52%
Distance Learning Courses Available.
Nursing Student Activities Sigma Theta Tau, Student Nurses' Association.
Nursing Student Resources Academic advising; academic or career counseling; assistance for students with disabilities; bookstore; campus computer network; career placement assistance; computer lab; computer-assisted instruction; e-mail services; employment services for current students; housing assistance; interactive nursing skills videos; Internet; learning resource lab; library services; nursing audiovisuals; skills, simulation, or other laboratory; tutoring.
Library Facilities 2.2 million volumes (253,595 in health, 2,806 in nursing); 74,116 periodical subscriptions (4,329 health-care related).

BACCALAUREATE PROGRAMS

Degree BSN
Available Programs Accelerated Baccalaureate for Second Degree; Generic Baccalaureate; RN Baccalaureate.
Site Options Owensboro, KY.
Study Options Full-time.
Online Degree Options Yes.
Program Entrance Requirements Minimum overall college GPA of 2.8, transcript of college record, CPR certification, written essay, health insurance, high school foreign language, 3 years high school math, 3 years high school science, high school transcript, immunizations, minimum high school GPA of 2.8, minimum GPA in nursing prerequisites of 2.8, professional liability insurance/malpractice insurance, prerequisite course work. Transfer students are accepted. *Application deadline:* 5/1 (fall), 9/15 (spring). *Application fee:* $40.
Advanced Placement Credit by examination available. Credit given for nursing courses completed elsewhere dependent upon specific evaluations.
Expenses (2010-11) *Tuition, state resident:* full-time $8424; part-time $351 per credit hour. *Tuition, nonresident:* full-time $20,242; part-time $851 per credit hour. *Room and board:* $7400; room only: $5400 per academic year. *Required fees:* full-time $845.
Financial Aid 87% of baccalaureate students in nursing programs received some form of financial aid in 2009-10. *Gift aid (need-based):* Federal Pell, FSEOG, state, private, college/university gift aid from institutional funds. *Loans:* Federal Nursing Student Loans, Federal Direct (Subsidized and Unsubsidized Stafford PLUS), Perkins. *Work-study:* Federal Work-Study. *Financial aid application deadline (priority):* 3/15.
Contact Trish Hart, Director of Student Services, School of Nursing, University of Louisville, 555 South Floyd Street, Louisville, KY 40202. *Telephone:* 502-852-8298. *Fax:* 502-852-8783. *E-mail:* p0hart01@louisville.edu.

GRADUATE PROGRAMS

Expenses (2010-11) *Tuition, state resident:* full-time $10,944; part-time $608 per credit hour. *Tuition, nonresident:* full-time $20,826; part-time $1157 per credit hour. *Room and board:* $7400; room only: $5400 per academic year. *Required fees:* full-time $1100.
Financial Aid 87% of graduate students in nursing programs received some form of financial aid in 2009-10. 2 fellowships with full tuition reimbursements available (averaging $20,000 per year), 5 research assistantships with full tuition reimbursements available (averaging $18,000 per year), 5 teaching assistantships with full tuition reimbursements available (averaging $18,000 per year) were awarded; institutionally sponsored loans, scholarships, traineeships, and unspecified assistantships also available. Aid available to part-time students. *Financial aid application deadline:* 4/15.
Contact Dr. Rosalie Mainous, Associate Dean for Graduate Academic Affairs, School of Nursing, University of Louisville, 555 South Floyd Street, Louisville, KY 40292. *Telephone:* 502-852-8387. *Fax:* 502-852-8783. *E-mail:* rosalie.mainous@louisville.edu.

MASTER'S DEGREE PROGRAM

Degree MSN
Available Programs Master's.
Concentrations Available Nursing education. *Clinical nurse specialist programs in:* psychiatric/mental health. *Nurse practitioner programs in:* adult health, family health, neonatal health, psychiatric/mental health.
Study Options Full-time and part-time.
Program Entrance Requirements Clinical experience, minimum overall college GPA of 3.0, transcript of college record, CPR certification, written essay, immunizations, 2 letters of recommendation, professional liability insurance/malpractice insurance, GRE General Test. *Application deadline:* 4/1 (fall), 10/1 (spring). *Application fee:* $50.
Advanced Placement Credit given for nursing courses completed elsewhere dependent upon specific evaluations.
Degree Requirements 45 total credit hours.

POST-MASTER'S PROGRAM

Areas of Study *Clinical nurse specialist programs in:* psychiatric/mental health. *Nurse practitioner programs in:* adult health, family health, neonatal health, psychiatric/mental health.

DOCTORAL DEGREE PROGRAM

Degree PhD
Available Programs Doctorate; Post-Baccalaureate Doctorate.
Areas of Study Faculty preparation, health policy, individualized study, nursing research, nursing science.
Program Entrance Requirements Minimum overall college GPA of 3.0, interview by faculty committee, 3 letters of recommendation, vita, writing sample, GRE General Test. Application deadline: 2/1 (fall). Application fee: $50.
Degree Requirements Dissertation, written exam.

POSTDOCTORAL PROGRAM

Areas of Study Family health.

Postdoctoral Program Contact Dr. Rosalie Mainous, Associate Dean for Graduate Academic Affairs, School of Nursing, University of Louisville, 555 South Floyd Street, Louisville, KY 40292. *Telephone:* 502-852-8387. *Fax:* 502-852-8783. *E-mail:* rosalie.mainous@louisville.edu.

CONTINUING EDUCATION PROGRAM

Contact Dr. Deborah Thomas, Director, School of Nursing, University of Louisville, 555 South Floyd Street, K-3019, Louisville, KY 40292. *Telephone:* 502-852-8392. *Fax:* 502-852-8783. *E-mail:* dvthom01@louisville.edu.

Western Kentucky University

School of Nursing
Bowling Green, Kentucky

http://www.wku.edu
Founded in 1906

DEGREES • BSN • MSN

Nursing Program Faculty 18 (58% with doctorates).
Baccalaureate Enrollment 163 **Women** 89% **Men** 11% **Minority** 3% **Part-time** 40%
Graduate Enrollment 34 **Women** 89% **Men** 11% **Minority** 2%
Nursing Student Activities Nursing Honor Society, Sigma Theta Tau, Student Nurses' Association.
Nursing Student Resources Academic advising; academic or career counseling; assistance for students with disabilities; bookstore; campus computer network; career placement assistance; computer lab; computer-assisted instruction; e-mail services; employment services for current students; externships; housing assistance; interactive nursing skills videos; Internet; learning resource lab; library services; nursing audiovisuals; paid internships; placement services for program completers; remedial services; resume preparation assistance; skills, simulation, or other laboratory; tutoring; unpaid internships.
Library Facilities 1.8 million volumes (17,880 in health, 1,697 in nursing); 3,931 periodical subscriptions (217 health-care related).

BACCALAUREATE PROGRAMS

Degree BSN
Study Options Full-time.
Program Entrance Requirements Minimum overall college GPA of 2.75, transcript of college record, CPR certification, health exam, health insurance, high school transcript, immunizations, professional liability insurance/malpractice insurance. Transfer students are accepted.
Advanced Placement Credit given for nursing courses completed elsewhere dependent upon specific evaluations.
Contact ***Telephone:*** 270-745-3391. *Fax:* 270-745-3392.

GRADUATE PROGRAMS

Contact ***Telephone:*** 270-745-3490. *Fax:* 270-745-3392.

MASTER'S DEGREE PROGRAM

Degree MSN
Concentrations Available Nursing administration; nursing education. *Nurse practitioner programs in:* primary care.
Study Options Full-time and part-time.
Program Entrance Requirements Computer literacy, minimum overall college GPA of 2.75, transcript of college record, CPR certification, written essay, immunizations, interview, 3 letters of recommendation, nursing research course, physical assessment course, professional liability insurance/malpractice insurance, statistics course, GRE General Test.
Advanced Placement Credit given for nursing courses completed elsewhere dependent upon specific evaluations.
Degree Requirements 45 total credit hours, thesis or project, comprehensive exam.

POST-MASTER'S PROGRAM

Areas of Study *Nurse practitioner programs in:* primary care.

CONTINUING EDUCATION PROGRAM

Contact ***Telephone:*** 270-745-3762. *Fax:* 270-745-3392.

LOUISIANA

Dillard University

Division of Nursing
New Orleans, Louisiana

http://www.dillard.edu/academic/nursing
Founded in 1869

DEGREE • BSN

Nursing Program Faculty 9 (44% with doctorates).
Baccalaureate Enrollment 58 **Women** 98% **Men** 2% **Minority** 99% **International** 2%
Nursing Student Activities Nursing Honor Society, Sigma Theta Tau, Student Nurses' Association.
Nursing Student Resources Academic advising; academic or career counseling; assistance for students with disabilities; bookstore; campus computer network; career placement assistance; computer lab; computer-assisted instruction; e-mail services; externships; interactive nursing skills videos; Internet; learning resource lab; library services; nursing audiovisuals; paid internships; placement services for program completers; remedial services; resume preparation assistance; skills, simulation, or other laboratory; tutoring.
Library Facilities 105,128 volumes; 295 periodical subscriptions (21 health-care related).

BACCALAUREATE PROGRAMS

Degree BSN
Available Programs Generic Baccalaureate; LPN to RN Baccalaureate; RN Baccalaureate.
Study Options Full-time.
Program Entrance Requirements Minimum overall college GPA of 2.5, transcript of college record, CPR certification, health exam, health insurance, high school transcript, immunizations, minimum high school GPA of 2.5, minimum GPA in nursing prerequisites of 2.5, professional liability insurance/malpractice insurance, prerequisite course work. Transfer students are accepted. *Application deadline:* 5/1 (fall), 5/15 (spring). Applications may be processed on a rolling basis for some programs.
Expenses (2010-11) *Tuition:* full-time $13,000; part-time $542 per contact hour. *Room and board:* $4608; room only: $3095 per academic year. *Required fees:* part-time $1040 per credit; part-time $520 per term.
Financial Aid 99% of baccalaureate students in nursing programs received some form of financial aid in 2009-10. *Gift aid (need-based):* Federal Pell, FSEOG, state, private, college/university gift aid from institutional funds, United Negro College Fund, Federal Nursing. *Loans:* Federal Nursing Student Loans, Federal Direct (Subsidized and Unsubsidized Stafford PLUS), Perkins, alternative loans. *Work-study:* Federal Work-Study, part-time campus jobs. *Financial aid application deadline (priority):* 3/1.
Contact Dr. Lenetra L. Jefferson, School of Nursing, Division of Nursing, Dillard University, 2601 Gentilly Boulevard, New Orleans, LA 70122. *Telephone:* 504-816-4717. *Fax:* 504-816-4861. *E-mail:* ljefferson@dillard.edu.

Grambling State University

School of Nursing
Grambling, Louisiana

Founded in 1901

DEGREES • BSN • MSN

Nursing Program Faculty 23 (20% with doctorates).
Baccalaureate Enrollment 600 **Women** 85% **Men** 15% **Minority** 68% **International** 9% **Part-time** 5%
Graduate Enrollment 41 **Women** 86% **Men** 14% **Minority** 66% **International** 12%
Distance Learning Courses Available.
Nursing Student Activities Student Nurses' Association.
Nursing Student Resources Academic advising; academic or career counseling; assistance for students with disabilities; bookstore; campus computer network; career placement assistance; computer lab; computer-assisted instruction; e-mail services; employment services for current students; interactive nursing skills videos; Internet; learning resource lab;

library services; nursing audiovisuals; skills, simulation, or other laboratory; tutoring.
Library Facilities 322,995 volumes (10,000 in health, 5,000 in nursing); 1.2 million periodical subscriptions (65 health-care related).

BACCALAUREATE PROGRAMS

Degree BSN
Available Programs Generic Baccalaureate; LPN to RN Baccalaureate; RN Baccalaureate.
Study Options Full-time.
Program Entrance Requirements Transcript of college record, CPR certification, health exam, high school foreign language, 3 years high school math, 3 years high school science, high school transcript, immunizations, minimum high school GPA of 2.0, minimum GPA in nursing prerequisites of 2.75, professional liability insurance/malpractice insurance, prerequisite course work. Transfer students are accepted. *Application deadline:* 6/1 (fall), 12/1 (spring). *Application fee:* $20.
Advanced Placement Credit given for nursing courses completed elsewhere dependent upon specific evaluations.
Contact *Telephone:* 318-274-2528. *Fax:* 318-274-3491.

GRADUATE PROGRAMS

Contact *Telephone:* 318-274-2897. *Fax:* 318-274-3491.

MASTER'S DEGREE PROGRAM

Degree MSN
Available Programs Master's.
Concentrations Available Nursing education. *Clinical nurse specialist programs in:* adult health, maternity-newborn, pediatric. *Nurse practitioner programs in:* family health, pediatric.
Study Options Full-time and part-time.
Program Entrance Requirements Clinical experience, minimum overall college GPA of 3.0, transcript of college record, CPR certification, immunizations, interview, 3 letters of recommendation, physical assessment course, professional liability insurance/malpractice insurance, prerequisite course work, statistics course, GRE. *Application deadline:* 6/1 (fall). *Application fee:* $20.
Advanced Placement Credit given for nursing courses completed elsewhere dependent upon specific evaluations.
Degree Requirements 49 total credit hours, thesis or project, comprehensive exam.

POST-MASTER'S PROGRAM

Areas of Study *Nurse practitioner programs in:* family health.

Louisiana College

Department of Nursing
Pineville, Louisiana

http://www.lacollege.edu
Founded in 1906

DEGREE • BSN
Nursing Program Faculty 6 (17% with doctorates).
Baccalaureate Enrollment 100
Nursing Student Activities Sigma Theta Tau, Student Nurses' Association.
Nursing Student Resources Academic advising; academic or career counseling; assistance for students with disabilities; bookstore; campus computer network; career placement assistance; computer lab; computer-assisted instruction; e-mail services; employment services for current students; externships; Internet; learning resource lab; library services; nursing audiovisuals; skills, simulation, or other laboratory; tutoring; unpaid internships.
Library Facilities 348,673 volumes (3,426 in health, 500 in nursing); 402 periodical subscriptions (142 health-care related).

BACCALAUREATE PROGRAMS

Degree BSN
Available Programs Generic Baccalaureate.
Study Options Full-time.
Program Entrance Requirements Minimum overall college GPA of 2.6, transcript of college record, CPR certification, health exam, health insurance, immunizations, interview, minimum high school GPA of 2.0, minimum high school rank 50%, minimum GPA in nursing prerequisites of 2.6, professional liability insurance/malpractice insurance, prerequisite course work. Transfer students are accepted.
Advanced Placement Credit given for nursing courses completed elsewhere dependent upon specific evaluations.
Contact *Telephone:* 318-487-7127. *Fax:* 318-487-7488.

Louisiana State University Health Sciences Center

School of Nursing
New Orleans, Louisiana

http://nursing.lsuhsc.edu/
Founded in 1931

DEGREES • BSN • DNS • MN
Nursing Program Faculty 70 (33% with doctorates).
Baccalaureate Enrollment 766 **Women** 82.5% **Men** 17.5% **Minority** 19.45% **International** .65% **Part-time** 22.1%
Graduate Enrollment 305 **Women** 78.7% **Men** 21.3% **Minority** 22.6% **International** .32% **Part-time** 46%
Nursing Student Activities Nursing Honor Society, Sigma Theta Tau, Student Nurses' Association.
Nursing Student Resources Academic advising; academic or career counseling; assistance for students with disabilities; bookstore; campus computer network; computer lab; computer-assisted instruction; e-mail services; housing assistance; interactive nursing skills videos; Internet; learning resource lab; library services; nursing audiovisuals; skills, simulation, or other laboratory.
Library Facilities 215,938 volumes in health, 4,487 volumes in nursing; 4,913 periodical subscriptions (8,233 health-care related).

BACCALAUREATE PROGRAMS

Degree BSN
Available Programs Accelerated Baccalaureate for Second Degree; Generic Baccalaureate; RN Baccalaureate.
Study Options Full-time and part-time.
Program Entrance Requirements Minimum overall college GPA of 2.8, transcript of college record, interview, prerequisite course work. Transfer students are accepted. *Application deadline:* 1/15 (fall), 8/15 (spring). *Application fee:* $50.
Expenses (2010-11) *Tuition, state resident:* full-time $3644; part-time $185 per semester. *Tuition, nonresident:* full-time $5986; part-time $302 per semester. *Room and board:* $6396 per academic year. *Required fees:* full-time $893; part-time $39 per credit.
Financial Aid 79% of baccalaureate students in nursing programs received some form of financial aid in 2009-10.
Contact Ms. Catherine Lopez, Nurse Recruiter, School of Nursing, Louisiana State University Health Sciences Center, 1900 Gravier Street, New Orleans, LA 70112. *Telephone:* 504-568-4180. *Fax:* 504-568-5853. *E-mail:* clopez@lsuhsc.edu.

GRADUATE PROGRAMS

Expenses (2010-11) *Tuition, state resident:* full-time $4634; part-time $206 per semester. *Tuition, nonresident:* full-time $8078; part-time $359 per semester. *Room and board:* $3396 per academic year. *Required fees:* full-time $834; part-time $37 per credit.
Financial Aid 66% of graduate students in nursing programs received some form of financial aid in 2009-10. 12 fellowships, 1 research assistantship were awarded; teaching assistantships, Federal Work-Study, institutionally sponsored loans, and unspecified assistantships also available. Aid available to part-time students.
Contact Ms. Catherine Lopez, Nurse Recruiter, School of Nursing, Louisiana State University Health Sciences Center, 1900 Gravier Street, New Orleans, LA 70112. *Telephone:* 504-568-4180. *Fax:* 504-568-5853. *E-mail:* clopez@lsuhsc.edu.

MASTER'S DEGREE PROGRAM

Degree MN
Available Programs Master's.
Concentrations Available Health-care administration; nurse anesthesia; nursing administration; nursing education. *Clinical nurse specialist programs in:* adult health, community health, parent-child, psychiatric/mental health. *Nurse practitioner programs in:* neonatal health, primary care.
Study Options Full-time and part-time.

Program Entrance Requirements Clinical experience, minimum overall college GPA of 3.0, transcript of college record, CPR certification, interview, 3 letters of recommendation, statistics course, GRE General Test, MAT. *Application deadline:* 1/15 (fall), 8/15 (spring). *Application fee:* $100.
Degree Requirements 38 total credit hours.

DOCTORAL DEGREE PROGRAM
Degree DNS
Available Programs Doctorate.
Areas of Study Clinical practice, nursing education.
Program Entrance Requirements Clinical experience, minimum overall college GPA of 3.5, 3 letters of recommendation, MSN or equivalent, scholarly papers, writing sample, GRE General Test. Application deadline: 2/1 (fall), 9/1 (spring). Application fee: $50.
Degree Requirements 54 total credit hours, dissertation, oral exam.

POSTDOCTORAL PROGRAM
Postdoctoral Program Contact Dr. Anita Hufft, Associate Dean, School of Nursing, Louisiana State University Health Sciences Center, 1900 Gravier Street, New Orleans, LA 70112. *Telephone:* 504-568-4107. *Fax:* 504-568-5853. *E-mail:* ahufft@lsuhsc.edu.

CONTINUING EDUCATION PROGRAM
Contact Dr. Demetrius J. Porche, Dean, School of Nursing, Louisiana State University Health Sciences Center, 1900 Gravier Street, New Orleans, LA 70112. *Telephone:* 504-568-4106. *Fax:* 504-568-5853. *E-mail:* dporch@lsuhsc.edu.

Loyola University New Orleans
School of Nursing
New Orleans, Louisiana

http://www.loyno.edu/~nursing
Founded in 1912

DEGREES • BSN • DNP • MSN
Nursing Program Faculty 42 (69% with doctorates).
Baccalaureate Enrollment 41 **Women** 100% **Minority** 26% **Part-time** 97.25%
Graduate Enrollment 635 **Women** 94% **Men** 6% **Minority** 23.77% **International** .01% **Part-time** 79.12%
Distance Learning Courses Available.
Nursing Student Activities Sigma Theta Tau.
Nursing Student Resources Academic advising; academic or career counseling; assistance for students with disabilities; bookstore; campus computer network; career placement assistance; computer lab; computer-assisted instruction; e-mail services; interactive nursing skills videos; Internet; learning resource lab; library services; nursing audiovisuals; skills, simulation, or other laboratory; tutoring.
Library Facilities 623,596 volumes (6,881 in health, 913 in nursing); 80,410 periodical subscriptions (6,716 health-care related).

BACCALAUREATE PROGRAMS
Degree BSN
Available Programs RN Baccalaureate.
Study Options Full-time and part-time.
Online Degree Options Yes (online only).
Program Entrance Requirements Minimum overall college GPA of 2.5, transcript of college record, written essay, immunizations, minimum GPA in nursing prerequisites of 2.0, professional liability insurance/malpractice insurance, RN licensure. Transfer students are accepted. *Application deadline:* Applications may be processed on a rolling basis for some programs.
Advanced Placement Credit by examination available. Credit given for nursing courses completed elsewhere dependent upon specific evaluations.
Expenses (2010-11) *Tuition:* part-time $434 per credit hour.
Financial Aid 98% of baccalaureate students in nursing programs received some form of financial aid in 2009-10. *Gift aid (need-based):* Federal Pell, FSEOG, state, private, college/university gift aid from institutional funds. *Loans:* Perkins. *Work-study:* Federal Work-Study. *Financial aid application deadline:* 6/1(priority: 2/15).
Contact Dr. Debra Copeland, BSN Program Coordinator, School of Nursing, Loyola University New Orleans, 6363 St. Charles Avenue, Campus Box 45, New Orleans, LA 70118. *Telephone:* 504-865-3253. *Fax:* 504-865-3254. *E-mail:* copeland@loyno.edu.

GRADUATE PROGRAMS
Expenses (2010-11) *Tuition:* part-time $702 per credit hour.
Financial Aid 100% of graduate students in nursing programs received some form of financial aid in 2009-10. Traineeships and Incumbent Workers Training Program grants available. *Financial aid application deadline:* 5/1.
Contact Dr. Ann H. Cary, Director, School of Nursing, School of Nursing, Loyola University New Orleans, 6363 St. Charles Avenue, Campus Box 45, New Orleans, LA 70118. *Telephone:* 504-865-3142. *Fax:* 504-865-3254. *E-mail:* nursing@loyno.edu.

MASTER'S DEGREE PROGRAM
Degree MSN
Available Programs Master's; Master's for Nurses with Non-Nursing Degrees; RN to Master's.
Concentrations Available Health-care administration; nurse case management. *Nurse practitioner programs in:* adult health, family health.
Study Options Full-time and part-time.
Online Degree Options Yes.
Program Entrance Requirements Clinical experience, minimum overall college GPA of 2.8, transcript of college record, CPR certification, written essay, immunizations, interview, 3 letters of recommendation, nursing research course, professional liability insurance/malpractice insurance, prerequisite course work, statistics course. *Application deadline:* 7/15 (fall), 11/19 (spring), 4/1 (summer).
Advanced Placement Credit given for nursing courses completed elsewhere dependent upon specific evaluations.
Degree Requirements 45 total credit hours, comprehensive exam.

POST-MASTER'S PROGRAM
Areas of Study *Nurse practitioner programs in:* adult health, family health.

DOCTORAL DEGREE PROGRAM
Degree DNP
Available Programs Doctorate; Post-Baccalaureate Doctorate.
Areas of Study Advanced practice nursing, clinical practice, faculty preparation, family health, nursing administration, nursing research.
Online Degree Options Yes (online only).
Program Entrance Requirements Clinical experience, minimum overall college GPA of 3.2, interview by faculty committee, interview, 3 letters of recommendation, MSN or equivalent, statistics course, writing sample. Application deadline: 11/1 (fall), 2/1 (spring). Application fee: $75.
Degree Requirements 38 total credit hours, dissertation, written exam, residency.

McNeese State University
College of Nursing
Lake Charles, Louisiana

http://www.mcneese.edu/
Founded in 1939

DEGREES • BSN • MSN
Nursing Program Faculty 51 (8% with doctorates).
Baccalaureate Enrollment 1,084 **Women** 79% **Men** 21% **Minority** 23% **International** 4% **Part-time** 14%
Graduate Enrollment 84 **Women** 76% **Men** 24% **Minority** 20% **Part-time** 90%
Distance Learning Courses Available.
Nursing Student Activities Sigma Theta Tau, Student Nurses' Association.
Nursing Student Resources Academic advising; academic or career counseling; assistance for students with disabilities; bookstore; campus computer network; career placement assistance; computer lab; computer-assisted instruction; daycare for children of students; e-mail services; employment services for current students; housing assistance; interactive nursing skills videos; Internet; learning resource lab; library services; nursing audiovisuals; placement services for program completers; resume preparation assistance; skills, simulation, or other laboratory; tutoring.
Library Facilities 41,000 volumes in health, 27,500 volumes in nursing; 120 periodical subscriptions health-care related.

BACCALAUREATE PROGRAMS
Degree BSN

Available Programs ADN to Baccalaureate; Generic Baccalaureate; LPN to Baccalaureate; LPN to RN Baccalaureate.
Study Options Full-time and part-time.
Program Entrance Requirements Minimum overall college GPA of 2.7, transcript of college record, CPR certification, health exam, health insurance, high school transcript, immunizations, minimum high school GPA of 2.5, minimum GPA in nursing prerequisites of 2.7, prerequisite course work. Transfer students are accepted. *Application deadline:* 10/15 (fall), 3/10 (spring). *Application fee:* $30.
Advanced Placement Credit by examination available. Credit given for nursing courses completed elsewhere dependent upon specific evaluations.
Expenses (2010-11) *Tuition, state resident:* full-time $2477; part-time $660 per semester. *Tuition, nonresident:* full-time $8378; part-time $1946 per semester. *Room and board:* $6800; room only: $4500 per academic year. *Required fees:* full-time $1094; part-time $91 per credit; part-time $547 per term.
Financial Aid 83% of baccalaureate students in nursing programs received some form of financial aid in 2009-10.
Contact Dr. Peggy L. Wolfe, Dean and Professor, College of Nursing, McNeese State University, PO Box 90415, Lake Charles, LA 70609-0415. *Telephone:* 337-475-5820. *Fax:* 337-475-5924. *E-mail:* pwolfe@mail.mcneese.edu.

GRADUATE PROGRAMS

Expenses (2010-11) *Tuition, state resident:* full-time $2918; part-time $200 per credit. *Tuition, nonresident:* full-time $5578; part-time $500 per credit. *International tuition:* $5578 full-time. *Room and board:* $6800; room only: $4500 per academic year. *Required fees:* full-time $1094; part-time $91 per credit; part-time $547 per term.
Financial Aid 38% of graduate students in nursing programs received some form of financial aid in 2009-10. *Application deadline:* 5/1.
Contact Dr. Valarie Waldmeier, MSN Coordinator, College of Nursing, McNeese State University, PO Box 90415, Lake Charles, LA 70609-0415. *Telephone:* 337-475-5753. *Fax:* 337-475-5702. *E-mail:* vwaldmei@mcneese.edu.

MASTER'S DEGREE PROGRAM

Degree MSN
Available Programs Master's.
Concentrations Available Health-care administration; nursing administration; nursing education. *Clinical nurse specialist programs in:* adult health, psychiatric/mental health. *Nurse practitioner programs in:* adult health, psychiatric/mental health.
Site Options Baton Rouge, LA; Lafayette, LA; Lake Charles, LA.
Study Options Full-time and part-time.
Online Degree Options Yes (online only).
Program Entrance Requirements Minimum overall college GPA of 3.2, transcript of college record, CPR certification, immunizations, physical assessment course, statistics course, GRE. *Application deadline:* 6/23 (fall), 11/18 (spring). *Application fee:* $20.
Advanced Placement Credit given for nursing courses completed elsewhere dependent upon specific evaluations.
Degree Requirements 42 total credit hours, thesis or project.

POST-MASTER'S PROGRAM

Areas of Study Health-care administration; nursing administration; nursing education. *Clinical nurse specialist programs in:* adult health, psychiatric/mental health. *Nurse practitioner programs in:* adult health, psychiatric/mental health.

CONTINUING EDUCATION PROGRAM

Contact Mrs. Patsy Trahan, Continuing Education Coordinator, College of Nursing, McNeese State University, PO Box 90415, Lake Charles, LA 70609-0415. *Telephone:* 337-475-5832. *Fax:* 337-475-5924. *E-mail:* ptrahan@mcneese.edu.

Nicholls State University

Department of Nursing
Thibodaux, Louisiana

http://www.nicholls.edu/nursing/
Founded in 1948

DEGREE • BSN

Nursing Program Faculty 19 (21% with doctorates).
Library Facilities 254,683 volumes; 1,259 periodical subscriptions.

BACCALAUREATE PROGRAMS

Degree BSN
Available Programs Generic Baccalaureate; LPN to Baccalaureate; RN Baccalaureate.
Program Entrance Requirements Minimum overall college GPA of 2.75, transcript of college record, minimum GPA in nursing prerequisites of 2.0, prerequisite course work. Transfer students are accepted.
Contact *Telephone:* 985-448-4696. *Fax:* 985-448-4932.

CONTINUING EDUCATION PROGRAM

Contact *Telephone:* 985-448-4696. *Fax:* 985-448-4932.

Northwestern State University of Louisiana

College of Nursing
Shreveport, Louisiana

http://www.nsula.edu/nursing
Founded in 1884

DEGREES • BSN • MSN

Nursing Program Faculty 54 (24% with doctorates).
Baccalaureate Enrollment 1,166 **Women** 85% **Men** 15% **Minority** 38% **Part-time** 37%
Graduate Enrollment 198 **Women** 89% **Men** 11% **Minority** 18% **International** 2% **Part-time** 95%
Distance Learning Courses Available.
Nursing Student Activities Sigma Theta Tau, Student Nurses' Association.
Nursing Student Resources Academic advising; academic or career counseling; assistance for students with disabilities; bookstore; campus computer network; computer lab; computer-assisted instruction; e-mail services; employment services for current students; interactive nursing skills videos; Internet; learning resource lab; library services; nursing audiovisuals; remedial services; skills, simulation, or other laboratory; tutoring.
Library Facilities 777,027 volumes (4,443 in health, 3,047 in nursing); 1,183 periodical subscriptions (1,359 health-care related).

BACCALAUREATE PROGRAMS

Degree BSN
Available Programs ADN to Baccalaureate; Generic Baccalaureate; LPN to Baccalaureate; RN Baccalaureate.
Site Options Alexandria, LA; Ferriday, LA.
Study Options Full-time and part-time.
Online Degree Options Yes.
Program Entrance Requirements Minimum overall college GPA of 2.0, transcript of college record, CPR certification, health exam, health insurance, high school transcript, immunizations, minimum GPA in nursing prerequisites of 2.7, prerequisite course work, RN licensure. Transfer students are accepted. *Application deadline:* 5/31 (fall), 8/31 (spring). *Application fee:* $20.
Advanced Placement Credit by examination available. Credit given for nursing courses completed elsewhere dependent upon specific evaluations.
Expenses (2010-11) *Tuition, state resident:* full-time $5646; part-time $170 per credit hour. *Tuition, nonresident:* full-time $15,675; part-time $278 per credit hour. *Required fees:* full-time $1275.
Financial Aid 80% of baccalaureate students in nursing programs received some form of financial aid in 2009-10. *Gift aid (need-based):* Federal Pell, FSEOG, state, private, college/university gift aid from institutional funds, United Negro College Fund, Federal Nursing, third party scholarships. *Loans:* Federal Direct (Subsidized and Unsubsidized Stafford PLUS), Perkins, alternative loans. *Work-study:* Federal Work-Study, part-time campus jobs. *Financial aid application deadline (priority):* 5/1.
Contact Ms. Linda Copple, Director, Undergraduate Studies in Nursing, College of Nursing, Northwestern State University of Louisiana, 1800 Line Avenue, Shreveport, LA 71101. *Telephone:* 318-677-3100. *Fax:* 318-677-3127. *E-mail:* copplel@nsula.edu.

GRADUATE PROGRAMS

Expenses (2010-11) *Tuition, state resident:* full-time $6486; part-time $201 per credit hour. *Tuition, nonresident:* full-time $16,512; part-time $412 per credit hour. *Required fees:* full-time $1275.

Financial Aid 20% of graduate students in nursing programs received some form of financial aid in 2009-10. Career-related internships or fieldwork and Federal Work-Study available. Aid available to part-time students. *Financial aid application deadline:* 7/15.
Contact Dr. Dana Roe, Director, Graduate Studies and Research in Nursing, College of Nursing, Northwestern State University of Louisiana, College of Nursing and Allied Health, 1800 Line Avenue, Shreveport, LA 71101. *Telephone:* 318-677-3100. *Fax:* 318-677-3127. *E-mail:* roed@nsula.edu.

MASTER'S DEGREE PROGRAM

Degree MSN
Available Programs Master's.
Concentrations Available Nursing administration; nursing education. *Clinical nurse specialist programs in:* adult health, critical care. *Nurse practitioner programs in:* acute care, family health, neonatal health, pediatric, women's health.
Site Options Alexandria, LA; Ferriday, LA.
Study Options Full-time and part-time.
Program Entrance Requirements Clinical experience, minimum overall college GPA of 3.0, transcript of college record, written essay, immunizations, 2 letters of recommendation, nursing research course, physical assessment course, professional liability insurance/malpractice insurance, statistics course, GRE General Test. *Application deadline:* 3/15 (fall), 10/15 (spring). *Application fee:* $20.
Advanced Placement Credit given for nursing courses completed elsewhere dependent upon specific evaluations.
Degree Requirements 42 total credit hours, thesis or project, comprehensive exam.

POST-MASTER'S PROGRAM

Areas of Study *Nurse practitioner programs in:* acute care, family health, neonatal health, pediatric, women's health.

CONTINUING EDUCATION PROGRAM

Contact Ms. Billie Bitowski, Director, Non-Traditional Studies in Nursing, College of Nursing, Northwestern State University of Louisiana, College of Nursing and Allied Health, 1800 Line Avenue, Shreveport, LA 71101. *Telephone:* 318-677-3100. *Fax:* 318-677-3127. *E-mail:* bitowskib@nsula.edu.

Our Lady of Holy Cross College
Division of Nursing
New Orleans, Louisiana

http://www.olhcc.edu
Founded in 1916

DEGREE • BSN
Nursing Program Faculty 16 (32% with doctorates).
Baccalaureate Enrollment 168 **Women** 90% **Men** 10% **Minority** 15% **Part-time** 11%
Nursing Student Activities Sigma Theta Tau, Student Nurses' Association, nursing club.
Nursing Student Resources Academic advising; academic or career counseling; assistance for students with disabilities; bookstore; campus computer network; career placement assistance; computer lab; computer-assisted instruction; e-mail services; interactive nursing skills videos; Internet; learning resource lab; library services; nursing audiovisuals; remedial services; resume preparation assistance; skills, simulation, or other laboratory; tutoring.
Library Facilities 83,631 volumes (5,000 in health, 3,100 in nursing); 1,002 periodical subscriptions (103 health-care related).

BACCALAUREATE PROGRAMS

Degree BSN
Available Programs Generic Baccalaureate.
Study Options Full-time.
Program Entrance Requirements Minimum overall college GPA of 2.5, transcript of college record, CPR certification, written essay, health exam, health insurance, high school transcript, immunizations, 3 letters of recommendation, minimum high school GPA of 2.0, minimum GPA in nursing prerequisites of 2.5, professional liability insurance/malpractice insurance, prerequisite course work. Transfer students are accepted.
Advanced Placement Credit by examination available. Credit given for nursing courses completed elsewhere dependent upon specific evaluations.
Contact *Telephone:* 504-398-2215. *Fax:* 504-391-2421.

Our Lady of the Lake College
Division of Nursing
Baton Rouge, Louisiana

http://www.ololcollege.edu
Founded in 1990

DEGREES • BSN • MSN
Nursing Program Faculty 44 (14% with doctorates).
Baccalaureate Enrollment 90 **Women** 90% **Men** 10% **Minority** 5% **Part-time** 45%
Graduate Enrollment 94 **Women** 55% **Men** 45% **Minority** 3%
Nursing Student Activities Nursing Honor Society, Student Nurses' Association.
Nursing Student Resources Academic advising; academic or career counseling; assistance for students with disabilities; bookstore; campus computer network; career placement assistance; computer lab; computer-assisted instruction; e-mail services; employment services for current students; interactive nursing skills videos; Internet; learning resource lab; library services; nursing audiovisuals; paid internships; remedial services; resume preparation assistance; skills, simulation, or other laboratory; tutoring.
Library Facilities 10,000 volumes in health, 1,000 volumes in nursing; 200 periodical subscriptions health-care related.

BACCALAUREATE PROGRAMS

Degree BSN
Available Programs RN Baccalaureate.
Site Options New Orleans, LA.
Study Options Full-time and part-time.
Program Entrance Requirements Minimum overall college GPA of 2.0, transcript of college record, CPR certification, written essay, health exam, health insurance, immunizations, minimum high school GPA of 2.0, professional liability insurance/malpractice insurance, prerequisite course work, RN licensure. Transfer students are accepted. *Application deadline:* 1/15 (fall), 8/15 (spring). *Application fee:* $35.
Advanced Placement Credit by examination available.
Expenses (2009-10) *Tuition:* full-time $7904; part-time $304 per credit hour. *Required fees:* full-time $775; part-time $12 per credit; part-time $125 per term.
Financial Aid 90% of baccalaureate students in nursing programs received some form of financial aid in 2008-09.
Contact Dr. Phyllis LeBlanc, RN-BSN Program Coordinator, Division of Nursing, Our Lady of the Lake College, 7434 Perkins Road, Baton Rouge, LA 70808. *Telephone:* 225-768-1793. *Fax:* 225-768-1760. *E-mail:* pleblanc@ololcollege.edu.

GRADUATE PROGRAMS

Expenses (2009-10) *Tuition:* full-time $23,220; part-time $645 per credit hour. *International tuition:* $23,220 full-time. *Required fees:* full-time $1392; part-time $12 per credit; part-time $475 per term.
Financial Aid 95% of graduate students in nursing programs received some form of financial aid in 2008-09.
Contact Dr. Melanie Green, Dean, School of Nursing, Division of Nursing, Our Lady of the Lake College, 7500 Hennessy Boulevard, Baton Rouge, LA 70808. *Telephone:* 225-768-1751. *Fax:* 225-768-1760. *E-mail:* Melanie.Green@ololcollege.edu.

MASTER'S DEGREE PROGRAM

Degree MSN
Available Programs Master's.
Concentrations Available Nurse anesthesia; nursing administration; nursing education.
Study Options Full-time and part-time.
Program Entrance Requirements Clinical experience, minimum overall college GPA of 3.3, transcript of college record, interview, letters of recommendation, nursing research course, physical assessment course, statistics course. *Application deadline:* 1/15 (fall), 8/15 (spring). *Application fee:* $35.
Advanced Placement Credit given for nursing courses completed elsewhere dependent upon specific evaluations.
Degree Requirements 42 total credit hours, thesis or project.

CONTINUING EDUCATION PROGRAM

Contact Mrs. Marie Kelley, Vice President, HCI, Division of Nursing, Our Lady of the Lake College, 7434 Perkins Road, Baton Rouge, LA 70808. *Telephone:* 225-768-1789. *Fax:* 225-214-1940. *E-mail:* mkelley@ololcollege.edu.

Southeastern Louisiana University

School of Nursing
Hammond, Louisiana

http://www.selu.edu/acad_research/depts/nurs
Founded in 1925

DEGREES • BS • MSN

Nursing Program Faculty 62 (27% with doctorates).
Baccalaureate Enrollment 1,771 **Women** 85.6% **Men** 14.4% **Minority** 23.7% **International** .8% **Part-time** 18.6%
Graduate Enrollment 103 **Women** 83.5% **Men** 16.5% **Minority** 9.7% **Part-time** 90%
Distance Learning Courses Available.
Nursing Student Activities Nursing Honor Society, Sigma Theta Tau, Student Nurses' Association.
Nursing Student Resources Academic advising; academic or career counseling; assistance for students with disabilities; bookstore; campus computer network; career placement assistance; computer lab; computer-assisted instruction; e-mail services; employment services for current students; interactive nursing skills videos; Internet; learning resource lab; library services; nursing audiovisuals; other; placement services for program completers; remedial services; resume preparation assistance; skills, simulation, or other laboratory; tutoring.
Library Facilities 714,423 volumes (11,818 in health, 6,813 in nursing); 3,997 periodical subscriptions (2,548 health-care related).

BACCALAUREATE PROGRAMS

Degree BS
Available Programs ADN to Baccalaureate; Accelerated Baccalaureate for Second Degree; Generic Baccalaureate; LPN to Baccalaureate; LPN to RN Baccalaureate; RN Baccalaureate.
Site Options Baton Rouge, LA.
Study Options Full-time and part-time.
Online Degree Options Yes.
Program Entrance Requirements CPR certification, health exam, immunizations, minimum GPA in nursing prerequisites of 3.0. Transfer students are accepted. *Application deadline:* 7/15 (fall), 12/1 (spring), 5/1 (summer). Applications may be processed on a rolling basis for some programs. *Application fee:* $20.
Advanced Placement Credit given for nursing courses completed elsewhere dependent upon specific evaluations.
Expenses (2010-11) *Tuition, state resident:* full-time $2993; part-time $167 per credit hour. *Tuition, nonresident:* full-time $11,462; part-time $520 per credit hour. *Room and board:* $6590; room only: $4140 per academic year. *Required fees:* full-time $1007; part-time $84 per credit.
Financial Aid 81% of baccalaureate students in nursing programs received some form of financial aid in 2009-10. *Gift aid (need-based):* Federal Pell, FSEOG, state, private, college/university gift aid from institutional funds, Federal Nursing. *Loans:* Perkins, college/university. *Work-study:* Federal Work-Study, part-time campus jobs. *Financial aid application deadline (priority):* 5/1.
Contact Dr. Susan Pryor, Interim Director, School of Nursing, Southeastern Louisiana University, SLU 10835, Hammond, LA 70402. *Telephone:* 985-549-2156. *Fax:* 985-549-2869. *E-mail:* nursing@selu.edu.

GRADUATE PROGRAMS

Expenses (2010-11) *Tuition, state resident:* full-time $3533; part-time $247 per credit hour. *Tuition, nonresident:* full-time $12,002; part-time $717 per credit hour. *International tuition:* $12,002 full-time. *Room and board:* $6590; room only: $4140 per academic year. *Required fees:* full-time $1195; part-time $133 per credit.
Financial Aid 38% of graduate students in nursing programs received some form of financial aid in 2009-10. 1 teaching assistantship (averaging $9,000 per year) was awarded; career-related internships or fieldwork, Federal Work-Study, institutionally sponsored loans, scholarships, and administrative assistantship also available. Aid available to part-time students. *Financial aid application deadline:* 5/1.
Contact Dr. Ann Carruth, Graduate Nursing Program Coordinator, School of Nursing, Southeastern Louisiana University, SLU 10835, Hammond, LA 70402. *Telephone:* 985-549-5045. *Fax:* 985-549-2869. *E-mail:* acarruth@selu.edu.

MASTER'S DEGREE PROGRAM

Degree MSN
Available Programs Master's.
Concentrations Available Nursing administration; nursing education. *Clinical nurse specialist programs in:* adult health, gerontology, psychiatric/mental health. *Nurse practitioner programs in:* adult health, gerontology, psychiatric/mental health.
Site Options Lafayette, LA; Baton Rouge, LA; Lake Charles, LA.
Study Options Full-time and part-time.
Program Entrance Requirements Clinical experience, minimum overall college GPA of 2.7, transcript of college record, immunizations, physical assessment course, resume, statistics course, GRE (verbal and quantitative). *Application deadline:* 7/15 (fall), 12/1 (spring), 5/1 (summer). Applications may be processed on a rolling basis for some programs. *Application fee:* $20.
Advanced Placement Credit given for nursing courses completed elsewhere dependent upon specific evaluations.
Degree Requirements 39 total credit hours, thesis or project.

Southern University and Agricultural and Mechanical College

School of Nursing
Baton Rouge, Louisiana

http://www.subr.edu/suson
Founded in 1880

DEGREES • BSN • MSN • PHD

Nursing Program Faculty 36 (3% with doctorates).
Baccalaureate Enrollment 1,020 **Women** 91% **Men** 9% **Minority** 96% **International** 1% **Part-time** 12%
Nursing Student Activities Nursing Honor Society, Student Nurses' Association, nursing club.
Nursing Student Resources Academic advising; academic or career counseling; assistance for students with disabilities; bookstore; campus computer network; computer lab; computer-assisted instruction; e-mail services; interactive nursing skills videos; Internet; learning resource lab; library services; nursing audiovisuals; resume preparation assistance; skills, simulation, or other laboratory; tutoring.
Library Facilities 880,098 volumes (4,220 in health, 716 in nursing); 8,882 periodical subscriptions (114 health-care related).

BACCALAUREATE PROGRAMS

Degree BSN
Available Programs Generic Baccalaureate.
Study Options Full-time and part-time.
Program Entrance Requirements Minimum overall college GPA of 2.6, CPR certification, health exam, immunizations, minimum GPA in nursing prerequisites, prerequisite course work. Transfer students are accepted.
Contact ***Telephone:*** 225-771-3416. *Fax:* 225-771-2651.

GRADUATE PROGRAMS

Contact ***Telephone:*** 225-771-2663. *Fax:* 225-771-3547.

MASTER'S DEGREE PROGRAM

Degree MSN
Available Programs Master's.
Concentrations Available Health-care administration; nursing education. *Clinical nurse specialist programs in:* family health. *Nurse practitioner programs in:* family health.
Study Options Full-time and part-time.
Program Entrance Requirements Minimum overall college GPA of 3.0, transcript of college record, 3 letters of recommendation, physical assessment course, statistics course, GRE General Test.
Degree Requirements 46 total credit hours, thesis or project, comprehensive exam.

POST-MASTER'S PROGRAM
Areas of Study *Nurse practitioner programs in:* family health.

DOCTORAL DEGREE PROGRAM
Degree PhD
Areas of Study Advanced practice nursing, nursing education, nursing research, women's health.
Program Entrance Requirements Clinical experience, minimum overall college GPA of 3.2, interview by faculty committee, 3 letters of recommendation, MSN or equivalent, scholarly papers, statistics course, vita, writing sample, GRE General Test.
Degree Requirements 60 total credit hours, dissertation, written exam.

University of Louisiana at Lafayette
College of Nursing
Lafayette, Louisiana

http://www.nursing.louisiana.edu
Founded in 1898

DEGREES • BSN • MSN
Nursing Program Faculty 47 (13% with doctorates).
Baccalaureate Enrollment 1,354 **Women** 83% **Men** 17% **Minority** 25% **Part-time** 10%
Distance Learning Courses Available.
Nursing Student Activities Nursing Honor Society, Sigma Theta Tau, Student Nurses' Association.
Nursing Student Resources Academic advising; academic or career counseling; assistance for students with disabilities; bookstore; campus computer network; career placement assistance; computer lab; computer-assisted instruction; daycare for children of students; e-mail services; employment services for current students; externships; housing assistance; interactive nursing skills videos; Internet; learning resource lab; library services; nursing audiovisuals; other; paid internships; placement services for program completers; remedial services; resume preparation assistance; skills, simulation, or other laboratory; tutoring; unpaid internships.
Library Facilities 999,913 volumes (6,883 in health, 4,593 in nursing); 2,851 periodical subscriptions (184 health-care related).

BACCALAUREATE PROGRAMS
Degree BSN
Available Programs ADN to Baccalaureate; Accelerated Baccalaureate for Second Degree; Generic Baccalaureate; LPN to Baccalaureate.
Study Options Full-time and part-time.
Online Degree Options Yes.
Program Entrance Requirements Minimum overall college GPA of 2.8, transcript of college record, CPR certification, health exam, health insurance, high school biology, high school chemistry, high school foreign language, 2 years high school math, 3 years high school science, high school transcript, immunizations, minimum high school GPA of 2.0, minimum high school rank 25%, minimum GPA in nursing prerequisites of 2.0, prerequisite course work. Transfer students are accepted. *Application deadline:* 4/1 (fall), 11/2 (spring).
Advanced Placement Credit by examination available. Credit given for nursing courses completed elsewhere dependent upon specific evaluations.
Contact ***Telephone:*** 337-482-5604. *Fax:* 337-482-5700.

GRADUATE PROGRAMS
Contact ***Telephone:*** 337-482-5639. *Fax:* 337-482-5650.

MASTER'S DEGREE PROGRAM
Degree MSN
Available Programs Master's; RN to Master's.
Concentrations Available Health-care administration; nursing administration; nursing education. *Clinical nurse specialist programs in:* adult health, psychiatric/mental health. *Nurse practitioner programs in:* adult health, psychiatric/mental health.
Site Options Hammond, LA; Baton Rouge, LA; Lake Charles, LA.
Study Options Full-time and part-time.
Online Degree Options Yes (online only).
Program Entrance Requirements Minimum overall college GPA of 2.75, transcript of college record, immunizations, 3 letters of recommendation, physical assessment course, statistics course, GRE General Test. *Application deadline:* Applications may be processed on a rolling basis for some programs. *Application fee:* $25.
Advanced Placement Credit given for nursing courses completed elsewhere dependent upon specific evaluations.
Degree Requirements 38 total credit hours, thesis or project.

POST-MASTER'S PROGRAM
Areas of Study *Clinical nurse specialist programs in:* adult health, psychiatric/mental health. *Nurse practitioner programs in:* adult health, psychiatric/mental health.

CONTINUING EDUCATION PROGRAM
Contact ***Telephone:*** 337-482-5648. *Fax:* 337-482-5053.

University of Louisiana at Monroe
Nursing
Monroe, Louisiana

http://www.ulm.edu/nursing
Founded in 1931

DEGREE • BS
Nursing Program Faculty 32 (2% with doctorates).
Baccalaureate Enrollment 220 **Women** 85% **Men** 15% **Minority** 20% **International** 1% **Part-time** 20%
Nursing Student Activities Sigma Theta Tau, Student Nurses' Association.
Nursing Student Resources Academic advising; academic or career counseling; assistance for students with disabilities; bookstore; campus computer network; computer lab; computer-assisted instruction; daycare for children of students; e-mail services; employment services for current students; interactive nursing skills videos; Internet; learning resource lab; library services; nursing audiovisuals; placement services for program completers; remedial services; resume preparation assistance; skills, simulation, or other laboratory; tutoring.
Library Facilities 639,133 volumes (20,924 in health, 3,000 in nursing); 140 periodical subscriptions (425 health-care related).

BACCALAUREATE PROGRAMS
Degree BS
Available Programs ADN to Baccalaureate; Accelerated Baccalaureate; Generic Baccalaureate; LPN to Baccalaureate; LPN to RN Baccalaureate; RN Baccalaureate.
Study Options Full-time and part-time.
Online Degree Options Yes (online only).
Program Entrance Requirements Transcript of college record, CPR certification, health exam, high school transcript, immunizations, minimum high school GPA of 2.0, minimum high school rank 50%, minimum GPA in nursing prerequisites of 2.8, professional liability insurance/malpractice insurance, prerequisite course work. Transfer students are accepted.
Advanced Placement Credit given for nursing courses completed elsewhere dependent upon specific evaluations.
Contact ***Telephone:*** 318-342-1640. *Fax:* 318-342-1567.

CONTINUING EDUCATION PROGRAM
Contact ***Telephone:*** 318-342-1679. *Fax:* 318-342-1567.

University of Phoenix–Louisiana Campus
College of Nursing
Metairie, Louisiana

Founded in 1976

DEGREE • BSN
Nursing Program Faculty 2 (50% with doctorates).
Baccalaureate Enrollment 9
Nursing Student Activities Sigma Theta Tau.
Nursing Student Resources Academic advising; academic or career counseling; assistance for students with disabilities; bookstore; campus computer network; computer lab; computer-assisted instruction; e-mail services; interactive nursing skills videos; Internet; learning resource lab; library services; nursing audiovisuals; remedial services; tutoring.

Library Facilities 16,781 periodical subscriptions (1,300 health-care related).

BACCALAUREATE PROGRAMS

Degree BSN
Available Programs Accelerated Baccalaureate; LPN to Baccalaureate.
Study Options Full-time.
Program Entrance Requirements Transcript of college record, CPR certification, immunizations, 1 letter of recommendation, RN licensure. Transfer students are accepted. *Application deadline:* Applications may be processed on a rolling basis for some programs.
Advanced Placement Credit by examination available. Credit given for nursing courses completed elsewhere dependent upon specific evaluations.
Expenses (2009-10) *Tuition:* full-time $8832. *International tuition:* $8832 full-time.
Contact Campus College Chair, Nursing, College of Nursing, University of Phoenix–Louisiana Campus, One Galleria Boulevard, Suite 725, Metairie, LA 70001-2082. *Telephone:* 504-461-8852.

MAINE

Husson University
School of Nursing
Bangor, Maine

http://www.husson.edu/
Founded in 1898

DEGREES • BSN • MSN
Nursing Program Faculty 14 (3% with doctorates).
Baccalaureate Enrollment 265 **Women** 92% **Men** 8% **Minority** 4% **International** 1%
Graduate Enrollment 48 **Women** 96% **Men** 4% **Part-time** 21%
Distance Learning Courses Available.
Nursing Student Activities Sigma Theta Tau, Student Nurses' Association, nursing club.
Nursing Student Resources Academic advising; academic or career counseling; assistance for students with disabilities; bookstore; campus computer network; career placement assistance; computer lab; computer-assisted instruction; e-mail services; employment services for current students; externships; interactive nursing skills videos; Internet; learning resource lab; library services; nursing audiovisuals; remedial services; resume preparation assistance; skills, simulation, or other laboratory; tutoring; unpaid internships.
Library Facilities 40,814 volumes (3,450 in health, 1,100 in nursing); 27,881 periodical subscriptions (183 health-care related).

BACCALAUREATE PROGRAMS

Degree BSN
Available Programs Generic Baccalaureate.
Study Options Full-time and part-time.
Program Entrance Requirements Minimum overall college GPA of 3.0, transcript of college record, written essay, health exam, health insurance, high school biology, high school chemistry, 2 years high school math, 2 years high school science, high school transcript, immunizations, 2 letters of recommendation, minimum high school GPA of 3.0, minimum GPA in nursing prerequisites of 3.0, prerequisite course work. Transfer students are accepted. *Application deadline:* Applications may be processed on a rolling basis for some programs. *Application fee:* $25.
Advanced Placement Credit by examination available. Credit given for nursing courses completed elsewhere dependent upon specific evaluations.
Expenses (2010-11) *Tuition:* full-time $13,140; part-time $438 per credit hour. *Room and board:* $7239 per academic year. *Required fees:* full-time $310; part-time $50 per credit.
Financial Aid 75% of baccalaureate students in nursing programs received some form of financial aid in 2009-10. *Gift aid (need-based):* Federal Pell, FSEOG, state, private, college/university gift aid from institutional funds. *Loans:* Federal Direct (Subsidized and Unsubsidized Stafford PLUS), Perkins, state, alternative loans. *Work-study:* Federal Work-Study. *Financial aid application deadline (priority):* 4/15.
Contact Gloria Brawn, Administrative Assistant, Undergraduate Nursing Program, School of Nursing, Husson University, 1 College Circle, Bangor, ME 04401-2999. *Telephone:* 207-941-7058. *Fax:* 207-941-7198. *E-mail:* brawng@husson.edu.

GRADUATE PROGRAMS

Expenses (2010-11) *Tuition:* part-time $458 per credit hour. *Room and board:* $7239 per academic year. *Required fees:* part-time $50 per credit.
Financial Aid 67% of graduate students in nursing programs received some form of financial aid in 2009-10.
Contact Ms. Jeanne Harvey, Administrative Assistant, School of Nursing, Husson University, 1 College Circle, Bangor, ME 04401. *Telephone:* 207-941-7166. *Fax:* 207-941-7198. *E-mail:* harveyj@husson.edu.

MASTER'S DEGREE PROGRAM

Degree MSN
Available Programs Master's; Master's for Nurses with Non-Nursing Degrees.
Concentrations Available Nursing education. *Clinical nurse specialist programs in:* psychiatric/mental health. *Nurse practitioner programs in:* family health.
Site Options South Portland, ME; Presque Isle, ME.
Study Options Full-time and part-time.
Program Entrance Requirements Clinical experience, minimum overall college GPA of 3.0, transcript of college record, written essay, immunizations, interview, 3 letters of recommendation, physical assessment course, prerequisite course work, statistics course. *Application deadline:* Applications may be processed on a rolling basis for some programs. *Application fee:* $25.
Advanced Placement Credit by examination available. Credit given for nursing courses completed elsewhere dependent upon specific evaluations.
Degree Requirements 44 total credit hours, thesis or project.

POST-MASTER'S PROGRAM

Areas of Study Nursing education. *Clinical nurse specialist programs in:* psychiatric/mental health. *Nurse practitioner programs in:* family health, psychiatric/mental health.

Saint Joseph's College of Maine
Department of Nursing
Standish, Maine

Founded in 1912

DEGREES • BSN • MSN • MSN/MHA
Nursing Program Faculty 65 (8% with doctorates).
Baccalaureate Enrollment 558 **Women** 95% **Men** 5% **Minority** 1% **Part-time** 48%
Graduate Enrollment 343 **Women** 93% **Men** 7% **Minority** 3% **Part-time** 100%
Distance Learning Courses Available.
Nursing Student Activities Sigma Theta Tau, Student Nurses' Association.
Nursing Student Resources Academic advising; academic or career counseling; assistance for students with disabilities; bookstore; campus computer network; computer lab; computer-assisted instruction; e-mail services; interactive nursing skills videos; Internet; learning resource lab; library services; nursing audiovisuals; remedial services; resume preparation assistance; skills, simulation, or other laboratory; tutoring.
Library Facilities 113,453 volumes (4,114 in health, 409 in nursing); 15,646 periodical subscriptions (108 health-care related).

BACCALAUREATE PROGRAMS

Degree BSN
Available Programs Generic Baccalaureate; RN Baccalaureate.
Study Options Full-time and part-time.
Program Entrance Requirements Minimum overall college GPA of 2.0, transcript of college record, written essay, health exam, health insurance, high school biology, high school chemistry, 3 years high school math, 2 years high school science, high school transcript, immunizations, 1 letter of recommendation, minimum high school GPA of 2.0. *Application deadline:* 5/1 (spring). *Application fee:* $250.
Advanced Placement Credit given for nursing courses completed elsewhere dependent upon specific evaluations.

Expenses (2009-10) *Tuition:* full-time $25,150; part-time $835 per credit. *Room and board:* $10,350 per academic year. *Required fees:* full-time $990; part-time $160 per term.
Financial Aid 98% of baccalaureate students in nursing programs received some form of financial aid in 2008-09. *Gift aid (need-based):* Federal Pell, FSEOG, state, private, college/university gift aid from institutional funds, Federal Nursing. *Loans:* Federal Nursing Student Loans, Federal Direct (Subsidized and Unsubsidized Stafford PLUS), Perkins, state. *Work-study:* Federal Work-Study. *Financial aid application deadline (priority):* 3/1.
Contact Admissions Department, Department of Nursing, Saint Joseph's College of Maine, 278 Whites Bridge Road, Standish, ME 04084-5263. *Telephone:* 207-893-7830. *Fax:* 207-892-7423. *E-mail:* info@sjcme.edu.

GRADUATE PROGRAMS

Expenses (2009-10) *Tuition:* part-time $400 per credit.
Financial Aid 1% of graduate students in nursing programs received some form of financial aid in 2008-09. Institutionally sponsored loans available. Aid available to part-time students.
Contact Dr. Lois Hamel, Director of Distance Nursing Education, Department of Nursing, Saint Joseph's College of Maine, 278 Whites Bridge Road, Standish, ME 04084-5263. *Telephone:* 207-893-7956. *Fax:* 207-893-7520. *E-mail:* lhamel@sjcme.edu.

MASTER'S DEGREE PROGRAM

Degrees MSN; MSN/MHA
Available Programs Master's; Master's for Nurses with Non-Nursing Degrees; RN to Master's.
Concentrations Available Nursing administration; nursing education.
Study Options Full-time and part-time.
Online Degree Options Yes (online only).
Program Entrance Requirements Clinical experience, computer literacy, minimum overall college GPA of 3.0, transcript of college record, prerequisite course work, resume, MAT. *Application deadline:* Applications may be processed on a rolling basis for some programs.
Advanced Placement Credit given for nursing courses completed elsewhere dependent upon specific evaluations.
Degree Requirements 42 total credit hours, thesis or project.

CONTINUING EDUCATION PROGRAM

Contact Dr. Lois Hamel, Director of Distance Nursing Education, Department of Nursing, Saint Joseph's College of Maine, 278 Whites Bridge Road, Standish, ME 04084-5263. *Telephone:* 207-893-7956. *Fax:* 207-893-7520. *E-mail:* lhamel@sjcme.edu.

University of Maine

School of Nursing
Orono, Maine

Founded in 1865

DEGREES • BSN • MSN

Nursing Program Faculty 20 (40% with doctorates).
Baccalaureate Enrollment 407 **Women** 90% **Men** 10% **Minority** .4% **International** .1% **Part-time** .5%
Graduate Enrollment 27 **Women** 99% **Men** 1% **Part-time** 50%
Distance Learning Courses Available.
Nursing Student Activities Sigma Theta Tau, Student Nurses' Association.
Nursing Student Resources Academic advising; academic or career counseling; assistance for students with disabilities; bookstore; campus computer network; computer lab; daycare for children of students; e-mail services; employment services for current students; housing assistance; interactive nursing skills videos; Internet; learning resource lab; library services; nursing audiovisuals; skills, simulation, or other laboratory; tutoring.
Library Facilities 1.1 million volumes (20,600 in health, 2,100 in nursing); 16,988 periodical subscriptions (3,750 health-care related).

BACCALAUREATE PROGRAMS

Degree BSN
Available Programs Generic Baccalaureate; RN Baccalaureate.
Site Options Presque Isle, ME; Augusta, ME; Portland, ME.
Study Options Full-time and part-time.
Program Entrance Requirements Minimum overall college GPA of 2.75, transcript of college record, CPR certification, written essay, health exam, high school biology, high school chemistry, high school foreign language, 3 years high school math, 3 years high school science, high school transcript, immunizations, interview, minimum high school rank 30%. Transfer students are accepted.
Advanced Placement Credit by examination available. Credit given for nursing courses completed elsewhere dependent upon specific evaluations.
Contact *Telephone:* 207-581-2588. *Fax:* 207-581-2585.

GRADUATE PROGRAMS

Contact *Telephone:* 207-581-2605. *Fax:* 207-581-2585.

MASTER'S DEGREE PROGRAM

Degree MSN
Available Programs Master's; RN to Master's.
Concentrations Available Health-care administration; nursing education. *Nurse practitioner programs in:* family health.
Study Options Full-time and part-time.
Program Entrance Requirements Clinical experience, minimum overall college GPA of 3.0, transcript of college record, CPR certification, written essay, immunizations, interview, 3 letters of recommendation, nursing research course, physical assessment course, statistics course, GRE General Test.
Advanced Placement Credit given for nursing courses completed elsewhere dependent upon specific evaluations.
Degree Requirements 47 total credit hours, thesis or project.

University of Maine at Fort Kent

Department of Nursing
Fort Kent, Maine

http://www.umfk.maine.edu/academics/programs/nursing/
Founded in 1878

DEGREE • BSN

Nursing Program Faculty 6 (16% with doctorates).
Baccalaureate Enrollment 246 **Women** 90% **Men** 10% **Minority** 2% **International** 2% **Part-time** 63%
Distance Learning Courses Available.
Nursing Student Activities Nursing Honor Society, Student Nurses' Association, nursing club.
Nursing Student Resources Academic advising; academic or career counseling; assistance for students with disabilities; bookstore; campus computer network; career placement assistance; computer lab; computer-assisted instruction; e-mail services; employment services for current students; externships; housing assistance; interactive nursing skills videos; Internet; learning resource lab; library services; nursing audiovisuals; paid internships; placement services for program completers; remedial services; resume preparation assistance; skills, simulation, or other laboratory; tutoring; unpaid internships.
Library Facilities 58,298 volumes (3,386 in health, 2,425 in nursing); 35,192 periodical subscriptions (73 health-care related).

BACCALAUREATE PROGRAMS

Degree BSN
Available Programs Accelerated Baccalaureate; Generic Baccalaureate; RN Baccalaureate.
Study Options Full-time and part-time.
Online Degree Options Yes.
Program Entrance Requirements Minimum overall college GPA of 2.5, CPR certification, written essay, health exam, health insurance, high school chemistry, high school foreign language, high school math, high school transcript, immunizations, minimum GPA in nursing prerequisites of 2.5, prerequisite course work. Transfer students are accepted. *Application deadline:* 8/15 (fall), 1/10 (spring). *Application fee:* $40.
Advanced Placement Credit given for nursing courses completed elsewhere dependent upon specific evaluations.
Expenses (2010-11) *Tuition, state resident:* full-time $6030; part-time $201 per credit. *Tuition, nonresident:* full-time $15,180; part-time $506 per credit. *Room and board:* $3500; room only: $2000 per academic year. *Required fees:* full-time $335; part-time $20 per credit.
Financial Aid 80% of baccalaureate students in nursing programs received some form of financial aid in 2009-10. *Gift aid (need-based):* Federal Pell, FSEOG, state, private, college/university gift aid from institutional funds. *Loans:* Federal Direct (Subsidized and Unsubsidized

Stafford PLUS), Perkins, state. *Work-study:* Federal Work-Study, part-time campus jobs. *Financial aid application deadline (priority):* 3/1.
Contact Ms. Diana White, Chair of Admission, Advisement, and Advancement Committee, Department of Nursing, University of Maine at Fort Kent, 23 University Drive, Fort Kent, ME 04743-1292. *Telephone:* 207-834-8607. *Fax:* 207-834-7577. *E-mail:* dianaw@maine.edu.

University of New England

Department of Nursing
Biddeford, Maine

http://www.une.edu/chp/nursing/
Founded in 1831

DEGREE • BSN
Nursing Program Faculty 16 (26% with doctorates).
Baccalaureate Enrollment 75 **Women** 73% **Men** 27%
Nursing Student Activities Nursing Honor Society, Sigma Theta Tau, Student Nurses' Association, nursing club.
Nursing Student Resources Academic advising; academic or career counseling; assistance for students with disabilities; bookstore; campus computer network; career placement assistance; computer lab; computer-assisted instruction; e-mail services; employment services for current students; housing assistance; interactive nursing skills videos; Internet; learning resource lab; library services; nursing audiovisuals; placement services for program completers; remedial services; resume preparation assistance; skills, simulation, or other laboratory; tutoring; unpaid internships.
Library Facilities 156,752 volumes (10,000 in health, 5,500 in nursing); 39,705 periodical subscriptions (1,300 health-care related).

BACCALAUREATE PROGRAMS

Degree BSN
Available Programs Accelerated RN Baccalaureate; Generic Baccalaureate; RN Baccalaureate.
Study Options Full-time and part-time.
Program Entrance Requirements Minimum overall college GPA of 2.5, transcript of college record, CPR certification, health exam, health insurance, high school biology, high school chemistry, 2 years high school math, 2 years high school science, high school transcript, immunizations, minimum high school GPA of 2.5, professional liability insurance/malpractice insurance. Transfer students are accepted. *Application deadline:* 2/15 (fall). *Application fee:* $100.
Advanced Placement Credit by examination available. Credit given for nursing courses completed elsewhere dependent upon specific evaluations.
Financial Aid 88% of baccalaureate students in nursing programs received some form of financial aid in 2009-10.
Contact Admissions Office, Department of Nursing, University of New England, 716 Stevens Avenue, Portland, ME 04103. *Telephone:* 800-477-4863. *E-mail:* admissions@une.edu.

CONTINUING EDUCATION PROGRAM

Contact Ms. Audrey Gup-Mathews, Director of Continuing Education, Department of Nursing, University of New England, 11 Hills Beach Road, Biddeford, ME 04005. *Telephone:* 207-602-2050. *Fax:* 207-602-5973.

University of Southern Maine

College of Nursing and Health Professions
Portland, Maine

http://www.usm.maine.edu/conhp
Founded in 1878

DEGREES • BS • DNP • MS • MS/MBA
Nursing Program Faculty 63 (24% with doctorates).
Baccalaureate Enrollment 436 **Women** 91% **Men** 9% **Minority** 8% **Part-time** 32%
Graduate Enrollment 102 **Women** 88% **Men** 12% **Minority** 3% **Part-time** 43%
Nursing Student Activities Sigma Theta Tau, Student Nurses' Association.
Nursing Student Resources Academic advising; academic or career counseling; assistance for students with disabilities; bookstore; campus computer network; computer lab; computer-assisted instruction; daycare for children of students; e-mail services; interactive nursing skills videos; Internet; learning resource lab; library services; nursing audiovisuals; remedial services; resume preparation assistance; skills, simulation, or other laboratory; tutoring.
Library Facilities 455,129 volumes (18,042 in health, 622 in nursing); 3,249 periodical subscriptions (230 health-care related).

BACCALAUREATE PROGRAMS

Degree BS
Available Programs ADN to Baccalaureate; Accelerated Baccalaureate for Second Degree; Generic Baccalaureate; RN Baccalaureate.
Site Options Lewiston, ME.
Study Options Full-time and part-time.
Program Entrance Requirements Minimum overall college GPA of 3.0, transcript of college record, written essay, high school biology, high school chemistry, 3 years high school math, 2 years high school science, high school transcript, immunizations, 2 letters of recommendation, minimum high school GPA of 3.0. Transfer students are accepted. *Application deadline:* 1/15 (fall). *Application fee:* $40.
Advanced Placement Credit by examination available. Credit given for nursing courses completed elsewhere dependent upon specific evaluations.
Expenses (2010-11) *Tuition, state resident:* full-time $7260; part-time $242 per credit hour. *Tuition, nonresident:* full-time $19,620; part-time $654 per credit hour. *Room and board:* $9394 per academic year. *Required fees:* full-time $1278; part-time $27 per credit; part-time $234 per term.
Financial Aid 96% of baccalaureate students in nursing programs received some form of financial aid in 2009-10. *Gift aid (need-based):* Federal Pell, FSEOG, state, college/university gift aid from institutional funds. *Loans:* Federal Nursing Student Loans, Federal Direct (Subsidized and Unsubsidized Stafford PLUS), Perkins, college/university. *Work-study:* Federal Work-Study. *Financial aid application deadline (priority):* 2/15.
Contact Ms. Brenda D. Webster, Coordinator of Nursing Student Services, College of Nursing and Health Professions, University of Southern Maine, School of Nursing, PO Box 9300, Portland, ME 04104-9300. *Telephone:* 207-780-4802. *Fax:* 207-228-8177. *E-mail:* bwebster@usm.maine.edu.

GRADUATE PROGRAMS

Expenses (2010-11) *Tuition, state resident:* full-time $8736; part-time $364 per credit hour. *Tuition, nonresident:* full-time $24,240; part-time $1010 per credit hour. *International tuition:* $24,240 full-time. *Room and board:* $9394 per academic year. *Required fees:* full-time $958; part-time $27 per credit; part-time $155 per term.
Financial Aid 90% of graduate students in nursing programs received some form of financial aid in 2009-10. 5 research assistantships with tuition reimbursements available (averaging $3,375 per year), 3 teaching assistantships with tuition reimbursements available (averaging $3,375 per year) were awarded; career-related internships or fieldwork, Federal Work-Study, scholarships, traineeships, tuition waivers (full and partial), and unspecified assistantships also available. Aid available to part-time students. *Financial aid application deadline:* 2/15.
Contact Ms. Brenda D. Webster, Coordinator of Nursing Student Services, College of Nursing and Health Professions, University of Southern Maine, School of Nursing, PO Box 9300, Portland, ME 04104-9300. *Telephone:* 207-780-4802. *Fax:* 207-228-8177. *E-mail:* bwebster@usm.maine.edu.

MASTER'S DEGREE PROGRAM

Degrees MS; MS/MBA
Available Programs Master's; Master's for Non-Nursing College Graduates; Master's for Nurses with Non-Nursing Degrees; RN to Master's.
Concentrations Available Clinical nurse leader. *Clinical nurse specialist programs in:* medical-surgical, psychiatric/mental health. *Nurse practitioner programs in:* adult health, family health, psychiatric/mental health.
Study Options Full-time and part-time.
Program Entrance Requirements Minimum overall college GPA of 3.0, transcript of college record, written essay, 2 letters of recommendation, physical assessment course, prerequisite course work, statistics course, GRE General Test or MAT. *Application deadline:* 4/1 (fall), 10/1 (spring), 11/1 (summer). *Application fee:* $50.
Advanced Placement Credit given for nursing courses completed elsewhere dependent upon specific evaluations.
Degree Requirements 54 total credit hours.

POST-MASTER'S PROGRAM

Areas of Study Clinical nurse leader. *Clinical nurse specialist programs in:* medical-surgical, psychiatric/mental health. *Nurse practitioner programs in:* adult health, family health, psychiatric/mental health.

DOCTORAL DEGREE PROGRAM

Degree DNP
Available Programs Doctorate.
Areas of Study Clinical practice, ethics, health policy, health-care systems, nursing policy.
Program Entrance Requirements Clinical experience, minimum overall college GPA of 3.25, interview by faculty committee, 3 letters of recommendation, MSN or equivalent, statistics course, vita, writing sample. Application deadline: 3/15 (fall). Application fee: $65.
Degree Requirements 43 total credit hours, residency.

CONTINUING EDUCATION PROGRAM

Contact Ms. Molly Morrell, Associate Director for Program Development, College of Nursing and Health Professions, University of Southern Maine, PO Box 9300, Center for Continuing Education, Portland, ME 04104-9300. *Telephone:* 207-780-5931. *Fax:* 207-780-5954. *E-mail:* mmorrell@usm.maine.edu.

MARYLAND

Bowie State University

Department of Nursing
Bowie, Maryland

http://www.bowiestate.edu/academics/nursing.htm
Founded in 1865

DEGREES • BSN • MSN

Nursing Program Faculty 20 (35% with doctorates).
Baccalaureate Enrollment 225 **Women** 88% **Men** 12% **Minority** 93% **International** 5% **Part-time** 25%
Graduate Enrollment 43 **Women** 87% **Men** 13% **Minority** 93% **International** 47% **Part-time** 5%
Distance Learning Courses Available.
Nursing Student Activities Nursing Honor Society, Student Nurses' Association.
Nursing Student Resources Academic advising; academic or career counseling; assistance for students with disabilities; bookstore; campus computer network; computer lab; computer-assisted instruction; housing assistance; interactive nursing skills videos; Internet; library services; nursing audiovisuals; skills, simulation, or other laboratory; tutoring.
Library Facilities 331,640 volumes; 3,152 periodical subscriptions.

BACCALAUREATE PROGRAMS

Degree BSN
Available Programs Accelerated Baccalaureate; Generic Baccalaureate; RN Baccalaureate.
Study Options Full-time.
Program Entrance Requirements Minimum overall college GPA of 2.75, transcript of college record, health exam, health insurance, high school biology, high school chemistry, 4 years high school math, 4 years high school science, high school transcript, immunizations, minimum high school GPA of 3.0, minimum GPA in nursing prerequisites of 2.75, prerequisite course work. Transfer students are accepted. *Application deadline:* 3/31 (fall).
Advanced Placement Credit given for nursing courses completed elsewhere dependent upon specific evaluations.
Expenses (2009-10) *Tuition, state resident:* full-time $4286; part-time $189 per credit. *Tuition, nonresident:* full-time $14,724; part-time $620 per credit. *Room and board:* $3342; room only: $1990 per academic year. *Required fees:* full-time $877; part-time $88 per credit.
Financial Aid 90% of baccalaureate students in nursing programs received some form of financial aid in 2008-09.
Contact Mr. Kenneth Dovale, Nursing Academic Adviser, Department of Nursing, Bowie State University, 14000 Jericho Park Road, Center for Learning Technology, Suite 202, Bowie, MD 20715. *Telephone:* 301-860-3202. *Fax:* 301-860-3222. *E-mail:* kdovale@bowiestate.edu.

GRADUATE PROGRAMS

Expenses (2009-10) *Tuition, state resident:* full-time $6030; part-time $335 per credit. *Tuition, nonresident:* full-time $11,520; part-time $640 per credit. *Room and board:* $7185; room only: $4480 per academic year. *Required fees:* full-time $1079; part-time $67 per credit; part-time $540 per term.
Financial Aid 20% of graduate students in nursing programs received some form of financial aid in 2008-09. Institutionally sponsored loans and traineeships available. *Financial aid application deadline:* 4/1.
Contact Mr. Kenneth Dovale, Nursing Academic Adviser, Department of Nursing, Bowie State University, 14000 Jericho Park Road, Center for Learning Technology, Suite 202, Bowie, MD 20715. *Telephone:* 301-860-3202. *Fax:* 301-860-3222. *E-mail:* kdovale@bowiestate.edu.

MASTER'S DEGREE PROGRAM

Degree MSN
Available Programs Master's.
Concentrations Available Nursing education. *Nurse practitioner programs in:* family health.
Study Options Full-time and part-time.
Program Entrance Requirements Clinical experience, minimum overall college GPA of 2.5, CPR certification, written essay, immunizations, 3 letters of recommendation, physical assessment course, professional liability insurance/malpractice insurance, resume, statistics course. *Application deadline:* 11/30 (fall), 4/30 (spring). Applications may be processed on a rolling basis for some programs.
Advanced Placement Credit by examination available. Credit given for nursing courses completed elsewhere dependent upon specific evaluations.
Degree Requirements 45 total credit hours, comprehensive exam.

College of Notre Dame of Maryland

Department of Nursing
Baltimore, Maryland

http://206.205.71.30/academics/departments/nd_aca_nursing.cfm
Founded in 1873

DEGREE • BS

Nursing Program Faculty 5 (60% with doctorates).
Nursing Student Resources Library services.
Library Facilities 999,295 volumes; 42,427 periodical subscriptions.

BACCALAUREATE PROGRAMS

Degree BS
Available Programs Accelerated RN Baccalaureate; RN Baccalaureate.
Site Options Frederick, MD; Aberdeen, MD.
Study Options Full-time and part-time.
Program Entrance Requirements Minimum overall college GPA of 2.5, transcript of college record, interview, minimum GPA in nursing prerequisites of 2.0, prerequisite course work, RN licensure. Transfer students are accepted.
Advanced Placement Credit by examination available. Credit given for nursing courses completed elsewhere dependent upon specific evaluations.
Contact ***Telephone:*** 410-532-5500.

Coppin State University

Helene Fuld School of Nursing
Baltimore, Maryland

http://www.coppin.edu/nursing
Founded in 1900

DEGREES • BSN • MSN

Nursing Program Faculty 45 (18% with doctorates).
Baccalaureate Enrollment 529 **Women** 91% **Men** 9% **Minority** 99% **International** 2% **Part-time** 33%
Graduate Enrollment 32 **Women** 94% **Men** 6% **Minority** 94% **Part-time** 22%
Distance Learning Courses Available.

Nursing Student Activities Nursing Honor Society, Sigma Theta Tau, Student Nurses' Association.
Nursing Student Resources Academic advising; academic or career counseling; assistance for students with disabilities; bookstore; campus computer network; career placement assistance; computer lab; computer-assisted instruction; e-mail services; externships; interactive nursing skills videos; Internet; learning resource lab; library services; nursing audiovisuals; other; placement services for program completers; remedial services; resume preparation assistance; skills, simulation, or other laboratory; tutoring; unpaid internships.
Library Facilities 134,983 volumes (1,339 in health, 1,298 in nursing); 665 periodical subscriptions (132 health-care related).

BACCALAUREATE PROGRAMS

Degree BSN
Available Programs Accelerated RN Baccalaureate; Baccalaureate for Second Degree; Generic Baccalaureate; RN Baccalaureate.
Site Options Baltimore, MD.
Study Options Full-time and part-time.
Program Entrance Requirements Written essay, health exam, high school biology, high school chemistry, high school foreign language, 3 years high school math, 2 years high school science, high school transcript, immunizations, 3 letters of recommendation, minimum high school GPA of 2.5, minimum GPA in nursing prerequisites of 2.5. Transfer students are accepted.
Contact *Telephone:* 410-951-3988. *Fax:* 410-400-5978.

GRADUATE PROGRAMS

Contact *Telephone:* 410-951-3988. *Fax:* 410-400-5978.

MASTER'S DEGREE PROGRAM

Degree MSN
Available Programs Master's.
Concentrations Available *Nurse practitioner programs in:* family health.
Site Options Baltimore, MD.
Study Options Full-time and part-time.
Program Entrance Requirements Clinical experience, computer literacy, minimum overall college GPA of 3.0, transcript of college record, CPR certification, written essay, immunizations, interview, 3 letters of recommendation, nursing research course, physical assessment course, statistics course.
Advanced Placement Credit given for nursing courses completed elsewhere dependent upon specific evaluations.
Degree Requirements 48 total credit hours, thesis or project, comprehensive exam.

POST-MASTER'S PROGRAM

Areas of Study *Nurse practitioner programs in:* family health.

The Johns Hopkins University
School of Nursing
Baltimore, Maryland

http://www.son.jhmi.edu
Founded in 1876

DEGREES • BS • MSN • MSN/MBA • MSN/MPH • MSN/PHD • PHD

Nursing Program Faculty 250 (45% with doctorates).
Baccalaureate Enrollment 380 **Women** 90% **Men** 10% **Minority** 26.3% **International** 4% **Part-time** 4.6%
Graduate Enrollment 240 **Women** 92.9% **Men** 7.1% **Minority** 21.8% **International** 3% **Part-time** 67.6%
Distance Learning Courses Available.
Nursing Student Activities Nursing Honor Society, Sigma Theta Tau, Student Nurses' Association, nursing club.
Nursing Student Resources Academic advising; academic or career counseling; assistance for students with disabilities; bookstore; campus computer network; career placement assistance; computer lab; computer-assisted instruction; e-mail services; employment services for current students; housing assistance; Internet; learning resource lab; library services; nursing audiovisuals; other; resume preparation assistance; skills, simulation, or other laboratory; tutoring.
Library Facilities 3.7 million volumes (412,000 in health); 76,000 periodical subscriptions (6,000 health-care related).

BACCALAUREATE PROGRAMS

Degree BS

Available Programs Accelerated Baccalaureate for Second Degree; Baccalaureate for Second Degree; Generic Baccalaureate; RN Baccalaureate.

Study Options Full-time and part-time.

Program Entrance Requirements Minimum overall college GPA of 3.0, transcript of college record, CPR certification, written essay, health exam, health insurance, immunizations, interview, 3 letters of recommendation, minimum GPA in nursing prerequisites of 3.0, prerequisite course work. Transfer students are accepted. *Application deadline:* 1/15 (fall), 11/15 (summer). *Application fee:* $75.

Advanced Placement Credit by examination available. Credit given for nursing courses completed elsewhere dependent upon specific evaluations.

Expenses (2009-10) *Tuition:* full-time $31,920; part-time $1330 per credit. *International tuition:* $31,920 full-time.

Financial Aid 80% of baccalaureate students in nursing programs received some form of financial aid in 2008-09. *Gift aid (need-based):* Federal Pell, FSEOG, state, private, college/university gift aid from institutional funds. *Loans:* Federal Direct (Subsidized and Unsubsidized Stafford PLUS), Perkins, college/university. *Work-study:* Federal Work-Study. *Financial aid application deadline:* 3/1.

Contact Office of Admissions and Student Services, School of Nursing, The Johns Hopkins University, 525 North Wolfe Street, Baltimore, MD 21205-2110. *Telephone:* 410-955-7548. *Fax:* 410-614-7086. *E-mail:* jhuson@son.jhmi.edu.

GRADUATE PROGRAMS

Expenses (2009-10) *Tuition:* full-time $31,416; part-time $1309 per credit. *International tuition:* $31,416 full-time.

Financial Aid 6 fellowships (averaging $23,272 per year) were awarded; research assistantships, teaching assistantships, career-related internships or fieldwork, Federal Work-Study, scholarships, traineeships, and tuition waivers (partial) also available.

Contact Ms. Mary O'Rourke, Director of Admissions and Student Services, School of Nursing, The Johns Hopkins University, 525 North Wolfe Street, Suite 113, Baltimore, MD 21205-2110. *Telephone:* 410-955-7548. *Fax:* 410-614-7086. *E-mail:* jhuson@son.jhmi.edu.

MASTER'S DEGREE PROGRAM

Degrees MSN; MSN/MBA; MSN/MPH; MSN/PhD

Available Programs Master's.

Concentrations Available Health-care administration; nurse case management; nurse-midwifery; nursing administration. *Clinical nurse specialist programs in:* acute care, adult health, cardiovascular, community health, critical care, family health, forensic nursing, gerontology, maternity-newborn, medical-surgical, oncology, palliative care, parent-child, pediatric, perinatal, public health, women's health. *Nurse practitioner programs in:* acute care, adult health, family health, pediatric, primary care.

Study Options Full-time and part-time.

Program Entrance Requirements Clinical experience, computer literacy, minimum overall college GPA of 3.0, transcript of college record, CPR certification, written essay, immunizations, interview, 3 letters of recommendation, nursing research course, physical assessment course, prerequisite course work, resume, statistics course, GRE. *Application deadline:* 8/1 (fall), 12/1 (winter), 12/1 (spring), 5/1 (summer). Applications may be processed on a rolling basis for some programs. *Application fee:* $75.

Advanced Placement Credit by examination available. Credit given for nursing courses completed elsewhere dependent upon specific evaluations.

Degree Requirements 36 total credit hours, thesis or project.

POST-MASTER'S PROGRAM

Areas of Study Nursing education. *Nurse practitioner programs in:* acute care, adult health, family health, pediatric, primary care.

DOCTORAL DEGREE PROGRAM

Degree PhD

Available Programs Doctorate.

Areas of Study Addiction/substance abuse, advanced practice nursing, aging, bio-behavioral research, biology of health and illness, clinical practice, community health, critical care, family health, forensic nursing, gerontology, health policy, health promotion/disease prevention, health-care systems, human health and illness, illness and transition, individualized study, nurse case management, nursing research, nursing science, oncology, urban health, women's health.

Program Entrance Requirements Clinical experience, minimum overall college GPA of 3.5, interview, 3 letters of recommendation, MSN or equivalent, scholarly papers, statistics course, vita, writing sample, GRE. Application deadline: 1/15 (fall). Applications may be processed on a rolling basis for some programs. Application fee: $100.

Degree Requirements Dissertation, oral exam, written exam.

POSTDOCTORAL PROGRAM

Areas of Study Health promotion/disease prevention, vulnerable population.

Postdoctoral Program Contact Dr. Gayle Page, Director of Center for Nursing Research and Sponsored Projects, School of Nursing, The Johns Hopkins University, 525 North Wolfe Street, Baltimore, MD 21205-2110. *Telephone:* 410-955-7548. *Fax:* 410-614-7086. *E-mail:* gpage@son.jhmi.edu.

CONTINUING EDUCATION PROGRAM

Contact Jane Shivnan, Director, Institute for Johns Hopkins Nursing, School of Nursing, The Johns Hopkins University, 525 North Wolfe Street, Baltimore, MD 21205-2110. *Telephone:* 443-287-4745. *Fax:* 410-614-8972. *E-mail:* ijhn@son.jhmi.edu.

See full description on page 480.

Salisbury University
Program in Nursing
Salisbury, Maryland

http://www.salisbury.edu/nursing

Founded in 1925

DEGREES • BS • MS

Nursing Program Faculty 30 (75% with doctorates).

Baccalaureate Enrollment 475 **Women** 90% **Men** 10% **Minority** 15% **International** 3% **Part-time** 10%

Graduate Enrollment 28 **Women** 90% **Men** 10% **Minority** 10% **International** 5% **Part-time** 85%

Distance Learning Courses Available.

Nursing Student Activities Nursing Honor Society, Sigma Theta Tau, Student Nurses' Association.

Nursing Student Resources Academic advising; academic or career counseling; assistance for students with disabilities; bookstore; campus computer network; career placement assistance; computer lab; computer-assisted instruction; e-mail services; employment services for current students; externships; housing assistance; interactive nursing skills videos; Internet; learning resource lab; library services; nursing audiovisuals; paid internships; placement services for program completers; remedial services; resume preparation assistance; skills, simulation, or other laboratory; tutoring; unpaid internships.

Library Facilities 442,682 volumes (6,850 in health, 1,025 in nursing); 1,241 periodical subscriptions (145 health-care related).

BACCALAUREATE PROGRAMS

Degree BS

Available Programs ADN to Baccalaureate; Accelerated Baccalaureate for Second Degree; Generic Baccalaureate; RN Baccalaureate.

Study Options Full-time.

Program Entrance Requirements Minimum overall college GPA of 2.75, transcript of college record, CPR certification, health exam, high school biology, high school chemistry, 2 years high school math, high school transcript, immunizations, minimum GPA in nursing prerequisites of 3.0, prerequisite course work. Transfer students are accepted. *Application deadline:* 2/1 (winter).

Advanced Placement Credit given for nursing courses completed elsewhere dependent upon specific evaluations.

Expenses (2010-11) *Tuition, state resident:* part-time $206 per credit hour. *Tuition, nonresident:* part-time $559 per credit hour. *Room and board:* $4439; room only: $2425 per academic year. *Required fees:* part-time $65 per credit; part-time $974 per term.

Financial Aid 80% of baccalaureate students in nursing programs received some form of financial aid in 2009-10.

Contact Dr. Lisa A. Seldomridge, Chair and Professor, Department of Nursing, Program in Nursing, Salisbury University, 1101 Camden Avenue, Salisbury, MD 21801. *Telephone:* 410-543-6413. *Fax:* 410-548-3313. *E-mail:* laseldomridge@salisbury.edu.

GRADUATE PROGRAMS

Expenses (2010-11) *Tuition, state resident:* part-time $290 per credit hour. *Tuition, nonresident:* part-time $587 per credit hour. *Required fees:* part-time $61 per credit.
Financial Aid Career-related internships or fieldwork, scholarships, and unspecified assistantships available.
Contact Dr. Mary T. Parsons, Director, Graduate and Second Degree Programs, Program in Nursing, Salisbury University, 1101 Camden Avenue, Salisbury, MD 21801. *Telephone:* 410-543-6416. *Fax:* 410-548-3313. *E-mail:* mtparsons@salisbury.edu.

MASTER'S DEGREE PROGRAM

Degree MS
Available Programs Master's; RN to Master's.
Concentrations Available Health-care administration; nursing education. *Nurse practitioner programs in:* family health.
Study Options Full-time and part-time.
Program Entrance Requirements Minimum overall college GPA of 3.0, transcript of college record, CPR certification, written essay, immunizations, interview, 2 letters of recommendation, nursing research course, physical assessment course, resume, statistics course. *Application deadline:* Applications may be processed on a rolling basis for some programs.
Advanced Placement Credit given for nursing courses completed elsewhere dependent upon specific evaluations.
Degree Requirements 43 total credit hours, thesis or project.

POST-MASTER'S PROGRAM

Areas of Study Health-care administration; nursing education. *Nurse practitioner programs in:* family health.

Stevenson University
Nursing Division
Stevenson, Maryland

http://www4.vjc.edu/Nursing
Founded in 1952

DEGREE • BS
Nursing Program Faculty 43 (35% with doctorates).
Baccalaureate Enrollment 428 **Women** 94% **Men** 6% **Minority** 25% **Part-time** 52%
Distance Learning Courses Available.
Nursing Student Activities Sigma Theta Tau, Student Nurses' Association.
Nursing Student Resources Academic advising; academic or career counseling; assistance for students with disabilities; bookstore; campus computer network; career placement assistance; computer lab; e-mail services; employment services for current students; Internet; learning resource lab; library services; nursing audiovisuals; placement services for program completers; remedial services; resume preparation assistance; skills, simulation, or other laboratory; tutoring.
Library Facilities 81,802 volumes (3,301 in health, 776 in nursing); 1,058 periodical subscriptions (635 health-care related).

BACCALAUREATE PROGRAMS

Degree BS
Available Programs ADN to Baccalaureate; Accelerated Baccalaureate for Second Degree; Accelerated RN Baccalaureate; Generic Baccalaureate; RN Baccalaureate.
Site Options Arnold, MD; Easton, MD; Westminster, MD.
Study Options Full-time and part-time.
Program Entrance Requirements Minimum overall college GPA of 3.0, transcript of college record, written essay, health exam, health insurance, high school biology, high school chemistry, 2 years high school math, high school transcript, immunizations, interview, minimum high school GPA of 3.0, minimum GPA in nursing prerequisites of 3.0. Transfer students are accepted.
Advanced Placement Credit by examination available. Credit given for nursing courses completed elsewhere dependent upon specific evaluations.
Contact ***Telephone:*** 443-334-2312. *Fax:* 443-334-2148.

Towson University
Department of Nursing
Towson, Maryland

http://www.towson.edu/nursing
Founded in 1866

DEGREES • BS • MS
Nursing Program Faculty 81 (17% with doctorates).
Baccalaureate Enrollment 300 **Women** 96% **Men** 4% **Minority** 24% **Part-time** 14%
Graduate Enrollment 115 **Women** 92% **Men** 8% **Minority** 21% **Part-time** 60%
Distance Learning Courses Available.
Nursing Student Activities Sigma Theta Tau, Student Nurses' Association.
Nursing Student Resources Academic advising; academic or career counseling; assistance for students with disabilities; bookstore; campus computer network; career placement assistance; computer lab; computer-assisted instruction; daycare for children of students; e-mail services; housing assistance; interactive nursing skills videos; Internet; learning resource lab; library services; nursing audiovisuals; remedial services; resume preparation assistance; skills, simulation, or other laboratory; tutoring.
Library Facilities 578,057 volumes (15,660 in health, 1,409 in nursing); 4,653 periodical subscriptions (665 health-care related).

BACCALAUREATE PROGRAMS

Degree BS
Available Programs Generic Baccalaureate; RN Baccalaureate.
Site Options Hagerstown, MD.
Study Options Full-time and part-time.
Program Entrance Requirements Minimum overall college GPA of 3.0, transcript of college record, CPR certification, health exam, health insurance, immunizations, prerequisite course work. Transfer students are accepted. *Application deadline:* 1/15 (fall), 8/15 (spring). *Application fee:* $50.
Advanced Placement Credit by examination available. Credit given for nursing courses completed elsewhere dependent upon specific evaluations.
Expenses (2010-11) *Tuition, state resident:* full-time $5336; part-time $232 per unit. *Tuition, nonresident:* full-time $16,794; part-time $641 per unit. *Room and board:* $10,550; room only: $6550 per academic year. *Required fees:* part-time $86 per credit; part-time $1043 per term.
Financial Aid ***Gift aid (need-based):*** Federal Pell, FSEOG, state, private, college/university gift aid from institutional funds. *Loans:* Federal Direct (Subsidized and Unsubsidized Stafford PLUS), Perkins. *Work-study:* Federal Work-Study. *Financial aid application deadline:* 2/10(priority: 1/31).
Contact Ms. Brook R. Necker, Admissions and Retention Coordinator, Department of Nursing, Towson University, 8000 York Road, Towson, MD 21252-0001. *Telephone:* 410-704-4170. *E-mail:* bnecker@towson.edu.

GRADUATE PROGRAMS

Expenses (2010-11) *Tuition, area resident:* part-time $324 per credit. *Tuition, state resident:* part-time $681 per credit. *Required fees:* part-time $97 per credit.
Contact Dr. Kathleen Ogle, Graduate Program Director, Department of Nursing, Towson University, 8000 York Road, Towson, MD 21252-0001. *Telephone:* 410-704-4389. *Fax:* 410-704-4325. *E-mail:* kogle@towson.edu.

MASTER'S DEGREE PROGRAM

Degree MS
Available Programs Master's.
Concentrations Available Health-care administration; nursing education.
Site Options Hagerstown, MD.
Study Options Full-time and part-time.
Program Entrance Requirements Minimum overall college GPA of 3.0, transcript of college record, nursing research course, physical assessment course, resume, statistics course. *Application deadline:* Applications may be processed on a rolling basis for some programs. *Application fee:* $50.
Degree Requirements 36 total credit hours.

University of Maryland, Baltimore

Master's Program in Nursing
Baltimore, Maryland

http://nursing.umaryland.edu/

DEGREES • BSN • DNP • MS • MSN/JD • MSN/MBA • MSN/MPH

Nursing Program Faculty 191 (82% with doctorates).

Baccalaureate Enrollment 637 **Women** 87% **Men** 13% **Minority** 27% **Part-time** 31%

Graduate Enrollment 855 **Women** 88% **Men** 12% **Minority** 25% **International** 1% **Part-time** 58%

Distance Learning Courses Available.

Nursing Student Activities Nursing Honor Society, Sigma Theta Tau, Student Nurses' Association.

Nursing Student Resources Academic advising; academic or career counseling; assistance for students with disabilities; bookstore; campus computer network; career placement assistance; computer lab; computer-assisted instruction; e-mail services; interactive nursing skills videos; Internet; learning resource lab; library services; nursing audiovisuals; remedial services; skills, simulation, or other laboratory; tutoring.

Library Facilities 360,000 volumes in health, 60 volumes in nursing; 2,400 periodical subscriptions health-care related.

BACCALAUREATE PROGRAMS

Degree BSN

Available Programs Generic Baccalaureate; RN Baccalaureate.

Site Options Baltimore-Shady Grove, MD.

Study Options Full-time and part-time.

Online Degree Options Yes.

Program Entrance Requirements Minimum overall college GPA of 3.0, transcript of college record, CPR certification, written essay, health exam, health insurance, immunizations, 2 letters of recommendation, minimum GPA in nursing prerequisites of 3.0, prerequisite course work. *Application deadline:* 2/1 (fall), 9/1 (spring). *Application fee:* $50.

Advanced Placement Credit by examination available. Credit given for nursing courses completed elsewhere dependent upon specific evaluations.

Expenses (2010-11) *Tuition, state resident:* full-time $7096; part-time $496 per credit. *Tuition, nonresident:* full-time $24,756; part-time $604 per credit. *Room and board:* room only: $850 per academic year. *Required fees:* part-time $310 per credit.

Financial Aid 90% of baccalaureate students in nursing programs received some form of financial aid in 2009-10.

Contact Mr. Kevin Nies, Associate Director of Admissions, Master's Program in Nursing, University of Maryland, Baltimore, 655 West Lombard Street, Room 102, Student Services, Baltimore, MD 21201. *Telephone:* 410-706-1281. *Fax:* 410-706-7238. *E-mail:* nies@son.umaryland.edu.

GRADUATE PROGRAMS

Expenses (2010-11) *Tuition, state resident:* full-time $22,302; part-time $531 per credit. *Tuition, nonresident:* full-time $41,034; part-time $977 per credit. *Required fees:* full-time $1266.

Financial Aid 50% of graduate students in nursing programs received some form of financial aid in 2009-10. Fellowships, research assistantships, teaching assistantships, career-related internships or fieldwork and traineeships available. Aid available to part-time students. *Financial aid application deadline:* 2/15.

Contact Mr. Kevin Nies, Assistant Director of Admissions, Master's Program in Nursing, University of Maryland, Baltimore, 655 West Lombard Street, Room 102, Baltimore, MD 21201-1579. *Telephone:* 410-706-1281. *Fax:* 410-706-7238. *E-mail:* knies001@son.umaryland.edu.

MASTER'S DEGREE PROGRAM

Degrees MS; MSN/JD; MSN/MBA; MSN/MPH

Available Programs Accelerated Master's for Non-Nursing College Graduates; Master's; RN to Master's.

Concentrations Available Clinical nurse leader; nurse anesthesia; nursing administration; nursing informatics. *Clinical nurse specialist programs in:* acute care, community health, critical care, psychiatric/mental health. *Nurse practitioner programs in:* acute care, adult health, family health, gerontology, pediatric, primary care, psychiatric/mental health.

Site Options Baltimore-Shady Grove, MD.

Study Options Full-time and part-time.

Online Degree Options Yes (online only).

Program Entrance Requirements Computer literacy, minimum overall college GPA of 3.0, transcript of college record, CPR certification, written essay, immunizations, interview, 2 letters of recommendation, nursing research course, physical assessment course, professional liability insurance/malpractice insurance, prerequisite course work, resume, statistics course, GRE General Test. *Application deadline:* 2/1 (fall), 9/1 (spring). *Application fee:* $50.

Advanced Placement Credit given for nursing courses completed elsewhere dependent upon specific evaluations.

Degree Requirements 36 total credit hours, thesis or project.

POST-MASTER'S PROGRAM

Areas of Study Nursing administration; nursing education; nursing informatics. *Clinical nurse specialist programs in:* community health, pediatric, psychiatric/mental health, public health. *Nurse practitioner programs in:* acute care, adult health, family health, gerontology, pediatric, primary care, psychiatric/mental health.

DOCTORAL DEGREE PROGRAM

Degree DNP

Available Programs Doctorate; Post-Baccalaureate Doctorate.

Areas of Study Aging, community health, critical care, family health, gerontology, health policy, nursing policy.

Program Entrance Requirements Clinical experience, minimum overall college GPA of 3.0, interview by faculty committee, 3 letters of recommendation, MSN or equivalent, statistics course, vita. Application deadline: 2/15 (fall), 11/1 (spring). Application fee: $50.

Degree Requirements 38 total credit hours, oral exam.

CONTINUING EDUCATION PROGRAM

Contact Sonia Smith, Program Coordinator, Master's Program in Nursing, University of Maryland, Baltimore, 655 West Lombard Street, Room 311G, Baltimore, MD 21201-1579. *Telephone:* 410-706-3768. *E-mail:* ssmith@son.umaryland.edu.

Washington Adventist University

Nursing Department
Takoma Park, Maryland

Founded in 1904

DEGREE • BS

Nursing Program Faculty 8 (14% with doctorates).

Baccalaureate Enrollment 240 **Women** 90% **Men** 10% **Minority** 75% **International** 1% **Part-time** 10%

Nursing Student Activities Student Nurses' Association, nursing club.

Nursing Student Resources Academic advising; academic or career counseling; bookstore; campus computer network; computer lab; e-mail services; externships; interactive nursing skills videos; Internet; learning resource lab; library services; nursing audiovisuals; remedial services; skills, simulation, or other laboratory; tutoring; unpaid internships.

BACCALAUREATE PROGRAMS

Degree BS

Available Programs Accelerated RN Baccalaureate; Generic Baccalaureate.

Study Options Full-time.

Program Entrance Requirements Minimum overall college GPA of 2.75, transcript of college record, CPR certification, written essay, health exam, immunizations, interview, 2 letters of recommendation, minimum GPA in nursing prerequisites of 2.75, prerequisite course work. Transfer students are accepted.

Advanced Placement Credit given for nursing courses completed elsewhere dependent upon specific evaluations.

Contact ***Telephone:*** 301-891-4144. *Fax:* 301-891-4191.

MASSACHUSETTS

American International College

Division of Nursing
Springfield, Massachusetts

http://www.aic.edu/pages/315.html
Founded in 1885

DEGREES • BSN • MSN

Nursing Program Faculty 11 (10% with doctorates).

Nursing Student Activities Nursing Honor Society, Student Nurses' Association.

Nursing Student Resources Academic advising; academic or career counseling; assistance for students with disabilities; bookstore; campus computer network; career placement assistance; computer lab; e-mail services; employment services for current students; externships; housing assistance; interactive nursing skills videos; Internet; learning resource lab; library services; nursing audiovisuals; other; placement services for program completers; resume preparation assistance; skills, simulation, or other laboratory; tutoring.

Library Facilities 70,741 volumes (750 in health, 275 in nursing); 7,211 periodical subscriptions (50 health-care related).

BACCALAUREATE PROGRAMS

Degree BSN

Available Programs Generic Baccalaureate; RN Baccalaureate.

Study Options Full-time and part-time.

Program Entrance Requirements Minimum overall college GPA of 2.75, transcript of college record, health exam, health insurance, high school biology, high school chemistry, 3 years high school math, 2 years high school science, high school transcript, immunizations, 1 letter of recommendation, minimum high school GPA of 2.5, minimum GPA in nursing prerequisites of 2.5, professional liability insurance/malpractice insurance. Transfer students are accepted.

Advanced Placement Credit by examination available. Credit given for nursing courses completed elsewhere dependent upon specific evaluations.

Contact ***Telephone:*** 413-205-3201. *Fax:* 413-205-3051.

GRADUATE PROGRAMS

Contact ***Telephone:*** 413-205-3519. *Fax:* 413-205-3957.

MASTER'S DEGREE PROGRAM

Degree MSN

Available Programs Master's.

Concentrations Available Nursing administration; nursing education.

Study Options Part-time.

Program Entrance Requirements Clinical experience, minimum overall college GPA of 3.0, transcript of college record, CPR certification, immunizations, interview, 2 letters of recommendation, nursing research course, professional liability insurance/malpractice insurance, prerequisite course work, resume, statistics course.

Advanced Placement Credit given for nursing courses completed elsewhere dependent upon specific evaluations.

Degree Requirements 36 total credit hours, thesis or project.

Anna Maria College

Department of Nursing
Paxton, Massachusetts

http://www.annamaria.edu
Founded in 1946

DEGREE • BSN

Nursing Program Faculty 6 (16% with doctorates).

Baccalaureate Enrollment 32 **Women** 94% **Men** 6% **Minority** 6% **Part-time** 100%

Nursing Student Activities Sigma Theta Tau.

Nursing Student Resources Academic advising; academic or career counseling; assistance for students with disabilities; bookstore; campus computer network; career placement assistance; computer lab; e-mail services; employment services for current students; Internet; learning resource lab; library services; nursing audiovisuals; placement services for program completers; remedial services; resume preparation assistance; skills, simulation, or other laboratory; tutoring; unpaid internships.

Library Facilities 3,000 volumes in health, 400 volumes in nursing; 22 periodical subscriptions health-care related.

BACCALAUREATE PROGRAMS

Degree BSN

Available Programs ADN to Baccalaureate; RN Baccalaureate.

Study Options Part-time.

Program Entrance Requirements Minimum overall college GPA of 2.5, transcript of college record, interview, 1 letter of recommendation, minimum high school GPA of 2.5, minimum GPA in nursing prerequisites of 2.5, RN licensure. Transfer students are accepted. *Application deadline:* Applications may be processed on a rolling basis for some programs. *Application fee:* $40.

Advanced Placement Credit by examination available. Credit given for nursing courses completed elsewhere dependent upon specific evaluations.

Contact ***Telephone:*** 508-829-3316 Ext. 316. *Fax:* 508-849-3343 Ext. 371.

CONTINUING EDUCATION PROGRAM

Contact ***Telephone:*** 508-849-3316 Ext. 316. *Fax:* 508-849-3343 Ext. 371.

Atlantic Union College

Department of Nursing
South Lancaster, Massachusetts

http://www.atlanticuc.edu
Founded in 1882

DEGREE • BS

Nursing Program Faculty 3 (20% with doctorates).

Baccalaureate Enrollment 32 **Women** 97% **Men** 3% **Minority** 53% **Part-time** 59%

Nursing Student Activities Nursing Honor Society, Sigma Theta Tau.

Nursing Student Resources Academic advising; academic or career counseling; campus computer network; computer lab; computer-assisted instruction; e-mail services; employment services for current students; interactive nursing skills videos; Internet; learning resource lab; library services; nursing audiovisuals; remedial services; skills, simulation, or other laboratory; tutoring.

Library Facilities 153,827 volumes (1,478 in health, 892 in nursing); 76 periodical subscriptions health-care related.

BACCALAUREATE PROGRAMS

Degree BS

Available Programs ADN to Baccalaureate; RN Baccalaureate.

Study Options Full-time and part-time.

Program Entrance Requirements Minimum overall college GPA of 2.75, transcript of college record, CPR certification, written essay, health exam, health insurance, high school biology, high school chemistry, high school foreign language, 3 years high school math, 2 years high school science, high school transcript, immunizations, 2 letters of recommendation, minimum high school GPA of 2.75, minimum GPA in nursing prerequisites of 2.75, professional liability insurance/malpractice insurance, prerequisite course work, RN licensure. Transfer students are accepted. *Application deadline:* 5/25 (fall), 12/15 (winter). Applications may be processed on a rolling basis for some programs.

Advanced Placement Credit by examination available. Credit given for nursing courses completed elsewhere dependent upon specific evaluations.

Contact ***Telephone:*** 978-368-2401. *Fax:* 978-368-2518.

Boston College
William F. Connell School of Nursing
Chestnut Hill, Massachusetts

http://www.bc.edu/nursing
Founded in 1863

DEGREES • BS • MS • MSN/MA • MSN/MBA • MSN/PHD • PHD

Nursing Program Faculty 83 (42% with doctorates).
Baccalaureate Enrollment 378 **Women** 96% **Men** 4% **Minority** 26% **International** 1%
Graduate Enrollment 330 **Women** 93% **Men** 7% **Minority** 16% **International** 3% **Part-time** 40%
Nursing Student Activities Nursing Honor Society, Sigma Theta Tau, Student Nurses' Association.
Nursing Student Resources Academic advising; academic or career counseling; assistance for students with disabilities; bookstore; campus computer network; career placement assistance; computer lab; computer-assisted instruction; e-mail services; employment services for current students; externships; housing assistance; interactive nursing skills videos; Internet; learning resource lab; library services; nursing audiovisuals; other; placement services for program completers; remedial services; resume preparation assistance; skills, simulation, or other laboratory; tutoring; unpaid internships.
Library Facilities 2.5 million volumes (65,000 in health, 20,000 in nursing); 36,553 periodical subscriptions (5,395 health-care related).

BACCALAUREATE PROGRAMS

Degree BS
Available Programs Generic Baccalaureate.
Study Options Full-time.
Program Entrance Requirements Transcript of college record, written essay, health exam, health insurance, high school biology, high school chemistry, high school foreign language, 4 years high school math, 3 years high school science, high school transcript, immunizations, 2 letters of recommendation. Transfer students are accepted. *Application deadline:* 1/1 (fall), 10/1 (winter). *Application fee:* $70.
Advanced Placement Credit given for nursing courses completed elsewhere dependent upon specific evaluations.
Expenses (2010-11) *Tuition:* full-time $39,880. *Room and board:* $12,082; room only: $7452 per academic year. *Required fees:* full-time $662.
Financial Aid 69% of baccalaureate students in nursing programs received some form of financial aid in 2009-10. *Gift aid (need-based):* Federal Pell, FSEOG, state, private, college/university gift aid from institutional funds. *Loans:* Federal Nursing Student Loans, Perkins, state. *Work-study:* Federal Work-Study. *Financial aid application deadline (priority):* 2/1.
Contact Ms. Christine Murphy, Undergraduate Program Assistant, William F. Connell School of Nursing, Boston College, 140 Commonwealth Avenue, Cushing Hall 202D, Chestnut Hill, MA 02467-3812. *Telephone:* 617-552-4925. *Fax:* 617-552-0745. *E-mail:* christine.murphy.1@bc.edu.

GRADUATE PROGRAMS

Expenses (2010-11) *Tuition:* full-time $12,600; part-time $1050 per credit. *International tuition:* $18,900 full-time. *Room and board:* room only: $8882 per academic year. *Required fees:* full-time $120; part-time $45 per term.
Financial Aid 85% of graduate students in nursing programs received some form of financial aid in 2009-10. 12 fellowships with partial tuition reimbursements available (averaging $15,000 per year), 5 teaching assistantships (averaging $13,746 per year) were awarded; research assistantships, Federal Work-Study, institutionally sponsored loans, scholarships, traineeships, and tuition waivers (partial) also available. Aid available to part-time students. *Financial aid application deadline:* 3/1.
Contact Ms. Marybeth Crowley, Graduate Programs Office, William F. Connell School of Nursing, Boston College, 140 Commonwealth Avenue, Cushing Hall, Chestnut Hill, MA 02467-3812. *Telephone:* 617-552-4928. *Fax:* 617-552-2121. *E-mail:* csongrad@bc.edu.

MASTER'S DEGREE PROGRAM

Degrees MS; MSN/MA; MSN/MBA; MSN/PhD
Available Programs Accelerated Master's; Accelerated Master's for Non-Nursing College Graduates; Accelerated Master's for Nurses with Non-Nursing Degrees; Master's; RN to Master's.
Concentrations Available Nurse anesthesia. *Clinical nurse specialist programs in:* adult health, community health, forensic nursing, gerontology, palliative care, pediatric, psychiatric/mental health. *Nurse practitioner programs in:* adult health, family health, gerontology, pediatric, psychiatric/mental health, women's health.
Study Options Full-time and part-time.
Program Entrance Requirements Minimum overall college GPA of 3.0, transcript of college record, written essay, 3 letters of recommendation, statistics course. *Application deadline:* 11/1 (fall), 9/15 (spring). Applications may be processed on a rolling basis for some programs. *Application fee:* $40.
Advanced Placement Credit given for nursing courses completed elsewhere dependent upon specific evaluations.
Degree Requirements 45 total credit hours, comprehensive exam.

POST-MASTER'S PROGRAM

Areas of Study Nurse anesthesia; nursing education. *Clinical nurse specialist programs in:* adult health, community health, forensic nursing, gerontology, palliative care, pediatric, psychiatric/mental health. *Nurse practitioner programs in:* adult health, family health, gerontology, pediatric, psychiatric/mental health, women's health.

DOCTORAL DEGREE PROGRAM

Degree PhD
Available Programs Doctorate; Post-Baccalaureate Doctorate.
Areas of Study Addiction/substance abuse, advanced practice nursing, aging, bio-behavioral research, biology of health and illness, clinical practice, community health, ethics, family health, forensic nursing, gerontology, health promotion/disease prevention, human health and illness, illness and transition, individualized study, maternity-newborn, neurobehavior, nurse case management, nursing research, nursing science, oncology, urban health, women's health.
Program Entrance Requirements Minimum overall college GPA of 3.0, interview by faculty committee, interview, 3 letters of recommendation, MSN or equivalent, statistics course, vita, writing sample, GRE General Test. Application deadline: 12/31 (fall). Application fee: $40.
Degree Requirements 46 total credit hours, dissertation, oral exam, written exam.

CONTINUING EDUCATION PROGRAM

Contact Dr. Jean Weyman, Assistant Dean, Continuing Education, William F. Connell School of Nursing, Boston College, 140 Commonwealth Avenue, Service Building, 211F, Chestnut Hill, MA 02467-3812. *Telephone:* 617-552-4256. *Fax:* 617-552-0745. *E-mail:* jean.weyman@bc.edu.

Curry College
Division of Nursing
Milton, Massachusetts

http://www.curry.edu
Founded in 1879

DEGREES • BS • MSN

Nursing Program Faculty 48 (33% with doctorates).
Baccalaureate Enrollment 611 **Women** 92% **Men** 8% **Minority** 15% **Part-time** 48%
Graduate Enrollment 31 **Women** 97% **Men** 3% **Minority** 20% **Part-time** 100%
Nursing Student Activities Sigma Theta Tau, Student Nurses' Association.
Nursing Student Resources Academic advising; academic or career counseling; assistance for students with disabilities; bookstore; campus computer network; career placement assistance; computer lab; computer-assisted instruction; daycare for children of students; e-mail services; employment services for current students; housing assistance; interactive nursing skills videos; Internet; learning resource lab; library services; nursing audiovisuals; placement services for program completers; remedial services; resume preparation assistance; skills, simulation, or other laboratory; tutoring.
Library Facilities 139,600 volumes (5,867 in health, 4,589 in nursing); 33,700 periodical subscriptions (162 health-care related).

BACCALAUREATE PROGRAMS

Degree BS
Available Programs Accelerated Baccalaureate for Second Degree; Generic Baccalaureate; RN Baccalaureate; RPN to Baccalaureate.

Site Options Boston, MA; Plymouth, MA.
Study Options Full-time.
Program Entrance Requirements Written essay, health exam, health insurance, high school biology, high school chemistry, high school foreign language, 4 years high school math, 4 years high school science, high school transcript, immunizations, 1 letter of recommendation, minimum high school GPA of 2.75, minimum GPA in nursing prerequisites of 3.0. Transfer students are accepted. *Application deadline:* 4/1 (fall). Applications may be processed on a rolling basis for some programs. *Application fee:* $50.
Advanced Placement Credit by examination available. Credit given for nursing courses completed elsewhere dependent upon specific evaluations.
Expenses (2009-10) *Tuition:* full-time $28,000; part-time $933 per credit. *Room and board:* $11,960; room only: $6210 per academic year. *Required fees:* full-time $1955.
Financial Aid 70% of baccalaureate students in nursing programs received some form of financial aid in 2008-09. *Gift aid (need-based):* Federal Pell, FSEOG, state, private, college/university gift aid from institutional funds. *Loans:* Federal Direct (Subsidized and Unsubsidized Stafford PLUS), Perkins, state. *Work-study:* Federal Work-Study. *Financial aid application deadline (priority):* 3/1.
Contact Miss Jane Fidler, Dean of Admission, Division of Nursing, Curry College, 1071 Blue Hill Avenue, Milton, MA 02186. *Telephone:* 800-669-0686. *Fax:* 617-333-2114. *E-mail:* jfidler0803@curry.edu.

GRADUATE PROGRAMS

Expenses (2009-10) *Tuition:* part-time $780 per credit.
Contact Judy Hammond, Division of Nursing, Curry College, 1071 Blue Hill Avenue, Milton, MA 02186. *Telephone:* 617-333-2243. *Fax:* 617-333-6680. *E-mail:* msn@curry.edu.

MASTER'S DEGREE PROGRAM

Degree MSN
Available Programs Master's; RN to Master's.
Concentrations Available Clinical nurse leader.
Site Options Boston, MA.
Program Entrance Requirements Minimum overall college GPA of 3.0, transcript of college record, written essay, immunizations, 2 letters of recommendation, nursing research course, physical assessment course, resume, statistics course. *Application deadline:* Applications may be processed on a rolling basis for some programs. *Application fee:* $50.
Degree Requirements 37 total credit hours, thesis or project.

Elms College
Division of Nursing
Chicopee, Massachusetts

http://www.elms.edu/
Founded in 1928

DEGREES • BS • MSN
Nursing Program Faculty 13 (46% with doctorates).
Baccalaureate Enrollment 200 **Women** 87% **Men** 13% **Minority** 11% **Part-time** 35%
Graduate Enrollment 42 **Women** 97% **Men** 3% **Minority** 5% **Part-time** 50%
Nursing Student Activities Nursing Honor Society, Sigma Theta Tau, Student Nurses' Association.
Nursing Student Resources Academic advising; academic or career counseling; assistance for students with disabilities; bookstore; campus computer network; career placement assistance; computer lab; computer-assisted instruction; e-mail services; employment services for current students; externships; interactive nursing skills videos; Internet; learning resource lab; library services; nursing audiovisuals; resume preparation assistance; skills, simulation, or other laboratory; tutoring.
Library Facilities 3,832 volumes in health, 3,000 volumes in nursing; 130 periodical subscriptions health-care related.

BACCALAUREATE PROGRAMS

Degree BS
Available Programs Generic Baccalaureate; RN Baccalaureate.
Study Options Full-time and part-time.
Program Entrance Requirements Minimum overall college GPA of 2.5, transcript of college record, CPR certification, written essay, health exam, health insurance, high school biology, high school chemistry, high school transcript, immunizations, interview, 2 letters of recommendation, minimum high school GPA of 3.3, minimum high school rank 25%, minimum GPA in nursing prerequisites of 2.5, professional liability insurance/malpractice insurance. Transfer students are accepted. *Application deadline:* Applications may be processed on a rolling basis for some programs. *Application fee:* $30.
Advanced Placement Credit given for nursing courses completed elsewhere dependent upon specific evaluations.
Expenses (2010-11) *Tuition:* full-time $25,780; part-time $524 per credit. *Room and board:* $9810 per academic year. *Required fees:* full-time $1400.
Financial Aid 90% of baccalaureate students in nursing programs received some form of financial aid in 2009-10.
Contact Dr. Kathleen B. Scoble, EdD, Director and Chair, Division of Nursing, Elms College, 291 Springfield Street, Chicopee, MA 01013. *Telephone:* 413-265-2237. *Fax:* 413-265-2335. *E-mail:* scoblek@elms.edu.

GRADUATE PROGRAMS

Expenses (2010-11) *Tuition:* full-time $3672; part-time $612 per credit. *Required fees:* full-time $75.
Financial Aid 10% of graduate students in nursing programs received some form of financial aid in 2009-10.
Contact Cynthia Dakin, PhD, Graduate Program Coordinator, Division of Nursing, Elms College, 291 Springfield Street, Chicopee, MA 01013. *Telephone:* 413-265-2455. *E-mail:* dakinc@elms.edu.

MASTER'S DEGREE PROGRAM

Degree MSN
Available Programs Master's; RN to Master's.
Concentrations Available Nursing administration; nursing education.
Study Options Full-time and part-time.
Program Entrance Requirements Minimum overall college GPA of 3.0, transcript of college record, CPR certification, written essay, immunizations, interview, 2 letters of recommendation, professional liability insurance/malpractice insurance, resume. *Application deadline:* Applications may be processed on a rolling basis for some programs. *Application fee:* $30.
Degree Requirements 36 total credit hours, thesis or project.

Emmanuel College
Department of Nursing
Boston, Massachusetts

http://www.emmanuel.edu/x11602.xml
Founded in 1919

DEGREES • BSN • MS
Nursing Program Faculty 14 (34% with doctorates).
Baccalaureate Enrollment 151 **Women** 97% **Men** 3% **Minority** 27% **International** 1% **Part-time** 100%
Distance Learning Courses Available.
Nursing Student Activities Sigma Theta Tau.
Nursing Student Resources Academic advising; academic or career counseling; assistance for students with disabilities; bookstore; campus computer network; computer lab; computer-assisted instruction; e-mail services; interactive nursing skills videos; Internet; library services; nursing audiovisuals; resume preparation assistance; skills, simulation, or other laboratory; tutoring.
Library Facilities 140,000 volumes (2,276 in health, 497 in nursing); 7,843 periodical subscriptions health-care related.

BACCALAUREATE PROGRAMS

Degree BSN
Available Programs RN Baccalaureate.
Site Options Woburn, MA; Boston, MA.
Program Entrance Requirements Transcript of college record, written essay, interview, 2 letters of recommendation, RN licensure. Transfer students are accepted. *Application deadline:* Applications may be processed on a rolling basis for some programs.
Expenses (2010-11) *Tuition:* part-time $1650 per course.
Financial Aid ***Gift aid (need-based):*** Federal Pell, FSEOG, state, private, college/university gift aid from institutional funds. *Loans:* Federal Direct (Subsidized and Unsubsidized Stafford PLUS), Perkins, state, alternative loans. *Work-study:* Federal Work-Study, part-time campus jobs. *Financial aid application deadline (priority):* 4/1.
Contact Dr. Mary Diane Arathuzik, Chair and Associate Professor, Department of Nursing, Emmanuel College, 400 The Fenway, Boston,

MA 02115. *Telephone:* 617-735-9945. *Fax:* 617-507-0434. *E-mail:* arathuzi@emmanuel.edu.

GRADUATE PROGRAMS

Contact Dr. Mary Diane Arathuzik, Chair and Associate Professor of Nursing, Department of Nursing, Emmanuel College, 400 The Fenway, Boston, MA 02115. *Telephone:* 617-735-9845. *Fax:* 617-507-0434. *E-mail:* arathuzi@emmanuel.edu.

MASTER'S DEGREE PROGRAM

Degree MS
Available Programs Master's.
Concentrations Available Nursing administration; nursing education.
Study Options Full-time.
Program Entrance Requirements Clinical experience, minimum overall college GPA of 3.0, transcript of college record, written essay, 2 letters of recommendation, resume. *Application deadline:* 4/30 (fall).
Degree Requirements 36 total credit hours, comprehensive exam.

Endicott College
Major in Nursing
Beverly, Massachusetts

http://www.endicott.edu/
Founded in 1939

DEGREES • BS • MSN

Nursing Program Faculty 24 (10% with doctorates).
Baccalaureate Enrollment 120 **Women** 95% **Men** 5% **Minority** 2%
Graduate Enrollment 12 **Women** 100% **Minority** 1%
Nursing Student Activities Nursing Honor Society, Student Nurses' Association.
Nursing Student Resources Academic advising; academic or career counseling; assistance for students with disabilities; bookstore; campus computer network; career placement assistance; computer lab; computer-assisted instruction; e-mail services; externships; interactive nursing skills videos; Internet; learning resource lab; library services; nursing audiovisuals; resume preparation assistance; skills, simulation, or other laboratory; tutoring; unpaid internships.
Library Facilities 121,485 volumes (2,828 in health, 624 in nursing); 84,970 periodical subscriptions (55 health-care related).

BACCALAUREATE PROGRAMS

Degree BS
Available Programs Generic Baccalaureate; RN Baccalaureate.
Site Options Beverly, MA.
Study Options Full-time.
Program Entrance Requirements Minimum overall college GPA of 2.5, transcript of college record, written essay, health exam, health insurance, high school biology, high school chemistry, 3 years high school math, 2 years high school science, high school transcript, immunizations, 1 letter of recommendation, minimum high school GPA of 2.5, minimum high school rank 50%, minimum GPA in nursing prerequisites of 2.5. Transfer students are accepted.
Advanced Placement Credit given for nursing courses completed elsewhere dependent upon specific evaluations.
Financial Aid 88% of baccalaureate students in nursing programs received some form of financial aid in 2009-10. *Gift aid (need-based):* Federal Pell, FSEOG, state, private, college/university gift aid from institutional funds. *Loans:* Federal Direct (Subsidized and Unsubsidized Stafford PLUS), Perkins. *Work-study:* Federal Work-Study. *Financial aid application deadline (priority):* 3/15.
Contact Mr. Thomas J. Redman, Vice President for Admissions and Financial Aid, Major in Nursing, Endicott College, 376 Hale Street, Beverly, MA 01915. *Telephone:* 978-232-2005. *Fax:* 978-232-2500. *E-mail:* admissio@endicott.edu.

GRADUATE PROGRAMS

Contact Dr. Kelly L. Fisher, Dean, School of Nursing, Major in Nursing, Endicott College, 375 Hale Street, Beverly, MA 01915. *E-mail:* kfisher@endicott.edu.

MASTER'S DEGREE PROGRAM

Degree MSN
Available Programs Master's.
Concentrations Available Nursing administration; nursing education.
Site Options Beverly, MA.
Study Options Full-time and part-time.
Program Entrance Requirements Clinical experience, transcript of college record, written essay, letters of recommendation, statistics course.
Advanced Placement Credit given for nursing courses completed elsewhere dependent upon specific evaluations.
Degree Requirements 33 total credit hours, thesis or project.

CONTINUING EDUCATION PROGRAM

Contact Dr. Kelly Fisher, Dean, School of Nursing, Major in Nursing, Endicott College, 376 Hale Street, Beverly, MA 01915. *Telephone:* 978-232-2328. *Fax:* 978-232-3100. *E-mail:* kfisher@endicott.edu.

Fitchburg State University
Department of Nursing
Fitchburg, Massachusetts

http://www.fsc.edu/nursing/
Founded in 1894

DEGREES • BS • M SC N

Nursing Program Faculty 18 (27% with doctorates).
Distance Learning Courses Available.
Nursing Student Activities Sigma Theta Tau, Student Nurses' Association.
Nursing Student Resources Academic advising; academic or career counseling; assistance for students with disabilities; bookstore; campus computer network; career placement assistance; computer lab; computer-assisted instruction; e-mail services; employment services for current students; housing assistance; interactive nursing skills videos; Internet; learning resource lab; library services; nursing audiovisuals; remedial services; resume preparation assistance; skills, simulation, or other laboratory; tutoring; unpaid internships.
Library Facilities 248,644 volumes (111 in health, 74 in nursing); 2,104 periodical subscriptions (1,218 health-care related).

BACCALAUREATE PROGRAMS

Degree BS
Available Programs ADN to Baccalaureate; RN Baccalaureate.
Study Options Full-time.
Program Entrance Requirements Minimum overall college GPA of 2.5, transcript of college record, CPR certification, written essay, health exam, health insurance, high school biology, high school chemistry, 3 years high school math, 3 years high school science, high school transcript, immunizations, minimum high school GPA of 3.0, minimum GPA in nursing prerequisites of 2.5, prerequisite course work. Transfer students are accepted. *Application deadline:* 1/1 (fall), 11/1 (spring). *Application fee:* $25.
Financial Aid 76% of baccalaureate students in nursing programs received some form of financial aid in 2008-09. *Gift aid (need-based):* Federal Pell, FSEOG, state, private, college/university gift aid from institutional funds. *Loans:* Federal Nursing Student Loans, Federal Direct (Subsidized and Unsubsidized Stafford PLUS), Perkins, state. *Work-study:* Federal Work-Study. *Financial aid application deadline (priority):* 3/1.
Contact Office of Admissions, Department of Nursing, Fitchburg State University, 160 Pearl Street, Fitchburg, MA 01420-2697. *Telephone:* 978-665-3144. *Fax:* 978-665-4540. *E-mail:* admissions@fsc.edu.

GRADUATE PROGRAMS

Expenses (2009-10) *Tuition, state resident:* part-time $150 per credit hour. *Tuition, nonresident:* part-time $150 per credit hour. *Required fees:* part-time $192 per credit.
Financial Aid 11% of graduate students in nursing programs received some form of financial aid in 2008-09.
Contact Dr. Rachel Boersma, RN, Chairperson, Department of Nursing, Fitchburg State University, 160 Pearl Street, Fitchburg, MA 01420-2697. *Telephone:* 978-665-3036. *Fax:* 978-665-3658. *E-mail:* rboersma@fsc.edu.

MASTER'S DEGREE PROGRAM

Degree M Sc N
Available Programs Master's.
Concentrations Available *Clinical nurse specialist programs in:* forensic nursing.
Study Options Part-time.

Online Degree Options Yes (online only).
Program Entrance Requirements Clinical experience, computer literacy, minimum overall college GPA of 2.8, transcript of college record, CPR certification, written essay, immunizations, 3 letters of recommendation, nursing research course, physical assessment course, prerequisite course work, resume, statistics course. *Application deadline:* 10/1 (fall), 2/15 (spring). *Application fee:* $25.
Degree Requirements 37 total credit hours, thesis or project.

POST-MASTER'S PROGRAM

Areas of Study *Clinical nurse specialist programs in:* forensic nursing.

Framingham State University

Department of Nursing
Framingham, Massachusetts

http://www.framingham.edu/nursing
Founded in 1839

DEGREES • BS • MSN
Nursing Program Faculty 8 (75% with doctorates).
Baccalaureate Enrollment 74 **Women** 85% **Men** 15% **Minority** 33% **International** 2% **Part-time** 90%
Graduate Enrollment 58 **Women** 98% **Men** 2% **Minority** 3% **International** 1% **Part-time** 100%
Nursing Student Activities Sigma Theta Tau.
Nursing Student Resources Academic advising; academic or career counseling; assistance for students with disabilities; bookstore; campus computer network; career placement assistance; computer lab; computer-assisted instruction; daycare for children of students; e-mail services; employment services for current students; housing assistance; interactive nursing skills videos; Internet; learning resource lab; library services; nursing audiovisuals; placement services for program completers; remedial services; resume preparation assistance; skills, simulation, or other laboratory; tutoring.
Library Facilities 216,518 volumes (5,338 in health, 5,338 in nursing); 423 periodical subscriptions (1,200 health-care related).

BACCALAUREATE PROGRAMS

Degree BS
Available Programs ADN to Baccalaureate.
Study Options Full-time and part-time.
Program Entrance Requirements Minimum overall college GPA of 3.0, transcript of college record, written essay, RN licensure. Transfer students are accepted. *Application deadline:* Applications may be processed on a rolling basis for some programs. *Application fee:* $50.
Advanced Placement Credit by examination available. Credit given for nursing courses completed elsewhere dependent upon specific evaluations.
Expenses (2009-10) *Tuition, state resident:* full-time $970; part-time $162 per course. *Tuition, nonresident:* full-time $7050; part-time $1175 per course. *International tuition:* $7050 full-time. *Room and board:* $8518; room only: $5248 per academic year. *Required fees:* part-time $232 per credit.
Financial Aid 60% of baccalaureate students in nursing programs received some form of financial aid in 2008-09.
Contact Dr. Susan L. Conrad, RN, Chairperson and Professor, Department of Nursing, Framingham State University, 100 State Street, H220, Framingham, MA 01701. *Telephone:* 508-626-4713. *Fax:* 508-626-4746. *E-mail:* sconrad@framingham.edu.

GRADUATE PROGRAMS

Expenses (2009-10) *Tuition, state resident:* part-time $995 per course. *Tuition, nonresident:* part-time $995 per course.
Contact Dr. Susan L. Conrad, RN, Chairperson and Professor, Department of Nursing, Framingham State University, 100 State Street, H220, Framingham, MA 01701. *Telephone:* 508-626-4713. *Fax:* 508-626-4746. *E-mail:* sconrad@framingham.edu.

MASTER'S DEGREE PROGRAM

Degree MSN
Available Programs Master's.
Concentrations Available Nursing administration; nursing education.
Study Options Part-time.
Program Entrance Requirements Minimum overall college GPA of 3.0, transcript of college record, written essay, interview, 3 letters of recommendation, nursing research course, resume, statistics course. *Application deadline:* 6/1 (fall). Applications may be processed on a rolling basis for some programs. *Application fee:* $50.
Degree Requirements 36 total credit hours, thesis or project.

CONTINUING EDUCATION PROGRAM

Contact Dr. Susan L. Conrad, RN, Chairperson and Professor, Department of Nursing, Framingham State University, 100 State Street, H220, Framingham, MA 01701. *Telephone:* 508-626-4713. *Fax:* 508-626-4746. *E-mail:* sconrad@framingham.edu.

Massachusetts College of Pharmacy and Health Sciences

School of Nursing
Boston, Massachusetts

Founded in 1823

DEGREE • BSN
Nursing Program Faculty 16 (44% with doctorates).
Baccalaureate Enrollment 358 **Women** 66.3% **Men** 33.7% **Minority** 35% **International** 3%
Distance Learning Courses Available.
Nursing Student Activities Nursing Honor Society, Sigma Theta Tau, Student Nurses' Association, nursing club.
Nursing Student Resources Academic advising; academic or career counseling; assistance for students with disabilities; bookstore; campus computer network; career placement assistance; computer lab; computer-assisted instruction; e-mail services; employment services for current students; housing assistance; interactive nursing skills videos; Internet; learning resource lab; library services; nursing audiovisuals; remedial services; resume preparation assistance; skills, simulation, or other laboratory; tutoring.
Library Facilities 17,400 volumes in health, 1,200 volumes in nursing; 10,000 periodical subscriptions health-care related.

BACCALAUREATE PROGRAMS

Degree BSN
Available Programs Accelerated Baccalaureate; Accelerated Baccalaureate for Second Degree.
Site Options Manchester , NH; Worcester , MA.
Study Options Full-time.
Program Entrance Requirements Minimum overall college GPA of 2.5, written essay, high school biology, high school chemistry, 3 years high school math, 2 years high school science, high school transcript, 2 letters of recommendation, prerequisite course work. Transfer students are accepted. *Application deadline:* 2/1 (fall), 10/1 (spring). *Application fee:* $70.
Contact ***Telephone:*** 800-225-5506.

CONTINUING EDUCATION PROGRAM

Contact ***Telephone:*** 617-735-1080.

MGH Institute of Health Professions

School of Nursing
Boston, Massachusetts

http://www.mghihp.edu/academics/nursing/#
Founded in 1977

DEGREES • BSN • DNP • MS
Nursing Program Faculty 49 (50% with doctorates).
Baccalaureate Enrollment 98 **Women** 91% **Men** 9% **Minority** 11%
Graduate Enrollment 348 **Women** 87% **Men** 13% **Minority** 10% **International** 1% **Part-time** 25%
Distance Learning Courses Available.
Nursing Student Activities Nursing Honor Society, Student Nurses' Association.
Nursing Student Resources Academic advising; academic or career counseling; assistance for students with disabilities; bookstore; campus computer network; career placement assistance; computer lab; computer-assisted instruction; daycare for children of students; e-mail services; Internet; learning resource lab; library services; nursing audiovisuals;

remedial services; resume preparation assistance; skills, simulation, or other laboratory; tutoring.
Library Facilities 35,000 volumes in health, 13,000 volumes in nursing; 1,400 periodical subscriptions health-care related.

BACCALAUREATE PROGRAMS

Degree BSN
Available Programs Accelerated Baccalaureate.
Site Options Boston, MA.
Study Options Full-time.
Program Entrance Requirements Transcript of college record, written essay, health insurance, immunizations, 3 letters of recommendation, minimum GPA in nursing prerequisites of 3.0, prerequisite course work. Transfer students are accepted. *Application deadline:* 11/1 (summer). *Application fee:* $65.
Advanced Placement Credit by examination available. Credit given for nursing courses completed elsewhere dependent upon specific evaluations.
Expenses (2010-11) *Tuition:* full-time $29,200. *Required fees:* full-time $1375.
Financial Aid 89% of baccalaureate students in nursing programs received some form of financial aid in 2009-10.
Contact Admissions, School of Nursing, MGH Institute of Health Professions, 36 1st Avenue, Boston, MA 02129. *Telephone:* 617-726-3140. *Fax:* 617-726-8010. *E-mail:* admissions@mghihp.edu.

GRADUATE PROGRAMS

Financial Aid 73% of graduate students in nursing programs received some form of financial aid in 2009-10. 4 research assistantships (averaging $1,200 per year), 17 teaching assistantships (averaging $1,200 per year) were awarded; career-related internships or fieldwork, scholarships, traineeships, and unspecified assistantships also available. Aid available to part-time students. *Financial aid application deadline:* 4/1.
Contact Office of Admissions, School of Nursing, MGH Institute of Health Professions, PO Box 6357, Boston, MA 02114. *Telephone:* 617-726-3140. *Fax:* 617-726-8010. *E-mail:* admissions@mghihp.edu.

MASTER'S DEGREE PROGRAM

Degree MS
Available Programs Master's; Master's for Non-Nursing College Graduates; Master's for Nurses with Non-Nursing Degrees; RN to Master's.
Concentrations Available Nursing education. *Clinical nurse specialist programs in:* acute care, adult health, family health, gerontology, pediatric, psychiatric/mental health. *Nurse practitioner programs in:* acute care, adult health, family health, gerontology, pediatric, primary care, psychiatric/mental health, women's health.
Site Options Boston, MA.
Study Options Full-time and part-time.
Program Entrance Requirements Minimum overall college GPA of 3.0, transcript of college record, CPR certification, written essay, immunizations, 3 letters of recommendation, professional liability insurance/malpractice insurance, prerequisite course work, resume, statistics course, GRE General Test. *Application deadline:* 1/10 (fall). *Application fee:* $65.
Advanced Placement Credit by examination available. Credit given for nursing courses completed elsewhere dependent upon specific evaluations.
Degree Requirements Thesis or project.

POST-MASTER'S PROGRAM

Areas of Study *Clinical nurse specialist programs in:* psychiatric/mental health. *Nurse practitioner programs in:* acute care, adult health, gerontology, pediatric, primary care, psychiatric/mental health, women's health.

DOCTORAL DEGREE PROGRAM

Degree DNP
Available Programs Doctorate; Doctorate for Nurses with Non-Nursing Degrees.
Site Options Boston, MA.
Program Entrance Requirements interview by faculty committee, 3 letters of recommendation, MSN or equivalent, vita. Application deadline: Applications may be processed on a rolling basis for some programs. Application fee: $65.
Degree Requirements 43 total credit hours, residency.

Northeastern University
School of Nursing
Boston, Massachusetts

http://www.northeastern.edu/bouve/nursing/index.html
Founded in 1898

DEGREES • BSN • DNP • MS • MSN/MBA • PHD

Nursing Program Faculty 76
Baccalaureate Enrollment 445 **Women** 94% **Men** 6% **Minority** 16% **International** 1%
Graduate Enrollment 436 **Women** 75% **Men** 25% **Minority** 21% **International** 1% **Part-time** 28%
Distance Learning Courses Available.
Nursing Student Activities Nursing Honor Society, Sigma Theta Tau, Student Nurses' Association.
Nursing Student Resources Academic advising; academic or career counseling; assistance for students with disabilities; bookstore; campus computer network; career placement assistance; computer lab; computer-assisted instruction; e-mail services; employment services for current students; externships; housing assistance; interactive nursing skills videos; Internet; learning resource lab; library services; nursing audiovisuals; other; paid internships; placement services for program completers; remedial services; resume preparation assistance; skills, simulation, or other laboratory; tutoring; unpaid internships.
Library Facilities 1.3 million volumes (66,364 in health, 2,125 in nursing); 41,950 periodical subscriptions (2,024 health-care related).

BACCALAUREATE PROGRAMS

Degree BSN
Available Programs ADN to Baccalaureate; Generic Baccalaureate; RN Baccalaureate.
Study Options Full-time.
Program Entrance Requirements Transcript of college record, written essay, health exam, high school biology, high school chemistry, 3 years high school math, 2 years high school science, high school transcript, immunizations, 2 letters of recommendation, prerequisite course work. *Application deadline:* 1/15 (fall). *Application fee:* $70.
Advanced Placement Credit given for nursing courses completed elsewhere dependent upon specific evaluations.
Expenses (2010-11) *Tuition:* full-time $36,380. *Room and board:* $12,760; room only: $6760 per academic year. *Required fees:* full-time $412.
Financial Aid ***Gift aid (need-based):*** Federal Pell, FSEOG, state, private, college/university gift aid from institutional funds. *Loans:* Federal Nursing Student Loans, Federal Direct (Subsidized and Unsubsidized Stafford PLUS), Perkins, state. *Work-study:* Federal Work-Study, part-time campus jobs. *Financial aid application deadline (priority):* 2/15.
Contact Undergraduate Admissions, School of Nursing, Northeastern University, 360 Huntington Avenue, 150 Richards Hall, Boston, MA 02115. *Telephone:* 617-373-2200. *Fax:* 617-373-8780. *E-mail:* admissions@neu.edu.

GRADUATE PROGRAMS

Expenses (2010-11) *Tuition:* full-time $26,400; part-time $1100 per credit hour. *Required fees:* full-time $256; part-time $37 per term.
Financial Aid Fellowships, research assistantships, teaching assistantships, career-related internships or fieldwork, institutionally sponsored loans, scholarships, traineeships, tuition waivers (full and partial), and unspecified assistantships available.
Contact Ms. Molly Schnabel, Director of Graduate Admissions and Student Services, School of Nursing, Northeastern University, 360 Huntington Avenue, 123 Behrakis Health Sciences Building, Boston, MA 02115. *Telephone:* 617-373-3501. *Fax:* 617-373-4701. *E-mail:* bouvegrad@neu.edu.

MASTER'S DEGREE PROGRAM

Degrees MS; MSN/MBA
Available Programs Accelerated Master's for Non-Nursing College Graduates; Master's; Master's for Non-Nursing College Graduates; RN to Master's.
Concentrations Available Nurse anesthesia; nursing administration. *Clinical nurse specialist programs in:* psychiatric/mental health. *Nurse practitioner programs in:* acute care, adult health, family health, neonatal health, pediatric, primary care, psychiatric/mental health.
Study Options Full-time and part-time.
Program Entrance Requirements Minimum overall college GPA of 3.0, transcript of college record, written essay, immunizations, 3 letters of

recommendation, professional liability insurance/malpractice insurance, resume, statistics course, GRE General Test. *Application deadline:* 5/1 (fall). Applications may be processed on a rolling basis for some programs. *Application fee:* $50.
Advanced Placement Credit given for nursing courses completed elsewhere dependent upon specific evaluations.
Degree Requirements 43 total credit hours.

POST-MASTER'S PROGRAM
Areas of Study Nurse anesthesia; nursing administration. *Clinical nurse specialist programs in:* psychiatric/mental health. *Nurse practitioner programs in:* acute care, adult health, family health, neonatal health, pediatric, primary care, psychiatric/mental health.

DOCTORAL DEGREE PROGRAM
Degree DNP
Available Programs Doctorate; Post-Baccalaureate Doctorate.
Areas of Study Advanced practice nursing, nursing administration, nursing research, nursing science, urban health.
Online Degree Options Yes (online only).
Program Entrance Requirements Minimum overall college GPA of 3.5, interview by faculty committee, interview, 3 letters of recommendation, MSN or equivalent. Application deadline: 3/1 (fall). Application fee: $50.
Degree Requirements 49 total credit hours.

Degree PhD
Available Programs Doctorate.
Areas of Study Nursing research, nursing science, urban health.
Program Entrance Requirements Minimum overall college GPA of 3.5, interview by faculty committee, interview, 3 letters of recommendation, MSN or equivalent, GRE. *Application deadline*: 3/1 (fall). *Application fee*: $50.
Degree Requirements 49 total credit hours, dissertation.

CONTINUING EDUCATION PROGRAM
Contact Anita Finkleman, Bouve College of Health Sciences, School of Nursing, Northeastern University, 360 Huntington Avenue, 102 Robinson Hall, Boston, MA 02115. *Telephone:* 617-373-3649. *E-mail:* a.finkelman@neu.edu.

Regis College
School of Nursing and Health Professions
Weston, Massachusetts

http://www.regiscollege.edu/graduate_programs/department.cfm?id=Nursing_Dept
Founded in 1927

DEGREES • BSN • DNP • MSN
Nursing Program Faculty 36 (75% with doctorates).
Baccalaureate Enrollment 78
Graduate Enrollment 496 **Women** 94% **Men** 6%
Nursing Student Activities Sigma Theta Tau, Student Nurses' Association, nursing club.
Nursing Student Resources Academic advising; academic or career counseling; assistance for students with disabilities; bookstore; campus computer network; computer lab; e-mail services; Internet; learning resource lab; library services; nursing audiovisuals; resume preparation assistance; skills, simulation, or other laboratory; tutoring.
Library Facilities 135,458 volumes (6,300 in health, 4,700 in nursing); 607 periodical subscriptions (228 health-care related).

BACCALAUREATE PROGRAMS
Degree BSN
Available Programs ADN to Baccalaureate; Accelerated Baccalaureate; Accelerated Baccalaureate for Second Degree; Accelerated RN Baccalaureate; Baccalaureate for Second Degree; Generic Baccalaureate; RN Baccalaureate.
Site Options Brighton, MA; Boston, MA; Medford, MA.
Study Options Full-time.
Program Entrance Requirements Written essay, health exam, health insurance, high school foreign language, 3 years high school math, 2 years high school science, high school transcript, immunizations, 2 letters of recommendation, minimum high school GPA of 3.0, minimum high school rank 40%, minimum GPA in nursing prerequisites. Transfer students are accepted. *Application deadline:* Applications may be processed on a rolling basis for some programs. *Application fee:* $50.
Advanced Placement Credit by examination available. Credit given for nursing courses completed elsewhere dependent upon specific evaluations.
Expenses (2010-11) *Tuition:* full-time $30,300; part-time $1480 per course. *Room and board:* $12,190 per academic year. *Required fees:* full-time $725.
Financial Aid 85% of baccalaureate students in nursing programs received some form of financial aid in 2009-10.
Contact Dr. Antionette Hays, Dean, School of Nursing and Health Professions, School of Nursing and Health Professions, Regis College, 235 Wellesley Street, Weston, MA 02493. *Telephone:* 781-768-7090. *Fax:* 781-768-7071. *E-mail:* antoinette.hays@regiscollege.edu.

GRADUATE PROGRAMS
Expenses (2010-11) *Tuition:* full-time $30,300; part-time $840 per credit. *Room and board:* $12,900 per academic year.
Financial Aid 52% of graduate students in nursing programs received some form of financial aid in 2009-10. 13 research assistantships were awarded; Federal Work-Study, scholarships, traineeships, and unspecified assistantships also available. Aid available to part-time students.
Contact Ms. Claudia C. Pouravelis, Director of Graduate Admission, School of Nursing and Health Professions, Regis College, 235 Wellesley Street, Weston, MA 02493. *Telephone:* 781-768-7058. *Fax:* 781-768-7071. *E-mail:* claudia.pouravelis@regiscollege.edu.

MASTER'S DEGREE PROGRAM
Degree MSN
Available Programs Accelerated AD/RN to Master's; Accelerated Master's; Accelerated Master's for Non-Nursing College Graduates; Accelerated Master's for Nurses with Non-Nursing Degrees; Accelerated RN to Master's; Master's; Master's for Non-Nursing College Graduates; Master's for Nurses with Non-Nursing Degrees; RN to Master's.
Concentrations Available Clinical nurse leader; health-care administration; nurse case management; nursing administration; nursing education. *Clinical nurse specialist programs in:* acute care. *Nurse practitioner programs in:* adult health, family health, pediatric, primary care, psychiatric/mental health, women's health.
Site Options Brighton, MA; Boston, MA; Medford, MA.
Study Options Full-time and part-time.
Program Entrance Requirements Computer literacy, minimum overall college GPA of 3.0, transcript of college record, CPR certification, written essay, immunizations, interview, 3 letters of recommendation, physical assessment course, professional liability insurance/malpractice insurance, prerequisite course work, resume, statistics course, GRE General Test or MAT. *Application deadline:* Applications may be processed on a rolling basis for some programs. *Application fee:* $50.
Advanced Placement Credit by examination available. Credit given for nursing courses completed elsewhere dependent upon specific evaluations.
Degree Requirements 44 total credit hours, thesis or project.

POST-MASTER'S PROGRAM
Areas of Study Clinical nurse leader; health-care administration; nurse case management; nursing administration; nursing education. *Nurse practitioner programs in:* adult health, family health, pediatric, primary care, psychiatric/mental health, women's health.

DOCTORAL DEGREE PROGRAM
Degree DNP
Available Programs Doctorate; Post-Baccalaureate Doctorate.
Areas of Study Gerontology, health policy, nursing administration, nursing education.
Program Entrance Requirements Clinical experience, minimum overall college GPA of 3.5, interview by faculty committee, interview, 2 letters of recommendation, MSN or equivalent, statistics course, vita, writing sample, MAT or GRE if GPA from master's lower than 3.5. Application deadline: Applications may be processed on a rolling basis for some programs. Application fee: $75.
Degree Requirements 50 total credit hours.

CONTINUING EDUCATION PROGRAM
Contact Dr. Antoinette Hays, Dean, School of Nursing and Health Professions, School of Nursing and Health Professions, Regis College, 235 Wellesley Street, Weston, MA 02493. *Telephone:* 781-768-7090. *Fax:* 781-768-7089. *E-mail:* antoinette.hays@regiscollege.edu.

Salem State University
Program in Nursing
Salem, Massachusetts

http://www.salemstate.edu/
Founded in 1854

DEGREES • BSN • MSN • MSN/MBA

Nursing Program Faculty 100 (25% with doctorates).
Distance Learning Courses Available.
Nursing Student Activities Nursing Honor Society, Sigma Theta Tau, Student Nurses' Association.
Nursing Student Resources Academic advising; academic or career counseling; assistance for students with disabilities; bookstore; campus computer network; career placement assistance; computer lab; computer-assisted instruction; daycare for children of students; e-mail services; employment services for current students; externships; housing assistance; interactive nursing skills videos; Internet; learning resource lab; library services; nursing audiovisuals; paid internships; remedial services; resume preparation assistance; skills, simulation, or other laboratory; tutoring.
Library Facilities 273,225 volumes (2,000 in health, 1,600 in nursing); 1,914 periodical subscriptions (50 health-care related).

BACCALAUREATE PROGRAMS

Degree BSN
Available Programs ADN to Baccalaureate; Accelerated Baccalaureate for Second Degree; Generic Baccalaureate; International Nurse to Baccalaureate; LPN to Baccalaureate; LPN to RN Baccalaureate.
Site Options Haverhill, MA.
Study Options Full-time.
Program Entrance Requirements Minimum overall college GPA of 3.5, transcript of college record, CPR certification, health exam, health insurance, high school biology, high school chemistry, 3 years high school math, 2 years high school science, high school transcript, immunizations, interview, minimum high school GPA of 3.5, professional liability insurance/malpractice insurance. Transfer students are accepted. *Application deadline:* 2/1 (fall), 10/1 (spring), 4/1 (summer). Applications may be processed on a rolling basis for some programs. *Application fee:* $30.
Advanced Placement Credit by examination available. Credit given for nursing courses completed elsewhere dependent upon specific evaluations.
Expenses (2010-11) *Tuition, state resident:* full-time $455; part-time $38 per credit hour. *Tuition, nonresident:* full-time $3525; part-time $294 per credit hour. *Room and board:* $12,000; room only: $9000 per academic year. *Required fees:* full-time $3130; part-time $120 per credit; part-time $120 per term.
Financial Aid 60% of baccalaureate students in nursing programs received some form of financial aid in 2009-10. *Gift aid (need-based):* Federal Pell, FSEOG, state, private, college/university gift aid from institutional funds, Scholarships for Disadvantaged Students Nursing Grants, MSCBA Housing Grants. *Loans:* Federal Nursing Student Loans, Perkins, state, MEFA Loans, CitiAssist Loans, Sallie Mae SMART Loans. *Work-study:* Federal Work-Study. *Financial aid application deadline (priority):* 3/1.
Contact Dr. Mary Dunn, Assistant Dean of Admissions, Program in Nursing, Salem State University, 352 Lafayette Street, Salem, MA 01970. *Telephone:* 978-542-6200. *E-mail:* admissions@salemstate.edu.

GRADUATE PROGRAMS

Expenses (2010-11) *Tuition, state resident:* full-time $7000; part-time $140 per credit hour. *Tuition, nonresident:* full-time $9500; part-time $230 per credit hour. *Room and board:* $13,000; room only: $9000 per academic year. *Required fees:* full-time $1800; part-time $120 per credit; part-time $360 per term.
Financial Aid 25% of graduate students in nursing programs received some form of financial aid in 2009-10. Career-related internships or fieldwork, Federal Work-Study, scholarships, and unspecified assistantships available. Aid available to part-time students. *Financial aid application deadline:* 5/1.
Contact Dr. Kathleen Skrabut, Coordinator, Graduate Program, Program in Nursing, Salem State University, 352 Lafayette Street, Salem, MA 01970. *Telephone:* 978-542-7018. *Fax:* 978-542-2016. *E-mail:* kskrabut@salemstate.edu.

MASTER'S DEGREE PROGRAM

Degrees MSN; MSN/MBA
Available Programs Accelerated Master's for Non-Nursing College Graduates; Master's; Master's for Nurses with Non-Nursing Degrees; RN to Master's.
Concentrations Available Clinical nurse leader; nursing administration; nursing education. *Clinical nurse specialist programs in:* community health, public health, rehabilitation.
Study Options Full-time and part-time.
Program Entrance Requirements Clinical experience, computer literacy, minimum overall college GPA of 3.0, transcript of college record, CPR certification, written essay, immunizations, interview, 3 letters of recommendation, professional liability insurance/malpractice insurance, resume, statistics course, GRE or MAT. *Application deadline:* 3/1 (fall), 10/1 (winter), 10/1 (spring), 3/1 (summer). Applications may be processed on a rolling basis for some programs. *Application fee:* $35.
Advanced Placement Credit given for nursing courses completed elsewhere dependent upon specific evaluations.
Degree Requirements 39 total credit hours, thesis or project.

CONTINUING EDUCATION PROGRAM

Contact Dr. Mary A. Farrell, Chairperson, School of Nursing, Program in Nursing, Salem State University, 352 Lafayette Street, Salem, MA 01970. *Telephone:* 978-542-6805. *Fax:* 978-542-2016. *E-mail:* mfarrell@salemstate.edu.

Simmons College
Department of Nursing
Boston, Massachusetts

http://www.simmons.edu/shs/academics/nursing/index.shtml
Founded in 1899

DEGREES • BS • DNP • MS

Nursing Program Faculty 135 (18% with doctorates).
Baccalaureate Enrollment 212 **Women** 100% **Minority** 19% **International** 6% **Part-time** 28%
Graduate Enrollment 189 **Women** 95% **Men** 5% **Minority** 13% **Part-time** 30%
Distance Learning Courses Available.
Nursing Student Activities Nursing Honor Society, Sigma Theta Tau, Student Nurses' Association, nursing club.
Nursing Student Resources Academic advising; academic or career counseling; assistance for students with disabilities; bookstore; campus computer network; career placement assistance; computer lab; computer-assisted instruction; e-mail services; employment services for current students; housing assistance; interactive nursing skills videos; Internet; learning resource lab; library services; nursing audiovisuals; placement services for program completers; remedial services; resume preparation assistance; skills, simulation, or other laboratory; tutoring; unpaid internships.
Library Facilities 206,238 volumes (5,005 in health, 1,562 in nursing); 49,808 periodical subscriptions (196 health-care related).

BACCALAUREATE PROGRAMS

Degree BS
Available Programs ADN to Baccalaureate; Accelerated Baccalaureate; Accelerated Baccalaureate for Second Degree; Baccalaureate for Second Degree; Generic Baccalaureate; LPN to Baccalaureate; RN Baccalaureate.
Site Options South Shore, MA.
Study Options Full-time and part-time.
Program Entrance Requirements Transcript of college record, written essay, health exam, health insurance, high school biology, high school chemistry, high school foreign language, 4 years high school math, 3 years high school science, high school transcript, immunizations, 2 letters of recommendation, minimum GPA in nursing prerequisites of 3.0, prerequisite course work. Transfer students are accepted. *Application deadline:* 2/1 (fall), 12/1 (spring), 4/1 (summer). *Application fee:* $55.
Advanced Placement Credit given for nursing courses completed elsewhere dependent upon specific evaluations.
Expenses (2010-11) *Tuition:* full-time $34,280; part-time $1071 per credit hour. *Room and board:* $12,470 per academic year. *Required fees:* full-time $950; part-time $475 per term.
Financial Aid ***Gift aid (need-based):*** Federal Pell, FSEOG, state, private, college/university gift aid from institutional funds. *Loans:* Federal Direct (Subsidized and Unsubsidized Stafford PLUS), Perkins, state, college/university. *Work-study:* Federal Work-Study. *Financial aid application deadline (priority):* 2/15.

Contact Ms. Catherine C. Capolupo, Director, Undergraduate Admission, Department of Nursing, Simmons College, 300 The Fenway, Boston, MA 02115. *Telephone:* 617-521-2051. *Fax:* 617-521-3190. *E-mail:* ugadm@simmons.edu.

GRADUATE PROGRAMS

Expenses (2010-11) *Tuition:* full-time $34,800; part-time $1015 per credit hour. *Room and board:* $13,970 per academic year. *Required fees:* full-time $2700; part-time $1350 per term.
Financial Aid 75% of graduate students in nursing programs received some form of financial aid in 2009-10.
Contact Ms. Carmen Fortin, Assistant Dean, Director of Admission, Department of Nursing, Simmons College, 300 The Fenway, Boston, MA 02115. *Telephone:* 617-521-2605. *Fax:* 617-521-3137. *E-mail:* carmen.fortin@simmons.edu.

MASTER'S DEGREE PROGRAM

Degree MS
Available Programs Accelerated AD/RN to Master's; Accelerated Master's; Accelerated Master's for Non-Nursing College Graduates; Accelerated Master's for Nurses with Non-Nursing Degrees; Accelerated RN to Master's; Master's; Master's for Non-Nursing College Graduates; Master's for Nurses with Non-Nursing Degrees; RN to Master's.
Concentrations Available Nursing administration. *Nurse practitioner programs in:* family health, primary care.
Site Options Longwood Medical, MA.
Study Options Full-time and part-time.
Program Entrance Requirements Clinical experience, computer literacy, minimum overall college GPA of 3.0, transcript of college record, written essay, 3 letters of recommendation, physical assessment course, resume, statistics course. *Application deadline:* 6/1 (fall), 11/1 (spring), 3/1 (summer).
Advanced Placement Credit given for nursing courses completed elsewhere dependent upon specific evaluations.
Degree Requirements 45 total credit hours, thesis or project.

POST-MASTER'S PROGRAM

Areas of Study *Nurse practitioner programs in:* family health, primary care.

DOCTORAL DEGREE PROGRAM

Degree DNP
Available Programs Doctorate.
Areas of Study Clinical practice, faculty preparation, nursing education.
Online Degree Options Yes (online only).
Program Entrance Requirements Clinical experience, minimum overall college GPA of 3.0, 3 letters of recommendation, MSN or equivalent, statistics course, vita, writing sample. Application deadline: 6/1 (fall), 11/1 (spring). Application fee: $50.
Degree Requirements 36 total credit hours.

University of Massachusetts Amherst

School of Nursing
Amherst, Massachusetts

http://www.umass.edu/nursing
Founded in 1863

DEGREES • BS • MS • PHD

Nursing Program Faculty 60 (30% with doctorates).
Baccalaureate Enrollment 382 **Women** 90% **Men** 10% **Minority** 21% **International** 3% **Part-time** 2%
Graduate Enrollment 218 **Women** 78% **Men** 22% **Minority** 22% **International** 4% **Part-time** 71%
Distance Learning Courses Available.
Nursing Student Activities Nursing Honor Society, Sigma Theta Tau, Student Nurses' Association.
Nursing Student Resources Academic advising; academic or career counseling; bookstore; campus computer network; career placement assistance; computer lab; computer-assisted instruction; e-mail services; employment services for current students; housing assistance; interactive nursing skills videos; Internet; learning resource lab; library services; nursing audiovisuals; paid internships; resume preparation assistance; skills, simulation, or other laboratory; tutoring; unpaid internships.
Library Facilities 3.7 million volumes (328,727 in health, 40,785 in nursing); 94,745 periodical subscriptions (3,808 health-care related).

BACCALAUREATE PROGRAMS

Degree BS
Available Programs Accelerated Baccalaureate for Second Degree; Accelerated RN Baccalaureate; Generic Baccalaureate.
Study Options Full-time.
Online Degree Options Yes.
Program Entrance Requirements Minimum overall college GPA of 3.0, transcript of college record, CPR certification, written essay, health exam, health insurance, high school foreign language, 3 years high school math, 3 years high school science, high school transcript, immunizations, 1 letter of recommendation, minimum high school GPA of 3.5, minimum GPA in nursing prerequisites of 2.5, professional liability insurance/malpractice insurance, prerequisite course work. *Application deadline:* 1/1 (fall). *Application fee:* $70.
Advanced Placement Credit given for nursing courses completed elsewhere dependent upon specific evaluations.
Expenses (2010-11) *Tuition, state resident:* full-time $11,732; part-time $3532 per semester. *Tuition, nonresident:* full-time $23,628; part-time $4756 per semester. *International tuition:* $39,900 full-time. *Room and board:* $8814 per academic year.
Financial Aid 78% of baccalaureate students in nursing programs received some form of financial aid in 2009-10.
Contact Ms. Elizabeth Theroux, Academic Secretary, Office for the Advancement of Nursing Education, School of Nursing, University of Massachusetts Amherst, 128 Skinner Hall, 651 North Pleasant Street, Amherst, MA 01003-9304. *Telephone:* 413-545-5096. *Fax:* 413-577-2550. *E-mail:* etheroux@acad.umass.edu.

GRADUATE PROGRAMS

Financial Aid 41% of graduate students in nursing programs received some form of financial aid in 2009-10. 8 fellowships with full tuition reimbursements available (averaging $5,175 per year), 1 research assistantship with full tuition reimbursement available (averaging $8,911 per year), 27 teaching assistantships with full tuition reimbursements available (averaging $7,250 per year) were awarded; career-related internships or fieldwork, Federal Work-Study, scholarships, traineeships, tuition waivers (full), and unspecified assistantships also available. Aid available to part-time students. *Financial aid application deadline:* 2/1.
Contact Ms. Karen Ayotte, Academic Services Graduate Program Assistant, School of Nursing, University of Massachusetts Amherst, 125 Skinner Hall, 651 North Pleasant Street, Amherst, MA 01003-9299. *Telephone:* 413-545-1302. *Fax:* 413-577-2550. *E-mail:* kayotte@nursing.umass.edu.

MASTER'S DEGREE PROGRAM

Degree MS
Available Programs Master's.
Concentrations Available Clinical nurse leader.
Study Options Full-time and part-time.
Online Degree Options Yes (online only).
Program Entrance Requirements Transcript of college record, CPR certification, written essay, immunizations, 2 letters of recommendation, physical assessment course, professional liability insurance/malpractice insurance, prerequisite course work, statistics course, GRE General Test. *Application deadline:* 2/1 (fall). Applications may be processed on a rolling basis for some programs. *Application fee:* $50.
Advanced Placement Credit given for nursing courses completed elsewhere dependent upon specific evaluations.
Degree Requirements 37 total credit hours.

DOCTORAL DEGREE PROGRAM

Degree PhD
Available Programs Doctorate; Post-Baccalaureate Doctorate.
Areas of Study Ethics, faculty preparation, health-care systems, individualized study, nursing education, nursing research, nursing science.
Program Entrance Requirements Minimum overall college GPA of 3.2, interview, 2 letters of recommendation, MSN or equivalent, scholarly papers, statistics course, vita, writing sample, GRE General Test. Application deadline: 2/1 (fall). Applications may be processed on a rolling basis for some programs. Application fee: $50.
Degree Requirements 57 total credit hours, dissertation, oral exam, written exam, residency.

CONTINUING EDUCATION PROGRAM

Contact Ms. Karen Ayotte, Academic Services Graduate Programs Assistant, School of Nursing, University of Massachusetts Amherst, 125 Skinner Hall, 651 North Pleasant Street, Amherst, MA 01003-9299. *Telephone:* 413-545-1302. *Fax:* 413-577-2550. *E-mail:* kayotte@nursing.umass.edu.

University of Massachusetts Boston

College of Nursing and Health Sciences
Boston, Massachusetts

http://www.cnhs.umb.edu/
Founded in 1964

DEGREES • BS • MS • PHD

Nursing Program Faculty 128 (27% with doctorates).
Baccalaureate Enrollment 1,776 **Women** 90% **Men** 10% **Minority** 41% **International** .5% **Part-time** 26%
Graduate Enrollment 185 **Women** 92% **Men** 8% **Minority** 19.5% **Part-time** 70%
Distance Learning Courses Available.
Nursing Student Activities Sigma Theta Tau, Student Nurses' Association.
Nursing Student Resources Academic advising; academic or career counseling; assistance for students with disabilities; bookstore; campus computer network; career placement assistance; computer lab; computer-assisted instruction; daycare for children of students; e-mail services; employment services for current students; housing assistance; interactive nursing skills videos; Internet; learning resource lab; library services; nursing audiovisuals; other; paid internships; remedial services; resume preparation assistance; skills, simulation, or other laboratory; tutoring.
Library Facilities 600,000 volumes (3,700 in health, 1,911 in nursing); 26,500 periodical subscriptions (5,027 health-care related).

BACCALAUREATE PROGRAMS

Degree BS
Available Programs Accelerated Baccalaureate for Second Degree; Generic Baccalaureate; RN Baccalaureate.
Study Options Full-time and part-time.
Online Degree Options Yes.
Program Entrance Requirements Minimum overall college GPA of 2.75, transcript of college record, written essay, health insurance, 3 years high school math, high school transcript, immunizations, 1 letter of recommendation, minimum high school GPA of 2.75, minimum GPA in nursing prerequisites of 3.0. Transfer students are accepted. *Application deadline:* 2/1 (fall), 11/1 (spring). *Application fee:* $60.
Advanced Placement Credit given for nursing courses completed elsewhere dependent upon specific evaluations.
Expenses (2010-11) *Tuition, state resident:* full-time $1714; part-time $72 per credit. *Tuition, nonresident:* full-time $9758; part-time $407 per credit. *Required fees:* full-time $8897; part-time $371 per credit; part-time $4449 per term.
Financial Aid 90% of baccalaureate students in nursing programs received some form of financial aid in 2009-10.
Contact Mr. Jon Hutton, Director of Enrollment Information Services, College of Nursing and Health Sciences, University of Massachusetts Boston, 100 Morrissey Boulevard, Boston, MA 02125. *Telephone:* 617-287-6000. *Fax:* 617-265-7173. *E-mail:* enrollment.information@umb.edu.

GRADUATE PROGRAMS

Expenses (2010-11) *Tuition, state resident:* full-time $2590; part-time $108 per credit. *Tuition, nonresident:* full-time $9758; part-time $406 per credit. *International tuition:* $9758 full-time. *Required fees:* full-time $9387; part-time $391 per credit; part-time $4694 per term.
Financial Aid 30% of graduate students in nursing programs received some form of financial aid in 2009-10. 3 research assistantships with full tuition reimbursements available (averaging $13,000 per year), 13 teaching assistantships with full tuition reimbursements available (averaging $13,000 per year) were awarded; career-related internships or fieldwork, Federal Work-Study, and unspecified assistantships also available. Aid available to part-time students. *Financial aid application deadline:* 3/1.
Contact Mr. Jon Hutton, Director of Enrollment Information Services, College of Nursing and Health Sciences, University of Massachusetts Boston, 100 Morrissey Boulevard, Boston, MA 02125. *Telephone:* 617-287-6000. *Fax:* 617-265-7173. *E-mail:* enrollment.information@umb.edu.

MASTER'S DEGREE PROGRAM

Degree MS
Available Programs Master's.
Concentrations Available *Clinical nurse specialist programs in:* acute care, critical care. *Nurse practitioner programs in:* adult health, family health, gerontology.
Study Options Full-time and part-time.
Program Entrance Requirements Clinical experience, minimum overall college GPA of 3.0, transcript of college record, CPR certification, written essay, immunizations, 3 letters of recommendation, nursing research course, physical assessment course, professional liability insurance/malpractice insurance, prerequisite course work, statistics course. *Application deadline:* 6/15 (fall), 11/1 (spring). Applications may be processed on a rolling basis for some programs. *Application fee:* $60.
Advanced Placement Credit given for nursing courses completed elsewhere dependent upon specific evaluations.
Degree Requirements 48 total credit hours, thesis or project.

POST-MASTER'S PROGRAM

Areas of Study *Nurse practitioner programs in:* adult health, family health, gerontology.

DOCTORAL DEGREE PROGRAM

Degree PhD
Available Programs Doctorate; Post-Baccalaureate Doctorate.
Areas of Study Health policy, oncology.
Program Entrance Requirements Clinical experience, minimum overall college GPA of 3.3, interview by faculty committee, interview, 3 letters of recommendation, MSN or equivalent, statistics course, vita, writing sample, GRE General Test. Application deadline: 2/15 (fall). Applications may be processed on a rolling basis for some programs. Application fee: $60.
Degree Requirements 60 total credit hours, dissertation, oral exam, written exam, residency.

POSTDOCTORAL PROGRAM

Postdoctoral Program Contact Dr. Laura L. Hayman, Associate Dean for Research, College of Nursing and Health Sciences, University of Massachusetts Boston, Boston, MA 02125. *Telephone:* 617-2877504. *E-mail:* laura.hayman@umb.edu.

CONTINUING EDUCATION PROGRAM

Contact Ms. Wanda Willard, Director of Credit Programs, College of Nursing and Health Sciences, University of Massachusetts Boston, 100 Morrissey Boulevard, Wheatley Building, 2nd Floor, Boston, MA 02125-3393. *Telephone:* 617-287-7874. *Fax:* 617-287-7922. *E-mail:* wanda.willard@umb.edu.

University of Massachusetts Dartmouth

College of Nursing
North Dartmouth, Massachusetts

http://www.umassd.edu/nursing
Founded in 1895

DEGREES • BSN • MS • PHD

Nursing Program Faculty 52 (33% with doctorates).
Nursing Student Activities Sigma Theta Tau, Student Nurses' Association, nursing club.
Nursing Student Resources Academic advising; academic or career counseling; assistance for students with disabilities; bookstore; campus computer network; career placement assistance; computer lab; computer-assisted instruction; daycare for children of students; e-mail services; employment services for current students; externships; housing assistance; interactive nursing skills videos; Internet; learning resource lab; library services; nursing audiovisuals; placement services for program completers; resume preparation assistance; skills, simulation, or other laboratory; tutoring; unpaid internships.
Library Facilities 461,338 volumes; 2,783 periodical subscriptions.

BACCALAUREATE PROGRAMS

Degree BSN
Available Programs Generic Baccalaureate; RN Baccalaureate.
Site Options Fall River, MA.
Study Options Full-time and part-time.
Program Entrance Requirements Transcript of college record, CPR certification, written essay, health exam, health insurance, high school biology, high school chemistry, high school foreign language, 3 years high school math, 3 years high school science, high school transcript, immunizations, letters of recommendation, minimum high school GPA of 3.0, minimum high school rank 66%, professional liability insurance/malpractice insurance. Transfer students are accepted.
Advanced Placement Credit by examination available. Credit given for nursing courses completed elsewhere dependent upon specific evaluations.
Contact *Telephone:* 508-999-8605. *Fax:* 508-999-8755.

GRADUATE PROGRAMS

Contact *Telephone:* 508-999-8251.

MASTER'S DEGREE PROGRAM

Degree MS
Available Programs Master's.
Concentrations Available *Clinical nurse specialist programs in:* adult health, community health. *Nurse practitioner programs in:* adult health.
Study Options Full-time and part-time.
Program Entrance Requirements Clinical experience, computer literacy, minimum overall college GPA of 3.0, transcript of college record, CPR certification, written essay, immunizations, interview, 3 letters of recommendation, nursing research course, physical assessment course, professional liability insurance/malpractice insurance, statistics course, GRE General Test.
Advanced Placement Credit given for nursing courses completed elsewhere dependent upon specific evaluations.
Degree Requirements 39 total credit hours, thesis or project.

POST-MASTER'S PROGRAM

Areas of Study *Nurse practitioner programs in:* adult health.

DOCTORAL DEGREE PROGRAM

Degree PhD
Available Programs Doctorate.
Areas of Study Nursing education.
Program Entrance Requirements Clinical experience, minimum overall college GPA of 3.3, 3 letters of recommendation, MSN or equivalent, statistics course, vita, writing sample, GRE General Test.
Degree Requirements 52 total credit hours.

CONTINUING EDUCATION PROGRAM

Contact *Telephone:* 508-999-8591.

University of Massachusetts Lowell

Department of Nursing
Lowell, Massachusetts

http://www.uml.edu/dept/nursing
Founded in 1894

DEGREES • BS • MS • PHD

Nursing Program Faculty 35 (100% with doctorates).
Baccalaureate Enrollment 291 **Women** 90% **Men** 10% **Minority** 13%
Graduate Enrollment 50 **Women** 90% **Men** 10%
Distance Learning Courses Available.
Nursing Student Activities Sigma Theta Tau, Student Nurses' Association.
Nursing Student Resources Academic advising; academic or career counseling; assistance for students with disabilities; bookstore; campus computer network; career placement assistance; computer lab; computer-assisted instruction; e-mail services; employment services for current students; housing assistance; interactive nursing skills videos; Internet; learning resource lab; library services; nursing audiovisuals; placement services for program completers; resume preparation assistance; skills, simulation, or other laboratory; tutoring.
Library Facilities 382,599 volumes (29,100 in health, 4,465 in nursing); 32,744 periodical subscriptions (350 health-care related).

BACCALAUREATE PROGRAMS

Degree BS
Available Programs Generic Baccalaureate; RN Baccalaureate.
Study Options Full-time.
Program Entrance Requirements Minimum overall college GPA of 2.7, transcript of college record, CPR certification, health exam, health insurance, high school chemistry, high school foreign language, 3 years high school math, 3 years high school science, high school transcript, immunizations, minimum high school GPA of 3.25, minimum GPA in nursing prerequisites of 2.7, professional liability insurance/malpractice insurance. Transfer students are accepted.
Advanced Placement Credit by examination available.
Contact *Telephone:* 800-410-4607.

GRADUATE PROGRAMS

Contact *Telephone:* 978-934-4426. *Fax:* 978-934-3006.

MASTER'S DEGREE PROGRAM

Degree MS
Available Programs Accelerated Master's; Accelerated RN to Master's; Master's.
Concentrations Available *Clinical nurse specialist programs in:* psychiatric/mental health. *Nurse practitioner programs in:* family health, gerontology, psychiatric/mental health.
Study Options Full-time and part-time.
Program Entrance Requirements Computer literacy, minimum overall college GPA of 3.0, transcript of college record, CPR certification, written essay, immunizations, interview, 3 letters of recommendation, professional liability insurance/malpractice insurance, statistics course, GRE General Test.
Advanced Placement Credit given for nursing courses completed elsewhere dependent upon specific evaluations.
Degree Requirements 42 total credit hours, thesis or project.

DOCTORAL DEGREE PROGRAM

Degree PhD
Available Programs Doctorate.
Areas of Study Health promotion/disease prevention.
Program Entrance Requirements Minimum overall college GPA of 3.4, interview by faculty committee, interview, 3 letters of recommendation, MSN or equivalent, scholarly papers, statistics course, writing sample, GRE General Test.
Degree Requirements 60 total credit hours, dissertation, oral exam, written exam.

University of Massachusetts Worcester

Graduate School of Nursing
Worcester, Massachusetts

http://www.umassmed.edu/gsn/

DEGREES • MS • PHD

Nursing Program Faculty 51 (40% with doctorates).
Graduate Enrollment 174 **Women** 87% **Men** 13% **Minority** 23% **International** 1% **Part-time** 4%.
Distance Learning Courses Available.
Nursing Student Activities Sigma Theta Tau, Student Nurses' Association.
Nursing Student Resources Academic advising; academic or career counseling; assistance for students with disabilities; bookstore; campus computer network; computer lab; computer-assisted instruction; e-mail services; interactive nursing skills videos; Internet; learning resource lab; library services; nursing audiovisuals; skills, simulation, or other laboratory; unpaid internships.
Library Facilities 207,500 volumes in health, 1,173 volumes in nursing; 5,400 periodical subscriptions health-care related.

GRADUATE PROGRAMS

Expenses (2010-11) *Tuition, state resident:* full-time $11,416; part-time $363 per credit. *Tuition, nonresident:* full-time $16,380; part-time $659

per credit. *International tuition:* $16,380 full-time. *Required fees:* full-time $1223.
Financial Aid 80% of graduate students in nursing programs received some form of financial aid in 2009-10. Scholarships and traineeships available. Aid available to part-time students. *Financial aid application deadline:* 5/18.
Contact Ms. Susan Young, Director of Student Affairs, Graduate School of Nursing, University of Massachusetts Worcester, 55 Lake Avenue North, S1-853, Worcester, MA 01655-0115. *Telephone:* 508-856-5756. *Fax:* 508-856-5756. *E-mail:* susan.young@umassmed.edu.

MASTER'S DEGREE PROGRAM

Degree MS
Available Programs Accelerated Master's for Non-Nursing College Graduates; Master's.
Concentrations Available Nursing education. *Nurse practitioner programs in:* acute care, family health, gerontology, primary care.
Site Options Shrewsbury, MA; Worcester, MA.
Study Options Full-time and part-time.
Program Entrance Requirements Clinical experience, computer literacy, minimum overall college GPA of 3.0, transcript of college record, CPR certification, written essay, immunizations, interview, 3 letters of recommendation, physical assessment course, prerequisite course work, resume, statistics course, GRE General Test. *Application deadline:* 3/15 (fall). Applications may be processed on a rolling basis for some programs.
Advanced Placement Credit given for nursing courses completed elsewhere dependent upon specific evaluations.
Degree Requirements 42 total credit hours.

POST-MASTER'S PROGRAM

Areas of Study Nursing education. *Nurse practitioner programs in:* acute care, gerontology, primary care.

DOCTORAL DEGREE PROGRAM

Degree PhD
Available Programs Doctorate.
Areas of Study Advanced practice nursing, bio-behavioral research, clinical practice, critical care, family health, health promotion/disease prevention, human health and illness, illness and transition, nursing research, nursing science, oncology.
Site Options Worcester, MA.
Program Entrance Requirements Minimum overall college GPA of 3.0, interview by faculty committee, interview, 3 letters of recommendation, MSN or equivalent, scholarly papers, statistics course, vita, writing sample, GRE General Test. Application deadline: 3/15 (fall). Applications may be processed on a rolling basis for some programs.
Degree Requirements 57 total credit hours, dissertation, oral exam, written exam.

CONTINUING EDUCATION PROGRAM

Contact Ms. Diane Brescia, Admissions Coordinator, Graduate School of Nursing, University of Massachusetts Worcester, S1-853, 55 Lake Avenue North, Worcester, MA 01655-0115. *Telephone:* 508-856-3488. *Fax:* 508-856-6552. *E-mail:* gsnadmissions@umassmed.edu.

Worcester State College

Department of Nursing
Worcester, Massachusetts

http://www.worcester.edu/
Founded in 1874

DEGREES • BS • MS

Nursing Program Faculty 25 (20% with doctorates).
Baccalaureate Enrollment 287 **Women** 95% **Men** 5% **Minority** 5%
Graduate Enrollment 56 **Women** 90% **Men** 10% **Minority** 15% **International** .5% **Part-time** 5%
Nursing Student Activities Sigma Theta Tau, Student Nurses' Association.
Nursing Student Resources Academic advising; academic or career counseling; assistance for students with disabilities; bookstore; campus computer network; career placement assistance; computer lab; computer-assisted instruction; e-mail services; employment services for current students; housing assistance; interactive nursing skills videos; Internet; learning resource lab; library services; nursing audiovisuals; paid internships; remedial services; resume preparation assistance; skills, simulation, or other laboratory; tutoring; unpaid internships.
Library Facilities 201,975 volumes (5,400 in health, 500 in nursing); 802 periodical subscriptions (85 health-care related).

BACCALAUREATE PROGRAMS

Degree BS
Available Programs Generic Baccalaureate; RN Baccalaureate.
Study Options Full-time.
Program Entrance Requirements Transcript of college record, high school foreign language, 3 years high school math, 3 years high school science, high school transcript, minimum high school GPA of 3.2. *Application deadline:* 1/15 (fall). Applications may be processed on a rolling basis for some programs. *Application fee:* $40.
Advanced Placement Credit by examination available.
Expenses (2010-11) *Tuition, state resident:* full-time $970. *Tuition, nonresident:* full-time $7050. *Room and board:* $9300 per academic year. *Required fees:* full-time $6185.
Financial Aid 80% of baccalaureate students in nursing programs received some form of financial aid in 2009-10.
Contact Ms. Elizabeth Axelson, Director, Admissions, Department of Nursing, Worcester State College, 486 Chandler Street, Worcester, MA 01602. *Telephone:* 508-929-8040. *Fax:* 508-929-8183. *E-mail:* baxelson@worcester.edu.

GRADUATE PROGRAMS

Expenses (2010-11) *Tuition, state resident:* full-time $1800; part-time $150 per credit. *Tuition, nonresident:* full-time $1800; part-time $150 per credit. *Required fees:* full-time $672; part-time $112 per credit.
Financial Aid 45% of graduate students in nursing programs received some form of financial aid in 2009-10.
Contact Dr. Stephanie Chalupka, Coordinator, Department of Nursing, Worcester State College, 486 Chandler Street, Worcester, MA 01602. *Telephone:* 508-929-8129. *Fax:* 508-929-8680. *E-mail:* schalupka@worcester.edu.

MASTER'S DEGREE PROGRAM

Degree MS
Available Programs Master's; Master's for Nurses with Non-Nursing Degrees; RN to Master's.
Concentrations Available Nursing education. *Clinical nurse specialist programs in:* community health, public health.
Study Options Full-time and part-time.
Program Entrance Requirements Clinical experience, computer literacy, minimum overall college GPA of 3.0, transcript of college record, CPR certification, written essay, immunizations, interview, 1 letter of recommendation, nursing research course, professional liability insurance/malpractice insurance, prerequisite course work, resume, statistics course. *Application deadline:* 4/1 (fall), 11/1 (winter). Applications may be processed on a rolling basis for some programs. *Application fee:* $40.
Advanced Placement Credit given for nursing courses completed elsewhere dependent upon specific evaluations.
Degree Requirements 42 total credit hours, thesis or project.

MICHIGAN

Andrews University

Department of Nursing
Berrien Springs, Michigan

Founded in 1874

DEGREES • BS • MS

Nursing Program Faculty 11 (50% with doctorates).
Baccalaureate Enrollment 106
Graduate Enrollment 10
Nursing Student Activities Nursing Honor Society, Sigma Theta Tau, Student Nurses' Association.
Nursing Student Resources Academic advising; academic or career counseling; assistance for students with disabilities; bookstore; campus computer network; career placement assistance; computer lab; computer-assisted instruction; daycare for children of students; e-mail services;

employment services for current students; externships; housing assistance; interactive nursing skills videos; Internet; learning resource lab; library services; nursing audiovisuals; paid internships; placement services for program completers; remedial services; resume preparation assistance; skills, simulation, or other laboratory; tutoring; unpaid internships.

Library Facilities 727,764 volumes (77,000 in health, 500 in nursing); 39,000 periodical subscriptions (700 health-care related).

BACCALAUREATE PROGRAMS

Degree BS

Available Programs ADN to Baccalaureate; Generic Baccalaureate.

Study Options Full-time.

Program Entrance Requirements Minimum overall college GPA of 2.5, transcript of college record, health exam, high school transcript, immunizations, minimum GPA in nursing prerequisites of 2.5. Transfer students are accepted.

Contact *Telephone:* 269-471-3192. *Fax:* 269-471-3454.

GRADUATE PROGRAMS

Contact *Telephone:* 269-471-3337. *Fax:* 269-471-3454.

MASTER'S DEGREE PROGRAM

Degree MS

Available Programs Master's.

Concentrations Available Nursing education.

Study Options Part-time.

Program Entrance Requirements Minimum overall college GPA of 3.0, transcript of college record, CPR certification, immunizations, 3 letters of recommendation, GRE.

Degree Requirements 38 total credit hours, thesis or project.

POST-MASTER'S PROGRAM

Areas of Study Nursing education.

Calvin College

Department of Nursing
Grand Rapids, Michigan

Founded in 1876

DEGREE • BSN

Nursing Program Faculty 20 (20% with doctorates).

Baccalaureate Enrollment 120 **Women** 95% **Men** 5% **Minority** 10% **International** 10%

Nursing Student Activities Sigma Theta Tau, Student Nurses' Association, nursing club.

Nursing Student Resources Academic advising; academic or career counseling; assistance for students with disabilities; bookstore; campus computer network; career placement assistance; computer lab; computer-assisted instruction; e-mail services; employment services for current students; externships; housing assistance; interactive nursing skills videos; Internet; learning resource lab; library services; nursing audiovisuals; paid internships; placement services for program completers; remedial services; resume preparation assistance; skills, simulation, or other laboratory; tutoring.

Library Facilities 493,213 volumes; 22,183 periodical subscriptions.

BACCALAUREATE PROGRAMS

Degree BSN

Available Programs Generic Baccalaureate.

Site Options Grand Rapids, MI.

Study Options Full-time.

Program Entrance Requirements Minimum overall college GPA of 2.5, transcript of college record, CPR certification, health exam, health insurance, immunizations, 2 letters of recommendation, minimum GPA in nursing prerequisites of 2.5, professional liability insurance/malpractice insurance, prerequisite course work. Transfer students are accepted.

Contact *Telephone:* 616-526-6268. *Fax:* 616-526-8567.

Davenport University

Division of Nursing
Grand Rapids, Michigan

Founded in 1866

DEGREE • BSN

Nursing Program Faculty 40

Baccalaureate Enrollment 215 **Women** 94% **Men** 6% **Minority** 30% **Part-time** 17%

Distance Learning Courses Available.

Nursing Student Activities Student Nurses' Association.

Nursing Student Resources Academic advising; academic or career counseling; assistance for students with disabilities; bookstore; campus computer network; career placement assistance; computer lab; computer-assisted instruction; e-mail services; employment services for current students; externships; housing assistance; interactive nursing skills videos; Internet; learning resource lab; library services; nursing audiovisuals; placement services for program completers; remedial services; resume preparation assistance; skills, simulation, or other laboratory; tutoring.

Library Facilities 82,078 volumes (100 in health, 50 in nursing); 571 periodical subscriptions (20 health-care related).

BACCALAUREATE PROGRAMS

Degree BSN

Available Programs ADN to Baccalaureate; Generic Baccalaureate; RN Baccalaureate.

Site Options Midland, MI; Warren, MI.

Study Options Full-time and part-time.

Online Degree Options Yes.

Program Entrance Requirements Minimum overall college GPA of 3.5, transcript of college record, CPR certification, written essay, health exam, health insurance, high school biology, high school chemistry, 2 years high school math, 3 years high school science, high school transcript, immunizations, 2 letters of recommendation, minimum high school GPA of 3.5, minimum GPA in nursing prerequisites. Transfer students are accepted. *Application deadline:* 1/31 (fall).

Advanced Placement Credit by examination available. Credit given for nursing courses completed elsewhere dependent upon specific evaluations.

Expenses (2009-10) *Tuition:* full-time $15,000; part-time $450 per credit hour. *Room and board:* $8500; room only: $6200 per academic year. *Required fees:* full-time $600; part-time $100 per credit.

Financial Aid 70% of baccalaureate students in nursing programs received some form of financial aid in 2008-09. *Gift aid (need-based):* Federal Pell, FSEOG, state, private, college/university gift aid from institutional funds. *Loans:* private alternative loans. *Work-study:* Federal Work-Study, part-time campus jobs. *Financial aid application deadline (priority):* 3/1.

Contact Division of Nursing, Division of Nursing, Davenport University, 415 Fulton Street East, Grand Rapids, MI 49503-5926. *Telephone:* 616-451-3511. *Fax:* 616-732-1145.

Davenport University

Bachelor of Science in Nursing Program
Kalamazoo, Michigan

Founded in 1977

DEGREE • BSN

BACCALAUREATE PROGRAMS

Degree BSN

Available Programs Generic Baccalaureate; RN Baccalaureate.

Contact Sandra Welling, Interim Director of Nursing, Bachelor of Science in Nursing Program, Davenport University, Kalamazoo, MI 49006. *Telephone:* 616-871-3977. *Fax:* 616-554-5225.

Eastern Michigan University

School of Nursing
Ypsilanti, Michigan

http://www.emich.edu/nursing
Founded in 1849

DEGREES • BSN • MSN

Nursing Program Faculty 53 (28% with doctorates).
Baccalaureate Enrollment 338 **Women** 87% **Men** 13% **Minority** 30% **International** 2% **Part-time** 58%
Graduate Enrollment 40 **Women** 98% **Men** 2% **Minority** 32% **International** 2% **Part-time** 95%
Nursing Student Activities Sigma Theta Tau, Student Nurses' Association.
Nursing Student Resources Academic advising; academic or career counseling; assistance for students with disabilities; bookstore; campus computer network; career placement assistance; computer lab; computer-assisted instruction; daycare for children of students; e-mail services; employment services for current students; housing assistance; interactive nursing skills videos; Internet; learning resource lab; library services; nursing audiovisuals; placement services for program completers; remedial services; resume preparation assistance; skills, simulation, or other laboratory; tutoring.
Library Facilities 995,386 volumes (24,200 in health, 5,300 in nursing); 13,146 periodical subscriptions (1,600 health-care related).

BACCALAUREATE PROGRAMS

Degree BSN
Available Programs Baccalaureate for Second Degree; Generic Baccalaureate; RN Baccalaureate.
Site Options Livonia, MI; Monroe, MI; Jackson, MI; Brighton, MI; Detroit, MI.
Study Options Full-time and part-time.
Program Entrance Requirements Transcript of college record, CPR certification, health exam, health insurance, immunizations, minimum GPA in nursing prerequisites of 3.0, prerequisite course work, RN licensure. Transfer students are accepted.
Advanced Placement Credit given for nursing courses completed elsewhere dependent upon specific evaluations.
Contact ***Telephone:*** 734-487-2340. *Fax:* 734-487-6946.

GRADUATE PROGRAMS

Contact ***Telephone:*** 734-487-3275. *Fax:* 734-487-6946.

MASTER'S DEGREE PROGRAM

Degree MSN
Available Programs Master's.
Concentrations Available *Clinical nurse specialist programs in:* adult health.
Site Options Livonia, MI; Monroe, MI.
Program Entrance Requirements Clinical experience, minimum overall college GPA of 2.5, transcript of college record, CPR certification, written essay, immunizations, interview, 3 letters of recommendation, physical assessment course, statistics course.
Degree Requirements 40 total credit hours, thesis or project.

Ferris State University

School of Nursing
Big Rapids, Michigan

http://www.ferris.edu/htmls/colleges/alliedhe/department_desc.cfm?DepartmentID=7
Founded in 1884

DEGREES • BSN • MSN • MSN/MBA

Nursing Program Faculty 24 (20% with doctorates).
Baccalaureate Enrollment 510 **Women** 87% **Men** 13% **Minority** 7% **Part-time** 72%
Graduate Enrollment 64 **Women** 90% **Men** 10% **Part-time** 98%
Distance Learning Courses Available.
Nursing Student Activities Sigma Theta Tau, Student Nurses' Association.
Nursing Student Resources Academic advising; academic or career counseling; assistance for students with disabilities; bookstore; campus computer network; career placement assistance; computer lab; computer-assisted instruction; daycare for children of students; e-mail services; employment services for current students; housing assistance; interactive nursing skills videos; Internet; library services; nursing audiovisuals; resume preparation assistance; skills, simulation, or other laboratory; tutoring.
Library Facilities 411,778 volumes (12,177 in health, 785 in nursing); 45,000 periodical subscriptions (515 health-care related).

BACCALAUREATE PROGRAMS

Degree BSN
Available Programs Accelerated Baccalaureate for Second Degree; Accelerated RN Baccalaureate; Generic Baccalaureate; RN Baccalaureate.
Site Options Midland, MI; Holland, MI; Traverse City, MI.
Study Options Full-time.
Online Degree Options Yes.
Program Entrance Requirements Minimum overall college GPA of 2.7, transcript of college record, CPR certification, health insurance, immunizations, minimum GPA in nursing prerequisites of 2.7, prerequisite course work. Transfer students are accepted. *Application deadline:* 1/15 (fall), 8/15 (spring).
Advanced Placement Credit by examination available. Credit given for nursing courses completed elsewhere dependent upon specific evaluations.
Expenses (2010-11) *Tuition, state resident:* full-time $9930; part-time $331 per credit. *Tuition, nonresident:* full-time $15,900; part-time $530 per credit. *Room and board:* $9180; room only: $8916 per academic year. *Required fees:* full-time $1150.
Financial Aid 87% of baccalaureate students in nursing programs received some form of financial aid in 2009-10. *Gift aid (need-based):* Federal Pell, FSEOG, state, private, college/university gift aid from institutional funds. *Loans:* Federal Nursing Student Loans, Federal Direct (Subsidized and Unsubsidized Stafford PLUS), Perkins, college/university, alternative loans. *Work-study:* Federal Work-Study, part-time campus jobs. *Financial aid application deadline (priority):* 3/1.
Contact Dr. Mary P. Alkire, Interim Director, School of Nursing, Ferris State University, 200 Ferris Drive, Room 400A, Big Rapids, MI 49307. *Telephone:* 231-591-2267. *Fax:* 231-591-2325. *E-mail:* alkire@ferris.edu.

GRADUATE PROGRAMS

Expenses (2010-11) *Tuition, state resident:* part-time $450 per credit. *Tuition, nonresident:* part-time $675 per credit.
Financial Aid 20% of graduate students in nursing programs received some form of financial aid in 2009-10.
Contact Dr. Marietta Bell-Scriber, Program Coordinator, School of Nursing, Ferris State University, 200 Ferris Drive, Big Rapids, MI 49307. *Telephone:* 231-591-3987. *Fax:* 231-591-2325. *E-mail:* bellscri@ferris.edu.

MASTER'S DEGREE PROGRAM

Degrees MSN; MSN/MBA
Available Programs Accelerated AD/RN to Master's; Master's.
Concentrations Available Nursing administration; nursing education; nursing informatics.
Study Options Full-time and part-time.
Online Degree Options Yes (online only).
Program Entrance Requirements Clinical experience, minimum overall college GPA of 3.0, transcript of college record, written essay, 3 letters of recommendation, resume. *Application deadline:* 8/1 (fall), 12/1 (winter), 12/2 (spring).
Advanced Placement Credit given for nursing courses completed elsewhere dependent upon specific evaluations.
Degree Requirements 36 total credit hours, thesis or project, comprehensive exam.

Finlandia University

College of Professional Studies
Hancock, Michigan

http://www.finlandia.edu/
Founded in 1896

DEGREE • BSN

Nursing Program Faculty 14 (7% with doctorates).
Baccalaureate Enrollment 86 **Women** 85% **Men** 15% **Minority** 2% **Part-time** 7%

Distance Learning Courses Available.
Nursing Student Activities Student Nurses' Association, nursing club.
Nursing Student Resources Academic advising; academic or career counseling; assistance for students with disabilities; bookstore; campus computer network; career placement assistance; computer lab; computer-assisted instruction; e-mail services; interactive nursing skills videos; Internet; learning resource lab; library services; nursing audiovisuals; placement services for program completers; remedial services; resume preparation assistance; skills, simulation, or other laboratory; tutoring.
Library Facilities 68,803 volumes (4,601 in health, 2,316 in nursing); 997 periodical subscriptions (97 health-care related).

BACCALAUREATE PROGRAMS

Degree BSN
Available Programs Generic Baccalaureate; RN Baccalaureate.
Study Options Full-time.
Online Degree Options Yes.
Program Entrance Requirements Minimum overall college GPA of 2.5, transcript of college record, CPR certification, health exam, high school biology, high school chemistry, 1 year of high school math, 2 years high school science, high school transcript, immunizations, minimum high school GPA of 2.5, minimum GPA in nursing prerequisites of 2.5, prerequisite course work. Transfer students are accepted. *Application deadline:* Applications may be processed on a rolling basis for some programs.
Advanced Placement Credit given for nursing courses completed elsewhere dependent upon specific evaluations.
Expenses (2010-11) *Tuition:* full-time $18,474; part-time $3696 per semester. *Room and board:* $6154 per academic year. *Required fees:* full-time $400.
Financial Aid 95% of baccalaureate students in nursing programs received some form of financial aid in 2009-10.
Contact Kitti Loukus, Admissions Office, College of Professional Studies, Finlandia University, 601 Quincy Street, Hancock, MI 49930. *Telephone:* 906-487-7274. *E-mail:* kitti.loukus@finlandia.edu.

Grand Valley State University

Kirkhof College of Nursing
Allendale, Michigan

http://www.gvsu.edu/kcon
Founded in 1960

DEGREES • BSN • DNP • MSN

Nursing Program Faculty 88 (32% with doctorates).
Baccalaureate Enrollment 373 **Women** 82% **Men** 18% **Minority** 6% **Part-time** 40%
Graduate Enrollment 60 **Women** 85% **Men** 15% **Part-time** 96%
Distance Learning Courses Available.
Nursing Student Activities Sigma Theta Tau, Student Nurses' Association.
Nursing Student Resources Academic advising; academic or career counseling; assistance for students with disabilities; bookstore; campus computer network; career placement assistance; computer lab; computer-assisted instruction; daycare for children of students; e-mail services; employment services for current students; housing assistance; interactive nursing skills videos; Internet; learning resource lab; library services; nursing audiovisuals; remedial services; resume preparation assistance; skills, simulation, or other laboratory; tutoring.
Library Facilities 664,000 volumes (23,000 in health, 1,800 in nursing); 8,000 periodical subscriptions (1,250 health-care related).

BACCALAUREATE PROGRAMS

Degree BSN
Available Programs ADN to Baccalaureate; Accelerated Baccalaureate for Second Degree; Baccalaureate for Second Degree; Generic Baccalaureate; RN Baccalaureate.
Site Options Grand Rapids, MI.
Study Options Full-time and part-time.
Program Entrance Requirements Minimum overall college GPA of 2.8, transcript of college record, CPR certification, written essay, health exam, health insurance, immunizations, minimum GPA in nursing prerequisites of 2.0, prerequisite course work. Transfer students are accepted. *Application deadline:* 3/1 (fall), 3/1 (winter), 11/1 (spring).
Advanced Placement Credit given for nursing courses completed elsewhere dependent upon specific evaluations.
Expenses (2010-11) *Tuition, state resident:* full-time $9088; part-time $395 per credit hour. *Tuition, nonresident:* full-time $13,402; part-time $571 per credit hour. *International tuition:* $13,500 full-time. *Room and board:* $7624 per academic year. *Required fees:* full-time $204; part-time $17 per credit.
Financial Aid 89% of baccalaureate students in nursing programs received some form of financial aid in 2009-10. *Gift aid (need-based):* Federal Pell, FSEOG, state, private, college/university gift aid from institutional funds. *Loans:* Federal Nursing Student Loans, Federal Direct (Subsidized and Unsubsidized Stafford PLUS), Perkins. *Work-study:* Federal Work-Study, part-time campus jobs. *Financial aid application deadline (priority):* 3/1.
Contact Ms. Cassonya Carter, Director of Student Services, Kirkhof College of Nursing, Grand Valley State University, Cook-DeVos Center for Health Sciences, 301 Michigan Street NE, Room 320, Grand Rapids, MI 49503-3314. *Telephone:* 616-331-5782. *Fax:* 616-331-2510. *E-mail:* carterc@gvsu.edu.

GRADUATE PROGRAMS

Expenses (2010-11) *Tuition, state resident:* part-time $471 per credit hour. *Tuition, nonresident:* part-time $646 per credit hour. *Room and board:* room only: $5406 per academic year. *Required fees:* full-time $306; part-time $17 per credit.
Financial Aid 69% of graduate students in nursing programs received some form of financial aid in 2009-10. 14 fellowships (averaging $3,207 per year), 9 research assistantships with full and partial tuition reimbursements available (averaging $8,053 per year) were awarded; career-related internships or fieldwork, Federal Work-Study, institutionally sponsored loans, and traineeships also available. *Financial aid application deadline:* 2/15.
Contact Ms. Linda Buck, Student Services Coordinator, Kirkhof College of Nursing, Grand Valley State University, Cook-DeVos Center for Health Sciences, 301 Michigan Street NE, Room 318, Grand Rapids, MI 49503-3314. *Telephone:* 616-331-5785. *Fax:* 616-331-2510. *E-mail:* buckli@gvsu.edu.

MASTER'S DEGREE PROGRAM

Degree MSN
Available Programs Master's.
Concentrations Available Clinical nurse leader.
Site Options Grand Rapids, MI.
Study Options Full-time and part-time.
Program Entrance Requirements Minimum overall college GPA of 3.0, transcript of college record, CPR certification, written essay, immunizations, interview, resume, GRE. *Application deadline:* 2/1 (fall). *Application fee:* $30.
Advanced Placement Credit given for nursing courses completed elsewhere dependent upon specific evaluations.
Degree Requirements 41 total credit hours, thesis or project.

DOCTORAL DEGREE PROGRAM

Degree DNP
Available Programs Post-Baccalaureate Doctorate.
Areas of Study Advanced practice nursing, nursing administration.
Site Options Grand Rapids, MI.
Program Entrance Requirements Minimum overall college GPA of 3.0, interview by faculty committee, vita, writing sample. Application deadline: 2/1 (fall). Application fee: $30.
Degree Requirements 93 total credit hours, dissertation.

CONTINUING EDUCATION PROGRAM

Contact Ms. Jan Coye, Academic Community Liaison, Kirkhof College of Nursing, Grand Valley State University, Cook-DeVos Center for Health Sciences, 301 Michigan Street NE, Room 350, Grand Rapids, MI 49503-3314. *Telephone:* 616-331-3558. *Fax:* 616-331-2510. *E-mail:* coyej@gvsu.edu.

Hope College

Department of Nursing
Holland, Michigan

Founded in 1866

DEGREE • BSN

Nursing Program Faculty 13 (23% with doctorates).
Baccalaureate Enrollment 120 **Women** 91% **Men** 9% **Minority** 9% **Part-time** 2%

Nursing Student Activities Sigma Theta Tau, Student Nurses' Association.
Nursing Student Resources Academic advising; academic or career counseling; assistance for students with disabilities; bookstore; campus computer network; career placement assistance; computer lab; computer-assisted instruction; e-mail services; employment services for current students; externships; housing assistance; interactive nursing skills videos; Internet; learning resource lab; library services; nursing audiovisuals; remedial services; resume preparation assistance; skills, simulation, or other laboratory; tutoring; unpaid internships.
Library Facilities 371,987 volumes; 12,573 periodical subscriptions.

BACCALAUREATE PROGRAMS

Degree BSN
Available Programs Generic Baccalaureate.
Study Options Full-time and part-time.
Program Entrance Requirements Minimum overall college GPA of 3.0, transcript of college record, written essay, 2 letters of recommendation, minimum GPA in nursing prerequisites of 2.5. Transfer students are accepted. *Application deadline:* 10/1 (fall), 2/1 (winter).
Financial Aid ***Gift aid (need-based):*** Federal Pell, FSEOG, state, private, college/university gift aid from institutional funds. *Loans:* Federal Direct (Subsidized and Unsubsidized Stafford PLUS), Perkins, college/university. *Work-study:* Federal Work-Study, part-time campus jobs. *Financial aid application deadline (priority):* 3/1.
Contact Nursing Contact, Department of Nursing, Hope College, 35 East 12th Street, Holland, MI 49422-9000. *Telephone:* 616-395-7420. *Fax:* 616-395-7163. *E-mail:* nursing@hope.edu.

Lake Superior State University
Department of Nursing
Sault Sainte Marie, Michigan

http://www.lssu.edu/academics/science/schools/nursing_health/nursdept/
Founded in 1946

DEGREE • BSN

Nursing Program Faculty 20 (15% with doctorates).
Baccalaureate Enrollment 115 **Women** 90% **Men** 10% **Minority** 10% **International** 3%
Distance Learning Courses Available.
Nursing Student Activities Nursing Honor Society, Student Nurses' Association, nursing club.
Nursing Student Resources Academic advising; academic or career counseling; assistance for students with disabilities; bookstore; campus computer network; career placement assistance; computer lab; computer-assisted instruction; daycare for children of students; e-mail services; employment services for current students; interactive nursing skills videos; Internet; learning resource lab; library services; nursing audiovisuals; placement services for program completers; remedial services; resume preparation assistance; skills, simulation, or other laboratory; tutoring.
Library Facilities 200,449 volumes (5,246 in health, 942 in nursing); 850 periodical subscriptions (1,196 health-care related).

BACCALAUREATE PROGRAMS

Degree BSN
Available Programs ADN to Baccalaureate; Generic Baccalaureate; LPN to Baccalaureate; LPN to RN Baccalaureate; RN Baccalaureate; RPN to Baccalaureate.
Site Options Escanaba, MI; Petoskey, MI.
Study Options Full-time and part-time.
Program Entrance Requirements Minimum overall college GPA of 2.5, transcript of college record, CPR certification, health exam, health insurance, high school biology, high school chemistry, high school transcript, immunizations, 1 letter of recommendation, minimum high school GPA of 2.0, minimum GPA in nursing prerequisites of 2.5, professional liability insurance/malpractice insurance, prerequisite course work. Transfer students are accepted. *Application deadline:* 2/1 (fall), 10/1 (spring).
Advanced Placement Credit given for nursing courses completed elsewhere dependent upon specific evaluations.
Contact ***Telephone:*** 906-635-2446. *Fax:* 906-635-2266.

Madonna University
College of Nursing and Health
Livonia, Michigan

http://www.madonna.edu/
Founded in 1947

DEGREES • BSN • DNP • M SC N • MSN/MBA

Nursing Program Faculty 59 (27% with doctorates).
Baccalaureate Enrollment 348 **Women** 87% **Men** 13% **Minority** 13% **International** 1.7% **Part-time** 28%
Graduate Enrollment 52 **Women** 94% **Men** 6% **Minority** 14% **International** 4% **Part-time** 94%
Distance Learning Courses Available.
Nursing Student Activities Sigma Theta Tau, Student Nurses' Association.
Nursing Student Resources Academic advising; academic or career counseling; assistance for students with disabilities; bookstore; campus computer network; career placement assistance; computer lab; computer-assisted instruction; e-mail services; interactive nursing skills videos; Internet; learning resource lab; library services; nursing audiovisuals; remedial services; resume preparation assistance; skills, simulation, or other laboratory; tutoring.
Library Facilities 108,000 volumes (3,632 in health); 515 periodical subscriptions (2,778 health-care related).

BACCALAUREATE PROGRAMS

Degree BSN
Available Programs ADN to Baccalaureate; Generic Baccalaureate; LPN to Baccalaureate; RN Baccalaureate.
Study Options Full-time and part-time.
Program Entrance Requirements Minimum overall college GPA of 2.75, transcript of college record, written essay, high school biology, high school chemistry. Transfer students are accepted. *Application deadline:* 1/31 (fall), 7/31 (winter). *Application fee:* $25.
Advanced Placement Credit by examination available. Credit given for nursing courses completed elsewhere dependent upon specific evaluations.
Expenses (2010-11) *Tuition:* full-time $14,990; part-time $458 per credit hour. *International tuition:* $17,175 full-time. *Room and board:* $5235; room only: $3375 per academic year. *Required fees:* full-time $390; part-time $140 per term.
Financial Aid 75% of baccalaureate students in nursing programs received some form of financial aid in 2009-10.
Contact Ms. Lauren Stemberger, Pre-Nursing Admissions Officer, College of Nursing and Health, Madonna University, 36600 Schoolcraft Road, Livonia, MI 48150-1173. *Telephone:* 734-432-5346. *E-mail:* lstemberger@madonna.edu.

GRADUATE PROGRAMS

Expenses (2010-11) *Tuition:* full-time $9460; part-time $520 per credit hour. *Room and board:* $7120; room only: $3200 per academic year. *Required fees:* full-time $300; part-time $10 per credit; part-time $100 per term.
Financial Aid 20% of graduate students in nursing programs received some form of financial aid in 2009-10.
Contact Dr. Nancy O'Connor, Chair of Graduate Nursing Program, College of Nursing and Health, Madonna University, 36600 Schoolcraft Road, Livonia, MI 48150-1173. *Telephone:* 734-432-5461. *Fax:* 734-432-5463. *E-mail:* noconnor@madonna.edu.

MASTER'S DEGREE PROGRAM

Degrees M Sc N; MSN/MBA
Available Programs Master's.
Concentrations Available Nursing administration. *Clinical nurse specialist programs in:* adult health. *Nurse practitioner programs in:* acute care, adult health, primary care.
Study Options Full-time and part-time.
Program Entrance Requirements Clinical experience, computer literacy, minimum overall college GPA of 3.0, transcript of college record, written essay, interview, 2 letters of recommendation, nursing research course, physical assessment course, prerequisite course work, resume, statistics course. *Application deadline:* 2/1 (fall), 9/30 (winter), 2/1 (spring), 2/1 (summer). Applications may be processed on a rolling basis for some programs.
Degree Requirements 48 total credit hours.

POST-MASTER'S PROGRAM

Areas of Study Nursing administration; nursing education. *Nurse practitioner programs in:* acute care, adult health, primary care.

DOCTORAL DEGREE PROGRAM

Degree DNP
Available Programs Doctorate.
Areas of Study Advanced practice nursing, individualized study, nursing administration.
Program Entrance Requirements Clinical experience, minimum overall college GPA of 3.0, interview by faculty committee, interview, 3 letters of recommendation, MSN or equivalent, scholarly papers, vita, writing sample. Application deadline: Applications may be processed on a rolling basis for some programs.
Degree Requirements 36 total credit hours, oral exam, written exam, residency.

CONTINUING EDUCATION PROGRAM

Contact Dr. Susan Hasenau, Coordinator of Nursing Continuing Education, College of Nursing and Health, Madonna University, 36600 Schoolcraft Road, Livonia, MI 48150-1173. *Telephone:* 734-432-5863. *Fax:* 734-432-5463. *E-mail:* shasenau@madonna.edu.

Michigan State University
College of Nursing
East Lansing, Michigan

http://www.nursing.msu.edu/
Founded in 1855

DEGREES • BSN • MSN • PHD

Nursing Program Faculty 83 (37% with doctorates).
Baccalaureate Enrollment 337 **Women** 86.05% **Men** 13.95% **Minority** 8.01% **International** .89% **Part-time** 9.2%
Graduate Enrollment 188 **Women** 89.36% **Men** 10.64% **Minority** 7.45% **International** 2.13% **Part-time** 59.04%
Distance Learning Courses Available.
Nursing Student Activities Sigma Theta Tau, Student Nurses' Association.
Nursing Student Resources Academic advising; academic or career counseling; assistance for students with disabilities; bookstore; campus computer network; career placement assistance; computer lab; computer-assisted instruction; daycare for children of students; e-mail services; externships; housing assistance; interactive nursing skills videos; Internet; learning resource lab; library services; nursing audiovisuals; placement services for program completers; remedial services; resume preparation assistance; skills, simulation, or other laboratory; tutoring.
Library Facilities 5 million volumes (147,194 in health, 3,702 in nursing); 98,469 periodical subscriptions (6,951 health-care related).

BACCALAUREATE PROGRAMS

Degree BSN
Available Programs Accelerated Baccalaureate for Second Degree; Generic Baccalaureate; RN Baccalaureate.
Study Options Full-time and part-time.
Online Degree Options Yes.
Program Entrance Requirements Minimum overall college GPA of 2.75, written essay, immunizations, 2 letters of recommendation, prerequisite course work. Transfer students are accepted. *Application deadline:* 10/1 (fall), 3/1 (spring), 12/15 (summer).
Financial Aid 74% of baccalaureate students in nursing programs received some form of financial aid in 2009-10. *Gift aid (need-based):* Federal Pell, FSEOG, state, private, college/university gift aid from institutional funds, United Negro College Fund. *Loans:* Federal Direct (Subsidized and Unsubsidized Stafford PLUS), Perkins, college/university. *Work-study:* Federal Work-Study, part-time campus jobs. *Financial aid application deadline:* Continuous.
Contact Office of Student Support Services, College of Nursing, Michigan State University, A117 Life Sciences Building, East Lansing, MI 48824-1317. *Telephone:* 517-353-4827. *Fax:* 517-432-8251. *E-mail:* nurse@hc.msu.edu.

GRADUATE PROGRAMS

Financial Aid 82% of graduate students in nursing programs received some form of financial aid in 2009-10. 1 research assistantship with tuition reimbursement available (averaging $6,110 per year), 2 teaching assistantships with tuition reimbursements available (averaging $7,076 per year) were awarded.
Contact Ms. Nikki O'Brien, Program Advisor, College of Nursing, Michigan State University, A117 Life Sciences Building, East Lansing, MI 48824-1317. *Telephone:* 517-353-4827. *Fax:* 517-432-8251. *E-mail:* obrienni@msu.edu.

MASTER'S DEGREE PROGRAM

Degree MSN
Available Programs Master's.
Concentrations Available Nurse anesthesia. *Clinical nurse specialist programs in:* adult health. *Nurse practitioner programs in:* adult health, family health, gerontology.
Study Options Full-time and part-time.
Online Degree Options Yes.
Program Entrance Requirements Clinical experience, minimum overall college GPA of 3.0, transcript of college record, CPR certification, written essay, immunizations, interview, 3 letters of recommendation, resume, statistics course. *Application deadline:* 2/15 (fall), 5/15 (winter). Applications may be processed on a rolling basis for some programs.
Advanced Placement Credit given for nursing courses completed elsewhere dependent upon specific evaluations.
Degree Requirements Comprehensive exam.

POST-MASTER'S PROGRAM

Areas of Study *Clinical nurse specialist programs in:* adult health. *Nurse practitioner programs in:* adult health, family health, gerontology.

DOCTORAL DEGREE PROGRAM

Degree PhD
Available Programs Doctorate; Doctorate for Nurses with Non-Nursing Degrees; Post-Baccalaureate Doctorate.
Areas of Study Family health, health promotion/disease prevention, human health and illness, individualized study, nursing research.
Site Options Grand Rapids, MI.
Program Entrance Requirements Minimum overall college GPA of 3.0, interview by faculty committee, interview, 3 letters of recommendation, statistics course, vita, writing sample. Application deadline: Applications may be processed on a rolling basis for some programs.
Degree Requirements 72 total credit hours, dissertation, written exam.

CONTINUING EDUCATION PROGRAM

Contact Katie Kessler, Director of Professional Education, College of Nursing, Michigan State University, A103 Life Sciences Building, East Lansing, MI 48824-1317. *Telephone:* 517-355-8539. *Fax:* 517-432-8131. *E-mail:* kathleen.kessler@hc.msu.edu.

Northern Michigan University
College of Nursing and Allied Health Science
Marquette, Michigan

http://www.nmu.edu/departments/nursing.html
Founded in 1899

DEGREES • BSN • MSN

Nursing Program Faculty 16 (69% with doctorates).
Baccalaureate Enrollment 221 **Women** 81% **Men** 19% **Minority** 4% **Part-time** 7%
Graduate Enrollment 16 **Women** 81% **Men** 19% **Part-time** 100%
Distance Learning Courses Available.
Nursing Student Activities Sigma Theta Tau, Student Nurses' Association.
Nursing Student Resources Academic advising; academic or career counseling; assistance for students with disabilities; bookstore; campus computer network; career placement assistance; computer lab; computer-assisted instruction; e-mail services; employment services for current students; housing assistance; interactive nursing skills videos; Internet; learning resource lab; library services; nursing audiovisuals; other; paid internships; remedial services; resume preparation assistance; skills, simulation, or other laboratory; tutoring.
Library Facilities 631,244 volumes (32,879 in health, 2,733 in nursing); 20,657 periodical subscriptions (5,000 health-care related).

BACCALAUREATE PROGRAMS

Degree BSN

Available Programs Accelerated Baccalaureate; Generic Baccalaureate; LPN to Baccalaureate; RN Baccalaureate.
Study Options Full-time.
Program Entrance Requirements Minimum overall college GPA of 2.75, transcript of college record, CPR certification, health exam, high school transcript, immunizations, minimum GPA in nursing prerequisites of 2.0, prerequisite course work. Transfer students are accepted. *Application deadline:* 2/1 (fall), 10/1 (winter).
Advanced Placement Credit by examination available. Credit given for nursing courses completed elsewhere dependent upon specific evaluations.
Expenses (2010-11) *Tuition, state resident:* full-time $7864; part-time $302 per credit hour. *Tuition, nonresident:* full-time $12,280; part-time $486 per credit hour. *Room and board:* $7668 per academic year. *Required fees:* full-time $150.
Financial Aid 85% of baccalaureate students in nursing programs received some form of financial aid in 2009-10.
Contact Dr. Kerri Durnell Schuiling, Associate Dean for Nursing Education/Department Head, Nursing, College of Nursing and Allied Health Science, Northern Michigan University, 2301 New Science Facility, Marquette, MI 49855. *Telephone:* 906-227-2834. *Fax:* 906-227-1658. *E-mail:* kschuili@nmu.edu.

GRADUATE PROGRAMS

Expenses (2010-11) *Tuition, state resident:* full-time $6504; part-time $368 per credit hour. *Tuition, nonresident:* full-time $9116; part-time $531 per credit hour. *Required fees:* full-time $150; part-time $75 per term.
Financial Aid Career-related internships or fieldwork, Federal Work-Study, institutionally sponsored loans, and unspecified assistantships available.
Contact Dr. Melissa M. Romero, Coordinator of MSN Program, College of Nursing and Allied Health Science, Northern Michigan University, 2131 New Science Facility, Marquette, MI 49855. *Telephone:* 906-227-2488. *Fax:* 906-227-1658. *E-mail:* mromero@nmu.edu.

MASTER'S DEGREE PROGRAM

Degree MSN
Available Programs Master's.
Concentrations Available *Nurse practitioner programs in:* family health.
Study Options Part-time.
Program Entrance Requirements Clinical experience, computer literacy, minimum overall college GPA of 3.0, transcript of college record, CPR certification, written essay, immunizations, 2 letters of recommendation, physical assessment course, professional liability insurance/malpractice insurance, GRE General Test. *Application deadline:* 2/1 (fall).
Advanced Placement Credit given for nursing courses completed elsewhere dependent upon specific evaluations.
Degree Requirements 45 total credit hours, thesis or project, comprehensive exam.

POST-MASTER'S PROGRAM

Areas of Study *Nurse practitioner programs in:* family health.

CONTINUING EDUCATION PROGRAM

Contact Dr. Terrance Seethoff, Associate Provost, AA/Dean, Grad Studies/Academic Affairs, Provost and Vice President, College of Nursing and Allied Health Science, Northern Michigan University, 610 Cohodas Hall, Marquette, MI 49855. *Telephone:* 906-227-2044. *Fax:* 906-227-2928. *E-mail:* tseethof@nmu.edu.

Oakland University

School of Nursing
Rochester, Michigan

http://www2.oakland.edu/nursing
Founded in 1957

DEGREES • BSN • MSN

Nursing Program Faculty 44 (50% with doctorates).
Baccalaureate Enrollment 462 **Women** 89% **Men** 11% **Minority** 12% **Part-time** 29%
Graduate Enrollment 123 **Women** 79% **Men** 21% **Minority** 11% **International** 1% **Part-time** 35%
Nursing Student Activities Nursing Honor Society, Sigma Theta Tau, Student Nurses' Association.
Nursing Student Resources Academic advising; academic or career counseling; assistance for students with disabilities; bookstore; campus computer network; career placement assistance; computer lab; computer-assisted instruction; e-mail services; employment services for current students; externships; housing assistance; interactive nursing skills videos; Internet; learning resource lab; library services; nursing audiovisuals; paid internships; placement services for program completers; remedial services; resume preparation assistance; skills, simulation, or other laboratory; tutoring; unpaid internships.
Library Facilities 856,760 volumes (12,652 in health, 2,780 in nursing); 20,490 periodical subscriptions (375 health-care related).

BACCALAUREATE PROGRAMS

Degree BSN
Available Programs Generic Baccalaureate; RN Baccalaureate.
Site Options Royal Oak, MI.
Study Options Full-time and part-time.
Program Entrance Requirements Minimum overall college GPA of 3.0, transcript of college record, CPR certification, health exam, high school biology, high school chemistry, 2 years high school math, 1 year of high school science, high school transcript, immunizations, minimum high school GPA of 3.0, minimum GPA in nursing prerequisites of 3.0, professional liability insurance/malpractice insurance, prerequisite course work. Transfer students are accepted.
Advanced Placement Credit given for nursing courses completed elsewhere dependent upon specific evaluations.
Contact ***Telephone:*** 248-370-4065. *Fax:* 248-370-4279.

GRADUATE PROGRAMS

Contact ***Telephone:*** 248-370-4082. *Fax:* 248-370-2996.

MASTER'S DEGREE PROGRAM

Degree MSN
Available Programs Master's.
Concentrations Available Nurse anesthesia; nursing education. *Nurse practitioner programs in:* adult health, family health, gerontology.
Site Options Royal Oak, MI.
Study Options Full-time and part-time.
Program Entrance Requirements Clinical experience, minimum overall college GPA of 3.0, transcript of college record, CPR certification, written essay, immunizations, interview, 2 letters of recommendation, professional liability insurance/malpractice insurance, prerequisite course work, GRE General Test.
Advanced Placement Credit given for nursing courses completed elsewhere dependent upon specific evaluations.
Degree Requirements 45 total credit hours, thesis or project.

POST-MASTER'S PROGRAM

Areas of Study Nurse anesthesia; nursing education. *Nurse practitioner programs in:* adult health, family health, gerontology.

CONTINUING EDUCATION PROGRAM

Contact ***Telephone:*** 248-370-4013. *Fax:* 248-370-4279.

Saginaw Valley State University

Crystal M. Lange College of Nursing and Health Sciences
University Center, Michigan

http://www.svsu.edu/acadprog/nhs/
Founded in 1963

DEGREES • BSN • MSN

Nursing Program Faculty 12 (50% with doctorates).
Nursing Student Activities Sigma Theta Tau, Student Nurses' Association.
Nursing Student Resources Academic advising; academic or career counseling; assistance for students with disabilities; bookstore; campus computer network; career placement assistance; computer lab; computer-assisted instruction; e-mail services; externships; interactive nursing skills videos; Internet; learning resource lab; library services; nursing audiovisuals; remedial services; resume preparation assistance; skills, simulation, or other laboratory; tutoring.
Library Facilities 241,661 volumes; 23,741 periodical subscriptions.

BACCALAUREATE PROGRAMS

Degree BSN
Available Programs Accelerated Baccalaureate for Second Degree; Baccalaureate for Second Degree; Generic Baccalaureate; RN Baccalaureate.
Study Options Full-time and part-time.
Program Entrance Requirements Minimum overall college GPA of 2.5, transcript of college record, CPR certification, written essay, health exam, immunizations, interview, minimum GPA in nursing prerequisites of 2.5, professional liability insurance/malpractice insurance, prerequisite course work. Transfer students are accepted.
Advanced Placement Credit by examination available. Credit given for nursing courses completed elsewhere dependent upon specific evaluations.
Contact ***Telephone:*** 989-964-4145 Ext. 4145. *Fax:* 989-964-4024.

GRADUATE PROGRAMS

Contact ***Telephone:*** 989-964-4145 Ext. 4145. *Fax:* 989-964-4024.

MASTER'S DEGREE PROGRAM

Degree MSN
Available Programs Master's; RN to Master's.
Concentrations Available Nursing administration; nursing education; nursing informatics. *Nurse practitioner programs in:* family health.
Study Options Full-time and part-time.
Program Entrance Requirements Clinical experience, minimum overall college GPA of 3.0, transcript of college record, written essay, interview, 3 letters of recommendation, professional liability insurance/malpractice insurance, resume, statistics course, GRE.
Advanced Placement Credit given for nursing courses completed elsewhere dependent upon specific evaluations.
Degree Requirements 39 total credit hours, thesis or project.

POST-MASTER'S PROGRAM

Areas of Study Nursing administration; nursing education; nursing informatics. *Nurse practitioner programs in:* family health.

CONTINUING EDUCATION PROGRAM

Contact ***Telephone:*** 989-964-4145.

Siena Heights University

Nursing Program
Adrian, Michigan

http://www.sienaheights.edu/
Founded in 1919

DEGREE • BSN

Nursing Program Faculty 7 (50% with doctorates).
Baccalaureate Enrollment 64 **Women** 90% **Men** 10% **Minority** 5% **International** 5% **Part-time** 20%
Distance Learning Courses Available.
Nursing Student Activities Student Nurses' Association.
Nursing Student Resources Academic advising; campus computer network; computer lab; computer-assisted instruction; e-mail services; interactive nursing skills videos; Internet; learning resource lab; skills, simulation, or other laboratory; tutoring.
Library Facilities 142,000 volumes (200 in health, 80 in nursing); 300 periodical subscriptions (150 health-care related).

BACCALAUREATE PROGRAMS

Degree BSN
Available Programs Generic Baccalaureate; RN Baccalaureate.
Study Options Full-time.
Program Entrance Requirements Minimum overall college GPA of 3.0, transcript of college record, CPR certification, written essay, health exam, health insurance, immunizations, interview, minimum GPA in nursing prerequisites of 3.0, professional liability insurance/malpractice insurance, prerequisite course work. *Application deadline:* 10/1 (fall).
Expenses (2010-11) *Tuition:* full-time $20,000; part-time $450 per credit hour. *Room and board:* $5000; room only: $2200 per academic year. *Required fees:* full-time $2000; part-time $40 per credit; part-time $400 per term.
Financial Aid 90% of baccalaureate students in nursing programs received some form of financial aid in 2009-10.
Contact Miss Sara Johnson, Director of Admissions, Nursing Program, Siena Heights University, 1247 East Siena Heights Drive, Adrian, MI 49221. *Telephone:* 517-264-7180. *E-mail:* sjohnson@sienaheights.edu.

Spring Arbor University

Program in Nursing
Spring Arbor, Michigan

http://www.arbor.edu/bsn
Founded in 1873

DEGREES • BSN • MSN • MSN/MBA

Nursing Program Faculty 19 (12% with doctorates).
Baccalaureate Enrollment 283 **Women** 92% **Men** 8% **Minority** 9% **International** 1% **Part-time** 75%
Graduate Enrollment 36 **Women** 94% **Men** 6% **Minority** 5%
Distance Learning Courses Available.
Nursing Student Resources Academic advising; bookstore; campus computer network; computer-assisted instruction; e-mail services; Internet; library services; nursing audiovisuals; other; tutoring.
Library Facilities 115,987 volumes (1,000 in health, 350 in nursing); 523 periodical subscriptions (25 health-care related).

BACCALAUREATE PROGRAMS

Degree BSN
Available Programs ADN to Baccalaureate.
Site Options Battle Creek, Gaylord, Jackson, Kalamazoo, Lansing, MI; Lambertville, MI.
Program Entrance Requirements Minimum overall college GPA of 2.5, transcript of college record, written essay, high school biology, high school chemistry, 1 year of high school math, 2 years high school science, high school transcript, minimum GPA in nursing prerequisites of 2.5, RN licensure. Transfer students are accepted. *Application deadline:* Applications may be processed on a rolling basis for some programs. *Application fee:* $40.
Financial Aid 80% of baccalaureate students in nursing programs received some form of financial aid in 2009-10. *Gift aid (need-based):* Federal Pell, FSEOG, state, private, college/university gift aid from institutional funds. *Loans:* Perkins, alternative loans. *Work-study:* Federal Work-Study, part-time campus jobs. *Financial aid application deadline (priority):* 3/1.
Contact Mr. Alvin V. Kauffman, Director of Nursing, Program in Nursing, Spring Arbor University, 106 East Main Street, Suite #3, Spring Arbor, MI 49283-9799. *Telephone:* 517-750-6579. *Fax:* 517-750-6602. *E-mail:* alvin.kauffman@arbor.edu.

GRADUATE PROGRAMS

Financial Aid 65% of graduate students in nursing programs received some form of financial aid in 2009-10.
Contact Mr. Jim Madden, Senior Admission Specialist, Program in Nursing, Spring Arbor University, 3497 South 9th Street, Suite A, Kalamazoo, MI 49009-9501. *Telephone:* 800-930-9754 Ext. 4058. *Fax:* 269-372-1840. *E-mail:* jmadden@arbor.edu.

MASTER'S DEGREE PROGRAM

Degrees MSN; MSN/MBA
Available Programs Master's.
Concentrations Available Nursing education. *Nurse practitioner programs in:* adult health, gerontology.
Study Options Full-time.
Online Degree Options Yes (online only).
Program Entrance Requirements Computer literacy, minimum overall college GPA of 3.0, transcript of college record, written essay, interview, 2 letters of recommendation, nursing research course, prerequisite course work, statistics course. *Application deadline:* 7/1 (fall). *Application fee:* $40.
Degree Requirements 63 total credit hours, thesis or project.

University of Detroit Mercy
McAuley School of Nursing
Detroit, Michigan

http://www.udmercy.edu/healthprof/nursing/
Founded in 1877

DEGREES • BSN • MSN

Nursing Program Faculty 80
Baccalaureate Enrollment 933 **Women** 88% **Men** 12% **Minority** 24% **International** 6% **Part-time** 46%
Graduate Enrollment 132 **Women** 95% **Men** 5% **Minority** 27% **International** 2% **Part-time** 96%
Distance Learning Courses Available.
Nursing Student Activities Sigma Theta Tau, Student Nurses' Association.
Nursing Student Resources Academic advising; academic or career counseling; bookstore; campus computer network; career placement assistance; computer lab; computer-assisted instruction; e-mail services; Internet; learning resource lab; library services; nursing audiovisuals; other; paid internships; placement services for program completers; remedial services; resume preparation assistance; skills, simulation, or other laboratory; tutoring.
Library Facilities 32,330 volumes in health, 3,404 volumes in nursing; 2,670 periodical subscriptions health-care related.

BACCALAUREATE PROGRAMS

Degree BSN
Available Programs Accelerated Baccalaureate for Second Degree; Generic Baccalaureate; RN Baccalaureate.
Site Options Dearborn, MI; Grand Rapids, MI; Wayne, MI.
Study Options Full-time and part-time.
Program Entrance Requirements Minimum overall college GPA of 2.5, transcript of college record, CPR certification, health exam, health insurance, high school biology, high school chemistry, 2 years high school math, 2 years high school science, high school transcript, immunizations, minimum high school GPA of 2.5, minimum GPA in nursing prerequisites of 2.5, prerequisite course work. Transfer students are accepted.
Advanced Placement Credit given for nursing courses completed elsewhere dependent upon specific evaluations.
Contact ***Telephone:*** 313-993-1245. *Fax:* 313-993-3325.

GRADUATE PROGRAMS

Contact ***Telephone:*** 313-993-6423. *Fax:* 313-993-6175.

MASTER'S DEGREE PROGRAM

Degree MSN
Available Programs Accelerated AD/RN to Master's; Master's; Master's for Nurses with Non-Nursing Degrees.
Concentrations Available Nursing administration; nursing education. *Nurse practitioner programs in:* family health.
Study Options Full-time and part-time.
Program Entrance Requirements Clinical experience, minimum overall college GPA of 3.0, transcript of college record, CPR certification, immunizations, interview, 3 letters of recommendation, resume.
Degree Requirements 50 total credit hours.

POST-MASTER'S PROGRAM

Areas of Study Nursing administration; nursing education. *Nurse practitioner programs in:* family health.

University of Michigan
School of Nursing
Ann Arbor, Michigan

http://www.nursing.umich.edu
Founded in 1817

DEGREES • BSN • MS • MSN/MBA • MSN/MPH • PHD

Nursing Program Faculty 130 (66% with doctorates).
Baccalaureate Enrollment 618 **Women** 90% **Men** 10% **Minority** 20% **International** 3% **Part-time** 13%
Graduate Enrollment 240 **Women** 95% **Men** 5% **Minority** 30% **International** 11% **Part-time** 40%
Distance Learning Courses Available.
Nursing Student Activities Nursing Honor Society, Sigma Theta Tau, Student Nurses' Association, nursing club.
Nursing Student Resources Academic advising; academic or career counseling; assistance for students with disabilities; bookstore; campus computer network; career placement assistance; computer lab; computer-assisted instruction; daycare for children of students; e-mail services; employment services for current students; externships; housing assistance; interactive nursing skills videos; Internet; learning resource lab; library services; nursing audiovisuals; paid internships; placement services for program completers; remedial services; resume preparation assistance; skills, simulation, or other laboratory; tutoring; unpaid internships.
Library Facilities 9.6 million volumes (1.2 million in nursing); 70,047 periodical subscriptions.

BACCALAUREATE PROGRAMS

Degree BSN
Available Programs Accelerated Baccalaureate for Second Degree; Generic Baccalaureate; RN Baccalaureate.
Site Options Kalamazoo, MI; Traverse City, MI.
Study Options Full-time and part-time.
Program Entrance Requirements Minimum overall college GPA of 3.0, transcript of college record, written essay, high school chemistry, 2 years high school math, 2 years high school science, high school transcript, minimum high school GPA of 3.0, prerequisite course work. Transfer students are accepted. *Application deadline:* 2/1 (fall). Applications may be processed on a rolling basis for some programs. *Application fee:* $80.
Advanced Placement Credit given for nursing courses completed elsewhere dependent upon specific evaluations.
Contact ***Telephone:*** 734-647-1443. *Fax:* 734-936-0740.

GRADUATE PROGRAMS

Contact ***Telephone:*** 734-764-7188. *Fax:* 734-647-1419.

MASTER'S DEGREE PROGRAM

Degrees MS; MSN/MBA; MSN/MPH
Available Programs Accelerated RN to Master's; Master's; RN to Master's.
Concentrations Available Health-care administration; nurse-midwifery; nursing administration; nursing informatics. *Clinical nurse specialist programs in:* community health, gerontology, home health care, medical-surgical, occupational health, psychiatric/mental health. *Nurse practitioner programs in:* acute care, adult health, family health, gerontology, pediatric, primary care, psychiatric/mental health.
Study Options Full-time and part-time.
Program Entrance Requirements Computer literacy, minimum overall college GPA of 3.0, transcript of college record, written essay, interview, 3 letters of recommendation, resume, GRE General Test (if undergraduate GPA less than 3.25). *Application deadline:* 2/1 (fall). Applications may be processed on a rolling basis for some programs. *Application fee:* $80.
Advanced Placement Credit given for nursing courses completed elsewhere dependent upon specific evaluations.
Degree Requirements 37 total credit hours, thesis or project.

POST-MASTER'S PROGRAM

Areas of Study Health-care administration; nurse-midwifery; nursing administration; nursing informatics. *Clinical nurse specialist programs in:* community health, gerontology, home health care, medical-surgical, occupational health, psychiatric/mental health, women's health. *Nurse practitioner programs in:* acute care, adult health, family health, gerontology, pediatric, primary care, psychiatric/mental health, women's health.

DOCTORAL DEGREE PROGRAM

Degree PhD
Available Programs Doctorate; Post-Baccalaureate Doctorate.
Areas of Study Advanced practice nursing, aging, bio-behavioral research, biology of health and illness, community health, critical care, ethics, family health, gerontology, health policy, health promotion/disease prevention, health-care systems, individualized study, information systems, neuro-behavior, nursing administration, nursing policy, nursing research, nursing science, women's health.
Program Entrance Requirements Minimum overall college GPA of 3.0, interview, 3 letters of recommendation, scholarly papers, vita, writing sample, GRE General Test. Application deadline: 12/11 (fall). Application fee: $80.

Degree Requirements 50 total credit hours, dissertation, oral exam, written exam, residency.

POSTDOCTORAL PROGRAM

Areas of Study Addiction/substance abuse, aging, chronic illness, community health, family health, gerontology, health promotion/disease prevention, individualized study, information systems, neuro-behavior, nursing interventions, nursing research, nursing science, vulnerable population, women's health.
Postdoctoral Program Contact *Telephone:* 734-764-9454. *Fax:* 734-763-6668.

University of Michigan–Flint

Department of Nursing
Flint, Michigan

http://www.umflint.edu/nur
Founded in 1956

DEGREES • BSN • DNP • MSN

Nursing Program Faculty 95 (18% with doctorates).
Baccalaureate Enrollment 407 **Women** 79.61% **Men** 20.39% **Minority** 11.55% **International** .98% **Part-time** 44.23%
Graduate Enrollment 135 **Women** 82.22% **Men** 17.78% **Minority** 6.67% **International** .02% **Part-time** 67.44%
Distance Learning Courses Available.
Nursing Student Activities Nursing Honor Society, Sigma Theta Tau, Student Nurses' Association.
Nursing Student Resources Academic advising; academic or career counseling; assistance for students with disabilities; bookstore; campus computer network; career placement assistance; computer lab; computer-assisted instruction; daycare for children of students; e-mail services; employment services for current students; externships; housing assistance; interactive nursing skills videos; Internet; library services; nursing audiovisuals; remedial services; resume preparation assistance; skills, simulation, or other laboratory; tutoring.
Library Facilities 273,881 volumes (8,300 in health, 5,440 in nursing); 905 periodical subscriptions (16,451 health-care related).

BACCALAUREATE PROGRAMS

Degree BSN
Available Programs Accelerated Baccalaureate for Second Degree; Generic Baccalaureate; RN Baccalaureate.
Site Options Lansing, MI; Flint, MI.
Study Options Full-time.
Online Degree Options Yes.
Program Entrance Requirements Minimum overall college GPA of 3.00, transcript of college record, CPR certification, written essay, health exam, health insurance, immunizations, 2 letters of recommendation, minimum GPA in nursing prerequisites of 3.00, prerequisite course work. Transfer students are accepted. *Application deadline:* 1/10 (fall), 9/1 (winter). *Application fee:* $30.
Advanced Placement Credit given for nursing courses completed elsewhere dependent upon specific evaluations.
Expenses (2010-11) *Tuition, state resident:* full-time $9208; part-time $384 per credit. *Tuition, nonresident:* full-time $18,418; part-time $767 per credit. *Room and board:* $7080; room only: $4402 per academic year. *Required fees:* full-time $536; part-time $210 per term.
Financial Aid 86% of baccalaureate students in nursing programs received some form of financial aid in 2009-10. *Gift aid (need-based):* Federal Pell, FSEOG, state, private, college/university gift aid from institutional funds, TEACH Grants. *Loans:* Federal Direct (Subsidized and Unsubsidized Stafford PLUS), Perkins. *Work-study:* Federal Work-Study, part-time campus jobs. *Financial aid application deadline (priority):* 3/1.
Contact Ms. Marge Hathaway, Administrative Specialist, Department of Nursing, University of Michigan–Flint, 303 East Kearsley, 2180 WSW, Flint, MI 48502-1950. *Telephone:* 810-762-3420. *Fax:* 810-766-6851. *E-mail:* mhath@umflint.edu.

GRADUATE PROGRAMS

Expenses (2010-11) *Tuition, state resident:* full-time $8062; part-time $448 per credit. *Tuition, nonresident:* full-time $12,096; part-time $672 per credit. *International tuition:* $12,096 full-time. *Room and board:* $7080; room only: $4402 per academic year. *Required fees:* full-time $536; part-time $210 per term.
Financial Aid 60% of graduate students in nursing programs received some form of financial aid in 2009-10.
Contact Ms. Marge Hathaway, Administrative Specialist, Department of Nursing, University of Michigan–Flint, 303 East Kearsley, Flint, MI 48502-1950. *Telephone:* 810-762-3420. *Fax:* 810-766-6851. *E-mail:* nursing@list.flint.umich.edu.

MASTER'S DEGREE PROGRAM

Degree MSN
Available Programs Accelerated RN to Master's.
Concentrations Available Nurse anesthesia. *Nurse practitioner programs in:* adult health, family health, psychiatric/mental health.
Site Options Flint, MI.
Study Options Full-time.
Online Degree Options Yes.
Program Entrance Requirements Minimum overall college GPA of 3.5, transcript of college record, written essay, 3 letters of recommendation, resume. *Application deadline:* 8/1 (fall), 12/1 (winter). *Application fee:* $65.
Advanced Placement Credit given for nursing courses completed elsewhere dependent upon specific evaluations.
Degree Requirements 43 total credit hours.

DOCTORAL DEGREE PROGRAM

Degree DNP
Available Programs Doctorate.
Areas of Study Clinical practice, family health.
Site Options Flint, MI.
Online Degree Options Yes (online only).
Program Entrance Requirements Minimum overall college GPA of 3.2, interview, 3 letters of recommendation, MSN or equivalent, statistics course, vita. Application deadline: 4/1 (fall). Application fee: $55.
Degree Requirements 36 total credit hours.

University of Phoenix–Metro Detroit Campus

College of Nursing
Southfield, Michigan

DEGREES • BSN • MSN

Nursing Program Faculty 15 (33% with doctorates).
Baccalaureate Enrollment 18 **Women** 94.4% **Men** 5.6% **Minority** 38.9%
Graduate Enrollment 4 **Women** 100%
Nursing Student Activities Sigma Theta Tau.
Nursing Student Resources Academic advising; academic or career counseling; assistance for students with disabilities; bookstore; campus computer network; computer lab; computer-assisted instruction; e-mail services; interactive nursing skills videos; Internet; learning resource lab; library services; nursing audiovisuals; skills, simulation, or other laboratory; tutoring.
Library Facilities 1,759 volumes; 692 periodical subscriptions (1,300 health-care related).

BACCALAUREATE PROGRAMS

Degree BSN
Available Programs Accelerated Baccalaureate.
Site Options Livonia, MI; Ann Arbor, MI; Southfield, MI.
Study Options Full-time.
Program Entrance Requirements Transcript of college record, CPR certification, immunizations, 1 letter of recommendation, RN licensure. Transfer students are accepted. *Application deadline:* Applications may be processed on a rolling basis for some programs.
Advanced Placement Credit by examination available. Credit given for nursing courses completed elsewhere dependent upon specific evaluations.
Expenses (2009-10) *Tuition:* full-time $10,560. *Required fees:* full-time $600.
Contact Campus College Chair, Nursing, College of Nursing, University of Phoenix–Metro Detroit Campus, 5480 Corporate Drive, Suite 240, Troy, MI 48098-2623. *Telephone:* 800-834-2438.

GRADUATE PROGRAMS

Expenses (2009-10) *Tuition:* full-time $13,200. *Required fees:* full-time $760.

Financial Aid Institutionally sponsored loans and scholarships available.
Contact Campus College Chair, Nursing, College of Nursing, University of Phoenix–Metro Detroit Campus, 5480 Corporate Drive, Suite 240, Troy, MI 48098-2623. *Telephone:* 800-834-2438.

MASTER'S DEGREE PROGRAM

Degree MSN
Available Programs Master's.
Concentrations Available Health-care administration; nursing administration; nursing education.
Site Options Livonia, MI; Ann Arbor, MI; Southfield, MI.
Study Options Full-time.
Program Entrance Requirements Clinical experience, computer literacy, minimum overall college GPA of 2.5, transcript of college record. *Application deadline:* Applications may be processed on a rolling basis for some programs. *Application fee:* $45.
Advanced Placement Credit given for nursing courses completed elsewhere dependent upon specific evaluations.
Degree Requirements 39 total credit hours, thesis or project.

University of Phoenix–West Michigan Campus

College of Health and Human Services
Walker, Michigan

Founded in 2000
Nursing Program Faculty 2
Nursing Student Activities Sigma Theta Tau.
Nursing Student Resources Academic advising; academic or career counseling; assistance for students with disabilities; bookstore; computer lab; computer-assisted instruction; e-mail services; interactive nursing skills videos; Internet; learning resource lab; library services; nursing audiovisuals; remedial services; resume preparation assistance; skills, simulation, or other laboratory.
Library Facilities 16,781 periodical subscriptions (1,300 health-care related).

Wayne State University

College of Nursing
Detroit, Michigan

http://www.nursing.wayne.edu
Founded in 1868

DEGREES • BSN • DNP • MSN

Nursing Program Faculty 86 (35% with doctorates).
Baccalaureate Enrollment 342 **Women** 74% **Men** 26% **Minority** 17% **International** 5% **Part-time** 28%
Graduate Enrollment 415 **Women** 91.5% **Men** 8.5% **Minority** 20% **International** 4.5% **Part-time** 70%
Distance Learning Courses Available.
Nursing Student Activities Nursing Honor Society, Sigma Theta Tau, Student Nurses' Association, nursing club.
Nursing Student Resources Academic advising; academic or career counseling; assistance for students with disabilities; bookstore; campus computer network; career placement assistance; computer lab; computer-assisted instruction; e-mail services; employment services for current students; interactive nursing skills videos; Internet; learning resource lab; library services; nursing audiovisuals; placement services for program completers; resume preparation assistance; skills, simulation, or other laboratory; tutoring.
Library Facilities 3.7 million volumes (156,000 in health, 6,600 in nursing); 16,068 periodical subscriptions (5,000 health-care related).

BACCALAUREATE PROGRAMS

Degree BSN
Available Programs Accelerated Baccalaureate for Second Degree; Generic Baccalaureate.
Study Options Full-time and part-time.
Program Entrance Requirements Minimum overall college GPA of 2.0, transcript of college record, minimum GPA in nursing prerequisites of 2.5, prerequisite course work. Transfer students are accepted. *Application deadline:* 3/31 (fall). *Application fee:* $50.
Expenses (2009-10) *Tuition, area resident:* full-time $8872. *Tuition, nonresident:* full-time $18,711. *International tuition:* $18,711 full-time. *Room and board:* $7659 per academic year. *Required fees:* full-time $2200.
Contact Office of Student Affairs, College of Nursing, Wayne State University, 5557 Cass Avenue, Detroit, MI 48202. *Telephone:* 313-577-4082. *Fax:* 313-577-6949.

GRADUATE PROGRAMS

Expenses (2009-10) *Tuition, area resident:* full-time $6671. *Tuition, nonresident:* full-time $12,188. *Room and board:* $7659 per academic year.
Financial Aid 2 fellowships (averaging $13,901 per year), 2 research assistantships (averaging $16,028 per year), 4 teaching assistantships (averaging $22,997 per year) were awarded; Federal Work-Study, institutionally sponsored loans, scholarships, and traineeships also available.
Contact Office of Student Affairs, College of Nursing, Wayne State University, 5557 Cass Avenue, Detroit, MI 48202. *Telephone:* 313-577-4082. *Fax:* 313-577-6949.

MASTER'S DEGREE PROGRAM

Degree MSN
Available Programs Master's.
Concentrations Available Nurse-midwifery. *Clinical nurse specialist programs in:* acute care, community health, critical care, psychiatric/mental health. *Nurse practitioner programs in:* acute care, gerontology, neonatal health, pediatric, primary care, psychiatric/mental health, women's health.
Study Options Full-time and part-time.
Program Entrance Requirements Minimum overall college GPA of 3.0, transcript of college record, written essay, 3 letters of recommendation, resume. *Application deadline:* 7/1 (fall), 11/1 (winter), 4/1 (spring), 4/1 (summer).
Advanced Placement Credit given for nursing courses completed elsewhere dependent upon specific evaluations.
Degree Requirements 47 total credit hours.

POST-MASTER'S PROGRAM

Areas of Study Nurse-midwifery; nursing education. *Clinical nurse specialist programs in:* psychiatric/mental health. *Nurse practitioner programs in:* acute care, gerontology, pediatric, primary care, psychiatric/mental health, women's health.

DOCTORAL DEGREE PROGRAM

Degree DNP
Available Programs Doctorate; Post-Baccalaureate Doctorate.
Areas of Study Advanced practice nursing, clinical practice.
Program Entrance Requirements Clinical experience, minimum overall college GPA of 3.0, interview by faculty committee, interview, 2 letters of recommendation, vita, writing sample, GRE General Test. Application deadline: 1/15 (fall). Applications may be processed on a rolling basis for some programs. Application fee: $50.
Degree Requirements 90 total credit hours, written exam, residency.

POSTDOCTORAL PROGRAM

Areas of Study Adolescent health, community health, individualized study, self-care.
Postdoctoral Program Contact Dennis Ross, Academic Services Officer, College of Nursing, Wayne State University, 5557 Cass Avenue, Detroit, MI 48202. *Telephone:* 313-577-4082. *Fax:* 313-577-6949. *E-mail:* nursinginfo@wayne.edu.

CONTINUING EDUCATION PROGRAM

Contact Office of the Dean, College of Nursing, Wayne State University, 5557 Cass Avenue, Detroit, MI 48202. *Telephone:* 313-577-4070. *E-mail:* nursinginfo@wayne.edu.

Western Michigan University

College of Health and Human Services
Kalamazoo, Michigan

Founded in 1903

DEGREES • BSN • MSN

Nursing Program Faculty 38 (26% with doctorates).
Baccalaureate Enrollment 383 **Women** 85% **Men** 15% **Minority** 11% **International** 1% **Part-time** 21%

Graduate Enrollment 7 **Women** 85% **Men** 15% **Minority** 15% **Part-time** 100%

Nursing Student Activities Sigma Theta Tau, Student Nurses' Association.

Nursing Student Resources Academic advising; academic or career counseling; assistance for students with disabilities; bookstore; campus computer network; career placement assistance; computer lab; computer-assisted instruction; daycare for children of students; e-mail services; employment services for current students; externships; housing assistance; interactive nursing skills videos; Internet; learning resource lab; library services; nursing audiovisuals; placement services for program completers; remedial services; resume preparation assistance; skills, simulation, or other laboratory.

Library Facilities 2.8 million volumes (766 in nursing); 37,826 periodical subscriptions (362 health-care related).

BACCALAUREATE PROGRAMS

Degree BSN

Available Programs ADN to Baccalaureate; Generic Baccalaureate.

Site Options St. Joseph, MI.

Study Options Full-time and part-time.

Program Entrance Requirements Minimum overall college GPA of 3.0, transcript of college record, CPR certification, high school biology, high school chemistry, 3 years high school math, 3 years high school science, high school transcript, immunizations, minimum high school GPA of 3.0, minimum GPA in nursing prerequisites of 3.0, prerequisite course work. Transfer students are accepted. *Application deadline:* Applications may be processed on a rolling basis for some programs. *Application fee:* $35.

Advanced Placement Credit given for nursing courses completed elsewhere dependent upon specific evaluations.

Expenses (2010-11) *Tuition, state resident:* full-time $8182. *Tuition, nonresident:* full-time $20,070. *Room and board:* $9942; room only: $6223 per academic year. *Required fees:* full-time $824; part-time $475 per term.

Financial Aid 43% of baccalaureate students in nursing programs received some form of financial aid in 2009-10.

Contact Mrs. Marsha Ann Mahan, Student Advisor, College of Health and Human Services, Western Michigan University, 1903 West Michigan Avenue, Kalamazoo, MI 49008. *Telephone:* 269-387-8150. *Fax:* 269-387-8170. *E-mail:* marsha.mahan@wmich.edu.

GRADUATE PROGRAMS

Expenses (2010-11) *Tuition, state resident:* part-time $429 per credit hour. *Tuition, nonresident:* part-time $909 per credit hour. *Required fees:* part-time $412 per term.

Financial Aid 100% of graduate students in nursing programs received some form of financial aid in 2009-10. 2 fellowships (averaging $4,056 per year), 8 research assistantships (averaging $9,839 per year), 14 teaching assistantships (averaging $4,802 per year) were awarded; Federal Work-Study also available. *Financial aid application deadline:* 2/15.

Contact Dr. Linda H. Zoeller, Director and Professor, College of Health and Human Services, Western Michigan University, 1903 West Michigan Avenue, Kalamazoo, MI 49008-5345. *Telephone:* 269-387-8162. *E-mail:* linda.zoeller@wmich.edu.

MASTER'S DEGREE PROGRAM

Degree MSN

Available Programs Master's.

Concentrations Available Nursing administration; nursing education.

Site Options St. Joseph, MI.

Study Options Part-time.

Program Entrance Requirements Minimum overall college GPA of 3.4, transcript of college record, interview, 3 letters of recommendation, resume. *Application deadline:* Applications may be processed on a rolling basis for some programs. *Application fee:* $40.

Degree Requirements 36 total credit hours, thesis or project, comprehensive exam.

CONTINUING EDUCATION PROGRAM

Contact Ms. Marsha Ann Mahan, Student Advisor, College of Health and Human Services, Western Michigan University, 1903 West Michigan Avenue, Kalamazoo, MI 49008-5345. *Telephone:* 269-387-8150. *E-mail:* marsha.mahan@wmich.edu.

MINNESOTA

Augsburg College
Program in Nursing
Minneapolis, Minnesota

http://www.augsburg.edu/nursing
Founded in 1869

DEGREES • BS • MA

Nursing Program Faculty 9 (50% with doctorates).

Baccalaureate Enrollment 169 **Women** 83% **Men** 17% **Part-time** 89%

Graduate Enrollment 42 **Women** 100% **Minority** 2% **Part-time** 90%

Nursing Student Resources Academic advising; academic or career counseling; assistance for students with disabilities; bookstore; campus computer network; computer lab; computer-assisted instruction; e-mail services; Internet; library services; tutoring.

Library Facilities 146,166 volumes (1,550 in health, 200 in nursing); 754 periodical subscriptions (70 health-care related).

BACCALAUREATE PROGRAMS

Degree BS

Available Programs ADN to Baccalaureate.

Site Options Rochester, MN; Saint Paul, MN.

Study Options Full-time and part-time.

Program Entrance Requirements Minimum overall college GPA of 2.5, transcript of college record, CPR certification, written essay, high school transcript, immunizations, letters of recommendation, prerequisite course work, RN licensure. Transfer students are accepted.

Contact *Telephone:* 612-330-1101. *Fax:* 612-330-1784.

GRADUATE PROGRAMS

Contact *Telephone:* 612-330-1101. *Fax:* 612-330-1784.

MASTER'S DEGREE PROGRAM

Degree MA

Available Programs Master's.

Concentrations Available *Clinical nurse specialist programs in:* community health.

Site Options Rochester, MN; Saint Paul, MN.

Study Options Full-time and part-time.

Program Entrance Requirements Computer literacy, minimum overall college GPA of 3.0, transcript of college record, written essay, immunizations, 3 letters of recommendation, prerequisite course work, statistics course.

Advanced Placement Credit given for nursing courses completed elsewhere dependent upon specific evaluations.

Degree Requirements 48 total credit hours, thesis or project.

Bemidji State University
Department of Nursing
Bemidji, Minnesota

http://www.bemidjistate.edu/academics/departments/nursing/
Founded in 1919

DEGREE • BS

Nursing Program Faculty 5 (60% with doctorates).

Baccalaureate Enrollment 62 **Women** 95% **Men** 5% **Minority** 3% **Part-time** 68%

Distance Learning Courses Available.

Nursing Student Resources Academic advising; academic or career counseling; assistance for students with disabilities; bookstore; campus computer network; career placement assistance; computer lab; computer-assisted instruction; daycare for children of students; e-mail services; employment services for current students; housing assistance; Internet; library services; nursing audiovisuals; remedial services; tutoring.

Library Facilities 554,087 volumes (9,000 in health, 1,000 in nursing); 991 periodical subscriptions (300 health-care related).

BACCALAUREATE PROGRAMS

Degree BS

Available Programs Generic Baccalaureate; RN Baccalaureate.

Study Options Full-time and part-time.

Program Entrance Requirements Minimum overall college GPA, transcript of college record, immunizations, professional liability insurance/malpractice insurance, RN licensure. Transfer students are accepted.
Contact *Telephone:* 218-755-3892. *Fax:* 218-755-4402.

CONTINUING EDUCATION PROGRAM

Contact *Telephone:* 218-755-3892. *Fax:* 218-755-4402.

Bethel University

Department of Nursing
St. Paul, Minnesota

http://www.bethel.edu/college/dept/nursing/index.html
Founded in 1871

DEGREES • BSN • MA
Nursing Program Faculty 36 (40% with doctorates).
Baccalaureate Enrollment 283 **Women** 93.6% **Men** 6.4% **Minority** 11%
Graduate Enrollment 66 **Women** 97% **Men** 3% **Minority** 9.1%
Distance Learning Courses Available.
Nursing Student Activities Sigma Theta Tau, nursing club.
Nursing Student Resources Academic advising; academic or career counseling; assistance for students with disabilities; bookstore; campus computer network; career placement assistance; computer lab; computer-assisted instruction; daycare for children of students; e-mail services; employment services for current students; interactive nursing skills videos; Internet; learning resource lab; library services; nursing audiovisuals; paid internships; placement services for program completers; remedial services; resume preparation assistance; skills, simulation, or other laboratory; tutoring.
Library Facilities 194,000 volumes (4,900 in nursing); 38,080 periodical subscriptions (1,006 health-care related).

BACCALAUREATE PROGRAMS

Degree BSN
Available Programs Generic Baccalaureate; RN Baccalaureate.
Site Options Brooklyn Park, MN.
Study Options Full-time and part-time.
Program Entrance Requirements Minimum overall college GPA of 2.5, transcript of college record, CPR certification, written essay, health exam, health insurance, high school transcript, immunizations, interview, 2 letters of recommendation, minimum GPA in nursing prerequisites of 2.5, professional liability insurance/malpractice insurance, prerequisite course work. Transfer students are accepted. *Application deadline:* 9/15 (fall).
Advanced Placement Credit given for nursing courses completed elsewhere dependent upon specific evaluations.
Expenses (2009-10) *Tuition:* full-time $26,900; part-time $1125 per credit. *International tuition:* $26,900 full-time. *Room and board:* $8920; room only: $5720 per academic year. *Required fees:* full-time $385; part-time $193 per term.
Financial Aid 80% of baccalaureate students in nursing programs received some form of financial aid in 2008-09. *Gift aid (need-based):* Federal Pell, FSEOG, state, private, college/university gift aid from institutional funds. *Loans:* Federal Direct (Subsidized and Unsubsidized Stafford PLUS), Perkins, state, alternative loans. *Work-study:* Federal Work-Study, part-time campus jobs. *Financial aid application deadline (priority):* 4/15.
Contact Dr. Elizabeth A. Peterson, RN, Director, Pre-Professional Program, Department of Nursing, Bethel University, 3900 Bethel Drive, St. Paul, MN 55112-6999. *Telephone:* 651-638-6455. *Fax:* 651-635-1965. *E-mail:* e-peterson@bethel.edu.

GRADUATE PROGRAMS

Expenses (2009-10) *Tuition:* part-time $450 per credit.
Financial Aid 50% of graduate students in nursing programs received some form of financial aid in 2008-09.
Contact Ms. Jeanne Shaw, Admissions Advisor, Department of Nursing, Bethel University, 3900 Bethel Drive, PO #2377, St. Paul, MN 55112. *Telephone:* 651-635-8080. *Fax:* 651-635-1965. *E-mail:* jeanne-shaw@bethel.edu.

MASTER'S DEGREE PROGRAM

Degree MA
Available Programs Master's.
Concentrations Available Nursing administration; nursing education.
Study Options Full-time and part-time.
Program Entrance Requirements Clinical experience, computer literacy, minimum overall college GPA of 3.0, transcript of college record, written essay, immunizations, interview, 3 letters of recommendation, professional liability insurance/malpractice insurance, resume, statistics course, MAT. *Application deadline:* Applications may be processed on a rolling basis for some programs. *Application fee:* $25.
Advanced Placement Credit given for nursing courses completed elsewhere dependent upon specific evaluations.
Degree Requirements 43 total credit hours, thesis or project.

College of Saint Benedict

Department of Nursing
Saint Joseph, Minnesota

http://www.csbsju.edu/nursing/
Founded in 1887

DEGREE • BS
Nursing Program Faculty 17 (35% with doctorates).
Baccalaureate Enrollment 136 **Women** 90.5% **Men** 9.5% **Minority** 1% **International** 1%
Nursing Student Activities Sigma Theta Tau, Student Nurses' Association, nursing club.
Nursing Student Resources Academic advising; academic or career counseling; assistance for students with disabilities; bookstore; campus computer network; career placement assistance; computer lab; computer-assisted instruction; e-mail services; employment services for current students; interactive nursing skills videos; Internet; learning resource lab; library services; nursing audiovisuals; paid internships; placement services for program completers; resume preparation assistance; skills, simulation, or other laboratory; tutoring; unpaid internships.
Library Facilities 658,438 volumes (7,300 in health, 700 in nursing); 71,720 periodical subscriptions (335 health-care related).

BACCALAUREATE PROGRAMS

Degree BS
Available Programs Generic Baccalaureate.
Study Options Full-time.
Program Entrance Requirements Transcript of college record, CPR certification, health exam, health insurance, immunizations, minimum GPA in nursing prerequisites of 2.75, professional liability insurance/malpractice insurance, prerequisite course work. *Application deadline:* 12/1 (fall).
Advanced Placement Credit given for nursing courses completed elsewhere dependent upon specific evaluations.
Expenses (2009-10) *Tuition:* full-time $30,000; part-time $350 per credit. *Required fees:* full-time $700.
Financial Aid 93% of baccalaureate students in nursing programs received some form of financial aid in 2008-09. *Gift aid (need-based):* Federal Pell, FSEOG, state, private, college/university gift aid from institutional funds. *Loans:* Federal Direct (Subsidized and Unsubsidized Stafford PLUS), Perkins, state, private alternative loans. *Work-study:* Federal Work-Study, part-time campus jobs. *Financial aid application deadline (priority):* 3/15.
Contact Dr. Carie Ann Braun, Associate Professor and Chair, Department of Nursing, College of Saint Benedict, 37 College Avenue South, St. Joseph, MN 56374. *Telephone:* 320-363-5223. *Fax:* 320-363-6099. *E-mail:* cbraun@csbsju.edu.

The College of St. Scholastica

Department of Nursing
Duluth, Minnesota

http://www.css.edu/nursing.xml
Founded in 1912

DEGREES • BS • DNP • MA
Nursing Program Faculty 33 (33% with doctorates).
Baccalaureate Enrollment 392 **Women** 90.1% **Men** 9.9% **Minority** 18.9% **International** .3% **Part-time** 23.7%
Graduate Enrollment 170 **Women** 95.3% **Men** 4.7% **Minority** 13% **International** 2.3% **Part-time** 76.5%

Distance Learning Courses Available.

Nursing Student Activities Sigma Theta Tau, Student Nurses' Association.

Nursing Student Resources Academic advising; academic or career counseling; assistance for students with disabilities; bookstore; campus computer network; career placement assistance; computer lab; computer-assisted instruction; e-mail services; Internet; learning resource lab; library services; nursing audiovisuals; paid internships; placement services for program completers; resume preparation assistance; skills, simulation, or other laboratory; tutoring; unpaid internships.

Library Facilities 152,843 volumes (7,280 in health, 1,150 in nursing); 48,087 periodical subscriptions (291 health-care related).

BACCALAUREATE PROGRAMS

Degree BS

Available Programs ADN to Baccalaureate; Accelerated Baccalaureate for Second Degree; Generic Baccalaureate.

Site Options Duluth, MN.

Study Options Full-time.

Online Degree Options Yes.

Program Entrance Requirements Minimum overall college GPA of 3.0, transcript of college record, CPR certification, health insurance, high school transcript, immunizations, minimum GPA in nursing prerequisites of 2.0, prerequisite course work. Transfer students are accepted. *Application deadline:* 9/25 (fall).

Expenses (2010-11) *Tuition:* full-time $28,200; part-time $881 per credit. *Room and board:* $7498; room only: $4824 per academic year. *Required fees:* full-time $450; part-time $265 per term.

Financial Aid 98% of baccalaureate students in nursing programs received some form of financial aid in 2009-10. *Gift aid (need-based):* Federal Pell, FSEOG, state, private, college/university gift aid from institutional funds. *Loans:* Federal Nursing Student Loans, Federal Direct (Subsidized and Unsubsidized Stafford PLUS), Perkins, state, private loans. *Work-study:* Federal Work-Study, part-time campus jobs. *Financial aid application deadline (priority):* 3/1.

Contact Ms. Paula Byrne, Chair, Department of Traditional Undergraduate Nursing, Department of Nursing, The College of St. Scholastica, 1200 Kenwood Avenue, Duluth, MN 55811. *Telephone:* 218-723-6020. *Fax:* 218-733-2221. *E-mail:* pbyrne@css.edu.

GRADUATE PROGRAMS

Expenses (2010-11) *Tuition:* part-time $695 per credit. *Required fees:* full-time $300; part-time $150 per term.

Financial Aid 90% of graduate students in nursing programs received some form of financial aid in 2009-10. Scholarships and traineeships available. Aid available to part-time students.

Contact Dr. Sally Fauchald, Chair, Graduate Nursing Department, Department of Nursing, The College of St. Scholastica, 1200 Kenwood Avenue, Duluth, MN 55811. *Telephone:* 218-723-6590. *Fax:* 218-733-2221. *E-mail:* sfauchal@css.edu.

MASTER'S DEGREE PROGRAM

Degree MA

Available Programs Master's.

Concentrations Available Nursing administration. *Clinical nurse specialist programs in:* adult health, gerontology. *Nurse practitioner programs in:* adult health, family health, gerontology, pediatric, psychiatric/mental health.

Site Options Duluth, MN.

Study Options Full-time and part-time.

Program Entrance Requirements Clinical experience, computer literacy, minimum overall college GPA of 3.0, transcript of college record, CPR certification, written essay, immunizations, interview, 3 letters of recommendation, nursing research course, physical assessment course, professional liability insurance/malpractice insurance, resume, statistics course, GRE General Test or MAT. *Application deadline:* 3/1 (spring). *Application fee:* $50.

Advanced Placement Credit given for nursing courses completed elsewhere dependent upon specific evaluations.

Degree Requirements 47 total credit hours, thesis or project.

POST-MASTER'S PROGRAM

Areas of Study Nursing administration; nursing informatics. *Clinical nurse specialist programs in:* adult health, gerontology. *Nurse practitioner programs in:* adult health, family health, gerontology, pediatric, psychiatric/mental health.

DOCTORAL DEGREE PROGRAM

Degree DNP

Available Programs Doctorate; Post-Baccalaureate Doctorate.

Areas of Study Advanced practice nursing, health policy, nursing administration, nursing education, nursing policy.

Site Options Duluth, MN.

Program Entrance Requirements Minimum overall college GPA of 3.0, interview by faculty committee, 3 letters of recommendation, MSN or equivalent, vita, writing sample. Application deadline: 3/1 (spring). Application fee: $50.

Degree Requirements 30 total credit hours, dissertation.

POSTDOCTORAL PROGRAM

Postdoctoral Program Contact Dr. Carleen A. Maynard, Chair, Graduate Nursing Department, Department of Nursing, The College of St. Scholastica, 1200 Kenwood Avenue, Duluth, MN 55811. *Telephone:* 218-723-6452. *Fax:* 218-733-2295. *E-mail:* cmaynard@css.edu.

Concordia College

Department of Nursing
Moorhead, Minnesota

http://www.cord.edu/dept/nursing/index.htm

Founded in 1891

DEGREES • BA • MS

Nursing Program Faculty 6 (33% with doctorates).

Baccalaureate Enrollment 75

Graduate Enrollment 2 **Women** 100%

Nursing Student Activities Sigma Theta Tau, Student Nurses' Association.

Nursing Student Resources Academic advising; academic or career counseling; assistance for students with disabilities; bookstore; campus computer network; career placement assistance; computer lab; computer-assisted instruction; e-mail services; employment services for current students; externships; housing assistance; interactive nursing skills videos; Internet; learning resource lab; library services; nursing audiovisuals; paid internships; placement services for program completers; remedial services; resume preparation assistance; skills, simulation, or other laboratory; tutoring; unpaid internships.

Library Facilities 346,108 volumes (2,135 in health, 837 in nursing); 3,425 periodical subscriptions (81 health-care related).

BACCALAUREATE PROGRAMS

Degree BA

Available Programs Accelerated Baccalaureate for Second Degree; Generic Baccalaureate.

Study Options Full-time.

Program Entrance Requirements Minimum overall college GPA of 2.9, transcript of college record, CPR certification, health exam, health insurance, immunizations, interview, 2 letters of recommendation, minimum GPA in nursing prerequisites of 2.7, professional liability insurance/malpractice insurance, prerequisite course work. Transfer students are accepted.

Advanced Placement Credit by examination available. Credit given for nursing courses completed elsewhere dependent upon specific evaluations.

Contact ***Telephone:*** 218-299-3879. *Fax:* 218-299-4309.

GRADUATE PROGRAMS

Contact ***Telephone:*** 218-299-3879. *Fax:* 218-299-4309.

MASTER'S DEGREE PROGRAM

Degree MS

Available Programs Master's.

Concentrations Available Nursing education.

Study Options Full-time and part-time.

Program Entrance Requirements Computer literacy, minimum overall college GPA of 3.0, transcript of college record, written essay, interview, 3 letters of recommendation.

Advanced Placement Credit given for nursing courses completed elsewhere dependent upon specific evaluations.

Degree Requirements 36 total credit hours, thesis or project, comprehensive exam.

Crown College
Nursing Department
St. Bonifacius, Minnesota

Founded in 1916

DEGREE • BSN

Nursing Program Faculty 6
Baccalaureate Enrollment 20 **Women** 100% **International** 10%
Distance Learning Courses Available.
Nursing Student Activities Student Nurses' Association.
Nursing Student Resources Academic advising; academic or career counseling; assistance for students with disabilities; bookstore; campus computer network; computer lab; computer-assisted instruction; e-mail services; employment services for current students; housing assistance; interactive nursing skills videos; Internet; learning resource lab; library services; nursing audiovisuals; remedial services; resume preparation assistance; skills, simulation, or other laboratory; tutoring; unpaid internships.
Library Facilities 104,859 volumes; 30,829 periodical subscriptions.

BACCALAUREATE PROGRAMS

Degree BSN
Available Programs Generic Baccalaureate.
Site Options Owatonna, MN.
Study Options Full-time.
Program Entrance Requirements CPR certification, written essay, health exam, immunizations, 2 letters of recommendation, minimum high school GPA, minimum GPA in nursing prerequisites of 2.5, prerequisite course work. Transfer students are accepted. *Application deadline:* 2/1 (spring).
Expenses (2009-10) *Tuition:* full-time $19,870. *Room and board:* $7366 per academic year. *Required fees:* full-time $200.
Financial Aid 90% of baccalaureate students in nursing programs received some form of financial aid in 2008-09. *Gift aid (need-based):* Federal Pell, FSEOG, state, private, college/university gift aid from institutional funds. *Loans:* Perkins, state, SELF Loans, CitiAssist Loans, Signature Loans, U.S. Bank No Fee Educational Loans, Wells Fargo Collegiate Loans. *Work-study:* Federal Work-Study, part-time campus jobs. *Financial aid application deadline:* 8/1(priority: 4/5).
Contact Nursing Department, Nursing Department, Crown College, 8700 College View Drive, St. Bonifacius, MN 55375-9001. *Telephone:* 952-446-4482. *E-mail:* nursing@crown.edu.

Globe University
Bachelor of Science in Nursing
Woodbury, Minnesota

Founded in 1885

DEGREE • BS

Nursing Program Faculty 16
Baccalaureate Enrollment 135
Nursing Student Activities Student Nurses' Association.
Nursing Student Resources Academic advising; academic or career counseling; assistance for students with disabilities; bookstore; campus computer network; career placement assistance; computer lab; computer-assisted instruction; e-mail services; employment services for current students; interactive nursing skills videos; Internet; learning resource lab; library services; nursing audiovisuals; placement services for program completers; remedial services; resume preparation assistance; skills, simulation, or other laboratory; tutoring; unpaid internships.
Library Facilities 7,512 volumes; 90 periodical subscriptions.

BACCALAUREATE PROGRAMS

Degree BS
Available Programs Generic Baccalaureate.
Study Options Full-time and part-time.
Program Entrance Requirements Minimum overall college GPA of 2.75, transcript of college record, CPR certification, written essay, health exam, high school biology, high school chemistry, 2 years high school science, high school transcript, immunizations, interview, 2 letters of recommendation, minimum high school GPA of 2.75, minimum high school rank 60%, minimum GPA in nursing prerequisites of 2.75, prerequisite course work. Transfer students are accepted. *Application deadline:* Applications may be processed on a rolling basis for some programs. *Application fee:* $50.
Advanced Placement Credit given for nursing courses completed elsewhere dependent upon specific evaluations.
Contact Karen Miller, Nursing Admissions Representative, Bachelor of Science in Nursing, Globe University, 1401 West 76th Street, Richfield, MN 55423. *Telephone:* 612-798-3762. *E-mail:* kmiller@msbcollege.edu.

Gustavus Adolphus College
Department of Nursing
St. Peter, Minnesota

Founded in 1862

DEGREE • BA

Nursing Program Faculty 9 (20% with doctorates).
Baccalaureate Enrollment 76 **Women** 92% **Men** 8% **Minority** 8% **International** 4%
Nursing Student Activities Sigma Theta Tau, Student Nurses' Association.
Nursing Student Resources Academic advising; academic or career counseling; assistance for students with disabilities; bookstore; campus computer network; career placement assistance; computer lab; computer-assisted instruction; e-mail services; employment services for current students; housing assistance; interactive nursing skills videos; Internet; learning resource lab; library services; nursing audiovisuals; paid internships; remedial services; resume preparation assistance; skills, simulation, or other laboratory; tutoring; unpaid internships.
Library Facilities 357,186 volumes; 23,619 periodical subscriptions.

BACCALAUREATE PROGRAMS

Degree BA
Available Programs Generic Baccalaureate.
Study Options Full-time.
Program Entrance Requirements Minimum overall college GPA of 2.7, transcript of college record, written essay, high school transcript, immunizations, interview, minimum GPA in nursing prerequisites, prerequisite course work. Transfer students are accepted.
Contact ***Telephone:*** 507-933-6126. *Fax:* 507-933-6153.

Metropolitan State University
College of Nursing and Health Sciences
St. Paul, Minnesota

http://www.metrostate.edu
Founded in 1971

DEGREES • BSN • MSN

Nursing Program Faculty 22 (18% with doctorates).
Baccalaureate Enrollment 230 **Women** 91% **Men** 9% **Minority** 9% **Part-time** 96%
Graduate Enrollment 40 **Women** 95% **Men** 5% **Minority** 8% **Part-time** 23%
Nursing Student Activities Sigma Theta Tau, Student Nurses' Association.
Nursing Student Resources Academic advising; academic or career counseling; assistance for students with disabilities; bookstore; campus computer network; computer lab; e-mail services; externships; Internet; library services; skills, simulation, or other laboratory.
Library Facilities 39,128 volumes; 242 periodical subscriptions.

BACCALAUREATE PROGRAMS

Degree BSN
Site Options Minneapolis, MN.
Study Options Full-time and part-time.
Program Entrance Requirements Minimum overall college GPA of 2.5, transcript of college record, health insurance, immunizations, minimum GPA in nursing prerequisites of 3.0, professional liability insurance/malpractice insurance, prerequisite course work. Transfer students are accepted.
Advanced Placement Credit given for nursing courses completed elsewhere dependent upon specific evaluations.
Contact ***Telephone:*** 651-793-1379. *Fax:* 651-793-1382.

GRADUATE PROGRAMS

Contact *Telephone:* 651-793-1378. *Fax:* 651-793-1382.

MASTER'S DEGREE PROGRAM

Degree MSN
Available Programs Master's for Nurses with Non-Nursing Degrees; RN to Master's.
Concentrations Available Nursing administration. *Nurse practitioner programs in:* adult health, family health.
Study Options Full-time and part-time.
Program Entrance Requirements Clinical experience, computer literacy, minimum overall college GPA of 3.0, transcript of college record, written essay, immunizations, interview, 3 letters of recommendation, professional liability insurance/malpractice insurance, resume, statistics course, GRE General Test.
Advanced Placement Credit given for nursing courses completed elsewhere dependent upon specific evaluations.
Degree Requirements 42 total credit hours, thesis or project.

POST-MASTER'S PROGRAM

Areas of Study *Nurse practitioner programs in:* adult health, family health.

Minnesota Intercollegiate Nursing Consortium

Minnesota Intercollegiate Nursing Consortium
Northfield, Minnesota

http://www.stolaf.edu/depts/nursing/

DEGREE • BA

Nursing Program Faculty 9 (67% with doctorates).
Baccalaureate Enrollment 98 **Women** 93% **Men** 7% **Minority** 7%
Nursing Student Activities Sigma Theta Tau, Student Nurses' Association.
Nursing Student Resources Academic advising; academic or career counseling; assistance for students with disabilities; bookstore; campus computer network; career placement assistance; computer lab; computer-assisted instruction; e-mail services; employment services for current students; externships; interactive nursing skills videos; Internet; learning resource lab; library services; nursing audiovisuals; paid internships; remedial services; resume preparation assistance; skills, simulation, or other laboratory; tutoring; unpaid internships.

BACCALAUREATE PROGRAMS

Degree BA
Available Programs Generic Baccalaureate.
Site Options St. Peter, MN; Northfield, MN.
Study Options Full-time.
Program Entrance Requirements Minimum overall college GPA of 2.85, transcript of college record, CPR certification, written essay, health exam, health insurance, immunizations, interview, minimum GPA in nursing prerequisites of 2.70, prerequisite course work. Transfer students are accepted. *Application deadline:* 10/31 (fall).
Expenses (2010-11) *Tuition:* full-time $34,950; part-time $3900 per course. *Room and board:* $8450 per academic year. *Required fees:* full-time $1350; part-time $675 per term.
Contact Dr. Rita S. Glazebrook, Director, Minnesota Intercollegiate Nursing Consortium, 1520 St. Olaf Avenue, Northfield, MN 55057-1098. *Telephone:* 507-786-3265. *Fax:* 507-786-3733. *E-mail:* glazebro@stolaf.edu.

Minnesota State University Mankato

School of Nursing
Mankato, Minnesota

http://www.mnsu.edu/nursing/
Founded in 1868

DEGREES • BS • DNP • MSN • MSN/MS

Nursing Program Faculty 48 (21% with doctorates).
Baccalaureate Enrollment 292 **Women** 90% **Men** 10% **Minority** 9% **International** 1% **Part-time** 1%
Graduate Enrollment 60 **Women** 96% **Men** 4% **Part-time** 48%
Distance Learning Courses Available.
Nursing Student Activities Nursing Honor Society, Sigma Theta Tau, Student Nurses' Association.
Nursing Student Resources Academic advising; academic or career counseling; assistance for students with disabilities; bookstore; campus computer network; career placement assistance; computer lab; computer-assisted instruction; daycare for children of students; e-mail services; employment services for current students; Internet; learning resource lab; library services; nursing audiovisuals; paid internships; placement services for program completers; resume preparation assistance; skills, simulation, or other laboratory; tutoring.
Library Facilities 1.2 million volumes (35,852 in health, 1,500 in nursing); 20,000 periodical subscriptions (156 health-care related).

BACCALAUREATE PROGRAMS

Degree BS
Available Programs Accelerated Baccalaureate for Second Degree; Generic Baccalaureate; RN Baccalaureate.
Study Options Full-time and part-time.
Program Entrance Requirements Minimum overall college GPA of 2.5, transcript of college record, health exam, health insurance, minimum GPA in nursing prerequisites of 2.0, prerequisite course work. Transfer students are accepted.
Advanced Placement Credit by examination available. Credit given for nursing courses completed elsewhere dependent upon specific evaluations.
Contact *Telephone:* 507-389-6828. *Fax:* 507-389-6516.

GRADUATE PROGRAMS

Contact *Telephone:* 507-389-1317. *Fax:* 507-389-6516.

MASTER'S DEGREE PROGRAM

Degrees MSN; MSN/MS
Available Programs Accelerated RN to Master's; Master's; Master's for Nurses with Non-Nursing Degrees; RN to Master's.
Concentrations Available Nursing education. *Clinical nurse specialist programs in:* adult health, family health, pediatric. *Nurse practitioner programs in:* family health.
Study Options Full-time and part-time.
Program Entrance Requirements Clinical experience, computer literacy, minimum overall college GPA of 3.0, transcript of college record, CPR certification, written essay, immunizations, 3 letters of recommendation, nursing research course, professional liability insurance/malpractice insurance, prerequisite course work, resume, statistics course.
Advanced Placement Credit given for nursing courses completed elsewhere dependent upon specific evaluations.
Degree Requirements 53 total credit hours, thesis or project.

POST-MASTER'S PROGRAM

Areas of Study Nursing education. *Clinical nurse specialist programs in:* family health. *Nurse practitioner programs in:* family health.

DOCTORAL DEGREE PROGRAM

Degree DNP
Available Programs Doctorate.
Degree Requirements 36 total credit hours.

CONTINUING EDUCATION PROGRAM

Contact *Telephone:* 507-389-5194. *Fax:* 507-389-6516.

Minnesota State University Moorhead

School of Nursing and Healthcare Leadership
Moorhead, Minnesota

http://www.mnstate.edu/nursing/
Founded in 1885

DEGREES • BSN • DNP • MS

Nursing Program Faculty 11 (36% with doctorates).
Baccalaureate Enrollment 296 **Women** 95% **Men** 5% **Minority** 3% **International** 3% **Part-time** 50%

Graduate Enrollment 33 **Women** 94% **Men** 6% **Minority** 6% **Part-time** 42%

Distance Learning Courses Available.

Nursing Student Activities Sigma Theta Tau, Student Nurses' Association.

Nursing Student Resources Academic advising; academic or career counseling; assistance for students with disabilities; bookstore; campus computer network; career placement assistance; computer lab; computer-assisted instruction; daycare for children of students; e-mail services; employment services for current students; Internet; library services; nursing audiovisuals; remedial services; resume preparation assistance; tutoring; unpaid internships.

Library Facilities 645,544 volumes (5,560 in health, 824 in nursing); 7,894 periodical subscriptions (50 health-care related).

BACCALAUREATE PROGRAMS

Degree BSN

Available Programs ADN to Baccalaureate; Generic Baccalaureate; RN Baccalaureate.

Study Options Full-time.

Program Entrance Requirements CPR certification, written essay, high school biology, high school chemistry, high school transcript, immunizations, 2 letters of recommendation, minimum high school GPA of 3.25. Transfer students are accepted.

Contact ***Telephone:*** 218-477-4699. *Fax:* 218-477-5990.

GRADUATE PROGRAMS

Contact ***Telephone:*** 218-477-4699. *Fax:* 218-477-5990.

MASTER'S DEGREE PROGRAM

Degree MS

Available Programs Master's; Master's for Nurses with Non-Nursing Degrees.

Concentrations Available Nursing education. *Clinical nurse specialist programs in:* adult health.

Study Options Full-time and part-time.

Program Entrance Requirements Computer literacy, minimum overall college GPA of 3.0, transcript of college record, written essay, interview, 3 letters of recommendation.

Advanced Placement Credit given for nursing courses completed elsewhere dependent upon specific evaluations.

Degree Requirements 44 total credit hours, thesis or project.

DOCTORAL DEGREE PROGRAM

Degree DNP

Available Programs Doctorate.

Areas of Study Individualized study.

Online Degree Options Yes (online only).

Program Entrance Requirements Minimum overall college GPA of 3.0, interview, letters of recommendation, MSN or equivalent, vita, writing sample.

Degree Requirements 36 total credit hours, dissertation, oral exam.

St. Catherine University

Department of Nursing
St. Paul, Minnesota

http://www.stkate.edu/academic/nursing.nsf

Founded in 1905

DEGREES • BS • DNP • MA

Nursing Program Faculty 54 (35% with doctorates).

Baccalaureate Enrollment 290 **Women** 97% **Men** 3% **Minority** 24% **International** 2% **Part-time** 22%

Graduate Enrollment 124 **Women** 95% **Men** 5% **Minority** 19% **International** 3% **Part-time** 52%

Distance Learning Courses Available.

Nursing Student Activities Nursing Honor Society, Sigma Theta Tau, Student Nurses' Association.

Nursing Student Resources Academic advising; academic or career counseling; assistance for students with disabilities; bookstore; campus computer network; career placement assistance; computer lab; computer-assisted instruction; daycare for children of students; e-mail services; employment services for current students; housing assistance; interactive nursing skills videos; Internet; learning resource lab; library services; nursing audiovisuals; paid internships; remedial services; resume preparation assistance; skills, simulation, or other laboratory; tutoring; unpaid internships.

Library Facilities 71,300 volumes in health, 18,200 volumes in nursing; 4,600 periodical subscriptions health-care related.

BACCALAUREATE PROGRAMS

Degree BS

Available Programs Baccalaureate for Second Degree; Generic Baccalaureate; RN Baccalaureate.

Site Options Minneapolis, MN.

Study Options Full-time.

Program Entrance Requirements Minimum overall college GPA of 2.75, transcript of college record, CPR certification, written essay, health insurance, immunizations, 2 letters of recommendation, minimum GPA in nursing prerequisites of 2.67, prerequisite course work. Transfer students are accepted. *Application deadline:* 3/1 (winter).

Expenses (2010-11) *Tuition:* full-time $29,888; part-time $934 per credit. *Room and board:* $8728; room only: $5350 per academic year. *Required fees:* full-time $800; part-time $75 per credit; part-time $400 per term.

Financial Aid 81% of baccalaureate students in nursing programs received some form of financial aid in 2009-10. *Gift aid (need-based):* Federal Pell, FSEOG, state, private, college/university gift aid from institutional funds. *Loans:* Federal Nursing Student Loans, Federal Direct (Subsidized and Unsubsidized Stafford PLUS), Perkins, state, alternative loans. *Work-study:* Federal Work-Study, part-time campus jobs. *Financial aid application deadline (priority):* 4/15.

Contact Dr. Vicki Schug, Baccalaureate Program Director, Department of Nursing, St. Catherine University, 2004 Randolph Avenue, St. Paul, MN 55105. *Telephone:* 651-690-6940. *Fax:* 651-690-6941. *E-mail:* vlschug@stkate.edu.

GRADUATE PROGRAMS

Expenses (2010-11) *Tuition:* part-time $763 per credit. *Room and board:* $8728; room only: $5350 per academic year. *Required fees:* full-time $60; part-time $30 per term.

Financial Aid 55% of graduate students in nursing programs received some form of financial aid in 2009-10.

Contact Dr. Margaret Dexheimer Pharris, Graduate Programs Director, Department of Nursing, St. Catherine University, 2004 Randolph Avenue, #4250, St. Paul, MN 55105. *Telephone:* 651-690-6572. *Fax:* 651-690-6941. *E-mail:* mdpharris@stkate.edu.

MASTER'S DEGREE PROGRAM

Degree MA

Available Programs Master's.

Concentrations Available Nursing education. *Nurse practitioner programs in:* adult health, gerontology, neonatal health, pediatric.

Study Options Full-time.

Program Entrance Requirements Clinical experience, minimum overall college GPA of 3.0, transcript of college record, CPR certification, written essay, immunizations, interview, 3 letters of recommendation, professional liability insurance/malpractice insurance, resume, statistics course. *Application deadline:* 1/15 (winter).

Advanced Placement Credit given for nursing courses completed elsewhere dependent upon specific evaluations.

Degree Requirements 38 total credit hours, thesis or project.

POST-MASTER'S PROGRAM

Areas of Study Nursing education. *Nurse practitioner programs in:* adult health, gerontology, neonatal health, pediatric.

DOCTORAL DEGREE PROGRAM

Degree DNP

Available Programs Doctorate.

Areas of Study Advanced practice nursing, health-care systems.

Program Entrance Requirements Minimum overall college GPA of 3.0, interview by faculty committee, 3 letters of recommendation, MSN or equivalent, vita, writing sample. Application deadline: 1/15 (winter).

Degree Requirements 28 total credit hours, dissertation.

St. Cloud State University
Department of Nursing Science
St. Cloud, Minnesota

Founded in 1869

DEGREE • BS

Nursing Program Faculty 12 (25% with doctorates).

Baccalaureate Enrollment 111

Nursing Student Activities Nursing club.

Nursing Student Resources Academic advising; academic or career counseling; assistance for students with disabilities; bookstore; campus computer network; career placement assistance; computer lab; computer-assisted instruction; daycare for children of students; e-mail services; interactive nursing skills videos; Internet; learning resource lab; library services; nursing audiovisuals; remedial services; resume preparation assistance; skills, simulation, or other laboratory; tutoring; unpaid internships.

Library Facilities 947,787 volumes (18,000 in health, 750 in nursing); 955 periodical subscriptions (100 health-care related).

BACCALAUREATE PROGRAMS

Degree BS

Available Programs Generic Baccalaureate.

Study Options Full-time.

Program Entrance Requirements Minimum overall college GPA of 2.75, transcript of college record, CPR certification, health exam, immunizations, 2 letters of recommendation, minimum GPA in nursing prerequisites of 2.75, prerequisite course work.

Contact ***Telephone:*** 320-308-1749.

St. Olaf College
Department of Nursing
Northfield, Minnesota

http://www.stolaf.edu/depts/nursing/

Founded in 1874

DEGREE • BA

Nursing Program Faculty 5 (100% with doctorates).

Baccalaureate Enrollment 48 **Women** 99% **Men** 1% **Minority** 1%

Nursing Student Activities Sigma Theta Tau, Student Nurses' Association.

Nursing Student Resources Academic advising; academic or career counseling; assistance for students with disabilities; bookstore; campus computer network; career placement assistance; computer lab; computer-assisted instruction; e-mail services; employment services for current students; externships; interactive nursing skills videos; Internet; learning resource lab; library services; nursing audiovisuals; paid internships; placement services for program completers; remedial services; resume preparation assistance; skills, simulation, or other laboratory; tutoring; unpaid internships.

Library Facilities 751,464 volumes; 4,610 periodical subscriptions.

BACCALAUREATE PROGRAMS

Degree BA

Available Programs Generic Baccalaureate.

Site Options St. Peter, MN.

Study Options Full-time.

Program Entrance Requirements Minimum overall college GPA of 2.85, transcript of college record, CPR certification, written essay, health exam, health insurance, immunizations, interview, minimum GPA in nursing prerequisites of 2.70, prerequisite course work. Transfer students are accepted. *Application deadline:* 10/31 (fall).

Expenses (2010-11) *Tuition:* full-time $36,800; part-time $4600 per course. *Room and board:* $8500 per academic year. *Required fees:* full-time $1350; part-time $675 per term.

Financial Aid ***Gift aid (need-based):*** Federal Pell, FSEOG, state, private, college/university gift aid from institutional funds. *Loans:* Federal Nursing Student Loans, Perkins, state, college/university. *Work-study:* Federal Work-Study, part-time campus jobs. *Financial aid application deadline:* 4/15(priority: 1/15).

Contact Dr. Rita S. Glazebrook, Chair, Department of Nursing, St. Olaf College, 1520 St. Olaf Avenue, Northfield, MN 55057-1098. *Telephone:* 507-786-3265. *Fax:* 507-786-3733. *E-mail:* glazebro@stolaf.edu.

University of Minnesota, Twin Cities Campus
School of Nursing
Minneapolis, Minnesota

http://www.nursing.umn.edu/

Founded in 1851

DEGREES • BSN • MS • MS/MPH • PHD

Nursing Program Faculty 85 (90% with doctorates).

Baccalaureate Enrollment 392 **Women** 87% **Men** 13% **Minority** 12% **Part-time** 8%

Graduate Enrollment 343 **Women** 98% **Men** 2% **Minority** 12% **International** 5% **Part-time** 44%

Nursing Student Activities Nursing Honor Society, Sigma Theta Tau, Student Nurses' Association.

Nursing Student Resources Academic advising; academic or career counseling; assistance for students with disabilities; bookstore; campus computer network; computer lab; computer-assisted instruction; daycare for children of students; e-mail services; employment services for current students; housing assistance; Internet; learning resource lab; library services; skills, simulation, or other laboratory.

Library Facilities 5.7 million volumes (4,000 in health, 1,500 in nursing); 45,000 periodical subscriptions (4,800 health-care related).

BACCALAUREATE PROGRAMS

Degree BSN

Available Programs Generic Baccalaureate.

Site Options Rochester, MN.

Study Options Full-time.

Program Entrance Requirements Minimum overall college GPA of 2.8, transcript of college record, CPR certification, written essay, health exam, health insurance, immunizations, minimum GPA in nursing prerequisites of 2.8, prerequisite course work. Transfer students are accepted.

Contact ***Telephone:*** 612-625-7980. *Fax:* 612-625-7727.

GRADUATE PROGRAMS

Contact ***Telephone:*** 612-625-7980. *Fax:* 612-625-7727.

MASTER'S DEGREE PROGRAM

Degrees MS; MS/MPH

Available Programs Master's.

Concentrations Available Nurse anesthesia; nurse-midwifery; nursing administration. *Clinical nurse specialist programs in:* adult health, gerontology, pediatric, psychiatric/mental health. *Nurse practitioner programs in:* family health, gerontology, pediatric, women's health.

Study Options Full-time and part-time.

Program Entrance Requirements Clinical experience, computer literacy, minimum overall college GPA of 3.0, transcript of college record, CPR certification, written essay, immunizations, interview, 2 letters of recommendation, statistics course, GRE General Test.

Degree Requirements 33 total credit hours, thesis or project.

DOCTORAL DEGREE PROGRAM

Degree PhD

Available Programs Doctorate; Doctorate for Nurses with Non-Nursing Degrees; Post-Baccalaureate Doctorate.

Program Entrance Requirements Minimum overall college GPA of 3.0, interview by faculty committee, interview, 2 letters of recommendation, GRE General Test.

Degree Requirements 30 total credit hours, dissertation, oral exam, written exam, residency.

CONTINUING EDUCATION PROGRAM

Contact ***Telephone:*** 612-625-7980. *Fax:* 612-625-7727.

Walden University
Nursing Programs
Minneapolis, Minnesota

http://www.waldenu.edu/Colleges-and-Schools/College-of-Health-Sciences/School-of-Nursing.htm
Founded in 1970

DEGREES • BSN • MSN
Nursing Program Faculty 142 (100% with doctorates).
Baccalaureate Enrollment 510 **Women** 93% **Men** 7% **Minority** 26% **International** 5% **Part-time** 85%
Graduate Enrollment 4,544 **Women** 93% **Men** 7% **Minority** 24% **International** 4% **Part-time** 27%
Distance Learning Courses Available.
Nursing Student Activities Nursing Honor Society.
Nursing Student Resources Academic advising; academic or career counseling; assistance for students with disabilities; bookstore; campus computer network; e-mail services; library services; nursing audiovisuals; remedial services; resume preparation assistance; tutoring.
Library Facilities 31,644 volumes; 34,403 periodical subscriptions (5,273 health-care related).

BACCALAUREATE PROGRAMS

Degree BSN
Available Programs RN Baccalaureate.
Study Options Full-time and part-time.
Online Degree Options Yes (online only).
Program Entrance Requirements Transcript of college record, high school transcript, prerequisite course work, RN licensure. Transfer students are accepted. *Application deadline:* Applications may be processed on a rolling basis for some programs. *Application fee:* $50.
Expenses (2010-11) *Tuition:* full-time $9360; part-time $260 per credit hour. *Required fees:* full-time $180; part-time $60 per term.
Contact Dr. Karen Ouzts, Program Director, Nursing Programs, Walden University, 155 5th Avenue South, Suite 100, Minneapolis, MN 55401. *Telephone:* 720-383-1356. *E-mail:* karen.ouzts@waldenu.edu.

GRADUATE PROGRAMS

Expenses (2010-11) *Tuition:* full-time $8910; part-time $495 per credit hour. *Required fees:* full-time $240; part-time $80 per term.
Contact Dr. Lorraine Rodrigues-Fisher, Academic Program Director, Nursing Programs, Walden University, 155 5th Avenue South, Suite 100, Minneapolis, MN 55401. *Telephone:* 616-895-3558. *Fax:* 616-895-2510. *E-mail:* lorraine.rodriguesfisher@waldenu.edu.

MASTER'S DEGREE PROGRAM

Degree MSN
Available Programs Master's; RN to Master's.
Concentrations Available Nursing administration; nursing education; nursing informatics.
Study Options Full-time and part-time.
Online Degree Options Yes (online only).
Program Entrance Requirements Minimum overall college GPA of 2.5, transcript of college record, written essay. *Application deadline:* Applications may be processed on a rolling basis for some programs. *Application fee:* $50.
Degree Requirements 59 total credit hours, thesis or project.

POST-MASTER'S PROGRAM

Areas of Study Nursing administration; nursing education; nursing informatics.

Winona State University
College of Nursing and Health Sciences
Winona, Minnesota

http://www.winona.edu/nursing/
Founded in 1858

DEGREES • BS • DNP • MS
Nursing Program Faculty 39 (46% with doctorates).
Baccalaureate Enrollment 400 **Women** 94% **Men** 6% **Minority** 3% **International** 2% **Part-time** 13%
Graduate Enrollment 110 **Women** 89% **Men** 11% **Minority** 5% **International** 1% **Part-time** 65%
Distance Learning Courses Available.
Nursing Student Activities Sigma Theta Tau, Student Nurses' Association, nursing club.
Nursing Student Resources Academic advising; academic or career counseling; assistance for students with disabilities; bookstore; campus computer network; career placement assistance; computer lab; computer-assisted instruction; daycare for children of students; e-mail services; employment services for current students; externships; housing assistance; Internet; learning resource lab; library services; nursing audiovisuals; paid internships; placement services for program completers; remedial services; resume preparation assistance; skills, simulation, or other laboratory; tutoring.
Library Facilities 350,000 volumes (6,132 in health, 3,920 in nursing); 1,000 periodical subscriptions (413 health-care related).

BACCALAUREATE PROGRAMS

Degree BS
Available Programs Generic Baccalaureate; RN Baccalaureate.
Site Options Rochester, MN.
Study Options Full-time and part-time.
Program Entrance Requirements Minimum overall college GPA of 3.0, transcript of college record, CPR certification, health exam, health insurance, immunizations, minimum GPA in nursing prerequisites of 3.3, professional liability insurance/malpractice insurance, prerequisite course work. Transfer students are accepted. *Application deadline:* 11/1 (fall), 1/31 (spring).
Expenses (2009-10) *Tuition, state resident:* full-time $2971; part-time $196 per credit. *Tuition, nonresident:* full-time $4456; part-time $294 per credit. *International tuition:* $5386 full-time. *Room and board:* $3340; room only: $2435 per academic year. *Required fees:* full-time $1267; part-time $199 per credit; part-time $634 per term.
Financial Aid 70% of baccalaureate students in nursing programs received some form of financial aid in 2008-09.
Contact Nursing Contact, College of Nursing and Health Sciences, Winona State University, PO Box 5838, Winona, MN 55987-5838. *Telephone:* 507-457-5120. *Fax:* 507-457-5550. *E-mail:* nursing@winona.edu.

GRADUATE PROGRAMS

Financial Aid 20% of graduate students in nursing programs received some form of financial aid in 2008-09. 3 research assistantships with partial tuition reimbursements available (averaging $6,000 per year) were awarded; Federal Work-Study, traineeships, and unspecified assistantships also available. Aid available to part-time students. *Financial aid application deadline:* 8/15.
Contact Dr. Julie Ponto, Interim Director, College of Nursing and Health Sciences, Winona State University, 859 SE 30th Avenue, Rochester, MN 55904. *Telephone:* 507-285-7135. *Fax:* 507-292-5127. *E-mail:* jponto@winona.edu.

MASTER'S DEGREE PROGRAM

Degree MS
Available Programs Master's; Master's for Nurses with Non-Nursing Degrees; RN to Master's.
Concentrations Available Nursing administration; nursing education. *Clinical nurse specialist programs in:* adult health. *Nurse practitioner programs in:* adult health, family health.
Site Options Rochester, MN.
Study Options Full-time and part-time.
Program Entrance Requirements Clinical experience, computer literacy, minimum overall college GPA of 3.0, transcript of college record, CPR certification, written essay, immunizations, interview, 3 letters of recommendation, nursing research course, physical assessment course, professional liability insurance/malpractice insurance, statistics course, GRE (if GPA less than 3.0). *Application deadline:* 12/1 (fall). *Application fee:* $20.
Advanced Placement Credit given for nursing courses completed elsewhere dependent upon specific evaluations.
Degree Requirements 43 total credit hours, thesis or project.

POST-MASTER'S PROGRAM

Areas of Study Nursing administration; nursing education. *Clinical nurse specialist programs in:* adult health. *Nurse practitioner programs in:* adult health, family health.

DOCTORAL DEGREE PROGRAM

Degree DNP
Available Programs Doctorate.

Areas of Study Advanced practice nursing, faculty preparation, nursing administration.
Site Options Rochester, MN.
Online Degree Options Yes (online only).
Program Entrance Requirements Clinical experience, minimum overall college GPA of 3.0, 2 letters of recommendation, MSN or equivalent, statistics course, vita, writing sample. Application deadline: 3/15 (spring). Application fee: $20.
Degree Requirements 36 total credit hours, oral exam.

MISSISSIPPI

Alcorn State University

School of Nursing
Natchez, Mississippi

http://www.alcorn.edu/academic/academ/nurses.htm
Founded in 1871

DEGREES • BSN • MSN
Nursing Program Faculty 21 (29% with doctorates).
Baccalaureate Enrollment 63 **Women** 88.8% **Men** 11.2% **Minority** 42.8% **Part-time** 7.9%
Graduate Enrollment 53 **Women** 89.3% **Men** 10.7% **Minority** 35.7% **Part-time** 78.6%
Distance Learning Courses Available.
Nursing Student Activities Nursing Honor Society, Sigma Theta Tau, Student Nurses' Association.
Nursing Student Resources Academic advising; campus computer network; computer lab; housing assistance; learning resource lab; library services; nursing audiovisuals; paid internships; skills, simulation, or other laboratory.
Library Facilities 335,252 volumes (2,082 in health, 1,385 in nursing); 1,046 periodical subscriptions (30 health-care related).

BACCALAUREATE PROGRAMS

Degree BSN
Available Programs Generic Baccalaureate; LPN to RN Baccalaureate; RN Baccalaureate.
Study Options Full-time.
Online Degree Options Yes.
Program Entrance Requirements Minimum overall college GPA of 2.5, transcript of college record, health exam, immunizations, minimum high school GPA of 2.5, professional liability insurance/malpractice insurance, prerequisite course work. Transfer students are accepted. *Application deadline:* 12/19 (fall).
Expenses (2010-11) *Tuition, state resident:* full-time $4848; part-time $202 per credit hour. *Tuition, nonresident:* full-time $11,952; part-time $498 per credit hour. *Room and board:* $5630 per academic year. *Required fees:* full-time $800.
Financial Aid 85% of baccalaureate students in nursing programs received some form of financial aid in 2009-10.
Contact Dr. Meg Brown, Chairperson, School of Nursing, Alcorn State University, 15 Campus Drive, PO Box 18399, Natchez, MS 39122. *Telephone:* 601-304-4305. *Fax:* 601-304-4398. *E-mail:* megbrown@alcorn.edu.

GRADUATE PROGRAMS

Expenses (2010-11) *Tuition, state resident:* full-time $4860; part-time $270 per credit hour. *Tuition, nonresident:* full-time $11,952; part-time $664 per credit hour. *International tuition:* $11,952 full-time. *Room and board:* $5630 per academic year. *Required fees:* full-time $900.
Financial Aid 85% of graduate students in nursing programs received some form of financial aid in 2009-10.
Contact Dr. Linda Godley, Chairperson, School of Nursing, Alcorn State University, 15 Campus Drive, PO Box 18399, Natchez, MS 39122. *Telephone:* 601-304-4303. *Fax:* 601-304-4398. *E-mail:* godley@alcorn.edu.

MASTER'S DEGREE PROGRAM

Degree MSN
Available Programs Master's.
Concentrations Available Nursing education. *Nurse practitioner programs in:* family health.
Study Options Full-time and part-time.
Online Degree Options Yes.
Program Entrance Requirements Computer literacy, minimum overall college GPA of 3.0, transcript of college record, written essay, 2 letters of recommendation, statistics course. *Application deadline:* 7/15 (fall). *Application fee:* $10.
Advanced Placement Credit given for nursing courses completed elsewhere dependent upon specific evaluations.
Degree Requirements 43 total credit hours, thesis or project.

POST-MASTER'S PROGRAM

Areas of Study Nursing education. *Nurse practitioner programs in:* family health.

Delta State University

School of Nursing
Cleveland, Mississippi

http://nursing.deltastate.edu/
Founded in 1924

DEGREES • BSN • MSN
Nursing Program Faculty 20 (40% with doctorates).
Baccalaureate Enrollment 115 **Women** 91% **Men** 9% **Minority** 18% **Part-time** 9%
Graduate Enrollment 78 **Women** 91% **Men** 9% **Minority** 27% **Part-time** 41%
Distance Learning Courses Available.
Nursing Student Activities Sigma Theta Tau, Student Nurses' Association.
Nursing Student Resources Academic advising; academic or career counseling; assistance for students with disabilities; bookstore; campus computer network; career placement assistance; computer lab; computer-assisted instruction; daycare for children of students; e-mail services; externships; housing assistance; interactive nursing skills videos; Internet; learning resource lab; library services; nursing audiovisuals; other; remedial services; resume preparation assistance; skills, simulation, or other laboratory; tutoring.
Library Facilities 430,857 volumes (5,000 in health, 1,000 in nursing); 25,507 periodical subscriptions (120 health-care related).

BACCALAUREATE PROGRAMS

Degree BSN
Available Programs ADN to Baccalaureate; Generic Baccalaureate.
Site Options Greenville, MS; Clarksdale, MS.
Study Options Full-time and part-time.
Online Degree Options Yes.
Program Entrance Requirements Transcript of college record, CPR certification, health exam, health insurance, immunizations, interview, 3 letters of recommendation, minimum GPA in nursing prerequisites of 2.5, professional liability insurance/malpractice insurance, prerequisite course work. Transfer students are accepted.
Advanced Placement Credit given for nursing courses completed elsewhere dependent upon specific evaluations.
Expenses (2010-11) *Tuition, state resident:* full-time $4852; part-time $202 per credit hour. *Tuition, nonresident:* full-time $12,558; part-time $523 per credit hour. *Room and board:* $5918; room only: $3500 per academic year. *Required fees:* full-time $912; part-time $35 per credit; part-time $456 per term.
Financial Aid 95% of baccalaureate students in nursing programs received some form of financial aid in 2009-10.
Contact Dr. Vicki L. Bingham, Chair of Academic Programs, School of Nursing, Delta State University, PO Box 3343, Cleveland, MS 38733. *Telephone:* 662-846-4255. *Fax:* 662-846-4267. *E-mail:* vbingham@deltastate.edu.

GRADUATE PROGRAMS

Expenses (2010-11) *Tuition, state resident:* full-time $4852; part-time $270 per credit hour. *Tuition, nonresident:* full-time $12,558; part-time $698 per credit hour. *International tuition:* $12,558 full-time. *Room and board:* $5918; room only: $3500 per academic year. *Required fees:* full-time $275; part-time $13 per credit; part-time $138 per term.
Financial Aid 70% of graduate students in nursing programs received some form of financial aid in 2009-10. Research assistantships, career-related internships or fieldwork, Federal Work-Study, and institutionally sponsored loans available. *Financial aid application deadline:* 6/1.

Contact Dr. Vicki L. Bingham, Chair of Academic Programs, School of Nursing, Delta State University, PO Box 3343, Cleveland, MS 38733. *Telephone:* 662-846-4255. *Fax:* 662-846-4267. *E-mail:* vbingham@deltastate.edu.

MASTER'S DEGREE PROGRAM

Degree MSN
Available Programs Accelerated Master's for Nurses with Non-Nursing Degrees; Master's.
Concentrations Available Nursing administration; nursing education. *Nurse practitioner programs in:* family health, gerontology, psychiatric/mental health.
Study Options Full-time and part-time.
Online Degree Options Yes (online only).
Program Entrance Requirements Clinical experience, computer literacy, minimum overall college GPA of 3.0, transcript of college record, CPR certification, written essay, immunizations, interview, 3 letters of recommendation, nursing research course, physical assessment course, professional liability insurance/malpractice insurance, prerequisite course work, resume, statistics course, GRE General Test. *Application deadline:* 4/1 (fall), 4/5 (spring).
Advanced Placement Credit given for nursing courses completed elsewhere dependent upon specific evaluations.
Degree Requirements 44 total credit hours, thesis or project, comprehensive exam.

POST-MASTER'S PROGRAM

Areas of Study Nursing education. *Nurse practitioner programs in:* family health, gerontology, psychiatric/mental health.

Mississippi College

School of Nursing
Clinton, Mississippi

http://www.mc.edu/
Founded in 1826

DEGREE • BSN

Nursing Program Faculty 20 (35% with doctorates).
Baccalaureate Enrollment 140 **Women** 90% **Men** 10% **Minority** 38% **International** 3% **Part-time** 9%
Distance Learning Courses Available.
Nursing Student Activities Sigma Theta Tau, Student Nurses' Association, nursing club.
Nursing Student Resources Academic advising; academic or career counseling; assistance for students with disabilities; bookstore; campus computer network; career placement assistance; computer lab; computer-assisted instruction; e-mail services; employment services for current students; externships; housing assistance; interactive nursing skills videos; Internet; learning resource lab; library services; nursing audiovisuals; other; paid internships; placement services for program completers; remedial services; resume preparation assistance; skills, simulation, or other laboratory; tutoring; unpaid internships.
Library Facilities 382,586 volumes (40,000 in health, 8,000 in nursing); 290 periodical subscriptions health-care related.

BACCALAUREATE PROGRAMS

Degree BSN
Available Programs Generic Baccalaureate; RN Baccalaureate.
Study Options Full-time and part-time.
Online Degree Options Yes.
Program Entrance Requirements Minimum overall college GPA of 2.5, transcript of college record, CPR certification, health exam, high school biology, high school chemistry, high school transcript, immunizations, 2 letters of recommendation, minimum GPA in nursing prerequisites of 2.5, professional liability insurance/malpractice insurance, prerequisite course work. Transfer students are accepted. *Application deadline:* 2/1 (fall), 9/1 (spring), 4/1 (summer).
Advanced Placement Credit given for nursing courses completed elsewhere dependent upon specific evaluations.
Expenses (2010-11) *Tuition:* full-time $12,900; part-time $405 per credit hour. *Room and board:* $7500 per academic year. *Required fees:* full-time $750; part-time $250 per term.
Financial Aid 93% of baccalaureate students in nursing programs received some form of financial aid in 2009-10. *Gift aid (need-based):* Federal Pell, FSEOG, state, private, college/university gift aid from institutional funds, Federal Nursing. *Loans:* Federal Nursing Student Loans, Perkins, college/university. *Work-study:* Federal Work-Study. *Financial aid application deadline (priority):* 3/1.
Contact Dr. Mary Jean Padgett, Dean, School of Nursing, Mississippi College, Box 4037, 200 South Capitol Street, Clinton, MS 39058. *Telephone:* 601-925-3278. *Fax:* 601-925-3379. *E-mail:* padgett@mc.edu.

Mississippi University for Women

College of Nursing and Speech Language Pathology
Columbus, Mississippi

http://www.muw.edu/nursing
Founded in 1884

DEGREES • BSN • MSN

Nursing Program Faculty 38 (25% with doctorates).
Baccalaureate Enrollment 332 **Women** 88% **Men** 12% **Minority** 20% **International** 1%
Graduate Enrollment 49 **Women** 90% **Men** 10% **Minority** 15% **Part-time** 2%
Distance Learning Courses Available.
Nursing Student Activities Sigma Theta Tau, Student Nurses' Association.
Nursing Student Resources Academic advising; academic or career counseling; assistance for students with disabilities; bookstore; campus computer network; career placement assistance; computer lab; computer-assisted instruction; daycare for children of students; e-mail services; employment services for current students; externships; housing assistance; interactive nursing skills videos; Internet; learning resource lab; library services; nursing audiovisuals; paid internships; placement services for program completers; remedial services; resume preparation assistance; skills, simulation, or other laboratory; tutoring; unpaid internships.
Library Facilities 21,859 volumes (27,340 in health, 26,420 in nursing); 3,603 periodical subscriptions (235 health-care related).

BACCALAUREATE PROGRAMS

Degree BSN
Available Programs ADN to Baccalaureate; Generic Baccalaureate.
Site Options Tupelo, MS.
Study Options Full-time.
Online Degree Options Yes.
Program Entrance Requirements Minimum overall college GPA of 2.5, transcript of college record, CPR certification, health exam, health insurance, immunizations, minimum GPA in nursing prerequisites of 2.5, professional liability insurance/malpractice insurance, prerequisite course work. Transfer students are accepted. *Application deadline:* 1/15 (fall), 1/15 (winter), 1/15 (summer).
Advanced Placement Credit given for nursing courses completed elsewhere dependent upon specific evaluations.
Expenses (2010-11) *Tuition, state resident:* full-time $4644; part-time $194 per credit hour. *Tuition, nonresident:* full-time $12,653; part-time $528 per credit hour. *Room and board:* $5483; room only: $3225 per academic year. *Required fees:* full-time $1000.
Financial Aid 90% of baccalaureate students in nursing programs received some form of financial aid in 2009-10.
Contact Dr. Tammie McCoy, Baccalaureate Nursing Department Chair, College of Nursing and Speech Language Pathology, Mississippi University for Women, 1100 College Street, MUW-910, Columbus, MS 39701-5800. *Telephone:* 662-329-7301. *Fax:* 662-329-8559. *E-mail:* tmccoy@nsgslp.muw.edu.

GRADUATE PROGRAMS

Expenses (2010-11) *Tuition, state resident:* full-time $4644; part-time $258 per credit hour. *Tuition, nonresident:* full-time $12,653; part-time $703 per credit hour. *International tuition:* $12,653 full-time. *Room and board:* $5483; room only: $3225 per academic year. *Required fees:* full-time $1000.
Financial Aid 95% of graduate students in nursing programs received some form of financial aid in 2009-10. Fellowships, Federal Work-Study, institutionally sponsored loans, and traineeships available. *Financial aid application deadline:* 4/1.
Contact Dr. Patsy Smyth, Director of Graduate Nursing Program, College of Nursing and Speech Language Pathology, Mississippi University for Women, 1100 College Street, MUW-910, Columbus, MS

39701-5800. *Telephone:* 662-329-7323. *Fax:* 662-329-7372. *E-mail:* psmyth@nsgslp.muw.edu.

MASTER'S DEGREE PROGRAM

Degree MSN
Available Programs Master's.
Concentrations Available *Nurse practitioner programs in:* family health, gerontology, pediatric, psychiatric/mental health.
Study Options Full-time.
Program Entrance Requirements Clinical experience, computer literacy, minimum overall college GPA of 3.0, transcript of college record, CPR certification, immunizations, interview, 3 letters of recommendation, nursing research course, physical assessment course, professional liability insurance/malpractice insurance, prerequisite course work, statistics course, GRE General Test. *Application deadline:* 4/1 (fall), 4/1 (spring).
Advanced Placement Credit given for nursing courses completed elsewhere dependent upon specific evaluations.
Degree Requirements 39 total credit hours, thesis or project, comprehensive exam.

POST-MASTER'S PROGRAM

Areas of Study *Nurse practitioner programs in:* family health, gerontology, pediatric, psychiatric/mental health.

University of Mississippi Medical Center

Program in Nursing
Jackson, Mississippi

http://son.umc.edu/
Founded in 1955

DEGREES • BSN • MSN • PHD

Nursing Program Faculty 65 (58% with doctorates).
Baccalaureate Enrollment 214 **Women** 87% **Men** 13% **Minority** 16% **Part-time** 7%
Graduate Enrollment 141 **Women** 90% **Men** 10% **Minority** 23% **Part-time** 53%
Distance Learning Courses Available.
Nursing Student Activities Nursing Honor Society, Sigma Theta Tau, Student Nurses' Association, nursing club.
Nursing Student Resources Academic advising; academic or career counseling; assistance for students with disabilities; bookstore; campus computer network; computer lab; computer-assisted instruction; e-mail services; employment services for current students; externships; interactive nursing skills videos; Internet; learning resource lab; library services; nursing audiovisuals; remedial services; skills, simulation, or other laboratory; tutoring; unpaid internships.
Library Facilities 310,016 volumes (72,557 in health, 8,170 in nursing); 2,732 periodical subscriptions (4,180 health-care related).

BACCALAUREATE PROGRAMS

Degree BSN
Available Programs Accelerated Baccalaureate for Second Degree; Generic Baccalaureate.
Site Options Oxford, MS.
Study Options Full-time and part-time.
Program Entrance Requirements Minimum overall college GPA of 2.5, transcript of college record, CPR certification, written essay, health exam, health insurance, immunizations, minimum GPA in nursing prerequisites of 2.5, professional liability insurance/malpractice insurance, prerequisite course work. Transfer students are accepted. *Application deadline:* 1/15 (spring). *Application fee:* $25.
Advanced Placement Credit given for nursing courses completed elsewhere dependent upon specific evaluations.
Expenses (2010-11) *Tuition, state resident:* full-time $7025; part-time $227 per credit hour. *Tuition, nonresident:* full-time $17,946; part-time $579 per credit hour. *Required fees:* full-time $600.
Financial Aid 92% of baccalaureate students in nursing programs received some form of financial aid in 2009-10.
Contact Dr. Patricia A. Waltman, Associate Dean for Academic Affairs, Program in Nursing, University of Mississippi Medical Center, 2500 North State Street, Jackson, MS 39216-4505. *Telephone:* 601-984-6211. *Fax:* 601-815-9309. *E-mail:* pwaltman@son.umsmed.edu.

GRADUATE PROGRAMS

Expenses (2010-11) *Tuition, state resident:* full-time $8158; part-time $302 per credit hour. *Tuition, nonresident:* full-time $20,840; part-time $772 per credit hour.
Financial Aid 75% of graduate students in nursing programs received some form of financial aid in 2009-10. Institutionally sponsored loans and traineeships available. Aid available to part-time students. *Financial aid application deadline:* 4/1.
Contact Dr. Marcia Rachel, Associate Dean for Graduate Studies, Program in Nursing, University of Mississippi Medical Center, 2500 North State Street, Jackson, MS 39216-4505. *Telephone:* 601-984-6228. *Fax:* 601-815-4067. *E-mail:* mrachel@umc.edu.

MASTER'S DEGREE PROGRAM

Degree MSN
Available Programs Accelerated AD/RN to Master's; Master's; RN to Master's.
Concentrations Available Nursing administration; nursing education. *Nurse practitioner programs in:* acute care, family health, gerontology, psychiatric/mental health.
Site Options Southaven, MS.
Study Options Full-time and part-time.
Program Entrance Requirements Computer literacy, minimum overall college GPA of 3.0, transcript of college record, CPR certification, immunizations, 3 letters of recommendation, professional liability insurance/malpractice insurance, resume, statistics course, GRE. *Application deadline:* 10/15 (fall), 3/31 (spring). Applications may be processed on a rolling basis for some programs. *Application fee:* $25.
Advanced Placement Credit given for nursing courses completed elsewhere dependent upon specific evaluations.
Degree Requirements 40 total credit hours, comprehensive exam.

POST-MASTER'S PROGRAM

Areas of Study Nursing administration; nursing education. *Nurse practitioner programs in:* acute care, family health, gerontology, psychiatric/mental health.

DOCTORAL DEGREE PROGRAM

Degree PhD
Available Programs Doctorate.
Areas of Study Bio-behavioral research, health policy, health promotion/disease prevention, health-care systems, human health and illness, nursing research, nursing science.
Program Entrance Requirements Minimum overall college GPA of 3.0, interview by faculty committee, interview, letters of recommendation, MSN or equivalent, statistics course, vita, GRE. Application deadline: 5/1 (fall). Application fee: $25.
Degree Requirements 60 total credit hours, dissertation, oral exam, written exam, residency.

CONTINUING EDUCATION PROGRAM

Contact Dr. Renee Williams, Director of Continuing Education, Program in Nursing, University of Mississippi Medical Center, 2500 North State Street, Jackson, MS 39216-4505. *Telephone:* 601-984-6227. *Fax:* 601-984-6214. *E-mail:* rwilliams@son.umsmed.edu.

University of Southern Mississippi

School of Nursing
Hattiesburg, Mississippi

http://www.usm.edu/nursing/
Founded in 1910

DEGREES • BSN • MSN • PHD

Nursing Program Faculty 47 (47% with doctorates).
Baccalaureate Enrollment 434 **Women** 82% **Men** 18% **Minority** 20% **Part-time** 4%
Graduate Enrollment 101 **Women** 91% **Men** 9% **Minority** 21% **Part-time** 39%
Distance Learning Courses Available.
Nursing Student Activities Nursing Honor Society, Sigma Theta Tau, Student Nurses' Association.
Nursing Student Resources Academic advising; academic or career counseling; assistance for students with disabilities; bookstore; campus computer network; career placement assistance; computer lab; computer-assisted instruction; e-mail services; externships; interactive nursing skills videos; Internet; learning resource lab; library services; nursing

audiovisuals; remedial services; resume preparation assistance; skills, simulation, or other laboratory.
Library Facilities 1.2 million volumes; 4,570 periodical subscriptions (170 health-care related).

BACCALAUREATE PROGRAMS

Degree BSN
Available Programs ADN to Baccalaureate; Generic Baccalaureate.
Site Options Meridian, MS; Long Beach, MS.
Study Options Full-time and part-time.
Online Degree Options Yes.
Program Entrance Requirements Minimum overall college GPA of 2.5, transcript of college record, CPR certification, written essay, health exam, health insurance, high school transcript, immunizations, minimum GPA in nursing prerequisites of 2.5, professional liability insurance/malpractice insurance, prerequisite course work. Transfer students are accepted. *Application deadline:* 2/1 (fall), 9/1 (spring).
Expenses (2009-10) *Tuition, state resident:* full-time $4916; part-time $213 per hour. *Tuition, nonresident:* full-time $7956; part-time $332 per hour. *International tuition:* $7956 full-time. *Room and board:* $4900; room only: $3200 per academic year. *Required fees:* full-time $300; part-time $10 per credit; part-time $150 per term.
Financial Aid 85% of baccalaureate students in nursing programs received some form of financial aid in 2008-09.
Contact Cindy Sheffield, Coordinator of Student Services, School of Nursing, University of Southern Mississippi, 118 College Drive, Box 5095, Hattiesburg, MS 39406-5095. *Telephone:* 601-266-5394. *Fax:* 601-266-5454. *E-mail:* Cynthia.Sheffield@usm.edu.

GRADUATE PROGRAMS

Expenses (2009-10) *Tuition, state resident:* full-time $5096; part-time $284 per hour. *Tuition, nonresident:* full-time $7956; part-time $442 per hour. *International tuition:* $7956 full-time.
Financial Aid 85% of graduate students in nursing programs received some form of financial aid in 2008-09. 14 research assistantships with full tuition reimbursements available (averaging $12,577 per year) were awarded; teaching assistantships, Federal Work-Study and traineeships also available. *Financial aid application deadline:* 3/15.
Contact Ms. Rosalind Hawthorn, Program Contact, School of Nursing, University of Southern Mississippi, 118 College Drive, Box 5095, Hattiesburg, MS 39406-5095. *Telephone:* 601-266-5457. *Fax:* 601-266-5927. *E-mail:* rosalind.hawthorn@usm.edu.

MASTER'S DEGREE PROGRAM

Degree MSN
Available Programs Master's; RN to Master's.
Concentrations Available Nursing administration. *Clinical nurse specialist programs in:* adult health, community health, psychiatric/mental health. *Nurse practitioner programs in:* family health, psychiatric/mental health.
Site Options Meridian, MS; Long Beach, MS.
Study Options Full-time and part-time.
Program Entrance Requirements Minimum overall college GPA of 3.0, transcript of college record, CPR certification, immunizations, 3 letters of recommendation, professional liability insurance/malpractice insurance, statistics course, GRE General Test. *Application deadline:* 7/15 (fall), 11/15 (spring), 4/15 (summer). *Application fee:* $30.
Degree Requirements 45 total credit hours, thesis or project, comprehensive exam.

POST-MASTER'S PROGRAM

Areas of Study Nursing administration. *Clinical nurse specialist programs in:* adult health, community health, psychiatric/mental health. *Nurse practitioner programs in:* family health, psychiatric/mental health.

DOCTORAL DEGREE PROGRAM

Degree PhD
Available Programs Doctorate.
Areas of Study Ethics, health policy, nursing administration, nursing education.
Program Entrance Requirements Clinical experience, minimum overall college GPA of 3.5, interview by faculty committee, 3 letters of recommendation, MSN or equivalent, statistics course, vita, writing sample, GRE General Test. Application deadline: 3/1 (fall). Application fee: $30.
Degree Requirements 72 total credit hours, dissertation, written exam, residency.

William Carey University
School of Nursing
Hattiesburg, Mississippi

Founded in 1906

DEGREES • BSN • MSN
Nursing Program Faculty 21 (42% with doctorates).
Baccalaureate Enrollment 198 **Women** 93% **Men** 7% **Minority** 33% **Part-time** 7%
Graduate Enrollment 22 **Women** 100% **Minority** 26% **Part-time** 11%
Distance Learning Courses Available.
Nursing Student Activities Sigma Theta Tau, Student Nurses' Association.
Nursing Student Resources Academic advising; academic or career counseling; assistance for students with disabilities; bookstore; campus computer network; computer lab; computer-assisted instruction; e-mail services; interactive nursing skills videos; Internet; learning resource lab; library services; nursing audiovisuals; resume preparation assistance; skills, simulation, or other laboratory; tutoring.
Library Facilities 450 volumes in health, 450 volumes in nursing; 50 periodical subscriptions health-care related.

BACCALAUREATE PROGRAMS

Degree BSN
Available Programs ADN to Baccalaureate; Generic Baccalaureate.
Site Options Gulfport, MS; New Orleans, LA.
Study Options Full-time and part-time.
Program Entrance Requirements Minimum overall college GPA of 2.5, transcript of college record, CPR certification, health exam, high school transcript, immunizations, minimum GPA in nursing prerequisites of 3.0, prerequisite course work. Transfer students are accepted. *Application deadline:* 4/10 (fall), 10/10 (spring). *Application fee:* $25.
Advanced Placement Credit given for nursing courses completed elsewhere dependent upon specific evaluations.
Contact ***Telephone:*** 601-318-6478. *Fax:* 601-318-6446.

GRADUATE PROGRAMS

Contact ***Telephone:*** 228-897-7200.

MASTER'S DEGREE PROGRAM

Degree MSN
Available Programs Master's.
Concentrations Available Nursing education.
Site Options Gulfport, MS.
Study Options Full-time and part-time.
Program Entrance Requirements Computer literacy, minimum overall college GPA of 3.0, transcript of college record, CPR certification, immunizations, nursing research course, professional liability insurance/malpractice insurance, prerequisite course work, statistics course. *Application deadline:* 8/15 (fall), 2/15 (spring). *Application fee:* $25.
Advanced Placement Credit given for nursing courses completed elsewhere dependent upon specific evaluations.
Degree Requirements 35 total credit hours, thesis or project.

MISSOURI

Avila University
School of Nursing
Kansas City, Missouri

http://www.avila.edu/nursing
Founded in 1916

DEGREE • BSN
Nursing Program Faculty 16 (19% with doctorates).
Baccalaureate Enrollment 108 **Women** 91% **Men** 9% **Minority** 18%
Nursing Student Activities Nursing Honor Society, Sigma Theta Tau, Student Nurses' Association.
Nursing Student Resources Academic advising; academic or career counseling; assistance for students with disabilities; bookstore; campus computer network; career placement assistance; computer lab; computer-assisted instruction; e-mail services; employment services for current stu-

dents; externships; interactive nursing skills videos; Internet; learning resource lab; library services; nursing audiovisuals; remedial services; resume preparation assistance; skills, simulation, or other laboratory; tutoring.
Library Facilities 80,845 volumes (1,092 in health, 556 in nursing); 22,464 periodical subscriptions (86 health-care related).

BACCALAUREATE PROGRAMS

Degree BSN
Available Programs Generic Baccalaureate.
Study Options Full-time.
Program Entrance Requirements Minimum overall college GPA of 2.7, transcript of college record, CPR certification, written essay, health exam, health insurance, immunizations, interview, minimum GPA in nursing prerequisites of 2.0, prerequisite course work. Transfer students are accepted. *Application deadline:* 1/10 (fall). *Application fee:* $45.
Advanced Placement Credit given for nursing courses completed elsewhere dependent upon specific evaluations.
Expenses (2010-11) *Tuition:* full-time $21,050; part-time $535 per credit hour. *Room and board:* $4950 per academic year. *Required fees:* full-time $1270; part-time $29 per credit.
Financial Aid 98% of baccalaureate students in nursing programs received some form of financial aid in 2009-10.
Contact Office of Admissions, School of Nursing, Avila University, 11901 Wornall Road, Kansas City, MO 64145-1698. *Telephone:* 816-501-2400. *Fax:* 816-501-2453. *E-mail:* admissions@avila.edu.

Central Methodist University

College of Liberal Arts and Sciences
Fayette, Missouri

Founded in 1854

DEGREES • BN • MSN
Nursing Program Faculty 7
Library Facilities 97,793 volumes; 316 periodical subscriptions.

BACCALAUREATE PROGRAMS

Degree BN
Available Programs Generic Baccalaureate.
Program Entrance Requirements Written essay, health exam, high school biology, high school chemistry, immunizations, minimum high school GPA of 2.75, prerequisite course work. Transfer students are accepted.
Contact ***Telephone:*** 660-248-6359.

GRADUATE PROGRAMS

Contact ***Telephone:*** 573-220-1378.

MASTER'S DEGREE PROGRAM

Degree MSN
Available Programs Master's.
Program Entrance Requirements CPR certification, written essay, immunizations, prerequisite course work, statistics course.

Chamberlain College of Nursing

Chamberlain College of Nursing
St. Louis, Missouri

http://www.chamberlain.edu/home.html
Founded in 1889

DEGREE • BSN
Nursing Program Faculty 80 (21% with doctorates).
Distance Learning Courses Available.
Nursing Student Activities Student Nurses' Association.
Nursing Student Resources Academic advising; academic or career counseling; assistance for students with disabilities; bookstore; campus computer network; career placement assistance; computer lab; computer-assisted instruction; e-mail services; employment services for current students; housing assistance; Internet; learning resource lab; library services; nursing audiovisuals; placement services for program completers; skills, simulation, or other laboratory; tutoring.
Library Facilities 8,700 volumes (3,287 in health, 957 in nursing); 233 periodical subscriptions (182 health-care related).

BACCALAUREATE PROGRAMS

Degree BSN
Available Programs ADN to Baccalaureate; Accelerated RN Baccalaureate; Generic Baccalaureate; LPN to RN Baccalaureate; RN Baccalaureate.
Site Options Columbus, OH; Phoenix, AZ; Addison, IL.
Study Options Full-time.
Online Degree Options Yes (online only).
Program Entrance Requirements Minimum overall college GPA of 2.75, transcript of college record, written essay, health exam, health insurance, high school biology, high school chemistry, 3 years high school math, 3 years high school science, high school transcript, immunizations, interview, minimum high school GPA of 2.75, minimum high school rank 33%. Transfer students are accepted.
Advanced Placement Credit by examination available. Credit given for nursing courses completed elsewhere dependent upon specific evaluations.
Contact ***Telephone:*** 800-942-4310 Ext. 1. *Fax:* 314-768-3044.

College of the Ozarks

Armstrong McDonald School of Nursing
Point Lookout, Missouri

http://www.cofo.edu/
Founded in 1906

DEGREE • BSN
Nursing Program Faculty 9
Baccalaureate Enrollment 60 **Women** 93.3% **Men** 6.7% **Minority** .6% **International** 2%
Nursing Student Activities Nursing club.
Nursing Student Resources Academic advising; academic or career counseling; assistance for students with disabilities; bookstore; campus computer network; career placement assistance; computer lab; computer-assisted instruction; daycare for children of students; e-mail services; employment services for current students; externships; interactive nursing skills videos; Internet; learning resource lab; library services; nursing audiovisuals; paid internships; remedial services; resume preparation assistance; skills, simulation, or other laboratory; tutoring; unpaid internships.
Library Facilities 112,550 volumes (30 in health, 30 in nursing); 441 periodical subscriptions (38 health-care related).

BACCALAUREATE PROGRAMS

Degree BSN
Available Programs RN Baccalaureate.
Study Options Full-time and part-time.
Program Entrance Requirements Minimum overall college GPA of 2.5, transcript of college record, health exam, 2 years high school math, high school transcript, immunizations, interview, 2 letters of recommendation, minimum high school GPA of 3.0, minimum GPA in nursing prerequisites of 2.5, professional liability insurance/malpractice insurance. Transfer students are accepted. *Application deadline:* 3/1 (spring).
Expenses (2010-11) *Tuition:* part-time $295 per credit hour. *Room and board:* $5300 per academic year. *Required fees:* full-time $1200.
Financial Aid 100% of baccalaureate students in nursing programs received some form of financial aid in 2009-10.
Contact Mrs. Deborah J. Lyon, Office Manager, Armstrong McDonald School of Nursing, College of the Ozarks, PO Box 17, Point Lookout, MO 65726. *Telephone:* 417-690-2421. *Fax:* 417-690-2422. *E-mail:* dlyon@cofo.edu.

Cox College

Department of Nursing
Springfield, Missouri

Founded in 1994

DEGREE • BSN
Nursing Program Faculty 20 (50% with doctorates).
Baccalaureate Enrollment 250 **Women** 95% **Men** 5% **Minority** 5% **International** 4% **Part-time** 80%

Nursing Student Activities Nursing Honor Society, Student Nurses' Association, nursing club.
Nursing Student Resources Academic advising; academic or career counseling; assistance for students with disabilities; bookstore; campus computer network; career placement assistance; computer lab; computer-assisted instruction; daycare for children of students; e-mail services; employment services for current students; externships; housing assistance; interactive nursing skills videos; Internet; learning resource lab; library services; nursing audiovisuals; placement services for program completers; remedial services; resume preparation assistance; skills, simulation, or other laboratory; tutoring.
Library Facilities 29,750 volumes (5,500 in health, 1,900 in nursing); 249 periodical subscriptions (250 health-care related).

BACCALAUREATE PROGRAMS

Degree BSN
Available Programs ADN to Baccalaureate; Accelerated Baccalaureate; Accelerated Baccalaureate for Second Degree; Baccalaureate for Second Degree; Generic Baccalaureate; LPN to Baccalaureate; LPN to RN Baccalaureate; RN Baccalaureate.
Site Options Springfield, MO.
Study Options Full-time and part-time.
Program Entrance Requirements Minimum overall college GPA of 3.0, transcript of college record, CPR certification, written essay, health exam, high school biology, high school chemistry, 2 years high school math, 2 years high school science, high school transcript, immunizations, interview, minimum high school GPA of 3.0, minimum GPA in nursing prerequisites of 3.0, prerequisite course work. Transfer students are accepted.
Advanced Placement Credit given for nursing courses completed elsewhere dependent upon specific evaluations.
Contact ***Telephone:*** 417-269-3038.

CONTINUING EDUCATION PROGRAM

Contact ***Telephone:*** 417-269-8450.

Goldfarb School of Nursing at Barnes-Jewish College

Goldfarb School of Nursing at Barnes-Jewish College
St. Louis, Missouri

Founded in 1902

DEGREES • BSN • MSN • PHD
Nursing Program Faculty 40 (55% with doctorates).
Baccalaureate Enrollment 513 **Women** 88% **Men** 12% **Minority** 18% **International** 1% **Part-time** 22%
Graduate Enrollment 130 **Women** 95% **Men** 5% **Minority** 37% **International** 1% **Part-time** 45%
Distance Learning Courses Available.
Nursing Student Activities Nursing Honor Society, Sigma Theta Tau, Student Nurses' Association.
Nursing Student Resources Academic advising; academic or career counseling; assistance for students with disabilities; bookstore; campus computer network; career placement assistance; computer lab; computer-assisted instruction; e-mail services; employment services for current students; externships; housing assistance; interactive nursing skills videos; Internet; learning resource lab; library services; nursing audiovisuals; placement services for program completers; remedial services; resume preparation assistance; skills, simulation, or other laboratory; tutoring.
Library Facilities 1,100 volumes (13,000 in health, 8,100 in nursing); 44 periodical subscriptions (250 health-care related).

BACCALAUREATE PROGRAMS

Degree BSN
Available Programs ADN to Baccalaureate; Accelerated Baccalaureate; Accelerated Baccalaureate for Second Degree; Generic Baccalaureate; RN Baccalaureate.
Study Options Full-time.
Program Entrance Requirements Minimum overall college GPA of 3.0, transcript of college record, CPR certification, health exam, high school biology, high school transcript, immunizations, 2 letters of recommendation, minimum high school GPA of 3.0, minimum GPA in nursing prerequisites of 3.0, prerequisite course work. Transfer students are accepted. *Application deadline:* 9/1 (fall), 1/2 (spring), 5/1 (summer). Applications may be processed on a rolling basis for some programs. *Application fee:* $50.
Advanced Placement Credit by examination available. Credit given for nursing courses completed elsewhere dependent upon specific evaluations.
Expenses (2010-11) *Tuition:* full-time $22,500; part-time $548 per credit hour. *Required fees:* full-time $943.
Financial Aid 95% of baccalaureate students in nursing programs received some form of financial aid in 2009-10.
Contact Dr. Connie Koch, Associate Dean for Academic Programs, Goldfarb School of Nursing at Barnes-Jewish College, 4483 Duncan, MS #90-36-697, St. Louis, MO 63110-1091. *Telephone:* 314-362-6289. *Fax:* 314-362-0984. *E-mail:* ckoch@bjc.org.

GRADUATE PROGRAMS

Expenses (2010-11) *Tuition:* full-time $12,300; part-time $575 per credit hour. *Required fees:* full-time $250.
Financial Aid 80% of graduate students in nursing programs received some form of financial aid in 2009-10.
Contact Dr. Connie Koch, Associate Dean for Academic Programs, Goldfarb School of Nursing at Barnes-Jewish College, 4483 Duncan, MS #90-36-697, St. Louis, MO 63110-1091. *Telephone:* 314-362-6289. *Fax:* 314-362-0984. *E-mail:* ckoch@bjc.org.

MASTER'S DEGREE PROGRAM

Degree MSN
Available Programs Master's.
Concentrations Available Health-care administration; nurse anesthesia; nursing administration; nursing education. *Nurse practitioner programs in:* acute care, adult health.
Study Options Full-time and part-time.
Program Entrance Requirements Clinical experience, computer literacy, minimum overall college GPA of 3.0, transcript of college record, CPR certification, immunizations, 2 letters of recommendation, nursing research course, physical assessment course, resume, statistics course. *Application deadline:* 9/1 (fall), 1/2 (spring), 5/1 (summer). Applications may be processed on a rolling basis for some programs. *Application fee:* $50.
Advanced Placement Credit given for nursing courses completed elsewhere dependent upon specific evaluations.
Degree Requirements 34 total credit hours, thesis or project.

POST-MASTER'S PROGRAM

Areas of Study Health-care administration; nursing administration; nursing education. *Nurse practitioner programs in:* acute care, adult health.

DOCTORAL DEGREE PROGRAM

Degree PhD
Available Programs Doctorate; Doctorate for Nurses with Non-Nursing Degrees; Post-Baccalaureate Doctorate.
Areas of Study Clinical practice, nursing administration, nursing education.
Program Entrance Requirements Minimum overall college GPA of 3, interview by faculty committee, 3 letters of recommendation, statistics course, vita, writing sample. Application deadline: 7/15 (fall). Applications may be processed on a rolling basis for some programs. Application fee: $50.
Degree Requirements 111 total credit hours, dissertation, oral exam, written exam, residency.

Graceland University

School of Nursing
Independence, Missouri

http://www.graceland.edu/nursing
Founded in 1895

DEGREES • BSN • MSN
Nursing Program Faculty 22 (50% with doctorates).
Baccalaureate Enrollment 259 **Women** 90% **Men** 10% **Minority** 8% **International** .7% **Part-time** 8.5%
Graduate Enrollment 262 **Women** 92.7% **Men** 7.3% **Minority** 7.3% **Part-time** 36.6%
Distance Learning Courses Available.

Nursing Student Activities Nursing Honor Society, Sigma Theta Tau, Student Nurses' Association, nursing club.

Nursing Student Resources Academic advising; academic or career counseling; assistance for students with disabilities; bookstore; campus computer network; computer lab; computer-assisted instruction; e-mail services; housing assistance; interactive nursing skills videos; Internet; learning resource lab; library services; nursing audiovisuals; resume preparation assistance; skills, simulation, or other laboratory; tutoring.

Library Facilities 123,990 volumes (1,902 in health, 790 in nursing); 558 periodical subscriptions (2,815 health-care related).

BACCALAUREATE PROGRAMS

Degree BSN

Available Programs ADN to Baccalaureate; Accelerated Baccalaureate; Generic Baccalaureate; RN Baccalaureate.

Site Options Independence, MO.

Study Options Full-time and part-time.

Program Entrance Requirements Minimum overall college GPA of 2.5, transcript of college record, written essay, health exam, high school chemistry, high school transcript, immunizations, interview, 2 letters of recommendation, minimum high school GPA of 2.0, minimum GPA in nursing prerequisites of 2.0, prerequisite course work. Transfer students are accepted. *Application deadline:* 11/30 (fall). *Application fee:* $50.

Advanced Placement Credit given for nursing courses completed elsewhere dependent upon specific evaluations.

Expenses (2010-11) *Tuition:* full-time $20,680; part-time $650 per credit hour. *Required fees:* full-time $1325; part-time $663 per term.

Financial Aid 36% of baccalaureate students in nursing programs received some form of financial aid in 2009-10. *Gift aid (need-based):* Federal Pell, FSEOG, state, private, college/university gift aid from institutional funds. *Loans:* Federal Direct (Subsidized and Unsubsidized Stafford PLUS), Perkins, state, college/university. *Work-study:* Federal Work-Study, part-time campus jobs. *Financial aid application deadline:* Continuous.

Contact Ms. Laurie Hale, Admissions Counselor, School of Nursing, Graceland University, 1401 West Truman Road, Independence, MO 64050-3434. *Telephone:* 800-833-0524 Ext. 4250. *Fax:* 816-833-2990. *E-mail:* lhale@graceland.edu.

GRADUATE PROGRAMS

Expenses (2010-11) *Tuition:* part-time $549 per credit hour. *Required fees:* part-time $1530 per term.

Financial Aid 72% of graduate students in nursing programs received some form of financial aid in 2009-10.

Contact Ms. Cara Hakes, Program Consultant, School of Nursing, Graceland University, 1401 West Truman Road, Independence, MO 64050-3434. *Telephone:* 816-833-0524 Ext. 4803. *Fax:* 816-833-2990. *E-mail:* chakes@graceland.edu.

MASTER'S DEGREE PROGRAM

Degree MSN

Available Programs Master's; RN to Master's.

Concentrations Available Nursing education. *Nurse practitioner programs in:* family health.

Site Options Independence, MO.

Study Options Full-time and part-time.

Online Degree Options Yes (online only).

Program Entrance Requirements Clinical experience, minimum overall college GPA of 3.0, transcript of college record, written essay, 3 letters of recommendation, nursing research course, physical assessment course, prerequisite course work, statistics course. *Application deadline:* 6/1 (fall), 10/1 (winter), 2/1 (spring). *Application fee:* $50.

Advanced Placement Credit given for nursing courses completed elsewhere dependent upon specific evaluations.

Degree Requirements 47 total credit hours, thesis or project, comprehensive exam.

POST-MASTER'S PROGRAM

Areas of Study Nursing education. *Nurse practitioner programs in:* family health.

Grantham University

Nursing Programs
Kansas City, Missouri

Founded in 1951

DEGREES • BSN • MSN

Nursing Program Faculty 21

Distance Learning Courses Available.

Nursing Student Resources Academic advising; academic or career counseling; bookstore; e-mail services; Internet; library services; tutoring.

Library Facilities 2,044 volumes; 18,139 periodical subscriptions.

BACCALAUREATE PROGRAMS

Degree BSN

Available Programs RN Baccalaureate.

Contact Dr. Susan Fairchild, Professor and Chair, Department of Nursing. *Telephone:* 800-955-2527 Ext. 206. *E-mail:* sfairchild@grantham.edu.

GRADUATE PROGRAMS

Contact Dr. Susan Fairchild, Professor and Chair, Department of Nursing. *Telephone:* 800-955-2527 Ext. 206. *E-mail:* sfairchild@grantham.edu.

MASTER'S DEGREE PROGRAM

Degree MSN

Available Programs Master's; RN to Master's.

Culver-Stockton College

Blessing–Rieman College of Nursing
Canton, Missouri

http://www.culver.edu/

See description of programs under
Blessing–Rieman College of Nursing (Quincy, Illinois).

Lincoln University

Department of Nursing
Jefferson City, Missouri

Founded in 1866

DEGREE • BSN

Library Facilities 204,948 volumes; 368 periodical subscriptions.

BACCALAUREATE PROGRAMS

Degree BSN

Available Programs RN Baccalaureate.

Contact ***Telephone:*** 573-681-5421.

Maryville University of Saint Louis

Nursing Program, School of Health Professions
St. Louis, Missouri

http://www.maryville.edu/academics-hp-nursing.htm

Founded in 1872

DEGREES • BSN • DNP • MSN

Nursing Program Faculty 65 (4% with doctorates).

Baccalaureate Enrollment 463 **Women** 95% **Men** 5% **Minority** 10% **International** 1% **Part-time** 45%

Graduate Enrollment 116 **Women** 92% **Men** 8% **Minority** 14% **Part-time** 79%

Nursing Student Activities Sigma Theta Tau, Student Nurses' Association.

Nursing Student Resources Academic advising; academic or career counseling; assistance for students with disabilities; bookstore; campus computer network; career placement assistance; computer lab; computer-assisted instruction; e-mail services; externships; interactive nursing skills videos; Internet; learning resource lab; library services; nursing audiovisuals; paid internships; remedial services; resume preparation assistance; skills, simulation, or other laboratory; tutoring.
Library Facilities 158,930 volumes (8,680 in health, 1,464 in nursing); 42,582 periodical subscriptions (4,315 health-care related).

BACCALAUREATE PROGRAMS

Degree BSN
Available Programs Accelerated Baccalaureate; Accelerated RN Baccalaureate; Generic Baccalaureate; LPN to Baccalaureate; RN Baccalaureate.
Study Options Full-time and part-time.
Program Entrance Requirements Minimum overall college GPA of 2.75, transcript of college record, health exam, high school transcript, immunizations, minimum high school GPA of 2.75, minimum GPA in nursing prerequisites of 2.75. Transfer students are accepted. *Application deadline:* 12/15 (fall). Applications may be processed on a rolling basis for some programs.
Advanced Placement Credit given for nursing courses completed elsewhere dependent upon specific evaluations.
Expenses (2010-11) *Tuition:* full-time $21,100; part-time $634 per credit hour. *Room and board:* $8500 per academic year. *Required fees:* full-time $810.
Financial Aid 69% of baccalaureate students in nursing programs received some form of financial aid in 2009-10. *Gift aid (need-based):* Federal Pell, FSEOG, state, private, college/university gift aid from institutional funds, Academic Competitiveness Grants, National SMART Grants, TEACH Grants. *Loans:* Federal Direct (Subsidized and Unsubsidized Stafford PLUS), Perkins, Sallie Mae Signature Loans, KeyBank Loans, TERI Loans, CitiAssist Loans, Campus Door Loans. *Work-study:* Federal Work-Study, part-time campus jobs. *Financial aid application deadline (priority):* 3/1.
Contact Dr. Elizabeth Buck, Director, Nursing Program, School of Health Professions, Maryville University of Saint Louis, 650 Maryville University Drive, St. Louis, MO 63141-7299. *Telephone:* 314-529-9453. *Fax:* 314-529-9495. *E-mail:* ebuck@maryville.edu.

GRADUATE PROGRAMS

Expenses (2010-11) *Tuition:* full-time $21,100; part-time $650 per credit hour. *Room and board:* $8500 per academic year. *Required fees:* full-time $810.
Financial Aid 66% of graduate students in nursing programs received some form of financial aid in 2009-10.
Contact Dr. Elizabeth Buck, Director, Nursing Program, School of Health Professions, Maryville University of Saint Louis, 650 Maryville University Drive, St. Louis, MO 63141-7299. *Telephone:* 314-529-9453. *Fax:* 314-529-9495. *E-mail:* ebuck@maryville.edu.

MASTER'S DEGREE PROGRAM

Degree MSN
Available Programs Accelerated RN to Master's; Master's; RN to Master's.
Concentrations Available Nursing education. *Nurse practitioner programs in:* adult health, family health.
Study Options Full-time and part-time.
Program Entrance Requirements Minimum overall college GPA of 3.0, transcript of college record, written essay, 3 letters of recommendation, resume, statistics course. *Application deadline:* Applications may be processed on a rolling basis for some programs.
Advanced Placement Credit by examination available. Credit given for nursing courses completed elsewhere dependent upon specific evaluations.
Degree Requirements 42 total credit hours, thesis or project.

DOCTORAL DEGREE PROGRAM

Degree DNP
Available Programs Doctorate.
Areas of Study Advanced practice nursing, ethics, health policy, nursing research.
Program Entrance Requirements Minimum overall college GPA of 3.5, 3 letters of recommendation, MSN or equivalent, vita, writing sample. Application deadline: Applications may be processed on a rolling basis for some programs.
Degree Requirements 30 total credit hours.

Missouri Southern State University

Department of Nursing
Joplin, Missouri

http://www.mssu.edu/nursing/
Founded in 1937

DEGREES • BSN • MSN
Nursing Program Faculty 10 (20% with doctorates).
Baccalaureate Enrollment 87 **Women** 82% **Men** 18% **Minority** 9%
Graduate Enrollment 15 **Women** 86% **Men** 14%
Distance Learning Courses Available.
Nursing Student Activities Nursing Honor Society, Student Nurses' Association.
Nursing Student Resources Academic advising; academic or career counseling; assistance for students with disabilities; bookstore; campus computer network; career placement assistance; computer lab; computer-assisted instruction; daycare for children of students; e-mail services; employment services for current students; housing assistance; interactive nursing skills videos; Internet; learning resource lab; library services; nursing audiovisuals; remedial services; resume preparation assistance; skills, simulation, or other laboratory; tutoring.
Library Facilities 4,872 volumes in health, 4,470 volumes in nursing; 4,412 periodical subscriptions health-care related.

BACCALAUREATE PROGRAMS

Degree BSN
Available Programs ADN to Baccalaureate; Accelerated Baccalaureate; Baccalaureate for Second Degree; Generic Baccalaureate; LPN to Baccalaureate; RN Baccalaureate.
Study Options Full-time.
Program Entrance Requirements Transcript of college record, CPR certification, health exam, health insurance, immunizations, minimum GPA in nursing prerequisites of 2.5, professional liability insurance/malpractice insurance, prerequisite course work, RN licensure. Transfer students are accepted. *Application deadline:* 1/31 (fall). *Application fee:* $50.
Advanced Placement Credit by examination available. Credit given for nursing courses completed elsewhere dependent upon specific evaluations.
Expenses (2010-11) *Tuition, area resident:* part-time $143 per credit hour. *Tuition, nonresident:* part-time $298 per credit hour. *Required fees:* full-time $3798.
Financial Aid 83% of baccalaureate students in nursing programs received some form of financial aid in 2009-10. *Gift aid (need-based):* Federal Pell, FSEOG, state, private. *Loans:* Federal Direct (Subsidized and Unsubsidized Stafford PLUS), Perkins. *Work-study:* Federal Work-Study, part-time campus jobs. *Financial aid application deadline (priority):* 4/1.
Contact Dr. J. Mari Beth Linder, Director, Department of Nursing, Missouri Southern State University, Health Sciences Building, Room 243, 3950 East Newman Road, Joplin, MO 64801-1595. *Telephone:* 417-625-9322. *Fax:* 417-625-3186. *E-mail:* linder-m@mssu.edu.

GRADUATE PROGRAMS

Financial Aid 50% of graduate students in nursing programs received some form of financial aid in 2009-10.
Contact Dr. Mari Beth Linder, Director, Department of Nursing, Missouri Southern State University, Health Sciences Building, Room 243, 3950 East Newman Road, Joplin, MO 64801. *Telephone:* 417-625-9322. *Fax:* 417-625-3186. *E-mail:* linder-m@mssu.edu.

MASTER'S DEGREE PROGRAM

Degree MSN
Available Programs Master's.
Concentrations Available Nursing education. *Clinical nurse specialist programs in:* family health.
Study Options Full-time.
Program Entrance Requirements Minimum overall college GPA of 3.0, transcript of college record, resume. *Application deadline:* 12/1 (fall). *Application fee:* $35.
Degree Requirements 43 total credit hours.

Missouri State University

Department of Nursing
Springfield, Missouri

http://www.smsu.edu/nursing
Founded in 1905

DEGREES • BSN • MSN

Nursing Program Faculty 14 (36% with doctorates).

Baccalaureate Enrollment 118 **Women** 90% **Men** 10% **Minority** 4% **International** 1% **Part-time** 68%

Graduate Enrollment 36 **Women** 98% **Men** 2% **Minority** 1% **Part-time** 39%

Distance Learning Courses Available.

Nursing Student Activities Sigma Theta Tau, Student Nurses' Association.

Nursing Student Resources Academic advising; academic or career counseling; assistance for students with disabilities; bookstore; campus computer network; career placement assistance; computer lab; computer-assisted instruction; daycare for children of students; e-mail services; employment services for current students; externships; housing assistance; interactive nursing skills videos; Internet; learning resource lab; library services; nursing audiovisuals; paid internships; placement services for program completers; remedial services; resume preparation assistance; skills, simulation, or other laboratory; tutoring; unpaid internships.

Library Facilities 1.8 million volumes (10,500 in health, 3,516 in nursing); 3,534 periodical subscriptions (370 health-care related).

BACCALAUREATE PROGRAMS

Degree BSN

Available Programs ADN to Baccalaureate; Accelerated RN Baccalaureate; Generic Baccalaureate; LPN to Baccalaureate; RN Baccalaureate.

Study Options Full-time.

Online Degree Options Yes.

Program Entrance Requirements Minimum overall college GPA of 2.75, transcript of college record, CPR certification, health insurance, immunizations, prerequisite course work. Transfer students are accepted. *Application deadline:* 1/31 (summer).

Advanced Placement Credit given for nursing courses completed elsewhere dependent upon specific evaluations.

Contact ***Telephone:*** 417-836-5310. *Fax:* 417-836-5484.

GRADUATE PROGRAMS

Contact ***Telephone:*** 417-836-5310. *Fax:* 417-836-5484.

MASTER'S DEGREE PROGRAM

Degree MSN

Available Programs Accelerated AD/RN to Master's; Master's; RN to Master's.

Concentrations Available Nursing education. *Nurse practitioner programs in:* family health.

Study Options Full-time and part-time.

Online Degree Options Yes (online only).

Program Entrance Requirements Computer literacy, minimum overall college GPA of 3.0, transcript of college record, written essay, immunizations, interview, nursing research course, physical assessment course, professional liability insurance/malpractice insurance, statistics course, GRE General Test. *Application deadline:* 2/15 (fall).

Advanced Placement Credit given for nursing courses completed elsewhere dependent upon specific evaluations.

Degree Requirements 51 total credit hours, thesis or project, comprehensive exam.

POST-MASTER'S PROGRAM

Areas of Study Nursing education. *Nurse practitioner programs in:* family health.

CONTINUING EDUCATION PROGRAM

Contact ***Telephone:*** 417-836-6660. *Fax:* 417-836-7674.

Missouri Western State University

Department of Nursing
St. Joseph, Missouri

http://www.missouriwestern.edu/nursing
Founded in 1915

DEGREES • BSN • MSN

Nursing Program Faculty 35 (23% with doctorates).

Baccalaureate Enrollment 190 **Women** 90.5% **Men** 9.5% **Minority** 6.3%

Graduate Enrollment 9 **Women** 100% **Part-time** 100%

Nursing Student Activities Sigma Theta Tau, Student Nurses' Association.

Nursing Student Resources Academic advising; academic or career counseling; assistance for students with disabilities; bookstore; campus computer network; career placement assistance; computer lab; computer-assisted instruction; daycare for children of students; e-mail services; employment services for current students; interactive nursing skills videos; Internet; learning resource lab; library services; nursing audiovisuals; paid internships; placement services for program completers; remedial services; resume preparation assistance; skills, simulation, or other laboratory; tutoring; unpaid internships.

Library Facilities 147,509 volumes (9,441 in health, 8,902 in nursing); 1,068 periodical subscriptions (21 health-care related).

BACCALAUREATE PROGRAMS

Degree BSN

Available Programs ADN to Baccalaureate; Generic Baccalaureate.

Site Options Kansas City, MO.

Study Options Full-time.

Program Entrance Requirements Minimum overall college GPA of 2.5, transcript of college record, CPR certification, written essay, health insurance, high school transcript, immunizations, minimum GPA in nursing prerequisites of 2.7, prerequisite course work. Transfer students are accepted. *Application deadline:* 1/15 (fall), 8/15 (spring). *Application fee:* $30.

Advanced Placement Credit by examination available. Credit given for nursing courses completed elsewhere dependent upon specific evaluations.

Expenses (2010-11) *Tuition, state resident:* full-time $5228; part-time $166 per hour. *Tuition, nonresident:* full-time $9533; part-time $320 per hour.

Contact Information Contact, Department of Nursing, Missouri Western State University, 4525 Downs Drive, St. Joseph, MO 64507. *Telephone:* 816-271-4415. *Fax:* 816-271-5849. *E-mail:* nursing@missouriwestern.edu.

GRADUATE PROGRAMS

Expenses (2010-11) *Tuition, state resident:* full-time $3640; part-time $280 per hour. *Tuition, nonresident:* full-time $4225; part-time $325 per hour.

Financial Aid 78% of graduate students in nursing programs received some form of financial aid in 2009-10.

Contact Dr. Kathleen E. O'Connor, Associate Professor and Chairperson, Department of Nursing, Missouri Western State University, 4525 Downs Drive, St. Joseph, MO 64507. *Telephone:* 816-271-4415. *Fax:* 816-271-5849. *E-mail:* koconnor5@missouriwestern.edu.

MASTER'S DEGREE PROGRAM

Degree MSN

Available Programs Master's.

Concentrations Available Health-care administration.

Study Options Part-time.

Program Entrance Requirements Minimum overall college GPA of 2.75, transcript of college record, written essay, interview, nursing research course, prerequisite course work, statistics course. *Application deadline:* 7/15 (fall), 10/15 (spring). *Application fee:* $30.

Degree Requirements 36 total credit hours, thesis or project.

Research College of Nursing
College of Nursing
Kansas City, Missouri

http://www.researchcollege.edu/
Founded in 1980

DEGREES • BSN • MSN

Nursing Program Faculty 37 (16% with doctorates).
Baccalaureate Enrollment 339 **Women** 92% **Men** 8% **Minority** 7% **International** 1%
Graduate Enrollment 124 **Women** 95% **Men** 5% **Minority** 13% **Part-time** 90%
Distance Learning Courses Available.
Nursing Student Activities Sigma Theta Tau, Student Nurses' Association.
Nursing Student Resources Academic advising; academic or career counseling; bookstore; campus computer network; career placement assistance; computer lab; computer-assisted instruction; daycare for children of students; e-mail services; housing assistance; Internet; learning resource lab; library services; resume preparation assistance; skills, simulation, or other laboratory; tutoring.
Library Facilities 150,000 volumes; 675 periodical subscriptions.

BACCALAUREATE PROGRAMS

Degree BSN
Available Programs Accelerated Baccalaureate; Accelerated Baccalaureate for Second Degree; Baccalaureate for Second Degree; Generic Baccalaureate.
Study Options Full-time.
Program Entrance Requirements Transcript of college record, high school chemistry, 3 years high school math, 2 years high school science, high school transcript, minimum high school rank 50%, minimum GPA in nursing prerequisites of 2.7. Transfer students are accepted. *Application deadline:* 3/1 (spring). *Application fee:* $20.
Advanced Placement Credit given for nursing courses completed elsewhere dependent upon specific evaluations.
Expenses (2010-11) *Tuition:* full-time $25,000. *Room and board:* $7500; room only: $5000 per academic year. *Required fees:* part-time $25 per credit.
Financial Aid 90% of baccalaureate students in nursing programs received some form of financial aid in 2009-10.
Contact Ms. Leslie Ann Mendenhall, Director of Transfer and Graduate Admissions, College of Nursing, Research College of Nursing, 2525 East Meyer Boulevard, Kansas City, MO 64132-1199. *Telephone:* 816-995-2820. *Fax:* 816-995-2813. *E-mail:* leslie.mendenhall@research-college.edu.

GRADUATE PROGRAMS

Expenses (2010-11) *Tuition:* part-time $400 per credit hour. *Room and board:* room only: $5000 per academic year. *Required fees:* part-time $25 per credit.
Financial Aid 15% of graduate students in nursing programs received some form of financial aid in 2009-10.
Contact Ms. Leslie Ann Mendenhall, Director of Transfer and Graduate Admissions, College of Nursing, Research College of Nursing, 2525 East Meyer Boulevard, Kansas City, MO 64132-1199. *Telephone:* 816-995-2820. *Fax:* 816-995-2813. *E-mail:* leslie.mendenhall@research-college.edu.

MASTER'S DEGREE PROGRAM

Degree MSN
Available Programs Master's.
Concentrations Available Nursing administration; nursing education. *Nurse practitioner programs in:* adult health, family health.
Study Options Full-time and part-time.
Online Degree Options Yes.
Program Entrance Requirements Minimum overall college GPA of 3.0, transcript of college record, CPR certification, written essay, immunizations, interview, 3 letters of recommendation, physical assessment course, professional liability insurance/malpractice insurance, resume, statistics course. *Application deadline:* 7/1 (fall), 10/1 (spring), 4/1 (summer). *Application fee:* $50.
Advanced Placement Credit given for nursing courses completed elsewhere dependent upon specific evaluations.
Degree Requirements 45 total credit hours, thesis or project.

Saint Louis University
School of Nursing
St. Louis, Missouri

http://nursing.slu.edu/
Founded in 1818

DEGREES • BSN • DNP • MN • MSN • PHD

Nursing Program Faculty 45 (67% with doctorates).
Baccalaureate Enrollment 635 **Women** 95% **Men** 5% **Minority** 12% **International** 1% **Part-time** 4%
Graduate Enrollment 602 **Women** 92% **Men** 8% **Minority** 11% **International** 1% **Part-time** 97%
Distance Learning Courses Available.
Nursing Student Activities Sigma Theta Tau, Student Nurses' Association.
Nursing Student Resources Academic advising; academic or career counseling; assistance for students with disabilities; bookstore; campus computer network; career placement assistance; computer lab; computer-assisted instruction; e-mail services; employment services for current students; housing assistance; interactive nursing skills videos; Internet; learning resource lab; library services; nursing audiovisuals; placement services for program completers; remedial services; resume preparation assistance; skills, simulation, or other laboratory; tutoring; unpaid internships.
Library Facilities 1.8 million volumes (156,689 in health, 7,738 in nursing); 18,018 periodical subscriptions (4,776 health-care related).

BACCALAUREATE PROGRAMS

Degree BSN
Available Programs Accelerated Baccalaureate; Accelerated Baccalaureate for Second Degree; Generic Baccalaureate; RN Baccalaureate.
Site Options St. Louis, MO.
Study Options Full-time and part-time.
Program Entrance Requirements Minimum overall college GPA of 3.0, transcript of college record, health exam, high school biology, high school chemistry, high school transcript, immunizations, minimum high school GPA of 3.0. Transfer students are accepted. *Application deadline:* Applications may be processed on a rolling basis for some programs.
Advanced Placement Credit by examination available. Credit given for nursing courses completed elsewhere dependent upon specific evaluations.
Expenses (2010-11) *Tuition:* full-time $32,180; part-time $1125 per credit hour. *Room and board:* $9432 per academic year. *Required fees:* part-time $20 per credit.
Financial Aid 75% of baccalaureate students in nursing programs received some form of financial aid in 2009-10.
Contact Mr. Scott Ragsdale, Recruitment Specialist, School of Nursing, Saint Louis University, 3525 Caroline Street, St. Louis, MO 63104. *Telephone:* 314-977-8995. *Fax:* 314-977-8949. *E-mail:* sragsda2@slu.edu.

GRADUATE PROGRAMS

Expenses (2010-11) *Tuition:* part-time $905–970 per credit hour. *Required fees:* part-time $20 per credit.
Financial Aid 50% of graduate students in nursing programs received some form of financial aid in 2009-10. 2 research assistantships (averaging $10,250 per year), 5 teaching assistantships with full tuition reimbursements available (averaging $11,000 per year) were awarded; Federal Work-Study, scholarships, traineeships, tuition waivers, and unspecified assistantships also available. Aid available to part-time students. *Financial aid application deadline:* 6/1.
Contact Dr. Mary Lee Barron, MSN/DNP Program Director, School of Nursing, Saint Louis University, 3525 Caroline Street, St. Louis, MO 63104. *Telephone:* 314-977-8978. *Fax:* 314-977-8949. *E-mail:* barronml@slu.edu.

MASTER'S DEGREE PROGRAM

Degree MN, MSN
Available Programs Accelerated Master's for Non-Nursing College Graduates; Master's; Master's for Nurses with Non-Nursing Degrees; RN to Master's.
Concentrations Available Nursing education. *Clinical nurse specialist programs in:* adult health, gerontology, pediatric, psychiatric/mental health. *Nurse practitioner programs in:* acute care, adult health, family health, gerontology, pediatric, psychiatric/mental health.
Site Options St. Louis, MO.
Study Options Full-time and part-time.
Online Degree Options Yes (online only).

Program Entrance Requirements Minimum overall college GPA of 3.2, transcript of college record, CPR certification, immunizations, 3 letters of recommendation, resume. *Application deadline:* 4/1 (fall), 9/1 (spring). *Application fee:* $40.

Advanced Placement Credit given for nursing courses completed elsewhere dependent upon specific evaluations.

Degree Requirements 3 total credit hours, comprehensive exam.

POST-MASTER'S PROGRAM

Areas of Study Nursing education. *Clinical nurse specialist programs in:* adult health, gerontology, pediatric, psychiatric/mental health. *Nurse practitioner programs in:* acute care, adult health, family health, gerontology, pediatric, psychiatric/mental health.

DOCTORAL DEGREE PROGRAM

Degree DNP, PhD

Available Programs Doctorate.

Areas of Study Advanced practice nursing, nursing research.

Site Options St. Louis, MO.

Program Entrance Requirements Minimum overall college GPA of 3.25, 3 letters of recommendation, MSN or equivalent, statistics course, vita, writing sample, GRE general test. Application deadline: 3/15 (fall) for DNP, 4/1 (fall) for PhD. Applications may be processed on a rolling basis for some programs. *Application fee*: $40.

Degree Requirements 28 total credit hours (DNP), 69 total credit hours (PhD), dissertation, oral exam, written exam, residency.

CONTINUING EDUCATION PROGRAM

Contact Mrs. Vicki Moran, Continuing Education Director, Interim, School of Nursing, Saint Louis University, 3525 Caroline Street, St. Louis, MO 63104. *Telephone:* 314-977-8953. *Fax:* 314-977-8949. *E-mail:* moranvl@slu.edu.

Saint Luke's College

Nursing College
Kansas City, Missouri

http://www.saintlukescollege.edu

Founded in 1903

DEGREE • BSN

Nursing Program Faculty 17 (18% with doctorates).

Baccalaureate Enrollment 115 **Women** 95% **Men** 5% **Minority** 10% **International** 1% **Part-time** 12%

Nursing Student Activities Student Nurses' Association.

Nursing Student Resources Academic advising; assistance for students with disabilities; bookstore; campus computer network; career placement assistance; computer lab; computer-assisted instruction; e-mail services; employment services for current students; interactive nursing skills videos; Internet; learning resource lab; library services; nursing audiovisuals; paid internships; skills, simulation, or other laboratory; tutoring.

BACCALAUREATE PROGRAMS

Degree BSN

Available Programs Generic Baccalaureate.

Site Options Kansas City, MO.

Study Options Full-time and part-time.

Program Entrance Requirements Transcript of college record, CPR certification, written essay, health exam, health insurance, high school transcript, immunizations, interview, 3 letters of recommendation, minimum GPA in nursing prerequisites of 2.7, prerequisite course work. Transfer students are accepted.

Advanced Placement Credit given for nursing courses completed elsewhere dependent upon specific evaluations.

Contact ***Telephone:*** 816-932-2367.

Southeast Missouri State University

Department of Nursing
Cape Girardeau, Missouri

http://www.semo.edu/nursing

Founded in 1873

DEGREES • BSN • MSN

Nursing Program Faculty 30 (45% with doctorates).

Baccalaureate Enrollment 495 **Women** 95% **Men** 5% **Minority** 7% **International** 3% **Part-time** 20%

Graduate Enrollment 50 **Women** 80% **Men** 20% **Minority** 2% **Part-time** 65%

Distance Learning Courses Available.

Nursing Student Activities Sigma Theta Tau, Student Nurses' Association.

Nursing Student Resources Academic advising; academic or career counseling; assistance for students with disabilities; bookstore; campus computer network; computer lab; computer-assisted instruction; e-mail services; employment services for current students; externships; housing assistance; interactive nursing skills videos; Internet; learning resource lab; library services; nursing audiovisuals; remedial services; resume preparation assistance; skills, simulation, or other laboratory; tutoring.

Library Facilities 432,199 volumes (450,750 in health, 16,145 in nursing); 52,819 periodical subscriptions (75 health-care related).

BACCALAUREATE PROGRAMS

Degree BSN

Available Programs Accelerated Baccalaureate for Second Degree; Generic Baccalaureate; RN Baccalaureate.

Site Options Poplar Bluff, MO; Sikeston, MO; Kennett, MO.

Study Options Full-time.

Online Degree Options Yes.

Program Entrance Requirements Minimum overall college GPA of 2.5, transcript of college record, CPR certification, health exam, health insurance, immunizations, minimum GPA in nursing prerequisites of 2.5, professional liability insurance/malpractice insurance, prerequisite course work. Transfer students are accepted. *Application deadline:* 3/1 (fall), 10/1 (spring).

Advanced Placement Credit given for nursing courses completed elsewhere dependent upon specific evaluations.

Expenses (2010-11) *Tuition, state resident:* part-time $185 per credit hour. *Tuition, nonresident:* part-time $349 per credit hour. *Required fees:* part-time $24 per credit.

Financial Aid 65% of baccalaureate students in nursing programs received some form of financial aid in 2009-10.

Contact Dr. Ann Sprengel, Chairperson of Student Affairs Committee, Department of Nursing, Southeast Missouri State University, One University Plaza, Mail Stop 8300, Cape Girardeau, MO 63701-4799. *Telephone:* 573-651-2956. *Fax:* 573-651-2142. *E-mail:* asprengel@semo.edu.

GRADUATE PROGRAMS

Expenses (2010-11) *Tuition, state resident:* part-time $237 per credit hour. *Tuition, nonresident:* part-time $442 per credit hour. *Required fees:* part-time $24 per credit.

Financial Aid 50% of graduate students in nursing programs received some form of financial aid in 2009-10. 5 teaching assistantships with full tuition reimbursements available (averaging $7,600 per year) were awarded; unspecified assistantships also available.

Contact Dr. Elaine Jackson, Director, Graduate Studies, Department of Nursing, Southeast Missouri State University, One University Plaza, Mail Stop 8300, Cape Girardeau, MO 63701-4799. *Telephone:* 573-651-2871. *Fax:* 573-651-2142. *E-mail:* ejackson@semo.edu.

MASTER'S DEGREE PROGRAM

Degree MSN

Available Programs Master's.

Concentrations Available Nursing education. *Clinical nurse specialist programs in:* adult health. *Nurse practitioner programs in:* family health.

Site Options Poplar Bluff, MO; Sikeston, MO; Kennett, MO.

Study Options Full-time and part-time.

Program Entrance Requirements Clinical experience, minimum overall college GPA of 3.0, transcript of college record, CPR certification, written essay, immunizations, 2 letters of recommendation,

physical assessment course, professional liability insurance/malpractice insurance, prerequisite course work, resume, statistics course.
Degree Requirements 45 total credit hours, thesis or project.

POST-MASTER'S PROGRAM

Areas of Study *Nurse practitioner programs in:* family health.

Southwest Baptist University
College of Nursing
Bolivar, Missouri

http://www.sbuniv.edu/collegeofnursing
Founded in 1878

DEGREE • BSN
Nursing Program Faculty 8 (25% with doctorates).
Baccalaureate Enrollment 141 **Women** 88.5% **Men** 11.5% **Minority** 2% **Part-time** 70%
Distance Learning Courses Available.
Nursing Student Activities Nursing Honor Society, Student Nurses' Association.
Nursing Student Resources Academic advising; bookstore; campus computer network; computer lab; computer-assisted instruction; e-mail services; interactive nursing skills videos; Internet; learning resource lab; library services; nursing audiovisuals; skills, simulation, or other laboratory.
Library Facilities 208,233 volumes; 40,321 periodical subscriptions.

BACCALAUREATE PROGRAMS

Degree BSN
Available Programs RN Baccalaureate.
Site Options Springfield, MO.
Study Options Full-time and part-time.
Online Degree Options Yes.
Program Entrance Requirements Minimum overall college GPA of 2.5, transcript of college record, CPR certification, high school transcript, immunizations, minimum GPA in nursing prerequisites of 2.5, prerequisite course work, RN licensure. Transfer students are accepted. *Application deadline:* 8/15 (fall), 1/1 (winter), 1/15 (spring), 6/1 (summer). Applications may be processed on a rolling basis for some programs. *Application fee:* $25.
Advanced Placement Credit given for nursing courses completed elsewhere dependent upon specific evaluations.
Expenses (2010-11) *Tuition:* full-time $16,500; part-time $280 per credit hour. *Room and board:* $3640; room only: $2860 per academic year. *Required fees:* full-time $3780; part-time $127 per term.
Financial Aid 50% of baccalaureate students in nursing programs received some form of financial aid in 2009-10. *Gift aid (need-based):* Federal Pell, FSEOG, state, private, college/university gift aid from institutional funds. *Loans:* Federal Nursing Student Loans, Federal Direct (Subsidized and Unsubsidized Stafford PLUS), Perkins, state, alternative loans. *Work-study:* Federal Work-Study. *Financial aid application deadline (priority):* 3/15.
Contact Ms. Dana Hunt, Director, BSN Program, College of Nursing, Southwest Baptist University, 4431 South Fremont Avenue, Springfield, MO 65804. *Telephone:* 417-820-5060. *Fax:* 417-887-4847. *E-mail:* dhunt@sbuniv.edu.

Truman State University
Program in Nursing
Kirksville, Missouri

http://nursing.truman.edu
Founded in 1867

DEGREE • BSN
Nursing Program Faculty 11 (18% with doctorates).
Baccalaureate Enrollment 172 **Women** 94% **Men** 6% **Minority** 5% **International** 5% **Part-time** 1%
Nursing Student Activities Nursing Honor Society, Sigma Theta Tau, Student Nurses' Association, nursing club.
Nursing Student Resources Academic advising; academic or career counseling; assistance for students with disabilities; bookstore; campus computer network; career placement assistance; computer lab; computer-assisted instruction; e-mail services; employment services for current students; externships; interactive nursing skills videos; Internet; learning resource lab; library services; nursing audiovisuals; paid internships; remedial services; resume preparation assistance; skills, simulation, or other laboratory; tutoring; unpaid internships.
Library Facilities 498,273 volumes (6,923 in health, 1,654 in nursing); 3,837 periodical subscriptions (900 health-care related).

BACCALAUREATE PROGRAMS

Degree BSN
Available Programs Generic Baccalaureate.
Study Options Full-time.
Program Entrance Requirements Minimum overall college GPA of 2.75, transcript of college record, written essay, high school biology, high school chemistry, high school foreign language, 3 years high school math, 3 years high school science, high school transcript, immunizations, minimum high school GPA of 3.3, minimum GPA in nursing prerequisites of 3.0. Transfer students are accepted.
Contact *Telephone:* 660-785-4557. *Fax:* 660-785-7424.

University of Central Missouri
Department of Nursing
Warrensburg, Missouri

http://www.ucmo.edu/nursing
Founded in 1871

DEGREES • BS • MS
Nursing Program Faculty 20 (30% with doctorates).
Baccalaureate Enrollment 144 **Women** 93% **Men** 7% **Minority** 10% **International** 4%
Graduate Enrollment 131 **Women** 93% **Men** 7% **Minority** 8% **Part-time** 87%
Distance Learning Courses Available.
Nursing Student Activities Nursing club.
Nursing Student Resources Academic advising; academic or career counseling; assistance for students with disabilities; bookstore; campus computer network; career placement assistance; computer lab; computer-assisted instruction; daycare for children of students; e-mail services; employment services for current students; externships; housing assistance; interactive nursing skills videos; Internet; learning resource lab; library services; nursing audiovisuals; placement services for program completers; remedial services; resume preparation assistance; skills, simulation, or other laboratory; tutoring.
Library Facilities 1.3 million volumes (17,000 in health, 1,000 in nursing); 1,338 periodical subscriptions (300 health-care related).

BACCALAUREATE PROGRAMS

Degree BS
Available Programs ADN to Baccalaureate; Generic Baccalaureate; RN Baccalaureate.
Site Options Warrensburg, MO; Lee's Summit, MO.
Study Options Full-time.
Online Degree Options Yes.
Program Entrance Requirements Minimum overall college GPA of 2.75, minimum GPA in nursing prerequisites of 2.0, prerequisite course work. Transfer students are accepted. *Application deadline:* 1/1 (fall), 7/1 (spring). *Application fee:* $45.
Advanced Placement Credit by examination available. Credit given for nursing courses completed elsewhere dependent upon specific evaluations.
Expenses (2010-11) *Tuition, state resident:* full-time $5859; part-time $195 per credit hour. *Tuition, nonresident:* full-time $11,718; part-time $391 per credit hour. *Room and board:* $5620; room only: $4520 per academic year. *Required fees:* full-time $400.
Financial Aid 86% of baccalaureate students in nursing programs received some form of financial aid in 2009-10.
Contact Dr. Julie Ann Clawson, Chair, Department of Nursing, University of Central Missouri, 600 South College, UHC 106A, Warrensburg, MO 64093. *Telephone:* 660-543-4775. *Fax:* 660-543-8304. *E-mail:* clawson@ucmo.edu.

GRADUATE PROGRAMS

Expenses (2010-11) *Tuition, state resident:* full-time $3038; part-time $253 per credit hour. *Tuition, nonresident:* full-time $6076; part-time $506 per credit hour. *International tuition:* $6076 full-time. *Room and board:* $5620; room only: $4520 per academic year.

Financial Aid 70% of graduate students in nursing programs received some form of financial aid in 2009-10.
Contact Dr. Joseph Vaughn, Dean, Department of Nursing, University of Central Missouri, Graduate Studies, WDE 1800, Warrensburg, MO 64093. *Telephone:* 660-543-4621. *E-mail:* vaughn@ucmo.edu.

MASTER'S DEGREE PROGRAM

Degree MS
Available Programs Master's.
Concentrations Available Nursing education. *Nurse practitioner programs in:* family health.
Site Options Warrensburg, MO; Lee's Summit, MO.
Study Options Part-time.
Online Degree Options Yes (online only).
Program Entrance Requirements Clinical experience, minimum overall college GPA of 3.0, transcript of college record, CPR certification, immunizations, professional liability insurance/malpractice insurance. *Application deadline:* Applications may be processed on a rolling basis for some programs. *Application fee:* $45.
Advanced Placement Credit given for nursing courses completed elsewhere dependent upon specific evaluations.
Degree Requirements 32 total credit hours, thesis or project.

POST-MASTER'S PROGRAM

Areas of Study Nursing education. *Nurse practitioner programs in:* family health.

See full description on page 496.

University of Missouri

Sinclair School of Nursing
Columbia, Missouri

http://nursing.missouri.edu
Founded in 1839

DEGREES • BSN • MSN • MSN/PHD • PHD

Baccalaureate Enrollment 380 **Women** 90% **Men** 10% **Minority** 6% **International** 3% **Part-time** 31%
Graduate Enrollment 200 **Women** 95% **Men** 5% **Minority** 8% **International** 2% **Part-time** 77%
Distance Learning Courses Available.
Nursing Student Activities Nursing Honor Society, Sigma Theta Tau, Student Nurses' Association, nursing club.
Nursing Student Resources Academic advising; academic or career counseling; assistance for students with disabilities; bookstore; campus computer network; career placement assistance; computer lab; computer-assisted instruction; daycare for children of students; e-mail services; employment services for current students; externships; housing assistance; interactive nursing skills videos; Internet; learning resource lab; library services; nursing audiovisuals; paid internships; remedial services; resume preparation assistance; skills, simulation, or other laboratory; tutoring; unpaid internships.
Library Facilities 3.5 million volumes (114,580 in health, 6,416 in nursing); 46,543 periodical subscriptions.

BACCALAUREATE PROGRAMS

Degree BSN
Available Programs ADN to Baccalaureate; Accelerated Baccalaureate; Accelerated Baccalaureate for Second Degree; Generic Baccalaureate; RN Baccalaureate.
Study Options Full-time and part-time.
Online Degree Options Yes.
Program Entrance Requirements Minimum overall college GPA of 2.5, transcript of college record, CPR certification, high school biology, high school chemistry, 4 years high school math, 3 years high school science, high school transcript, immunizations, interview, minimum GPA in nursing prerequisites of 2.5, prerequisite course work. Transfer students are accepted.
Advanced Placement Credit by examination available. Credit given for nursing courses completed elsewhere dependent upon specific evaluations.
Contact ***Telephone:*** 573-882-0277. *Fax:* 573-884-4544.

GRADUATE PROGRAMS

Contact ***Telephone:*** 573-882-0277.

MASTER'S DEGREE PROGRAM

Degrees MSN; MSN/PhD
Available Programs Master's.
Concentrations Available Nursing administration; nursing education. *Clinical nurse specialist programs in:* acute care, adult health, cardiovascular, community health, critical care, home health care, maternity-newborn, oncology, palliative care, pediatric, public health, rehabilitation, school health, women's health. *Nurse practitioner programs in:* family health, gerontology, pediatric, primary care, psychiatric/mental health.
Study Options Full-time and part-time.
Online Degree Options Yes (online only).
Program Entrance Requirements Computer literacy, minimum overall college GPA of 3.0, transcript of college record, CPR certification, immunizations, interview, 2 letters of recommendation, nursing research course, prerequisite course work, statistics course, GRE General Test.
Advanced Placement Credit given for nursing courses completed elsewhere dependent upon specific evaluations.
Degree Requirements 43 total credit hours, comprehensive exam.

POST-MASTER'S PROGRAM

Areas of Study Nursing administration; nursing education. *Clinical nurse specialist programs in:* acute care, adult health, cardiovascular, community health, critical care, home health care, maternity-newborn, oncology, palliative care, pediatric, public health, rehabilitation, school health, women's health. *Nurse practitioner programs in:* family health, gerontology, pediatric, primary care, psychiatric/mental health.

DOCTORAL DEGREE PROGRAM

Degree PhD
Available Programs Doctorate; Post-Baccalaureate Doctorate.
Areas of Study Aging, family health, gerontology, health promotion/disease prevention, health-care systems, human health and illness, nursing research, oncology, women's health.
Program Entrance Requirements Minimum overall college GPA of 3.5, interview by faculty committee, 3 letters of recommendation, vita, writing sample.
Degree Requirements 72 total credit hours, dissertation, oral exam, written exam, residency.

CONTINUING EDUCATION PROGRAM

Contact *Telephone:* 573-882-0215. *Fax:* 573-884-4544.

University of Missouri–Kansas City

School of Nursing
Kansas City, Missouri

http://www.umkc.edu/nursing
Founded in 1929

DEGREES • BSN • MSN • PHD

Nursing Program Faculty 48 (44% with doctorates).
Baccalaureate Enrollment 462 **Women** 90% **Men** 10% **Minority** 19% **International** .01% **Part-time** 27%
Graduate Enrollment 381 **Women** 93% **Men** 7% **Minority** 10% **Part-time** 87%
Distance Learning Courses Available.
Nursing Student Activities Sigma Theta Tau, Student Nurses' Association.
Nursing Student Resources Academic advising; academic or career counseling; assistance for students with disabilities; bookstore; campus computer network; career placement assistance; computer lab; computer-assisted instruction; e-mail services; employment services for current students; housing assistance; interactive nursing skills videos; Internet; learning resource lab; library services; nursing audiovisuals; other; placement services for program completers; remedial services; resume preparation assistance; skills, simulation, or other laboratory; tutoring.
Library Facilities 1.8 million volumes (111,108 in health, 15,000 in nursing); 48,869 periodical subscriptions (60,000 health-care related).

BACCALAUREATE PROGRAMS

Degree BSN
Available Programs Accelerated Baccalaureate; Generic Baccalaureate; RN Baccalaureate.
Study Options Full-time.
Program Entrance Requirements Minimum overall college GPA of 2.75, transcript of college record, CPR certification, written essay, health insurance, high school foreign language, 4 years high school math, 4 years high school science, high school transcript, immunizations, 1 letter of recommendation, minimum GPA in nursing prerequisites of 2.75, professional liability insurance/malpractice insurance, prerequisite course work. Transfer students are accepted. *Application deadline:* 1/31 (fall).
Expenses (2010-11) *Tuition, state resident:* full-time $7358; part-time $246 per credit hour. *Tuition, nonresident:* full-time $18,459; part-time $615 per credit hour. *International tuition:* $27,098 full-time. *Room and board:* $16,320 per academic year. *Required fees:* full-time $2553; part-time $48 per credit; part-time $696 per term.
Financial Aid 76% of baccalaureate students in nursing programs received some form of financial aid in 2009-10. *Gift aid (need-based):* Federal Pell, FSEOG, state, private, college/university gift aid from institutional funds, United Negro College Fund. *Loans:* Federal Nursing Student Loans, Federal Direct (Subsidized and Unsubsidized Stafford PLUS), Perkins, state, college/university. *Work-study:* Federal Work-Study. *Financial aid application deadline (priority):* 3/1.
Contact Ms. Judy A. Jellison, Director, Nursing Student Services, School of Nursing, University of Missouri–Kansas City, 2464 Charlotte Street, Kansas City, MO 64108. *Telephone:* 816-235-1740. *Fax:* 816-235-6593. *E-mail:* jellisonj@umkc.edu.

GRADUATE PROGRAMS

Expenses (2010-11) *Tuition, state resident:* full-time $7363; part-time $307 per credit hour. *Tuition, nonresident:* full-time $19,008; part-time $792 per credit hour. *Room and board:* $16,320 per academic year. *Required fees:* full-time $2054; part-time $48 per credit; part-time $578 per term.
Financial Aid 62% of graduate students in nursing programs received some form of financial aid in 2009-10. 6 teaching assistantships with partial tuition reimbursements available (averaging $4,402 per year) were awarded; fellowships, research assistantships, career-related internships or fieldwork, Federal Work-Study, institutionally sponsored loans, and tuition waivers (full and partial) also available. Aid available to part-time students. *Financial aid application deadline:* 3/1.
Contact Ms. Judy A. Jellison, Director, Nursing Student Services, School of Nursing, University of Missouri–Kansas City, 2464 Charlotte Street, Kansas City, MO 64108. *Telephone:* 816-235-1740. *Fax:* 816-235-6593. *E-mail:* jellisonj@umkc.edu.

MASTER'S DEGREE PROGRAM

Degree MSN
Available Programs Master's.
Concentrations Available Nursing education. *Nurse practitioner programs in:* adult health, family health, neonatal health, pediatric, women's health.
Site Options Joplin, MO; St. Joseph, MO.
Study Options Full-time and part-time.
Program Entrance Requirements Clinical experience, computer literacy, minimum overall college GPA of 3.2, transcript of college record, CPR certification, written essay, immunizations, 3 letters of recommendation, physical assessment course, professional liability insurance/malpractice insurance, resume, statistics course. *Application deadline:* 12/1 (fall), 12/1 (summer). *Application fee:* $35.
Degree Requirements 43 total credit hours.

POST-MASTER'S PROGRAM

Areas of Study Nursing education. *Nurse practitioner programs in:* adult health, family health, neonatal health, pediatric, women's health.

DOCTORAL DEGREE PROGRAM

Degree PhD
Available Programs Doctorate; Post-Baccalaureate Doctorate.
Areas of Study Health promotion/disease prevention, health-care systems.
Program Entrance Requirements Minimum overall college GPA of 3.5, interview by faculty committee, interview, 3 letters of recommendation, MSN or equivalent, vita, writing sample, GRE. Application deadline: 2/1 (summer). Application fee: $35.
Degree Requirements 61 total credit hours, dissertation, oral exam, written exam, residency.

CONTINUING EDUCATION PROGRAM

Contact Jodi M. Baker, Continuing Education Coordinator, School of Nursing, University of Missouri–Kansas City, 2464 Charlotte Street,

Kansas City, MO 64108. *Telephone:* 816-235-6463. *Fax:* 816-235-1701. *E-mail:* bakerjm@umkc.edu.

University of Missouri–St. Louis
College of Nursing
St. Louis, Missouri

http://www.umsl.edu/divisions/nursing/
Founded in 1963

DEGREES • BSN • DNP • MSN
Nursing Program Faculty 72 (32% with doctorates).
Baccalaureate Enrollment 652 **Women** 89% **Men** 11% **Minority** 22% **International** 1% **Part-time** 32%
Graduate Enrollment 260 **Women** 94% **Men** 6% **Minority** 12% **Part-time** 98%
Distance Learning Courses Available.
Nursing Student Activities Nursing Honor Society, Sigma Theta Tau, Student Nurses' Association.
Nursing Student Resources Academic advising; academic or career counseling; assistance for students with disabilities; bookstore; campus computer network; career placement assistance; computer lab; computer-assisted instruction; daycare for children of students; e-mail services; employment services for current students; externships; interactive nursing skills videos; Internet; learning resource lab; library services; nursing audiovisuals; resume preparation assistance; skills, simulation, or other laboratory; tutoring; unpaid internships.
Library Facilities 1.2 million volumes (85,320 in health, 17,577 in nursing); 3,149 periodical subscriptions (6,000 health-care related).

BACCALAUREATE PROGRAMS

Degree BSN
Available Programs Accelerated Baccalaureate; Baccalaureate for Second Degree; Generic Baccalaureate; RN Baccalaureate.
Site Options Bridgeton, Creve Coeur, St. Louis, MO; St. Charles, MO.
Study Options Full-time and part-time.
Online Degree Options Yes.
Program Entrance Requirements Minimum overall college GPA of 2.5, transcript of college record, CPR certification, health exam, 4 years high school math, 3 years high school science, high school transcript, immunizations, minimum high school GPA of 2.5, minimum GPA in nursing prerequisites, professional liability insurance/malpractice insurance. Transfer students are accepted. *Application deadline:* 2/1 (fall), 10/1 (spring). *Application fee:* $35.
Advanced Placement Credit given for nursing courses completed elsewhere dependent upon specific evaluations.
Expenses (2010-11) *Tuition, state resident:* full-time $7368; part-time $246 per credit hour. *Tuition, nonresident:* full-time $18,957; part-time $632 per credit hour. *Room and board:* $8620; room only: $4804 per academic year. *Required fees:* full-time $1263; part-time $49 per credit; part-time $12 per term.
Financial Aid 73% of baccalaureate students in nursing programs received some form of financial aid in 2009-10. *Gift aid (need-based):* Federal Pell, FSEOG, state, private, college/university gift aid from institutional funds, United Negro College Fund, Federal Nursing, Academic Competitiveness Grants, National Smart Grants, Federal TEACH Grants. *Loans:* Federal Nursing Student Loans, Federal Direct (Subsidized and Unsubsidized Stafford PLUS), Perkins. *Work-study:* Federal Work-Study. *Financial aid application deadline (priority):* 4/1.
Contact Dr. Sandra J. Lindquist, Associate Dean for the Undergraduate Program, College of Nursing, University of Missouri–St. Louis, One University Boulevard, 233 Nursing Administration Building, St. Louis, MO 63121-4499. *Telephone:* 314-516-6066. *Fax:* 314-516-7519. *E-mail:* sandy_lindquist@umsl.edu.

GRADUATE PROGRAMS

Expenses (2010-11) *Tuition, state resident:* full-time $7363; part-time $307 per credit hour. *Tuition, nonresident:* full-time $19,008; part-time $792 per credit hour. *Room and board:* $8620; room only: $4804 per academic year. *Required fees:* full-time $1190; part-time $49 per credit; part-time $12 per term.
Financial Aid 62% of graduate students in nursing programs received some form of financial aid in 2009-10. 1 research assistantship with full and partial tuition reimbursement available (averaging $12,339 per year), 4 teaching assistantships with full and partial tuition reimbursements available (averaging $12,339 per year) were awarded. *Financial aid application deadline:* 4/1.
Contact Dr. Nancy Magnuson, Acting Associate Dean for Advanced Nursing Education, College of Nursing, University of Missouri–St. Louis, One University Boulevard, Nursing Administration Building, St. Louis, MO 63121-4499. *Telephone:* 314-516-6066. *Fax:* 314-516-7519. *E-mail:* magnusonn@umsl.edu.

MASTER'S DEGREE PROGRAM

Degree MSN
Available Programs Master's.
Concentrations Available Nursing education. *Nurse practitioner programs in:* adult health, family health, neonatal health, pediatric, women's health.
Site Options St. Charles, MO; Park Hills, Town & Country, MO.
Study Options Full-time and part-time.
Online Degree Options Yes.
Program Entrance Requirements Clinical experience, minimum overall college GPA of 3.0, transcript of college record, CPR certification, immunizations, 2 letters of recommendation, physical assessment course, statistics course, GRE. *Application deadline:* 2/15 (fall), 10/1 (spring). *Application fee:* $35.
Advanced Placement Credit given for nursing courses completed elsewhere dependent upon specific evaluations.
Degree Requirements 43 total credit hours.

POST-MASTER'S PROGRAM

Areas of Study *Nurse practitioner programs in:* adult health, family health, pediatric, women's health.

DOCTORAL DEGREE PROGRAM

Degree DNP
Available Programs Doctorate.
Areas of Study Advanced practice nursing.
Program Entrance Requirements Minimum overall college GPA of 3.0, interview, 2 letters of recommendation, MSN or equivalent, statistics course, writing sample, GRE. Application deadline: 4/1 (fall). Application fee: $35.
Degree Requirements 30 total credit hours, dissertation.

CONTINUING EDUCATION PROGRAM

Contact Vanessa Loyd, Director of Continuing Education and Outreach, College of Nursing, University of Missouri–St. Louis, One University Boulevard, St. Louis, MO 63121-4400. *Telephone:* 314-516-6066. *Fax:* 314-516-6730. *E-mail:* loydv@umsl.edu.

Webster University
Department of Nursing
St. Louis, Missouri

http://www.webster.edu/depts/artsci/nursing/nursing.html
Founded in 1915

DEGREES • BSN • MSN
Nursing Program Faculty 12 (72% with doctorates).
Baccalaureate Enrollment 150 **Women** 93% **Men** 7% **Minority** 14% **International** 1% **Part-time** 90%
Graduate Enrollment 75 **Women** 90% **Men** 10% **Minority** 20% **International** 10% **Part-time** 100%
Nursing Student Activities Nursing Honor Society, Sigma Theta Tau.
Nursing Student Resources Academic advising; academic or career counseling; assistance for students with disabilities; bookstore; campus computer network; career placement assistance; computer lab; e-mail services; employment services for current students; Internet; learning resource lab; library services; nursing audiovisuals; placement services for program completers; remedial services; resume preparation assistance; skills, simulation, or other laboratory; tutoring.
Library Facilities 279,928 volumes (7,030 in health, 3,114 in nursing); 1,536 periodical subscriptions (108 health-care related).

BACCALAUREATE PROGRAMS

Degree BSN
Available Programs ADN to Baccalaureate; RN Baccalaureate.
Site Options Kansas City, MO.
Program Entrance Requirements Minimum overall college GPA of 2.5, transcript of college record, immunizations, interview, prerequisite course work, RN licensure. Transfer students are accepted.

Contact *Telephone:* 314-968-7483. *Fax:* 314-963-6101.

GRADUATE PROGRAMS

Contact *Telephone:* 314-968-7483. *Fax:* 314-963-6101.

MASTER'S DEGREE PROGRAM

Degree MSN
Available Programs Master's; RN to Master's.
Concentrations Available Nursing administration; nursing education. *Clinical nurse specialist programs in:* family health.
Site Options Kansas City, MO.
Study Options Part-time.
Program Entrance Requirements Clinical experience, computer literacy, minimum overall college GPA of 3.0, transcript of college record, written essay, immunizations, interview, 3 letters of recommendation, nursing research course, physical assessment course, resume, statistics course.
Advanced Placement Credit given for nursing courses completed elsewhere dependent upon specific evaluations.
Degree Requirements 36 total credit hours, thesis or project.

William Jewell College

Department of Nursing
Liberty, Missouri

http://www.jewell.edu/
Founded in 1849

DEGREE • BS

Nursing Program Faculty 36 (25% with doctorates).
Baccalaureate Enrollment 150 **Women** 89% **Men** 11% **Minority** 3% **International** 1%
Nursing Student Activities Nursing Honor Society, Sigma Theta Tau, Student Nurses' Association.
Nursing Student Resources Academic advising; academic or career counseling; assistance for students with disabilities; bookstore; campus computer network; career placement assistance; computer lab; computer-assisted instruction; e-mail services; employment services for current students; externships; housing assistance; interactive nursing skills videos; Internet; learning resource lab; library services; nursing audiovisuals; paid internships; placement services for program completers; resume preparation assistance; skills, simulation, or other laboratory; tutoring; unpaid internships.
Library Facilities 191,798 volumes (4,000 in health, 1,000 in nursing); 323 periodical subscriptions (250 health-care related).

BACCALAUREATE PROGRAMS

Degree BS
Available Programs Accelerated Baccalaureate; Generic Baccalaureate.
Study Options Full-time.
Program Entrance Requirements Minimum overall college GPA of 2.7, transcript of college record, CPR certification, written essay, health insurance, high school foreign language, high school transcript, immunizations, interview, 2 letters of recommendation, minimum high school GPA of 3.0, minimum GPA in nursing prerequisites of 2.7, professional liability insurance/malpractice insurance, prerequisite course work. Transfer students are accepted. *Application deadline:* 6/1 (spring), 8/1 (summer). *Application fee:* $25.
Advanced Placement Credit given for nursing courses completed elsewhere dependent upon specific evaluations.
Expenses (2010-11) *Tuition:* full-time $28,450; part-time $825 per contact hour. *Room and board:* $7200; room only: $4000 per academic year. *Required fees:* full-time $825.
Financial Aid 90% of baccalaureate students in nursing programs received some form of financial aid in 2009-10. *Gift aid (need-based):* Federal Pell, FSEOG, state, college/university gift aid from institutional funds. *Loans:* Federal Nursing Student Loans, Perkins, alternative loans. *Work-study:* Federal Work-Study, part-time campus jobs. *Financial aid application deadline (priority):* 3/1.
Contact Ms. Katie A. Stiles, Nursing Admissions Counselor, Department of Nursing, William Jewell College, 500 College Hill, Box 2002, Liberty, MO 64068. *Telephone:* 816-415-5072. *Fax:* 816-415-5024. *E-mail:* stilesk@william.jewell.edu.

MONTANA

Carroll College

Department of Nursing
Helena, Montana

http://www.carroll.edu/
Founded in 1909

DEGREE • BSN

Nursing Program Faculty 24 (13% with doctorates).
Baccalaureate Enrollment 128 **Women** 91% **Men** 9% **Minority** 4% **Part-time** 4%
Nursing Student Activities Nursing Honor Society, Sigma Theta Tau, Student Nurses' Association.
Nursing Student Resources Academic advising; academic or career counseling; assistance for students with disabilities; bookstore; campus computer network; career placement assistance; computer lab; computer-assisted instruction; e-mail services; employment services for current students; externships; housing assistance; interactive nursing skills videos; Internet; learning resource lab; library services; nursing audiovisuals; paid internships; placement services for program completers; remedial services; resume preparation assistance; skills, simulation, or other laboratory; tutoring; unpaid internships.
Library Facilities 89,003 volumes (1,300 in health, 700 in nursing); 2,721 periodical subscriptions (1,000 health-care related).

BACCALAUREATE PROGRAMS

Degree BSN
Available Programs Generic Baccalaureate.
Study Options Full-time.
Program Entrance Requirements Minimum overall college GPA of 2.75, transcript of college record, high school transcript, immunizations, minimum GPA in nursing prerequisites of 2.75, prerequisite course work. Transfer students are accepted. *Application deadline:* 2/15 (spring).
Expenses (2010-11) *Tuition:* full-time $23,144; part-time $772 per credit. *Room and board:* $7518 per academic year. *Required fees:* full-time $920.
Financial Aid 97% of baccalaureate students in nursing programs received some form of financial aid in 2009-10.
Contact Mr. Scott Knickerbocker, Associate Director, Admissions, Department of Nursing, Carroll College, 1601 North Benton Avenue, Helena, MT 59625. *Telephone:* 406-447-4387. *Fax:* 406-447-4533. *E-mail:* sknicker@carroll.edu.

Montana State University

College of Nursing
Bozeman, Montana

http://www.montana.edu/nursing
Founded in 1893

DEGREES • BSN • MN

Nursing Program Faculty 90 (23% with doctorates).
Baccalaureate Enrollment 872 **Women** 88.6% **Men** 11.4% **Minority** 8.4% **International** .01% **Part-time** 23.3%
Graduate Enrollment 78 **Women** 97.4% **Men** 2.6% **Minority** 7.7% **Part-time** 53.8%
Distance Learning Courses Available.
Nursing Student Activities Sigma Theta Tau, Student Nurses' Association.
Nursing Student Resources Academic advising; academic or career counseling; assistance for students with disabilities; bookstore; campus computer network; career placement assistance; computer lab; computer-assisted instruction; daycare for children of students; e-mail services; employment services for current students; housing assistance; Internet; library services; nursing audiovisuals; paid internships; placement services for program completers; remedial services; resume preparation assistance; skills, simulation, or other laboratory; tutoring; unpaid internships.
Library Facilities 744,989 volumes (80,389 in health, 11,535 in nursing); 10,131 periodical subscriptions (1,690 health-care related).

BACCALAUREATE PROGRAMS

Degree BSN

Available Programs Accelerated Baccalaureate; Generic Baccalaureate; LPN to Baccalaureate.

Site Options Billings, MT; Missoula, MT; Great Falls, MT.

Study Options Full-time and part-time.

Program Entrance Requirements Minimum overall college GPA of 2.5, transcript of college record, CPR certification, health exam, health insurance, high school transcript, immunizations, minimum high school GPA of 2.5, minimum high school rank 50%, minimum GPA in nursing prerequisites of 2.5, prerequisite course work. Transfer students are accepted. *Application deadline:* 7/1 (fall), 12/1 (spring), 5/1 (summer). Applications may be processed on a rolling basis for some programs. *Application fee:* $30.

Advanced Placement Credit by examination available. Credit given for nursing courses completed elsewhere dependent upon specific evaluations.

Expenses (2010-11) *Tuition, state resident:* full-time $4836; part-time $202 per credit. *Tuition, nonresident:* full-time $16,872; part-time $703 per credit. *Room and board:* $7200 per academic year. *Required fees:* full-time $1718; part-time $118 per credit; part-time $859 per term.

Financial Aid 70% of baccalaureate students in nursing programs received some form of financial aid in 2009-10.

Contact Ms. Melissa Gutzman, Undergraduate Student Services Coordinator, College of Nursing, Montana State University, Sherrick Hall, PO Box 173560, Bozeman, MT 59717-3560. *Telephone:* 406-994-3783. *Fax:* 406-994-6020. *E-mail:* melissak@montana.edu.

GRADUATE PROGRAMS

Expenses (2010-11) *Tuition, state resident:* full-time $5803; part-time $242 per credit. *Tuition, nonresident:* full-time $17,839; part-time $743 per credit. *Room and board:* $7200 per academic year. *Required fees:* full-time $2655; part-time $158 per credit; part-time $1328 per term.

Financial Aid 70% of graduate students in nursing programs received some form of financial aid in 2009-10. 3 fellowships with full tuition reimbursements available (averaging $15,000 per year), 1 research assistantship (averaging $7,000 per year), 8 teaching assistantships with partial tuition reimbursements available (averaging $7,050 per year) were awarded; traineeships and tuition waivers (partial) also available. *Financial aid application deadline:* 3/1.

Contact Ms. Lynn Taylor, Graduate Program Assistant, College of Nursing, Montana State University, Sherrick Hall, PO Box 173560, Bozeman, MT 59717-3560. *Telephone:* 406-994-3500. *Fax:* 406-994-6020. *E-mail:* lynnt@montana.edu.

MASTER'S DEGREE PROGRAM

Degree MN

Available Programs Master's.

Concentrations Available Clinical nurse leader. *Nurse practitioner programs in:* family health, psychiatric/mental health.

Site Options Billings, MT; Missoula, MT; Great Falls, MT.

Study Options Full-time and part-time.

Program Entrance Requirements Computer literacy, minimum overall college GPA of 3.0, transcript of college record, CPR certification, written essay, immunizations, interview, 3 letters of recommendation, nursing research course, physical assessment course, prerequisite course work, statistics course, GRE General Test. *Application deadline:* 2/15 (fall). *Application fee:* $50.

Advanced Placement Credit given for nursing courses completed elsewhere dependent upon specific evaluations.

Degree Requirements 35 total credit hours, thesis or project, comprehensive exam.

POST-MASTER'S PROGRAM

Areas of Study Nursing education. *Nurse practitioner programs in:* family health, psychiatric/mental health.

Montana State University–Northern

College of Nursing
Havre, Montana

http://www.msun.edu/academics/nursing
Founded in 1929

DEGREE • BSN

Nursing Program Faculty 12 (8% with doctorates).
Baccalaureate Enrollment 53 **Women** 96% **Men** 4% **Part-time** 92%
Distance Learning Courses Available.
Nursing Student Activities Nursing club.
Nursing Student Resources Academic advising; academic or career counseling; assistance for students with disabilities; bookstore; campus computer network; career placement assistance; computer lab; computer-assisted instruction; e-mail services; employment services for current students; housing assistance; interactive nursing skills videos; Internet; learning resource lab; library services; nursing audiovisuals; remedial services; resume preparation assistance; skills, simulation, or other laboratory; tutoring.
Library Facilities 128,000 volumes (2,600 in health, 1,300 in nursing); 1,729 periodical subscriptions (40 health-care related).

BACCALAUREATE PROGRAMS

Degree BSN
Available Programs ADN to Baccalaureate; RN Baccalaureate.
Site Options Great Falls, MT; Lewistown, MT.
Study Options Full-time and part-time.
Online Degree Options Yes (online only).
Program Entrance Requirements Minimum overall college GPA of 2.25, transcript of college record, CPR certification, health exam, health insurance, immunizations, professional liability insurance/malpractice insurance, prerequisite course work, RN licensure. Transfer students are accepted. *Application deadline:* 8/1 (fall), 1/10 (winter), 5/2 (summer). Applications may be processed on a rolling basis for some programs. *Application fee:* $30.
Advanced Placement Credit given for nursing courses completed elsewhere dependent upon specific evaluations.
Expenses (2010-11) *Tuition, state resident:* full-time $11,200; part-time $250 per credit. *Tuition, nonresident:* full-time $22,000; part-time $500 per credit. *Room and board:* $6000 per academic year. *Required fees:* full-time $500; part-time $25 per credit; part-time $150 per term.
Financial Aid 60% of baccalaureate students in nursing programs received some form of financial aid in 2009-10.
Contact Ms. Judy Bricker, Administrative Associate II, College of Nursing, Montana State University–Northern, Havre, MT 59501. *Telephone:* 406-265-4196 Ext. 4196. *Fax:* 406-265-3772. *E-mail:* bricker@msun.edu.

Salish Kootenai College

Nursing Department
Pablo, Montana

Founded in 1977

DEGREE • BS

Nursing Program Faculty 7
Nursing Student Activities Nursing club.
Nursing Student Resources Academic advising; academic or career counseling; bookstore; computer lab; daycare for children of students; employment services for current students; Internet; library services.
Library Facilities 24,000 volumes; 200 periodical subscriptions.

BACCALAUREATE PROGRAMS

Degree BS
Available Programs RN Baccalaureate.
Study Options Full-time and part-time.
Program Entrance Requirements Transcript of college record, CPR certification, health exam, health insurance, high school biology, high school chemistry, 2 years high school math, 2 years high school science, high school transcript, immunizations, minimum high school GPA of 2.5, professional liability insurance/malpractice insurance, prerequisite course work, RN licensure.
Contact *Telephone:* 406-275-4800.

NEBRASKA

BryanLGH College of Health Sciences

School of Nursing
Lincoln, Nebraska

http://www.bryanlghcollege.edu/

DEGREES • BSN • MS

Nursing Program Faculty 29 (10% with doctorates).
Baccalaureate Enrollment 414 **Women** 91% **Men** 9% **Minority** 7% **Part-time** 47%
Graduate Enrollment 39 **Women** 54% **Men** 46% **Minority** 13%
Distance Learning Courses Available.
Nursing Student Activities Sigma Theta Tau, Student Nurses' Association.
Nursing Student Resources Academic advising; academic or career counseling; assistance for students with disabilities; bookstore; campus computer network; career placement assistance; computer lab; computer-assisted instruction; e-mail services; employment services for current students; housing assistance; Internet; learning resource lab; library services; nursing audiovisuals; remedial services; resume preparation assistance; skills, simulation, or other laboratory; tutoring.
Library Facilities 4,000 volumes in health, 3,500 volumes in nursing; 95 periodical subscriptions health-care related.

BACCALAUREATE PROGRAMS

Degree BSN
Available Programs Generic Baccalaureate; RN Baccalaureate.
Study Options Full-time.
Program Entrance Requirements Minimum overall college GPA of 2.0, transcript of college record, written essay, health exam, health insurance, high school transcript, immunizations, interview, 3 letters of recommendation, minimum high school GPA of 2.75. Transfer students are accepted. *Application deadline:* 2/1 (fall), 6/1 (spring). *Application fee:* $40.
Advanced Placement Credit given for nursing courses completed elsewhere dependent upon specific evaluations.
Expenses (2010-11) *Tuition:* full-time $10,660; part-time $410 per credit hour. *Required fees:* full-time $735; part-time $368 per term.
Financial Aid 83% of baccalaureate students in nursing programs received some form of financial aid in 2009-10.
Contact Kelli Backman, Admissions Counselor, School of Nursing, BryanLGH College of Health Sciences, 5035 Everett Street, Lincoln, NE 68505. *Telephone:* 402-481-8698. *Fax:* 402-481-8621. *E-mail:* kelli.backman@bryanlgh.org.

GRADUATE PROGRAMS

Expenses (2010-11) *Tuition:* full-time $11,680; part-time $640 per credit hour. *Required fees:* full-time $894; part-time $37 per credit; part-time $200 per term.
Financial Aid 97% of graduate students in nursing programs received some form of financial aid in 2009-10.
Contact Mr. James D. Cuddeford, Program Administrator/Dean of Nurse Anesthesia, School of Nursing, BryanLGH College of Health Sciences, 1600 South 48th Street, Lincoln, NE 68506. *Telephone:* 402-481-3135. *Fax:* 402-481-8404. *E-mail:* james.cuddeford@bryanlgh.org.

MASTER'S DEGREE PROGRAM

Degree MS
Available Programs Master's; Master's for Nurses with Non-Nursing Degrees.
Concentrations Available Nurse anesthesia.
Study Options Full-time.
Program Entrance Requirements Clinical experience, computer literacy, minimum overall college GPA of 3.0, transcript of college record, CPR certification, written essay, immunizations, interview, 4 letters of recommendation, prerequisite course work, resume. *Application deadline:* 10/30 (fall). *Application fee:* $75.
Degree Requirements 71 total credit hours, thesis or project.

Clarkson College

Master of Science in Nursing Program
Omaha, Nebraska

http://www.clarksoncollege.edu/Programs/Nursing/
Founded in 1888

DEGREES • BSN • MSN

Nursing Program Faculty 42 (6% with doctorates).
Baccalaureate Enrollment 500 **Women** 90% **Men** 10% **Minority** 10% **Part-time** 15%
Graduate Enrollment 200 **Women** 90% **Men** 10% **Minority** 10% **Part-time** 50%
Distance Learning Courses Available.
Nursing Student Activities Sigma Theta Tau, Student Nurses' Association.
Nursing Student Resources Academic advising; academic or career counseling; assistance for students with disabilities; bookstore; campus computer network; career placement assistance; computer lab; computer-assisted instruction; daycare for children of students; e-mail services; employment services for current students; interactive nursing skills videos; Internet; learning resource lab; library services; nursing audiovisuals; placement services for program completers; resume preparation assistance; skills, simulation, or other laboratory; tutoring.
Library Facilities 8,807 volumes (7,500 in health, 2,200 in nursing); 262 periodical subscriptions (600 health-care related).

BACCALAUREATE PROGRAMS

Degree BSN
Available Programs ADN to Baccalaureate; Accelerated RN Baccalaureate; Baccalaureate for Second Degree; Generic Baccalaureate; LPN to Baccalaureate; LPN to RN Baccalaureate; RN Baccalaureate.
Study Options Full-time and part-time.
Online Degree Options Yes.
Program Entrance Requirements Minimum overall college GPA of 2.5, transcript of college record, CPR certification, written essay, health exam, health insurance, 2 years high school math, 2 years high school science, high school transcript, immunizations, minimum high school GPA of 2.5, minimum high school rank 50%. Transfer students are accepted. *Application fee:* $35.
Advanced Placement Credit given for nursing courses completed elsewhere dependent upon specific evaluations.
Expenses (2010-11) *Tuition:* part-time $420 per credit hour. *Required fees:* part-time $25 per credit.
Financial Aid 90% of baccalaureate students in nursing programs received some form of financial aid in 2009-10.
Contact Ms. Denise A. Work, Director of Admissions, Master of Science in Nursing Program, Clarkson College, 101 South 42nd Street, Omaha, NE 68131-2739. *Telephone:* 402-552-3100. *Fax:* 402-552-6057. *E-mail:* admiss@clarksoncollege.edu.

GRADUATE PROGRAMS

Expenses (2010-11) *Tuition:* part-time $468 per credit hour. *Required fees:* part-time $59 per credit.
Financial Aid 65% of graduate students in nursing programs received some form of financial aid in 2009-10. Federal Work-Study, institutionally sponsored loans, and scholarships available. Aid available to part-time students. *Financial aid application deadline:* 3/1.
Contact Ms. Denise A. Work, Director of Admissions, Master of Science in Nursing Program, Clarkson College, 101 South 42nd Street, Omaha, NE 68131-2739. *Telephone:* 800-647-5500. *Fax:* 402-552-6057. *E-mail:* admiss@clarksoncollege.edu.

MASTER'S DEGREE PROGRAM

Degree MSN
Available Programs Master's; RN to Master's.
Concentrations Available Health-care administration; nurse anesthesia; nursing administration; nursing education. *Nurse practitioner programs in:* adult health, family health.
Study Options Full-time and part-time.
Online Degree Options Yes (online only).
Program Entrance Requirements Clinical experience, minimum overall college GPA of 3.0, transcript of college record, written essay, 2 letters of recommendation, resume. *Application deadline:* 7/1 (fall), 11/15 (spring), 4/1 (summer). *Application fee:* $35.

Advanced Placement Credit given for nursing courses completed elsewhere dependent upon specific evaluations.
Degree Requirements 46 total credit hours, thesis or project.

POST-MASTER'S PROGRAM

Areas of Study Health-care administration; nurse anesthesia; nursing administration; nursing education. *Nurse practitioner programs in:* adult health, family health.

CONTINUING EDUCATION PROGRAM

Contact Ms. Denise A. Work, Director of Admissions, Master of Science in Nursing Program, Clarkson College, 101 South 42nd Street, Omaha, NE 68131-2739. *Telephone:* 402-552-3100. *Fax:* 402-552-6057. *E-mail:* workdenise@clarksoncollege.edu.

College of Saint Mary

Division of Health Care Professions
Omaha, Nebraska

Founded in 1923

DEGREE • BSN

Nursing Program Faculty 18 (6% with doctorates).
Baccalaureate Enrollment 45 **Women** 100% **Minority** 10% **Part-time** 65%
Graduate Enrollment 8
Nursing Student Activities Nursing Honor Society, Sigma Theta Tau, Student Nurses' Association, nursing club.
Nursing Student Resources Academic advising; academic or career counseling; bookstore; campus computer network; career placement assistance; computer lab; computer-assisted instruction; e-mail services; interactive nursing skills videos; Internet; learning resource lab; library services; nursing audiovisuals; other; placement services for program completers; resume preparation assistance; skills, simulation, or other laboratory; tutoring.
Library Facilities 89,216 volumes; 224 periodical subscriptions (100 health-care related).

BACCALAUREATE PROGRAMS

Degree BSN
Available Programs ADN to Baccalaureate; Generic Baccalaureate.
Study Options Full-time and part-time.
Program Entrance Requirements Minimum overall college GPA of 2.5, transcript of college record, CPR certification, health exam, immunizations, 2 letters of recommendation, minimum high school GPA, minimum GPA in nursing prerequisites of 2.5, prerequisite course work. Transfer students are accepted.
Advanced Placement Credit given for nursing courses completed elsewhere dependent upon specific evaluations.
Contact ***Telephone:*** 402-399-2658. *Fax:* 402-399-2654.

GRADUATE PROGRAMS

Contact ***Telephone:*** 402-399-2482. *Fax:* 402-399-2414.

Creighton University

School of Nursing
Omaha, Nebraska

http://www.creighton.edu/nursing/
Founded in 1878

DEGREES • BSN • DNP • MSN

Nursing Program Faculty 54 (46% with doctorates).
Baccalaureate Enrollment 548 **Women** 90.7% **Men** 9.3% **Minority** 20.4% **International** .3% **Part-time** 3.2%
Graduate Enrollment 165 **Women** 95.8% **Men** 4.2% **Minority** 7.9% **Part-time** 54.5%
Distance Learning Courses Available.
Nursing Student Activities Nursing Honor Society, Sigma Theta Tau, Student Nurses' Association.
Nursing Student Resources Academic advising; academic or career counseling; assistance for students with disabilities; bookstore; campus computer network; career placement assistance; computer lab; computer-assisted instruction; daycare for children of students; e-mail services; employment services for current students; Internet; learning resource lab; library services; nursing audiovisuals; remedial services; resume preparation assistance; skills, simulation, or other laboratory; tutoring; unpaid internships.
Library Facilities 816,843 volumes (184,619 in health, 3,861 in nursing); 40,505 periodical subscriptions (10,376 health-care related).

BACCALAUREATE PROGRAMS

Degree BSN
Available Programs Accelerated Baccalaureate for Second Degree; Generic Baccalaureate; RN Baccalaureate.
Site Options Hastings, NE.
Study Options Full-time and part-time.
Online Degree Options Yes.
Program Entrance Requirements Minimum overall college GPA of 2.0, transcript of college record, written essay, health exam, health insurance, high school chemistry, 3 years high school math, 2 years high school science, high school transcript, immunizations, 1 letter of recommendation, minimum high school GPA of 3.0, minimum high school rank 50%. Transfer students are accepted. *Application deadline:* Applications may be processed on a rolling basis for some programs. *Application fee:* $50.
Advanced Placement Credit given for nursing courses completed elsewhere dependent upon specific evaluations.
Expenses (2010-11) *Tuition:* full-time $29,226; part-time $912 per credit hour. *Room and board:* $9502; room only: $6476 per academic year. *Required fees:* full-time $1802; part-time $356 per term.
Financial Aid 85% of baccalaureate students in nursing programs received some form of financial aid in 2009-10. *Gift aid (need-based):* Federal Pell, FSEOG, state, private, college/university gift aid from institutional funds, Federal Nursing. *Loans:* Federal Nursing Student Loans, Federal Direct (Subsidized and Unsubsidized Stafford PLUS), Perkins, college/university. *Work-study:* Federal Work-Study. *Financial aid application deadline (priority):* 3/1.
Contact Mrs. Erron M. Holland, Recruitment Counselor, School of Nursing, Creighton University, 2500 California Plaza, Omaha, NE 68178. *Telephone:* 402-280-2067. *Fax:* 402-280-2045. *E-mail:* erronholland@creighton.edu.

GRADUATE PROGRAMS

Expenses (2010-11) *Tuition:* full-time $10,816; part-time $676 per credit hour. *Required fees:* full-time $1543; part-time $1385 per term.
Financial Aid 85% of graduate students in nursing programs received some form of financial aid in 2009-10. Career-related internships or fieldwork, Federal Work-Study, institutionally sponsored loans, and traineeships available.
Contact Mrs. Erron M. Holland, Recruitment Coordinator, School of Nursing, Creighton University, 2500 California Plaza, Omaha, NE 68178. *Telephone:* 402-280-2067. *Fax:* 402-280-2045. *E-mail:* erronholland@creighton.edu.

MASTER'S DEGREE PROGRAM

Degree MSN
Available Programs Master's.
Concentrations Available Clinical nurse leader; nursing administration; nursing education. *Clinical nurse specialist programs in:* adult health, cardiovascular, family health, gerontology, maternity-newborn, oncology, pediatric. *Nurse practitioner programs in:* acute care, adult health, family health, gerontology, neonatal health, oncology, pediatric, psychiatric/mental health.
Site Options Hastings, NE.
Study Options Full-time and part-time.
Program Entrance Requirements Clinical experience, minimum overall college GPA of 3.0, transcript of college record, CPR certification, written essay, immunizations, 3 letters of recommendation, physical assessment course, prerequisite course work, resume, statistics course. *Application deadline:* Applications may be processed on a rolling basis for some programs. *Application fee:* $50.
Advanced Placement Credit given for nursing courses completed elsewhere dependent upon specific evaluations.
Degree Requirements 36 total credit hours, thesis or project.

POST-MASTER'S PROGRAM

Areas of Study Clinical nurse leader; nursing administration; nursing education. *Clinical nurse specialist programs in:* adult health, cardiovascular, family health, gerontology, maternity-newborn, oncology, pediatric. *Nurse practitioner programs in:* acute care, adult health, family health, gerontology, neonatal health, oncology, pediatric, psychiatric/mental health.

DOCTORAL DEGREE PROGRAM

Degree DNP
Available Programs Doctorate; Post-Baccalaureate Doctorate.
Areas of Study Advanced practice nursing, clinical practice, critical care, family health, gerontology, health promotion/disease prevention, maternity-newborn, neuro-behavior, nursing administration, nursing education, oncology.
Site Options Hastings, NE.
Program Entrance Requirements Clinical experience, minimum overall college GPA of 3.0, 3 letters of recommendation, statistics course, vita. Application deadline: Applications may be processed on a rolling basis for some programs. Application fee: $50.
Degree Requirements 32 total credit hours, residency.

Midland Lutheran College

Department of Nursing
Fremont, Nebraska

http://www.mlc.edu
Founded in 1883

DEGREE • BSN

Nursing Program Faculty 12 (25% with doctorates).
Baccalaureate Enrollment 130 **Women** 93% **Men** 7% **Minority** 4% **International** 3% **Part-time** 9%
Distance Learning Courses Available.
Nursing Student Activities Sigma Theta Tau, Student Nurses' Association.
Nursing Student Resources Academic advising; academic or career counseling; assistance for students with disabilities; bookstore; campus computer network; career placement assistance; computer lab; computer-assisted instruction; e-mail services; employment services for current students; housing assistance; interactive nursing skills videos; Internet; learning resource lab; library services; nursing audiovisuals; paid internships; placement services for program completers; remedial services; resume preparation assistance; skills, simulation, or other laboratory; tutoring; unpaid internships.
Library Facilities 110,000 volumes (4,700 in health, 2,000 in nursing); 900 periodical subscriptions (550 health-care related).

BACCALAUREATE PROGRAMS

Degree BSN
Available Programs ADN to Baccalaureate; Generic Baccalaureate; LPN to RN Baccalaureate; RN Baccalaureate.
Site Options Columbus, NE.
Study Options Full-time and part-time.
Program Entrance Requirements Minimum overall college GPA of 2.5, transcript of college record, CPR certification, written essay, health exam, high school transcript, immunizations, interview, 2 letters of recommendation, minimum GPA in nursing prerequisites of 2.5, prerequisite course work. Transfer students are accepted. *Application deadline:* 3/1 (spring). Applications may be processed on a rolling basis for some programs.
Advanced Placement Credit given for nursing courses completed elsewhere dependent upon specific evaluations.
Expenses (2009-10) *Tuition:* full-time $22,684; part-time $330 per credit hour. *International tuition:* $22,684 full-time. *Room and board:* $5612 per academic year. *Required fees:* full-time $622.
Financial Aid 98% of baccalaureate students in nursing programs received some form of financial aid in 2008-09.
Contact Ms. Amy Poggendorf, Director of Admissions, Department of Nursing, Midland Lutheran College, 900 North Clarkson, Fremont, NE 68025. *Telephone:* 402-941-6505. *Fax:* 402-941-6513. *E-mail:* poggendorf@mlc.edu.

Nebraska Methodist College

Department of Nursing
Omaha, Nebraska

http://www.methodistcollege.edu/
Founded in 1891

DEGREES • BSN • MSN

Nursing Program Faculty 48 (21% with doctorates).
Baccalaureate Enrollment 495 **Women** 92% **Men** 8% **Minority** 11% **Part-time** 36%
Graduate Enrollment 58 **Women** 98% **Men** 2% **Minority** 7% **Part-time** 31%
Distance Learning Courses Available.
Nursing Student Activities Nursing Honor Society, Sigma Theta Tau, Student Nurses' Association.
Nursing Student Resources Academic advising; academic or career counseling; assistance for students with disabilities; bookstore; campus computer network; career placement assistance; computer lab; computer-assisted instruction; e-mail services; employment services for current students; interactive nursing skills videos; Internet; learning resource lab; library services; nursing audiovisuals; remedial services; resume preparation assistance; skills, simulation, or other laboratory; tutoring.
Library Facilities 10,300 volumes (3,300 in health, 1,200 in nursing); 164 periodical subscriptions (13,600 health-care related).

BACCALAUREATE PROGRAMS

Degree BSN
Available Programs ADN to Baccalaureate; Accelerated Baccalaureate for Second Degree; Generic Baccalaureate; LPN to Baccalaureate.
Study Options Full-time and part-time.
Program Entrance Requirements Minimum overall college GPA of 2.5, transcript of college record, written essay, high school biology, high school chemistry, 2 years high school math, 2 years high school science, high school transcript, interview, minimum high school GPA of 2.5, minimum GPA in nursing prerequisites of 2.5. Transfer students are accepted. *Application deadline:* Applications may be processed on a rolling basis for some programs. *Application fee:* $25.
Advanced Placement Credit given for nursing courses completed elsewhere dependent upon specific evaluations.
Expenses (2010-11) *Tuition:* full-time $11,640; part-time $485 per credit hour. *Room and board:* room only: $5770 per academic year. *Required fees:* full-time $130.
Financial Aid 95% of baccalaureate students in nursing programs received some form of financial aid in 2009-10. *Gift aid (need-based):* Federal Pell, FSEOG, state, private, college/university gift aid from institutional funds. *Loans:* Federal Nursing Student Loans, Perkins, college/university, alternative loans. *Work-study:* Federal Work-Study. *Financial aid application deadline (priority):* 4/1.
Contact Dr. Marilyn Valerio, Chairperson, Department of Nursing, Nebraska Methodist College, 720 North 87th Street, Omaha, NE 68114-3426. *Telephone:* 402-354-7027. *Fax:* 402-354-7020. *E-mail:* marilyn.valerio@methodistcollege.edu.

GRADUATE PROGRAMS

Expenses (2010-11) *Tuition:* full-time $10,604; part-time $564 per credit hour. *Room and board:* $5770 per academic year. *Required fees:* full-time $450; part-time $25 per credit.
Financial Aid 72% of graduate students in nursing programs received some form of financial aid in 2009-10.
Contact Dr. Linda Foley, Associate Chairperson, Department of Nursing, Nebraska Methodist College, 720 North 87th Street, Omaha, NE 68114-3426. *Telephone:* 402-354-7050. *Fax:* 402-354-7020. *E-mail:* linda.foley@methodistcollege.edu.

MASTER'S DEGREE PROGRAM

Degree MSN
Available Programs Master's; Master's for Nurses with Non-Nursing Degrees; RN to Master's.
Concentrations Available Nursing administration; nursing education.
Study Options Full-time and part-time.
Online Degree Options Yes (online only).
Program Entrance Requirements Computer literacy, minimum overall college GPA of 3.0, transcript of college record, CPR certification, written essay, immunizations, interview, 2 letters of recommendation, nursing research course, physical assessment course, prerequisite course work, resume, statistics course. *Application deadline:* Applications may be processed on a rolling basis for some programs. *Application fee:* $25.
Advanced Placement Credit given for nursing courses completed elsewhere dependent upon specific evaluations.
Degree Requirements 36 total credit hours, thesis or project.

POST-MASTER'S PROGRAM

Areas of Study Nursing education.

CONTINUING EDUCATION PROGRAM

Contact Ms. Rose Leavitt, Associate Dean for Professional Development, Department of Nursing, Nebraska Methodist College, 720 North 87th Street, Omaha, NE 68114-3426. *Telephone:* 402-354-7137. *Fax:* 402-354-7020. *E-mail:* rose.leavitt@methodistcollege.edu.

Nebraska Wesleyan University

Department of Nursing
Lincoln, Nebraska

http://www.nebrwesleyan.edu
Founded in 1887

DEGREES • BSN • MSN

Nursing Program Faculty 15 (50% with doctorates).
Baccalaureate Enrollment 87 **Women** 92% **Men** 8% **Minority** 7% **International** 11% **Part-time** 40%
Graduate Enrollment 54 **Women** 96% **Men** 4% **Minority** 12% **International** 2% **Part-time** 50%
Distance Learning Courses Available.
Nursing Student Activities Sigma Theta Tau.
Nursing Student Resources Academic advising; academic or career counseling; assistance for students with disabilities; bookstore; campus computer network; career placement assistance; computer lab; e-mail services; Internet; library services; nursing audiovisuals; resume preparation assistance; unpaid internships.
Library Facilities 221,084 volumes (5,000 in health, 3,700 in nursing); 832 periodical subscriptions (470 health-care related).

BACCALAUREATE PROGRAMS

Degree BSN
Available Programs ADN to Baccalaureate; Accelerated RN Baccalaureate; International Nurse to Baccalaureate; RN Baccalaureate.
Site Options Omaha, NE.
Study Options Full-time and part-time.
Program Entrance Requirements Transfer students are accepted. *Application deadline:* Applications may be processed on a rolling basis for some programs. *Application fee:* $100.
Advanced Placement Credit by examination available. Credit given for nursing courses completed elsewhere dependent upon specific evaluations.
Expenses (2009-10) *Tuition:* full-time $7350; part-time $245 per credit hour. *International tuition:* $7350 full-time.
Financial Aid 90% of baccalaureate students in nursing programs received some form of financial aid in 2008-09. *Gift aid (need-based):* Federal Pell, FSEOG, state, private, college/university gift aid from institutional funds. *Loans:* Federal Direct (Subsidized and Unsubsidized Stafford PLUS), Perkins. *Work-study:* Federal Work-Study, part-time campus jobs. *Financial aid application deadline:* Continuous.
Contact Ms. Melissa Green, Recruiter, Department of Nursing, Nebraska Wesleyan University, 5000 St. Paul Avenue, Lincoln, NE 68504. *Telephone:* 800-541-3818 Ext. 2330. *Fax:* 402-465-2479. *E-mail:* jlb@nebrwesleyan.edu.

GRADUATE PROGRAMS

Expenses (2009-10) *Tuition:* full-time $6800; part-time $340 per credit hour. *International tuition:* $6800 full-time.
Financial Aid 60% of graduate students in nursing programs received some form of financial aid in 2008-09.
Contact Dr. Jeri L. Brandt, RN, Program Director, Department of Nursing, Nebraska Wesleyan University, 5000 St. Paul Avenue, Lincoln, NE 68504. *Telephone:* 402-465-2336. *Fax:* 402-465-2179. *E-mail:* jlb@nebrwesleyan.edu.

MASTER'S DEGREE PROGRAM

Degree MSN
Available Programs Accelerated AD/RN to Master's; Accelerated Master's; Accelerated RN to Master's; Master's; RN to Master's.
Concentrations Available Nursing administration; nursing education.
Site Options Omaha, NE.
Study Options Full-time and part-time.
Program Entrance Requirements Clinical experience, computer literacy, minimum overall college GPA of 3.0, transcript of college record, written essay, immunizations, 2 letters of recommendation, nursing research course, resume, statistics course. *Application deadline:* 8/1 (fall), 12/10 (spring). Applications may be processed on a rolling basis for some programs. *Application fee:* $100.
Advanced Placement Credit by examination available. Credit given for nursing courses completed elsewhere dependent upon specific evaluations.
Degree Requirements 40 total credit hours, thesis or project, comprehensive exam.

POST-MASTER'S PROGRAM

Areas of Study Nursing administration; nursing education.

Union College

Division of Health Sciences
Lincoln, Nebraska

http://www.ucollege.edu
Founded in 1891

DEGREE • BSN

Nursing Program Faculty 10
Baccalaureate Enrollment 162 **Women** 80% **Men** 20% **Minority** 5% **International** 9% **Part-time** 5%
Nursing Student Activities Sigma Theta Tau, nursing club.
Nursing Student Resources Academic advising; academic or career counseling; assistance for students with disabilities; bookstore; campus computer network; career placement assistance; computer lab; computer-assisted instruction; e-mail services; employment services for current students; externships; interactive nursing skills videos; Internet; learning resource lab; library services; nursing audiovisuals; placement services for program completers; remedial services; resume preparation assistance; skills, simulation, or other laboratory; tutoring; unpaid internships.
Library Facilities 147,813 volumes (450 in health, 350 in nursing); 1,357 periodical subscriptions (50 health-care related).

BACCALAUREATE PROGRAMS

Degree BSN
Available Programs ADN to Baccalaureate; Generic Baccalaureate; LPN to Baccalaureate.
Study Options Full-time and part-time.
Program Entrance Requirements Minimum overall college GPA of 2.75, transcript of college record, CPR certification, written essay, health exam, health insurance, high school transcript, immunizations, 3 letters of recommendation, minimum GPA in nursing prerequisites of 2.75, professional liability insurance/malpractice insurance, prerequisite course work. Transfer students are accepted. *Application deadline:* 4/1 (fall), 11/1 (spring). *Application fee:* $25.
Advanced Placement Credit by examination available. Credit given for nursing courses completed elsewhere dependent upon specific evaluations.
Expenses (2009-10) *Tuition:* full-time $16,930; part-time $710 per credit. *International tuition:* $21,930 full-time. *Room and board:* $1645 per academic year. *Required fees:* full-time $465; part-time $465 per term.
Financial Aid 83% of baccalaureate students in nursing programs received some form of financial aid in 2008-09.
Contact Mrs. Stacie Laursen, Office Manager, Division of Health Sciences, Union College, 3800 South 48th Street, Lincoln, NE 68506. *Telephone:* 402-486-2524. *Fax:* 402-486-2559. *E-mail:* stlaurse@ucollege.edu.

University of Nebraska Medical Center

College of Nursing
Omaha, Nebraska

http://www.unmc.edu/nursing/
Founded in 1869

DEGREES • BSN • MSN • PHD

Nursing Program Faculty 112 (60% with doctorates).
Baccalaureate Enrollment 600
Graduate Enrollment 300
Nursing Student Activities Nursing Honor Society, Sigma Theta Tau, Student Nurses' Association, nursing club.

Nursing Student Resources Academic advising; academic or career counseling; assistance for students with disabilities; bookstore; campus computer network; career placement assistance; computer lab; computer-assisted instruction; daycare for children of students; e-mail services; employment services for current students; externships; housing assistance; interactive nursing skills videos; Internet; learning resource lab; library services; nursing audiovisuals; other; paid internships; placement services for program completers; remedial services; resume preparation assistance; skills, simulation, or other laboratory; tutoring.

Library Facilities 238,074 volumes (240,000 in health, 3,500 in nursing); 6,403 periodical subscriptions (2,200 health-care related).

BACCALAUREATE PROGRAMS

Degree BSN

Available Programs ADN to Baccalaureate; Accelerated Baccalaureate; Accelerated Baccalaureate for Second Degree; Accelerated RN Baccalaureate; Baccalaureate for Second Degree; Generic Baccalaureate; International Nurse to Baccalaureate; LPN to Baccalaureate; LPN to RN Baccalaureate; RN Baccalaureate; RPN to Baccalaureate.

Study Options Full-time.

Program Entrance Requirements Minimum overall college GPA of 2.5, transcript of college record, CPR certification, health insurance, high school transcript, immunizations, 2 letters of recommendation, prerequisite course work. Transfer students are accepted.

Advanced Placement Credit by examination available. Credit given for nursing courses completed elsewhere dependent upon specific evaluations.

Contact *Telephone:* 402-559-5184.

GRADUATE PROGRAMS

Contact *Telephone:* 402-559-5184.

MASTER'S DEGREE PROGRAM

Degree MSN

Available Programs Master's; Master's for Non-Nursing College Graduates; RN to Master's.

Concentrations Available Health-care administration; nurse case management; nursing administration; nursing education; nursing informatics. *Clinical nurse specialist programs in:* acute care, adult health, cardiovascular, community health, critical care, family health, gerontology, maternity-newborn, medical-surgical, oncology, parent-child, pediatric, perinatal, psychiatric/mental health, public health, women's health. *Nurse practitioner programs in:* acute care, adult health, community health, family health, gerontology, neonatal health, oncology, pediatric, primary care, psychiatric/mental health, women's health.

Study Options Full-time and part-time.

Program Entrance Requirements Computer literacy, minimum overall college GPA of 3.0, transcript of college record, CPR certification, immunizations, interview, 3 letters of recommendation, nursing research course, statistics course.

Advanced Placement Credit given for nursing courses completed elsewhere dependent upon specific evaluations.

Degree Requirements 45 total credit hours.

POST-MASTER'S PROGRAM

Areas of Study Health-care administration; nurse case management; nursing administration; nursing education; nursing informatics. *Clinical nurse specialist programs in:* acute care, adult health, cardiovascular, community health, critical care, family health, gerontology, maternity-newborn, medical-surgical, oncology, parent-child, pediatric, perinatal, psychiatric/mental health, public health, women's health. *Nurse practitioner programs in:* acute care, adult health, community health, family health, gerontology, neonatal health, oncology, pediatric, primary care, psychiatric/mental health, women's health.

DOCTORAL DEGREE PROGRAM

Degree PhD

Available Programs Doctorate; Doctorate for Nurses with Non-Nursing Degrees; Post-Baccalaureate Doctorate.

Areas of Study Advanced practice nursing, aging, bio-behavioral research, biology of health and illness, clinical practice, community health, critical care, faculty preparation, family health, gerontology, health policy, health promotion/disease prevention, health-care systems, human health and illness, illness and transition, individualized study, information systems, maternity-newborn, neuro-behavior, nurse case management, nursing administration, nursing policy, nursing research, nursing science, oncology, women's health.

Program Entrance Requirements Minimum overall college GPA of 3.2, interview by faculty committee, interview, 3 letters of recommendation, scholarly papers, statistics course, vita, writing sample.

Degree Requirements Dissertation, oral exam, written exam.

POSTDOCTORAL PROGRAM

Postdoctoral Program Contact *Telephone:* 402-559-7457. *Fax:* 410-706-0945.

CONTINUING EDUCATION PROGRAM

Contact *Telephone:* 402-559-7487.

NEVADA

Great Basin College
BSN Program
Elko, Nevada

Founded in 1967

DEGREE • BSN

BACCALAUREATE PROGRAMS

Degree BSN

Available Programs RN Baccalaureate.

Program Entrance Requirements RN licensure.

Contact *Telephone:* 775-738-8493.

Nevada State College at Henderson
Nursing Program
Henderson, Nevada

http://www.nsc.nevada.edu/academics/programs/nursing/

Founded in 2002

DEGREE • BSN

Nursing Program Faculty 27 (26% with doctorates).

Baccalaureate Enrollment 207 **Women** 88% **Men** 12% **Minority** 34% **Part-time** 28%

Distance Learning Courses Available.

Nursing Student Activities Sigma Theta Tau, Student Nurses' Association.

Nursing Student Resources Academic advising; academic or career counseling; assistance for students with disabilities; bookstore; campus computer network; computer lab; computer-assisted instruction; e-mail services; interactive nursing skills videos; Internet; learning resource lab; library services; nursing audiovisuals; skills, simulation, or other laboratory; tutoring.

Library Facilities 12,905 volumes; 47 periodical subscriptions.

BACCALAUREATE PROGRAMS

Degree BSN

Available Programs Accelerated Baccalaureate for Second Degree; Generic Baccalaureate; RN Baccalaureate.

Study Options Full-time.

Program Entrance Requirements Minimum overall college GPA of 2.5, transcript of college record, CPR certification, health exam, health insurance, high school transcript, immunizations, minimum GPA in nursing prerequisites of 3.0, prerequisite course work. Transfer students are accepted. *Application deadline:* 3/1 (fall), 8/1 (spring).

Advanced Placement Credit given for nursing courses completed elsewhere dependent upon specific evaluations.

Contact *Telephone:* 702-992-2850. *Fax:* 702-992-2851.

Touro University
School of Nursing
Henderson, Nevada

http://tun.touro.edu/

DEGREES • BSN • DNP • MSN

Nursing Program Faculty 25 (30% with doctorates).
Baccalaureate Enrollment 150 **Women** 70% **Men** 30% **Minority** 68% **International** 6% **Part-time** 6%
Graduate Enrollment 25 **Women** 84% **Men** 16% **Minority** 40% **International** 4% **Part-time** 100%
Distance Learning Courses Available.
Nursing Student Activities Sigma Theta Tau, Student Nurses' Association.
Nursing Student Resources Academic advising; academic or career counseling; assistance for students with disabilities; bookstore; campus computer network; computer lab; e-mail services; interactive nursing skills videos; Internet; library services; nursing audiovisuals; remedial services; skills, simulation, or other laboratory; tutoring.

BACCALAUREATE PROGRAMS

Degree BSN
Available Programs ADN to Baccalaureate; Accelerated Baccalaureate; Accelerated Baccalaureate for Second Degree; Accelerated RN Baccalaureate; Baccalaureate for Second Degree; Generic Baccalaureate; RN Baccalaureate.
Study Options Full-time.
Online Degree Options Yes.
Program Entrance Requirements Minimum overall college GPA of 3.0, transcript of college record, CPR certification, health exam, health insurance, immunizations, minimum GPA in nursing prerequisites of 3.0, prerequisite course work. Transfer students are accepted. *Application deadline:* Applications may be processed on a rolling basis for some programs. *Application fee:* $50.
Advanced Placement Credit given for nursing courses completed elsewhere dependent upon specific evaluations.
Financial Aid 90% of baccalaureate students in nursing programs received some form of financial aid in 2009-10.
Contact Gladys Easterling, Admissions Counselor, School of Nursing, Touro University, 874 American Pacific Drive, Henderson, NV 89014. *Telephone:* 702-777-4748. *Fax:* 702-777-1752. *E-mail:* gladys.easterling@tun.touro.edu.

GRADUATE PROGRAMS

Financial Aid 70% of graduate students in nursing programs received some form of financial aid in 2009-10.
Contact Gladys Easterling, Admissions Counselor, School of Nursing, Touro University, 874 American Pacific Drive, Henderson, NV 89014. *Telephone:* 702-777-4748. *Fax:* 702-777-1752. *E-mail:* gladys.easterling@tun.touro.edu.

MASTER'S DEGREE PROGRAM

Degree MSN
Available Programs Master's; Master's for Nurses with Non-Nursing Degrees.
Concentrations Available Clinical nurse leader. *Nurse practitioner programs in:* family health.
Study Options Part-time.
Online Degree Options Yes (online only).
Program Entrance Requirements Clinical experience, computer literacy, minimum overall college GPA of 3.0, transcript of college record, CPR certification, immunizations, 2 letters of recommendation, statistics course. *Application deadline:* Applications may be processed on a rolling basis for some programs. *Application fee:* $50.
Advanced Placement Credit given for nursing courses completed elsewhere dependent upon specific evaluations.
Degree Requirements Thesis or project, comprehensive exam.

POST-MASTER'S PROGRAM

Areas of Study Clinical nurse leader; nursing education. *Nurse practitioner programs in:* family health.

DOCTORAL DEGREE PROGRAM

Degree DNP
Available Programs Doctorate; Post-Baccalaureate Doctorate.
Areas of Study Advanced practice nursing, clinical practice, health policy, health-care systems, individualized study, information systems, nursing administration.
Online Degree Options Yes (online only).
Program Entrance Requirements Clinical experience, minimum overall college GPA of 3.0, 3 letters of recommendation, MSN or equivalent, statistics course. Application deadline: Applications may be processed on a rolling basis for some programs. Application fee: $50.
Degree Requirements 39 total credit hours, dissertation.

CONTINUING EDUCATION PROGRAM

Contact Peggy Taylor, Director, Continuing Professional Education, School of Nursing, Touro University, 874 American Pacific Drive, Henderson, NV 89014. *Telephone:* 702-777-1788. *Fax:* 702-777-4834. *E-mail:* peggy.taylor@tun.touro.edu.

University of Nevada, Las Vegas
School of Nursing
Las Vegas, Nevada

http://nursing.unlv.edu/
Founded in 1957

DEGREES • BSN • MSN • PHD

Nursing Program Faculty 30 (48% with doctorates).
Baccalaureate Enrollment 170 **Women** 82% **Men** 18% **Minority** 43%
Graduate Enrollment 101 **Women** 79% **Men** 21% **Minority** 36% **International** 11% **Part-time** 58%
Distance Learning Courses Available.
Nursing Student Activities Nursing Honor Society, Sigma Theta Tau, Student Nurses' Association.
Nursing Student Resources Academic advising; academic or career counseling; assistance for students with disabilities; bookstore; campus computer network; career placement assistance; computer lab; computer-assisted instruction; daycare for children of students; e-mail services; employment services for current students; interactive nursing skills videos; Internet; learning resource lab; library services; nursing audiovisuals; remedial services; resume preparation assistance; skills, simulation, or other laboratory; tutoring.
Library Facilities 1.5 million volumes (35,800 in health, 12,000 in nursing); 31,847 periodical subscriptions (305 health-care related).

BACCALAUREATE PROGRAMS

Degree BSN
Available Programs Accelerated Baccalaureate; Generic Baccalaureate.
Study Options Full-time.
Program Entrance Requirements Minimum overall college GPA of 3.0, transcript of college record, CPR certification, health exam, health insurance, high school transcript, immunizations, minimum GPA in nursing prerequisites of 3.0, prerequisite course work. Transfer students are accepted. *Application deadline:* Applications may be processed on a rolling basis for some programs.
Advanced Placement Credit by examination available. Credit given for nursing courses completed elsewhere dependent upon specific evaluations.
Expenses (2010-11) *Tuition, state resident:* full-time $4283; part-time $143 per credit. *Tuition, nonresident:* full-time $17,573; part-time $143 per credit. *International tuition:* $19,067 full-time. *Room and board:* $5228; room only: $3273 per academic year. *Required fees:* full-time $891; part-time $96 per term.
Financial Aid 65% of baccalaureate students in nursing programs received some form of financial aid in 2009-10. *Gift aid (need-based):* Federal Pell, FSEOG, state, private, college/university gift aid from institutional funds. *Loans:* Federal Nursing Student Loans, Federal Direct (Subsidized and Unsubsidized Stafford PLUS), Perkins, state, college/university. *Work-study:* Federal Work-Study, part-time campus jobs. *Financial aid application deadline (priority):* 2/1.
Contact Ms. Cheryl Perna, Undergraduate Coordinator, School of Nursing, University of Nevada, Las Vegas, 4505 Maryland Parkway, Las Vegas, NV 89154-3018. *Telephone:* 702-895-0167. *Fax:* 702-895-4807. *E-mail:* cheryl.perna@unlv.edu.

GRADUATE PROGRAMS

Expenses (2010-11) *Tuition, state resident:* full-time $3919; part-time $218 per credit. *Tuition, nonresident:* full-time $17,209; part-time $218 per credit. *International tuition:* $18,703 full-time. *Room and board:*

$5228; room only: $3273 per academic year. *Required fees:* full-time $744; part-time $206 per term.
Financial Aid 40% of graduate students in nursing programs received some form of financial aid in 2009-10. 8 research assistantships with partial tuition reimbursements available (averaging $14,275 per year), 1 teaching assistantship (averaging $12,000 per year) were awarded; institutionally sponsored loans, scholarships, and unspecified assistantships also available. *Financial aid application deadline:* 3/1.
Contact Ms. Cheryl Maes, Coordinator, Graduate Programs, School of Nursing, University of Nevada, Las Vegas, Las Vegas, NV 89154-3018. *Telephone:* 702-895-2947. *Fax:* 702-895-4807. *E-mail:* cheryl.maes@unlv.edu.

MASTER'S DEGREE PROGRAM
Degree MSN
Available Programs Master's.
Concentrations Available Nursing education. *Nurse practitioner programs in:* family health.
Study Options Full-time and part-time.
Online Degree Options Yes (online only).
Program Entrance Requirements Clinical experience, computer literacy, minimum overall college GPA of 3.0, transcript of college record, CPR certification, written essay, immunizations, interview, 2 letters of recommendation, nursing research course, professional liability insurance/malpractice insurance, prerequisite course work, resume, statistics course. *Application deadline:* 2/1 (spring).
Advanced Placement Credit given for nursing courses completed elsewhere dependent upon specific evaluations.
Degree Requirements 46 total credit hours, thesis or project.

POST-MASTER'S PROGRAM
Areas of Study Nursing education. *Nurse practitioner programs in:* family health.

DOCTORAL DEGREE PROGRAM
Degree PhD
Available Programs Doctorate.
Areas of Study Nursing education, urban health.
Online Degree Options Yes (online only).
Program Entrance Requirements Clinical experience, minimum overall college GPA of 3.5, interview by faculty committee, 2 letters of recommendation, MSN or equivalent, statistics course, vita, writing sample, GRE General Test. Application deadline: 2/1 (spring).
Degree Requirements 65 total credit hours, dissertation, oral exam, written exam.

CONTINUING EDUCATION PROGRAM
Contact Dr. Tish M. Smyer, Continuing Education Coordinator, School of Nursing, University of Nevada, Las Vegas, 4505 Maryland Parkway, Las Vegas, NV 89154-3018. *Telephone:* 702-895-5952. *Fax:* 702-895-4807. *E-mail:* tish.smyer@unlv.edu.

University of Nevada, Reno
Orvis School of Nursing
Reno, Nevada

http://www.unr.edu/hcs/osn
Founded in 1874

DEGREES • BSN • MSN • MSN/MPH
Nursing Program Faculty 30 (40% with doctorates).
Baccalaureate Enrollment 144 **Women** 60% **Men** 40% **Minority** 16% **International** 5%
Graduate Enrollment 67 **Women** 90% **Men** 10% **Minority** 1% **Part-time** 90%
Distance Learning Courses Available.
Nursing Student Activities Nursing Honor Society, Sigma Theta Tau, Student Nurses' Association.
Nursing Student Resources Academic advising; academic or career counseling; assistance for students with disabilities; bookstore; campus computer network; computer lab; computer-assisted instruction; e-mail services; housing assistance; Internet; learning resource lab; library services; nursing audiovisuals; resume preparation assistance; skills, simulation, or other laboratory.
Library Facilities 5,000 volumes in health, 3,000 volumes in nursing; 172 periodical subscriptions health-care related.

BACCALAUREATE PROGRAMS
Degree BSN
Available Programs ADN to Baccalaureate; Accelerated Baccalaureate; Generic Baccalaureate; RN Baccalaureate.
Site Options Reno , NV.
Study Options Full-time.
Program Entrance Requirements Transcript of college record, CPR certification, health exam, health insurance, immunizations, minimum GPA in nursing prerequisites of 3.0, professional liability insurance/malpractice insurance, prerequisite course work. Transfer students are accepted. *Application deadline:* 2/12 (fall), 9/17 (spring).
Advanced Placement Credit given for nursing courses completed elsewhere dependent upon specific evaluations.
Expenses (2009-10) *Tuition, area resident:* full-time $11,299. *Tuition, state resident:* full-time $6589. *Tuition, nonresident:* full-time $19,879. *Room and board:* $10,595; room only: $6100 per academic year.
Financial Aid 50% of baccalaureate students in nursing programs received some form of financial aid in 2008-09.
Contact Mary Ann Lambert, Coordinator, Undergraduate Program, Orvis School of Nursing, University of Nevada, Reno, Mail Stop 134, Reno, NV 89557. *Telephone:* 775-682-7150. *Fax:* 775-784-4262. *E-mail:* lambert@unr.edu.

GRADUATE PROGRAMS
Expenses (2009-10) *Tuition, area resident:* part-time $247 per credit. *Tuition, state resident:* part-time $510 per credit. *Tuition, nonresident:* full-time $13,290; part-time $264 per credit. *Required fees:* full-time $155.
Financial Aid Research assistantships, teaching assistantships, Federal Work-Study, institutionally sponsored loans, scholarships, and unspecified assistantships available.
Contact Elizabeth Amos, PhD, Coordinator, Graduate Program, Orvis School of Nursing, University of Nevada, Reno, 1664 North Virginia Street, Reno, NV 89557-0052. *Telephone:* 775-682-7156. *Fax:* 775-784-4262. *E-mail:* eamos@unr.edu.

MASTER'S DEGREE PROGRAM
Degrees MSN; MSN/MPH
Available Programs Master's.
Concentrations Available Clinical nurse leader; nursing education. *Clinical nurse specialist programs in:* school health. *Nurse practitioner programs in:* family health.
Site Options Reno, NV.
Study Options Full-time and part-time.
Program Entrance Requirements Computer literacy, minimum overall college GPA of 3.0, transcript of college record, CPR certification, written essay, immunizations, 3 letters of recommendation, physical assessment course, professional liability insurance/malpractice insurance, prerequisite course work, resume, statistics course. *Application deadline:* 3/1 (fall).
Advanced Placement Credit given for nursing courses completed elsewhere dependent upon specific evaluations.
Degree Requirements 35 total credit hours, thesis or project, comprehensive exam.

POST-MASTER'S PROGRAM
Areas of Study Clinical nurse leader; nursing education. *Nurse practitioner programs in:* family health.

University of Southern Nevada
College of Nursing
Henderson, Nevada

http://www.usn.edu/
Founded in 1999

DEGREE • BSN
Nursing Program Faculty 19 (22% with doctorates).
Baccalaureate Enrollment 203 **Women** 70% **Men** 30% **Minority** 80% **International** 2%
Distance Learning Courses Available.
Nursing Student Activities Nursing Honor Society, Student Nurses' Association.
Nursing Student Resources Academic advising; academic or career counseling; assistance for students with disabilities; campus computer network; career placement assistance; computer lab; computer-assisted instruction; e-mail services; interactive nursing skills videos; Internet;

learning resource lab; library services; nursing audiovisuals; remedial services; resume preparation assistance; skills, simulation, or other laboratory; unpaid internships.

BACCALAUREATE PROGRAMS

Degree BSN
Available Programs Accelerated Baccalaureate; Generic Baccalaureate.
Study Options Full-time.
Program Entrance Requirements Transcript of college record, written essay, interview, minimum GPA in nursing prerequisites of 2.75, prerequisite course work. Transfer students are accepted. *Application deadline:* 8/10 (fall), 12/15 (spring). Applications may be processed on a rolling basis for some programs. *Application fee:* $100.
Advanced Placement Credit given for nursing courses completed elsewhere dependent upon specific evaluations.
Expenses (2010-11) *Tuition:* full-time $32,000. *Required fees:* full-time $2500.
Financial Aid 85% of baccalaureate students in nursing programs received some form of financial aid in 2009-10.
Contact Ms. Imelda C. Revuelto, Recruiter, Admissions and Enrollment Coordinator, College of Nursing, University of Southern Nevada, 11 Sunset Way, Henderson, NV 89014. *Telephone:* 702-968-2075. *Fax:* 702-968-2097. *E-mail:* irevuelto@usn.edu.

NEW HAMPSHIRE

Colby-Sawyer College

Department of Nursing
New London, New Hampshire

http://www.colby-sawyer.edu/academic/nursing
Founded in 1837

DEGREE • BSN
Nursing Program Faculty 14 (.14% with doctorates).
Baccalaureate Enrollment 169 **Women** 93% **Men** 7% **Minority** 4% **International** 1% **Part-time** 1%
Nursing Student Activities Nursing Honor Society, Student Nurses' Association.
Nursing Student Resources Academic advising; academic or career counseling; assistance for students with disabilities; bookstore; campus computer network; career placement assistance; computer lab; computer-assisted instruction; e-mail services; employment services for current students; housing assistance; interactive nursing skills videos; Internet; learning resource lab; library services; nursing audiovisuals; remedial services; resume preparation assistance; skills, simulation, or other laboratory; tutoring; unpaid internships.
Library Facilities 93,696 volumes (12,050 in health, 760 in nursing); 27,072 periodical subscriptions (135 health-care related).

BACCALAUREATE PROGRAMS

Degree BSN
Available Programs Generic Baccalaureate.
Study Options Full-time and part-time.
Program Entrance Requirements Minimum overall college GPA of 2.7, transcript of college record, CPR certification, written essay, health exam, health insurance, high school biology, high school chemistry, high school foreign language, 3 years high school math, 3 years high school science, high school transcript, immunizations, 2 letters of recommendation, minimum high school GPA of 2.75, minimum GPA in nursing prerequisites of 2.7, prerequisite course work. Transfer students are accepted. *Application deadline:* Applications may be processed on a rolling basis for some programs.
Advanced Placement Credit by examination available. Credit given for nursing courses completed elsewhere dependent upon specific evaluations.
Expenses (2009-10) *Tuition:* full-time $31,090; part-time $1040 per credit hour. *Room and board:* $10,860 per academic year. *Required fees:* full-time $395; part-time $395 per term.
Financial Aid 96% of baccalaureate students in nursing programs received some form of financial aid in 2008-09.
Contact Prof. Susan Anne Reeves, RN, Chair/Director, Nursing Department, Department of Nursing, Colby-Sawyer College, 541 Main Street, New London, NH 03257-7835. *Telephone:* 603-526-3795. *Fax:* 603-526-3159. *E-mail:* sreeves@colby-sawyer.edu.

Franklin Pierce University

Master of Science in Nursing
Rindge, New Hampshire

Founded in 1962

DEGREES • BS • MSN
Nursing Program Faculty 4 (50% with doctorates).
Baccalaureate Enrollment 110 **Women** 97% **Men** 3% **Minority** 3% **Part-time** 100%
Graduate Enrollment 24 **Women** 96% **Men** 4% **Minority** 8% **Part-time** 100%
Distance Learning Courses Available.
Nursing Student Resources Academic advising; assistance for students with disabilities; bookstore; campus computer network; computer lab; library services.
Library Facilities 137,458 volumes; 19,414 periodical subscriptions (200 health-care related).

BACCALAUREATE PROGRAMS

Degree BS
Available Programs ADN to Baccalaureate; RN Baccalaureate.
Site Options Concord, NH; Lebanon, NH; Portsmouth, NH.
Study Options Part-time.
Program Entrance Requirements RN licensure. Transfer students are accepted. *Application deadline:* Applications may be processed on a rolling basis for some programs.
Advanced Placement Credit by examination available.
Expenses (2009-10) *Tuition:* full-time $8640; part-time $240 per credit. *International tuition:* $8640 full-time.
Financial Aid 95% of baccalaureate students in nursing programs received some form of financial aid in 2008-09.
Contact Dr. Judith Ann Evans, RN, Director of Nursing. *Telephone:* 603-433-2000 Ext. 2000. *Fax:* 603-899-1067 Ext. 1067. *E-mail:* evansj@franklinpierce.edu.

GRADUATE PROGRAMS

Expenses (2009-10) *Tuition:* full-time $8400; part-time $700 per credit. *International tuition:* $8400 full-time.
Financial Aid 90% of graduate students in nursing programs received some form of financial aid in 2008-09.
Contact Dr. Judith Ann Evans, RN, Director of Nursing, Master of Science in Nursing, Franklin Pierce University, 73 Corporate Drive, Portsmouth, NH 03801. *Telephone:* 603-322-2000. *Fax:* 603-899-1067. *E-mail:* evansj@franklinpierce.edu.

MASTER'S DEGREE PROGRAM

Degree MSN
Available Programs Master's; Master's for Nurses with Non-Nursing Degrees; RN to Master's.
Concentrations Available Nursing administration; nursing education.
Site Options Concord, NH; Lebanon, NH; Portsmouth, NH.
Study Options Part-time.
Program Entrance Requirements Computer literacy, minimum overall college GPA of 2.8, transcript of college record, written essay, interview, 3 letters of recommendation, resume, statistics course. *Application deadline:* Applications may be processed on a rolling basis for some programs.
Degree Requirements 34 total credit hours, thesis or project.

Rivier College

Division of Nursing
Nashua, New Hampshire

http://www.rivier.edu/
Founded in 1933

DEGREES • BS • MS
Nursing Program Faculty 26 (20% with doctorates).
Baccalaureate Enrollment 200 **Women** 93% **Men** 7% **Minority** 8% **Part-time** 50%

Graduate Enrollment 76 **Women** 94% **Men** 6% **Minority** 5% **Part-time** 85%
Distance Learning Courses Available.
Nursing Student Activities Nursing Honor Society, Sigma Theta Tau, Student Nurses' Association.
Nursing Student Resources Academic advising; academic or career counseling; assistance for students with disabilities; bookstore; campus computer network; career placement assistance; computer lab; computer-assisted instruction; e-mail services; employment services for current students; externships; housing assistance; interactive nursing skills videos; Internet; learning resource lab; library services; nursing audiovisuals; other; placement services for program completers; remedial services; resume preparation assistance; skills, simulation, or other laboratory; tutoring.
Library Facilities 9,805 volumes in health, 949 volumes in nursing; 2,004 periodical subscriptions health-care related.

BACCALAUREATE PROGRAMS

Degree BS
Available Programs ADN to Baccalaureate; Generic Baccalaureate; LPN to Baccalaureate; LPN to RN Baccalaureate; RN Baccalaureate.
Study Options Full-time and part-time.
Online Degree Options Yes.
Program Entrance Requirements Minimum overall college GPA of 2.5, transcript of college record, written essay, health exam, health insurance, high school chemistry, high school foreign language, 2 years high school math, 2 years high school science, high school transcript, immunizations, 2 letters of recommendation, minimum high school GPA of 3.0, minimum high school rank 80%, prerequisite course work. Transfer students are accepted. *Application deadline:* Applications may be processed on a rolling basis for some programs. *Application fee:* $25.
Advanced Placement Credit by examination available. Credit given for nursing courses completed elsewhere dependent upon specific evaluations.
Expenses (2010-11) *Tuition:* full-time $24,420. *Room and board:* $9522; room only: $5294 per academic year. *Required fees:* full-time $800.
Financial Aid 94% of baccalaureate students in nursing programs received some form of financial aid in 2009-10. *Gift aid (need-based):* Federal Pell, FSEOG, state, private, college/university gift aid from institutional funds. *Loans:* Federal Direct (Subsidized and Unsubsidized Stafford PLUS), Perkins, college/university. *Work-study:* Federal Work-Study, part-time campus jobs. *Financial aid application deadline (priority):* 3/1.
Contact Anne Parks, Senior Associate Director of Admissions, Division of Nursing, Rivier College, 420 South Main Street, Nashua, NH 03060-5086. *Telephone:* 603-897-8515. *Fax:* 603-897-8808. *E-mail:* aparks@rivier.edu.

GRADUATE PROGRAMS

Contact Pamela A. Slawinowski, Assistant to Program Director, Division of Nursing, Rivier College, 420 South Main Street, Nashua, NH 03060-5086. *Telephone:* 603-897-8528. *Fax:* 603-897-8884. *E-mail:* pslawinowski@rivier.edu.

MASTER'S DEGREE PROGRAM

Degree MS
Available Programs Master's; Master's for Nurses with Non-Nursing Degrees; RN to Master's.
Concentrations Available Nursing education. *Clinical nurse specialist programs in:* psychiatric/mental health. *Nurse practitioner programs in:* family health, psychiatric/mental health.
Study Options Full-time and part-time.
Program Entrance Requirements Clinical experience, minimum overall college GPA of 3.0, transcript of college record, written essay, immunizations, interview, 2 letters of recommendation, resume, statistics course, GRE, MAT. *Application deadline:* Applications may be processed on a rolling basis for some programs. *Application fee:* $25.
Advanced Placement Credit by examination available. Credit given for nursing courses completed elsewhere dependent upon specific evaluations.
Degree Requirements 43 total credit hours, thesis or project.

POST-MASTER'S PROGRAM

Areas of Study Nursing education. *Clinical nurse specialist programs in:* psychiatric/mental health. *Nurse practitioner programs in:* family health, psychiatric/mental health.

Saint Anselm College

Department of Nursing
Manchester, New Hampshire

http://www.anselm.edu/academics/depts/nursing
Founded in 1889

DEGREE • BSN

Nursing Program Faculty 25 (35% with doctorates).
Baccalaureate Enrollment 250 **Women** 96% **Men** 4% **Minority** 2% **International** 1% **Part-time** 1%
Nursing Student Activities Sigma Theta Tau, Student Nurses' Association, nursing club.
Nursing Student Resources Academic advising; academic or career counseling; assistance for students with disabilities; bookstore; campus computer network; career placement assistance; computer lab; computer-assisted instruction; e-mail services; employment services for current students; externships; housing assistance; interactive nursing skills videos; Internet; learning resource lab; library services; nursing audiovisuals; resume preparation assistance; skills, simulation, or other laboratory; tutoring.
Library Facilities 222,000 volumes (7,127 in health); 1,900 periodical subscriptions (292 health-care related).

BACCALAUREATE PROGRAMS

Degree BSN
Available Programs RN Baccalaureate.
Study Options Full-time and part-time.
Program Entrance Requirements Transcript of college record, written essay, health exam, health insurance, high school biology, high school chemistry, high school foreign language, 3 years high school math, 3 years high school science, high school transcript, immunizations, 2 letters of recommendation, professional liability insurance/malpractice insurance. *Application deadline:* 11/15 (fall). *Application fee:* $55.
Advanced Placement Credit by examination available. Credit given for nursing courses completed elsewhere dependent upon specific evaluations.
Expenses (2009-10) *Tuition:* full-time $29,720. *International tuition:* $29,720 full-time. *Room and board:* $11,240 per academic year. *Required fees:* full-time $1200.
Financial Aid 86% of baccalaureate students in nursing programs received some form of financial aid in 2008-09. *Gift aid (need-based):* Federal Pell, FSEOG, state, private, college/university gift aid from institutional funds. *Loans:* Federal Direct (Subsidized and Unsubsidized Stafford PLUS), Perkins. *Work-study:* Federal Work-Study, part-time campus jobs. *Financial aid application deadline:* 3/15.
Contact Nancy Davis Griffin, Dean of Admission, Department of Nursing, Saint Anselm College, 100 Saint Anselm Drive, Manchester, NH 03102-1310. *Telephone:* 603-641-7500. *Fax:* 603-641-7550. *E-mail:* ngriffin@anselm.edu.

CONTINUING EDUCATION PROGRAM

Contact Sharon George, Dean of Nursing, Department of Nursing, Saint Anselm College, 100 Saint Anselm Drive, #1745, Manchester, NH 03102-1310. *Telephone:* 603-641-7083. *Fax:* 603-641-7089. *E-mail:* sgeorge@ansel.edu.

University of New Hampshire

Department of Nursing
Durham, New Hampshire

http://www.unh.edu/ur-nurs.html
Founded in 1866

DEGREES • BS • MS

Nursing Program Faculty 13 (75% with doctorates).
Baccalaureate Enrollment 268 **Women** 91% **Men** 9% **Minority** 1%
Graduate Enrollment 54 **Women** 95% **Men** 5% **Minority** 1%
Nursing Student Activities Nursing Honor Society, Sigma Theta Tau, Student Nurses' Association.
Nursing Student Resources Academic advising; academic or career counseling; assistance for students with disabilities; bookstore; campus computer network; computer lab; computer-assisted instruction; daycare for children of students; e-mail services; housing assistance; interactive nursing skills videos; Internet; learning resource lab; nursing audiovi-

suals; paid internships; resume preparation assistance; skills, simulation, or other laboratory; tutoring.

Library Facilities 2.2 million volumes; 50,043 periodical subscriptions.

BACCALAUREATE PROGRAMS

Degree BS

Available Programs Generic Baccalaureate; RN Baccalaureate.

Study Options Full-time and part-time.

Program Entrance Requirements High school transcript, prerequisite course work. Transfer students are accepted.

Contact ***Telephone:*** 603-862-4715. *Fax:* 603-862-4771.

GRADUATE PROGRAMS

Contact ***Telephone:*** 603-862-2285. *Fax:* 603-862-4771.

MASTER'S DEGREE PROGRAM

Degree MS

Available Programs Master's; Master's for Nurses with Non-Nursing Degrees.

Concentrations Available *Clinical nurse specialist programs in:* adult health. *Nurse practitioner programs in:* adult health, family health.

Program Entrance Requirements GRE General Test or MAT.

Degree Requirements 45 total credit hours, thesis or project, comprehensive exam.

POST-MASTER'S PROGRAM

Areas of Study *Clinical nurse specialist programs in:* adult health. *Nurse practitioner programs in:* adult health, family health.

NEW JERSEY

Bloomfield College

Division of Nursing
Bloomfield, New Jersey

http://www.bloomfield.edu/

Founded in 1868

DEGREE • BS

Nursing Program Faculty 16 (31% with doctorates).

Baccalaureate Enrollment 140 **Women** 88% **Men** 12% **Minority** 65% **International** 3% **Part-time** 20%

Distance Learning Courses Available.

Nursing Student Activities Student Nurses' Association.

Nursing Student Resources Academic advising; academic or career counseling; assistance for students with disabilities; bookstore; campus computer network; career placement assistance; computer lab; computer-assisted instruction; e-mail services; employment services for current students; interactive nursing skills videos; Internet; learning resource lab; library services; nursing audiovisuals; placement services for program completers; remedial services; resume preparation assistance; skills, simulation, or other laboratory; tutoring; unpaid internships.

Library Facilities 65,000 volumes (1,500 in health, 1,500 in nursing); 560 periodical subscriptions (44 health-care related).

BACCALAUREATE PROGRAMS

Degree BS

Available Programs Generic Baccalaureate; RN Baccalaureate.

Study Options Full-time and part-time.

Program Entrance Requirements Transcript of college record, CPR certification, health exam, minimum GPA in nursing prerequisites of 2.5, prerequisite course work. Transfer students are accepted. *Application deadline:* 8/1 (fall), 12/15 (spring), 5/1 (summer). Applications may be processed on a rolling basis for some programs. *Application fee:* $40.

Advanced Placement Credit by examination available. Credit given for nursing courses completed elsewhere dependent upon specific evaluations.

Expenses (2010-11) *Tuition:* full-time $21,200; part-time $2230 per course. *Room and board:* $10,600; room only: $5300 per academic year. *Required fees:* full-time $1200; part-time $150 per credit.

Financial Aid 87% of baccalaureate students in nursing programs received some form of financial aid in 2009-10. *Gift aid (need-based):* Federal Pell, FSEOG, state, private, college/university gift aid from institutional funds. *Work-study:* Federal Work-Study, part-time campus jobs. *Financial aid application deadline:* 6/1(priority: 3/15).

Contact Dr. Neddie Serra, Chair, Division of Nursing, Bloomfield College, Bloomfield, NJ 07003. *Telephone:* 973-748-9000 Ext. 120. *Fax:* 973-743-3998. *E-mail:* neddie_serra@bloomfield.edu.

The College of New Jersey

School of Nursing, Health and Exercise Science
Ewing, New Jersey

http://www.tcnj.edu/~nursing

Founded in 1855

DEGREES • BSN • MSN

Nursing Program Faculty 15 (60% with doctorates).

Baccalaureate Enrollment 273 **Women** 93% **Men** 7% **Minority** 34% **Part-time** 1%

Graduate Enrollment 47 **Women** 98% **Men** 2% **Minority** 23% **Part-time** 2%

Nursing Student Activities Sigma Theta Tau, Student Nurses' Association.

Nursing Student Resources Academic advising; academic or career counseling; assistance for students with disabilities; bookstore; campus computer network; career placement assistance; computer lab; computer-assisted instruction; daycare for children of students; e-mail services; employment services for current students; externships; interactive nursing skills videos; Internet; learning resource lab; library services; nursing audiovisuals; paid internships; resume preparation assistance; skills, simulation, or other laboratory; tutoring; unpaid internships.

Library Facilities 561,250 volumes (30,000 in health, 18,800 in nursing); 6,194 periodical subscriptions (228 health-care related).

BACCALAUREATE PROGRAMS

Degree BSN

Available Programs Generic Baccalaureate.

Study Options Full-time and part-time.

Program Entrance Requirements Written essay, health exam, high school transcript, immunizations. Transfer students are accepted.

Advanced Placement Credit by examination available. Credit given for nursing courses completed elsewhere dependent upon specific evaluations.

Contact ***Telephone:*** 609-771-2669. *Fax:* 609-637-5159.

GRADUATE PROGRAMS

Contact ***Telephone:*** 609-771-2591. *Fax:* 609-637-5159.

MASTER'S DEGREE PROGRAM

Degree MSN

Available Programs Master's; Master's for Nurses with Non-Nursing Degrees; RN to Master's.

Concentrations Available Nursing administration. *Clinical nurse specialist programs in:* adult health. *Nurse practitioner programs in:* family health, neonatal health.

Study Options Full-time and part-time.

Program Entrance Requirements Computer literacy, minimum overall college GPA of 3.0, transcript of college record, written essay, immunizations, interview, 3 letters of recommendation, physical assessment course, statistics course, GRE General Test.

Advanced Placement Credit given for nursing courses completed elsewhere dependent upon specific evaluations.

Degree Requirements 47 total credit hours, comprehensive exam.

POST-MASTER'S PROGRAM

Areas of Study Nursing administration. *Clinical nurse specialist programs in:* adult health. *Nurse practitioner programs in:* family health, neonatal health.

College of Saint Elizabeth

Department of Nursing
Morristown, New Jersey

http://www.cse.edu/sgcs_continuingstudies.htm
Founded in 1899

DEGREE • BSN

Nursing Program Faculty 13 (25% with doctorates).
Baccalaureate Enrollment 231 **Women** 95% **Men** 5% **Minority** 48% **Part-time** 99%
Nursing Student Activities Nursing Honor Society, Sigma Theta Tau, nursing club.
Nursing Student Resources Academic advising; academic or career counseling; assistance for students with disabilities; bookstore; campus computer network; career placement assistance; computer lab; computer-assisted instruction; e-mail services; employment services for current students; interactive nursing skills videos; Internet; learning resource lab; library services; nursing audiovisuals; other; remedial services; resume preparation assistance; skills, simulation, or other laboratory; tutoring.
Library Facilities 119,438 volumes (4,246 in health, 702 in nursing); 977 periodical subscriptions (194 health-care related).

BACCALAUREATE PROGRAMS

Degree BSN
Available Programs ADN to Baccalaureate; Accelerated RN Baccalaureate; International Nurse to Baccalaureate; RN Baccalaureate.
Site Options Randolph, NJ; Elizabeth , NJ; Hoboken, NJ.
Study Options Part-time.
Program Entrance Requirements Minimum overall college GPA of 2.0, transcript of college record, CPR certification, health exam, immunizations, prerequisite course work, RN licensure. Transfer students are accepted.
Advanced Placement Credit by examination available. Credit given for nursing courses completed elsewhere dependent upon specific evaluations.
Contact ***Telephone:*** 973-290-4056. *Fax:* 973-290-4177.

CONTINUING EDUCATION PROGRAM

Contact ***Telephone:*** 973-290-4073. *Fax:* 973-290-4177.

Fairleigh Dickinson University, Metropolitan Campus

Henry P. Becton School of Nursing and Allied Health
Teaneck, New Jersey

http://fduinfo.com/depts/ucnah.php
Founded in 1942

DEGREES • BSN • DNP • MSN

Nursing Program Faculty 18 (61% with doctorates).
Baccalaureate Enrollment 410 **Women** 88% **Men** 12% **Minority** 57% **International** 1.4% **Part-time** 30%
Graduate Enrollment 320 **Women** 93.2% **Men** 6.8% **Minority** 46% **Part-time** 92.5%
Distance Learning Courses Available.
Nursing Student Activities Nursing Honor Society, Sigma Theta Tau, Student Nurses' Association.
Nursing Student Resources Academic advising; academic or career counseling; assistance for students with disabilities; bookstore; campus computer network; career placement assistance; computer lab; computer-assisted instruction; e-mail services; employment services for current students; externships; housing assistance; interactive nursing skills videos; Internet; learning resource lab; library services; nursing audiovisuals; other; placement services for program completers; remedial services; resume preparation assistance; skills, simulation, or other laboratory; tutoring; unpaid internships.
Library Facilities 196,703 volumes (2,166 in nursing); 1,601 periodical subscriptions (1,196 health-care related).

BACCALAUREATE PROGRAMS

Degree BSN
Available Programs Accelerated Baccalaureate for Second Degree; Generic Baccalaureate; RN Baccalaureate.
Site Options Sewell, NJ; Teaneck, NJ; Morristown, NJ.
Study Options Full-time and part-time.
Program Entrance Requirements Minimum overall college GPA of 3.0, transcript of college record, health exam, health insurance, high school biology, high school chemistry, 2 years high school math, 2 years high school science, high school transcript, immunizations, 2 letters of recommendation. Transfer students are accepted. *Application deadline:* Applications may be processed on a rolling basis for some programs. *Application fee:* $40.
Advanced Placement Credit given for nursing courses completed elsewhere dependent upon specific evaluations.
Expenses (2010-11) *Tuition:* full-time $31,140. *Room and board:* $11,618; room only: $7782 per academic year. *Required fees:* full-time $370.
Financial Aid 91% of baccalaureate students in nursing programs received some form of financial aid in 2009-10.
Contact Ms. Sylvia Cabassa, Associate Director, Undergraduate Nursing, Henry P. Becton School of Nursing and Allied Health, Fairleigh Dickinson University, Metropolitan Campus, 1000 River Road, H-DH4-02, Teaneck, NJ 07666-1914. *Telephone:* 201-692-2880. *Fax:* 201-692-2388. *E-mail:* scabassa@fdu.edu.

GRADUATE PROGRAMS

Expenses (2010-11) *Tuition:* part-time $1070 per credit. *Required fees:* full-time $370; part-time $241 per term.
Financial Aid 91% of graduate students in nursing programs received some form of financial aid in 2009-10.
Contact Dr. Elizabeth S. Parietti, Associate Director of Graduate Programs, Henry P. Becton School of Nursing and Allied Health, Fairleigh Dickinson University, Metropolitan Campus, 1000 River Road, H-DH4-02, Teaneck, NJ 07666-1914. *Telephone:* 201-692-2881. *Fax:* 201-692-2388. *E-mail:* parietti@fdu.edu.

MASTER'S DEGREE PROGRAM

Degree MSN
Available Programs Accelerated RN to Master's; Master's; Master's for Nurses with Non-Nursing Degrees; RN to Master's.
Concentrations Available Nursing administration; nursing education; nursing informatics. *Clinical nurse specialist programs in:* forensic nursing. *Nurse practitioner programs in:* adult health, family health, psychiatric/mental health.
Site Options Sewell, NJ; Teaneck, NJ; Morristown, NJ.
Study Options Full-time and part-time.
Program Entrance Requirements Computer literacy, minimum overall college GPA of 3.0, transcript of college record, CPR certification, written essay, immunizations, 2 letters of recommendation, nursing research course, physical assessment course, professional liability insurance/malpractice insurance, statistics course. *Application deadline:* Applications may be processed on a rolling basis for some programs. *Application fee:* $40.
Advanced Placement Credit given for nursing courses completed elsewhere dependent upon specific evaluations.
Degree Requirements 30 total credit hours, thesis or project.

POST-MASTER'S PROGRAM

Areas of Study Nursing administration; nursing education; nursing informatics. *Clinical nurse specialist programs in:* forensic nursing. *Nurse practitioner programs in:* adult health, family health, psychiatric/mental health.

DOCTORAL DEGREE PROGRAM

Degree DNP
Available Programs Doctorate.
Areas of Study Advanced practice nursing, clinical practice, faculty preparation, health-care systems, information systems, nursing administration, nursing education, nursing policy, nursing research, nursing science.
Program Entrance Requirements Minimum overall college GPA of 3.0, interview by faculty committee, 3 letters of recommendation, MSN or equivalent. Application deadline: Applications may be processed on a rolling basis for some programs. Application fee: $40.
Degree Requirements 36 total credit hours, residency.

CONTINUING EDUCATION PROGRAM

Contact Mrs. Marian L. Rutherford, Administrator for Clinical Affairs, Henry P. Becton School of Nursing and Allied Health, Fairleigh Dickinson University, Metropolitan Campus, 1000 River Road, H-DH4-02,

Teaneck, NJ 07666-1914. *Telephone:* 201-692-2520. *Fax:* 201-692-2388. *E-mail:* marian@fdu.edu.

Felician College
Division of Nursing and Health Management
Lodi, New Jersey

http://www.felician.edu/academics/nahp/
Founded in 1942

DEGREES • BSN • MA/MSM • MSN
Nursing Program Faculty 25 (32% with doctorates).
Baccalaureate Enrollment 512 **Women** 92% **Men** 8% **Minority** 32% **International** 2% **Part-time** 20%
Graduate Enrollment 93 **Women** 89% **Men** 11% **Minority** 33% **Part-time** 88%
Distance Learning Courses Available.
Nursing Student Activities Nursing Honor Society, Sigma Theta Tau, Student Nurses' Association.
Nursing Student Resources Academic advising; academic or career counseling; assistance for students with disabilities; bookstore; campus computer network; career placement assistance; computer lab; computer-assisted instruction; daycare for children of students; e-mail services; interactive nursing skills videos; Internet; learning resource lab; library services; nursing audiovisuals; placement services for program completers; remedial services; resume preparation assistance; skills, simulation, or other laboratory; tutoring.
Library Facilities 105,000 volumes (12,519 in health, 12,519 in nursing); 434 periodical subscriptions (21 health-care related).

BACCALAUREATE PROGRAMS
Degree BSN
Available Programs Accelerated Baccalaureate for Second Degree; Generic Baccalaureate.
Site Options East Orange, NJ; Long Branch, NJ; Edison, NJ.
Study Options Full-time and part-time.
Program Entrance Requirements Minimum overall college GPA of 3.0, transcript of college record, written essay, health exam, health insurance, high school biology, high school chemistry, 2 years high school math, 2 years high school science, high school transcript, immunizations, minimum high school GPA of 3.0, minimum GPA in nursing prerequisites of 2.8, professional liability insurance/malpractice insurance. Transfer students are accepted. *Application deadline:* 8/15 (fall), 1/10 (spring). Applications may be processed on a rolling basis for some programs. *Application fee:* $30.
Advanced Placement Credit by examination available. Credit given for nursing courses completed elsewhere dependent upon specific evaluations.
Expenses (2010-11) *Tuition:* full-time $26,350; part-time $780 per credit. *Room and board:* $10,750 per academic year. *Required fees:* full-time $24,950; part-time $820 per credit; part-time $238 per term.
Financial Aid 80% of baccalaureate students in nursing programs received some form of financial aid in 2009-10. *Gift aid (need-based):* Federal Pell, FSEOG, state, private, college/university gift aid from institutional funds. *Loans:* state. *Work-study:* Federal Work-Study, part-time campus jobs. *Financial aid application deadline:* Continuous.
Contact Office of Undergraduate Admissions, Division of Nursing and Health Management, Felician College, 262 South Main Street, Lodi, NJ 07644-2117. *Telephone:* 201-559-6131. *Fax:* 201-559-6138. *E-mail:* admissions@felician.edu.

GRADUATE PROGRAMS
Expenses (2010-11) *Tuition:* part-time $875 per credit. *Room and board:* $10,750 per academic year. *Required fees:* full-time $1575; part-time $263 per term.
Financial Aid 27% of graduate students in nursing programs received some form of financial aid in 2009-10.
Contact Dr. Wendy Lin-Cook, Dean of Adult and Graduate Admissions, Division of Nursing and Health Management, Felician College, 262 South Main Street, Lodi, NJ 07644-2117. *Telephone:* 201-559-6077. *Fax:* 201-559-6138. *E-mail:* adultandgraduate@felician.edu.

MASTER'S DEGREE PROGRAM
Degrees MA/MSM; MSN
Available Programs Accelerated RN to Master's; Master's.
Concentrations Available Nursing administration; nursing education. *Nurse practitioner programs in:* adult health, family health.
Study Options Full-time and part-time.
Online Degree Options Yes.
Program Entrance Requirements Clinical experience, computer literacy, minimum overall college GPA of 3.0, transcript of college record, CPR certification, written essay, immunizations, 2 letters of recommendation, nursing research course, physical assessment course, professional liability insurance/malpractice insurance, prerequisite course work, statistics course. *Application deadline:* Applications may be processed on a rolling basis for some programs. *Application fee:* $40.
Advanced Placement Credit given for nursing courses completed elsewhere dependent upon specific evaluations.
Degree Requirements 46 total credit hours, thesis or project.

POST-MASTER'S PROGRAM
Areas of Study Nursing administration; nursing education. *Nurse practitioner programs in:* adult health, family health.

Kean University
Department of Nursing
Union, New Jersey

http://www.kean.edu/~nursing/
Founded in 1855

DEGREES • BSN • MSN • MSN/MPA
Nursing Program Faculty 31 (32% with doctorates).
Baccalaureate Enrollment 313 **Women** 93% **Men** 7% **Minority** 45% **International** 35% **Part-time** 90%
Graduate Enrollment 102 **Women** 93% **Men** 7% **Minority** 40% **International** 20% **Part-time** 95%
Nursing Student Activities Nursing Honor Society, Sigma Theta Tau, nursing club.
Nursing Student Resources Academic advising; academic or career counseling; assistance for students with disabilities; bookstore; campus computer network; career placement assistance; computer lab; computer-assisted instruction; daycare for children of students; e-mail services; employment services for current students; housing assistance; interactive nursing skills videos; Internet; learning resource lab; library services; nursing audiovisuals; placement services for program completers; remedial services; resume preparation assistance; tutoring.
Library Facilities 375,186 volumes; 32,675 periodical subscriptions.

BACCALAUREATE PROGRAMS
Degree BSN
Available Programs ADN to Baccalaureate; RN Baccalaureate.
Site Options Branchburg, NJ; Toms River, NJ.
Study Options Full-time and part-time.
Program Entrance Requirements Minimum overall college GPA of 2.0, written essay, 2 letters of recommendation, prerequisite course work, RN licensure. Transfer students are accepted. *Application deadline:* Applications may be processed on a rolling basis for some programs.
Advanced Placement Credit by examination available. Credit given for nursing courses completed elsewhere dependent upon specific evaluations.
Expenses (2010-11) *Tuition, state resident:* full-time $3200; part-time $230 per credit. *Tuition, nonresident:* full-time $6000; part-time $400 per credit.
Financial Aid 50% of baccalaureate students in nursing programs received some form of financial aid in 2009-10. *Gift aid (need-based):* Federal Pell, FSEOG, state, private, college/university gift aid from institutional funds. *Loans:* Federal Direct (Subsidized and Unsubsidized Stafford PLUS), Perkins. *Work-study:* Federal Work-Study. *Financial aid application deadline (priority):* 3/15.
Contact ***Telephone:*** 908-737-3390. *Fax:* 908-737-3393. *E-mail:* nursing@kean.edu.

GRADUATE PROGRAMS
Expenses (2010-11) *Tuition, state resident:* full-time $5436; part-time $500 per credit. *Tuition, nonresident:* full-time $7368; part-time $614 per credit. *Required fees:* full-time $1370; part-time $125 per credit.
Financial Aid 50% of graduate students in nursing programs received some form of financial aid in 2009-10. Research assistantships with full tuition reimbursements available available.
Contact Graduate Nursing contact, Department of Nursing, Kean University, 1000 Morris Avenue, Townsend 116, Union, NJ 07083-0411. *Telephone:* 908-737-3390. *Fax:* 908-737-3393. *E-mail:* nursing@kean.edu.

MASTER'S DEGREE PROGRAM

Degrees MSN; MSN/MPA
Available Programs Accelerated Master's for Nurses with Non-Nursing Degrees; Master's; Master's for Nurses with Non-Nursing Degrees.
Concentrations Available Health-care administration; nursing administration. *Clinical nurse specialist programs in:* community health, school health.
Site Options Toms River, NJ.
Study Options Full-time and part-time.
Program Entrance Requirements Clinical experience, computer literacy, minimum overall college GPA of 3.0, transcript of college record, written essay, immunizations, interview, 2 letters of recommendation, nursing research course, physical assessment course, professional liability insurance/malpractice insurance, statistics course.
Advanced Placement Credit given for nursing courses completed elsewhere dependent upon specific evaluations.
Degree Requirements 36 total credit hours, thesis or project.

Monmouth University

Marjorie K. Unterberg School of Nursing
West Long Branch, New Jersey

http://www.monmouth.edu/
Founded in 1933

DEGREES • BSN • MSN

Nursing Program Faculty 17 (67% with doctorates).
Baccalaureate Enrollment 71 **Women** 93% **Men** 7% **Minority** 23% **Part-time** 98%
Graduate Enrollment 245 **Women** 97% **Men** 3% **Minority** 25% **International** .08% **Part-time** 92%
Distance Learning Courses Available.
Nursing Student Activities Sigma Theta Tau, Student Nurses' Association.
Nursing Student Resources Academic advising; academic or career counseling; assistance for students with disabilities; bookstore; campus computer network; career placement assistance; computer lab; computer-assisted instruction; e-mail services; employment services for current students; interactive nursing skills videos; Internet; learning resource lab; library services; nursing audiovisuals; paid internships; remedial services; resume preparation assistance; skills, simulation, or other laboratory; tutoring.
Library Facilities 263,000 volumes (250,000 in health, 25,000 in nursing); 38,200 periodical subscriptions (98 health-care related).

BACCALAUREATE PROGRAMS

Degree BSN
Available Programs ADN to Baccalaureate; RN Baccalaureate.
Site Options Red Bank, NJ; Freehold, NJ.
Study Options Full-time and part-time.
Program Entrance Requirements Transcript of college record, health exam, immunizations, 2 letters of recommendation, minimum GPA in nursing prerequisites of 2.0, professional liability insurance/malpractice insurance, prerequisite course work, RN licensure. Transfer students are accepted. *Application deadline:* 7/15 (fall), 11/15 (spring), 5/1 (summer). Applications may be processed on a rolling basis for some programs. *Application fee:* $50.
Advanced Placement Credit by examination available. Credit given for nursing courses completed elsewhere dependent upon specific evaluations.
Expenses (2010-11) *Tuition:* full-time $12,864; part-time $745 per credit. *Room and board:* $10,000; room only: $6000 per academic year. *Required fees:* full-time $730; part-time $157 per term.
Financial Aid 80% of baccalaureate students in nursing programs received some form of financial aid in 2009-10. *Gift aid (need-based):* Federal Pell, FSEOG, state, private, college/university gift aid from institutional funds, Federal Nursing. *Loans:* Federal Direct (Subsidized and Unsubsidized Stafford PLUS), Perkins, state, college/university, alternative private loans. *Work-study:* Federal Work-Study. *Financial aid application deadline:* Continuous.
Contact Dr. Cira Fraser, Associate Professor, Marjorie K. Unterberg School of Nursing, Monmouth University, West Long Branch, NJ 07764. *Telephone:* 732-571-3443. *Fax:* 732-263-5131. *E-mail:* cfraser@monmouth.edu.

GRADUATE PROGRAMS

Expenses (2010-11) *Tuition:* part-time $816 per credit. *Room and board:* $10,000; room only: $6000 per academic year. *Required fees:* full-time $720; part-time $314 per term.
Financial Aid 80% of graduate students in nursing programs received some form of financial aid in 2009-10.
Contact Dr. Laura Jannone, Director of MSN Program, Marjorie K. Unterberg School of Nursing, Monmouth University, 400 Cedar Avenue, West Long Branch, NJ 07764. *Telephone:* 732-571-3443. *Fax:* 732-263-5131. *E-mail:* ljannone@monmouth.edu.

MASTER'S DEGREE PROGRAM

Degree MSN
Available Programs Master's; Master's for Nurses with Non-Nursing Degrees; RN to Master's.
Concentrations Available Nursing administration; nursing education. *Clinical nurse specialist programs in:* forensic nursing, school health. *Nurse practitioner programs in:* adult health, family health, psychiatric/mental health.
Site Options Edison, NJ.
Study Options Full-time and part-time.
Program Entrance Requirements Minimum overall college GPA of 2.75, transcript of college record, immunizations, 2 letters of recommendation, professional liability insurance/malpractice insurance. *Application deadline:* 7/15 (fall), 11/15 (spring), 5/1 (summer). Applications may be processed on a rolling basis for some programs. *Application fee:* $50.
Advanced Placement Credit by examination available. Credit given for nursing courses completed elsewhere dependent upon specific evaluations.
Degree Requirements 42 total credit hours.

POST-MASTER'S PROGRAM

Areas of Study Nursing administration; nursing education. *Clinical nurse specialist programs in:* forensic nursing, school health. *Nurse practitioner programs in:* adult health, family health, psychiatric/mental health.

CONTINUING EDUCATION PROGRAM

Contact Ms. Barbara Paskewich, Special Projects Coordinator, Marjorie K. Unterberg School of Nursing, Monmouth University, 400 Cedar Avenue, West Long Branch, NJ 07764. *Telephone:* 732-571-3694. *Fax:* 732-263-5131. *E-mail:* bpaskewi@monmouth.edu.

New Jersey City University

Department of Nursing
Jersey City, New Jersey

http://www.njcu.edu/dept/ProfStudies/nursing2/rnbsn.htm
Founded in 1927

DEGREE • BSN

Nursing Program Faculty 7 (50% with doctorates).
Baccalaureate Enrollment 110 **Women** 85% **Men** 15% **Minority** 75% **International** 15% **Part-time** 40%
Nursing Student Activities Nursing Honor Society, Sigma Theta Tau, Student Nurses' Association.
Nursing Student Resources Academic advising; academic or career counseling; assistance for students with disabilities; bookstore; campus computer network; computer lab; computer-assisted instruction; daycare for children of students; e-mail services; interactive nursing skills videos; Internet; learning resource lab; library services; nursing audiovisuals; other; remedial services; skills, simulation, or other laboratory.
Library Facilities 319,360 volumes; 25,214 periodical subscriptions.

BACCALAUREATE PROGRAMS

Degree BSN
Available Programs Accelerated Baccalaureate for Second Degree; RN Baccalaureate.
Site Options Wall Township, NJ; East Orange, NJ.
Study Options Full-time.
Program Entrance Requirements Minimum overall college GPA of 3.0, transcript of college record, CPR certification, written essay, health exam, immunizations, 2 letters of recommendation, professional liability insurance/malpractice insurance, prerequisite course work, RN licensure. Transfer students are accepted. *Application fee:* $35.

Advanced Placement Credit by examination available. Credit given for nursing courses completed elsewhere dependent upon specific evaluations.
Financial Aid 40% of baccalaureate students in nursing programs received some form of financial aid in 2008-09.
Contact Dr. Kevin J. O'Neill, Assistant Professor, Department of Nursing, New Jersey City University, 2039 Kennedy Boulevard, R404, Jersey City, NJ 07305. *Telephone:* 201-200-3157. *Fax:* 201-200-3222. *E-mail:* koneill@njcu.edu.

Ramapo College of New Jersey

Master of Science in Nursing Program
Mahwah, New Jersey

Founded in 1969

DEGREES • BSN • MSN

Nursing Program Faculty 29 (20% with doctorates).
Baccalaureate Enrollment 435 **Women** 90% **Men** 10% **Minority** 35% **International** 7% **Part-time** 15%
Graduate Enrollment 41 **Women** 95% **Men** 5% **Minority** 17% **Part-time** 90%
Distance Learning Courses Available.
Nursing Student Activities Nursing Honor Society, Student Nurses' Association.
Nursing Student Resources Academic advising; academic or career counseling; assistance for students with disabilities; bookstore; campus computer network; career placement assistance; computer lab; computer-assisted instruction; e-mail services; employment services for current students; externships; housing assistance; interactive nursing skills videos; Internet; learning resource lab; library services; nursing audiovisuals; placement services for program completers; remedial services; resume preparation assistance; skills, simulation, or other laboratory; tutoring; unpaid internships.
Library Facilities 280,588 volumes (3,500 in nursing); 487 periodical subscriptions (200 health-care related).

BACCALAUREATE PROGRAMS

Degree BSN
Available Programs Generic Baccalaureate; RN Baccalaureate.
Site Options Englewood, NJ.
Study Options Full-time.
Online Degree Options Yes.
Program Entrance Requirements CPR certification, health exam, 3 years high school science, immunizations, minimum high school GPA of 2.5, minimum high school rank 20%, professional liability insurance/malpractice insurance. Transfer students are accepted. *Application deadline:* 3/1 (fall), 3/1 (spring). Applications may be processed on a rolling basis for some programs. *Application fee:* $60.
Advanced Placement Credit given for nursing courses completed elsewhere dependent upon specific evaluations.
Expenses (2009-10) *Tuition, state resident:* part-time $240 per credit. *Tuition, nonresident:* part-time $480 per credit. *Room and board:* $9950; room only: $7550 per academic year. *Required fees:* part-time $350 per term.
Financial Aid ***Gift aid (need-based):*** Federal Pell, FSEOG, state, private, college/university gift aid from institutional funds, Federal Nursing. *Loans:* Federal Direct (Subsidized and Unsubsidized Stafford PLUS), Perkins, state. *Work-study:* Federal Work-Study, part-time campus jobs. *Financial aid application deadline (priority):* 3/1.
Contact Kathleen M. Burke, Assistant Dean in Charge of Nursing, Master of Science in Nursing Program, Ramapo College of New Jersey, 505 Ramapo Valley Road, Mahwah, NJ 07430. *Telephone:* 201-684-7737. *Fax:* 201-684-7934. *E-mail:* kmburke@ramapo.edu.

GRADUATE PROGRAMS

Expenses (2009-10) *Tuition, state resident:* part-time $525 per credit. *Tuition, nonresident:* part-time $675 per credit. *Room and board:* $9950; room only: $7550 per academic year. *Required fees:* part-time $100 per term.
Financial Aid 10 fellowships (averaging $1,992 per year) were awarded; traineeships also available.
Contact Kathleen M. Burke, Assistant Dean in Charge of Nursing, Master of Science in Nursing Program, Ramapo College of New Jersey, 505 Ramapo Valley Road, Mahwah, NJ 07430. *Telephone:* 201-684-7737. *Fax:* 201-684-7934. *E-mail:* kmburke@ramapo.edu.

MASTER'S DEGREE PROGRAM

Degree MSN
Available Programs Master's.
Concentrations Available Nursing education.
Study Options Full-time and part-time.
Online Degree Options Yes (online only).
Program Entrance Requirements Clinical experience, computer literacy, minimum overall college GPA of 3.0, transcript of college record, CPR certification, 2 letters of recommendation, nursing research course, professional liability insurance/malpractice insurance, statistics course. *Application deadline:* Applications may be processed on a rolling basis for some programs. *Application fee:* $60.
Advanced Placement Credit given for nursing courses completed elsewhere dependent upon specific evaluations.
Degree Requirements 32 total credit hours.

POST-MASTER'S PROGRAM

Areas of Study Nursing education.

CONTINUING EDUCATION PROGRAM

Contact Dr. Margaret Greene, Associate Professor, Master of Science in Nursing Program, Ramapo College of New Jersey, 505 Ramapo Valley Road, Mahwah, NJ 07430. *Telephone:* 201-684-7206. *Fax:* 201-684-7954. *E-mail:* mgreene1@ramapo.edu.

The Richard Stockton College of New Jersey

Program in Nursing
Pomona, New Jersey

http://intraweb.stockton.edu/eyos/page.cfm?siteID=168&pageID=1
Founded in 1969

DEGREES • BSN • MSN

Nursing Program Faculty 6 (66% with doctorates).
Baccalaureate Enrollment 69 **Women** 98% **Men** 2% **Minority** 10% **Part-time** 80%
Graduate Enrollment 20 **Women** 90% **Men** 10% **Minority** 15% **Part-time** 95%
Nursing Student Activities Sigma Theta Tau.
Nursing Student Resources Academic advising; academic or career counseling; assistance for students with disabilities; bookstore; campus computer network; computer lab; computer-assisted instruction; daycare for children of students; e-mail services; housing assistance; Internet; learning resource lab; library services; nursing audiovisuals; resume preparation assistance; skills, simulation, or other laboratory; tutoring.
Library Facilities 281,155 volumes (9,761 in health, 1,258 in nursing); 37,050 periodical subscriptions (83 health-care related).

BACCALAUREATE PROGRAMS

Degree BSN
Available Programs RN Baccalaureate.
Study Options Full-time and part-time.
Program Entrance Requirements Transfer students are accepted.
Advanced Placement Credit given for nursing courses completed elsewhere dependent upon specific evaluations.
Contact ***Telephone:*** 609-652-4837.

GRADUATE PROGRAMS

Contact ***Telephone:*** 609-652-4501.

MASTER'S DEGREE PROGRAM

Degree MSN
Concentrations Available *Nurse practitioner programs in:* adult health.
Study Options Full-time and part-time.
Program Entrance Requirements Clinical experience, computer literacy, minimum overall college GPA of 3.0, transcript of college record, CPR certification, written essay, immunizations, 2 letters of recommendation, nursing research course, physical assessment course, professional liability insurance/malpractice insurance, statistics course, GRE General Test.
Advanced Placement Credit given for nursing courses completed elsewhere dependent upon specific evaluations.

Degree Requirements 42 total credit hours, thesis or project.

Rutgers, The State University of New Jersey, Camden College of Arts and Sciences

Department of Nursing
Camden, New Jersey

http://nursing.camden.rutgers.edu/
Founded in 1927

DEGREE • BS

Nursing Program Faculty 22 (40% with doctorates).
Baccalaureate Enrollment 230 **Women** 88% **Men** 12% **Minority** 55% **Part-time** 27%
Distance Learning Courses Available.
Nursing Student Activities Sigma Theta Tau, Student Nurses' Association.
Nursing Student Resources Academic advising; academic or career counseling; assistance for students with disabilities; bookstore; campus computer network; computer lab; computer-assisted instruction; e-mail services; employment services for current students; externships; housing assistance; interactive nursing skills videos; Internet; learning resource lab; library services; nursing audiovisuals; remedial services; resume preparation assistance; skills, simulation, or other laboratory; tutoring.
Library Facilities 6.4 million volumes; 28,934 periodical subscriptions.

BACCALAUREATE PROGRAMS

Degree BS
Available Programs Accelerated RN Baccalaureate; Generic Baccalaureate; RN Baccalaureate.
Site Options Atlantic City, NJ.
Study Options Full-time.
Program Entrance Requirements CPR certification, written essay, health exam, health insurance, high school biology, high school chemistry, high school foreign language, 2 years high school math, high school science, high school transcript, immunizations, minimum high school GPA of 2.5, minimum GPA in nursing prerequisites of 3.0, professional liability insurance/malpractice insurance, prerequisite course work. Transfer students are accepted. *Application deadline:* 2/28 (fall).
Contact Dr. Joanne Robinson, Clinical Associate Professor and Acting Chair, Department of Nursing, Rutgers, The State University of New Jersey, Camden College of Arts and Sciences, 311 North Fifth Street, Armitage Hall, Room 448, Camden, NJ 08102. *Telephone:* 856-225-6226. *Fax:* 856-225-6250. *E-mail:* nursecam@camden.rutgers.edu.

Rutgers, The State University of New Jersey, College of Nursing

Rutgers, The State University of New Jersey, College of Nursing
Newark, New Jersey

http://www.rutgers.edu/
Founded in 1956

DEGREES • BS • MS • MS/MPH • PHD

Nursing Program Faculty 31 (80% with doctorates).
Baccalaureate Enrollment 567 **Women** 90% **Men** 10% **Minority** 52% **International** 1% **Part-time** 20%
Graduate Enrollment 176 **Women** 98% **Men** 2% **Minority** 30% **Part-time** 90%
Distance Learning Courses Available.
Nursing Student Activities Sigma Theta Tau, Student Nurses' Association, nursing club.
Nursing Student Resources Academic advising; academic or career counseling; assistance for students with disabilities; bookstore; campus computer network; career placement assistance; computer lab; computer-assisted instruction; e-mail services; employment services for current students; externships; housing assistance; interactive nursing skills videos; Internet; learning resource lab; library services; nursing audiovisuals; paid internships; remedial services; resume preparation assistance; skills, simulation, or other laboratory; tutoring; unpaid internships.
Library Facilities 6.4 million volumes; 28,934 periodical subscriptions.

BACCALAUREATE PROGRAMS

Degree BS
Available Programs Accelerated Baccalaureate for Second Degree; Baccalaureate for Second Degree; Generic Baccalaureate; RN Baccalaureate.
Site Options Freehold, NJ; New Brunswick, NJ.
Study Options Full-time and part-time.
Program Entrance Requirements Minimum overall college GPA of 3.2, transcript of college record, health exam, high school biology, high school chemistry, 3 years high school math, 2 years high school science, high school transcript, immunizations, minimum high school GPA of 3.2, minimum high school rank, professional liability insurance/malpractice insurance. Transfer students are accepted. *Application deadline:* 12/1 (fall). *Application fee:* $65.
Advanced Placement Credit by examination available. Credit given for nursing courses completed elsewhere dependent upon specific evaluations.
Expenses (2009-10) *Tuition, area resident:* full-time $4773; part-time $307 per credit. *Tuition, nonresident:* full-time $10,089; part-time $654 per credit. *International tuition:* $10,089 full-time. *Room and board:* $10,498; room only: $7064 per academic year. *Required fees:* full-time $925.
Financial Aid 15% of baccalaureate students in nursing programs received some form of financial aid in 2008-09.
Contact Admissions Office, Rutgers, The State University of New Jersey, College of Nursing, 249 University Avenue, Newark, NJ 07102-1803. *Telephone:* 973-353-5205.

GRADUATE PROGRAMS

Expenses (2009-10) *Tuition, area resident:* full-time $7656; part-time $638 per credit. *Tuition, nonresident:* full-time $11,448; part-time $954 per credit. *International tuition:* $11,448 full-time. *Room and board:* $10,399; room only: $6965 per academic year. *Required fees:* full-time $753; part-time $335 per term.
Financial Aid 74% of graduate students in nursing programs received some form of financial aid in 2008-09.
Contact Dr. Mary Ann Scoloveno, Interim Associate Dean for Graduate Education, Rutgers, The State University of New Jersey, College of Nursing, 180 University Avenue, Newark, NJ 07102-1803. *Telephone:* 973-353-5060. *Fax:* 973-353-1277. *E-mail:* scoloven@rutgers.edu.

MASTER'S DEGREE PROGRAM

Degrees MS; MS/MPH
Available Programs Master's.
Concentrations Available *Clinical nurse specialist programs in:* adult health, community health, oncology, parent-child, psychiatric/mental health. *Nurse practitioner programs in:* acute care, adult health, family health, pediatric, psychiatric/mental health, women's health.
Site Options Freehold, NJ; Camden, NJ.
Study Options Full-time and part-time.
Program Entrance Requirements Minimum overall college GPA of 3.0, transcript of college record, written essay, immunizations, 3 letters of recommendation, physical assessment course, professional liability insurance/malpractice insurance, resume, statistics course. *Application deadline:* 6/1 (fall), 10/1 (spring). *Application fee:* $65.
Advanced Placement Credit given for nursing courses completed elsewhere dependent upon specific evaluations.
Degree Requirements 42 total credit hours.

POST-MASTER'S PROGRAM

Areas of Study Nursing education. *Clinical nurse specialist programs in:* adult health, community health, oncology, parent-child, psychiatric/mental health. *Nurse practitioner programs in:* acute care, adult health, family health, pediatric, psychiatric/mental health, women's health.

DOCTORAL DEGREE PROGRAM

Degree PhD
Available Programs Doctorate.
Areas of Study Nursing research.
Program Entrance Requirements Minimum overall college GPA of 3.2, interview by faculty committee, 3 letters of recommendation, MSN or equivalent, scholarly papers, statistics course, vita, writing sample. Application deadline: 3/15 (fall). Application fee: $65.
Degree Requirements 59 total credit hours, dissertation, written exam, residency.

CONTINUING EDUCATION PROGRAM

Contact Dr. Gayle Pearson, Assistant Dean, Center for Professional Development, Rutgers, The State University of New Jersey, College of Nursing, 175 University Avenue, Newark, NJ 07102. *Telephone:* 973-353-1061. *Fax:* 973-353-1700. *E-mail:* gaylep@rutgers.edu.

Saint Peter's College

Nursing Program
Jersey City, New Jersey

Founded in 1872

DEGREES • BSN • MSN

Nursing Program Faculty 15 (73% with doctorates).

Baccalaureate Enrollment 161 **Women** 85% **Men** 15% **Minority** 40%

Graduate Enrollment 55 **Women** 99% **Men** 1% **Minority** 45%

Distance Learning Courses Available.

Nursing Student Activities Nursing Honor Society, Sigma Theta Tau, Student Nurses' Association.

Nursing Student Resources Academic advising; academic or career counseling; assistance for students with disabilities; bookstore; campus computer network; career placement assistance; computer lab; computer-assisted instruction; e-mail services; externships; interactive nursing skills videos; Internet; learning resource lab; library services; nursing audiovisuals; remedial services; resume preparation assistance; skills, simulation, or other laboratory; tutoring.

Library Facilities 178,587 volumes (7,200 in health); 1,741 periodical subscriptions (1,586 health-care related).

BACCALAUREATE PROGRAMS

Degree BSN

Available Programs ADN to Baccalaureate; Generic Baccalaureate; RN Baccalaureate.

Site Options Englewood Cliffs, NJ.

Study Options Full-time.

Program Entrance Requirements Minimum overall college GPA of 2.7, transcript of college record, written essay, high school biology, high school chemistry, high school foreign language, 3 years high school math, 3 years high school science, high school transcript, immunizations, 2 letters of recommendation, minimum high school GPA of 3.0. Transfer students are accepted. *Application deadline:* Applications may be processed on a rolling basis for some programs.

Contact ***Telephone:*** 201-761-7113. *Fax:* 201-761-7105.

GRADUATE PROGRAMS

Contact ***Telephone:*** 201-761-6272. *Fax:* 201-761-6271.

MASTER'S DEGREE PROGRAM

Degree MSN

Available Programs Master's; Master's for Nurses with Non-Nursing Degrees.

Concentrations Available Nurse case management; nursing administration. *Nurse practitioner programs in:* adult health.

Site Options Englewood Cliffs, NJ.

Study Options Part-time.

Program Entrance Requirements Clinical experience, minimum overall college GPA of 3.0, transcript of college record, written essay, immunizations, 3 letters of recommendation, nursing research course, physical assessment course, professional liability insurance/malpractice insurance, statistics course. *Application deadline:* 8/25 (fall), 10/24 (winter), 12/15 (spring), 5/5 (summer). *Application fee:* $40.

Degree Requirements 39 total credit hours, thesis or project.

POST-MASTER'S PROGRAM

Areas of Study *Nurse practitioner programs in:* adult health.

Seton Hall University

College of Nursing
South Orange, New Jersey

http://nursing.shu.edu/

Founded in 1856

DEGREES • BSN • DNP • MSN • MSN/MA • MSN/MBA

Nursing Program Faculty 43 (50% with doctorates).

Baccalaureate Enrollment 730 **Women** 89% **Men** 11% **Minority** 43% **International** 1% **Part-time** 10%

Graduate Enrollment 190 **Women** 87% **Men** 13% **Minority** 17% **Part-time** 46%

Distance Learning Courses Available.

Nursing Student Activities Sigma Theta Tau, Student Nurses' Association.

Nursing Student Resources Academic advising; academic or career counseling; assistance for students with disabilities; bookstore; campus computer network; career placement assistance; computer lab; computer-assisted instruction; e-mail services; externships; housing assistance; interactive nursing skills videos; Internet; learning resource lab; library services; nursing audiovisuals; paid internships; remedial services; resume preparation assistance; skills, simulation, or other laboratory; tutoring.

Library Facilities 506,042 volumes; 1,475 periodical subscriptions.

BACCALAUREATE PROGRAMS

Degree BSN

Available Programs Accelerated Baccalaureate for Second Degree; Baccalaureate for Second Degree; Generic Baccalaureate; RN Baccalaureate.

Site Options Camden, NJ; Brick/Toms River, NJ; Lakewood, NJ.

Study Options Full-time and part-time.

Program Entrance Requirements Minimum overall college GPA of 3.0, transcript of college record, CPR certification, written essay, high school biology, high school chemistry, high school foreign language, 3 years high school math, 2 years high school science, high school transcript, minimum high school GPA of 3.0, professional liability insurance/malpractice insurance. Transfer students are accepted.

Financial Aid 75% of baccalaureate students in nursing programs received some form of financial aid in 2009-10.

Contact Ms. Kristyn Kent-Wuillermin, Director of Strategic Alliances, Marketing, and Enrollment, College of Nursing, Seton Hall University, 400 South Orange Avenue, South Orange, NJ 07079-2697. *Telephone:* 973-761-9291. *Fax:* 973-761-9607. *E-mail:* kristyn.kent@shu.edu.

GRADUATE PROGRAMS

Financial Aid 31% of graduate students in nursing programs received some form of financial aid in 2009-10. Institutionally sponsored loans, scholarships, traineeships, tuition waivers (partial), and unspecified assistantships available. Aid available to part-time students.

Contact Ms. Kristyn Kent-Wuillermin, Director of Strategic Alliances, Marketing, and Enrollment, College of Nursing, Seton Hall University, 400 South Orange Avenue, South Orange, NJ 07079-2697. *Telephone:* 973-761-9291. *Fax:* 973-761-9607. *E-mail:* kristyn.kent@shu.edu.

MASTER'S DEGREE PROGRAM

Degrees MSN; MSN/MA; MSN/MBA

Available Programs Accelerated Master's for Nurses with Non-Nursing Degrees; Master's; Master's for Nurses with Non-Nursing Degrees; RN to Master's.

Concentrations Available Clinical nurse leader; health-care administration; nurse case management; nursing administration; nursing education. *Clinical nurse specialist programs in:* school health. *Nurse practitioner programs in:* adult health, gerontology, pediatric, school health.

Study Options Full-time and part-time.

Online Degree Options Yes (online only).

Program Entrance Requirements Clinical experience, computer literacy, minimum overall college GPA of 3.0, transcript of college record, CPR certification, written essay, immunizations, interview, 2 letters of recommendation, nursing research course, physical assessment course, professional liability insurance/malpractice insurance, prerequisite course work, resume, statistics course. *Application deadline:* Applications may be processed on a rolling basis for some programs.

Advanced Placement Credit by examination available. Credit given for nursing courses completed elsewhere dependent upon specific evaluations.

Degree Requirements 43 total credit hours, thesis or project.

POST-MASTER'S PROGRAM

Areas of Study Health-care administration; nurse case management; nursing administration; nursing education. *Nurse practitioner programs in:* adult health, gerontology, pediatric, school health.

DOCTORAL DEGREE PROGRAM

Degree DNP
Available Programs Doctorate; Post-Baccalaureate Doctorate.
Areas of Study Advanced practice nursing, nursing administration, nursing research.
Program Entrance Requirements Clinical experience, minimum overall college GPA of 3.0, interview, 2 letters of recommendation, MSN or equivalent, scholarly papers, statistics course, vita, writing sample, GRE.
Degree Requirements 46 total credit hours, dissertation.

Thomas Edison State College

W. Cary Edwards School of Nursing
Trenton, New Jersey

http://www.tesc.edu/nursing
Nursing program founded in 1983

DEGREES • RN TO BSN • RN TO BSN/MSN • BSN TO MSN

Nursing Student Resources Students in the W. Cary Edwards School of Nursing have the opportunity to earn degrees through traditional and non-traditional methods, which take into consideration the individual needs and interests of each student. All nursing courses are designed and delivered as mentored, independent study courses via the Internet using myEdison®, the College's online course management system that utilizes the Blackboard platform. Students in these courses communicate with mentors and fellow students using e-mail and submit assignments to mentors through the Internet. Students may earn credit toward a degree by demonstrating college-level knowledge through testing and assessment of prior learning; by transfer credit for courses taken through other regionally accredited institutions; through the College's *e*-Pack® courses; and for licenses, certificates, and courses taken at work or through military training, if approved and recommended for academic credit.
W. Cary Edwards School of Nursing Faculty The School utilizes off-site nurse educators from a variety of nursing education and service settings to develop, implement, and evaluate the program. All nurse educators have a minimum of a master's degree in nursing, with approximately 75% prepared at the doctoral level and many tenured at their home institution. With its courses offered by distance learning, the School has the opportunity to draw nurse educators from throughout the United States, resulting in a very diverse and experienced group of online nurse educators. The W. Cary Edwards School of Nursing has accreditation through the New Jersey Board of Nursing, the National League for Nursing Accrediting Commission (NLNAC) and, most recently, the Commission on Collegiate Nursing Education (CCNE).

BACHELOR'S AND MASTER'S DEGREE PROGRAMS

Degrees RN to BSN, RN to BSN/MSN, BSN to MSN. Master's degree has three specialties: Nurse Educator, Nursing Informatics and Nursing Administration
Certificate Programs Three 12–18 credit graduate nursing certificate programs—Nurse Educator; Nursing Informatics; and Nursing Administration—are available to RNs with a master's degree in another area of nursing specialty.
Study Options Self-paced programs; online nursing courses offered quarterly; multiple options for credit earning; no time limit for degree completion; no residency requirement with maximum flexibility in transfer credit.
Program Entrance Requirements Admission is open and rolling. RNs can enroll any day of the year. In addition to the documentation of their current RN license valid in the United States, all applicants must submit a completed online application with $75 fee and have official transcripts of all completed course work sent to the Office of the Registrar (undergraduate students) or Office of Admissions for graduate students. All RNs will have 20 credits applied from previous nursing course work toward the 48-credit nursing requirement in the BSN degree. A total of 80 credits may be accepted from a community college, and up to 60 credits, including the 20 credits used in the nursing requirement, will be awarded to diploma graduates based on current licensure. There is no age restriction on credits transferred in to meet general education requirements or lower-division nursing requirements. All upper-division nursing credits must be from an accredited baccalaureate or higher degree nursing program, and newer than ten years if completed prior to application to the W. Cary Edwards School of Nursing. All credits used in the nursing requirement must have a grade equivalent of C or better. All previously completed graduate credits transferred in to meet MSN degree and graduate certificate requirements must be newer than seven years at the time of enrollment in the W. Carey Edwards School of Nursing, have a grade equivalent of B or better, and be from a regionally accredited college or university or recognized international institution. Applicants to the BSN/MSN (BSNM) program will be enrolled in the MSN degree on certification for graduation from the BSN degree. Nine graduate credits required in the BSN degree will be applied to the MSN degree requirements.
Expenses (2010–11) *Tuition, state resident:* $340 per credit. *Tuition, nonresident:* $410 per credit for the BSN degree program; $505 for the MSN degree and Graduate Nursing certificate programs.
Financial Aid 4% of the RNs in the undergraduate nursing program and 5% in the graduate nursing program received some form of financial aid in 2009–10.
Contact Thomas Edison State College, 101 W. State Street, Trenton, NJ 08608-1176. *Telephone*: 888-442-8372. *E-mail*: nursinginfo@tesc.edu.
Degree Requirements 46 total credit hours, dissertation.

University of Medicine and Dentistry of New Jersey

School of Nursing
Newark, New Jersey

http://sn.umdnj.edu/
Founded in 1970

DEGREES • BSN • DNP • MSN

Nursing Program Faculty 150 (30% with doctorates).
Baccalaureate Enrollment 493 **Women** 85% **Men** 15% **Minority** 48%
Graduate Enrollment 720 **Women** 80% **Men** 20% **Minority** 30% **Part-time** 80%
Distance Learning Courses Available.
Nursing Student Activities Nursing Honor Society, Sigma Theta Tau, Student Nurses' Association.
Nursing Student Resources Academic advising; academic or career counseling; assistance for students with disabilities; bookstore; campus computer network; computer lab; computer-assisted instruction; daycare for children of students; e-mail services; housing assistance; interactive nursing skills videos; Internet; learning resource lab; library services; nursing audiovisuals; remedial services; resume preparation assistance; skills, simulation, or other laboratory; tutoring.
Library Facilities 91,446 volumes in health, 3,273 volumes in nursing; 4,350 periodical subscriptions health-care related.

BACCALAUREATE PROGRAMS

Degree BSN
Available Programs Accelerated Baccalaureate for Second Degree; RN Baccalaureate.
Site Options Stratford, NJ; Glassboro, NJ.
Study Options Full-time and part-time.
Program Entrance Requirements Minimum overall college GPA of 3.0, transcript of college record, CPR certification, written essay, health exam, health insurance, immunizations, 3 letters of recommendation, minimum GPA in nursing prerequisites of 2.75, prerequisite course work. *Application deadline:* 5/20 (fall), 11/1 (spring), 3/15 (summer). Applications may be processed on a rolling basis for some programs. *Application fee:* $45.
Advanced Placement Credit given for nursing courses completed elsewhere dependent upon specific evaluations.
Expenses (2010-11) *Tuition, state resident:* full-time $15,744; part-time $359 per credit. *Tuition, nonresident:* full-time $24,160; part-time $510 per credit. *Required fees:* full-time $2377.
Financial Aid 88% of baccalaureate students in nursing programs received some form of financial aid in 2009-10.
Contact Dr. Denise Tate, Assistant Dean, Prelicensure Programs, School of Nursing, University of Medicine and Dentistry of New Jersey, 65 Bergen Street, Newark, NJ 07101. *Telephone:* 973-972-0509. *E-mail:* tatedm@umdnj.edu.

GRADUATE PROGRAMS

Expenses (2010-11) *Tuition, state resident:* part-time $564 per credit. *Tuition, nonresident:* part-time $814 per credit. *Room and board:* room only: $11,700 per academic year. *Required fees:* full-time $620.
Financial Aid 28% of graduate students in nursing programs received some form of financial aid in 2009-10. Teaching assistantships, institutionally sponsored loans and scholarships available. Aid available to part-time students. *Financial aid application deadline:* 5/1.
Contact Dr. Patricia Hindin, PhD, Assistant Dean, Graduate Programs, School of Nursing, University of Medicine and Dentistry of New Jersey, 65 Bergen Street, SSB 1130, Newark, NJ 07101. *Telephone:* 973-972-4211. *Fax:* 973-972-7904. *E-mail:* hindinpk@umdnj.edu.

MASTER'S DEGREE PROGRAM

Degree MSN
Available Programs Master's; Master's for Nurses with Non-Nursing Degrees; RN to Master's.
Concentrations Available Clinical nurse leader; nurse anesthesia; nurse-midwifery; nursing education; nursing informatics. *Clinical nurse specialist programs in:* psychiatric/mental health. *Nurse practitioner programs in:* acute care, adult health, community health, family health, gerontology, psychiatric/mental health, women's health.
Site Options Stratford, NJ.
Study Options Full-time and part-time.
Online Degree Options Yes.
Program Entrance Requirements Clinical experience, minimum overall college GPA of 3.0, transcript of college record, CPR certification, immunizations, interview, 2 letters of recommendation, physical assessment course, statistics course, GRE. *Application deadline:* 7/1 (fall), 11/1 (spring), 3/15 (summer). Applications may be processed on a rolling basis for some programs. *Application fee:* $50.
Advanced Placement Credit given for nursing courses completed elsewhere dependent upon specific evaluations.
Degree Requirements 40 total credit hours.

POST-MASTER'S PROGRAM

Areas of Study Clinical nurse leader; nurse anesthesia; nurse-midwifery; nursing informatics. *Clinical nurse specialist programs in:* psychiatric/mental health. *Nurse practitioner programs in:* acute care, adult health, family health, gerontology, psychiatric/mental health, women's health.

DOCTORAL DEGREE PROGRAM

Degree DNP
Available Programs Doctorate; Doctorate for Nurses with Non-Nursing Degrees; Post-Baccalaureate Doctorate.
Areas of Study Clinical practice, nursing administration.
Site Options Stratford, NJ.
Program Entrance Requirements Clinical experience, minimum overall college GPA of 3.0, interview by faculty committee, interview, 2 letters of recommendation, MSN or equivalent, statistics course, vita, writing sample. Application deadline: 7/1 (fall), 11/1 (spring). Applications may be processed on a rolling basis for some programs. Application fee: $50.
Degree Requirements 32 total credit hours, dissertation.

CONTINUING EDUCATION PROGRAM

Contact Dr. Donna Cill, Assistant Dean & Director of the Center for Lifelong Learning, School of Nursing, University of Medicine and Dentistry of New Jersey, 65 Bergen Street, Room 1132-A, Newark, NJ 07101-1709. *Telephone:* 973-972-9793. *Fax:* 973-972-7904. *E-mail:* cilldm@umdnj.edu.

William Paterson University of New Jersey

Department of Nursing
Wayne, New Jersey

http://www.wpunj.edu/cos/nursing/
Founded in 1855

DEGREES • BSN • DNP • MSN

Nursing Program Faculty 29 (64% with doctorates).
Baccalaureate Enrollment 400 **Women** 82% **Men** 18% **Minority** 55% **International** 5% **Part-time** 25%
Graduate Enrollment 52 **Women** 95% **Men** 5% **Minority** 20% **International** 5% **Part-time** 90%
Distance Learning Courses Available.
Nursing Student Activities Sigma Theta Tau, Student Nurses' Association.
Nursing Student Resources Academic advising; academic or career counseling; assistance for students with disabilities; bookstore; campus computer network; career placement assistance; computer lab; computer-assisted instruction; daycare for children of students; e-mail services; employment services for current students; housing assistance; interactive nursing skills videos; Internet; learning resource lab; library services; nursing audiovisuals; placement services for program completers; remedial services; resume preparation assistance; skills, simulation, or other laboratory; tutoring.
Library Facilities 338,573 volumes (15,000 in health, 12,700 in nursing); 6,569 periodical subscriptions (150 health-care related).

BACCALAUREATE PROGRAMS

Degree BSN
Available Programs ADN to Baccalaureate; Accelerated Baccalaureate for Second Degree; Generic Baccalaureate; LPN to Baccalaureate; RN Baccalaureate.
Study Options Full-time.
Program Entrance Requirements Minimum overall college GPA of 2.5, transcript of college record, CPR certification, health exam, health insurance, high school biology, high school chemistry, 1 year of high school math, 2 years high school science, high school transcript, immunizations, minimum high school GPA of 3.25, professional liability insurance/malpractice insurance, prerequisite course work. Transfer students are accepted. *Application deadline:* 5/1 (fall). Applications may be processed on a rolling basis for some programs. *Application fee:* $50.
Expenses (2010-11) *Tuition, state resident:* full-time $6830; part-time $219 per credit. *Tuition, nonresident:* full-time $13,854; part-time $449 per credit. *Room and board:* $9860; room only: $7840 per academic year. *Required fees:* full-time $4408; part-time $142 per credit; part-time $2204 per term.
Financial Aid 67% of baccalaureate students in nursing programs received some form of financial aid in 2009-10. *Gift aid (need-based):* Federal Pell, FSEOG, state, private, college/university gift aid from institutional funds. *Loans:* Federal Nursing Student Loans, Federal Direct (Subsidized and Unsubsidized Stafford PLUS), Perkins, state. *Work-study:* Federal Work-Study, part-time campus jobs. *Financial aid application deadline (priority):* 4/1.
Contact Dr. Julie Bliss, Chairperson, Department of Nursing, William Paterson University of New Jersey, 300 Pompton Road, W106, Wayne, NJ 07470. *Telephone:* 973-720-2673. *Fax:* 973-720-2668. *E-mail:* blissj@wpunj.edu.

GRADUATE PROGRAMS

Expenses (2010-11) *Tuition, state resident:* part-time $475 per credit. *Tuition, nonresident:* part-time $811 per credit. *Room and board:* room only: $7840 per academic year. *Required fees:* part-time $135 per credit.
Financial Aid 15% of graduate students in nursing programs received some form of financial aid in 2009-10. Research assistantships with tuition reimbursements available, unspecified assistantships available. *Financial aid application deadline:* 4/1.
Contact Dr. Kem Louie, Director, Graduate Program, Department of Nursing, William Paterson University of New Jersey, 300 Pompton Road, W240, Wayne, NJ 07470. *Telephone:* 973-720-3511. *Fax:* 973-720-3517. *E-mail:* louiek@wpunj.edu.

MASTER'S DEGREE PROGRAM

Degree MSN
Available Programs Master's; Master's for Nurses with Non-Nursing Degrees.
Concentrations Available Nursing administration; nursing education. *Clinical nurse specialist programs in:* community health. *Nurse practitioner programs in:* adult health, family health.
Site Options Englewood, NJ; Paramus, NJ.
Study Options Full-time and part-time.
Program Entrance Requirements Computer literacy, minimum overall college GPA of 3.0, transcript of college record, CPR certification, written essay, 2 letters of recommendation, nursing research course, physical assessment course, professional liability insurance/malpractice insurance, resume, statistics course, GRE General Test. *Application deadline:* Applications may be processed on a rolling basis for some programs. *Application fee:* $50.
Advanced Placement Credit given for nursing courses completed elsewhere dependent upon specific evaluations.

Degree Requirements 42 total credit hours, thesis or project.

POST-MASTER'S PROGRAM

Areas of Study *Clinical nurse specialist programs in:* school health. *Nurse practitioner programs in:* adult health, family health.

DOCTORAL DEGREE PROGRAM

Degree DNP
Available Programs Doctorate.
Areas of Study Advanced practice nursing, clinical practice, health-care systems, individualized study.
Program Entrance Requirements Clinical experience, minimum overall college GPA of 3.3, interview by faculty committee, letters of recommendation, MSN or equivalent, statistics course, vita, writing sample. Application deadline: 4/15 (fall). Application fee: $75.
Degree Requirements 42 total credit hours.

NEW MEXICO

Eastern New Mexico University

Department of Allied Health–Nursing
Portales, New Mexico

http://www.enmu.edu/academics/undergrad/colleges/las/disorders-nursing
Founded in 1934

DEGREE • BSN

Nursing Program Faculty 5 (2% with doctorates).
Baccalaureate Enrollment 198 **Women** 90% **Men** 10% **Minority** 45% **International** 5% **Part-time** 95%
Distance Learning Courses Available.
Nursing Student Activities Nursing Honor Society, Student Nurses' Association.
Nursing Student Resources Academic advising; academic or career counseling; assistance for students with disabilities; bookstore; campus computer network; career placement assistance; computer lab; computer-assisted instruction; e-mail services; housing assistance; Internet; library services; other; resume preparation assistance; tutoring.
Library Facilities 782,076 volumes (100 in health, 50 in nursing); 55,586 periodical subscriptions (15 health-care related).

BACCALAUREATE PROGRAMS

Degree BSN
Available Programs RPN to Baccalaureate.
Study Options Full-time and part-time.
Online Degree Options Yes (online only).
Program Entrance Requirements Minimum overall college GPA of 2.0, transcript of college record, CPR certification, high school biology, high school chemistry, 2 years high school math, 2 years high school science, high school transcript, immunizations, interview, 3 letters of recommendation, minimum high school GPA of 2.5, minimum GPA in nursing prerequisites of 2.0, professional liability insurance/malpractice insurance, prerequisite course work, RN licensure. Transfer students are accepted. *Application deadline:* 9/4 (fall), 9/4 (winter), 1/19 (spring), 6/1 (summer).
Advanced Placement Credit given for nursing courses completed elsewhere dependent upon specific evaluations.
Expenses (2010-11) *Tuition, area resident:* part-time $113 per credit hour. *Tuition, state resident:* part-time $163 per credit hour. *Tuition, nonresident:* part-time $393 per credit hour. *Required fees:* full-time $51.
Financial Aid 100% of baccalaureate students in nursing programs received some form of financial aid in 2009-10. *Gift aid (need-based):* Federal Pell, FSEOG, state, private, college/university gift aid from institutional funds. *Loans:* Federal Direct (Subsidized and Unsubsidized Stafford PLUS), Perkins, state, college/university. *Work-study:* Federal Work-Study, part-time campus jobs. *Financial aid application deadline:* Continuous.
Contact Dr. Leslie Paternoster, Nursing Program Director, Department of Allied Health–Nursing, Eastern New Mexico University, 1500 South Avenue K, Station 12, Portales, NM 88130. *Telephone:* 575-562-2773. *Fax:* 575-562-2293. *E-mail:* leslie.paternoster@enmu.edu.

New Mexico Highlands University

Department of Nursing
Las Vegas, New Mexico

Founded in 1893

DEGREE • BSN

Library Facilities 436,742 volumes; 40,316 periodical subscriptions.

BACCALAUREATE PROGRAMS

Degree BSN
Available Programs RN Baccalaureate.
Program Entrance Requirements Minimum overall college GPA of 2.5, RN licensure.
Contact Susan Williams, Director of RN-BSN Program, Department of Nursing, New Mexico Highlands University, Box 9000, Las Vegas, NV 87701. *Telephone:* 505-426-2116. *Fax:* 405-325-4216. *E-mail:* sdwilliams@nmhu.edu.

New Mexico State University

School of Nursing
Las Cruces, New Mexico

http://www.nmsu.edu/~nursing
Founded in 1888

DEGREES • BSN • MSN

Nursing Program Faculty 36 (37% with doctorates).
Baccalaureate Enrollment 292 **Women** 84% **Men** 16% **Minority** 49% **International** 1% **Part-time** 15%
Graduate Enrollment 42 **Women** 88% **Men** 12% **Minority** 24% **International** 1% **Part-time** 69%
Nursing Student Activities Sigma Theta Tau, Student Nurses' Association.
Nursing Student Resources Academic advising; academic or career counseling; assistance for students with disabilities; bookstore; campus computer network; computer lab; computer-assisted instruction; daycare for children of students; e-mail services; housing assistance; interactive nursing skills videos; Internet; learning resource lab; library services; nursing audiovisuals; paid internships; remedial services; skills, simulation, or other laboratory; tutoring.
Library Facilities 1.8 million volumes (33,000 in health, 17,500 in nursing); 4,402 periodical subscriptions (620 health-care related).

BACCALAUREATE PROGRAMS

Degree BSN
Available Programs Accelerated Baccalaureate for Second Degree; Generic Baccalaureate; RN Baccalaureate.
Study Options Full-time.
Program Entrance Requirements Minimum overall college GPA of 3.0, transcript of college record, CPR certification, immunizations, minimum GPA in nursing prerequisites of 2.0, prerequisite course work. Transfer students are accepted.
Advanced Placement Credit given for nursing courses completed elsewhere dependent upon specific evaluations.
Contact *Telephone:* 505-646-3534. *Fax:* 505-646-6166.

GRADUATE PROGRAMS

Contact *Telephone:* 505-646-8170. *Fax:* 505-646-2167.

MASTER'S DEGREE PROGRAM

Degree MSN
Available Programs Master's.
Concentrations Available Nursing administration. *Clinical nurse specialist programs in:* community health, medical-surgical, psychiatric/mental health. *Nurse practitioner programs in:* psychiatric/mental health.
Study Options Full-time and part-time.
Program Entrance Requirements Minimum overall college GPA of 3.0, transcript of college record, CPR certification, written essay, immunizations, 3 letters of recommendation, resume, statistics course, NCLEX exam.
Advanced Placement Credit given for nursing courses completed elsewhere dependent upon specific evaluations.
Degree Requirements 50 total credit hours, comprehensive exam.

DOCTORAL DEGREE PROGRAM
Program Entrance Requirements NCLEX exam.

CONTINUING EDUCATION PROGRAM
Contact *Telephone:* 505-646-3812. *Fax:* 505-646-2167.

University of New Mexico
College of Nursing
Albuquerque, New Mexico

http://hsc.unm.edu/consg/
Founded in 1889

DEGREES • BSN • MSN • MSN/MALAS • MSN/MPA • MSN/MPH • PHD

Nursing Program Faculty 51 (57% with doctorates).
Baccalaureate Enrollment 239 **Women** 87% **Men** 13% **Minority** 47% **Part-time** 41%
Graduate Enrollment 188 **Women** 91% **Men** 9% **Minority** 33% **Part-time** 73%
Distance Learning Courses Available.
Nursing Student Activities Sigma Theta Tau, Student Nurses' Association.
Nursing Student Resources Academic advising; assistance for students with disabilities; bookstore; campus computer network; career placement assistance; computer lab; computer-assisted instruction; daycare for children of students; e-mail services; housing assistance; interactive nursing skills videos; Internet; learning resource lab; library services; nursing audiovisuals; remedial services; skills, simulation, or other laboratory.
Library Facilities 3.1 million volumes (152,411 in health, 12,600 in nursing); 77,094 periodical subscriptions (2,000 health-care related).

BACCALAUREATE PROGRAMS
Degree BSN
Available Programs Accelerated Baccalaureate for Second Degree; Generic Baccalaureate; RN Baccalaureate.
Study Options Full-time.
Program Entrance Requirements Minimum overall college GPA of 3.0, transcript of college record, written essay, 2 letters of recommendation, minimum GPA in nursing prerequisites of 3.0, prerequisite course work. Transfer students are accepted. *Application deadline:* 2/15 (fall), 9/15 (spring). *Application fee:* $50.
Advanced Placement Credit given for nursing courses completed elsewhere dependent upon specific evaluations.
Expenses (2010-11) *Tuition, state resident:* full-time $13,875. *Required fees:* full-time $200.
Financial Aid 70% of baccalaureate students in nursing programs received some form of financial aid in 2009-10.
Contact Ms. Ann Marie Oechsler, Director of Student Services, College of Nursing, University of New Mexico, MSC09 5350, 1 University of New Mexico, Albuquerque, NM 87131-0001. *Telephone:* 505-272-4223. *Fax:* 505-272-3970. *E-mail:* aoechsler@salud.unm.edu.

GRADUATE PROGRAMS
Financial Aid 40% of graduate students in nursing programs received some form of financial aid in 2009-10. 5 teaching assistantships with partial tuition reimbursements available (averaging $6,750 per year) were awarded; research assistantships with partial tuition reimbursements available, scholarships and traineeships also available. *Financial aid application deadline:* 3/1.
Contact Ms. Karen Wells, Senior Academic Advisor, College of Nursing, University of New Mexico, MSC09 5350, NRPH Building, Room 152, 1 University of New Mexico, Albuquerque, NM 87131-0001. *Telephone:* 505-272-4223. *Fax:* 505-272-3970. *E-mail:* kwells@salud.unm.edu.

MASTER'S DEGREE PROGRAM
Degrees MSN; MSN/MALAS; MSN/MPA; MSN/MPH
Available Programs Master's.
Concentrations Available Nurse-midwifery; nursing administration; nursing education. *Nurse practitioner programs in:* acute care, family health, pediatric.
Study Options Full-time and part-time.
Online Degree Options Yes (online only).
Program Entrance Requirements Clinical experience, minimum overall college GPA of 3.0, transcript of college record, interview, 3 letters of recommendation, resume. *Application deadline:* 2/15 (fall), 10/15 (spring). *Application fee:* $50.
Advanced Placement Credit given for nursing courses completed elsewhere dependent upon specific evaluations.
Degree Requirements 32 total credit hours, thesis or project, comprehensive exam.

POST-MASTER'S PROGRAM
Areas of Study Nurse-midwifery; nursing administration; nursing education. *Nurse practitioner programs in:* acute care, family health, pediatric.

DOCTORAL DEGREE PROGRAM
Degree PhD
Available Programs Doctorate.
Areas of Study Health policy, nursing research.
Online Degree Options Yes.
Program Entrance Requirements Clinical experience, minimum overall college GPA of 3.0, interview by faculty committee, 3 letters of recommendation, MSN or equivalent, vita, writing sample. Application deadline: 2/15 (summer). Application fee: $50.
Degree Requirements 69 total credit hours, dissertation.

University of Phoenix–New Mexico Campus
College of Nursing
Albuquerque, New Mexico

DEGREES • BSN • MSN • MSN/ED D

Nursing Program Faculty 18 (13% with doctorates).
Baccalaureate Enrollment 24 **Women** 100% **Minority** 33.3%
Graduate Enrollment 14 **Women** 100% **Minority** 21.43%
Nursing Student Activities Sigma Theta Tau.
Nursing Student Resources Academic advising; academic or career counseling; assistance for students with disabilities; bookstore; campus computer network; computer lab; computer-assisted instruction; e-mail services; interactive nursing skills videos; Internet; learning resource lab; library services; nursing audiovisuals; remedial services; skills, simulation, or other laboratory; tutoring.
Library Facilities 16,781 periodical subscriptions (1,300 health-care related).

BACCALAUREATE PROGRAMS
Degree BSN
Available Programs Accelerated Baccalaureate.
Site Options Santa Fe, NM; Santa Teresa, NM.
Study Options Full-time.
Program Entrance Requirements Transcript of college record, CPR certification, immunizations, 1 letter of recommendation, RN licensure. Transfer students are accepted.
Advanced Placement Credit by examination available. Credit given for nursing courses completed elsewhere dependent upon specific evaluations.
Expenses (2009-10) *Tuition:* full-time $8640. *Required fees:* full-time $600.
Contact Campus College Chair, Nursing, College of Nursing, University of Phoenix–New Mexico Campus, 7471 Pan American Freeway NE, Albuquerque, NM 87109-4645. *Telephone:* 505-821-4800.

GRADUATE PROGRAMS
Expenses (2009-10) *Tuition:* full-time $11,640. *Required fees:* full-time $760.
Financial Aid Institutionally sponsored loans and scholarships available.
Contact Campus College Chair, Nursing, College of Nursing, University of Phoenix–New Mexico Campus, 7471 Pan American Freeway NE, Albuquerque, NM 87109-4645. *Telephone:* 505-821-4800.

MASTER'S DEGREE PROGRAM
Degrees MSN; MSN/Ed D
Available Programs Master's.
Concentrations Available Nursing administration; nursing education.
Site Options Santa Fe, NM; Santa Teresa, NM.
Study Options Full-time.

Online Degree Options Yes.
Program Entrance Requirements Clinical experience, computer literacy, minimum overall college GPA of 2.5, transcript of college record. *Application deadline:* Applications may be processed on a rolling basis for some programs. *Application fee:* $45.
Advanced Placement Credit given for nursing courses completed elsewhere dependent upon specific evaluations.
Degree Requirements 39 total credit hours, thesis or project.

Western New Mexico University
Nursing Department
Silver City, New Mexico

Founded in 1893

DEGREE • BSN

Library Facilities 245,146 volumes; 236 periodical subscriptions.

BACCALAUREATE PROGRAMS

Degree BSN
Available Programs RN Baccalaureate.
Program Entrance Requirements Minimum overall college GPA of 2.75, CPR certification, professional liability insurance/malpractice insurance, RN licensure. Transfer students are accepted.
Contact ***Telephone:*** 575-574-5140.

NEW YORK

Adelphi University
School of Nursing
Garden City, New York

http://www.adelphi.edu/
Founded in 1896

DEGREES • BS • MS • MS/MBA • PHD

Nursing Program Faculty 135 (33% with doctorates).
Baccalaureate Enrollment 920 **Women** 90% **Men** 10% **Minority** 40% **International** 1% **Part-time** 21%
Graduate Enrollment 175 **Women** 88% **Men** 12% **Minority** 55% **Part-time** 100%
Distance Learning Courses Available.
Nursing Student Activities Nursing Honor Society, Sigma Theta Tau, Student Nurses' Association, nursing club.
Nursing Student Resources Academic advising; academic or career counseling; assistance for students with disabilities; bookstore; campus computer network; career placement assistance; computer lab; computer-assisted instruction; daycare for children of students; e-mail services; employment services for current students; externships; housing assistance; interactive nursing skills videos; Internet; learning resource lab; library services; nursing audiovisuals; paid internships; placement services for program completers; remedial services; resume preparation assistance; skills, simulation, or other laboratory; tutoring; unpaid internships.
Library Facilities 593,920 volumes (29,918 in health, 2,666 in nursing); 31,883 periodical subscriptions (364 health-care related).

BACCALAUREATE PROGRAMS

Degree BS
Available Programs ADN to Baccalaureate; Accelerated Baccalaureate; Accelerated Baccalaureate for Second Degree; Baccalaureate for Second Degree; Generic Baccalaureate; LPN to Baccalaureate; LPN to RN Baccalaureate; RN Baccalaureate.
Site Options Manhattan, NY.
Study Options Full-time and part-time.
Program Entrance Requirements Minimum overall college GPA of 3.0, transcript of college record, written essay, health exam, high school foreign language, 3 years high school math, 3 years high school science, high school transcript, immunizations, interview, 2 letters of recommendation, minimum high school GPA of 3.0, minimum GPA in nursing prerequisites of 2.7. Transfer students are accepted. *Application deadline:* 11/30 (spring). Applications may be processed on a rolling basis for some programs. *Application fee:* $35.
Advanced Placement Credit by examination available.
Expenses (2010-11) *Tuition:* full-time $28,150; part-time $820 per credit. *Room and board:* $13,100; room only: $10,560 per academic year. *Required fees:* full-time $900.
Financial Aid 90% of baccalaureate students in nursing programs received some form of financial aid in 2009-10. *Gift aid (need-based):* Federal Pell, FSEOG, state, private, college/university gift aid from institutional funds, United Negro College Fund, endowed-donor scholarships. *Loans:* Federal Nursing Student Loans, Perkins, New York HELP Program (private alternative loans). *Work-study:* Federal Work-Study, part-time campus jobs. *Financial aid application deadline (priority):* 3/1.
Contact Mrs. Christine Murphy, Director of Admissions, School of Nursing, Adelphi University, One South Avenue, Levermore Hall, Garden City, NY 11530. *Telephone:* 516-877-3050. *E-mail:* murphy2@adelphi.edu.

GRADUATE PROGRAMS

Expenses (2010-11) *Tuition:* full-time $29,000; part-time $905 per credit. *Room and board:* $13,100; room only: $10,560 per academic year. *Required fees:* full-time $1100; part-time $550 per term.
Financial Aid 50% of graduate students in nursing programs received some form of financial aid in 2009-10. 15 teaching assistantships (averaging $4,512 per year) were awarded; career-related internships or fieldwork, unspecified assistantships, and graduate achievement awards also available. Aid available to part-time students. *Financial aid application deadline:* 2/15.
Contact Mrs. Christine Murphy, Director of Admissions, School of Nursing, Adelphi University, One South Avenue, Levermore Hall, Garden City, NY 11530. *Telephone:* 516-877-3050. *Fax:* 516-877-3039. *E-mail:* murphy2@adelphi.edu.

MASTER'S DEGREE PROGRAM

Degrees MS; MS/MBA
Available Programs Master's.
Concentrations Available Health-care administration; nursing administration; nursing education. *Nurse practitioner programs in:* adult health.
Site Options Manhattan, NY.
Study Options Full-time and part-time.
Program Entrance Requirements Clinical experience, computer literacy, minimum overall college GPA of 3.0, transcript of college record, CPR certification, written essay, immunizations, interview, 2 letters of recommendation, nursing research course, professional liability insurance/malpractice insurance, resume, statistics course. *Application deadline:* 3/1 (fall), 11/30 (spring). Applications may be processed on a rolling basis for some programs. *Application fee:* $50.
Advanced Placement Credit given for nursing courses completed elsewhere dependent upon specific evaluations.
Degree Requirements 42 total credit hours, thesis or project, comprehensive exam.

POST-MASTER'S PROGRAM

Areas of Study Health-care administration; nursing administration; nursing education. *Nurse practitioner programs in:* adult health.

DOCTORAL DEGREE PROGRAM

Degree PhD
Available Programs Doctorate; Doctorate for Nurses with Non-Nursing Degrees.
Areas of Study Faculty preparation, health-care systems, nursing administration, nursing education, nursing research.
Program Entrance Requirements Minimum overall college GPA of 3.5, interview by faculty committee, interview, 3 letters of recommendation, MSN or equivalent, statistics course, vita, writing sample, GRE. Application deadline: 2/15 (fall). Application fee: $50.
Degree Requirements 54 total credit hours, dissertation, oral exam, written exam.

CONTINUING EDUCATION PROGRAM

Contact Mrs. Karen Pappas, Director, Professional Development and Lifelong Learning, School of Nursing, Adelphi University, One South Avenue, Garden City, NY 11530. *Telephone:* 516-877-4554. *Fax:* 516-877-4558. *E-mail:* pappas@adelphi.edu.

The College at Brockport, State University of New York

Department of Nursing
Brockport, New York

http://www.brockport.edu/
Founded in 1867

DEGREE • BSN

Nursing Program Faculty 15 (50% with doctorates).
Baccalaureate Enrollment 180 **Women** 93% **Men** 7% **Minority** 15% **International** 2% **Part-time** 9%
Distance Learning Courses Available.
Nursing Student Activities Nursing Honor Society, Sigma Theta Tau, Student Nurses' Association.
Nursing Student Resources Academic advising; academic or career counseling; assistance for students with disabilities; bookstore; campus computer network; career placement assistance; computer lab; computer-assisted instruction; daycare for children of students; e-mail services; interactive nursing skills videos; Internet; learning resource lab; library services; nursing audiovisuals; remedial services; resume preparation assistance; skills, simulation, or other laboratory; tutoring.
Library Facilities 18,952 volumes in health, 1,065 volumes in nursing; 257 periodical subscriptions health-care related.

BACCALAUREATE PROGRAMS

Degree BSN
Available Programs ADN to Baccalaureate; Generic Baccalaureate.
Site Options Rochester, NY.
Study Options Full-time and part-time.
Program Entrance Requirements Minimum overall college GPA of 2.75, transcript of college record, CPR certification, health exam, health insurance, high school transcript, immunizations, minimum GPA in nursing prerequisites of 2.0, prerequisite course work. Transfer students are accepted. *Application deadline:* 1/20 (fall).
Advanced Placement Credit given for nursing courses completed elsewhere dependent upon specific evaluations.
Expenses (2010-11) *Tuition, state resident:* full-time $4970; part-time $207 per credit. *Tuition, nonresident:* full-time $12,870; part-time $536 per credit. *Room and board:* $9200; room only: $6040 per academic year. *Required fees:* full-time $1138.
Financial Aid 66% of baccalaureate students in nursing programs received some form of financial aid in 2009-10. *Gift aid (need-based):* Federal Pell, FSEOG, state, private, college/university gift aid from institutional funds. *Loans:* Federal Nursing Student Loans, Federal Direct (Subsidized and Unsubsidized Stafford PLUS), Perkins, alternative loans. *Work-study:* Federal Work-Study, part-time campus jobs. *Financial aid application deadline (priority):* 2/15.
Contact Dr. Kathleen Peterson, Chairperson, Department of Nursing, The College at Brockport, State University of New York, 350 New Campus Drive, Brockport, NY 14420-2988. *Telephone:* 585-395-2355. *Fax:* 585-395-5312. *E-mail:* kpeterso@brockport.edu.

College of Mount Saint Vincent

Department of Nursing
Riverdale, New York

http://www.mountsaintvincent.edu/academics/majors_and_programs/nursing2/nursing.htm
Founded in 1911

DEGREES • BS • MSN

Nursing Program Faculty 30 (90% with doctorates).
Baccalaureate Enrollment 520 **Women** 80% **Men** 20% **Minority** 80% **International** 10% **Part-time** 10%
Graduate Enrollment 100 **Women** 90% **Men** 10% **Minority** 80% **International** 10% **Part-time** 100%
Nursing Student Activities Sigma Theta Tau, Student Nurses' Association.
Nursing Student Resources Academic advising; academic or career counseling; bookstore; campus computer network; computer lab; computer-assisted instruction; e-mail services; employment services for current students; housing assistance; interactive nursing skills videos; Internet; learning resource lab; library services; nursing audiovisuals; paid internships; remedial services; resume preparation assistance; skills, simulation, or other laboratory; tutoring.
Library Facilities 104,158 volumes (5,304 in nursing).

BACCALAUREATE PROGRAMS

Degree BS
Available Programs Baccalaureate for Second Degree; Generic Baccalaureate; International Nurse to Baccalaureate; LPN to Baccalaureate; LPN to RN Baccalaureate.
Site Options Manhattan, NY.
Study Options Full-time and part-time.
Program Entrance Requirements Minimum overall college GPA of 2.7, transcript of college record, CPR certification, written essay, health exam, health insurance, high school biology, high school chemistry, high school foreign language, 3 years high school math, 3 years high school science, high school transcript, immunizations, 1 letter of recommendation, minimum high school GPA of 2.7, minimum GPA in nursing prerequisites of 3.0, prerequisite course work. Transfer students are accepted. *Application deadline:* 8/1 (fall), 1/5 (spring). Applications may be processed on a rolling basis for some programs. *Application fee:* $35.
Expenses (2010-11) *Tuition:* full-time $24,400; part-time $750 per credit. *Room and board:* $10,600 per academic year. *Required fees:* full-time $2000.
Financial Aid 90% of baccalaureate students in nursing programs received some form of financial aid in 2009-10.
Contact Ms. Harriet Rothman, Recruitment and Advisement Coordinator, Department of Nursing, College of Mount Saint Vincent, 6301 Riverdale Avenue, Riverdale, NY 10471-1093. *Telephone:* 718-405-3365. *Fax:* 718-405-3286. *E-mail:* harriet.rothman@mountsaintvincent.edu.

GRADUATE PROGRAMS

Expenses (2010-11) *Tuition:* part-time $675 per credit.
Financial Aid 90% of graduate students in nursing programs received some form of financial aid in 2009-10. Career-related internships or fieldwork available. *Financial aid application deadline:* 6/1.
Contact Dr. Carol Vicino, Director, Graduate Program of Nursing, Department of Nursing, College of Mount Saint Vincent, 6301 Riverdale Avenue, Riverdale, NY 10471-1093. *Telephone:* 718-405-3351. *Fax:* 718-405-3286. *E-mail:* carol.vicino@mountsaintvincent.edu.

MASTER'S DEGREE PROGRAM

Degree MSN
Available Programs Master's; Master's for Nurses with Non-Nursing Degrees.
Concentrations Available Nursing administration; nursing education. *Nurse practitioner programs in:* adult health, family health.
Study Options Part-time.
Program Entrance Requirements Clinical experience, computer literacy, minimum overall college GPA of 3.0, transcript of college record, CPR certification, written essay, immunizations, interview, 2 letters of recommendation, nursing research course, physical assessment course, professional liability insurance/malpractice insurance, prerequisite course work, statistics course. *Application deadline:* 8/1 (fall), 1/5 (spring). *Application fee:* $35.
Degree Requirements 43 total credit hours, thesis or project.

POST-MASTER'S PROGRAM

Areas of Study Nursing education. *Nurse practitioner programs in:* adult health, family health.

The College of New Rochelle

School of Nursing
New Rochelle, New York

Founded in 1904

DEGREES • BSN • MS

Nursing Program Faculty 15 (75% with doctorates).
Baccalaureate Enrollment 521 **Women** 90% **Men** 10% **Minority** 67% **International** 1% **Part-time** 50%
Graduate Enrollment 121 **Women** 90% **Men** 10% **Minority** 18% **International** 1% **Part-time** 100%
Nursing Student Activities Nursing Honor Society, Sigma Theta Tau, Student Nurses' Association, nursing club.
Nursing Student Resources Academic advising; academic or career counseling; assistance for students with disabilities; bookstore; campus

computer network; career placement assistance; computer lab; computer-assisted instruction; e-mail services; housing assistance; interactive nursing skills videos; Internet; learning resource lab; library services; nursing audiovisuals; other; remedial services; resume preparation assistance; skills, simulation, or other laboratory; tutoring.
Library Facilities 220,000 volumes (8,700 in health, 8,700 in nursing); 1,450 periodical subscriptions (165 health-care related).

BACCALAUREATE PROGRAMS

Degree BSN
Available Programs Accelerated Baccalaureate for Second Degree; Accelerated RN Baccalaureate; Baccalaureate for Second Degree; Generic Baccalaureate; RN Baccalaureate.
Site Options Bronx, NY.
Study Options Full-time and part-time.
Program Entrance Requirements Transcript of college record, CPR certification, written essay, health exam, health insurance, high school biology, high school chemistry, high school transcript, immunizations. Transfer students are accepted. *Application deadline:* 3/1 (fall), 10/1 (spring). *Application fee:* $35.
Advanced Placement Credit by examination available. Credit given for nursing courses completed elsewhere dependent upon specific evaluations.
Contact *Telephone:* 914-654-5803. *Fax:* 914-654-5994.

GRADUATE PROGRAMS

Contact *Telephone:* 914-654-5803. *Fax:* 914-654-5994.

MASTER'S DEGREE PROGRAM

Degree MS
Available Programs Master's; RN to Master's.
Concentrations Available Health-care administration; nursing administration; nursing education. *Nurse practitioner programs in:* family health.
Site Options New Rochelle, NY.
Study Options Full-time and part-time.
Program Entrance Requirements Clinical experience, minimum overall college GPA of 3.0, transcript of college record, written essay, immunizations, interview, 2 letters of recommendation, physical assessment course, professional liability insurance/malpractice insurance, resume, statistics course.*Application fee:* $35.
Advanced Placement Credit given for nursing courses completed elsewhere dependent upon specific evaluations.
Degree Requirements 40 total credit hours, thesis or project.

POST-MASTER'S PROGRAM

Areas of Study Health-care administration; nursing administration; nursing education. *Clinical nurse specialist programs in:* palliative care. *Nurse practitioner programs in:* family health.

College of Staten Island of the City University of New York

Department of Nursing
Staten Island, New York

http://www.csi.cuny.edu/nursing
Founded in 1955

DEGREES • BS • MS
Nursing Program Faculty 61 (23% with doctorates).
Baccalaureate Enrollment 182 **Women** 87% **Men** 13% **Minority** 40% **Part-time** 74%
Graduate Enrollment 52 **Women** 99% **Men** 1% **Minority** 43% **International** 7% **Part-time** 93%
Nursing Student Activities Nursing Honor Society, Sigma Theta Tau.
Nursing Student Resources Academic advising; academic or career counseling; assistance for students with disabilities; bookstore; campus computer network; career placement assistance; computer lab; computer-assisted instruction; daycare for children of students; e-mail services; externships; Internet; learning resource lab; library services; nursing audiovisuals; remedial services; resume preparation assistance; skills, simulation, or other laboratory; tutoring.
Library Facilities 250,000 volumes (3,700 in health, 1,500 in nursing); 28,000 periodical subscriptions (4,900 health-care related).

BACCALAUREATE PROGRAMS

Degree BS
Available Programs RN Baccalaureate.
Site Options Brooklyn, NY.
Study Options Full-time and part-time.
Program Entrance Requirements Minimum overall college GPA of 2.5, transcript of college record, CPR certification, health exam, health insurance, high school transcript, immunizations, minimum GPA in nursing prerequisites, professional liability insurance/malpractice insurance, prerequisite course work, RN licensure. Transfer students are accepted. *Application fee:* $65.
Advanced Placement Credit given for nursing courses completed elsewhere dependent upon specific evaluations.
Expenses (2010-11) *Tuition, area resident:* full-time $4830; part-time $205 per credit. *Tuition, state resident:* full-time $10,440; part-time $435 per credit. *Tuition, nonresident:* full-time $10,440; part-time $435 per credit. *Required fees:* full-time $378; part-time $226 per term.
Financial Aid 40% of baccalaureate students in nursing programs received some form of financial aid in 2009-10. *Gift aid (need-based):* Federal Pell, FSEOG, state, private, college/university gift aid from institutional funds. *Loans:* Federal Direct (Subsidized and Unsubsidized Stafford PLUS), Perkins. *Work-study:* Federal Work-Study, part-time campus jobs. *Financial aid application deadline (priority):* 3/31.
Contact Dr. Mary E. O'Donnell, Chairperson, Department of Nursing, College of Staten Island of the City University of New York, 2800 Victory Boulevard, Marcus Hall, 5S-213, Staten Island, NY 10314. *Telephone:* 718-982-3810. *Fax:* 718-982-3813. *E-mail:* odonnellm@mail.csi.cuny.edu.

GRADUATE PROGRAMS

Expenses (2010-11) *Tuition, area resident:* full-time $7730; part-time $325 per credit. *Tuition, state resident:* full-time $14,520; part-time $605 per credit. *Tuition, nonresident:* full-time $14,520; part-time $605 per credit. *International tuition:* $605 full-time. *Required fees:* full-time $378; part-time $226 per term.
Financial Aid 20% of graduate students in nursing programs received some form of financial aid in 2009-10.
Contact Dr. Margaret Lunney, Director, Graduate Program, Department of Nursing, College of Staten Island of the City University of New York, 2800 Victory Boulevard, Staten Island, NY 10314. *Telephone:* 718-982-3845. *Fax:* 718-982-3813. *E-mail:* lunney@mail.csi.cuny.edu.

MASTER'S DEGREE PROGRAM

Degree MS
Available Programs Master's.
Concentrations Available *Clinical nurse specialist programs in:* adult health, gerontology. *Nurse practitioner programs in:* adult health, gerontology.
Site Options Brooklyn, NY.
Study Options Full-time and part-time.
Program Entrance Requirements Clinical experience, minimum overall college GPA of 3.0, transcript of college record, written essay, immunizations, interview, 2 letters of recommendation, nursing research course, physical assessment course, professional liability insurance/malpractice insurance, prerequisite course work, statistics course. *Application deadline:* Applications may be processed on a rolling basis for some programs. *Application fee:* $65.
Advanced Placement Credit given for nursing courses completed elsewhere dependent upon specific evaluations.
Degree Requirements 48 total credit hours, thesis or project.

POST-MASTER'S PROGRAM

Areas of Study *Nurse practitioner programs in:* adult health, gerontology.

Columbia University

School of Nursing
New York, New York

http://www.nursing.columbia.edu/
Founded in 1754

DEGREES • BS • MS • MSN/MBA • MSN/MPH • PHD
Nursing Program Faculty 68 (73% with doctorates).
Baccalaureate Enrollment 150 **Women** 92% **Men** 8% **Minority** 26% **International** 1%
Graduate Enrollment 348 **Women** 92% **Men** 8% **Minority** 27% **International** 2% **Part-time** 53%
Nursing Student Activities Sigma Theta Tau, nursing club.

Nursing Student Resources Academic advising; academic or career counseling; assistance for students with disabilities; bookstore; campus computer network; computer lab; computer-assisted instruction; daycare for children of students; e-mail services; employment services for current students; housing assistance; interactive nursing skills videos; Internet; learning resource lab; library services; resume preparation assistance; skills, simulation, or other laboratory.
Library Facilities 9.5 million volumes (469,000 in health, 8,220 in nursing); 117,264 periodical subscriptions.

BACCALAUREATE PROGRAMS

Degree BS
Available Programs Accelerated Baccalaureate; Accelerated Baccalaureate for Second Degree.
Study Options Full-time.
Program Entrance Requirements Transcript of college record, written essay, 3 letters of recommendation, prerequisite course work. *Application deadline:* 11/17 (summer). *Application fee:* $65.
Expenses (2010-11) *Tuition:* part-time $1212 per credit. *Room and board:* room only: $8000 per academic year. *Required fees:* full-time $675; part-time $225 per term.
Financial Aid 97% of baccalaureate students in nursing programs received some form of financial aid in 2009-10. *Gift aid (need-based):* Federal Pell, FSEOG, state, private, college/university gift aid from institutional funds. *Loans:* Perkins, alternative loans. *Work-study:* Federal Work-Study, part-time campus jobs. *Financial aid application deadline:* 3/1.
Contact Office of Admissions, School of Nursing, Columbia University, 617 West 168th Street, Suite 134, New York, NY 10032. *Telephone:* 212-305-5756. *Fax:* 212-305-3680. *E-mail:* nursing@columbia.edu.

GRADUATE PROGRAMS

Expenses (2010-11) *Tuition:* part-time $1212 per credit. *Required fees:* full-time $675; part-time $225 per term.
Financial Aid 97% of graduate students in nursing programs received some form of financial aid in 2009-10. Research assistantships, teaching assistantships, Federal Work-Study and institutionally sponsored loans available. Aid available to part-time students.
Contact Office of Admissions, School of Nursing, Columbia University, 630 West 168th Street, Box 6, New York, NY 10032. *Telephone:* 212-305-5756. *Fax:* 212-305-3680. *E-mail:* nursing@columbia.edu.

MASTER'S DEGREE PROGRAM

Degrees MS; MSN/MBA; MSN/MPH
Available Programs Accelerated Master's for Non-Nursing College Graduates; Master's; Master's for Non-Nursing College Graduates.
Concentrations Available Nurse anesthesia; nurse-midwifery. *Nurse practitioner programs in:* acute care, adult health, family health, gerontology, neonatal health, oncology, pediatric, psychiatric/mental health, women's health.
Study Options Full-time and part-time.
Program Entrance Requirements Transcript of college record, written essay, interview, 3 letters of recommendation, physical assessment course, prerequisite course work, resume, statistics course, GRE General Test. *Application deadline:* 4/15 (fall), 12/15 (summer). *Application fee:* $65.
Advanced Placement Credit by examination available. Credit given for nursing courses completed elsewhere dependent upon specific evaluations.
Degree Requirements 45 total credit hours, thesis or project, comprehensive exam.

POST-MASTER'S PROGRAM

Areas of Study Nurse anesthesia. *Nurse practitioner programs in:* acute care, adult health, family health, gerontology, neonatal health, oncology, pediatric, psychiatric/mental health, women's health.

DOCTORAL DEGREE PROGRAM

Degree PhD
Available Programs Doctorate; Post-Baccalaureate Doctorate.
Areas of Study Addiction/substance abuse, advanced practice nursing, clinical practice, information systems, maternity-newborn, nursing education, nursing research, nursing science.
Program Entrance Requirements Minimum overall college GPA of 3.00, interview by faculty committee, interview, 3 letters of recommendation, statistics course, vita, writing sample, GRE General Test. Application deadline: 2/1 (fall). Application fee: $75.
Degree Requirements 60 total credit hours, dissertation.

POSTDOCTORAL PROGRAM

Areas of Study Nursing informatics, nursing research.
Postdoctoral Program Contact Sarah Cook, Vice Dean, School of Nursing, Columbia University, 630 West 168th Street, Box 6, New York,

NY 10032. *Telephone:* 212-305-3582. *Fax:* 212-305-1116. *E-mail:* ssc3@columbia.edu.

CONTINUING EDUCATION PROGRAM

Contact Sarah Cook, Vice Dean, School of Nursing, Columbia University, 630 West 168th Street, Box 6, New York, NY 10032. *Telephone:* 212-305-3582. *Fax:* 212-305-1116. *E-mail:* ssc3@columbia.edu.

See full description on page 468.

Concordia College–New York

Nursing Program
Bronxville, New York

http://www.concordia-ny.edu/
Founded in 1881

DEGREE • BS

Nursing Program Faculty 6 (50% with doctorates).
Baccalaureate Enrollment 40 **Women** 80% **Men** 20% **Minority** 48% **International** 2%
Nursing Student Activities Student Nurses' Association.
Nursing Student Resources Academic advising; academic or career counseling; assistance for students with disabilities; bookstore; campus computer network; career placement assistance; computer lab; computer-assisted instruction; e-mail services; housing assistance; interactive nursing skills videos; Internet; learning resource lab; library services; nursing audiovisuals; resume preparation assistance; skills, simulation, or other laboratory; tutoring.
Library Facilities 71,500 volumes; 467 periodical subscriptions.

BACCALAUREATE PROGRAMS

Degree BS
Available Programs Accelerated Baccalaureate for Second Degree; Generic Baccalaureate.
Study Options Full-time.
Program Entrance Requirements Minimum overall college GPA of 3.2, transcript of college record, written essay, health exam, health insurance, high school biology, high school chemistry, 3 years high school science, high school transcript, immunizations, interview, 2 letters of recommendation, minimum high school GPA, minimum GPA in nursing prerequisites of 3.0, professional liability insurance/malpractice insurance, prerequisite course work. Transfer students are accepted. *Application deadline:* 4/1 (winter). *Application fee:* $50.
Advanced Placement Credit given for nursing courses completed elsewhere dependent upon specific evaluations.
Expenses (2010-11) *Tuition:* full-time $25,000; part-time $400 per credit. *Room and board:* $10,000 per academic year. *Required fees:* full-time $1000.
Financial Aid 20% of baccalaureate students in nursing programs received some form of financial aid in 2009-10.
Contact ***Telephone:*** 914-337-9300.

Daemen College

Department of Nursing
Amherst, New York

http://www.daemen.edu/
Founded in 1947

DEGREES • BS • DNP • MS

Nursing Program Faculty 15 (75% with doctorates).
Baccalaureate Enrollment 250 **Women** 96% **Men** 4% **Minority** 3% **International** 2% **Part-time** 15%
Graduate Enrollment 150 **Women** 96% **Men** 4% **Minority** 8% **International** 6% **Part-time** 90%
Distance Learning Courses Available.
Nursing Student Activities Sigma Theta Tau, nursing club.
Nursing Student Resources Academic advising; academic or career counseling; assistance for students with disabilities; bookstore; campus computer network; career placement assistance; computer lab; computer-assisted instruction; e-mail services; Internet; learning resource lab; library services; nursing audiovisuals; placement services for program completers; remedial services; resume preparation assistance; skills, simulation, or other laboratory; tutoring.
Library Facilities 136,883 volumes (10,000 in health, 4,000 in nursing); 31,925 periodical subscriptions (250 health-care related).

BACCALAUREATE PROGRAMS

Degree BS
Available Programs ADN to Baccalaureate; Accelerated RN Baccalaureate; International Nurse to Baccalaureate; RN Baccalaureate.
Site Options Jamestown, NY; Olean, NY.
Study Options Full-time and part-time.
Program Entrance Requirements Minimum overall college GPA of 2.0, transcript of college record, 2 years high school math, 2 years high school science, high school transcript, immunizations, minimum high school GPA of 3, minimum GPA in nursing prerequisites of 2.0. Transfer students are accepted. *Application deadline:* Applications may be processed on a rolling basis for some programs.
Advanced Placement Credit given for nursing courses completed elsewhere dependent upon specific evaluations.
Expenses (2010-11) *Tuition:* full-time $5237; part-time $350 per credit hour. *International tuition:* $10,475 full-time. *Room and board:* $4600 per academic year. *Required fees:* full-time $255; part-time $6 per credit.
Financial Aid 100% of baccalaureate students in nursing programs received some form of financial aid in 2009-10.
Contact Dr. Mary Lou Rusin, Professor and Chair, Department of Nursing, Daemen College, 4380 Main Street, Amherst, NY 14226. *Telephone:* 716-839-8387. *Fax:* 716-839-8403. *E-mail:* mrusin@daemen.edu.

GRADUATE PROGRAMS

Expenses (2010-11) *Tuition:* part-time $795 per credit hour.
Financial Aid 75% of graduate students in nursing programs received some form of financial aid in 2009-10. Institutionally sponsored loans and scholarships available. *Financial aid application deadline:* 2/15.
Contact Dr. Mary Lou Rusin, Professor and Chair, Department of Nursing, Daemen College, 4380 Main Street, Amherst, NY 14226. *Telephone:* 716-839-8387. *Fax:* 716-839-8403. *E-mail:* mrusin@daemen.edu.

MASTER'S DEGREE PROGRAM

Degree MS
Available Programs Accelerated AD/RN to Master's; Accelerated RN to Master's; Master's; Master's for Nurses with Non-Nursing Degrees; RN to Master's.
Concentrations Available Health-care administration; nursing education. *Clinical nurse specialist programs in:* palliative care. *Nurse practitioner programs in:* adult health.
Study Options Full-time and part-time.
Program Entrance Requirements Clinical experience, minimum overall college GPA of 3.25, transcript of college record, written essay, immunizations, interview, 3 letters of recommendation, statistics course. *Application deadline:* Applications may be processed on a rolling basis for some programs. *Application fee:* $25.
Advanced Placement Credit given for nursing courses completed elsewhere dependent upon specific evaluations.
Degree Requirements 30 total credit hours, thesis or project.

POST-MASTER'S PROGRAM

Areas of Study Health-care administration; nursing education. *Clinical nurse specialist programs in:* palliative care. *Nurse practitioner programs in:* adult health.

DOCTORAL DEGREE PROGRAM

Degree DNP
Available Programs Doctorate.
Areas of Study Advanced practice nursing.
Program Entrance Requirements Minimum overall college GPA of 3.25, interview, 3 letters of recommendation, statistics course, vita, writing sample. Application deadline: Applications may be processed on a rolling basis for some programs. Application fee: $25.
Degree Requirements 36 total credit hours, dissertation.

Dominican College

Department of Nursing
Orangeburg, New York

Founded in 1952

DEGREES • BSN • M SC N

Nursing Program Faculty 14 (21% with doctorates).

Baccalaureate Enrollment 182 **Women** 87% **Men** 13% **Minority** 44% **International** 40% **Part-time** 43%

Graduate Enrollment 37 **Women** 100% **Minority** 66% **International** 60% **Part-time** 100%

Nursing Student Activities Nursing Honor Society, Sigma Theta Tau, Student Nurses' Association.

Nursing Student Resources Academic advising; academic or career counseling; assistance for students with disabilities; bookstore; campus computer network; career placement assistance; computer lab; computer-assisted instruction; e-mail services; externships; Internet; learning resource lab; library services; nursing audiovisuals; paid internships; remedial services; resume preparation assistance; skills, simulation, or other laboratory; tutoring.

Library Facilities 125,000 volumes (5,650 in health); 450 periodical subscriptions (235 health-care related).

BACCALAUREATE PROGRAMS

Degree BSN

Available Programs Accelerated Baccalaureate for Second Degree; Accelerated LPN to Baccalaureate; Accelerated RN Baccalaureate; Generic Baccalaureate; LPN to Baccalaureate; RN Baccalaureate.

Study Options Full-time and part-time.

Program Entrance Requirements Minimum overall college GPA of 2.7, transcript of college record, CPR certification, health exam, health insurance, high school transcript, immunizations, minimum GPA in nursing prerequisites of 2.0, professional liability insurance/malpractice insurance, prerequisite course work. Transfer students are accepted.

Advanced Placement Credit by examination available. Credit given for nursing courses completed elsewhere dependent upon specific evaluations.

Contact ***Telephone:*** 845-848-6051. *Fax:* 845-398-4891.

GRADUATE PROGRAMS

Contact ***Telephone:*** 845-848-6026. *Fax:* 845-398-4891.

MASTER'S DEGREE PROGRAM

Degree M Sc N

Available Programs Master's.

Concentrations Available *Nurse practitioner programs in:* family health.

Study Options Full-time and part-time.

Program Entrance Requirements Clinical experience, minimum overall college GPA of 3.0, transcript of college record, written essay, immunizations, 3 letters of recommendation, nursing research course, physical assessment course, professional liability insurance/malpractice insurance, prerequisite course work, statistics course.

Degree Requirements 42 total credit hours, thesis or project.

D'Youville College

Department of Nursing
Buffalo, New York

http://www.dyc.edu/academics/nursing/

Founded in 1908

DEGREES • BSN • MS

Nursing Program Faculty 41 (20% with doctorates).

Baccalaureate Enrollment 492 **Women** 90% **Men** 10% **Minority** 20% **International** 10% **Part-time** 30%

Graduate Enrollment 115 **Women** 96% **Men** 4% **Minority** 10% **International** 35% **Part-time** 40%

Distance Learning Courses Available.

Nursing Student Activities Sigma Theta Tau, Student Nurses' Association.

Nursing Student Resources Academic advising; academic or career counseling; assistance for students with disabilities; bookstore; campus computer network; career placement assistance; computer lab; computer-assisted instruction; e-mail services; externships; interactive nursing skills videos; Internet; learning resource lab; library services; nursing audiovisuals; paid internships; placement services for program com-

pleters; remedial services; resume preparation assistance; skills, simulation, or other laboratory; tutoring.
Library Facilities 116,237 volumes (100,000 in health, 17,000 in nursing); 725 periodical subscriptions (171 health-care related).

BACCALAUREATE PROGRAMS

Degree BSN
Available Programs Generic Baccalaureate; RN Baccalaureate.
Site Options Buffalo, NY.
Study Options Full-time and part-time.
Program Entrance Requirements Minimum overall college GPA of 2.5, transcript of college record, health exam, health insurance, high school biology, high school chemistry, 1 year of high school math, 1 year of high school science, high school transcript, immunizations, minimum high school GPA of 2.0, minimum high school rank 50%, minimum GPA in nursing prerequisites of 2.0, professional liability insurance/malpractice insurance, prerequisite course work. Transfer students are accepted.
Advanced Placement Credit given for nursing courses completed elsewhere dependent upon specific evaluations.
Contact ***Telephone:*** 716-881-7600. *Fax:* 716-515-0679.

GRADUATE PROGRAMS

Contact ***Telephone:*** 716-881-7744. *Fax:* 716-515-0679.

MASTER'S DEGREE PROGRAM

Degree MS
Available Programs Master's; RN to Master's.
Concentrations Available Nursing education. *Clinical nurse specialist programs in:* community health, palliative care. *Nurse practitioner programs in:* family health.
Study Options Full-time and part-time.
Program Entrance Requirements Clinical experience, computer literacy, minimum overall college GPA of 3.0, transcript of college record, CPR certification, written essay, immunizations, interview, 2 letters of recommendation, nursing research course, physical assessment course, professional liability insurance/malpractice insurance, prerequisite course work, resume, statistics course.
Advanced Placement Credit given for nursing courses completed elsewhere dependent upon specific evaluations.
Degree Requirements 41 total credit hours, thesis or project.

POST-MASTER'S PROGRAM

Areas of Study *Nurse practitioner programs in:* family health.

See full description on page 474.

Elmira College

Program in Nursing Education
Elmira, New York

http://www.elmira.edu/
Founded in 1855

DEGREE • BS

Nursing Program Faculty 23 (13% with doctorates).
Baccalaureate Enrollment 191 **Women** 91% **Men** 9% **Minority** 7% **International** 1% **Part-time** 23%
Nursing Student Activities Sigma Theta Tau, Student Nurses' Association, nursing club.
Nursing Student Resources Academic advising; academic or career counseling; assistance for students with disabilities; bookstore; campus computer network; career placement assistance; computer lab; computer-assisted instruction; e-mail services; housing assistance; interactive nursing skills videos; Internet; learning resource lab; library services; nursing audiovisuals; placement services for program completers; resume preparation assistance; skills, simulation, or other laboratory; tutoring; unpaid internships.
Library Facilities 203,343 volumes (7,461 in health, 5,200 in nursing); 337 periodical subscriptions (72 health-care related).

BACCALAUREATE PROGRAMS

Degree BS
Available Programs ADN to Baccalaureate; Generic Baccalaureate; RN Baccalaureate.
Study Options Full-time and part-time.
Program Entrance Requirements Minimum overall college GPA of 2.0, transcript of college record, CPR certification, written essay, health exam, health insurance, high school biology, high school chemistry, 3 years high school math, 3 years high school science, high school transcript, immunizations, 2 letters of recommendation, minimum high school GPA of 2.5. Transfer students are accepted. *Application deadline:* Applications may be processed on a rolling basis for some programs. *Application fee:* $100.
Advanced Placement Credit by examination available. Credit given for nursing courses completed elsewhere dependent upon specific evaluations.
Expenses (2010-11) *Tuition:* full-time $34,500; part-time $300 per credit hour. *Room and board:* $11,150; room only: $6100 per academic year. *Required fees:* full-time $1600; part-time $100 per term.
Financial Aid 80% of baccalaureate students in nursing programs received some form of financial aid in 2009-10. *Gift aid (need-based):* Federal Pell, FSEOG, state, private, college/university gift aid from institutional funds. *Loans:* Federal Direct (Subsidized and Unsubsidized Stafford PLUS), Perkins, college/university. *Work-study:* Federal Work-Study, part-time campus jobs. *Financial aid application deadline (priority):* 2/1.
Contact Mrs. Julianna Baumann, Dean, Program in Nursing Education, Elmira College, One Park Place, Elmira, NY 14901. *Telephone:* 607-735-1724. *Fax:* 607-735-1718. *E-mail:* admissions@elmira.edu.

CONTINUING EDUCATION PROGRAM

Contact Dr. Lois Schoener, Director of Nurse Education, Program in Nursing Education, Elmira College, One Park Place, Elmira, NY 14901. *Telephone:* 607-735-1890. *Fax:* 607-735-1159. *E-mail:* lschoener@elmira.edu.

Excelsior College

School of Nursing
Albany, New York

Founded in 1970

DEGREES • BS • MS

Distance Learning Courses Available.
Nursing Student Activities Sigma Theta Tau.
Nursing Student Resources Academic advising; academic or career counseling; assistance for students with disabilities; bookstore; computer-assisted instruction; e-mail services; Internet; learning resource lab; library services; nursing audiovisuals; other; resume preparation assistance; skills, simulation, or other laboratory; tutoring.

BACCALAUREATE PROGRAMS

Degree BS
Available Programs RN Baccalaureate.
Study Options Part-time.
Program Entrance Requirements Transcript of college record, high school transcript, RN licensure. Transfer students are accepted. *Application deadline:* Applications may be processed on a rolling basis for some programs.
Advanced Placement Credit by examination available. Credit given for nursing courses completed elsewhere dependent upon specific evaluations.
Contact ***Telephone:*** 518-464-8500. *Fax:* 518-464-8777.

GRADUATE PROGRAMS

Contact ***Telephone:*** 518-464-8500. *Fax:* 518-464-8777.

MASTER'S DEGREE PROGRAM

Degree MS
Available Programs Master's; RN to Master's.
Concentrations Available Nursing administration; nursing education; nursing informatics.
Study Options Full-time and part-time.
Online Degree Options Yes (online only).
Program Entrance Requirements Computer literacy, minimum overall college GPA of 3, transcript of college record, written essay, resume. *Application deadline:* Applications may be processed on a rolling basis for some programs.
Advanced Placement Credit given for nursing courses completed elsewhere dependent upon specific evaluations.
Degree Requirements 39 total credit hours, thesis or project.

POST-MASTER'S PROGRAM
Areas of Study Nursing education.

Farmingdale State College
Nursing Department
Farmingdale, New York

Founded in 1912

DEGREE • BS

Library Facilities 125,000 volumes; 800 periodical subscriptions.

BACCALAUREATE PROGRAMS
Degree BS
Available Programs Generic Baccalaureate; RN Baccalaureate.
Contact Kathleen Walsh. *Telephone:* 631-420-2229. *Fax:* 631-420-2269. *E-mail:* kathleen.walsh@farmingdale.edu.

Hartwick College
Department of Nursing
Oneonta, New York

http://www.hartwick.edu
Founded in 1797

DEGREE • BS

Nursing Program Faculty 11 (18% with doctorates).
Baccalaureate Enrollment 145 **Women** 93% **Men** 7% **Minority** 9% **International** 1% **Part-time** 12%
Nursing Student Activities Sigma Theta Tau, Student Nurses' Association.
Nursing Student Resources Academic advising; academic or career counseling; assistance for students with disabilities; bookstore; campus computer network; career placement assistance; computer lab; computer-assisted instruction; e-mail services; employment services for current students; externships; housing assistance; interactive nursing skills videos; Internet; learning resource lab; library services; nursing audiovisuals; placement services for program completers; remedial services; resume preparation assistance; skills, simulation, or other laboratory; tutoring; unpaid internships.
Library Facilities 311,063 volumes (5,697 in health, 1,199 in nursing); 400 periodical subscriptions (30 health-care related).

BACCALAUREATE PROGRAMS
Degree BS
Available Programs Accelerated Baccalaureate; Accelerated Baccalaureate for Second Degree; Generic Baccalaureate; RN Baccalaureate.
Site Options Cooperstown, NY; Albany, NY.
Study Options Full-time and part-time.
Program Entrance Requirements Minimum overall college GPA of 2.5, transcript of college record, CPR certification, written essay, health exam, high school biology, high school chemistry, high school foreign language, 3 years high school math, 2 years high school science, high school transcript, immunizations, 2 letters of recommendation, minimum GPA in nursing prerequisites of 2.5, professional liability insurance/malpractice insurance. Transfer students are accepted. *Application deadline:* Applications may be processed on a rolling basis for some programs. *Application fee:* $35.
Advanced Placement Credit given for nursing courses completed elsewhere dependent upon specific evaluations.
Expenses (2009-10) *Tuition:* full-time $32,550; part-time $1030 per credit. *Room and board:* $9075; room only: $4700 per academic year.
Financial Aid 96% of baccalaureate students in nursing programs received some form of financial aid in 2008-09. *Gift aid (need-based):* Federal Pell, FSEOG, state, private, college/university gift aid from institutional funds. *Loans:* Federal Nursing Student Loans, Perkins, college/university, alternative loans. *Work-study:* Federal Work-Study. *Financial aid application deadline:* Continuous.
Contact Dr. Jeanne-Marie E. Havener, RN, Chair and Associate Professor of Nursing, Department of Nursing, Hartwick College, Johnstone Science Center, 1 Hartwick Drive, Oneonta, NY 13820. *Telephone:* 607-431-4780. *Fax:* 607-431-4850. *E-mail:* havenerj@hartwick.edu.

Hunter College of the City University of New York
Hunter-Bellevue School of Nursing
New York, New York

http://www.hunter.cuny.edu/schoolhp/nursing
Founded in 1870

DEGREES • BS • MS • MS/MPH

Nursing Program Faculty 22 (56% with doctorates).
Nursing Student Activities Sigma Theta Tau.
Nursing Student Resources Academic advising; academic or career counseling; assistance for students with disabilities; bookstore; campus computer network; computer lab; computer-assisted instruction; e-mail services; interactive nursing skills videos; Internet; learning resource lab; library services; nursing audiovisuals.
Library Facilities 815,668 volumes (39,245 in health, 4,295 in nursing); 6,260 periodical subscriptions (375 health-care related).

BACCALAUREATE PROGRAMS
Degree BS
Available Programs Generic Baccalaureate; RN Baccalaureate.
Study Options Full-time.
Program Entrance Requirements Minimum overall college GPA of 2.5, CPR certification, health exam, immunizations, professional liability insurance/malpractice insurance, prerequisite course work. Transfer students are accepted.
Contact ***Telephone:*** 212-481-7598. *Fax:* 212-481-4427.

GRADUATE PROGRAMS
Contact ***Telephone:*** 212-481-4465. *Fax:* 212-481-4427.

MASTER'S DEGREE PROGRAM
Degrees MS; MS/MPH
Available Programs Master's.
Concentrations Available *Clinical nurse specialist programs in:* community health, medical-surgical, parent-child, psychiatric/mental health. *Nurse practitioner programs in:* adult health, gerontology, pediatric.
Study Options Full-time and part-time.
Program Entrance Requirements Clinical experience, minimum overall college GPA of 3.0, transcript of college record, written essay, immunizations, 2 letters of recommendation, resume, statistics course.
Degree Requirements 42 total credit hours, thesis or project.

POST-MASTER'S PROGRAM
Areas of Study *Nurse practitioner programs in:* pediatric.

CONTINUING EDUCATION PROGRAM
Contact ***Telephone:*** 212-650-3850. *Fax:* 212-772-3402.

Keuka College
Division of Nursing
Keuka Park, New York

http://www.keuka.edu/asap/nursing.htm
Founded in 1890

DEGREE • BS

Nursing Program Faculty 5 (20% with doctorates).
Baccalaureate Enrollment 238 **Women** 94% **Men** 6% **Minority** 4%
Distance Learning Courses Available.
Nursing Student Activities Sigma Theta Tau.
Nursing Student Resources Academic advising; academic or career counseling; assistance for students with disabilities; bookstore; campus computer network; computer lab; computer-assisted instruction; e-mail services; employment services for current students; interactive nursing skills videos; Internet; learning resource lab; library services; nursing audiovisuals; resume preparation assistance; tutoring.
Library Facilities 112,541 volumes (986 in health, 532 in nursing); 384 periodical subscriptions (48 health-care related).

BACCALAUREATE PROGRAMS
Degree BS
Available Programs Accelerated RN Baccalaureate.

Site Options Geneva, NY; Rochester, NY; Canandaigua, NY.
Study Options Full-time and part-time.
Program Entrance Requirements Minimum overall college GPA of 2.5, transcript of college record, CPR certification, health exam, immunizations, minimum GPA in nursing prerequisites of 2.5, prerequisite course work, RN licensure. Transfer students are accepted.
Advanced Placement Credit by examination available. Credit given for nursing courses completed elsewhere dependent upon specific evaluations.
Contact *Telephone:* 315-279-5393. *Fax:* 315-279-5407.

Lehman College of the City University of New York

Department of Nursing
Bronx, New York

http://www.lehman.cuny.edu/nursing
Founded in 1931

DEGREES • BS • DNS • MS

Nursing Program Faculty 43 (35% with doctorates).
Baccalaureate Enrollment 300 **Women** 80% **Men** 20% **Minority** 85% **International** 40% **Part-time** 50%
Graduate Enrollment 200 **Women** 90% **Men** 10% **Minority** 75% **International** 25% **Part-time** 75%
Distance Learning Courses Available.
Nursing Student Activities Nursing Honor Society, Sigma Theta Tau, Student Nurses' Association, nursing club.
Nursing Student Resources Academic advising; academic or career counseling; assistance for students with disabilities; bookstore; campus computer network; career placement assistance; computer lab; computer-assisted instruction; daycare for children of students; e-mail services; employment services for current students; externships; interactive nursing skills videos; Internet; learning resource lab; library services; nursing audiovisuals; paid internships; placement services for program completers; resume preparation assistance; skills, simulation, or other laboratory; tutoring; unpaid internships.
Library Facilities 595,952 volumes (1,000 in health, 500 in nursing); 5,738 periodical subscriptions (200 health-care related).

BACCALAUREATE PROGRAMS

Degree BS
Available Programs ADN to Baccalaureate; Accelerated Baccalaureate for Second Degree; Accelerated RN Baccalaureate; Baccalaureate for Second Degree; Generic Baccalaureate; International Nurse to Baccalaureate; RN Baccalaureate.
Site Options New York, NY; Queens, NY.
Study Options Full-time.
Online Degree Options Yes.
Program Entrance Requirements Minimum overall college GPA of 2.0, transcript of college record, health exam, high school transcript, immunizations, minimum GPA in nursing prerequisites of 2.75, professional liability insurance/malpractice insurance, prerequisite course work. Transfer students are accepted. *Application deadline:* 3/15 (fall).
Advanced Placement Credit given for nursing courses completed elsewhere dependent upon specific evaluations.
Expenses (2010-11) *Tuition, state resident:* full-time $5910; part-time $205 per credit. *Tuition, nonresident:* full-time $10,440; part-time $435 per credit. *Required fees:* full-time $248; part-time $208 per credit.
Financial Aid 70% of baccalaureate students in nursing programs received some form of financial aid in 2009-10. *Gift aid (need-based):* Federal Pell, FSEOG, state, college/university gift aid from institutional funds. *Loans:* Federal Direct (Subsidized and Unsubsidized Stafford PLUS), Perkins. *Work-study:* Federal Work-Study. *Financial aid application deadline:* Continuous.
Contact Alice Akan, Director of Undergraduate Programs, Department of Nursing, Lehman College of the City University of New York, 250 Bedford Park Boulevard West, T-3 201, Bronx, NY 10468. *Telephone:* 718-960-8214. *Fax:* 718-960-8488. *E-mail:* alice.akan@lehman.cuny.edu.

GRADUATE PROGRAMS

Expenses (2010-11) *Tuition, state resident:* full-time $10,220; part-time $325 per credit. *Tuition, nonresident:* full-time $16,440; part-time $605 per credit. *International tuition:* $16,440 full-time. *Required fees:* full-time $248; part-time $208 per credit.
Financial Aid 25% of graduate students in nursing programs received some form of financial aid in 2009-10. Career-related internships or fieldwork, Federal Work-Study, and tuition waivers (partial) available. Aid available to part-time students. *Financial aid application deadline:* 5/15.
Contact Dr. Catherine Alicia Georges, Graduate Program, Department of Nursing, Lehman College of the City University of New York, 250 Bedford Park Boulevard West, Bronx, NY 10468. *Telephone:* 718-960-8213. *Fax:* 718-960-8488. *E-mail:* nursing@lehman.cuny.edu.

MASTER'S DEGREE PROGRAM

Degree MS
Available Programs Master's; Master's for Nurses with Non-Nursing Degrees.
Concentrations Available Nursing administration; nursing education. *Clinical nurse specialist programs in:* adult health, gerontology, parent-child. *Nurse practitioner programs in:* family health, pediatric.
Site Options New York, NY.
Study Options Full-time and part-time.
Program Entrance Requirements Clinical experience, minimum overall college GPA of 3.0, transcript of college record, written essay, immunizations, interview, 2 letters of recommendation, professional liability insurance/malpractice insurance, prerequisite course work. *Application deadline:* 4/1 (fall), 11/1 (spring). Applications may be processed on a rolling basis for some programs. *Application fee:* $125.
Degree Requirements 43 total credit hours.

POST-MASTER'S PROGRAM

Areas of Study *Nurse practitioner programs in:* family health, pediatric.

DOCTORAL DEGREE PROGRAM

Degree DNS
Available Programs Doctorate.
Areas of Study Urban health.
Site Options New York, NY.
Program Entrance Requirements Clinical experience, minimum overall college GPA of 3.5, interview by faculty committee, interview, letters of recommendation, MSN or equivalent, statistics course, vita, writing sample. Application deadline: 4/1 (fall).
Degree Requirements 51 total credit hours, dissertation, oral exam, written exam, residency.

CONTINUING EDUCATION PROGRAM

Contact Dr. Catherine Alicia Georges, Chairperson, Department of Nursing, Lehman College of the City University of New York, T-3 Room 201, 250 Bedford Park Boulevard West, Bronx, NY 10468. *Telephone:* 718-960-8799. *E-mail:* catherine.georges@lehman.cuny.edu.

Le Moyne College

Nursing Programs
Syracuse, New York

Founded in 1946

DEGREES • BS • MS

Nursing Program Faculty 7 (50% with doctorates).
Baccalaureate Enrollment 175 **Women** 90% **Men** 10% **Minority** 5% **Part-time** 20%
Graduate Enrollment 40 **Women** 99% **Men** 1% **Minority** 1% **Part-time** 100%
Distance Learning Courses Available.
Nursing Student Activities Nursing Honor Society.
Nursing Student Resources Academic advising; academic or career counseling; assistance for students with disabilities; bookstore; campus computer network; career placement assistance; computer lab; computer-assisted instruction; e-mail services; employment services for current students; housing assistance; interactive nursing skills videos; Internet; learning resource lab; library services; nursing audiovisuals; placement services for program completers; remedial services; resume preparation assistance; skills, simulation, or other laboratory; tutoring.
Library Facilities 270,763 volumes; 122,165 periodical subscriptions.

BACCALAUREATE PROGRAMS

Degree BS
Available Programs ADN to Baccalaureate; RN Baccalaureate.
Study Options Full-time.

Program Entrance Requirements Minimum overall college GPA of 2.6, transcript of college record, CPR certification, written essay, health exam, health insurance, high school biology, high school chemistry, high school foreign language, 3 years high school math, 3 years high school science, high school transcript, immunizations, 2 letters of recommendation, minimum high school GPA of 3.0, minimum high school rank 85%, minimum GPA in nursing prerequisites of 2.5, RN licensure. Transfer students are accepted. *Application deadline:* 1/1 (fall), 8/1 (spring), 5/1 (summer). Applications may be processed on a rolling basis for some programs. *Application fee:* $50.

Advanced Placement Credit by examination available. Credit given for nursing courses completed elsewhere dependent upon specific evaluations.

Expenses (2010-11) *Tuition:* full-time $25,000; part-time $552 per credit. *Room and board:* $7000 per academic year. *Required fees:* full-time $200; part-time $100 per term.

Financial Aid 90% of baccalaureate students in nursing programs received some form of financial aid in 2009-10.

Contact Dr. Susan B. Bastable, Chair and Professor, Nursing Programs, Le Moyne College, 1419 Salt Springs Road, Syracuse, NY 13214. *Telephone:* 315-445-5435. *Fax:* 315-445-4602. *E-mail:* bastabsb@lemoyne.edu.

GRADUATE PROGRAMS

Expenses (2010-11) *Tuition:* part-time $575 per credit. *Required fees:* full-time $150; part-time $150 per credit.

Financial Aid 50% of graduate students in nursing programs received some form of financial aid in 2009-10.

Contact Mrs. Kristen P. Trapasso, Director of Graduate Admissions, Nursing Programs, Le Moyne College, 1419 Salt Springs Road, Syracuse, NY 13214. *Telephone:* 315-445-4265. *Fax:* 315-445-6027. *E-mail:* trapaskp@lemoyne.edu.

MASTER'S DEGREE PROGRAM

Degree MS

Available Programs Master's; Master's for Nurses with Non-Nursing Degrees.

Concentrations Available Nursing administration; nursing education.

Study Options Full-time and part-time.

Program Entrance Requirements Computer literacy, minimum overall college GPA of 3.0, transcript of college record, written essay, immunizations, interview, 2 letters of recommendation, nursing research course, physical assessment course, resume, statistics course. *Application deadline:* 8/1 (fall), 12/15 (spring), 5/1 (summer). Applications may be processed on a rolling basis for some programs. *Application fee:* $50.

Advanced Placement Credit given for nursing courses completed elsewhere dependent upon specific evaluations.

Degree Requirements 39 total credit hours, thesis or project.

POST-MASTER'S PROGRAM

Areas of Study Nursing administration; nursing education.

Long Island University, Brooklyn Campus

School of Nursing
Brooklyn, New York

http://www.liunet.edu/

Founded in 1926

DEGREES • BS • MS

Nursing Program Faculty 95 (25% with doctorates).

Baccalaureate Enrollment 1,200 **Women** 88% **Men** 12% **Minority** 85% **Part-time** 20%

Graduate Enrollment 200 **Women** 90% **Men** 10% **Minority** 85% **Part-time** 83%

Distance Learning Courses Available.

Nursing Student Activities Nursing Honor Society, Student Nurses' Association.

Nursing Student Resources Academic advising; academic or career counseling; assistance for students with disabilities; bookstore; campus computer network; computer lab; computer-assisted instruction; daycare for children of students; e-mail services; employment services for current students; interactive nursing skills videos; Internet; learning resource lab; library services; nursing audiovisuals; paid internships; remedial services; skills, simulation, or other laboratory; tutoring.

Library Facilities 314,565 volumes (11,000 in health, 850 in nursing); 329,366 periodical subscriptions (230 health-care related).

BACCALAUREATE PROGRAMS

Degree BS

Available Programs Accelerated Baccalaureate; Generic Baccalaureate; International Nurse to Baccalaureate; RN Baccalaureate.

Site Options Brooklyn, NY.

Study Options Full-time and part-time.

Program Entrance Requirements Minimum overall college GPA of 2.75, transcript of college record, CPR certification, health exam, health insurance, high school biology, high school chemistry, 2 years high school math, 2 years high school science, high school transcript, immunizations, interview, minimum high school GPA of 3.0, minimum GPA in nursing prerequisites of 2.75, professional liability insurance/malpractice insurance, prerequisite course work. Transfer students are accepted. *Application deadline:* Applications may be processed on a rolling basis for some programs. *Application fee:* $30.

Advanced Placement Credit given for nursing courses completed elsewhere dependent upon specific evaluations.

Expenses (2010-11) *Tuition:* full-time $19,200; part-time $640 per credit. *Room and board:* $7500 per academic year. *Required fees:* full-time $2320; part-time $320 per term.

Financial Aid 96% of baccalaureate students in nursing programs received some form of financial aid in 2009-10. *Gift aid (need-based):* Federal Pell, FSEOG, state, private, college/university gift aid from institutional funds, Scholarships for Disadvantaged Students (Nursing and Pharmacy). *Loans:* Federal Direct (Subsidized and Unsubsidized Stafford PLUS), Perkins, Federal Health Professions Student Loans, alternative loans. *Work-study:* Federal Work-Study, part-time campus jobs. *Financial aid application deadline:* Continuous.

Contact Prof. Dawn F. Kilts, Dean, School of Nursing, Long Island University, Brooklyn Campus, 1 University Plaza, Brooklyn, NY 11201. *Telephone:* 718-488-1509. *Fax:* 718-780-4019. *E-mail:* dawn.kilts@liu.edu.

GRADUATE PROGRAMS

Expenses (2010-11) *Tuition:* full-time $8838; part-time $982 per credit. *Room and board:* $7500 per academic year.

Financial Aid 75% of graduate students in nursing programs received some form of financial aid in 2009-10. Scholarships and unspecified assistantships available. Aid available to part-time students.

Contact Prof. Susanne Flower, Director, School of Nursing, Long Island University, Brooklyn Campus, 1 University Plaza, Brooklyn, NY 11201. *Telephone:* 718-488-1059. *Fax:* 718-780-4019. *E-mail:* susanne.flower@liu.edu.

MASTER'S DEGREE PROGRAM

Degree MS

Available Programs Master's; RN to Master's.

Concentrations Available Nursing administration; nursing education. *Nurse practitioner programs in:* adult health, family health, gerontology.

Site Options Brooklyn, NY.

Study Options Full-time and part-time.

Program Entrance Requirements Clinical experience, minimum overall college GPA of 3.0, transcript of college record, immunizations, interview, 3 letters of recommendation, nursing research course, physical assessment course, professional liability insurance/malpractice insurance, prerequisite course work, resume, statistics course. *Application deadline:* Applications may be processed on a rolling basis for some programs. *Application fee:* $30.

Advanced Placement Credit given for nursing courses completed elsewhere dependent upon specific evaluations.

Degree Requirements 43 total credit hours, thesis or project.

POST-MASTER'S PROGRAM

Areas of Study *Nurse practitioner programs in:* adult health, family health, gerontology.

Long Island University, C.W. Post Campus

Department of Nursing
Brookville, New York

http://www.liu.edu/cwpost/nursing

Founded in 1954

DEGREES • BS • MS

Nursing Program Faculty 13 (46% with doctorates).
Baccalaureate Enrollment 60 **Women** 97% **Men** 3% **Minority** 30% **Part-time** 100%
Graduate Enrollment 64 **Women** 94% **Men** 6% **Minority** 30% **Part-time** 100%
Nursing Student Activities Student Nurses' Association.
Nursing Student Resources Academic advising; academic or career counseling; assistance for students with disabilities; bookstore; campus computer network; career placement assistance; computer lab; computer-assisted instruction; e-mail services; employment services for current students; housing assistance; interactive nursing skills videos; Internet; library services; nursing audiovisuals; placement services for program completers; remedial services; resume preparation assistance; skills, simulation, or other laboratory; tutoring.
Library Facilities 177,108 volumes (20,000 in health, 15,000 in nursing); 3,100 periodical subscriptions health-care related.

BACCALAUREATE PROGRAMS

Degree BS
Available Programs RN Baccalaureate.
Site Options Manhasset, NY.
Study Options Part-time.
Program Entrance Requirements Minimum overall college GPA of 2.5, transcript of college record, health exam, health insurance, immunizations, minimum GPA in nursing prerequisites of 2.5, professional liability insurance/malpractice insurance, prerequisite course work, RN licensure. Transfer students are accepted. *Application deadline:* Applications may be processed on a rolling basis for some programs. *Application fee:* $30.
Advanced Placement Credit by examination available. Credit given for nursing courses completed elsewhere dependent upon specific evaluations.
Expenses (2010-11) *Tuition:* full-time $28,710; part-time $896 per credit. *Room and board:* $10,980; room only: $7180 per academic year. *Required fees:* full-time $1500; part-time $7 per credit; part-time $405 per term.
Financial Aid 10% of baccalaureate students in nursing programs received some form of financial aid in 2009-10. *Gift aid (need-based):* Federal Pell, FSEOG, state, private, college/university gift aid from institutional funds. *Loans:* Federal Direct (Subsidized and Unsubsidized Stafford PLUS), Perkins, college/university. *Work-study:* Federal Work-Study, part-time campus jobs. *Financial aid application deadline:* 3/1.
Contact Dr. Mary Infantino, Chairperson and Associate Professor, Department of Nursing, Long Island University, C.W. Post Campus, Life Science, Room 270, 720 Northern Boulevard, Brookville, NY 11548-1300. *Telephone:* 516-299-2320. *Fax:* 516-299-2352. *E-mail:* mary.infantino@liu.edu.

GRADUATE PROGRAMS

Expenses (2010-11) *Tuition:* full-time $11,784; part-time $982 per credit. *Room and board:* $10,980; room only: $7180 per academic year. *Required fees:* full-time $1500; part-time $7 per credit; part-time $405 per term.
Financial Aid 10% of graduate students in nursing programs received some form of financial aid in 2009-10. Federal Work-Study and unspecified assistantships available. Aid available to part-time students. *Financial aid application deadline:* 5/15.
Contact Dr. Mary Infantino, Chairperson and Associate Professor, Department of Nursing, Long Island University, C.W. Post Campus, Life Science, Room 270, 720 Northern Boulevard, Brookville, NY 11548-1300. *Telephone:* 516-299-2320. *Fax:* 516-299-2352. *E-mail:* mary.infantino@liu.edu.

MASTER'S DEGREE PROGRAM

Degree MS
Available Programs Master's; Master's for Nurses with Non-Nursing Degrees.
Concentrations Available Nursing education. *Clinical nurse specialist programs in:* adult health. *Nurse practitioner programs in:* family health.
Study Options Part-time.
Program Entrance Requirements Clinical experience, minimum overall college GPA of 3.0, transcript of college record, written essay, immunizations, interview, 2 letters of recommendation, physical assessment course, professional liability insurance/malpractice insurance, prerequisite course work. *Application deadline:* Applications may be processed on a rolling basis for some programs. *Application fee:* $30.
Advanced Placement Credit given for nursing courses completed elsewhere dependent upon specific evaluations.
Degree Requirements 46 total credit hours, thesis or project.

POST-MASTER'S PROGRAM

Areas of Study Nursing education. *Nurse practitioner programs in:* family health.

Medgar Evers College of the City University of New York

Department of Nursing
Brooklyn, New York

http://www.mec.cuny.edu/academic_affairs/science_tech_school/nursing/nurse_home.htm

Founded in 1969

DEGREE • BSN

Nursing Program Faculty 7 (85% with doctorates).
Baccalaureate Enrollment 60 **Women** 98% **Men** 2% **Minority** 99% **Part-time** 90%
Nursing Student Activities Student Nurses' Association, nursing club.
Nursing Student Resources Academic advising; academic or career counseling; assistance for students with disabilities; bookstore; campus computer network; computer lab; computer-assisted instruction; daycare for children of students; e-mail services; interactive nursing skills videos; Internet; learning resource lab; library services; nursing audiovisuals; remedial services; resume preparation assistance; skills, simulation, or other laboratory; tutoring; unpaid internships.
Library Facilities 120,000 volumes; 24,410 periodical subscriptions.

BACCALAUREATE PROGRAMS

Degree BSN
Available Programs ADN to Baccalaureate; Accelerated RN Baccalaureate.
Study Options Full-time and part-time.
Program Entrance Requirements Minimum overall college GPA of 2.5, transcript of college record, CPR certification, health exam, health insurance, immunizations, professional liability insurance/malpractice insurance, prerequisite course work, RN licensure. Transfer students are accepted.
Advanced Placement Credit given for nursing courses completed elsewhere dependent upon specific evaluations.
Contact *Telephone:* 718-270-6230. *Fax:* 718-270-6235.

Mercy College

Program in Nursing
Dobbs Ferry, New York

Founded in 1951

DEGREES • BS • MS

Nursing Program Faculty 5 (2% with doctorates).
Baccalaureate Enrollment 333 **Women** 96% **Men** 4% **Minority** 75% **International** 1% **Part-time** 88%
Graduate Enrollment 100 **Women** 99% **Men** 1% **Minority** 50% **International** 10% **Part-time** 75%
Distance Learning Courses Available.
Nursing Student Activities Sigma Theta Tau, Student Nurses' Association.
Nursing Student Resources Academic advising; academic or career counseling; assistance for students with disabilities; bookstore; campus computer network; career placement assistance; computer lab; computer-assisted instruction; e-mail services; employment services for current students; Internet; learning resource lab; library services; nursing audiovi-

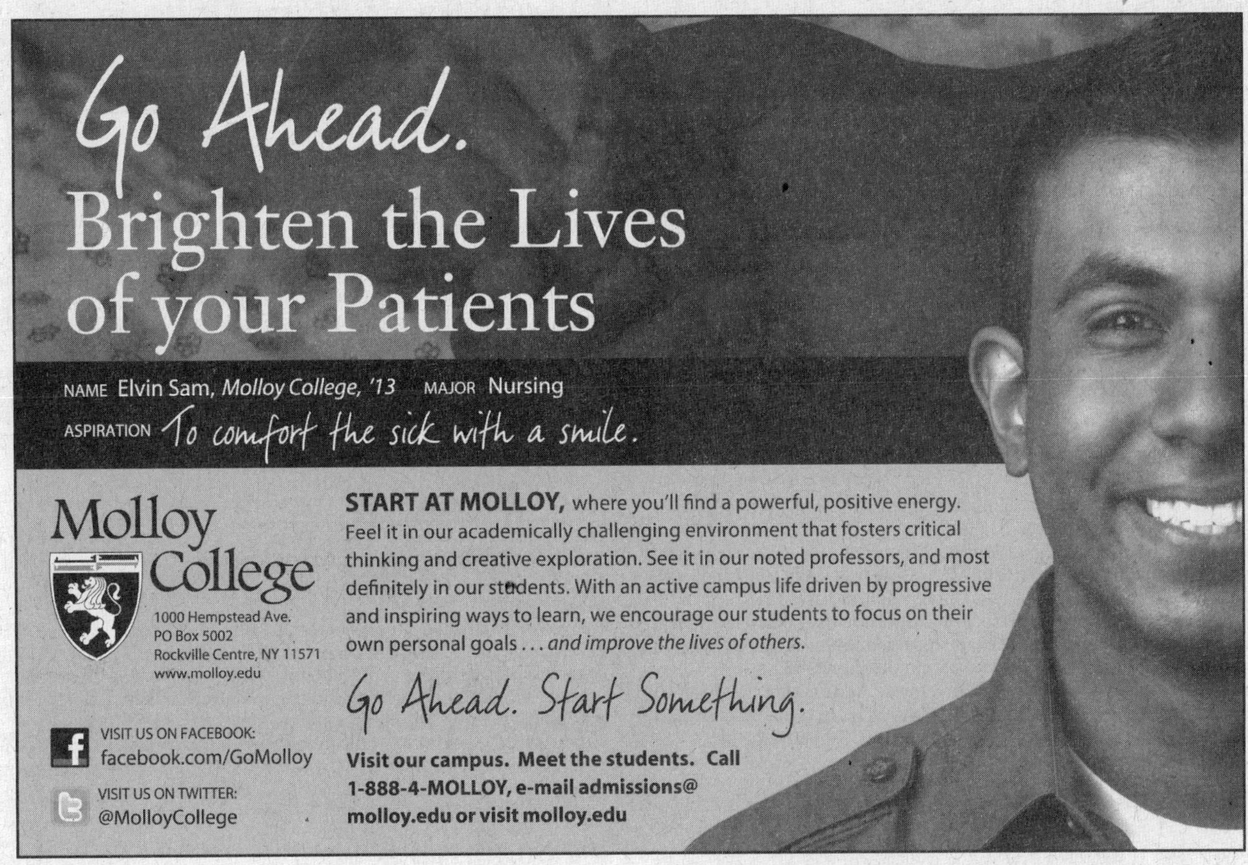

suals; remedial services; resume preparation assistance; skills, simulation, or other laboratory; tutoring.
Library Facilities 401,714 volumes (10,000 in health, 550 in nursing); 642 periodical subscriptions (180 health-care related).

BACCALAUREATE PROGRAMS

Degree BS
Available Programs Accelerated RN Baccalaureate; RN Baccalaureate.
Site Options Dobbs Ferry, NY.
Study Options Full-time and part-time.
Online Degree Options Yes.
Program Entrance Requirements Minimum overall college GPA, transcript of college record, written essay, immunizations, interview, minimum GPA in nursing prerequisites, prerequisite course work, RN licensure. Transfer students are accepted. *Application deadline:* Applications may be processed on a rolling basis for some programs.
Advanced Placement Credit given for nursing courses completed elsewhere dependent upon specific evaluations.
Contact ***Telephone:*** 914-674-7865. *Fax:* 914-674-7623.

GRADUATE PROGRAMS

Contact ***Telephone:*** 914-674-7867. *Fax:* 914-674-7623.

MASTER'S DEGREE PROGRAM

Degree MS
Available Programs Accelerated Master's for Non-Nursing College Graduates; Accelerated Master's for Nurses with Non-Nursing Degrees; Accelerated RN to Master's; Master's; Master's for Non-Nursing College Graduates; Master's for Nurses with Non-Nursing Degrees.
Concentrations Available Health-care administration; nursing administration; nursing education.
Site Options Dobbs Ferry, NY.
Study Options Full-time and part-time.
Online Degree Options Yes.
Program Entrance Requirements Clinical experience, minimum overall college GPA of 3.0, transcript of college record, written essay, immunizations, interview, 2 letters of recommendation, professional liability insurance/malpractice insurance, resume. *Application deadline:* Applications may be processed on a rolling basis for some programs.
Advanced Placement Credit given for nursing courses completed elsewhere dependent upon specific evaluations.
Degree Requirements 36 total credit hours, thesis or project.

POST-MASTER'S PROGRAM

Areas of Study Nursing administration; nursing education.

Molloy College
Division of Nursing
Rockville Centre, New York

http://www.molloy.edu/
Founded in 1955

DEGREES • BS • MS • PHD

Nursing Program Faculty 181 (17% with doctorates).
Baccalaureate Enrollment 1,243 **Women** 88% **Men** 12% **Minority** 45% **Part-time** 32%
Graduate Enrollment 464 **Women** 93% **Men** 7% **Minority** 49% **Part-time** 96%
Nursing Student Activities Sigma Theta Tau, Student Nurses' Association.
Nursing Student Resources Academic advising; academic or career counseling; assistance for students with disabilities; bookstore; campus computer network; computer lab; computer-assisted instruction; e-mail services; interactive nursing skills videos; Internet; learning resource lab; library services; nursing audiovisuals; tutoring.
Library Facilities 110,000 volumes (2,883 in health, 1,489 in nursing); 720 periodical subscriptions (145 health-care related).

BACCALAUREATE PROGRAMS

Degree BS
Available Programs ADN to Baccalaureate; Accelerated Baccalaureate for Second Degree; Accelerated RN Baccalaureate; Baccalaureate for Second Degree; Generic Baccalaureate; LPN to Baccalaureate; LPN to RN Baccalaureate; RN Baccalaureate.
Site Options Plainview, NY; New Hyde Park, NY.
Study Options Full-time and part-time.
Program Entrance Requirements Minimum overall college GPA of 3.0, transcript of college record, written essay, health exam, high school biology, high school chemistry, high school foreign language, 3 years

high school math, high school transcript, immunizations, minimum high school GPA of 3.0. Transfer students are accepted. *Application deadline:* Applications may be processed on a rolling basis for some programs.
Advanced Placement Credit given for nursing courses completed elsewhere dependent upon specific evaluations.
Expenses (2010-11) *Tuition:* full-time $19,970; part-time $660 per credit. *Required fees:* full-time $1626.
Financial Aid 29% of baccalaureate students in nursing programs received some form of financial aid in 2009-10. *Gift aid (need-based):* Federal Pell, FSEOG, state, private, college/university gift aid from institutional funds, Federal Nursing, Academic Competitiveness Grants, National SMART Grants, TRiO Scholarships, TEACH Grants. *Loans:* Federal Nursing Student Loans, Federal Direct (Subsidized and Unsubsidized Stafford PLUS), Perkins, state, alternative loans. *Work-study:* Federal Work-Study. *Financial aid application deadline:* 5/1.
Contact Marguerite Lane, Director of Admissions, Division of Nursing, Molloy College, 1000 Hempstead Avenue, PO Box 5002, Rockville Centre, NY 11571-5002. *Telephone:* 516-678-5000 Ext. 6233. *E-mail:* mlane@molloy.edu.

GRADUATE PROGRAMS

Expenses (2010-11) *Tuition:* full-time $14,580; part-time $810 per credit. *Required fees:* full-time $1730.
Financial Aid 70% of graduate students in nursing programs received some form of financial aid in 2009-10. Research assistantships with partial tuition reimbursements available, teaching assistantships with partial tuition reimbursements available, institutionally sponsored loans, scholarships, and unspecified assistantships available. Aid available to part-time students. *Financial aid application deadline:* 4/1.
Contact Ms. Alina Haitz, Assistant Director of Admissions, Division of Nursing, Molloy College, 1000 Hempstead Avenue, PO Box 5002, Rockville Centre, NY 11571-5002. *Telephone:* 516-678-5000 Ext. 6399. *E-mail:* ahaitz@molloy.edu.

MASTER'S DEGREE PROGRAM

Degree MS
Available Programs Master's.
Concentrations Available Nursing administration; nursing education; nursing informatics. *Clinical nurse specialist programs in:* adult health. *Nurse practitioner programs in:* adult health, family health, pediatric, psychiatric/mental health.
Site Options Plainview, NY; Farmingdale, NY; New Hyde Park, NY.
Study Options Full-time and part-time.
Program Entrance Requirements Clinical experience, minimum overall college GPA of 3.0, transcript of college record, written essay, interview, 3 letters of recommendation, nursing research course, prerequisite course work, statistics course. *Application deadline:* Applications may be processed on a rolling basis for some programs. *Application fee:* $30.
Advanced Placement Credit given for nursing courses completed elsewhere dependent upon specific evaluations.
Degree Requirements 48 total credit hours, thesis or project.

POST-MASTER'S PROGRAM

Areas of Study Nursing administration; nursing education; nursing informatics. *Clinical nurse specialist programs in:* adult health. *Nurse practitioner programs in:* adult health, family health, pediatric, psychiatric/mental health.

DOCTORAL DEGREE PROGRAM

Degree PhD
Available Programs Doctorate.
Areas of Study Health policy, nursing education, nursing research.
Program Entrance Requirements Clinical experience, minimum overall college GPA of 3.5, interview by faculty committee, interview, 3 letters of recommendation, MSN or equivalent, scholarly papers, statistics course, vita, writing sample. Application deadline: 2/1 (fall). Application fee: $75.
Degree Requirements 45 total credit hours, dissertation.

CONTINUING EDUCATION PROGRAM

Contact Anna Jansson, Associate Director, Continuing Education, Division of Nursing, Molloy College, 1000 Hempstead Avenue, Rockville Centre, NY 11571-5002. *Telephone:* 516-678-5000 Ext. 6106. *Fax:* 516-678-7295. *E-mail:* ajansson@molloy.edu.

See full description on page 488.

Mount Saint Mary College
Division of Nursing
Newburgh, New York

Founded in 1960

DEGREES • BSN • MS
Nursing Program Faculty 36 (50% with doctorates).
Nursing Student Activities Sigma Theta Tau, Student Nurses' Association, nursing club.
Nursing Student Resources Academic advising; academic or career counseling; assistance for students with disabilities; bookstore; campus computer network; career placement assistance; computer lab; computer-assisted instruction; e-mail services; employment services for current students; externships; housing assistance; interactive nursing skills videos; Internet; learning resource lab; library services; nursing audiovisuals; paid internships; remedial services; resume preparation assistance; skills, simulation, or other laboratory; tutoring.
Library Facilities 105,999 volumes (2,443 in health, 1,723 in nursing); 29,775 periodical subscriptions (114 health-care related).

BACCALAUREATE PROGRAMS

Degree BSN
Available Programs Accelerated Baccalaureate; Accelerated RN Baccalaureate; Generic Baccalaureate; RN Baccalaureate.
Study Options Full-time and part-time.
Program Entrance Requirements Minimum overall college GPA of 2.75, transcript of college record, CPR certification, health exam, high school biology, high school chemistry, 3 years high school math, high school transcript, immunizations, interview. Transfer students are accepted.
Advanced Placement Credit by examination available. Credit given for nursing courses completed elsewhere dependent upon specific evaluations.
Contact ***Telephone:*** 845-569-3248.

GRADUATE PROGRAMS

Contact ***Telephone:*** 845-569-3248.

MASTER'S DEGREE PROGRAM

Degree MS
Available Programs Master's.
Concentrations Available *Clinical nurse specialist programs in:* adult health. *Nurse practitioner programs in:* adult health.
Study Options Full-time and part-time.
Program Entrance Requirements Clinical experience, computer literacy, minimum overall college GPA of 3.0, transcript of college record, written essay, immunizations, interview, 3 letters of recommendation, nursing research course, physical assessment course, professional liability insurance/malpractice insurance, resume, statistics course.
Degree Requirements 42 total credit hours, thesis or project.

POST-MASTER'S PROGRAM

Areas of Study Nursing administration; nursing education.

Nazareth College of Rochester
Department of Nursing
Rochester, New York

http://www.naz.edu/dept/nursing/
Founded in 1924

DEGREES • BS • MS
Nursing Program Faculty 20 (50% with doctorates).
Baccalaureate Enrollment 173 **Women** 92% **Men** 8% **Minority** 11% **International** .5% **Part-time** 22%
Graduate Enrollment 20 **Women** 95% **Men** 5% **Minority** 10% **Part-time** 90%
Distance Learning Courses Available.
Nursing Student Activities Nursing Honor Society, Sigma Theta Tau, nursing club.
Nursing Student Resources Academic advising; academic or career counseling; assistance for students with disabilities; bookstore; campus computer network; career placement assistance; computer lab; computer-assisted instruction; daycare for children of students; e-mail services; employment services for current students; externships; housing assis-

tance; interactive nursing skills videos; Internet; learning resource lab; library services; nursing audiovisuals; resume preparation assistance; skills, simulation, or other laboratory; tutoring.

Library Facilities 283,248 volumes (267,000 in health, 66,000 in nursing); 16,102 periodical subscriptions (44,000 health-care related).

BACCALAUREATE PROGRAMS

Degree BS

Available Programs Generic Baccalaureate; LPN to Baccalaureate; RN Baccalaureate.

Site Options Geneva, NY; Rochester, NY.

Study Options Full-time and part-time.

Program Entrance Requirements Minimum overall college GPA of 2.5, transcript of college record, CPR certification, written essay, health exam, high school chemistry,, high school transcript, immunizations, minimum high school GPA of 2.5, minimum GPA in nursing prerequisites of 2.5, prerequisite course work. Transfer students are accepted.

Advanced Placement Credit by examination available. Credit given for nursing courses completed elsewhere dependent upon specific evaluations.

Contact ***Telephone:*** 585-389-2865.

GRADUATE PROGRAMS

Contact ***Telephone:*** 585-389-2713. *Fax:* 585-389-2714.

MASTER'S DEGREE PROGRAM

Degree MS

Available Programs Master's.

Concentrations Available *Nurse practitioner programs in:* gerontology.

Site Options Rochester, NY.

Study Options Full-time and part-time.

Program Entrance Requirements Minimum overall college GPA of 3.0, transcript of college record, written essay, immunizations, interview, 2 letters of recommendation, physical assessment course, statistics course.

Advanced Placement Credit given for nursing courses completed elsewhere dependent upon specific evaluations.

Degree Requirements 42 total credit hours, thesis or project.

POST-MASTER'S PROGRAM

Areas of Study Nursing education. *Nurse practitioner programs in:* gerontology.

CONTINUING EDUCATION PROGRAM

Contact ***Telephone:*** 585-389-2709. *Fax:* 585-389-2714.

New York City College of Technology of the City University of New York

Department of Nursing
Brooklyn, New York

Founded in 1946

DEGREE • BS

Nursing Program Faculty 22

Library Facilities 179,062 volumes; 54,021 periodical subscriptions.

BACCALAUREATE PROGRAMS

Degree BS

Available Programs RN Baccalaureate.

Program Entrance Requirements Minimum overall college GPA of 2.5, immunizations, professional liability insurance/malpractice insurance, RN licensure. Transfer students are accepted.

Contact ***Telephone:*** 718-260-5660. *Fax:* 718-260-5662.

New York Institute of Technology

Department of Nursing
Old Westbury, New York

Founded in 1955

DEGREE • BSN

Library Facilities 157,763 volumes; 1,224 periodical subscriptions.

BACCALAUREATE PROGRAMS

Degree BSN

Available Programs Generic Baccalaureate.

Contact Susan Neville, Chairperson and Associate Professor, Department of Nursing, New York Institute of Technology, Old Westbury, NY 11568. *Telephone:* 516-686-7516. *E-mail:* sneville@nyit.edu.

New York University

College of Nursing
New York, New York

http://www.nyu.edu/nursing/index.html

Founded in 1831

DEGREES • BS • DNP • MS • MS/MPH • PHD

Nursing Program Faculty 185 (24% with doctorates).

Baccalaureate Enrollment 845 **Women** 90.3% **Men** 9.7% **Minority** 63% **International** 1% **Part-time** 6.4%

Graduate Enrollment 521 **Women** 93.9% **Men** 6.1% **Minority** 63.53% **International** 2.3% **Part-time** 94.81%

Nursing Student Activities Sigma Theta Tau, Student Nurses' Association, nursing club.

Nursing Student Resources Academic advising; academic or career counseling; assistance for students with disabilities; bookstore; campus computer network; career placement assistance; computer lab; computer-assisted instruction; e-mail services; employment services for current students; externships; housing assistance; interactive nursing skills videos; Internet; learning resource lab; library services; nursing audiovisuals; resume preparation assistance; skills, simulation, or other laboratory; tutoring.

Library Facilities 5.8 million volumes (102,448 in health, 62,781 in nursing); 108,454 periodical subscriptions (4,658 health-care related).

BACCALAUREATE PROGRAMS

Degree BS

Available Programs Accelerated Baccalaureate; Accelerated Baccalaureate for Second Degree; Accelerated RN Baccalaureate; Baccalaureate for Second Degree; Generic Baccalaureate; RN Baccalaureate.

Study Options Full-time and part-time.

Program Entrance Requirements Minimum overall college GPA of 3.0, transcript of college record, CPR certification, written essay, health exam, health insurance, high school biology, high school chemistry, high school foreign language, 4 years high school math, 4 years high school science, high school transcript, immunizations, 2 letters of recommendation, minimum high school GPA of 3.3, minimum GPA in nursing prerequisites of 2.7. Transfer students are accepted. *Application deadline:* 1/1 (fall), 11/1 (spring). Applications may be processed on a rolling basis for some programs. *Application fee:* $65.

Advanced Placement Credit given for nursing courses completed elsewhere dependent upon specific evaluations.

Expenses (2010-11) *Tuition:* full-time $37,866; part-time $1116 per credit. *Room and board:* room only: $12,988 per academic year. *Required fees:* full-time $2216; part-time $409 per term.

Financial Aid 88% of baccalaureate students in nursing programs received some form of financial aid in 2009-10.

Contact Ms. Lindsay J. Sutton, Assistant Director of Undergraduate Student Affairs and Admissions, College of Nursing, New York University, 726 Broadway, 10th Floor, New York, NY 10003-6677. *Telephone:* 212-998-5336. *Fax:* 212-995-4302. *E-mail:* ljs333@nyu.edu.

GRADUATE PROGRAMS

Expenses (2010-11) *Tuition:* full-time $30,936; part-time $1289 per credit. *Required fees:* part-time $409 per term.

Financial Aid 54% of graduate students in nursing programs received some form of financial aid in 2009-10. 2 research assistantships with full

and partial tuition reimbursements available were awarded; fellowships with full and partial tuition reimbursements available, career-related internships or fieldwork, institutionally sponsored loans, scholarships, and tuition waivers (partial) also available. Aid available to part-time students. *Financial aid application deadline:* 2/1.
Contact Ms. Gail Wolfmeyer, Assistant Director of Graduate Student Affairs and Admissions, College of Nursing, New York University, 726 Broadway, 10th Floor, New York, NY 10003-6677. *Telephone:* 212-992-7653. *Fax:* 212-995-4302. *E-mail:* gew227@nyu.edu.

MASTER'S DEGREE PROGRAM
Degrees MS; MS/MPH
Available Programs Master's; RN to Master's.
Concentrations Available Nurse-midwifery; nursing administration; nursing education; nursing informatics. *Nurse practitioner programs in:* acute care, gerontology, pediatric, primary care, psychiatric/mental health.
Study Options Full-time and part-time.
Program Entrance Requirements Clinical experience, minimum overall college GPA of 3.0, transcript of college record, CPR certification, written essay, immunizations, 2 letters of recommendation, nursing research course, resume, statistics course. *Application deadline:* 7/1 (fall), 12/1 (spring). Applications may be processed on a rolling basis for some programs. *Application fee:* $75.
Advanced Placement Credit given for nursing courses completed elsewhere dependent upon specific evaluations.
Degree Requirements 48 total credit hours, thesis or project.

POST-MASTER'S PROGRAM
Areas of Study Nurse-midwifery; nursing administration; nursing education; nursing informatics. *Nurse practitioner programs in:* acute care, gerontology, pediatric, primary care, psychiatric/mental health.

DOCTORAL DEGREE PROGRAM
Degree DNP
Available Programs Doctorate.
Areas of Study Adult primary care, adult primary care/geriatrics, adult primary care/palliative care, adult primary care/holistic, geriatrics, pediatrics, adult acute care, mental health, nurse midwifery.
Program Entrance Requirements Minimum overall college GPA of 3.5, 3 letters of recommendation, transcripts, resume, standardized test scores, essay. *Application deadline*: 3/1 (fall). Applications accepted on a rolling basis.
Degree Requirements 40 total credits (post-MS NP/CNM), 58-64 total credits (post-MS non-NP/CNM), Capstone project, Capstone project defense.

Degree PhD
Available Programs Doctorate.
Areas of Study Addiction/substance abuse, aging, bio-behavioral research, gerontology, health policy, health-care systems, illness and transition, nursing administration, nursing education, nursing policy, nursing research, oncology, urban health.
Program Entrance Requirements Minimum overall college GPA of 3.0, interview by faculty committee, interview, 3 letters of recommendation, MSN or equivalent, vita, writing sample, GRE General Test. Application deadline: 1/15 (fall). Applications may be processed on a rolling basis for some programs. Application fee: $75.
Degree Requirements 45 total credit hours, dissertation, oral exam, residency.

CONTINUING EDUCATION PROGRAM
Contact Dr. Hila Richardson, Continuing Education Director, College of Nursing, New York University, 726 Broadway, 10th Floor, New York, NY 10003-6677. *Telephone:* 212-998-5329. *Fax:* 212-995-4302. *E-mail:* nursing.programs@nyu.edu.

Niagara University
Department of Nursing
Niagara Falls, Niagara University, New York

Founded in 1856
DEGREE • BS
Nursing Program Faculty 6
Baccalaureate Enrollment 32 **Women** 97% **Men** 3% **Minority** 19% **International** 6% **Part-time** 84%
Distance Learning Courses Available.
Nursing Student Activities Sigma Theta Tau.
Nursing Student Resources Academic advising; academic or career counseling; assistance for students with disabilities; bookstore; campus computer network; computer lab; computer-assisted instruction; e-mail services; externships; Internet; library services; nursing audiovisuals; tutoring; unpaid internships.
Library Facilities 297,813 volumes; 164 periodical subscriptions.

BACCALAUREATE PROGRAMS
Degree BS
Available Programs RN Baccalaureate.
Contact *Telephone:* 716-286-8155. *Fax:* 716-286-8079.

Pace University
Lienhard School of Nursing
New York, New York

http://www.pace.edu/pace/lienhard
Founded in 1906
DEGREES • BS • DNP • MS
Nursing Program Faculty 99 (21% with doctorates).
Baccalaureate Enrollment 438 **Women** 91% **Men** 9% **Minority** 37% **International** 1% **Part-time** 13%
Graduate Enrollment 594 **Women** 90% **Men** 10% **Minority** 29% **International** 1% **Part-time** 83%
Distance Learning Courses Available.
Nursing Student Activities Nursing Honor Society, Sigma Theta Tau, Student Nurses' Association.
Nursing Student Resources Academic advising; academic or career counseling; assistance for students with disabilities; bookstore; campus computer network; career placement assistance; computer lab; computer-assisted instruction; e-mail services; employment services for current students; housing assistance; interactive nursing skills videos; Internet; learning resource lab; library services; nursing audiovisuals; placement services for program completers; resume preparation assistance; skills, simulation, or other laboratory.
Library Facilities 808,429 volumes (17,304 in health, 2,357 in nursing); 79,103 periodical subscriptions (4,788 health-care related).

BACCALAUREATE PROGRAMS
Degree BS
Available Programs Accelerated Baccalaureate for Second Degree; Generic Baccalaureate.
Site Options New York, NY; Pleasantville, NY.
Study Options Full-time and part-time.
Program Entrance Requirements Transcript of college record, CPR certification, written essay, health exam, health insurance, high school biology, high school chemistry, high school foreign language, 4 years high school math, 2 years high school science, high school transcript, immunizations, 2 letters of recommendation, minimum GPA in nursing prerequisites of 2.75. Transfer students are accepted. *Application deadline:* 2/15 (fall). *Application fee:* $50.
Advanced Placement Credit by examination available. Credit given for nursing courses completed elsewhere dependent upon specific evaluations.
Expenses (2010-11) *Tuition:* full-time $32,656; part-time $937 per credit. *Room and board:* $11,900 per academic year. *Required fees:* full-time $614.
Financial Aid 93% of baccalaureate students in nursing programs received some form of financial aid in 2009-10. *Gift aid (need-based):* Federal Pell, FSEOG, state, private, college/university gift aid from institutional funds, Federal Nursing, endowed and restricted scholarships and grants. *Loans:* Federal Nursing Student Loans, Federal Direct (Subsidized and Unsubsidized Stafford PLUS), Perkins. *Work-study:* Federal Work-Study. *Financial aid application deadline (priority):* 2/15.
Contact Dr. Martha Greenberg, Associate Professor and Chairperson, Undergraduate Department, Lienhard School of Nursing, Pace University, 861 Bedford Road, Pleasantville, NY 10570. *Telephone:* 914-773-3325. *Fax:* 914-773-3345. *E-mail:* mgreenberg@pace.edu.

GRADUATE PROGRAMS
Expenses (2010-11) *Tuition:* part-time $830 per credit. *Room and board:* $11,900 per academic year. *Required fees:* full-time $614.
Financial Aid 54% of graduate students in nursing programs received some form of financial aid in 2009-10. Research assistantships, career-

related internships or fieldwork, Federal Work-Study, and tuition waivers (partial) available. Aid available to part-time students.
Contact Dr. Joanne K. Singleton, Chair of the Department of Graduate Studies/Director, Doctor of Nursing Program, Lienhard School of Nursing, Pace University, 41 Park Row, New York, NY 10038. *Telephone:* 212-346-1903. *Fax:* 212-346-1587. *E-mail:* jsingleton@pace.edu.

MASTER'S DEGREE PROGRAM
Degree MS
Available Programs Master's; Master's for Nurses with Non-Nursing Degrees.
Concentrations Available Nursing education. *Nurse practitioner programs in:* family health.
Site Options New York, NY; Pleasantville, NY.
Study Options Full-time and part-time.
Online Degree Options Yes (online only).
Program Entrance Requirements Computer literacy, minimum overall college GPA of 3.0, transcript of college record, CPR certification, immunizations, 2 letters of recommendation, nursing research course, professional liability insurance/malpractice insurance, prerequisite course work, resume, statistics course, GRE General Test or MAT. *Application deadline:* 6/1 (fall). *Application fee:* $70.
Advanced Placement Credit by examination available. Credit given for nursing courses completed elsewhere dependent upon specific evaluations.
Degree Requirements 42 total credit hours, comprehensive exam.

POST-MASTER'S PROGRAM
Areas of Study Nursing education. *Nurse practitioner programs in:* family health.

DOCTORAL DEGREE PROGRAM
Degree DNP
Available Programs Doctorate.
Areas of Study Family health.
Site Options New York, NY.
Program Entrance Requirements Clinical experience, minimum overall college GPA of 3.3, 2 letters of recommendation, MSN or equivalent, writing sample. Application deadline: 5/1 (fall). Application fee: $70.
Degree Requirements 37 total credit hours, residency.

Roberts Wesleyan College
Division of Nursing
Rochester, New York

http://www.roberts.edu/Nursing/
Founded in 1866

DEGREES • BSCN • M SC N
Nursing Program Faculty 15 (20% with doctorates).
Baccalaureate Enrollment 289 **Women** 92% **Men** 8% **Minority** 11% **International** 2% **Part-time** 3%
Graduate Enrollment 66 **Women** 97% **Men** 3% **Minority** 8%
Distance Learning Courses Available.
Nursing Student Activities Sigma Theta Tau, nursing club.
Nursing Student Resources Academic advising; academic or career counseling; assistance for students with disabilities; bookstore; campus computer network; career placement assistance; computer lab; computer-assisted instruction; e-mail services; employment services for current students; externships; housing assistance; interactive nursing skills videos; Internet; learning resource lab; library services; nursing audiovisuals; placement services for program completers; remedial services; resume preparation assistance; skills, simulation, or other laboratory; tutoring; unpaid internships.
Library Facilities 134,798 volumes (7,552 in health, 5,000 in nursing); 1,845 periodical subscriptions (247 health-care related).

BACCALAUREATE PROGRAMS
Degree BScN
Available Programs Accelerated RN Baccalaureate; Generic Baccalaureate; RN Baccalaureate.
Site Options Buffalo, NY; Rochester, NY; Weedsport, NY; Rochester, NY; Dansville, NY; Clifton Springs, NY.
Study Options Full-time and part-time.
Online Degree Options Yes.
Program Entrance Requirements Minimum overall college GPA of 2.5, transcript of college record, CPR certification, written essay, health exam, health insurance, high school biology, high school chemistry, high school transcript, immunizations, 2 letters of recommendation, minimum GPA in nursing prerequisites of 2.5, prerequisite course work. Transfer students are accepted. *Application deadline:* 2/1 (fall). Applications may be processed on a rolling basis for some programs. *Application fee:* $35.
Expenses (2010-11) *Tuition:* full-time $23,460; part-time $978 per credit hour. *Room and board:* $8826; room only: $5932 per academic year. *Required fees:* full-time $900.
Financial Aid 98% of baccalaureate students in nursing programs received some form of financial aid in 2009-10. *Gift aid (need-based):* Federal Pell, FSEOG, state, private, college/university gift aid from institutional funds, Academic Competitiveness Grants, National SMART Grants, TEACH Grants. *Loans:* Federal Direct (Subsidized and Unsubsidized Stafford PLUS), Perkins. *Work-study:* Federal Work-Study, part-time campus jobs. *Financial aid application deadline (priority):* 3/15.
Contact Mr. Kirk Kettinger, Director of Admissions, Division of Nursing, Roberts Wesleyan College, 2301 Westside Drive, Rochester, NY 14624. *Telephone:* 585-594-6400. *Fax:* 585-549-6371. *E-mail:* admissions@roberts.edu.

GRADUATE PROGRAMS
Expenses (2010-11) *Tuition:* full-time $12,762. *Required fees:* full-time $150.
Financial Aid 97% of graduate students in nursing programs received some form of financial aid in 2009-10.
Contact Mrs. Christine S. Lee, Assistant to the Chairperson, Division of Nursing, Roberts Wesleyan College, 2301 Westside Drive, Rochester, NY 14624-1997. *Telephone:* 585-594-6668. *Fax:* 585-594-6593. *E-mail:* lee_christine@roberts.edu.

MASTER'S DEGREE PROGRAM
Degree M Sc N
Available Programs Accelerated Master's; Accelerated Master's for Nurses with Non-Nursing Degrees.
Concentrations Available Nursing administration; nursing education.
Study Options Full-time.
Program Entrance Requirements Clinical experience, computer literacy, minimum overall college GPA of 3.0, transcript of college record, written essay, immunizations, interview, 2 letters of recommendation, nursing research course, prerequisite course work, resume, statistics course. *Application deadline:* Applications may be processed on a rolling basis for some programs. *Application fee:* $35.
Degree Requirements 39 total credit hours, thesis or project.

POST-MASTER'S PROGRAM
Areas of Study Nursing administration; nursing education.

The Sage Colleges
Department of Nursing
Troy, New York

http://www.sage.edu/academics/health-sciences/programs/nursing/

DEGREES • BS • DNS • MS • MS/MBA
Nursing Program Faculty 17 (41% with doctorates).
Baccalaureate Enrollment 244 **Women** 98% **Men** 2% **Minority** 22% **International** .5% **Part-time** 25%
Graduate Enrollment 174 **Women** 97% **Men** 3% **Minority** 13% **International** 3% **Part-time** 79%
Distance Learning Courses Available.
Nursing Student Activities Nursing Honor Society, Sigma Theta Tau, nursing club.
Nursing Student Resources Academic advising; academic or career counseling; assistance for students with disabilities; bookstore; campus computer network; career placement assistance; computer lab; computer-assisted instruction; e-mail services; employment services for current students; externships; interactive nursing skills videos; Internet; learning resource lab; library services; remedial services; resume preparation assistance; skills, simulation, or other laboratory; tutoring.
Library Facilities 4,003 volumes in health, 2,516 volumes in nursing; 400 periodical subscriptions health-care related.

BACCALAUREATE PROGRAMS
Degree BS

Available Programs ADN to Baccalaureate; Accelerated Baccalaureate; Accelerated Baccalaureate for Second Degree; Baccalaureate for Second Degree; Generic Baccalaureate; International Nurse to Baccalaureate; LPN to Baccalaureate; RN Baccalaureate.
Study Options Full-time and part-time.
Program Entrance Requirements Minimum overall college GPA of 2.75, transcript of college record, written essay, health exam, health insurance, high school biology, high school chemistry, 3 years high school math, 3 years high school science, high school transcript, immunizations, interview, 2 letters of recommendation, minimum high school GPA of 2.75, professional liability insurance/malpractice insurance. Transfer students are accepted. *Application deadline:* Applications may be processed on a rolling basis for some programs. *Application fee:* $30.
Advanced Placement Credit by examination available. Credit given for nursing courses completed elsewhere dependent upon specific evaluations.
Expenses (2010-11) *Tuition:* full-time $27,000; part-time $900 per credit hour. *Room and board:* $10,150; room only: $5350 per academic year. *Required fees:* full-time $850.
Financial Aid 86% of baccalaureate students in nursing programs received some form of financial aid in 2009-10.
Contact Michelle Hayward, MS, Program Contact, Department of Nursing, The Sage Colleges, Troy, NY 12180-4115. *Telephone:* 518-244-4520. *Fax:* 518-244-2009. *E-mail:* nursing@sage.edu.

GRADUATE PROGRAMS

Expenses (2010-11) *Tuition:* full-time $10,980; part-time $610 per credit hour. *Room and board:* $10,150; room only: $5350 per academic year.
Financial Aid 82% of graduate students in nursing programs received some form of financial aid in 2009-10. Fellowships, research assistantships, Federal Work-Study, scholarships, and unspecified assistantships available. Aid available to part-time students. *Financial aid application deadline:* 3/1.
Contact Dr. Arlene Pericak, MS Program, Department of Nursing, The Sage Colleges, Troy, NY 12180-4115. *Telephone:* 518-244-2012. *Fax:* 518-244-2009. *E-mail:* nursing@sage.edu.

MASTER'S DEGREE PROGRAM

Degrees MS; MS/MBA
Available Programs Accelerated Master's; Accelerated RN to Master's; Master's.
Concentrations Available Health-care administration; nursing administration; nursing education. *Clinical nurse specialist programs in:* acute care, adult health, cardiovascular, community health, critical care, family health, gerontology, medical-surgical, oncology, palliative care, psychiatric/mental health. *Nurse practitioner programs in:* acute care, adult health, community health, family health, gerontology, psychiatric/mental health.
Study Options Full-time and part-time.
Program Entrance Requirements Minimum overall college GPA of 2.75, transcript of college record, CPR certification, written essay, 2 letters of recommendation, physical assessment course, professional liability insurance/malpractice insurance, resume.
Advanced Placement Credit given for nursing courses completed elsewhere dependent upon specific evaluations.
Degree Requirements 42 total credit hours, thesis or project.

POST-MASTER'S PROGRAM

Areas of Study Health-care administration; nursing administration; nursing education. *Clinical nurse specialist programs in:* acute care, adult health, cardiovascular, community health, critical care, family health, gerontology, medical-surgical, oncology, palliative care, psychiatric/mental health. *Nurse practitioner programs in:* acute care, adult health, community health, family health, gerontology, psychiatric/mental health.

DOCTORAL DEGREE PROGRAM

Degree DNS
Available Programs Doctorate.
Areas of Study Faculty preparation, health-care systems, nursing administration, nursing education, nursing policy, nursing research, nursing science.
Program Entrance Requirements Minimum overall college GPA of 3.5, interview by faculty committee, 3 letters of recommendation, MSN or equivalent, statistics course, vita, writing sample.
Degree Requirements 42 total credit hours, dissertation.

CONTINUING EDUCATION PROGRAM

Contact Wendy Nelson, Program Contact. *Telephone:* 518-244-3149. *Fax:* 518-244-2009. *E-mail:* nelsow@sage.edu.

St. Francis College
Department of Nursing
Brooklyn Heights, New York

Founded in 1884

DEGREE • BS

Nursing Program Faculty 6
Baccalaureate Enrollment 76 **Women** 98% **Men** 2% **Minority** 63% **International** 25% **Part-time** 56%
Nursing Student Resources Academic advising; academic or career counseling; assistance for students with disabilities; bookstore; campus computer network; career placement assistance; computer lab; computer-assisted instruction; e-mail services; employment services for current students; interactive nursing skills videos; learning resource lab; library services; nursing audiovisuals; placement services for program completers; remedial services; resume preparation assistance; skills, simulation, or other laboratory; tutoring.
Library Facilities 116,716 volumes (5,531 in health, 186 in nursing); 31,391 periodical subscriptions (558 health-care related).

BACCALAUREATE PROGRAMS

Degree BS
Available Programs ADN to Baccalaureate; International Nurse to Baccalaureate; RPN to Baccalaureate.
Site Options Brooklyn, NY; New York, NY; Brooklyn, NY.
Study Options Full-time and part-time.
Program Entrance Requirements Minimum overall college GPA of 2.0, transcript of college record, written essay, health exam, health insurance, high school transcript, immunizations, interview, 2 letters of recommendation, professional liability insurance/malpractice insurance, prerequisite course work, RN licensure. Transfer students are accepted.
Advanced Placement Credit by examination available. Credit given for nursing courses completed elsewhere dependent upon specific evaluations.
Contact *Telephone:* 718-489-5267 Ext. 5267. *Fax:* 718-489-5408.

St. John Fisher College
Advanced Practice Nursing Program
Rochester, New York

http://www.sjfc.edu/
Founded in 1948

DEGREES • BS • DNP • MS

Nursing Program Faculty 49 (25% with doctorates).
Baccalaureate Enrollment 470 **Women** 90% **Men** 10% **Minority** 12% **Part-time** 6%
Graduate Enrollment 95 **Women** 94% **Men** 6% **Minority** 9% **Part-time** 95%
Distance Learning Courses Available.
Nursing Student Activities Sigma Theta Tau, Student Nurses' Association.
Nursing Student Resources Academic advising; academic or career counseling; assistance for students with disabilities; bookstore; campus computer network; career placement assistance; computer lab; computer-assisted instruction; daycare for children of students; e-mail services; employment services for current students; interactive nursing skills videos; Internet; learning resource lab; library services; nursing audiovisuals; resume preparation assistance; skills, simulation, or other laboratory; tutoring.
Library Facilities 214,834 volumes (30,000 in health, 5,000 in nursing); 22,428 periodical subscriptions (200 health-care related).

BACCALAUREATE PROGRAMS

Degree BS
Available Programs ADN to Baccalaureate; Accelerated RN Baccalaureate; Baccalaureate for Second Degree; Generic Baccalaureate; RN Baccalaureate.
Site Options Geneva, NY; Rochester, NY.

Study Options Full-time.
Program Entrance Requirements Minimum overall college GPA of 2.75, transcript of college record, CPR certification, written essay, health exam, health insurance, high school transcript, immunizations, 2 letters of recommendation, minimum high school GPA of 2.0, minimum GPA in nursing prerequisites of 2.75, prerequisite course work. Transfer students are accepted. *Application deadline:* 3/1 (fall), 10/1 (spring). Applications may be processed on a rolling basis for some programs. *Application fee:* $30.
Advanced Placement Credit given for nursing courses completed elsewhere dependent upon specific evaluations.
Expenses (2010-11) *Tuition:* full-time $24,800; part-time $675 per credit hour. *Room and board:* $10,290; room only: $6680 per academic year. *Required fees:* full-time $470; part-time $50 per term.
Financial Aid 95% of baccalaureate students in nursing programs received some form of financial aid in 2009-10. *Gift aid (need-based):* Federal Pell, FSEOG, state, private, college/university gift aid from institutional funds, Federal Nursing. *Loans:* Federal Direct (Subsidized and Unsubsidized Stafford PLUS), Perkins. *Work-study:* Federal Work-Study. *Financial aid application deadline (priority):* 2/15.
Contact Dr. Marilyn Dollinger, Chairperson, Advanced Practice Nursing Program, St. John Fisher College, 3690 East Avenue, Rochester, NY 14618. *Telephone:* 585-385-8476. *Fax:* 585-385-8466. *E-mail:* mdollinger@sjfc.edu.

GRADUATE PROGRAMS

Expenses (2010-11) *Tuition:* full-time $8460; part-time $705 per credit hour. *Required fees:* full-time $50; part-time $50 per term.
Financial Aid 20% of graduate students in nursing programs received some form of financial aid in 2009-10. Federal Work-Study, scholarships, and traineeships available.
Contact Dr. Cynthia Ricci McCloskey, Graduate Program Director, Advanced Practice Nursing Program, St. John Fisher College, 3690 East Avenue, Rochester, NY 14618. *Telephone:* 585-385-8471. *Fax:* 585-385-8466. *E-mail:* cmccloskey@sjfc.edu.

MASTER'S DEGREE PROGRAM
Degree MS
Available Programs Master's; RN to Master's.
Concentrations Available Nursing education. *Clinical nurse specialist programs in:* adult health, gerontology, pediatric, women's health. *Nurse practitioner programs in:* family health.
Study Options Full-time and part-time.
Program Entrance Requirements Computer literacy, minimum overall college GPA of 3.0, transcript of college record, CPR certification, written essay, immunizations, 2 letters of recommendation, nursing research course, physical assessment course, resume, statistics course. *Application deadline:* Applications may be processed on a rolling basis for some programs. *Application fee:* $30.
Advanced Placement Credit given for nursing courses completed elsewhere dependent upon specific evaluations.
Degree Requirements 46 total credit hours, thesis or project.

POST-MASTER'S PROGRAM
Areas of Study Nursing education. *Nurse practitioner programs in:* family health.

DOCTORAL DEGREE PROGRAM
Degree DNP
Available Programs Doctorate; Post-Baccalaureate Doctorate.
Areas of Study Advanced practice nursing.
Program Entrance Requirements Clinical experience, minimum overall college GPA of 3.0, interview by faculty committee, letters of recommendation, scholarly papers, vita, writing sample. Application deadline: Applications may be processed on a rolling basis for some programs. Application fee: $30.
Degree Requirements 48 total credit hours, residency.

St. Joseph's College, New York
Department of Nursing
Brooklyn, New York

http://www.sjcny.edu/
Founded in 1916

DEGREES • BSN • MS
Nursing Program Faculty 16 (44% with doctorates).
Baccalaureate Enrollment 240 **Women** 93% **Men** 7% **Minority** 53% **Part-time** 95%
Graduate Enrollment 77 **Women** 95% **Men** 5% **Minority** 69% **Part-time** 100%
Nursing Student Activities Nursing Honor Society, nursing club.
Nursing Student Resources Academic advising; academic or career counseling; assistance for students with disabilities; bookstore; campus computer network; computer lab; computer-assisted instruction; e-mail services; Internet; learning resource lab; library services; nursing audio-visuals; remedial services; resume preparation assistance; skills, simulation, or other laboratory; tutoring.
Library Facilities 156,570 volumes (10,857 in health, 924 in nursing); 7,816 periodical subscriptions (2,952 health-care related).

BACCALAUREATE PROGRAMS

Degree BSN
Available Programs RN Baccalaureate.
Site Options Patchogue, NY.
Study Options Full-time and part-time.
Program Entrance Requirements Minimum overall college GPA of 2.5, transcript of college record, CPR certification, written essay, health exam, health insurance, immunizations, 2 letters of recommendation, minimum GPA in nursing prerequisites of 2.5, professional liability insurance/malpractice insurance, prerequisite course work, RN licensure. Transfer students are accepted. *Application deadline:* 8/31 (fall), 1/15 (spring). Applications may be processed on a rolling basis for some programs. *Application fee:* $25.
Advanced Placement Credit by examination available. Credit given for nursing courses completed elsewhere dependent upon specific evaluations.
Expenses (2010-11) *Tuition:* full-time $8500; part-time $555 per credit. *Required fees:* full-time $575; part-time $96 per credit; part-time $289 per term.
Financial Aid 37% of baccalaureate students in nursing programs received some form of financial aid in 2009-10. *Gift aid (need-based):* Federal Pell, FSEOG, state, private, college/university gift aid from institutional funds. *Loans:* Perkins. *Work-study:* Federal Work-Study, part-time campus jobs. *Financial aid application deadline (priority):* 2/25.
Contact Dr. Barbara L. Sands, Director, Department of Nursing, St. Joseph's College, New York, 245 Clinton Avenue, Brooklyn, NY 11205-3688. *Telephone:* 718-940-5892. *Fax:* 718-638-8839. *E-mail:* bsands@sjcny.edu.

GRADUATE PROGRAMS

Expenses (2010-11) *Tuition:* part-time $650 per credit. *Required fees:* part-time $96 per credit; part-time $289 per term.
Financial Aid 62% of graduate students in nursing programs received some form of financial aid in 2009-10.
Contact Dr. Barbara L. Sands, Director, Department of Nursing, St. Joseph's College, New York, 245 Clinton Avenue, Brooklyn, NY 11205-3688. *Telephone:* 718-940-5892. *Fax:* 718-638-8839. *E-mail:* bsands@sjcny.edu.

MASTER'S DEGREE PROGRAM
Degree MS
Available Programs Master's.
Concentrations Available Nursing education. *Clinical nurse specialist programs in:* adult health.
Site Options Patchogue, NY.
Study Options Part-time.
Program Entrance Requirements Clinical experience, minimum overall college GPA of 3.0, transcript of college record, CPR certification, written essay, immunizations, interview, 2 letters of recommendation, nursing research course, physical assessment course, professional liability insurance/malpractice insurance, prerequisite course work, resume, statistics course. *Application deadline:* 5/15 (fall). Applications may be processed on a rolling basis for some programs. *Application fee:* $25.
Advanced Placement Credit given for nursing courses completed elsewhere dependent upon specific evaluations.
Degree Requirements 38 total credit hours, comprehensive exam.

State University of New York at Binghamton

Decker School of Nursing
Binghamton, New York

http://dson.binghamton.edu
Founded in 1946

DEGREES • BS • MS • PHD

Nursing Program Faculty 43 (40% with doctorates).
Baccalaureate Enrollment 300
Graduate Enrollment 150
Nursing Student Activities Sigma Theta Tau, Student Nurses' Association.
Nursing Student Resources Campus computer network; computer lab; skills, simulation, or other laboratory.
Library Facilities 2.4 million volumes (7,000 in health); 81,959 periodical subscriptions (9,300 health-care related).

BACCALAUREATE PROGRAMS

Degree BS
Available Programs Accelerated RN Baccalaureate; Generic Baccalaureate.
Study Options Full-time and part-time.
Program Entrance Requirements Minimum overall college GPA of 2.7, transcript of college record, CPR certification, written essay, health exam, high school biology, high school chemistry, high school foreign language, 3 years high school math, 2 years high school science, high school transcript, minimum high school GPA of 3.0, prerequisite course work. Transfer students are accepted.
Advanced Placement Credit by examination available. Credit given for nursing courses completed elsewhere dependent upon specific evaluations.
Contact ***Telephone:*** 607-777-4954. *Fax:* 607-777-4440.

GRADUATE PROGRAMS

Contact ***Telephone:*** 607-777-4964. *Fax:* 607-777-4440.

MASTER'S DEGREE PROGRAM

Degree MS
Available Programs Master's.
Concentrations Available Nursing administration; nursing education. *Clinical nurse specialist programs in:* community health, family health, gerontology. *Nurse practitioner programs in:* community health, family health, gerontology, primary care.
Study Options Full-time and part-time.
Program Entrance Requirements Minimum overall college GPA of 3.0, transcript of college record, written essay, 2 letters of recommendation, statistics course, GRE General Test.
Advanced Placement Credit given for nursing courses completed elsewhere dependent upon specific evaluations.
Degree Requirements 48 total credit hours, thesis or project, comprehensive exam.

POST-MASTER'S PROGRAM

Areas of Study *Nurse practitioner programs in:* community health, family health, gerontology.

DOCTORAL DEGREE PROGRAM

Degree PhD
Available Programs Doctorate.
Program Entrance Requirements Clinical experience, interview by faculty committee, interview, 3 letters of recommendation, MSN or equivalent, scholarly papers, statistics course, vita, writing sample.
Degree Requirements 66 total credit hours, dissertation, written exam.

CONTINUING EDUCATION PROGRAM

Contact ***Telephone:*** 607-777-4954. *Fax:* 607-777-4440.

State University of New York at Plattsburgh

Department of Nursing
Plattsburgh, New York

http://www.plattsburgh.edu/nursing
Founded in 1889

DEGREE • BS

Nursing Program Faculty 18 (25% with doctorates).
Baccalaureate Enrollment 280 **Women** 90% **Men** 10% **Minority** 25% **International** 4% **Part-time** 25%
Distance Learning Courses Available.
Nursing Student Activities Nursing Honor Society, Sigma Theta Tau, Student Nurses' Association.
Nursing Student Resources Academic advising; academic or career counseling; assistance for students with disabilities; bookstore; campus computer network; career placement assistance; computer lab; computer-assisted instruction; e-mail services; employment services for current students; interactive nursing skills videos; Internet; learning resource lab; library services; nursing audiovisuals; remedial services; resume preparation assistance; skills, simulation, or other laboratory; tutoring.
Library Facilities 592,543 volumes (19,450 in health, 200 in nursing); 3,379 periodical subscriptions (174 health-care related).

BACCALAUREATE PROGRAMS

Degree BS
Available Programs ADN to Baccalaureate; Generic Baccalaureate; RN Baccalaureate.
Study Options Full-time.
Online Degree Options Yes.
Program Entrance Requirements Minimum overall college GPA of 2.5, transcript of college record, CPR certification, health exam, high school biology, high school chemistry, high school foreign language, 3 years high school math, 3 years high school science, high school transcript, immunizations, minimum GPA in nursing prerequisites of 2.5, professional liability insurance/malpractice insurance, prerequisite course work. Transfer students are accepted. *Application deadline:* Applications may be processed on a rolling basis for some programs.
Expenses (2010-11) *Tuition, state resident:* full-time $4970. *Tuition, nonresident:* full-time $13,386. *Room and board:* $9094; room only: $5894 per academic year. *Required fees:* full-time $1174.
Financial Aid ***Gift aid (need-based):*** Federal Pell, FSEOG, state, private, college/university gift aid from institutional funds. *Loans:* Federal Nursing Student Loans, Federal Direct (Subsidized and Unsubsidized Stafford PLUS), Perkins, state, alternative loans. *Work-study:* Federal Work-Study, part-time campus jobs. *Financial aid application deadline (priority):* 2/15.
Contact Dr. JoAnn Gleeson-Kreig, Chairperson, Department of Nursing, State University of New York at Plattsburgh, 101 Broad Street, Plattsburgh, NY 12901. *Telephone:* 518-564-3124. *Fax:* 518-564-3100. *E-mail:* joann.gleeson-kreig@plattsburgh.edu.

State University of New York College of Agriculture and Technology at Morrisville

Division of Nursing
Morrisville, New York

Founded in 1908

DEGREE • BS

Library Facilities 100,000 volumes; 2,500 periodical subscriptions.

BACCALAUREATE PROGRAMS

Degree BS
Available Programs RN Baccalaureate.
Contact Nursing Program, Division of Nursing, State University of New York College of Agriculture and Technology at Morrisville, 80 Eaton Street, PO Box 901, Morrisville, NY 13408. *Telephone:* 800-258-0111.

State University of New York College of Technology at Delhi

Bachelor of Science in Nursing Program
Delhi, New York

Founded in 1913

DEGREE • BSN

BACCALAUREATE PROGRAMS

Degree BSN
Available Programs RN Baccalaureate.
Study Options Full-time and part-time.
Online Degree Options Yes (online only).
Program Entrance Requirements RN licensure.
Contact Misty Fields, Online Enrollment Counselor, Bachelor of Science in Nursing Program, State University of New York College of Technology at Delhi, Delhi, NY 13753. *Telephone:* 607-746-4519. *E-mail:* fieldsmr@delhi.edu.

State University of New York Downstate Medical Center

College of Nursing
Brooklyn, New York

http://sls.downstate.edu/admissions/nursing/index.html
Founded in 1858

DEGREES • BS • MS • MS/MPH

Nursing Program Faculty 17 (53% with doctorates).
Baccalaureate Enrollment 133 **Women** 93% **Men** 7% **Minority** 80% **Part-time** 77%
Graduate Enrollment 192 **Women** 83% **Men** 17% **Minority** 79% **Part-time** 74%
Nursing Student Activities Student Nurses' Association, nursing club.
Nursing Student Resources Academic advising; academic or career counseling; assistance for students with disabilities; bookstore; campus computer network; computer lab; computer-assisted instruction; e-mail services; housing assistance; interactive nursing skills videos; Internet; learning resource lab; library services; nursing audiovisuals; paid internships; skills, simulation, or other laboratory.
Library Facilities 357,209 volumes in health, 2,679 volumes in nursing; 619 periodical subscriptions health-care related.

BACCALAUREATE PROGRAMS

Degree BS
Available Programs Accelerated Baccalaureate for Second Degree; RN Baccalaureate.
Study Options Full-time.
Program Entrance Requirements Minimum overall college GPA of 3.0, transcript of college record, written essay, health exam, 2 letters of recommendation, professional liability insurance/malpractice insurance, prerequisite course work. Transfer students are accepted.
Contact *Telephone:* 718-270-7617. *Fax:* 718-270-7641.

GRADUATE PROGRAMS

Contact *Telephone:* 718-270-7605. *Fax:* 718-270-7636.

MASTER'S DEGREE PROGRAM

Degrees MS; MS/MPH
Available Programs Master's.
Concentrations Available Nurse anesthesia; nurse-midwifery. *Clinical nurse specialist programs in:* adult health, maternity-newborn. *Nurse practitioner programs in:* family health, women's health.
Study Options Full-time and part-time.
Program Entrance Requirements Clinical experience, minimum overall college GPA of 3.0, transcript of college record, CPR certification, written essay, interview, 2 letters of recommendation, nursing research course, physical assessment course, professional liability insurance/malpractice insurance, prerequisite course work, resume, statistics course, GRE.
Advanced Placement Credit by examination available. Credit given for nursing courses completed elsewhere dependent upon specific evaluations.
Degree Requirements Thesis or project.

POST-MASTER'S PROGRAM

Areas of Study *Nurse practitioner programs in:* family health, women's health.

CONTINUING EDUCATION PROGRAM

Contact *Telephone:* 718-270-7616. *Fax:* 718-270-7641.

State University of New York Empire State College

Bachelor of Science in Nursing Program
Saratoga Springs, New York

http://www.esc.edu/nursing
Founded in 1971

DEGREE • BS

Nursing Program Faculty 6 (33% with doctorates).
Baccalaureate Enrollment 192 **Women** 92.4% **Men** 7.6% **Minority** 17.4% **Part-time** 85.9%
Distance Learning Courses Available.
Nursing Student Activities Nursing club.
Nursing Student Resources Academic advising; academic or career counseling; assistance for students with disabilities; bookstore; computer-assisted instruction; e-mail services; interactive nursing skills videos; Internet; library services; nursing audiovisuals; resume preparation assistance; tutoring.
Library Facilities 70,000 volumes; 57,000 periodical subscriptions.

BACCALAUREATE PROGRAMS

Degree BS
Available Programs RN Baccalaureate.
Study Options Full-time and part-time.
Online Degree Options Yes (online only).
Program Entrance Requirements Minimum overall college GPA of 3.0, transcript of college record, written essay, immunizations, 2 letters of recommendation, RN licensure. Transfer students are accepted. *Application deadline:* 4/1 (fall), 10/1 (spring). *Application fee:* $50.
Advanced Placement Credit by examination available. Credit given for nursing courses completed elsewhere dependent upon specific evaluations.
Expenses (2010-11) *Tuition, state resident:* part-time $207 per credit. *Tuition, nonresident:* part-time $558 per credit. *Required fees:* full-time $342.
Financial Aid 27% of baccalaureate students in nursing programs received some form of financial aid in 2009-10.
Contact Ms. Erin White, Coordinator of Student Services, Bachelor of Science in Nursing Program, State University of New York Empire State College, 113 West Avenue, Saratoga Springs, NY 12866. *Telephone:* 518-587-2100 Ext. 2812. *Fax:* 518-587-5126. *E-mail:* erin.white@esc.edu.

State University of New York Institute of Technology

School of Nursing and Health Systems
Utica, New York

http://www.sunyit.edu
Founded in 1966

DEGREES • BS • MS

Nursing Program Faculty 8 (70% with doctorates).
Baccalaureate Enrollment 280 **Women** 96% **Men** 4% **Minority** 5% **Part-time** 82%
Graduate Enrollment 36 **Women** 96.5% **Men** 3.5% **Minority** 10% **Part-time** 70%
Nursing Student Activities Nursing Honor Society, Sigma Theta Tau, Student Nurses' Association, nursing club.
Nursing Student Resources Academic advising; academic or career counseling; assistance for students with disabilities; bookstore; campus computer network; career placement assistance; computer lab; computer-assisted instruction; e-mail services; employment services for current stu-

dents; externships; housing assistance; interactive nursing skills videos; Internet; learning resource lab; library services; nursing audiovisuals; other; placement services for program completers; remedial services; resume preparation assistance; skills, simulation, or other laboratory; tutoring; unpaid internships.

Library Facilities 200,730 volumes (14,000 in health, 8,500 in nursing); 372 periodical subscriptions (335 health-care related).

BACCALAUREATE PROGRAMS

Degree BS

Available Programs ADN to Baccalaureate; Accelerated RN Baccalaureate; RN Baccalaureate.

Study Options Full-time and part-time.

Program Entrance Requirements Minimum overall college GPA of 2.0, transcript of college record, CPR certification, minimum GPA in nursing prerequisites of 2.0, prerequisite course work. Transfer students are accepted.

Advanced Placement Credit given for nursing courses completed elsewhere dependent upon specific evaluations.

Contact *Telephone:* 315-792-7500. *Fax:* 315-792-7837.

GRADUATE PROGRAMS

Contact *Telephone:* 315-792-7297. *Fax:* 315-792-7555.

MASTER'S DEGREE PROGRAM

Degree MS

Available Programs Accelerated AD/RN to Master's; Accelerated RN to Master's; Master's.

Concentrations Available Nursing administration. *Nurse practitioner programs in:* adult health, family health.

Study Options Full-time and part-time.

Program Entrance Requirements Clinical experience, computer literacy, minimum overall college GPA of 3.0, transcript of college record, written essay, interview, 2 letters of recommendation, nursing research course, physical assessment course, prerequisite course work, statistics course, GRE General Test (if undergraduate GPA less than 3.3).

Advanced Placement Credit given for nursing courses completed elsewhere dependent upon specific evaluations.

Degree Requirements 45 total credit hours, thesis or project, comprehensive exam.

POST-MASTER'S PROGRAM

Areas of Study Nursing administration. *Nurse practitioner programs in:* adult health, family health.

CONTINUING EDUCATION PROGRAM

Contact *Telephone:* 315-792-7295. *Fax:* 315-792-7555.

State University of New York Upstate Medical University

College of Nursing
Syracuse, New York

http://www.upstate.edu/con

Founded in 1950

DEGREES • BS • MS

Nursing Program Faculty 21 (40% with doctorates).

Baccalaureate Enrollment 182 **Women** 99% **Men** 1% **Minority** 1% **Part-time** 68%

Graduate Enrollment 168 **Women** 99% **Men** 1% **Minority** 1% **International** 1% **Part-time** 60%

Distance Learning Courses Available.

Nursing Student Activities Sigma Theta Tau, Student Nurses' Association.

Nursing Student Resources Academic advising; academic or career counseling; assistance for students with disabilities; bookstore; campus computer network; career placement assistance; computer lab; computer-assisted instruction; daycare for children of students; e-mail services; Internet; learning resource lab; library services; skills, simulation, or other laboratory; tutoring.

Library Facilities 226,060 volumes (220,382 in health, 1,241 in nursing); 3,200 periodical subscriptions (4,928 health-care related).

BACCALAUREATE PROGRAMS

Degree BS

Available Programs ADN to Baccalaureate.

Site Options Ithaca, NY.

Study Options Full-time and part-time.

Program Entrance Requirements Transcript of college record, CPR certification, written essay, health exam, immunizations, 2 letters of recommendation, prerequisite course work, RN licensure. *Application deadline:* 7/1 (fall), 10/1 (spring). *Application fee:* $50.

Advanced Placement Credit by examination available. Credit given for nursing courses completed elsewhere dependent upon specific evaluations.

Expenses (2010-11) *Tuition, state resident:* full-time $4970; part-time $207 per credit. *Tuition, nonresident:* full-time $13,380; part-time $558 per credit. *Room and board:* room only: $5000 per academic year. *Required fees:* part-time $1 per credit.

Financial Aid 35% of baccalaureate students in nursing programs received some form of financial aid in 2009-10. *Gift aid (need-based):* Federal Pell, FSEOG, state, college/university gift aid from institutional funds. *Loans:* Federal Direct (Subsidized and Unsubsidized Stafford PLUS), Perkins. *Work-study:* Federal Work-Study. *Financial aid application deadline (priority):* 3/1.

Contact Mrs. Debora E. Kirsch, Director, Undergraduate Program, College of Nursing, State University of New York Upstate Medical University, 750 East Adams Street, Syracuse, NY 13210. *Telephone:* 315-464-4276. *Fax:* 315-464-5168. *E-mail:* kirschde@upstate.edu.

GRADUATE PROGRAMS

Expenses (2010-11) *Tuition, state resident:* full-time $8370; part-time $349 per course. *Tuition, nonresident:* full-time $13,780; part-time $574 per course. *Room and board:* room only: $5000 per academic year.

Financial Aid 30% of graduate students in nursing programs received some form of financial aid in 2009-10. Federal Work-Study, institutionally sponsored loans, scholarships, and traineeships available. Aid available to part-time students. *Financial aid application deadline:* 3/1.

Contact Dr. Carol Gavan, Associate Professor/Associate Dean and Director, Graduate Program, College of Nursing, State University of New York Upstate Medical University, 750 East Adams Street, Syracuse, NY 13210. *Telephone:* 315-464-4276. *Fax:* 315-464-5168. *E-mail:* gavanc@upstate.edu.

MASTER'S DEGREE PROGRAM

Degree MS

Available Programs Accelerated RN to Master's; Master's; Master's for Nurses with Non-Nursing Degrees; RN to Master's.

Concentrations Available *Clinical nurse specialist programs in:* medical-surgical. *Nurse practitioner programs in:* adult health, family health, pediatric, psychiatric/mental health.

Site Options Watertown, NY.

Study Options Full-time and part-time.

Program Entrance Requirements Clinical experience, minimum overall college GPA of 3.0, transcript of college record, CPR certification, written essay, immunizations, 3 letters of recommendation, nursing research course, physical assessment course, statistics course. *Application deadline:* 7/1 (fall), 10/1 (spring). *Application fee:* $50.

Advanced Placement Credit by examination available. Credit given for nursing courses completed elsewhere dependent upon specific evaluations.

Degree Requirements 47 total credit hours, thesis or project.

POST-MASTER'S PROGRAM

Areas of Study *Clinical nurse specialist programs in:* medical-surgical. *Nurse practitioner programs in:* adult health, family health, pediatric, psychiatric/mental health.

CONTINUING EDUCATION PROGRAM

Contact Ms. Barbara A. Black, Director, Continuing Nursing Education, College of Nursing, State University of New York Upstate Medical University, 750 East Adams Street, Syracuse, NY 13210. *Telephone:* 315-464-4276. *Fax:* 315-464-5168. *E-mail:* blackb@upstate.edu.

Stony Brook University, State University of New York

School of Nursing
Stony Brook, New York

Founded in 1957

DEGREES • BS • DNP • MS

Nursing Program Faculty 64 (68% with doctorates).
Baccalaureate Enrollment 493 **Women** 83% **Men** 17% **Minority** 46% **International** 12% **Part-time** 71%
Graduate Enrollment 557 **Women** 91% **Men** 9% **Minority** 41% **International** 7% **Part-time** 95%
Distance Learning Courses Available.
Nursing Student Activities Nursing Honor Society, Sigma Theta Tau, Student Nurses' Association, nursing club.
Nursing Student Resources Academic advising; academic or career counseling; assistance for students with disabilities; bookstore; campus computer network; career placement assistance; computer lab; computer-assisted instruction; daycare for children of students; e-mail services; employment services for current students; housing assistance; interactive nursing skills videos; Internet; learning resource lab; library services; nursing audiovisuals; placement services for program completers; resume preparation assistance; skills, simulation, or other laboratory.
Library Facilities 2.5 million volumes (11,022 in health, 5,075 in nursing); 64,803 periodical subscriptions (280,000 health-care related).

BACCALAUREATE PROGRAMS

Degree BS
Available Programs Accelerated Baccalaureate; Generic Baccalaureate; RN Baccalaureate.
Study Options Full-time and part-time.
Program Entrance Requirements Minimum overall college GPA of 2.5, transcript of college record, CPR certification, written essay, health insurance, immunizations, 3 letters of recommendation, minimum GPA in nursing prerequisites of 2.5, professional liability insurance/malpractice insurance. *Application deadline:* 1/5 (fall), 11/2 (summer). *Application fee:* $40.
Advanced Placement Credit by examination available. Credit given for nursing courses completed elsewhere dependent upon specific evaluations.
Expenses (2010-11) *Tuition, state resident:* full-time $7552; part-time $207 per credit. *Tuition, nonresident:* full-time $15,962; part-time $558 per credit. *Room and board:* room only: $8000 per academic year. *Required fees:* part-time $79 per credit.
Financial Aid 56% of baccalaureate students in nursing programs received some form of financial aid in 2009-10. *Gift aid (need-based):* Federal Pell, FSEOG, state, private, college/university gift aid from institutional funds. *Loans:* Federal Direct (Subsidized and Unsubsidized Stafford PLUS), Perkins. *Work-study:* Federal Work-Study, part-time campus jobs. *Financial aid application deadline (priority):* 3/1.
Contact Kathy Miller, Staff Assistant, School of Nursing, Stony Brook University, State University of New York, Health Sciences Center, Level 2, Stony Brook, NY 11974-8240. *Telephone:* 631-444-3241. *Fax:* 631-444-3136. *E-mail:* kathy.miller@stonybrook.edu.

GRADUATE PROGRAMS

Expenses (2010-11) *Tuition, state resident:* full-time $10,701; part-time $349 per credit. *Tuition, nonresident:* full-time $16,111; part-time $574 per credit. *Room and board:* room only: $11,000 per academic year. *Required fees:* part-time $55 per credit.
Financial Aid 57% of graduate students in nursing programs received some form of financial aid in 2009-10. Fellowships, research assistantships, teaching assistantships, career-related internships or fieldwork, Federal Work-Study, institutionally sponsored loans, and traineeships available. *Financial aid application deadline:* 3/15.
Contact Dolores Bilges, Senior Staff Assistant, School of Nursing, Stony Brook University, State University of New York, Health Sciences Center, Level 2, Stony Brook, NY 11794-8240. *Telephone:* 631-444-2644. *Fax:* 631-444-3136. *E-mail:* dolores.bilges@stonybrook.edu.

MASTER'S DEGREE PROGRAM

Degree MS
Available Programs Master's; RN to Master's.
Concentrations Available Nurse-midwifery. *Clinical nurse specialist programs in:* adult health, community health, critical care, parent-child, pediatric, perinatal, psychiatric/mental health, women's health. *Nurse practitioner programs in:* adult health, neonatal health, pediatric, psychiatric/mental health, women's health.
Study Options Full-time and part-time.
Program Entrance Requirements Clinical experience, computer literacy, minimum overall college GPA of 3.0, transcript of college record, CPR certification, written essay, immunizations, interview, 3 letters of recommendation, physical assessment course, professional liability insurance/malpractice insurance, prerequisite course work, resume, statistics course. *Application deadline:* 4/1 (fall), 1/20 (summer). *Application fee:* $40.
Advanced Placement Credit given for nursing courses completed elsewhere dependent upon specific evaluations.
Degree Requirements 45 total credit hours.

POST-MASTER'S PROGRAM

Areas of Study Nurse-midwifery. *Clinical nurse specialist programs in:* adult health, community health, critical care, parent-child, pediatric, perinatal, psychiatric/mental health, women's health. *Nurse practitioner programs in:* adult health, neonatal health, pediatric, psychiatric/mental health, women's health.

DOCTORAL DEGREE PROGRAM

Degree DNP
Available Programs Doctorate.
Areas of Study Advanced practice nursing, biology of health and illness, clinical practice, ethics, health policy, health promotion/disease prevention, health-care systems, individualized study, nursing policy, nursing research.
Program Entrance Requirements Clinical experience, minimum overall college GPA of 3.0, interview by faculty committee, interview, 3 letters of recommendation, MSN or equivalent, vita, writing sample. Application deadline: 12/1 (summer). Application fee: $60.
Degree Requirements 42 total credit hours.

CONTINUING EDUCATION PROGRAM

Contact Dr. Philip Tarantino, Assistant Dean for Business Affairs, School of Nursing, Stony Brook University, State University of New York, Health Sciences Center, Level 2, Room 226, Stony Brook, NY 11794-8240. *Telephone:* 631-444-3259. *Fax:* 631-444-3136. *E-mail:* philip.tarantino@stonybrook.edu.

University at Buffalo, the State University of New York

School of Nursing
Buffalo, New York

http://nursing.buffalo.edu/
Founded in 1846

DEGREES • BS • MS • PHD

Nursing Program Faculty 60 (52% with doctorates).
Baccalaureate Enrollment 423 **Women** 91% **Men** 9% **Minority** 36% **International** 4% **Part-time** 4%
Graduate Enrollment 197 **Women** 81% **Men** 19% **Minority** 26% **International** 7.6% **Part-time** 35%
Nursing Student Activities Sigma Theta Tau, Student Nurses' Association, nursing club.
Nursing Student Resources Academic advising; academic or career counseling; assistance for students with disabilities; bookstore; campus computer network; career placement assistance; computer-assisted instruction; daycare for children of students; e-mail services; employment services for current students; externships; housing assistance; interactive nursing skills videos; Internet; learning resource lab; library services; nursing audiovisuals; paid internships; placement services for program completers; remedial services; resume preparation assistance; skills, simulation, or other laboratory; tutoring; unpaid internships.
Library Facilities 3.9 million volumes (250,000 in health, 25,000 in nursing); 79,944 periodical subscriptions (2,500 health-care related).

BACCALAUREATE PROGRAMS

Degree BS
Available Programs Accelerated Baccalaureate for Second Degree; Generic Baccalaureate.
Study Options Full-time.

Program Entrance Requirements Minimum overall college GPA of 3.0, transcript of college record, written essay, health exam, health insurance, high school chemistry, high school transcript, immunizations, minimum GPA in nursing prerequisites of 3.0, prerequisite course work. Transfer students are accepted. *Application deadline:* 2/28 (fall).

Advanced Placement Credit by examination available. Credit given for nursing courses completed elsewhere dependent upon specific evaluations.

Expenses (2010-11) *Tuition, state resident:* full-time $4970; part-time $207 per credit hour. *Tuition, nonresident:* full-time $13,380; part-time $558 per credit hour. *Room and board:* $10,442; room only: $6342 per academic year. *Required fees:* full-time $2166; part-time $95 per credit; part-time $1083 per term.

Financial Aid 80% of baccalaureate students in nursing programs received some form of financial aid in 2009-10.

Contact Dr. David J. Lang, Director of Student Affairs, School of Nursing, University at Buffalo, the State University of New York, 103 Wende Hall, 3435 Main Street, Buffalo, NY 14214. *Telephone:* 716-829-2537. *Fax:* 716-829-2067. *E-mail:* nursing@buffalo.edu.

GRADUATE PROGRAMS

Expenses (2010-11) *Tuition, state resident:* full-time $8370; part-time $349 per credit hour. *Tuition, nonresident:* full-time $13,780; part-time $574 per credit hour. *Room and board:* $11,948; room only: $7848 per academic year. *Required fees:* full-time $1608; part-time $120 per credit.

Financial Aid 65% of graduate students in nursing programs received some form of financial aid in 2009-10. 14 fellowships with full tuition reimbursements available (averaging $8,200 per year), 5 research assistantships with full tuition reimbursements available (averaging $16,794 per year), 13 teaching assistantships with full tuition reimbursements available (averaging $10,636 per year) were awarded; scholarships, traineeships, and unspecified assistantships also available. *Financial aid application deadline:* 3/15.

Contact Dr. David J. Lang, Director of Student Affairs, School of Nursing, University at Buffalo, the State University of New York, 103 Wende Hall, 3435 Main Street, Buffalo, NY 14214. *Telephone:* 716-829-2537. *Fax:* 716-829-2067. *E-mail:* nursing@buffalo.edu.

MASTER'S DEGREE PROGRAM

Degree MS

Available Programs Master's.

Concentrations Available Nurse anesthesia. *Clinical nurse specialist programs in:* adult health. *Nurse practitioner programs in:* adult health, family health, psychiatric/mental health.

Study Options Full-time and part-time.

Program Entrance Requirements Computer literacy, minimum overall college GPA of 3.0, transcript of college record, CPR certification, written essay, immunizations, interview, 3 letters of recommendation, physical assessment course, resume, statistics course, GRE General Test (if overall GPA less than 3.0). *Application deadline:* 8/15 (fall), 1/1 (spring), 4/15 (summer). *Application fee:* $75.

Advanced Placement Credit given for nursing courses completed elsewhere dependent upon specific evaluations.

Degree Requirements 45 total credit hours, thesis or project, comprehensive exam.

POST-MASTER'S PROGRAM

Areas of Study Nursing education.

DOCTORAL DEGREE PROGRAM

Degree PhD

Available Programs Doctorate.

Areas of Study Addiction/substance abuse, advanced practice nursing, aging, clinical practice, critical care, ethics, faculty preparation, family health, gerontology, health policy, health promotion/disease prevention, health-care systems, individualized study, information systems, maternity-newborn, nurse case management, nursing administration, nursing education, nursing policy, nursing research, nursing science, oncology, women's health.

Program Entrance Requirements Minimum overall college GPA of 3.25, interview, 3 letters of recommendation, MSN or equivalent, vita, writing sample, GRE General Test, MAT. Application deadline: Applications may be processed on a rolling basis for some programs. Application fee: $75.

Degree Requirements 57 total credit hours, dissertation, written exam, residency.

University of Rochester

School of Nursing
Rochester, New York

http://www.son.rochester.edu/
Founded in 1850

DEGREES • BS • DNP • MS • MSN/PHD • PHD

Nursing Program Faculty 102 (41% with doctorates).

Baccalaureate Enrollment 200 **Women** 90% **Men** 10% **Minority** 17% **International** 1% **Part-time** 43%

Graduate Enrollment 208 **Women** 92% **Men** 8% **Minority** 16% **International** 5% **Part-time** 76%

Distance Learning Courses Available.

Nursing Student Activities Sigma Theta Tau, Student Nurses' Association.

Nursing Student Resources Academic advising; academic or career counseling; assistance for students with disabilities; bookstore; campus computer network; career placement assistance; computer lab; computer-assisted instruction; e-mail services; housing assistance; interactive nursing skills videos; Internet; learning resource lab; library services; nursing audiovisuals; resume preparation assistance; skills, simulation, or other laboratory; tutoring.

Library Facilities 3.7 million volumes (240,000 in health); 27,240 periodical subscriptions (2,000 health-care related).

BACCALAUREATE PROGRAMS

Degree BS

Available Programs ADN to Baccalaureate; Accelerated Baccalaureate for Second Degree; Accelerated RN Baccalaureate; RN Baccalaureate.

Study Options Full-time.

Program Entrance Requirements Transcript of college record, CPR certification, written essay, health exam, health insurance, immunizations, 2 letters of recommendation, prerequisite course work. *Application deadline:* 7/1 (winter), 11/1 (summer). Applications may be processed on a rolling basis for some programs. *Application fee:* $50.

Advanced Placement Credit by examination available.

Financial Aid 95% of baccalaureate students in nursing programs received some form of financial aid in 2009-10. *Financial aid application deadline (priority):* 2/1.

Contact Ms. Elaine M. Andolina, Director of Admissions, School of Nursing, University of Rochester, Box SON, 601 Elmwood Avenue, Rochester, NY 14642. *Telephone:* 585-275-2375. *Fax:* 585-756-8299. *E-mail:* son_admissions@urmc.rochester.edu.

GRADUATE PROGRAMS

Financial Aid 95% of graduate students in nursing programs received some form of financial aid in 2009-10. *Financial aid application deadline:* 6/30.

Contact Ms. Elaine M. Andolina, Director of Admissions, School of Nursing, University of Rochester, Box SON, 601 Elmwood Avenue, Rochester, NY 14642. *Telephone:* 585-275-2375. *Fax:* 585-756-8299. *E-mail:* son_admissions@urmc.rochester.edu.

MASTER'S DEGREE PROGRAM

Degrees MS; MSN/PhD

Available Programs Accelerated AD/RN to Master's; Accelerated Master's for Non-Nursing College Graduates; Accelerated RN to Master's; Master's.

Concentrations Available Clinical nurse leader; health-care administration. *Nurse practitioner programs in:* acute care, adult health, family health, gerontology, neonatal health, pediatric, psychiatric/mental health.

Study Options Full-time and part-time.

Online Degree Options Yes.

Program Entrance Requirements Minimum overall college GPA of 3.0, transcript of college record, CPR certification, written essay, immunizations, interview, 2 letters of recommendation, resume, statistics course. *Application deadline:* Applications may be processed on a rolling basis for some programs. *Application fee:* $50.

Advanced Placement Credit given for nursing courses completed elsewhere dependent upon specific evaluations.

Degree Requirements 42–62 total credit hours, comprehensive exam.

POST-MASTER'S PROGRAM

Areas of Study *Nurse practitioner programs in:* acute care, adult health, family health, gerontology, neonatal health, pediatric, psychiatric/mental health.

DOCTORAL DEGREE PROGRAM

Degree DNP, PhD

Available Programs Doctorate; Post-Baccalaureate Doctorate.

Areas of Study Bio-behavioral research, nursing research.

Program Entrance Requirements Minimum overall college GPA of 3.5, interview, 3 letters of recommendation, MSN or equivalent, statistics course, vita, writing sample, GRE General Test. Application deadline: 2/1 (fall). Application fee: $50.

Degree Requirements 60 total credit hours, dissertation, oral exam, written exam, residency.

POSTDOCTORAL PROGRAM

Areas of Study Addiction/substance abuse, adolescent health, aging, cancer care, chronic illness, community health, family health, gerontology, individualized study, nursing interventions, nursing research, outcomes, vulnerable population.

Postdoctoral Program Contact Dr. Harriet Kitzman, Associate Dean for Research, School of Nursing, University of Rochester, Box SON, 601 Elmwood Avenue, Rochester, NY 14642. *Telephone:* 585-275-8874. *Fax:* 585-273-1258. *E-mail:* harriet_kitzman@urmc.rochester.edu.

CONTINUING EDUCATION PROGRAM

Contact Ms. Nadine Taylor, Administrative Assistant, Center for Lifelong Learning, School of Nursing, University of Rochester, Box SON, 601 Elmwood Avenue, Rochester, NY 14642. *Telephone:* 585-273-0446. *Fax:* 585-461-4488. *E-mail:* nadine_taylor@urmc.rochester.edu.

Utica College

Department of Nursing
Utica, New York

http://www.utica.edu/

Founded in 1946

DEGREE • BS

Nursing Program Faculty 30 (6% with doctorates).

Baccalaureate Enrollment 419 **Women** 90% **Men** 10% **Minority** 21% **International** .01% **Part-time** 40%

Distance Learning Courses Available.

Nursing Student Activities Sigma Theta Tau, Student Nurses' Association.

Nursing Student Resources Academic advising; academic or career counseling; assistance for students with disabilities; bookstore; campus computer network; career placement assistance; computer lab; computer-assisted instruction; e-mail services; employment services for current students; externships; housing assistance; interactive nursing skills videos; Internet; learning resource lab; library services; nursing audiovisuals; paid internships; placement services for program completers; remedial services; resume preparation assistance; skills, simulation, or other laboratory; tutoring; unpaid internships.

Library Facilities 17,884 volumes (2,652 in health, 1,122 in nursing); 1,480 periodical subscriptions (118 health-care related).

BACCALAUREATE PROGRAMS

Degree BS

Available Programs Generic Baccalaureate; RN Baccalaureate.

Study Options Full-time and part-time.

Online Degree Options Yes.

Program Entrance Requirements Minimum overall college GPA of 2.5, transcript of college record, written essay, health exam, health insurance, high school biology, high school chemistry, 3 years high school math, 3 years high school science, high school transcript, immunizations, 3 letters of recommendation, minimum high school GPA of 2.5, minimum high school rank 25%, minimum GPA in nursing prerequisites of 2.0. Transfer students are accepted. *Application deadline:* 1/15 (fall), 10/15 (spring). Applications may be processed on a rolling basis for some programs. *Application fee:* $40.

Advanced Placement Credit by examination available. Credit given for nursing courses completed elsewhere dependent upon specific evaluations.

Expenses (2010-11) *Tuition:* full-time $28,100; part-time $345 per credit hour. *Room and board:* $11,290; room only: $5000 per academic year. *Required fees:* full-time $165; part-time $80 per term.

Financial Aid 97% of baccalaureate students in nursing programs received some form of financial aid in 2009-10. *Gift aid (need-based):* Federal Pell, FSEOG, state, private, college/university gift aid from institutional funds, Federal Nursing. *Loans:* Federal Direct (Subsidized and Unsubsidized Stafford PLUS), Perkins. *Work-study:* Federal Work-Study, part-time campus jobs. *Financial aid application deadline (priority):* 2/15.

Contact Mr. Patrick A. Quinn, Vice President for Enrollment Management, Department of Nursing, Utica College, 1600 Burrstone Road, Utica, NY 13502-4892. *Telephone:* 315-792-3006. *Fax:* 315-792-3003. *E-mail:* pquinn@utica.edu.

Wagner College

Department of Nursing
Staten Island, New York

http://www.wagner.edu/programs/nursing.html

Founded in 1883

DEGREES • BS • MSN

Nursing Program Faculty 17 (90% with doctorates).

Baccalaureate Enrollment 60 **Women** 82% **Men** 18% **Minority** 20% **International** 10% **Part-time** 5%

Graduate Enrollment 63 **Women** 90% **Men** 10% **Minority** 10% **Part-time** 95%

Nursing Student Activities Nursing Honor Society, Sigma Theta Tau, Student Nurses' Association.

Nursing Student Resources Academic advising; academic or career counseling; assistance for students with disabilities; bookstore; campus computer network; career placement assistance; computer lab; computer-assisted instruction; e-mail services; externships; housing assistance; interactive nursing skills videos; Internet; learning resource lab; library services; nursing audiovisuals; remedial services; skills, simulation, or other laboratory; tutoring; unpaid internships.

Library Facilities 175,344 volumes (4,505 in health, 859 in nursing); 20,600 periodical subscriptions (87 health-care related).

BACCALAUREATE PROGRAMS

Degree BS

Available Programs Baccalaureate for Second Degree; Generic Baccalaureate.

Study Options Full-time.

Program Entrance Requirements Minimum overall college GPA of 3.0, written essay, health exam, health insurance, high school chemistry, high school transcript, immunizations, letters of recommendation, minimum high school GPA of 2.7, minimum GPA in nursing prerequisites of 3.0, prerequisite course work. Transfer students are accepted.

Advanced Placement Credit by examination available. Credit given for nursing courses completed elsewhere dependent upon specific evaluations.

Contact ***Telephone:*** 718-390-3452. *Fax:* 718-420-4009.

GRADUATE PROGRAMS

Contact ***Telephone:*** 718-390-3444. *Fax:* 718-420-4009.

MASTER'S DEGREE PROGRAM

Degree MSN

Concentrations Available Nursing education. *Nurse practitioner programs in:* family health.

Study Options Full-time and part-time.

Program Entrance Requirements Clinical experience, minimum overall college GPA of 2.7, transcript of college record, CPR certification, immunizations, interview, 2 letters of recommendation, nursing research course, professional liability insurance/malpractice insurance, resume.

Degree Requirements 44 total credit hours.

POST-MASTER'S PROGRAM

Areas of Study *Nurse practitioner programs in:* family health.

York College of the City University of New York
Program in Nursing
Jamaica, New York

http://www.york.cuny.edu/~healthsci/nuprogram.html
Founded in 1967

DEGREE • BS

Nursing Program Faculty 9 (20% with doctorates).

Baccalaureate Enrollment 80 **Women** 85% **Men** 15% **Minority** 80% **Part-time** 50%

Nursing Student Activities Nursing club.

Nursing Student Resources Academic advising; academic or career counseling; assistance for students with disabilities; bookstore; campus computer network; career placement assistance; computer lab; computer-assisted instruction; daycare for children of students; e-mail services; employment services for current students; Internet; library services; resume preparation assistance; skills, simulation, or other laboratory; tutoring.

Library Facilities 424,049 volumes (8,714 in health, 567 in nursing); 13,433 periodical subscriptions.

BACCALAUREATE PROGRAMS

Degree BS

Available Programs ADN to Baccalaureate; RN Baccalaureate.

Program Entrance Requirements Minimum overall college GPA of 3.0, transcript of college record, CPR certification, health exam, immunizations, minimum GPA in nursing prerequisites of 3.0, professional liability insurance/malpractice insurance, prerequisite course work, RN licensure. Transfer students are accepted.

Advanced Placement Credit by examination available. Credit given for nursing courses completed elsewhere dependent upon specific evaluations.

Contact Admissions Office, Program in Nursing, York College of the City University of New York, 94-20 Guy R. Brewer Boulevard, Jamaica, NY 11451. *Telephone:* 718-262-2165. *E-mail:* admissions@york.cuny.edu.

NORTH CAROLINA

Appalachian State University
Department of Nursing
Boone, North Carolina

http://www.nursing.appstate.edu/
Founded in 1899

DEGREE • BSN

Nursing Program Faculty 7 (86% with doctorates).

Baccalaureate Enrollment 60 **Women** 83% **Men** 17% **Minority** 5%

Nursing Student Activities Nursing Honor Society, Student Nurses' Association, nursing club.

Nursing Student Resources Academic advising; academic or career counseling; assistance for students with disabilities; bookstore; campus computer network; career placement assistance; computer lab; computer-assisted instruction; e-mail services; interactive nursing skills videos; Internet; learning resource lab; library services; nursing audiovisuals; remedial services; skills, simulation, or other laboratory; tutoring.

Library Facilities 955,717 volumes (3.2 million in health, 541,000 in nursing); 7,488 periodical subscriptions (6,764 health-care related).

BACCALAUREATE PROGRAMS

Degree BSN

Available Programs Generic Baccalaureate; RN Baccalaureate.

Site Options Boone, NC; Hickory, NC; Morganton, NC.

Study Options Full-time and part-time.

Program Entrance Requirements Minimum overall college GPA of 2.75, transcript of college record, CPR certification, health exam, immunizations, minimum GPA in nursing prerequisites of 2.5, professional liability insurance/malpractice insurance, prerequisite course work, RN licensure. Transfer students are accepted. *Application deadline:* 7/15 (fall), 4/1 (spring), 2/15 (summer). Applications may be processed on a rolling basis for some programs. *Application fee:* $50.

Expenses (2010-11) *Tuition, state resident:* full-time $5461; part-time $744 per credit. *Tuition, nonresident:* full-time $16,773; part-time $2158 per credit. *Room and board:* $2000; room only: $1850 per academic year.

Financial Aid 50% of baccalaureate students in nursing programs received some form of financial aid in 2009-10. *Gift aid (need-based):* Federal Pell, FSEOG, state, private, college/university gift aid from institutional funds. *Loans:* Perkins. *Work-study:* Federal Work-Study. *Financial aid application deadline (priority):* 3/1.

Contact Ms. Teri Goodman, Administrative Assistant, Department of Nursing, Appalachian State University, 400 University Hall Drive, Boone, NC 28608. *Telephone:* 828-262-8039. *Fax:* 828-262-8066. *E-mail:* goodmantk@appstate.edu.

Barton College
School of Nursing
Wilson, North Carolina

http://www.barton.edu/nursing
Founded in 1902

DEGREE • BSN

Nursing Program Faculty 10 (10% with doctorates).

Baccalaureate Enrollment 98 **Women** 94.8% **Men** 5.2% **Minority** 17.9% **International** 2.5% **Part-time** 3.8%

Nursing Student Activities Sigma Theta Tau, Student Nurses' Association, nursing club.

Nursing Student Resources Academic advising; academic or career counseling; assistance for students with disabilities; bookstore; campus computer network; career placement assistance; computer lab; computer-assisted instruction; e-mail services; employment services for current students; externships; interactive nursing skills videos; Internet; learning resource lab; library services; nursing audiovisuals; paid internships; placement services for program completers; remedial services; resume preparation assistance; skills, simulation, or other laboratory; tutoring; unpaid internships.

Library Facilities 3,500 volumes in health, 2,250 volumes in nursing; 100 periodical subscriptions health-care related.

BACCALAUREATE PROGRAMS

Degree BSN

Available Programs ADN to Baccalaureate; Generic Baccalaureate; RN Baccalaureate.

Study Options Full-time and part-time.

Program Entrance Requirements Minimum overall college GPA of 2.5, transcript of college record, CPR certification, health exam, health insurance, high school biology, high school chemistry, high school transcript, immunizations, minimum GPA in nursing prerequisites of 2.7, professional liability insurance/malpractice insurance, prerequisite course work. Transfer students are accepted. *Application deadline:* 11/1 (fall).

Advanced Placement Credit given for nursing courses completed elsewhere dependent upon specific evaluations.

Expenses (2010-11) *Tuition:* full-time $21,000. *Room and board:* $3500 per academic year. *Required fees:* full-time $200.

Financial Aid 92% of baccalaureate students in nursing programs received some form of financial aid in 2009-10. *Gift aid (need-based):* Federal Pell, FSEOG, state, private, college/university gift aid from institutional funds. *Loans:* Perkins, alternative loans. *Work-study:* Federal Work-Study. *Financial aid application deadline (priority):* 4/1.

Contact Ms. Joan Taylor, Department Administrator, School of Nursing, Barton College, PO Box 5000, Wilson, NC 27893-7000. *Telephone:* 252-399-6400. *Fax:* 252-399-6416. *E-mail:* jtaylor@barton.edu.

Cabarrus College of Health Sciences

Louise Harkey School of Nursing
Concord, North Carolina

http://www.cabarruscollege.edu
Founded in 1942

DEGREE • BSN

Nursing Program Faculty 3 (25% with doctorates).
Baccalaureate Enrollment 35 **Women** 90% **Men** 10% **Minority** 10% **Part-time** 50%
Distance Learning Courses Available.
Nursing Student Activities Sigma Theta Tau, Student Nurses' Association, nursing club.
Nursing Student Resources Academic advising; academic or career counseling; assistance for students with disabilities; bookstore; campus computer network; career placement assistance; computer lab; computer-assisted instruction; e-mail services; interactive nursing skills videos; Internet; library services; resume preparation assistance; skills, simulation, or other laboratory.
Library Facilities 500 volumes in health, 300 volumes in nursing; 300 periodical subscriptions health-care related.

BACCALAUREATE PROGRAMS

Degree BSN
Available Programs RN Baccalaureate.
Study Options Full-time and part-time.
Program Entrance Requirements Minimum overall college GPA of 2.5, transcript of college record, CPR certification, written essay, health exam, health insurance, 4 years high school math, immunizations, 2 letters of recommendation, RN licensure. Transfer students are accepted. *Application deadline:* 5/1 (fall), 10/1 (spring). Applications may be processed on a rolling basis for some programs. *Application fee:* $35.
Advanced Placement Credit by examination available.
Contact ***Telephone:*** 704-403-1756. *Fax:* 704-403-2077.

Duke University

School of Nursing
Durham, North Carolina

http://www.nursing.duke.edu
Founded in 1838

DEGREES • BSN • MSN • MSN/MBA • PHD

Nursing Program Faculty 48 (71% with doctorates).
Baccalaureate Enrollment 138 **Women** 88% **Men** 12% **Minority** 11% **International** 1%
Graduate Enrollment 360 **Women** 85% **Men** 15% **Minority** 13% **International** 1% **Part-time** 68%
Distance Learning Courses Available.
Nursing Student Activities Sigma Theta Tau, Student Nurses' Association.
Nursing Student Resources Academic advising; academic or career counseling; assistance for students with disabilities; bookstore; campus computer network; career placement assistance; computer lab; computer-assisted instruction; e-mail services; Internet; library services; nursing audiovisuals; skills, simulation, or other laboratory.
Library Facilities 6 million volumes (280,606 in health, 12,366 in nursing); 62,639 periodical subscriptions (3,948 health-care related).

BACCALAUREATE PROGRAMS

Degree BSN
Available Programs Accelerated Baccalaureate for Second Degree.
Site Options Durham, NC.
Study Options Full-time.
Program Entrance Requirements Minimum overall college GPA of 3.0, transcript of college record, CPR certification, written essay, health exam, health insurance, immunizations, interview, 3 letters of recommendation, prerequisite course work. *Application deadline:* 1/1 (fall). *Application fee:* $50.
Contact ***Telephone:*** 919-684-9161. *Fax:* 919-668-4693.

GRADUATE PROGRAMS

Contact ***Telephone:*** 919-684-9163. *Fax:* 919-668-4693.

MASTER'S DEGREE PROGRAM

Degrees MSN; MSN/MBA
Available Programs Master's; RN to Master's.
Concentrations Available Health-care administration; nurse anesthesia; nurse case management; nursing administration; nursing education; nursing informatics. *Clinical nurse specialist programs in:* critical care, gerontology, maternity-newborn, oncology, pediatric. *Nurse practitioner programs in:* acute care, adult health, family health, gerontology, neonatal health, oncology, pediatric, primary care.
Site Options Durham, NC.
Study Options Full-time and part-time.
Online Degree Options Yes.
Program Entrance Requirements Clinical experience, computer literacy, minimum overall college GPA of 3.0, transcript of college record, CPR certification, written essay, immunizations, interview, 3 letters of recommendation, prerequisite course work, resume, statistics course, GRE General Test. *Application deadline:* 7/1 (fall), 12/1 (spring), 4/1 (summer). Applications may be processed on a rolling basis for some programs. *Application fee:* $50.
Advanced Placement Credit given for nursing courses completed elsewhere dependent upon specific evaluations.
Degree Requirements 39 total credit hours.

POST-MASTER'S PROGRAM

Areas of Study Health-care administration; nurse anesthesia; nurse case management; nursing administration; nursing education; nursing informatics. *Clinical nurse specialist programs in:* critical care, gerontology, maternity-newborn, oncology, pediatric. *Nurse practitioner programs in:* acute care, adult health, family health, gerontology, neonatal health, oncology, pediatric, primary care.

DOCTORAL DEGREE PROGRAM

Degree PhD
Available Programs Doctorate; Post-Baccalaureate Doctorate.
Areas of Study Health-care systems, illness and transition.
Site Options Durham, NC.
Program Entrance Requirements Minimum overall college GPA of 3.5, interview by faculty committee, interview, 3 letters of recommendation, MSN or equivalent, statistics course, vita. Application deadline: 12/15 (fall). Application fee: $75.
Degree Requirements 54 total credit hours, dissertation, oral exam.

See full description on page 470.

East Carolina University

College of Nursing
Greenville, North Carolina

http://www.nursing.ecu.edu/
Founded in 1907

DEGREES • BSN • MSN • PHD

Nursing Program Faculty 104 (40% with doctorates).
Baccalaureate Enrollment 628 **Women** 90.6% **Men** 9.4% **Minority** 13.4% **International** .4% **Part-time** 16.2%
Graduate Enrollment 559 **Women** 90.8% **Men** 9.2% **Minority** 14.6% **Part-time** 73.2%
Distance Learning Courses Available.
Nursing Student Activities Nursing Honor Society, Sigma Theta Tau, Student Nurses' Association.
Nursing Student Resources Academic advising; academic or career counseling; assistance for students with disabilities; bookstore; campus computer network; career placement assistance; computer lab; computer-assisted instruction; e-mail services; employment services for current students; externships; housing assistance; interactive nursing skills videos; Internet; learning resource lab; library services; nursing audiovisuals; remedial services; resume preparation assistance; skills, simulation, or other laboratory; tutoring; unpaid internships.
Library Facilities 135,271 volumes in health, 4,000 volumes in nursing; 16,000 periodical subscriptions health-care related.

BACCALAUREATE PROGRAMS

Degree BSN
Available Programs ADN to Baccalaureate; Generic Baccalaureate.

Study Options Full-time.
Online Degree Options Yes.
Program Entrance Requirements Minimum overall college GPA of 2.5, transcript of college record, CPR certification, health exam, health insurance, immunizations, professional liability insurance/malpractice insurance, prerequisite course work. Transfer students are accepted. *Application deadline:* 2/1 (fall), 9/1 (spring).
Advanced Placement Credit given for nursing courses completed elsewhere dependent upon specific evaluations.
Expenses (2010-11) *Tuition, state resident:* full-time $4885; part-time $2443 per semester. *Tuition, nonresident:* full-time $16,871; part-time $8436 per semester. *Room and board:* $7950; room only: $5130 per academic year.
Financial Aid 60% of baccalaureate students in nursing programs received some form of financial aid in 2009-10. *Gift aid (need-based):* Federal Pell, FSEOG, state, private, college/university gift aid from institutional funds, Federal Nursing. *Loans:* Federal Nursing Student Loans, Perkins, state. *Work-study:* Federal Work-Study, part-time campus jobs. *Financial aid application deadline (priority):* 3/1.
Contact Ms. Erin Rogers, Executive Director of Student Services, College of Nursing, East Carolina University, Health Sciences Building, Suite 2150, Greenville, NC 27858-4353. *Telephone:* 252-744-6477. *Fax:* 252-744-6391. *E-mail:* ecunursestudentsvc@ecu.edu.

GRADUATE PROGRAMS

Expenses (2010-11) *Tuition, state resident:* full-time $4601; part-time $2300 per semester. *Tuition, nonresident:* full-time $14,917; part-time $7459 per semester. *Room and board:* $7950; room only: $5130 per academic year.
Financial Aid 45% of graduate students in nursing programs received some form of financial aid in 2009-10. Research assistantships with partial tuition reimbursements available, teaching assistantships with partial tuition reimbursements available, Federal Work-Study available. Aid available to part-time students. *Financial aid application deadline:* 6/1.
Contact Ms. Erin Rogers, Executive Director of Student Services, College of Nursing, East Carolina University, Health Sciences Building, Room 2150, Greenville, NC 27858-4353. *Telephone:* 252-744-6477. *Fax:* 252-744-6391. *E-mail:* rogerse@ecu.edu.

MASTER'S DEGREE PROGRAM

Degree MSN
Available Programs Accelerated Master's for Non-Nursing College Graduates; Accelerated Master's for Nurses with Non-Nursing Degrees; Master's; RN to Master's.
Concentrations Available Nurse anesthesia; nurse-midwifery; nursing administration; nursing education. *Clinical nurse specialist programs in:* adult health. *Nurse practitioner programs in:* adult health, family health, neonatal health.
Study Options Full-time and part-time.
Online Degree Options Yes.
Program Entrance Requirements Clinical experience, computer literacy, minimum overall college GPA of 3.0, transcript of college record, CPR certification, written essay, immunizations, interview, 3 letters of recommendation, nursing research course, professional liability insurance/malpractice insurance, prerequisite course work, statistics course, GRE General Test or MAT. *Application deadline:* Applications may be processed on a rolling basis for some programs.
Advanced Placement Credit given for nursing courses completed elsewhere dependent upon specific evaluations.
Degree Requirements Comprehensive exam.

POST-MASTER'S PROGRAM

Areas of Study Nurse anesthesia; nurse-midwifery; nursing administration; nursing education. *Clinical nurse specialist programs in:* adult health. *Nurse practitioner programs in:* adult health, family health, neonatal health.

DOCTORAL DEGREE PROGRAM

Degree PhD
Available Programs Doctorate; Post-Baccalaureate Doctorate.
Areas of Study Nursing science.
Program Entrance Requirements Minimum overall college GPA of 3.2, interview by faculty committee, interview, 3 letters of recommendation, MSN or equivalent, scholarly papers, statistics course, vita, writing sample. Application deadline: 3/1 (fall).
Degree Requirements 54 total credit hours, dissertation, oral exam, written exam.

Gardner-Webb University

School of Nursing
Boiling Springs, North Carolina

http://www.nursing.gardner-webb.edu/index.html
Founded in 1905

DEGREES • BSN • MSN • MSN/MBA
Nursing Student Activities Nursing Honor Society, Student Nurses' Association.
Library Facilities 238,861 volumes; 28,797 periodical subscriptions.

BACCALAUREATE PROGRAMS

Degree BSN
Available Programs RN Baccalaureate.
Site Options Statesville, NC; Charlotte, NC; Cabarrus, NC.
Study Options Full-time and part-time.
Program Entrance Requirements Minimum overall college GPA of 2.5, transcript of college record, minimum GPA in nursing prerequisites of 2.5, prerequisite course work, RN licensure. Transfer students are accepted.
Contact ***Telephone:*** 704-406-4360. *Fax:* 704-406-3919.

GRADUATE PROGRAMS

Contact ***Telephone:*** 704-406-4358. *Fax:* 704-406-3919.

MASTER'S DEGREE PROGRAM

Degrees MSN; MSN/MBA
Available Programs Master's; RN to Master's.
Concentrations Available Nursing administration; nursing education.
Program Entrance Requirements Minimum overall college GPA of 2.7, transcript of college record, immunizations, 3 letters of recommendation, statistics course.
Degree Requirements 30 total credit hours.

Lees-McRae College

Nursing Program
Banner Elk, North Carolina

http://www.lmc.edu/sites/Academics/OffCampusPrograms/nursing.htm
Founded in 1900

DEGREE • BSN
Nursing Program Faculty 3
Baccalaureate Enrollment 51 **Women** 88% **Men** 12% **Minority** 2% **International** 2%
Distance Learning Courses Available.
Nursing Student Resources Academic advising; academic or career counseling; bookstore; computer lab; computer-assisted instruction; e-mail services; Internet; learning resource lab; library services; nursing audiovisuals; skills, simulation, or other laboratory.

BACCALAUREATE PROGRAMS

Degree BSN
Available Programs ADN to Baccalaureate.
Site Options Spruce Pine, NC.
Study Options Full-time.
Program Entrance Requirements Transcript of college record, immunizations, 2 letters of recommendation, RN licensure. Transfer students are accepted. *Application deadline:* Applications may be processed on a rolling basis for some programs.
Financial Aid 100% of baccalaureate students in nursing programs received some form of financial aid in 2008-09. *Gift aid (need-based):* Federal Pell, FSEOG, state, private, college/university gift aid from institutional funds. *Loans:* Perkins, state, college/university. *Work-study:* Federal Work-Study, part-time campus jobs. *Financial aid application deadline:* Continuous.
Contact Ms. Martha P. Hartley, RN, Director of RN to BSN Completion Program, Nursing Program, Lees-McRae College, 375 College Drive, PO Box 128, Banner Elk, NC 28604. *Telephone:* 828-898-8752. *Fax:* 866-774-4280. *E-mail:* Hartley@lmc.edu.

Lenoir-Rhyne University

Program in Nursing
Hickory, North Carolina

http://nur.lr.edu/
Founded in 1891

DEGREE • BS

Nursing Program Faculty 30 (4% with doctorates).
Baccalaureate Enrollment 122 **Women** 90% **Men** 10% **Minority** 11% **International** 2%
Distance Learning Courses Available.
Nursing Student Activities Sigma Theta Tau, Student Nurses' Association.
Nursing Student Resources Academic advising; academic or career counseling; assistance for students with disabilities; bookstore; campus computer network; career placement assistance; computer lab; computer-assisted instruction; e-mail services; employment services for current students; externships; housing assistance; interactive nursing skills videos; Internet; learning resource lab; library services; nursing audiovisuals; placement services for program completers; remedial services; resume preparation assistance; skills, simulation, or other laboratory; tutoring; unpaid internships.
Library Facilities 275,961 volumes (5,000 in health, 4,200 in nursing); 445 periodical subscriptions (220 health-care related).

BACCALAUREATE PROGRAMS

Degree BS
Available Programs ADN to Baccalaureate; Generic Baccalaureate.
Study Options Full-time and part-time.
Program Entrance Requirements Minimum overall college GPA of 3.0, transcript of college record, CPR certification, written essay, health exam, high school chemistry, high school foreign language, 3 years high school math, high school transcript, immunizations, minimum high school GPA of 3.0, minimum GPA in nursing prerequisites of 2.7, prerequisite course work. Transfer students are accepted. *Application deadline:* 3/1 (fall), 4/1 (summer). Applications may be processed on a rolling basis for some programs. *Application fee:* $35.
Advanced Placement Credit by examination available. Credit given for nursing courses completed elsewhere dependent upon specific evaluations.
Expenses (2010-11) *Tuition:* full-time $12,645; part-time $395 per credit hour. *Room and board:* $4465 per academic year. *Required fees:* full-time $250.
Financial Aid 100% of baccalaureate students in nursing programs received some form of financial aid in 2009-10.
Contact Dr. Kerry C. Thompson, Chair, School of Nursing, Program in Nursing, Lenoir-Rhyne University, PO Box 7292, Hickory, NC 28603. *Telephone:* 828-328-7282. *Fax:* 828-328-7284. *E-mail:* thompsonk@lr.edu.

North Carolina Agricultural and Technical State University

School of Nursing
Greensboro, North Carolina

http://www.ncat.edu/~nursing/index.html
Founded in 1891

DEGREE • BSN

Nursing Program Faculty 28 (32% with doctorates).
Baccalaureate Enrollment 418 **Women** 99% **Men** 1% **Minority** 91% **Part-time** 1%
Distance Learning Courses Available.
Nursing Student Activities Nursing Honor Society, Sigma Theta Tau, Student Nurses' Association, nursing club.
Nursing Student Resources Academic advising; academic or career counseling; assistance for students with disabilities; bookstore; campus computer network; career placement assistance; computer lab; computer-assisted instruction; e-mail services; employment services for current students; externships; housing assistance; interactive nursing skills videos; Internet; learning resource lab; library services; nursing audiovisuals; other; paid internships; placement services for program completers; remedial services; resume preparation assistance; skills, simulation, or other laboratory; tutoring; unpaid internships.
Library Facilities 597,093 volumes (19,510 in health, 3,232 in nursing); 40,425 periodical subscriptions (85 health-care related).

BACCALAUREATE PROGRAMS

Degree BSN
Available Programs Generic Baccalaureate; LPN to Baccalaureate; LPN to RN Baccalaureate; RN Baccalaureate.
Site Options Greensboro, NC.
Study Options Full-time and part-time.
Program Entrance Requirements Minimum overall college GPA of 2.8, transcript of college record, CPR certification, written essay, health exam, health insurance, high school biology, high school foreign language, 3 years high school math, 3 years high school science, high school transcript, immunizations, minimum high school GPA of 3.0, minimum GPA in nursing prerequisites of 2.8, professional liability insurance/malpractice insurance, prerequisite course work. Transfer students are accepted. *Application deadline:* 2/15 (spring). *Application fee:* $45.
Advanced Placement Credit by examination available. Credit given for nursing courses completed elsewhere dependent upon specific evaluations.
Contact *Telephone:* 336-334-7752. *Fax:* 336-334-7637.

North Carolina Central University

Department of Nursing
Durham, North Carolina

http://www.nccu.edu/artsci/nursing/
Founded in 1910

DEGREE • BSN

Nursing Program Faculty 30 (4% with doctorates).
Nursing Student Activities Sigma Theta Tau.
Nursing Student Resources Academic advising; academic or career counseling; assistance for students with disabilities; bookstore; campus computer network; career placement assistance; computer lab; computer-assisted instruction; e-mail services; employment services for current students; externships; housing assistance; interactive nursing skills videos; Internet; learning resource lab; library services; nursing audiovisuals; paid internships; placement services for program completers; resume preparation assistance; skills, simulation, or other laboratory; tutoring.
Library Facilities 2,027 periodical subscriptions.

BACCALAUREATE PROGRAMS

Degree BSN
Available Programs Generic Baccalaureate.
Study Options Full-time.
Program Entrance Requirements Minimum overall college GPA of 2.0, transcript of college record, health exam, immunizations, minimum GPA in nursing prerequisites of 2.5, professional liability insurance/malpractice insurance, prerequisite course work. Transfer students are accepted.
Advanced Placement Credit given for nursing courses completed elsewhere dependent upon specific evaluations.
Contact *Telephone:* 919-530-5336. *Fax:* 919-530-5343.

Queens University of Charlotte

Presbyterian School of Nursing
Charlotte, North Carolina

http://www.queens.edu/nursing/
Founded in 1857

DEGREES • BSN • MSN • MSN/MBA

Nursing Program Faculty 60 (20% with doctorates).
Baccalaureate Enrollment 260 **Women** 95% **Men** 5% **Minority** 25% **International** 5% **Part-time** 10%
Graduate Enrollment 55 **Women** 95% **Men** 5% **Minority** 25% **International** 5% **Part-time** 50%
Distance Learning Courses Available.
Nursing Student Activities Nursing Honor Society, Sigma Theta Tau, Student Nurses' Association.
Nursing Student Resources Academic advising; academic or career counseling; assistance for students with disabilities; bookstore; campus

computer network; career placement assistance; computer lab; computer-assisted instruction; e-mail services; employment services for current students; externships; housing assistance; interactive nursing skills videos; Internet; learning resource lab; library services; nursing audiovisuals; placement services for program completers; remedial services; resume preparation assistance; skills, simulation, or other laboratory; tutoring; unpaid internships.

Library Facilities 126,242 volumes (1,703 in health, 713 in nursing); 592 periodical subscriptions (516 health-care related).

BACCALAUREATE PROGRAMS

Degree BSN

Available Programs ADN to Baccalaureate; Accelerated Baccalaureate; Accelerated Baccalaureate for Second Degree; Baccalaureate for Second Degree; Generic Baccalaureate; RN Baccalaureate.

Site Options Charlotte, NC.

Study Options Full-time.

Online Degree Options Yes.

Program Entrance Requirements Minimum overall college GPA of 2.5, transcript of college record, CPR certification, written essay, health exam, health insurance, high school biology, high school chemistry, 2 years high school math, 1 year of high school science, high school transcript, immunizations, minimum high school GPA of 3.0, minimum GPA in nursing prerequisites of 2.5, prerequisite course work. Transfer students are accepted. *Application deadline:* 3/15 (fall), 9/21 (spring). *Application fee:* $40.

Advanced Placement Credit given for nursing courses completed elsewhere dependent upon specific evaluations.

Expenses (2010-11) *Tuition:* full-time $23,752; part-time $425 per credit hour. *Room and board:* $8608 per academic year.

Financial Aid 85% of baccalaureate students in nursing programs received some form of financial aid in 2009-10.

Contact Danielle Dupree, Director of Admissions, Presbyterian School of Nursing, Queens University of Charlotte, 1900 Selwyn Avenue, Charlotte, NC 28274. *Telephone:* 704-688-2780. *Fax:* 704-714-1027. *E-mail:* dupreed@queens.edu.

GRADUATE PROGRAMS

Expenses (2010-11) *Tuition:* part-time $425 per credit hour.

Financial Aid 25% of graduate students in nursing programs received some form of financial aid in 2009-10.

Contact Dr. Janice Janken, Chair and Professor, Presbyterian School of Nursing, Queens University of Charlotte, 1900 Selwyn Avenue, Charlotte, NC 28274. *Telephone:* 704-337-2382. *Fax:* 704-337-2477. *E-mail:* jankenj@queens.edu.

MASTER'S DEGREE PROGRAM

Degrees MSN; MSN/MBA

Available Programs Master's; RN to Master's.

Concentrations Available Clinical nurse leader; nursing administration; nursing education.

Site Options Charlotte, NC.

Study Options Full-time and part-time.

Program Entrance Requirements Minimum overall college GPA of 3.0, transcript of college record, 2 letters of recommendation, professional liability insurance/malpractice insurance, resume. *Application deadline:* Applications may be processed on a rolling basis for some programs. *Application fee:* $40.

Advanced Placement Credit given for nursing courses completed elsewhere dependent upon specific evaluations.

Degree Requirements 36 total credit hours, thesis or project.

CONTINUING EDUCATION PROGRAM

Contact Heather Roberts, Coordinator of Nursing and Health Programs, Presbyterian School of Nursing, Queens University of Charlotte, 1900 Selwyn Avenue, Center for Lifelong Learning, Charlotte, NC 28274. *Telephone:* 704-337-2491. *E-mail:* robertsh@queens.edu.

The University of North Carolina at Chapel Hill

School of Nursing
Chapel Hill, North Carolina

http://nursing.unc.edu/

Founded in 1789

DEGREES • BSN • MSN • PHD

Baccalaureate Enrollment 376 **Women** 86.7% **Men** 13.3% **Minority** 28.5% **International** 1.3% **Part-time** 6.1%

Graduate Enrollment 294 **Women** 93.5% **Men** 6.5% **Minority** 69.1% **International** 3.7% **Part-time** 50.7%

Distance Learning Courses Available.

Nursing Student Activities Sigma Theta Tau, Student Nurses' Association, nursing club.

Nursing Student Resources Academic advising; academic or career counseling; assistance for students with disabilities; bookstore; campus computer network; career placement assistance; computer lab; computer-assisted instruction; daycare for children of students; e-mail services; employment services for current students; housing assistance; interactive nursing skills videos; Internet; learning resource lab; library services; nursing audiovisuals; other; remedial services; resume preparation assistance; skills, simulation, or other laboratory; tutoring.

Library Facilities 6.7 million volumes; 80,132 periodical subscriptions.

BACCALAUREATE PROGRAMS

Degree BSN

Available Programs ADN to Baccalaureate; Accelerated Baccalaureate for Second Degree; Generic Baccalaureate; RN Baccalaureate.

Study Options Full-time.

Online Degree Options Yes (online only).

Program Entrance Requirements Minimum overall college GPA, transcript of college record, CPR certification, written essay, health exam, health insurance, high school transcript, immunizations, minimum GPA in nursing prerequisites of 2.5, professional liability insurance/malpractice insurance, prerequisite course work. Transfer students are accepted. *Application deadline:* 8/10 (spring), 12/22 (summer). *Application fee:* $77.

Advanced Placement Credit by examination available. Credit given for nursing courses completed elsewhere dependent upon specific evaluations.

Expenses (2010-11) *Tuition, state resident:* full-time $4815. *Tuition, nonresident:* full-time $23,430. *Room and board:* $9306; room only: $5408 per academic year. *Required fees:* full-time $925.

Contact Ms. Amy Burdette, Assistant Director for Undergraduate Admissions, School of Nursing, The University of North Carolina at Chapel Hill, CB #7460, Chapel Hill, NC 27599-7460. *Telephone:* 919-966-4260. *Fax:* 919-966-3540. *E-mail:* amy_burdette@unc.edu.

GRADUATE PROGRAMS

Expenses (2010-11) *Tuition, state resident:* full-time $6363. *Tuition, nonresident:* full-time $21,093. *Room and board:* $14,714; room only: $10,816 per academic year. *Required fees:* full-time $1834; part-time $917 per term.

Financial Aid 8 fellowships, 6 research assistantships (averaging $8,000 per year), 10 teaching assistantships (averaging $8,000 per year) were awarded; scholarships, traineeships, and unspecified assistantships also available.

Contact Ms. Jennifer Moore, Admissions Counselor for Graduate Program and RN Options, School of Nursing, The University of North Carolina at Chapel Hill, CB #7460, Chapel Hill, NC 27599-7460. *Telephone:* 919-966-4260. *Fax:* 919-966-3540. *E-mail:* jennifer.j.moore@unc.edu.

MASTER'S DEGREE PROGRAM

Degree MSN

Available Programs Master's; Master's for Nurses with Non-Nursing Degrees; RN to Master's.

Concentrations Available Clinical nurse leader; nurse case management; nursing administration; nursing education; nursing informatics. *Clinical nurse specialist programs in:* psychiatric/mental health. *Nurse practitioner programs in:* adult health, family health, gerontology, oncology, pediatric, primary care, psychiatric/mental health, women's health.

Study Options Full-time and part-time.

Program Entrance Requirements Clinical experience, minimum overall college GPA of 3.0, transcript of college record, CPR certification, written essay, immunizations, 3 letters of recommendation, physical assessment course, professional liability insurance/malpractice insurance, resume, statistics course, GRE General Test. *Application deadline:* 1/15 (fall), 10/1 (spring). *Application fee:* $77.
Advanced Placement Credit given for nursing courses completed elsewhere dependent upon specific evaluations.
Degree Requirements 40 total credit hours, thesis or project, comprehensive exam.

POST-MASTER'S PROGRAM

Areas of Study Clinical nurse leader; nurse case management; nursing administration; nursing education; nursing informatics. *Clinical nurse specialist programs in:* psychiatric/mental health. *Nurse practitioner programs in:* adult health, family health, gerontology, oncology, pediatric, primary care, psychiatric/mental health, women's health.

DOCTORAL DEGREE PROGRAM

Degree PhD
Available Programs Doctorate; Post-Baccalaureate Doctorate.
Areas of Study Addiction/substance abuse, advanced practice nursing, aging, bio-behavioral research, biology of health and illness, clinical practice, community health, critical care, ethics, family health, forensic nursing, gerontology, health policy, health promotion/disease prevention, health-care systems, human health and illness, illness and transition, individualized study, information systems, maternity-newborn, neurobehavior, nurse case management, nursing administration, nursing education, nursing policy, nursing research, nursing science, oncology, urban health, women's health.
Program Entrance Requirements Minimum overall college GPA of 3.0, interview by faculty committee, 3 letters of recommendation, scholarly papers, statistics course, vita, writing sample, GRE General Test. Application deadline: 1/3 (fall), 10/1 (spring). Applications may be processed on a rolling basis for some programs. Application fee: $77.
Degree Requirements 48 total credit hours, dissertation, oral exam, written exam, residency.

POSTDOCTORAL PROGRAM

Areas of Study Addiction/substance abuse, adolescent health, aging, cancer care, chronic illness, community health, family health, gerontology, health promotion/disease prevention, individualized study, infection prevention/skin care, information systems, neuro-behavior, nursing informatics, nursing interventions, nursing research, nursing science, outcomes, self-care, vulnerable population, women's health.
Postdoctoral Program Contact Dr. Merle Mishel, Professor, School of Nursing, The University of North Carolina at Chapel Hill, 1002 Carrington Hall, CB #7460, Chapel Hill, NC 27599-7460. *Telephone:* 919-966-5294. *Fax:* 919-966-3540. *E-mail:* mishel@email.unc.edu.

CONTINUING EDUCATION PROGRAM

Contact Dr. Sonda Oppewal, Director, Center for Lifelong Learning, School of Nursing, The University of North Carolina at Chapel Hill, L400 Carrington Hall, CB #7460, Chapel Hill, NC 27599-7460. *Telephone:* 919-966-3638. *Fax:* 919-966-7298. *E-mail:* oppewal@email.unc.edu.

The University of North Carolina at Charlotte

School of Nursing
Charlotte, North Carolina

http://www.health.uncc.edu
Founded in 1946

DEGREES • BSN • MSN
Nursing Program Faculty 51 (50% with doctorates).
Baccalaureate Enrollment 330 **Women** 92% **Men** 8% **Minority** 8% **Part-time** 5%
Graduate Enrollment 200 **Women** 80% **Men** 20% **Minority** 10% **Part-time** 65%
Distance Learning Courses Available.
Nursing Student Activities Sigma Theta Tau, Student Nurses' Association.
Nursing Student Resources Academic advising; academic or career counseling; assistance for students with disabilities; bookstore; campus computer network; career placement assistance; computer lab; computer-assisted instruction; e-mail services; externships; interactive nursing skills videos; Internet; learning resource lab; library services; nursing audiovisuals; resume preparation assistance; skills, simulation, or other laboratory; tutoring.
Library Facilities 1.1 million volumes (39,000 in health, 2,400 in nursing); 52,621 periodical subscriptions (160 health-care related).

BACCALAUREATE PROGRAMS

Degree BSN
Available Programs ADN to Baccalaureate; Generic Baccalaureate; RN Baccalaureate.
Study Options Full-time.
Program Entrance Requirements Minimum overall college GPA of 2.5, transcript of college record, CPR certification, written essay, health exam, health insurance, high school biology, high school chemistry, high school foreign language, 3 years high school math, 3 years high school science, high school transcript, immunizations, 3 letters of recommendation, minimum GPA in nursing prerequisites of 2.5, prerequisite course work. Transfer students are accepted. *Application deadline:* 1/31 (fall), 8/31 (winter).
Contact *Telephone:* 704-687-4676. *Fax:* 704-687-3180.

GRADUATE PROGRAMS

Contact *Telephone:* 704-687-7992. *Fax:* 704-687-6017.

MASTER'S DEGREE PROGRAM

Degree MSN
Available Programs Master's; RN to Master's.
Concentrations Available Nurse anesthesia; nursing administration; nursing education. *Clinical nurse specialist programs in:* community health. *Nurse practitioner programs in:* adult health, family health.
Study Options Full-time and part-time.
Online Degree Options Yes.
Program Entrance Requirements Clinical experience, computer literacy, minimum overall college GPA of 3.0, transcript of college record, CPR certification, written essay, immunizations, interview, 3 letters of recommendation, nursing research course, professional liability insurance/malpractice insurance, resume, statistics course.

POST-MASTER'S PROGRAM

Areas of Study Nurse anesthesia; nursing administration; nursing education. *Nurse practitioner programs in:* family health.

The University of North Carolina at Greensboro

School of Nursing
Greensboro, North Carolina

http://www.uncg.edu/nur/
Founded in 1891

DEGREES • BSN • MSN • MSN/MBA • PHD
Nursing Program Faculty 60 (60% with doctorates).
Baccalaureate Enrollment 1,138 **Women** 93% **Men** 7% **Minority** 29% **International** 4% **Part-time** 33%
Graduate Enrollment 275 **Women** 80% **Men** 20% **Minority** 18% **International** 4% **Part-time** 30%
Nursing Student Activities Nursing Honor Society, Sigma Theta Tau, Student Nurses' Association.
Nursing Student Resources Academic advising; academic or career counseling; assistance for students with disabilities; bookstore; campus computer network; career placement assistance; computer lab; computer-assisted instruction; e-mail services; externships; Internet; learning resource lab; library services; nursing audiovisuals; paid internships; placement services for program completers; remedial services; resume preparation assistance; skills, simulation, or other laboratory; tutoring; unpaid internships.
Library Facilities 2 million volumes; 4,648 periodical subscriptions.

BACCALAUREATE PROGRAMS

Degree BSN
Available Programs ADN to Baccalaureate; Baccalaureate for Second Degree; Generic Baccalaureate; LPN to Baccalaureate; LPN to RN Baccalaureate; RN Baccalaureate.
Site Options Hickory, NC; Greensboro, NC.

Study Options Full-time.
Program Entrance Requirements Minimum overall college GPA of 2.7, transcript of college record, CPR certification, health exam, immunizations, minimum GPA in nursing prerequisites of 3.0, professional liability insurance/malpractice insurance, prerequisite course work. Transfer students are accepted.
Contact ***Telephone:*** 336-334-5280. *Fax:* 336-334-3628.

GRADUATE PROGRAMS

Contact ***Telephone:*** 336-334-5561. *Fax:* 336-334-3628.

MASTER'S DEGREE PROGRAM

Degrees MSN; MSN/MBA
Available Programs Master's.
Concentrations Available Nurse anesthesia; nursing administration; nursing education. *Nurse practitioner programs in:* adult health, gerontology.
Site Options Hickory, NC.
Study Options Full-time and part-time.
Program Entrance Requirements Clinical experience, minimum overall college GPA of 3.0, transcript of college record, CPR certification, immunizations, 3 letters of recommendation, physical assessment course, professional liability insurance/malpractice insurance, prerequisite course work, statistics course, GRE General Test or MAT.
Advanced Placement Credit given for nursing courses completed elsewhere dependent upon specific evaluations.
Degree Requirements 36 total credit hours, thesis or project, comprehensive exam.

POST-MASTER'S PROGRAM

Areas of Study Nurse anesthesia. *Nurse practitioner programs in:* adult health, gerontology.

DOCTORAL DEGREE PROGRAM

Degree PhD
Available Programs Doctorate.
Areas of Study Aging, faculty preparation, gerontology, health policy, health promotion/disease prevention, nursing administration, nursing education, nursing research, nursing science, women's health.
Program Entrance Requirements Minimum overall college GPA of 3.0, interview by faculty committee, interview, 3 letters of recommendation, MSN or equivalent, writing sample.
Degree Requirements 57 total credit hours, dissertation, oral exam, written exam, residency.

The University of North Carolina at Pembroke

Nursing Program
Pembroke, North Carolina

Founded in 1887

DEGREE • BSN

Nursing Program Faculty 20 (5% with doctorates).
Baccalaureate Enrollment 139
Distance Learning Courses Available.
Nursing Student Activities Student Nurses' Association.
Nursing Student Resources Academic advising; academic or career counseling; assistance for students with disabilities; bookstore; campus computer network; computer lab; computer-assisted instruction; e-mail services; housing assistance; interactive nursing skills videos; Internet; learning resource lab; library services; nursing audiovisuals; remedial services; resume preparation assistance; skills, simulation, or other laboratory; tutoring.
Library Facilities 367,565 volumes; 48,331 periodical subscriptions.

BACCALAUREATE PROGRAMS

Degree BSN
Available Programs Generic Baccalaureate; RN Baccalaureate.
Site Options Southern Pines, NC; Fayetteville, NC; Hamlet, NC.
Study Options Full-time.
Program Entrance Requirements Minimum overall college GPA, health exam, minimum GPA in nursing prerequisites, prerequisite course work, RN licensure. Transfer students are accepted. *Application deadline:* 1/15 (spring).
Advanced Placement Credit given for nursing courses completed elsewhere dependent upon specific evaluations.
Contact ***Telephone:*** 910-521-6522. *Fax:* 910-521-6178.

The University of North Carolina Wilmington

School of Nursing
Wilmington, North Carolina

http://www.uncw.edu/son
Founded in 1947

DEGREES • BS • MSN

Nursing Program Faculty 36 (47% with doctorates).
Baccalaureate Enrollment 264 **Women** 89% **Men** 11% **Minority** 11% **International** 9% **Part-time** 19%
Graduate Enrollment 74 **Women** 97% **Men** 3% **Minority** 27% **Part-time** 49%
Distance Learning Courses Available.
Nursing Student Activities Sigma Theta Tau, Student Nurses' Association.
Nursing Student Resources Academic advising; academic or career counseling; assistance for students with disabilities; bookstore; campus computer network; career placement assistance; computer lab; computer-assisted instruction; e-mail services; employment services for current students; externships; housing assistance; interactive nursing skills videos; Internet; learning resource lab; library services; nursing audiovisuals; remedial services; resume preparation assistance; skills, simulation, or other laboratory; tutoring; unpaid internships.
Library Facilities 1.1 million volumes (18,288 in health, 917 in nursing); 30,000 periodical subscriptions (2,681 health-care related).

BACCALAUREATE PROGRAMS

Degree BS
Available Programs Generic Baccalaureate; RN Baccalaureate.
Site Options Burgaw, Bolton, Southport, Whiteville, NC; Jacksonville, Supply, Elizabethtown, Kenansville , NC.
Study Options Full-time.
Online Degree Options Yes.
Program Entrance Requirements Minimum overall college GPA of 2.5, transcript of college record, CPR certification, written essay, health exam, health insurance, immunizations, minimum GPA in nursing prerequisites of 2.0, professional liability insurance/malpractice insurance, prerequisite course work. Transfer students are accepted. *Application deadline:* 1/10 (fall), 8/10 (spring).
Advanced Placement Credit given for nursing courses completed elsewhere dependent upon specific evaluations.
Expenses (2010-11) *Tuition, state resident:* full-time $3029; part-time $102 per credit hour. *Tuition, nonresident:* full-time $14,128; part-time $477 per credit hour. *Room and board:* $7608 per academic year. *Required fees:* full-time $2387; part-time $27 per term.
Financial Aid 70% of baccalaureate students in nursing programs received some form of financial aid in 2009-10.
Contact Ms. Marta Medina, Student Service Cordinator, School of Nursing, The University of North Carolina Wilmington, 601 South College Road, Wilmington, NC 28403-5995. *Telephone:* 910-962-7211. *Fax:* 910-962-7656. *E-mail:* medinam@uncw.edu.

GRADUATE PROGRAMS

Expenses (2010-11) *Tuition, state resident:* full-time $3421; part-time $168 per credit hour. *Tuition, nonresident:* full-time $14,348; part-time $703 per credit hour. *Room and board:* $9150 per academic year. *Required fees:* full-time $2387; part-time $39 per term.
Financial Aid 59% of graduate students in nursing programs received some form of financial aid in 2009-10. 2 teaching assistantships with full and partial tuition reimbursements available (averaging $9,500 per year) were awarded. *Financial aid application deadline:* 3/15.
Contact Dr. Julie S. Taylor, Graduate Coordinator, School of Nursing, The University of North Carolina Wilmington, 601 South College Road, Wilmington, NC 28403-5995. *Telephone:* 910-962-7927. *Fax:* 910-962-4921. *E-mail:* taylorjs@uncw.edu.

MASTER'S DEGREE PROGRAM

Degree MSN
Available Programs Master's.

Concentrations Available Nursing education. *Nurse practitioner programs in:* family health.
Site Options Burgaw, Bolton, Southport, Whiteville, NC; Raleigh, NC; Jacksonville, Supply, Elizabethtown, Kenansville , NC.
Study Options Full-time and part-time.
Program Entrance Requirements Clinical experience, computer literacy, minimum overall college GPA of 3.0, transcript of college record, CPR certification, written essay, immunizations, 3 letters of recommendation, nursing research course, physical assessment course, professional liability insurance/malpractice insurance, prerequisite course work, resume, statistics course, GRE General Test. *Application deadline:* 3/1 (fall).
Advanced Placement Credit given for nursing courses completed elsewhere dependent upon specific evaluations.
Degree Requirements 47 total credit hours, thesis or project, comprehensive exam.

POST-MASTER'S PROGRAM

Areas of Study Nursing education. *Nurse practitioner programs in:* family health.

CONTINUING EDUCATION PROGRAM

Contact Ms. Linda Ferrell, Executive Assistant, School of Nursing, The University of North Carolina Wilmington, 601 South College Road, Wilmington, NC 28403-5995. *Telephone:* 910-962-3200. *Fax:* 910-962-3723. *E-mail:* ferrell@uncw.edu.

Western Carolina University

School of Nursing
Cullowhee, North Carolina

Founded in 1889

DEGREES • BSN • MS

Nursing Program Faculty 31 (50% with doctorates).
Baccalaureate Enrollment 200 **Women** 94% **Men** 6% **Minority** 2%
Graduate Enrollment 122 **Women** 90% **Men** 10% **Minority** 2%
Distance Learning Courses Available.
Nursing Student Activities Sigma Theta Tau, Student Nurses' Association.
Nursing Student Resources Academic advising; academic or career counseling; assistance for students with disabilities; bookstore; campus computer network; career placement assistance; computer lab; computer-assisted instruction; daycare for children of students; e-mail services; externships; housing assistance; interactive nursing skills videos; Internet; learning resource lab; library services; nursing audiovisuals; resume preparation assistance; skills, simulation, or other laboratory; tutoring.
Library Facilities 625,730 volumes (10,000 in health, 900 in nursing); 47,928 periodical subscriptions (70 health-care related).

BACCALAUREATE PROGRAMS

Degree BSN
Available Programs Accelerated Baccalaureate; Generic Baccalaureate; RN Baccalaureate.
Site Options Enka, NC.
Study Options Full-time.
Online Degree Options Yes.
Program Entrance Requirements Minimum overall college GPA of 3.0, transcript of college record, CPR certification, health exam, high school transcript, immunizations, minimum GPA in nursing prerequisites of 2.0, professional liability insurance/malpractice insurance, prerequisite course work. Transfer students are accepted. *Application deadline:* 2/2 (fall). *Application fee:* $40.
Advanced Placement Credit given for nursing courses completed elsewhere dependent upon specific evaluations.
Financial Aid 75% of baccalaureate students in nursing programs received some form of financial aid in 2008-09. *Gift aid (need-based):* Federal Pell, FSEOG, state, private, college/university gift aid from institutional funds. *Loans:* Federal Direct (Subsidized and Unsubsidized Stafford PLUS), Perkins. *Work-study:* Federal Work-Study. *Financial aid application deadline (priority):* 3/15.
Contact Dr. Vincent P. Hall, RN, Director, School of Nursing, Western Carolina University, 209 Moore Building, Cullowhee, NC 28723. *Telephone:* 828-227-7467. *Fax:* 828-227-7052. *E-mail:* hallv@email.wcu.edu.

GRADUATE PROGRAMS

Financial Aid 75% of graduate students in nursing programs received some form of financial aid in 2008-09.
Contact Ms. Jessica Shirley, Director of Student Services, School of Nursing, School of Nursing, Western Carolina University, 1459 Sand Hill Road, AB Tech Campus, Suite 33, Enka, NC 28715. *Telephone:* 828-670-8810 Ext. 247. *E-mail:* jshirley@email.wcu.edu.

MASTER'S DEGREE PROGRAM

Degree MS
Available Programs Master's.
Concentrations Available Nurse anesthesia; nursing administration; nursing education. *Nurse practitioner programs in:* family health.
Site Options Enka, NC.
Study Options Full-time and part-time.
Online Degree Options Yes.
Program Entrance Requirements Clinical experience, minimum overall college GPA of 3.0, transcript of college record, CPR certification, written essay, immunizations, interview, 3 letters of recommendation, nursing research course, physical assessment course, professional liability insurance/malpractice insurance, resume, statistics course. *Application deadline:* 4/15 (fall), 10/15 (winter). *Application fee:* $40.
Advanced Placement Credit given for nursing courses completed elsewhere dependent upon specific evaluations.
Degree Requirements Thesis or project, comprehensive exam.

POST-MASTER'S PROGRAM

Areas of Study Nursing administration; nursing education. *Nurse practitioner programs in:* family health.

POSTDOCTORAL PROGRAM

Postdoctoral Program Contact Dr. Sandra Grenwicki, Head, School of Nursing, Western Carolina University, Cullowhee, NC 28723. *Telephone:* 828-227-7467. *Fax:* 828-227-7071. *E-mail:* grenwicki@wcu.edu.

Winston-Salem State University

Department of Nursing
Winston-Salem, North Carolina

http://www.wssu.edu
Founded in 1892

DEGREES • BSN • MSN

Nursing Program Faculty 34 (13% with doctorates).
Baccalaureate Enrollment 252 **Women** 77% **Men** 23% **Minority** 61%
Graduate Enrollment 15
Nursing Student Activities Nursing Honor Society, Sigma Theta Tau, Student Nurses' Association.
Nursing Student Resources Academic advising; academic or career counseling; assistance for students with disabilities; bookstore; campus computer network; computer lab; interactive nursing skills videos; learning resource lab; nursing audiovisuals; skills, simulation, or other laboratory.
Library Facilities 4,381 volumes in health, 2,691 volumes in nursing; 2,205 periodical subscriptions health-care related.

BACCALAUREATE PROGRAMS

Degree BSN
Available Programs ADN to Baccalaureate; Accelerated RN Baccalaureate; Baccalaureate for Second Degree; Generic Baccalaureate; LPN to Baccalaureate; RN Baccalaureate.
Site Options Wilkesboro, NC; Salisbury, NC; Boone, NC.
Study Options Full-time.
Program Entrance Requirements Minimum overall college GPA of 2.6, transcript of college record, CPR certification, health exam, immunizations, professional liability insurance/malpractice insurance, prerequisite course work. Transfer students are accepted.
Advanced Placement Credit by examination available. Credit given for nursing courses completed elsewhere dependent upon specific evaluations.
Contact ***Telephone:*** 336-750-2560. *Fax:* 336-750-2599.

GRADUATE PROGRAMS

Contact ***Telephone:*** 336-750-2275. *Fax:* 336-750-2007.

MASTER'S DEGREE PROGRAM

Degree MSN
Available Programs Master's.
Concentrations Available Nursing education. *Nurse practitioner programs in:* family health, psychiatric/mental health.
Study Options Full-time and part-time.
Program Entrance Requirements Clinical experience, transcript of college record, CPR certification, immunizations, interview, 3 letters of recommendation, nursing research course, physical assessment course, professional liability insurance/malpractice insurance, resume, statistics course.
Advanced Placement Credit given for nursing courses completed elsewhere dependent upon specific evaluations.
Degree Requirements 50 total credit hours, thesis or project.

CONTINUING EDUCATION PROGRAM

Contact *Telephone:* 336-750-2665. *Fax:* 336-750-2599.

NORTH DAKOTA

Dickinson State University

Department of Nursing
Dickinson, North Dakota

http://www.dickinsonstate.edu/d_nursing.asp
Founded in 1918

DEGREE • BSN

Nursing Program Faculty 7 (14% with doctorates).
Baccalaureate Enrollment 38 **Women** 97% **Men** 3% **Minority** 3% **International** 3% **Part-time** 11%
Nursing Student Activities Student Nurses' Association.
Nursing Student Resources Academic advising; academic or career counseling; assistance for students with disabilities; bookstore; campus computer network; career placement assistance; computer lab; computer-assisted instruction; e-mail services; employment services for current students; externships; housing assistance; interactive nursing skills videos; Internet; learning resource lab; library services; nursing audiovisuals; other; placement services for program completers; remedial services; resume preparation assistance; skills, simulation, or other laboratory; tutoring; unpaid internships.
Library Facilities 105,713 volumes (3,151 in health, 867 in nursing); 823 periodical subscriptions (2,898 health-care related).

BACCALAUREATE PROGRAMS

Degree BSN
Available Programs ADN to Baccalaureate; LPN to Baccalaureate; LPN to RN Baccalaureate; RN Baccalaureate.
Study Options Full-time and part-time.
Program Entrance Requirements Minimum overall college GPA of 2.50, transcript of college record, health exam, immunizations, minimum GPA in nursing prerequisites of 2.50, prerequisite course work. Transfer students are accepted. *Application deadline:* 2/1 (fall).
Advanced Placement Credit given for nursing courses completed elsewhere dependent upon specific evaluations.
Expenses (2010-11) *Tuition, state resident:* full-time $4306; part-time $179 per credit hour. *Tuition, nonresident:* full-time $12,584; part-time $475 per credit hour. *Room and board:* $4718; room only: $1690 per academic year. *Required fees:* full-time $1088; part-time $49 per credit; part-time $479 per term.
Financial Aid 85% of baccalaureate students in nursing programs received some form of financial aid in 2009-10. *Gift aid (need-based):* Federal Pell, FSEOG, state, college/university gift aid from institutional funds, National Guard tuition waivers, staff waivers. *Loans:* Federal Nursing Student Loans, Perkins, state, college/university, Alaska Loans, alternative loans. *Work-study:* Federal Work-Study, part-time campus jobs. *Financial aid application deadline (priority):* 3/15.
Contact Dr. Mary Anne Marsh, Chair, Department of Nursing, Dickinson State University, 291 Campus Drive, Dickinson, ND 58601-4896. *Telephone:* 800-279-4295 Ext. 2133. *Fax:* 701-483-2524. *E-mail:* maryanne.marsh@dickinsonstate.edu.

Jamestown College

Department of Nursing
Jamestown, North Dakota

Founded in 1883

DEGREE • BSN

Nursing Program Faculty 11 (9% with doctorates).
Baccalaureate Enrollment 80
Nursing Student Activities Sigma Theta Tau, Student Nurses' Association.
Nursing Student Resources Academic advising; academic or career counseling; bookstore; campus computer network; computer lab; computer-assisted instruction; e-mail services; externships; interactive nursing skills videos; Internet; learning resource lab; library services; nursing audiovisuals; resume preparation assistance; skills, simulation, or other laboratory; tutoring.
Library Facilities 107,732 volumes (990 in health, 983 in nursing); 20,226 periodical subscriptions (163 health-care related).

BACCALAUREATE PROGRAMS

Degree BSN
Study Options Full-time and part-time.
Program Entrance Requirements Minimum overall college GPA of 3.0, transcript of college record, written essay, high school transcript, immunizations, prerequisite course work. Transfer students are accepted.
Advanced Placement Credit given for nursing courses completed elsewhere dependent upon specific evaluations.
Contact *Telephone:* 701-252-3467 Ext. 2562. *Fax:* 701-253-4318.

Medcenter One College of Nursing

Medcenter One College of Nursing
Bismarck, North Dakota

http://www.medcenterone.com/college of nursing
Founded in 1988

DEGREE • BSN

Nursing Program Faculty 13 (8% with doctorates).
Baccalaureate Enrollment 91 **Women** 91% **Men** 9% **Minority** 10% **Part-time** 1%
Nursing Student Activities Sigma Theta Tau, Student Nurses' Association.
Nursing Student Resources Academic advising; bookstore; computer lab; computer-assisted instruction; e-mail services; Internet; library services; nursing audiovisuals; paid internships; placement services for program completers; resume preparation assistance; skills, simulation, or other laboratory; tutoring.
Library Facilities 26,078 volumes (2,498 in health, 1,725 in nursing); 446 periodical subscriptions (426 health-care related).

BACCALAUREATE PROGRAMS

Degree BSN
Available Programs RN Baccalaureate.
Study Options Full-time and part-time.
Program Entrance Requirements Minimum overall college GPA of 2.5, transcript of college record, written essay, health exam, high school transcript, immunizations, interview, minimum GPA in nursing prerequisites of 2.5, prerequisite course work. Transfer students are accepted. *Application deadline:* 11/1 (fall). *Application fee:* $40.
Advanced Placement Credit given for nursing courses completed elsewhere dependent upon specific evaluations.
Expenses (2010-11) *Tuition:* full-time $10,012; part-time $417 per credit. *Required fees:* full-time $839; part-time $35 per credit.
Financial Aid 97% of baccalaureate students in nursing programs received some form of financial aid in 2009-10.
Contact Ms. Mary Smith, Director of Student Services, Medcenter One College of Nursing, 512 North 7th Street, Bismarck, ND 58501. *Telephone:* 701-323-6271. *Fax:* 701-323-6289. *E-mail:* msmith@mohs.org.

Minot State University
Department of Nursing
Minot, North Dakota

http://www.minotstateu.edu/nursing/
Founded in 1913

DEGREE • BSN

Nursing Program Faculty 21 (19% with doctorates).
Baccalaureate Enrollment 106 **Women** 92% **Men** 8% **Minority** 23% **International** 5% **Part-time** 20%
Distance Learning Courses Available.
Nursing Student Activities Sigma Theta Tau, Student Nurses' Association.
Nursing Student Resources Academic advising; academic or career counseling; assistance for students with disabilities; bookstore; campus computer network; career placement assistance; computer lab; computer-assisted instruction; e-mail services; housing assistance; interactive nursing skills videos; Internet; learning resource lab; library services; nursing audiovisuals; paid internships; remedial services; resume preparation assistance; skills, simulation, or other laboratory; tutoring; unpaid internships.
Library Facilities 8,489 volumes in health, 1,731 volumes in nursing; 37 periodical subscriptions health-care related.

BACCALAUREATE PROGRAMS

Degree BSN
Available Programs Generic Baccalaureate; RN Baccalaureate.
Study Options Full-time.
Online Degree Options Yes.
Program Entrance Requirements Minimum overall college GPA of 2.75, transcript of college record, CPR certification, written essay, immunizations, 2 letters of recommendation, minimum GPA in nursing prerequisites of 2.8, prerequisite course work. Transfer students are accepted. *Application deadline:* 10/1 (fall), 2/1 (spring). *Application fee:* $25.
Advanced Placement Credit given for nursing courses completed elsewhere dependent upon specific evaluations.
Expenses (2010-11) *Tuition, state resident:* full-time $4476. *Tuition, nonresident:* full-time $4476. *Room and board:* $2976; room only: $1880 per academic year. *Required fees:* full-time $3161.
Financial Aid 76% of baccalaureate students in nursing programs received some form of financial aid in 2009-10.
Contact Ms. Kelly Buettner-Schmidt, Chair, Department of Nursing, Minot State University, 500 University Avenue West, Minot, ND 58707-0002. *Telephone:* 701-858-3101. *Fax:* 701-858-4309. *E-mail:* kelly.schmidt@minotstateu.edu.

North Dakota State University
Department of Nursing
Fargo, North Dakota

http://www.ndsu.edu/ndsu/nursing/
Founded in 1890

DEGREES • BSN • DNP • MS

Nursing Program Faculty 15 (49% with doctorates).
Baccalaureate Enrollment 195 **Women** 90% **Men** 10% **Minority** 5% **International** 3% **Part-time** 10%
Graduate Enrollment 24 **Women** 95% **Men** 5% **Minority** 1% **Part-time** 45%
Nursing Student Activities Sigma Theta Tau, Student Nurses' Association.
Nursing Student Resources Academic advising; academic or career counseling; assistance for students with disabilities; bookstore; campus computer network; career placement assistance; computer lab; computer-assisted instruction; daycare for children of students; e-mail services; employment services for current students; interactive nursing skills videos; Internet; learning resource lab; library services; nursing audiovisuals; paid internships; placement services for program completers; remedial services; resume preparation assistance; skills, simulation, or other laboratory; tutoring.
Library Facilities 8,631 volumes in health, 1,841 volumes in nursing; 121 periodical subscriptions health-care related.

BACCALAUREATE PROGRAMS

Degree BSN
Available Programs ADN to Baccalaureate; Generic Baccalaureate; LPN to Baccalaureate.
Study Options Full-time.
Program Entrance Requirements Minimum overall college GPA of 3.0, transcript of college record, CPR certification, health exam, health insurance, immunizations, 2 letters of recommendation, minimum GPA in nursing prerequisites of 3.0, prerequisite course work. Transfer students are accepted.
Advanced Placement Credit by examination available. Credit given for nursing courses completed elsewhere dependent upon specific evaluations.
Contact *Telephone:* 701-231-7395. *Fax:* 701-231-7606.

GRADUATE PROGRAMS

Contact *Telephone:* 701-231-8355. *Fax:* 701-231-7606.

MASTER'S DEGREE PROGRAM

Degree MS
Available Programs Master's.
Concentrations Available Nursing education. *Clinical nurse specialist programs in:* adult health. *Nurse practitioner programs in:* family health.
Study Options Full-time and part-time.
Program Entrance Requirements Computer literacy, minimum overall college GPA of 3.0, transcript of college record, CPR certification, immunizations, interview, 3 letters of recommendation, nursing research course, physical assessment course, professional liability insurance/malpractice insurance, resume, statistics course.
Advanced Placement Credit given for nursing courses completed elsewhere dependent upon specific evaluations.
Degree Requirements 58 total credit hours, thesis or project, comprehensive exam.

DOCTORAL DEGREE PROGRAM

Degree DNP
Available Programs Post-Baccalaureate Doctorate.
Areas of Study Advanced practice nursing, family health.
Online Degree Options Yes.
Program Entrance Requirements Clinical experience, minimum overall college GPA of 3.0, interview by faculty committee, 2 letters of recommendation, statistics course, vita, writing sample.
Degree Requirements 86 total credit hours, dissertation, oral exam.

University of Mary
Division of Nursing
Bismarck, North Dakota

http://www.umary.edu/AcadInfo/NurDiv
Founded in 1959

DEGREES • BS • MSN • MSN/MBA

Nursing Program Faculty 37 (26% with doctorates).
Baccalaureate Enrollment 125 **Women** 94% **Men** 6% **Minority** 6%
Graduate Enrollment 198 **Women** 98% **Men** 2% **Minority** 14% **Part-time** 23%
Distance Learning Courses Available.
Nursing Student Activities Sigma Theta Tau, Student Nurses' Association.
Nursing Student Resources Academic advising; academic or career counseling; assistance for students with disabilities; bookstore; campus computer network; career placement assistance; computer lab; computer-assisted instruction; e-mail services; employment services for current students; externships; housing assistance; interactive nursing skills videos; Internet; library services; nursing audiovisuals; placement services for program completers; resume preparation assistance; skills, simulation, or other laboratory; unpaid internships.
Library Facilities 64,524 volumes (4,350 in health, 800 in nursing); 210 periodical subscriptions (70 health-care related).

BACCALAUREATE PROGRAMS

Degree BS
Available Programs Generic Baccalaureate; LPN to Baccalaureate; RN Baccalaureate.
Study Options Full-time and part-time.
Online Degree Options Yes.
Program Entrance Requirements Minimum overall college GPA of 2.75, transcript of college record, CPR certification, written essay, health exam, high school transcript, immunizations, interview, 2 letters of rec-

ommendation, minimum GPA in nursing prerequisites of 2.0, professional liability insurance/malpractice insurance, prerequisite course work. Transfer students are accepted. *Application deadline:* 3/27 (spring).
Advanced Placement Credit by examination available. Credit given for nursing courses completed elsewhere dependent upon specific evaluations.
Expenses (2010-11) *Tuition:* full-time $12,800; part-time $420 per credit hour. *Room and board:* $5000; room only: $2400 per academic year. *Required fees:* full-time $220.
Financial Aid 100% of baccalaureate students in nursing programs received some form of financial aid in 2009-10. *Gift aid (need-based):* Federal Pell, FSEOG, state, private, college/university gift aid from institutional funds, Academic Competitiveness Grants, National SMART Grants, TEACH Grants. *Loans:* Federal Nursing Student Loans, Federal Direct (Subsidized and Unsubsidized Stafford PLUS), Perkins, alternative private loans. *Work-study:* Federal Work-Study, part-time campus jobs. *Financial aid application deadline (priority):* 3/15.
Contact Admissions Office, Division of Nursing, University of Mary, 7500 University Drive, Bismarck, ND 58504. *Telephone:* 701-255-7500. *Fax:* 701-255-7687.

GRADUATE PROGRAMS

Expenses (2010-11) *Tuition:* full-time $12,150; part-time $450 per credit. *Required fees:* full-time $3450; part-time $250 per term.
Financial Aid 95% of graduate students in nursing programs received some form of financial aid in 2009-10. 14 fellowships with partial tuition reimbursements available, 3 teaching assistantships with partial tuition reimbursements available were awarded; institutionally sponsored loans also available. Aid available to part-time students. *Financial aid application deadline:* 7/1.
Contact Dr. Billie Madler, Graduate Program Director, Division of Nursing, University of Mary, 7500 University Drive, Bismarck, ND 58504. *Telephone:* 701-355-8266. *Fax:* 701-255-7687. *E-mail:* bmadler@umary.edu.

MASTER'S DEGREE PROGRAM

Degrees MSN; MSN/MBA
Available Programs Master's; RN to Master's.
Concentrations Available Nursing administration; nursing education. *Nurse practitioner programs in:* family health.
Site Options Kansas City, MO; Billings, MT; Gillette, WY.
Study Options Full-time and part-time.
Online Degree Options Yes.
Program Entrance Requirements Clinical experience, minimum overall college GPA of 2.75, transcript of college record, CPR certification, written essay, immunizations, interview, 2 letters of recommendation, physical assessment course, prerequisite course work, resume. *Application deadline:* Applications may be processed on a rolling basis for some programs.
Degree Requirements 39 total credit hours, thesis or project, comprehensive exam.

University of North Dakota

College of Nursing
Grand Forks, North Dakota

http://www.nursing.und.edu/
Founded in 1883

DEGREES • BSN • MS • PHD
Nursing Program Faculty 79 (33% with doctorates).
Baccalaureate Enrollment 304 **Women** 85% **Men** 15% **Minority** 8% **Part-time** 9%
Graduate Enrollment 109 **Women** 88.1% **Men** 11.9% **Minority** 12.8% **Part-time** 52.3%
Distance Learning Courses Available.
Nursing Student Activities Nursing Honor Society, Sigma Theta Tau, Student Nurses' Association.
Nursing Student Resources Academic advising; academic or career counseling; assistance for students with disabilities; bookstore; career placement assistance; computer lab; computer-assisted instruction; daycare for children of students; e-mail services; employment services for current students; externships; housing assistance; interactive nursing skills videos; Internet; learning resource lab; library services; nursing audiovisuals; paid internships; placement services for program completers; remedial services; resume preparation assistance; skills, simulation, or other laboratory; tutoring.
Library Facilities 1.1 million volumes (105,982 in health, 15,000 in nursing); 42,291 periodical subscriptions (8,000 health-care related).

BACCALAUREATE PROGRAMS

Degree BSN
Available Programs ADN to Baccalaureate; Accelerated Baccalaureate; Accelerated Baccalaureate for Second Degree; Baccalaureate for Second Degree; Generic Baccalaureate; International Nurse to Baccalaureate; LPN to Baccalaureate; RN Baccalaureate.
Study Options Full-time and part-time.
Online Degree Options Yes.
Program Entrance Requirements Minimum overall college GPA of 2.5, transcript of college record, CPR certification, written essay, health insurance, immunizations, interview, 2 letters of recommendation, minimum GPA in nursing prerequisites of 2.5, prerequisite course work, RN licensure. Transfer students are accepted. *Application deadline:* 2/1 (fall), 7/1 (spring).
Advanced Placement Credit by examination available. Credit given for nursing courses completed elsewhere dependent upon specific evaluations.
Expenses (2010-11) *Tuition, area resident:* full-time $6726; part-time $289 per credit. *Tuition, nonresident:* full-time $15,845; part-time $682 per credit. *Room and board:* $3075; room only: $2919 per academic year. *Required fees:* full-time $1000; part-time $40 per credit; part-time $500 per term.
Financial Aid 90% of baccalaureate students in nursing programs received some form of financial aid in 2009-10. *Gift aid (need-based):* Federal Pell, FSEOG, state, private, college/university gift aid from institutional funds, Federal Nursing. *Loans:* Federal Nursing Student Loans, Perkins, alternative commercial loans. *Work-study:* Federal Work-Study. *Financial aid application deadline (priority):* 3/15.
Contact Ms. Marlys K. Escobar, Director of Student and Alumni Affairs, College of Nursing, University of North Dakota, 430 Oxford Street, Stop 9025, Room 301, Grand Forks, ND 58202-9025. *Telephone:* 701-777-4534. *Fax:* 701-777-4096. *E-mail:* marlysescobar@mail.und.nodak.edu.

GRADUATE PROGRAMS

Expenses (2010-11) *Tuition, state resident:* full-time $7139; part-time $253 per credit. *Tuition, nonresident:* full-time $7139; part-time $253 per credit. *Room and board:* $7500; room only: $6000 per academic year. *Required fees:* full-time $4500; part-time $135 per credit; part-time $1500 per term.
Financial Aid 75% of graduate students in nursing programs received some form of financial aid in 2009-10. 4 research assistantships with tuition reimbursements available (averaging $10,498 per year), 7 teaching assistantships with full tuition reimbursements available (averaging $10,669 per year) were awarded; fellowships with tuition reimbursements available, Federal Work-Study, institutionally sponsored loans, scholarships, traineeships, and tuition waivers (full and partial) also available. Aid available to part-time students. *Financial aid application deadline:* 3/15.
Contact Dr. Darla J. Adams, Associate Dean for Graduate Studies, College of Nursing, University of North Dakota, 430 Oxford Street, Box 9025, Room 361, Grand Forks, ND 58202-9025. *Telephone:* 701-777-4543. *Fax:* 701-777-4096. *E-mail:* darla,adams@email.und.edu.

MASTER'S DEGREE PROGRAM

Degree MS
Available Programs Master's; RN to Master's.
Concentrations Available Nurse anesthesia; nursing education. *Clinical nurse specialist programs in:* community health, gerontology, psychiatric/mental health, public health. *Nurse practitioner programs in:* family health, gerontology, psychiatric/mental health.
Study Options Full-time and part-time.
Online Degree Options Yes.
Program Entrance Requirements Clinical experience, minimum overall college GPA of 3.0, transcript of college record, CPR certification, written essay, immunizations, interview, 3 letters of recommendation, prerequisite course work, resume, statistics course. *Application deadline:* 8/1 (fall), 12/1 (spring). *Application fee:* $35.
Advanced Placement Credit given for nursing courses completed elsewhere dependent upon specific evaluations.
Degree Requirements 48 total credit hours, thesis or project.

POST-MASTER'S PROGRAM

Areas of Study Nurse anesthesia; nursing education. *Clinical nurse specialist programs in:* psychiatric/mental health. *Nurse practitioner programs in:* family health, psychiatric/mental health.

DOCTORAL DEGREE PROGRAM

Degree PhD
Available Programs Doctorate.
Areas of Study Faculty preparation, health promotion/disease prevention, nursing education, nursing research.
Online Degree Options Yes (online only).
Program Entrance Requirements Minimum overall college GPA of 3.5, interview by faculty committee, interview, 3 letters of recommendation, MSN or equivalent, statistics course, vita, GRE or MAT. Application deadline: 2/1 (fall). Application fee: $35.
Degree Requirements 90 total credit hours, dissertation, oral exam, written exam, residency.

OHIO

Ashland University

Dwight Schar College of Nursing
Ashland, Ohio

http://www.ashland.edu/nursing
Founded in 1878

DEGREE • BSN

Nursing Program Faculty 22 (18% with doctorates).
Baccalaureate Enrollment 325 **Women** 83% **Men** 17% **Minority** 6% **Part-time** 3%
Distance Learning Courses Available.
Nursing Student Activities Nursing Honor Society, Sigma Theta Tau, Student Nurses' Association, nursing club.
Nursing Student Resources Academic advising; academic or career counseling; assistance for students with disabilities; bookstore; campus computer network; career placement assistance; computer lab; computer-assisted instruction; e-mail services; employment services for current students; interactive nursing skills videos; Internet; learning resource lab; library services; nursing audiovisuals; remedial services; resume preparation assistance; skills, simulation, or other laboratory; tutoring; unpaid internships.
Library Facilities 205,200 volumes; 1,625 periodical subscriptions.

BACCALAUREATE PROGRAMS

Degree BSN
Available Programs ADN to Baccalaureate; Accelerated Baccalaureate for Second Degree; Accelerated RN Baccalaureate; Baccalaureate for Second Degree; RN Baccalaureate.
Study Options Full-time and part-time.
Online Degree Options Yes (online only).
Program Entrance Requirements Minimum overall college GPA of 2.0, transcript of college record, CPR certification, high school transcript, immunizations, minimum GPA in nursing prerequisites of 2.5, professional liability insurance/malpractice insurance, prerequisite course work, RN licensure. Transfer students are accepted. *Application deadline:* Applications may be processed on a rolling basis for some programs.
Advanced Placement Credit by examination available. Credit given for nursing courses completed elsewhere dependent upon specific evaluations.
Expenses (2010-11) *Tuition:* part-time $451 per credit hour.
Financial Aid 95% of baccalaureate students in nursing programs received some form of financial aid in 2009-10. *Gift aid (need-based):* Federal Pell, FSEOG, state, private, college/university gift aid from institutional funds. *Loans:* Federal Direct (Subsidized and Unsubsidized Stafford PLUS), Perkins, college/university. *Work-study:* Federal Work-Study. *Financial aid application deadline (priority):* 3/15.
Contact Dr. Lori Brohm, Administrator, Dwight Schar College of Nursing, Ashland University, 325 Glessner Avenue, Mansfield, OH 44903. *Telephone:* 419-520-2630. *Fax:* 419-520-2626. *E-mail:* lbrohm@ashland.edu.

Capital University

School of Nursing
Columbus, Ohio

http://www.capital.edu/nursing/nurshome.shtml
Founded in 1830

DEGREES • BSN • MN/MBA • MSN • MSN/JD • MSN/MDIV

Nursing Program Faculty 30 (30% with doctorates).
Baccalaureate Enrollment 464 **Women** 82% **Men** 18% **Minority** 9% **International** 1% **Part-time** 19%
Graduate Enrollment 45 **Women** 87% **Men** 13% **Minority** 31% **International** 2% **Part-time** 98%
Nursing Student Activities Sigma Theta Tau, Student Nurses' Association.
Nursing Student Resources Academic advising; academic or career counseling; assistance for students with disabilities; bookstore; campus computer network; computer lab; computer-assisted instruction; e-mail services; interactive nursing skills videos; Internet; learning resource lab; library services; nursing audiovisuals; remedial services; resume preparation assistance; skills, simulation, or other laboratory; tutoring; unpaid internships.
Library Facilities 209,524 volumes (6,209 in health); 8,523 periodical subscriptions (82 health-care related).

BACCALAUREATE PROGRAMS

Degree BSN
Available Programs ADN to Baccalaureate; Accelerated Baccalaureate for Second Degree; Generic Baccalaureate; RN Baccalaureate.
Study Options Full-time and part-time.
Program Entrance Requirements Minimum overall college GPA of 3.0, transcript of college record, health exam, high school biology, high school chemistry, high school foreign language, 3 years high school math, 3 years high school science, high school transcript, immunizations, minimum high school GPA of 3.1. Transfer students are accepted. *Application deadline:* 5/1 (fall). Applications may be processed on a rolling basis for some programs. *Application fee:* $25.
Advanced Placement Credit by examination available. Credit given for nursing courses completed elsewhere dependent upon specific evaluations.
Expenses (2010-11) *Tuition:* full-time $29,310; part-time $977 per contact hour. *Room and board:* $7864; room only: $3460 per academic year. *Required fees:* full-time $875.
Financial Aid 100% of baccalaureate students in nursing programs received some form of financial aid in 2009-10.
Contact Dr. Judi Macke, Program Coordinator, School of Nursing, Capital University, 1 College and Main, Columbus, OH 43209-2394. *Telephone:* 614-236-6339. *Fax:* 614-236-6157. *E-mail:* jmacke@capital.edu.

GRADUATE PROGRAMS

Expenses (2010-11) *Tuition:* full-time $5400; part-time $450 per credit. *International tuition:* $5400 full-time. *Room and board:* $11,240; room only: $6800 per academic year.
Financial Aid 30% of graduate students in nursing programs received some form of financial aid in 2009-10. Career-related internships or fieldwork and traineeships available.
Contact Dr. Sharon Stout-Shaffer, Program Coordinator, School of Nursing, Capital University, 1 College and Main, Columbus, OH 43209-2394. *Telephone:* 614-236-6363. *Fax:* 614-236-6703. *E-mail:* sstoutsh@capital.edu.

MASTER'S DEGREE PROGRAM

Degrees MN/MBA; MSN; MSN/JD; MSN/MDIV
Available Programs Master's; RN to Master's.
Concentrations Available Legal nurse consultant; nursing administration; nursing education.
Study Options Full-time and part-time.
Program Entrance Requirements Computer literacy, minimum overall college GPA of 3.0, transcript of college record, CPR certification, written essay, immunizations, 3 letters of recommendation, nursing research course, physical assessment course, professional liability insurance/malpractice insurance, prerequisite course work, resume, statistics course. *Application deadline:* 5/1 (fall), 12/1 (winter), 12/1 (spring), 5/1 (summer). Applications may be processed on a rolling basis for some programs. *Application fee:* $25.
Advanced Placement Credit given for nursing courses completed elsewhere dependent upon specific evaluations.

Degree Requirements 36 total credit hours, thesis or project, comprehensive exam.

POST-MASTER'S PROGRAM

Areas of Study Legal nurse consultant; nursing education.

Case Western Reserve University

Frances Payne Bolton School of Nursing
Cleveland, Ohio

http://fpb.case.edu
Founded in 1826

DEGREES • BSN • MSN • MSN/MA • MSN/MBA • MSN/MPH • PHD

Nursing Program Faculty 108 (54% with doctorates).
Baccalaureate Enrollment 352 **Women** 91% **Men** 9% **Minority** 26% **International** 2.6% **Part-time** .28%
Graduate Enrollment 533 **Women** 89% **Men** 11% **Minority** 19% **International** 5.3% **Part-time** 64%
Nursing Student Activities Sigma Theta Tau, Student Nurses' Association.
Nursing Student Resources Academic advising; academic or career counseling; assistance for students with disabilities; bookstore; campus computer network; career placement assistance; computer lab; computer-assisted instruction; e-mail services; employment services for current students; housing assistance; interactive nursing skills videos; Internet; learning resource lab; library services; nursing audiovisuals; other; placement services for program completers; remedial services; resume preparation assistance; skills, simulation, or other laboratory; tutoring.
Library Facilities 2.8 million volumes (475,000 in health); 75,083 periodical subscriptions (2,500 health-care related).

BACCALAUREATE PROGRAMS

Degree BSN
Available Programs ADN to Baccalaureate; Generic Baccalaureate; RN Baccalaureate.
Study Options Full-time.
Program Entrance Requirements Written essay, high school biology, high school chemistry, 2 years high school science, high school transcript, 2 letters of recommendation, minimum high school GPA of 3.0. Transfer students are accepted. *Application deadline:* 1/15 (fall). *Application fee:* $35.
Advanced Placement Credit given for nursing courses completed elsewhere dependent upon specific evaluations.
Contact ***Telephone:*** 216-368-2529. *Fax:* 216-368-0124.

GRADUATE PROGRAMS

Contact ***Telephone:*** 216-368-2529. *Fax:* 216-368-0124.

MASTER'S DEGREE PROGRAM

Degrees MSN; MSN/MA; MSN/MBA; MSN/MPH
Available Programs Accelerated AD/RN to Master's; Master's; RN to Master's.
Concentrations Available Nurse anesthesia; nurse-midwifery; nursing informatics. *Clinical nurse specialist programs in:* gerontology, medical-surgical, psychiatric/mental health, public health. *Nurse practitioner programs in:* acute care, adult health, family health, gerontology, neonatal health, oncology, pediatric, psychiatric/mental health, women's health.
Study Options Full-time and part-time.
Program Entrance Requirements Minimum overall college GPA of 3.0, transcript of college record, written essay, 3 letters of recommendation, resume, statistics course, MAT or GRE General Test. *Application deadline:* 6/1 (fall), 10/1 (spring), 3/1 (summer). Applications may be processed on a rolling basis for some programs. *Application fee:* $75.
Advanced Placement Credit given for nursing courses completed elsewhere dependent upon specific evaluations.
Degree Requirements 40 total credit hours.

POST-MASTER'S PROGRAM

Areas of Study Nurse anesthesia; nurse-midwifery; nursing informatics. *Clinical nurse specialist programs in:* medical-surgical, public health. *Nurse practitioner programs in:* acute care, adult health, family health, gerontology, neonatal health, oncology, pediatric, psychiatric/mental health, women's health.

DOCTORAL DEGREE PROGRAM

Degree PhD
Available Programs Doctorate; Doctorate for Nurses with Non-Nursing Degrees; Post-Baccalaureate Doctorate.
Areas of Study Aging, bio-behavioral research, community health, critical care, ethics, faculty preparation, family health, gerontology, health policy, health promotion/disease prevention, human health and illness, illness and transition, individualized study, maternity-newborn, nursing education, nursing research, nursing science, oncology, women's health.
Program Entrance Requirements Minimum overall college GPA of 3.0, interview by faculty committee, 3 letters of recommendation, statistics course, vita, writing sample, GRE General Test, MAT (DNP). Application deadline: 1/1 (fall), 10/1 (spring), 3/1 (summer). Applications may be processed on a rolling basis for some programs. Application fee: $75.
Degree Requirements 57 total credit hours, dissertation, oral exam, residency.

POSTDOCTORAL PROGRAM

Areas of Study Aging, cancer care, chronic illness, community health, family health, gerontology, health promotion/disease prevention, individualized study, information systems, nursing interventions, nursing research, nursing science, outcomes, self-care, vulnerable population, women's health.
Postdoctoral Program Contact ***Telephone:*** 216-368-5978. *Fax:* 216-368-3542.

CONTINUING EDUCATION PROGRAM

Contact ***Telephone:*** 216-368-6302. *Fax:* 216-368-5303.

Cedarville University

Department of Nursing
Cedarville, Ohio

http://www.cedarville.edu/academics/nursing
Founded in 1887

DEGREE • BSN

Nursing Program Faculty 23 (39% with doctorates).
Baccalaureate Enrollment 352 **Women** 90.3% **Men** 9.7% **Minority** 6.3% **International** .9% **Part-time** .9%
Nursing Student Activities Nursing Honor Society, Student Nurses' Association.
Nursing Student Resources Academic advising; academic or career counseling; assistance for students with disabilities; bookstore; campus computer network; career placement assistance; computer lab; computer-assisted instruction; e-mail services; employment services for current students; housing assistance; interactive nursing skills videos; Internet; library services; nursing audiovisuals; paid internships; resume preparation assistance; skills, simulation, or other laboratory.
Library Facilities 184,296 volumes (6,137 in health, 1,140 in nursing); 20,851 periodical subscriptions (87 health-care related).

BACCALAUREATE PROGRAMS

Degree BSN
Available Programs RN Baccalaureate.
Study Options Full-time.
Program Entrance Requirements Minimum overall college GPA of 2.8, transcript of college record, CPR certification, written essay, health exam, health insurance, high school biology, high school chemistry, high school foreign language, 4 years high school math, 4 years high school science, high school transcript, immunizations, 1 letter of recommendation, minimum high school GPA of 3.0, minimum high school rank 50%, minimum GPA in nursing prerequisites of 2.8, professional liability insurance/malpractice insurance, prerequisite course work. Transfer students are accepted. *Application deadline:* 5/1 (spring). *Application fee:* $30.
Advanced Placement Credit given for nursing courses completed elsewhere dependent upon specific evaluations.
Expenses (2010-11) *Tuition:* full-time $23,500; part-time $870 per credit hour. *Room and board:* $5086 per academic year.
Financial Aid 91% of baccalaureate students in nursing programs received some form of financial aid in 2009-10. *Gift aid (need-based):* Federal Pell, FSEOG, state, private, college/university gift aid from institutional funds. *Loans:* Federal Nursing Student Loans, Perkins,

college/university. *Work-study:* Federal Work-Study, part-time campus jobs. *Financial aid application deadline (priority):* 3/1.
Contact Mr. Mark Weinstein, Director of Admissions, Department of Nursing, Cedarville University, 251 North Main Street, Cedarville, OH 45314-0601. *Telephone:* 800-233-2784. *Fax:* 937-766-7575. *E-mail:* admissions@cedarville.edu.

Chamberlain College of Nursing
Chamberlain College of Nursing
Columbus, Ohio

DEGREES • BSN • MSN
Distance Learning Courses Available.

BACCALAUREATE PROGRAMS

Degree BSN
Available Programs Accelerated Baccalaureate; Accelerated Baccalaureate for Second Degree; RN Baccalaureate.
Contact Admissions, Chamberlain College of Nursing, 1350 Alum Creek Drive, Columbus, OH 43209. *Telephone:* 888-556-8226.

GRADUATE PROGRAMS

Contact Admissions, Chamberlain College of Nursing, 1350 Alum Creek Drive, Columbus, OH 43209. *Telephone:* 888-556-8226.

MASTER'S DEGREE PROGRAM
Degree MSN
Available Programs Master's.

Cleveland State University
School of Nursing
Cleveland, Ohio

http://www.csuohio.edu/nursing
Founded in 1964

DEGREES • BSN • MSN • MSN/MBA
Nursing Program Faculty 69 (17% with doctorates).
Baccalaureate Enrollment 190 **Women** 79.5% **Men** 20.5% **Minority** 18.4% **International** .5%
Graduate Enrollment 92 **Women** 96.6% **Men** 3.4% **Minority** 13.6% **Part-time** 100%
Distance Learning Courses Available.
Nursing Student Activities Sigma Theta Tau, Student Nurses' Association.
Nursing Student Resources Academic advising; academic or career counseling; assistance for students with disabilities; bookstore; campus computer network; computer lab; computer-assisted instruction; daycare for children of students; e-mail services; employment services for current students; interactive nursing skills videos; Internet; learning resource lab; library services; nursing audiovisuals; remedial services; resume preparation assistance; skills, simulation, or other laboratory.
Library Facilities 6,000 volumes in health, 300 volumes in nursing; 70 periodical subscriptions health-care related.

BACCALAUREATE PROGRAMS

Degree BSN
Available Programs Accelerated Baccalaureate for Second Degree; Generic Baccalaureate; RN Baccalaureate.
Study Options Full-time.
Online Degree Options Yes.
Program Entrance Requirements Minimum overall college GPA of 2.5, transcript of college record, CPR certification, written essay, health exam, health insurance, high school transcript, immunizations, interview, 2 letters of recommendation, minimum GPA in nursing prerequisites of 2.75, professional liability insurance/malpractice insurance, prerequisite course work. Transfer students are accepted. *Application deadline:* 3/1 (fall). *Application fee:* $15.
Advanced Placement Credit given for nursing courses completed elsewhere dependent upon specific evaluations.
Expenses (2010-11) *Tuition, state resident:* part-time $353 per contact hour. *Tuition, nonresident:* part-time $657 per contact hour. *Room and board:* $10,285; room only: $6985 per academic year. *Required fees:* full-time $358.
Financial Aid 80% of baccalaureate students in nursing programs received some form of financial aid in 2009-10. *Gift aid (need-based):* Federal Pell, FSEOG, state, private, college/university gift aid from institutional funds. *Loans:* Perkins, state, alternative loans. *Work-study:* Federal Work-Study, part-time campus jobs. *Financial aid application deadline (priority):* 2/15.
Contact Mrs. Mary Leanza Manzuk, Recruiter and Advisor, School of Nursing, Cleveland State University, 2121 Euclid Avenue, JH 240, Cleveland, OH 44115. *Telephone:* 216-687-3810. *Fax:* 216-687-3556. *E-mail:* sonadvising@csuohio.edu.

GRADUATE PROGRAMS

Expenses (2010-11) *Tuition, state resident:* part-time $469 per contact hour. *Tuition, nonresident:* part-time $890 per contact hour. *Room and board:* $10,285; room only: $6985 per academic year.
Financial Aid 50% of graduate students in nursing programs received some form of financial aid in 2009-10.
Contact Mrs. Carol Ivan, Recruiter Advisor, School of Nursing, Cleveland State University, 2121 Euclid Avenue, JH 239, Cleveland, OH 44115. *Telephone:* 216-687-5517. *Fax:* 216-687-3556. *E-mail:* sonadvising@csuohio.edu.

MASTER'S DEGREE PROGRAM
Degrees MSN; MSN/MBA
Available Programs Master's.
Concentrations Available Clinical nurse leader; health-care administration; legal nurse consultant; nursing administration; nursing education. *Clinical nurse specialist programs in:* community health, forensic nursing.
Study Options Part-time.
Online Degree Options Yes (online only).
Program Entrance Requirements Clinical experience, computer literacy, minimum overall college GPA of 3.0, transcript of college record, CPR certification, written essay, immunizations, 2 letters of recommendation, professional liability insurance/malpractice insurance, prerequisite course work, resume, statistics course. *Application deadline:* 3/1 (fall).
Advanced Placement Credit given for nursing courses completed elsewhere dependent upon specific evaluations.
Degree Requirements 38 total credit hours, thesis or project.

POST-MASTER'S PROGRAM
Areas of Study Clinical nurse leader; nursing education.

CONTINUING EDUCATION PROGRAM

Contact Jeanine Carroll, Director, Continuing Education Programs for Health Care Professionals, School of Nursing, Cleveland State University, 2121 Euclid Avenue, Division of Continuing Education, Cleveland, OH 44115. *Telephone:* 216-687-4843. *Fax:* 216-687-9399. *E-mail:* j.a.carroll@csuohio.edu.

College of Mount St. Joseph
Department of Nursing
Cincinnati, Ohio

Founded in 1920

DEGREES • BSN • MN
Nursing Program Faculty 32 (4% with doctorates).
Baccalaureate Enrollment 287 **Women** 97% **Men** 3% **Minority** 5% **Part-time** 60%
Graduate Enrollment 21 **Women** 90% **Men** 10% **Minority** 5%
Nursing Student Activities Nursing Honor Society, Sigma Theta Tau, Student Nurses' Association.
Nursing Student Resources Academic advising; academic or career counseling; assistance for students with disabilities; bookstore; campus computer network; career placement assistance; computer lab; computer-assisted instruction; daycare for children of students; e-mail services; employment services for current students; externships; housing assistance; interactive nursing skills videos; Internet; learning resource lab; library services; nursing audiovisuals; placement services for program completers; remedial services; resume preparation assistance; skills, simulation, or other laboratory; tutoring.
Library Facilities 97,165 volumes (1,800 in health, 1,200 in nursing); 9,362 periodical subscriptions (300 health-care related).

BACCALAUREATE PROGRAMS

Degree BSN
Available Programs Accelerated RN Baccalaureate; Generic Baccalaureate.
Site Options Cincinnati, OH; Covington, KY.
Study Options Full-time and part-time.
Program Entrance Requirements Minimum overall college GPA of 2.75, transcript of college record, CPR certification, health exam, health insurance, high school chemistry, 2 years high school math, 2 years high school science, high school transcript, immunizations, interview, minimum high school GPA of 2.75, minimum high school rank 60%, minimum GPA in nursing prerequisites of 2.75, professional liability insurance/malpractice insurance, prerequisite course work. Transfer students are accepted. *Application deadline:* Applications may be processed on a rolling basis for some programs. *Application fee:* $25.
Advanced Placement Credit by examination available. Credit given for nursing courses completed elsewhere dependent upon specific evaluations.
Contact *Telephone:* 513-244-4511. *Fax:* 513-451-2547.

GRADUATE PROGRAMS

Contact *Telephone:* 513-244-4503. *Fax:* 513-451-2547.

MASTER'S DEGREE PROGRAM

Degree MN
Available Programs Accelerated Master's for Non-Nursing College Graduates.
Study Options Full-time.
Program Entrance Requirements Minimum overall college GPA of 3.0, transcript of college record, CPR certification, written essay, immunizations, interview, professional liability insurance/malpractice insurance, prerequisite course work, statistics course. *Application deadline:* Applications may be processed on a rolling basis for some programs. *Application fee:* $50.
Advanced Placement Credit by examination available. Credit given for nursing courses completed elsewhere dependent upon specific evaluations.
Degree Requirements 64 total credit hours, thesis or project.

Defiance College

Bachelor's Degree in Nursing
Defiance, Ohio

Founded in 1850

DEGREE • BSN

Library Facilities 146,344 volumes; 7,088 periodical subscriptions.

BACCALAUREATE PROGRAMS

Degree BSN
Available Programs Generic Baccalaureate; RN Baccalaureate.
Program Entrance Requirements Transcript of college record, minimum GPA in nursing prerequisites of 2.75, RN licensure.
Contact Kathy Holloway, Program Director. *Telephone:* 419-783-2448. *E-mail:* kholloway@defiance.edu.

Franciscan University of Steubenville

Department of Nursing
Steubenville, Ohio

Founded in 1946

DEGREES • BSN • MSN

Nursing Program Faculty 15 (20% with doctorates).
Baccalaureate Enrollment 177 **Women** 91% **Men** 9% **Minority** 5% **International** 1% **Part-time** 5%
Graduate Enrollment 23 **Women** 78% **Men** 22% **Minority** 4% **Part-time** 83%
Nursing Student Activities Student Nurses' Association.
Nursing Student Resources Academic advising; academic or career counseling; assistance for students with disabilities; bookstore; campus computer network; computer lab; e-mail services; Internet; learning resource lab; library services; resume preparation assistance; tutoring.
Library Facilities 29,761 volumes in health, 8,946 volumes in nursing; 410 periodical subscriptions (178 health-care related).

BACCALAUREATE PROGRAMS

Degree BSN
Available Programs Generic Baccalaureate; RN Baccalaureate; RPN to Baccalaureate.
Study Options Full-time and part-time.
Program Entrance Requirements Minimum overall college GPA of 2.5, transcript of college record, health exam, health insurance, high school biology, high school chemistry, 2 years high school science, high school transcript, immunizations, 2 letters of recommendation, minimum high school GPA of 2.4, minimum GPA in nursing prerequisites of 2.5, professional liability insurance/malpractice insurance, prerequisite course work. Transfer students are accepted.
Advanced Placement Credit by examination available. Credit given for nursing courses completed elsewhere dependent upon specific evaluations.
Contact *Telephone:* 740-283-6324. *Fax:* 740-283-6449.

GRADUATE PROGRAMS

Contact *Telephone:* 740-284-7245. *Fax:* 740-283-6449.

MASTER'S DEGREE PROGRAM

Degree MSN
Available Programs Master's; RN to Master's.
Concentrations Available Nursing education. *Nurse practitioner programs in:* family health.
Study Options Full-time and part-time.
Program Entrance Requirements Clinical experience, minimum overall college GPA of 3.0, transcript of college record, interview, 2 letters of recommendation, nursing research course, physical assessment course, professional liability insurance/malpractice insurance, prerequisite course work, statistics course.
Advanced Placement Credit given for nursing courses completed elsewhere dependent upon specific evaluations.
Degree Requirements 48 total credit hours, thesis or project.

Hiram College

Nursing Department
Hiram, Ohio

Founded in 1850

DEGREE • BSN

Nursing Program Faculty 14 (14% with doctorates).
Baccalaureate Enrollment 83 **Women** 89% **Men** 11% **Minority** 18% **International** 2%
Nursing Student Activities Student Nurses' Association.
Nursing Student Resources Academic advising; academic or career counseling; assistance for students with disabilities; bookstore; campus computer network; career placement assistance; computer lab; computer-assisted instruction; e-mail services; employment services for current students; externships; interactive nursing skills videos; Internet; learning resource lab; library services; nursing audiovisuals; resume preparation assistance; skills, simulation, or other laboratory; tutoring.
Library Facilities 506,792 volumes (3,208 in health, 533 in nursing); 8,890 periodical subscriptions (557 health-care related).

BACCALAUREATE PROGRAMS

Degree BSN
Available Programs Generic Baccalaureate.
Study Options Full-time.
Program Entrance Requirements Transcript of college record, written essay, health exam, high school biology, high school chemistry, high school foreign language, high school transcript, immunizations, minimum high school GPA of 2.75. Transfer students are accepted. *Application deadline:* Applications may be processed on a rolling basis for some programs.
Advanced Placement Credit given for nursing courses completed elsewhere dependent upon specific evaluations.
Expenses (2010-11) *Tuition:* full-time $26,435. *International tuition:* $28,000 full-time. *Room and board:* $9460; room only: $4620 per academic year. *Required fees:* full-time $700.
Financial Aid 100% of baccalaureate students in nursing programs received some form of financial aid in 2009-10.

Contact Jennifer LaBenne, Nurse Recruiter, Nursing Department, Hiram College, PO Box 96, Hiram, OH 44234. *Telephone:* 330-569-6104. *Fax:* 330-569-6136. *E-mail:* labenneja@hiram.edu.

Kent State University
College of Nursing
Kent, Ohio

http://www.kent.edu/nursing
Founded in 1910

DEGREES • BSN • DNP • MSN • MSN/MBA • MSN/MPA • PHD

Nursing Program Faculty 120 (20% with doctorates).
Baccalaureate Enrollment 1,178 **Women** 84% **Men** 16% **Minority** 10% **International** 2% **Part-time** 16%
Graduate Enrollment 462 **Women** 95% **Men** 5% **Minority** 12% **International** 2% **Part-time** 85%
Distance Learning Courses Available.
Nursing Student Activities Nursing Honor Society, Sigma Theta Tau, Student Nurses' Association.
Nursing Student Resources Academic advising; academic or career counseling; assistance for students with disabilities; bookstore; campus computer network; career placement assistance; computer lab; computer-assisted instruction; e-mail services; employment services for current students; externships; housing assistance; interactive nursing skills videos; Internet; learning resource lab; library services; nursing audiovisuals; other; paid internships; placement services for program completers; remedial services; resume preparation assistance; skills, simulation, or other laboratory; tutoring.
Library Facilities 2.3 million volumes; 12,000 periodical subscriptions (300 health-care related).

BACCALAUREATE PROGRAMS

Degree BSN
Available Programs ADN to Baccalaureate; Accelerated Baccalaureate; Accelerated Baccalaureate for Second Degree; Accelerated RN Baccalaureate; Baccalaureate for Second Degree; Generic Baccalaureate; LPN to Baccalaureate; RN Baccalaureate.
Site Options Salem, OH; Burton, OH; Warren, OH; Canton, OH.
Study Options Full-time and part-time.
Program Entrance Requirements Minimum overall college GPA of 2.75, transcript of college record, CPR certification, written essay, health exam, high school biology, high school transcript, immunizations, 2 letters of recommendation, minimum high school GPA of 2.75, minimum GPA in nursing prerequisites of 2.75, prerequisite course work. Transfer students are accepted. *Application deadline:* 3/15 (fall), 11/30 (spring).
Advanced Placement Credit given for nursing courses completed elsewhere dependent upon specific evaluations.
Expenses (2010-11) *Tuition, state resident:* full-time $9030; part-time $411 per credit hour. *Tuition, nonresident:* full-time $16,990; part-time $773 per credit hour. *Room and board:* $4504; room only: $2909 per academic year. *Required fees:* full-time $366.
Financial Aid 91% of baccalaureate students in nursing programs received some form of financial aid in 2009-10. *Gift aid (need-based):* Federal Pell, FSEOG, state, private, college/university gift aid from institutional funds. *Loans:* Federal Nursing Student Loans, Federal Direct (Subsidized and Unsubsidized Stafford PLUS), Perkins, state, college/university, alternative loans. *Work-study:* Federal Work-Study. *Financial aid application deadline (priority):* 3/1.
Contact Mr. Curtis Good, Director of Student Services, College of Nursing, Kent State University, Henderson Hall, Kent, OH 44242-0001. *Telephone:* 330-672-9972. *Fax:* 330-672-7911. *E-mail:* cjgood@kent.edu.

GRADUATE PROGRAMS

Expenses (2010-11) *Tuition, state resident:* full-time $9030; part-time $437 per credit hour. *Tuition, nonresident:* full-time $16,990; part-time $779 per credit hour. *Room and board:* $8376 per academic year. *Required fees:* full-time $268.
Financial Aid 85% of graduate students in nursing programs received some form of financial aid in 2009-10. 10 research assistantships with full tuition reimbursements available, 10 teaching assistantships with full tuition reimbursements available were awarded; Federal Work-Study, institutionally sponsored loans, traineeships, tuition waivers (full), and unspecified assistantships also available. *Financial aid application deadline:* 2/1.

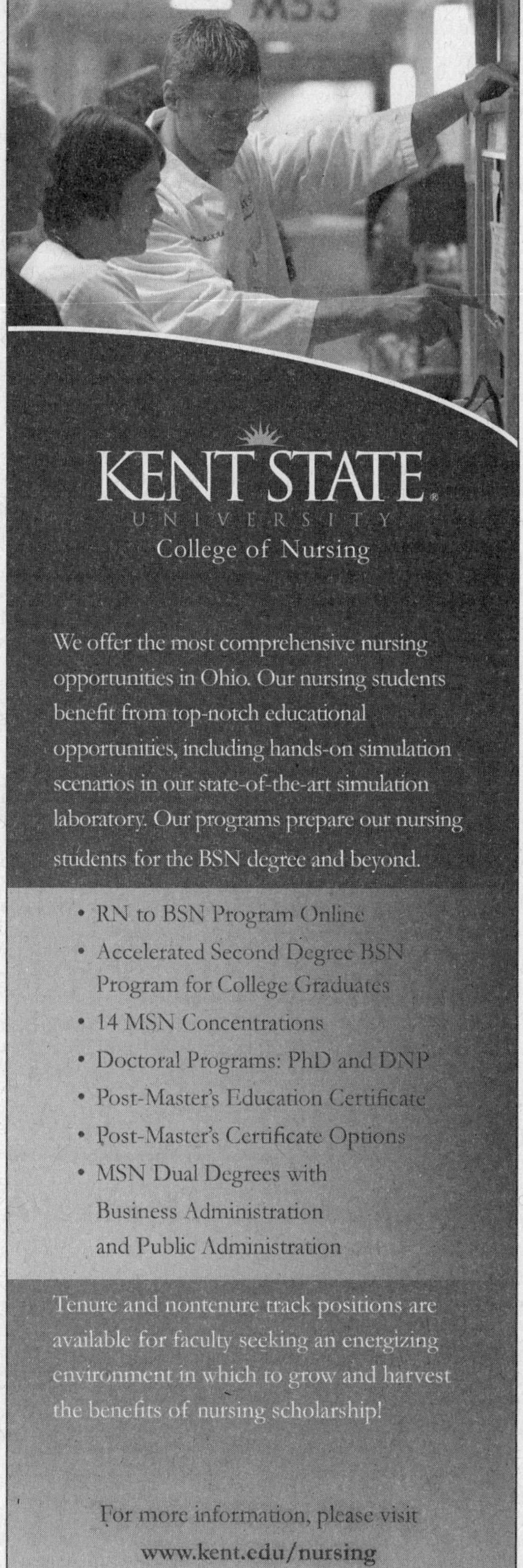

Contact Dr. Karen W. Budd, Director, Graduate Programs, College of Nursing, Kent State University, 214 Henderson Hall, PO Box 5190, Kent, OH 44242-0001. *Telephone:* 330-672-8776. *Fax:* 330-672-6387. *E-mail:* kbudd@kent.edu.

MASTER'S DEGREE PROGRAM

Degrees MSN; MSN/MBA; MSN/MPA
Available Programs Accelerated RN to Master's; Master's.
Concentrations Available Health-care administration; nursing administration; nursing education. *Clinical nurse specialist programs in:* adult health, gerontology, pediatric, psychiatric/mental health, women's health. *Nurse practitioner programs in:* acute care, adult health, family health, gerontology, pediatric, primary care, psychiatric/mental health, women's health.
Study Options Full-time and part-time.
Program Entrance Requirements Clinical experience, computer literacy, minimum overall college GPA of 3.0, transcript of college record, CPR certification, written essay, immunizations, interview, 3 letters of recommendation, professional liability insurance/malpractice insurance, resume, statistics course, GRE (if undergraduate GPA less than 3.0). *Application deadline:* 3/1 (fall), 11/1 (spring). Applications may be processed on a rolling basis for some programs. *Application fee:* $30.
Advanced Placement Credit given for nursing courses completed elsewhere dependent upon specific evaluations.
Degree Requirements 46 total credit hours.

POST-MASTER'S PROGRAM

Areas of Study Health-care administration; nursing education. *Clinical nurse specialist programs in:* adult health, pediatric, psychiatric/mental health. *Nurse practitioner programs in:* acute care, adult health, family health, gerontology, pediatric, primary care, psychiatric/mental health, women's health.

DOCTORAL DEGREE PROGRAM

Degree DNP, PhD
Available Programs Doctorate; Post-Baccalaureate Doctorate.
Areas of Study Aging, clinical practice, ethics, gerontology, health policy, health promotion/disease prevention, maternity-newborn, nurse case management, nursing administration, nursing education, nursing research, nursing science, women's health.
Program Entrance Requirements Minimum overall college GPA of 3.0, interview, 3 letters of recommendation, MSN or equivalent, scholarly papers, statistics course, writing sample, GRE. Application deadline: 7/15 (fall). Applications may be processed on a rolling basis for some programs. Application fee: $30.
Degree Requirements 72 total credit hours, dissertation, residency.

CONTINUING EDUCATION PROGRAM

Contact Betty Freund, Coordinator of Continuing Nursing Education, College of Nursing, Kent State University, PO Box 5190, Kent, OH 44242-0001. *Telephone:* 330-672-8810. *Fax:* 330-672-2433. *E-mail:* bfreund@kent.edu.

See full description on page 482.

Kettering College of Medical Arts
Division of Nursing
Kettering, Ohio

http://www.kcma.edu/
Founded in 1967

DEGREE • BSN

Nursing Program Faculty 20 (15% with doctorates).
Baccalaureate Enrollment 60 **Women** 95% **Part-time** 100%
Distance Learning Courses Available.
Nursing Student Activities Student Nurses' Association.
Nursing Student Resources Academic advising; academic or career counseling; assistance for students with disabilities; bookstore; campus computer network; computer lab; computer-assisted instruction; e-mail services; externships; interactive nursing skills videos; Internet; learning resource lab; library services; nursing audiovisuals; remedial services; resume preparation assistance; skills, simulation, or other laboratory; tutoring.
Library Facilities 29,390 volumes (4,060 in health, 1,073 in nursing); 266 periodical subscriptions (173 health-care related).

BACCALAUREATE PROGRAMS

Degree BSN
Available Programs Generic Baccalaureate; RN Baccalaureate.
Study Options Full-time and part-time.
Online Degree Options Yes (online only).
Program Entrance Requirements Minimum overall college GPA of 2.5, transcript of college record, CPR certification, health insurance, immunizations, minimum high school GPA of 2.75, minimum GPA in nursing prerequisites of 2.5, prerequisite course work. Transfer students are accepted. *Application deadline:* 5/15 (spring).
Advanced Placement Credit given for nursing courses completed elsewhere dependent upon specific evaluations.
Expenses (2010-11) *Tuition:* part-time $366 per credit hour.
Financial Aid 42% of baccalaureate students in nursing programs received some form of financial aid in 2009-10. *Gift aid (need-based):* Federal Pell, state, private, college/university gift aid from institutional funds. *Loans:* Federal Nursing Student Loans, Federal Direct (Subsidized and Unsubsidized Stafford PLUS), Perkins, college/university. *Work-study:* Federal Work-Study, part-time campus jobs. *Financial aid application deadline (priority):* 3/31.
Contact Dr. Cherie R. Rebar, Chair, BSN Completion Program, Division of Nursing, Kettering College of Medical Arts, 3737 Southern Boulevard, Kettering, OH 45429. *Telephone:* 937-395-8642. *Fax:* 937-395-8810. *E-mail:* cherie.rebar@kcma.edu.

Lourdes College
School of Nursing
Sylvania, Ohio

http://www.lourdes.edu
Founded in 1958

DEGREE • BSN

Nursing Program Faculty 15 (20% with doctorates).
Baccalaureate Enrollment 298 **Women** 95% **Men** 5% **Minority** 17% **Part-time** 24%
Nursing Student Activities Sigma Theta Tau, Student Nurses' Association.
Nursing Student Resources Academic advising; academic or career counseling; assistance for students with disabilities; bookstore; campus computer network; computer lab; computer-assisted instruction; e-mail services; employment services for current students; interactive nursing skills videos; Internet; learning resource lab; library services; nursing audiovisuals; remedial services; resume preparation assistance; skills, simulation, or other laboratory; tutoring.
Library Facilities 66,068 volumes (1,200 in health, 700 in nursing); 7,340 periodical subscriptions (101 health-care related).

BACCALAUREATE PROGRAMS

Degree BSN
Available Programs Generic Baccalaureate; LPN to Baccalaureate; RN Baccalaureate.
Site Options Sandusky, OH.
Study Options Full-time and part-time.
Program Entrance Requirements Minimum overall college GPA of 2.0, transcript of college record, CPR certification, health exam, health insurance, high school biology, high school chemistry, high school transcript, immunizations, 3 letters of recommendation, minimum GPA in nursing prerequisites of 2.5, professional liability insurance/malpractice insurance, prerequisite course work. Transfer students are accepted.
Advanced Placement Credit by examination available. Credit given for nursing courses completed elsewhere dependent upon specific evaluations.
Contact *Telephone:* 419-824-3793. *Fax:* 419-824-3985.

Malone University
School of Nursing
Canton, Ohio

http://www.malone.edu/
Founded in 1892

DEGREES • BSN • MSN

Nursing Program Faculty 39 (20% with doctorates).

Baccalaureate Enrollment 328 **Women** 85.7% **Men** 14.3% **Minority** 5.2% **International** .6% **Part-time** 18.3%
Graduate Enrollment 60 **Women** 88.3% **Men** 11.7% **Minority** 3.3% **Part-time** 100%
Nursing Student Activities Sigma Theta Tau, Student Nurses' Association.
Nursing Student Resources Academic advising; academic or career counseling; assistance for students with disabilities; bookstore; campus computer network; career placement assistance; computer lab; computer-assisted instruction; e-mail services; employment services for current students; interactive nursing skills videos; Internet; learning resource lab; library services; nursing audiovisuals; placement services for program completers; remedial services; resume preparation assistance; skills, simulation, or other laboratory; tutoring.
Library Facilities 181,420 volumes (3,919 in health, 295 in nursing); 49,418 periodical subscriptions (316 health-care related).

BACCALAUREATE PROGRAMS

Degree BSN
Available Programs ADN to Baccalaureate; Generic Baccalaureate; RN Baccalaureate.
Study Options Full-time and part-time.
Program Entrance Requirements Minimum overall college GPA of 2.5, transcript of college record, CPR certification, health exam, health insurance, high school biology, high school chemistry, 2 years high school math, 3 years high school science, high school transcript, immunizations, 2 letters of recommendation, minimum high school GPA of 2.5, minimum GPA in nursing prerequisites of 2.0, professional liability insurance/malpractice insurance, prerequisite course work. Transfer students are accepted. *Application deadline:* Applications may be processed on a rolling basis for some programs. *Application fee:* $20.
Advanced Placement Credit given for nursing courses completed elsewhere dependent upon specific evaluations.
Expenses (2010-11) *Tuition:* full-time $21,954; part-time $425 per credit hour. *Room and board:* $7548; room only: $3848 per academic year. *Required fees:* full-time $750; part-time $350 per term.
Financial Aid 96% of baccalaureate students in nursing programs received some form of financial aid in 2009-10. *Gift aid (need-based):* Federal Pell, FSEOG, state, private, college/university gift aid from institutional funds, Academic Competitiveness Grants, National SMART Grants, Teach Grant. *Loans:* Federal Direct (Subsidized and Unsubsidized Stafford PLUS), Perkins, state, college/university, alternative loans. *Work-study:* Federal Work-Study, part-time campus jobs. *Financial aid application deadline:* 7/31(priority: 3/1).
Contact Dr. Brock Schroeder, Vice President for Enrollment Management, School of Nursing, Malone University, 2600 Cleveland Avenue NW, Canton, OH 44709. *Telephone:* 330-471-8145. *Fax:* 330-471-8149. *E-mail:* admissions@malone.edu.

GRADUATE PROGRAMS

Expenses (2010-11) *Tuition:* full-time $16,602. *Required fees:* full-time $3725.
Financial Aid 100% of graduate students in nursing programs received some form of financial aid in 2009-10.
Contact Ms. Jean Yanok, Administrative Assistant, School of Nursing, Malone University, 2600 Cleveland Avenue NW, Canton, OH 44709. *Telephone:* 330-471-8366. *Fax:* 330-471-8607. *E-mail:* jyanok@malone.edu.

MASTER'S DEGREE PROGRAM

Degree MSN
Available Programs Master's.
Concentrations Available *Clinical nurse specialist programs in:* adult health, medical-surgical. *Nurse practitioner programs in:* family health.
Study Options Full-time and part-time.
Program Entrance Requirements Clinical experience, computer literacy, minimum overall college GPA of 3.0, transcript of college record, CPR certification, written essay, immunizations, interview, 2 letters of recommendation, nursing research course, physical assessment course, professional liability insurance/malpractice insurance, resume, statistics course. *Application deadline:* Applications may be processed on a rolling basis for some programs. *Application fee:* $25.
Advanced Placement Credit given for nursing courses completed elsewhere dependent upon specific evaluations.
Degree Requirements 56 total credit hours, thesis or project.

Mercy College of Northwest Ohio

Division of Nursing
Toledo, Ohio

http://www.mercycollege.edu
Founded in 1993

DEGREE • BSN

Nursing Program Faculty 14 (20% with doctorates).
Baccalaureate Enrollment 228 **Women** 88% **Men** 12% **Minority** 12% **Part-time** 13%
Distance Learning Courses Available.
Nursing Student Activities Sigma Theta Tau, Student Nurses' Association.
Nursing Student Resources Academic advising; academic or career counseling; assistance for students with disabilities; campus computer network; career placement assistance; computer lab; computer-assisted instruction; e-mail services; employment services for current students; housing assistance; Internet; learning resource lab; library services; nursing audiovisuals; placement services for program completers; remedial services; resume preparation assistance; skills, simulation, or other laboratory; tutoring.
Library Facilities 6,000 volumes; 129 periodical subscriptions.

BACCALAUREATE PROGRAMS

Degree BSN
Available Programs ADN to Baccalaureate; Generic Baccalaureate; RN Baccalaureate.
Study Options Full-time and part-time.
Online Degree Options Yes.
Program Entrance Requirements Minimum overall college GPA of 2.7, transcript of college record, CPR certification, health exam, high school biology, high school chemistry, 2 years high school math, high school transcript, immunizations, minimum high school GPA of 2.7. Transfer students are accepted. *Application deadline:* 8/1 (fall). *Application fee:* $25.
Advanced Placement Credit by examination available.
Expenses (2009-10) *Tuition:* full-time $8850; part-time $326 per credit hour. *Required fees:* full-time $500.
Financial Aid 80% of baccalaureate students in nursing programs received some form of financial aid in 2008-09.
Contact Susan O'Dell, RN, Program Chair, BS Nursing, Division of Nursing, Mercy College of Northwest Ohio, 2221 Madison Avenue, Toledo, OH 43604. *Telephone:* 888-806-3729. *Fax:* 419-251-1570. *E-mail:* susan.odell@mercycollege.edu.

CONTINUING EDUCATION PROGRAM

Contact Cheryl Nutter, Manager, Continiuing Professional Education, Division of Nursing, Mercy College of Northwest Ohio, 2221 Madison Avenue, Toledo, OH 43606. *Telephone:* 419-251-1519. *E-mail:* Cheryl.Nutter@mercycollege.edu.

Miami University

Department of Nursing
Hamilton, Ohio

http://www.eas.muohio.edu/nsg
Founded in 1809

DEGREE • BSN

Nursing Program Faculty 13 (23% with doctorates).
Baccalaureate Enrollment 106 **Women** 98% **Men** 2% **Minority** 7% **Part-time** 56%
Distance Learning Courses Available.
Nursing Student Activities Sigma Theta Tau, Student Nurses' Association.
Nursing Student Resources Academic advising; academic or career counseling; assistance for students with disabilities; bookstore; campus computer network; computer lab; daycare for children of students; e-mail services; interactive nursing skills videos; Internet; learning resource lab; library services; nursing audiovisuals; resume preparation assistance; tutoring.
Library Facilities 3.7 million volumes (29,000 in nursing); 91,229 periodical subscriptions (852 health-care related).

BACCALAUREATE PROGRAMS

Degree BSN
Available Programs ADN to Baccalaureate; Generic Baccalaureate; RN Baccalaureate.
Site Options Hamilton, OH; Middletown, OH.
Study Options Full-time and part-time.
Program Entrance Requirements Minimum overall college GPA of 2.5, transcript of college record, health exam, health insurance, high school chemistry, 2 years high school math, 1 year of high school science, high school transcript, immunizations, minimum high school GPA of 3.0, minimum GPA in nursing prerequisites of 2.5, professional liability insurance/malpractice insurance. Transfer students are accepted.
Advanced Placement Credit given for nursing courses completed elsewhere dependent upon specific evaluations.
Contact *Telephone:* 513-785-7751. *Fax:* 513-785-7767.

Miami University Hamilton

Bachelor of Science in Nursing Program
Hamilton, Ohio

Founded in 1968

DEGREE • BSN

Nursing Program Faculty 27 (15% with doctorates).
Baccalaureate Enrollment 116
Distance Learning Courses Available.
Nursing Student Activities Sigma Theta Tau, Student Nurses' Association.
Nursing Student Resources Academic advising; academic or career counseling; assistance for students with disabilities; bookstore; campus computer network; career placement assistance; computer lab; computer-assisted instruction; daycare for children of students; e-mail services; employment services for current students; interactive nursing skills videos; Internet; learning resource lab; library services; nursing audiovisuals; placement services for program completers; remedial services; resume preparation assistance; skills, simulation, or other laboratory; tutoring.
Library Facilities 68,000 volumes; 400 periodical subscriptions.

BACCALAUREATE PROGRAMS

Degree BSN
Available Programs Generic Baccalaureate; RN Baccalaureate.
Site Options West Chester, OH; Middletown, OH.
Contact Department of Nursing, Bachelor of Science in Nursing Program, Miami University Hamilton, 1601 University Boulevard, Hamilton, OH 45011-3399. *Telephone:* 513-785-7772. *Fax:* 513-785-7767. *E-mail:* nsginfo@muohio.edu.

Mount Carmel College of Nursing

Nursing Programs
Columbus, Ohio

http://www.mccn.edu/index.html
Founded in 1903

DEGREES • BSN • MS

Nursing Program Faculty 76
Baccalaureate Enrollment 746 **Women** 91% **Men** 9% **Minority** 13% **Part-time** 22%
Graduate Enrollment 72 **Women** 96% **Men** 4% **Minority** 11% **Part-time** 75%
Distance Learning Courses Available.
Nursing Student Activities Sigma Theta Tau, Student Nurses' Association.
Nursing Student Resources Academic advising; academic or career counseling; assistance for students with disabilities; bookstore; campus computer network; computer lab; computer-assisted instruction; e-mail services; housing assistance; interactive nursing skills videos; Internet; learning resource lab; library services; nursing audiovisuals; resume preparation assistance; skills, simulation, or other laboratory; tutoring.
Library Facilities 4,630 volumes in health, 1,972 volumes in nursing; 5,373 periodical subscriptions health-care related.

BACCALAUREATE PROGRAMS

Degree BSN
Available Programs Accelerated Baccalaureate for Second Degree; Generic Baccalaureate; RN Baccalaureate.
Site Options Lancaster, OH.
Study Options Full-time and part-time.
Program Entrance Requirements Minimum overall college GPA of 2.80, transcript of college record, written essay, health exam, high school biology, high school chemistry, high school foreign language, 3 years high school math, 3 years high school science, high school transcript, immunizations, minimum high school GPA of 3.00. Transfer students are accepted. *Application deadline:* 4/1 (fall), 11/1 (winter). Applications may be processed on a rolling basis for some programs. *Application fee:* $30.
Advanced Placement Credit given for nursing courses completed elsewhere dependent upon specific evaluations.
Expenses (2010-11) *Tuition:* full-time $17,090; part-time $323 per credit. *Room and board:* room only: $5400 per academic year. *Required fees:* full-time $443.
Financial Aid 86% of baccalaureate students in nursing programs received some form of financial aid in 2009-10.
Contact Kim M. Campbell, Director, Admissions and Recruitment, Nursing Programs, Mount Carmel College of Nursing, 127 South Davis Avenue, Columbus, OH 43222-1504. *Telephone:* 614-234-5144. *Fax:* 614-234-2875. *E-mail:* kcampbell@mccn.edu.

GRADUATE PROGRAMS

Expenses (2010-11) *Tuition:* full-time $6435; part-time $390 per credit. *Room and board:* room only: $5400 per academic year.
Financial Aid 20% of graduate students in nursing programs received some form of financial aid in 2009-10.
Contact Kip Sexton, MS Program Coordinator, Nursing Programs, Mount Carmel College of Nursing, 127 South Davis Avenue, Columbus, OH 43222-1504. *Telephone:* 614-234-5169. *Fax:* 614-234-2875. *E-mail:* ksexton@mccn.edu.

MASTER'S DEGREE PROGRAM

Degree MS
Available Programs Master's.
Concentrations Available Nursing administration; nursing education. *Clinical nurse specialist programs in:* adult health. *Nurse practitioner programs in:* family health.
Study Options Full-time and part-time.
Program Entrance Requirements Minimum overall college GPA of 3.0, transcript of college record, CPR certification, written essay, 3 letters of recommendation, professional liability insurance/malpractice insurance, resume. *Application deadline:* 7/1 (fall), 11/1 (spring), 4/1 (summer). Applications may be processed on a rolling basis for some programs. *Application fee:* $30.
Degree Requirements 33 total credit hours, thesis or project.

POST-MASTER'S PROGRAM

Areas of Study Nursing education. *Nurse practitioner programs in:* family health.

Mount Vernon Nazarene University

School of Nursing and Health Sciences
Mount Vernon, Ohio

Founded in 1964

DEGREE • BSN

Library Facilities 162,643 volumes; 8,710 periodical subscriptions.

BACCALAUREATE PROGRAMS

Degree BSN
Available Programs RN Baccalaureate.
Program Entrance Requirements Transcript of college record, immunizations, professional liability insurance/malpractice insurance, RN licensure.
Contact Nursing Program, School of Nursing and Health Sciences, Mount Vernon Nazarene University, 800 Martinsburg Road, Mount Vernon, OH 43050. *Telephone:* 740-392-6868.

Muskingum University

Department of Nursing
New Concord, Ohio

Founded in 1837

DEGREE • BSN

Library Facilities 233,000 volumes; 900 periodical subscriptions.

BACCALAUREATE PROGRAMS

Degree BSN
Available Programs Generic Baccalaureate.
Contact Dr. Elaine Haynes, RN, Director of Nursing, Chair and Professor, Department of Nursing, Muskingum University, New Concord, OH 43762. *Telephone:* 740-826-6151. *E-mail:* ehaynes@muskingum.edu.

Notre Dame College

Nursing Department
South Euclid, Ohio

Founded in 1922

DEGREE • BSN

BACCALAUREATE PROGRAMS

Degree BSN
Available Programs Generic Baccalaureate; RN Baccalaureate.
Contact Nursing Division, Nursing Department, Notre Dame College, 4545 College Road, South Euclid, OH 44121-4293. *Telephone:* 216-373-5183.

Ohio Northern University

Nursing Program
Ada, Ohio

Founded in 1871

DEGREE • BSN

BACCALAUREATE PROGRAMS

Degree BSN
Available Programs RN Baccalaureate.
Contact Nursing Program, Nursing Program, Ohio Northern University, 525 North Main Street, Ada, OH 45810. *Telephone:* 419-772-2000.

The Ohio State University

College of Nursing
Columbus, Ohio

http://www.nursing.osu.edu/
Founded in 1870

DEGREES • BSN • DNP • MS • MS/MPH

Nursing Program Faculty 79 (42% with doctorates).
Baccalaureate Enrollment 572 **Women** 88% **Men** 12% **Minority** 11% **International** 2% **Part-time** 20%
Graduate Enrollment 408 **Women** 91% **Men** 9% **Minority** 11% **International** 2% **Part-time** 43%
Distance Learning Courses Available.
Nursing Student Activities Nursing Honor Society, Sigma Theta Tau, Student Nurses' Association, nursing club.
Nursing Student Resources Academic advising; academic or career counseling; assistance for students with disabilities; bookstore; campus computer network; career placement assistance; computer lab; computer-assisted instruction; daycare for children of students; e-mail services; employment services for current students; externships; housing assistance; interactive nursing skills videos; Internet; learning resource lab; library services; nursing audiovisuals; other; paid internships; placement services for program completers; remedial services; resume preparation assistance; skills, simulation, or other laboratory; tutoring; unpaid internships.
Library Facilities 6.2 million volumes (188,602 in health, 4,198 in nursing); 79,751 periodical subscriptions (5,060 health-care related).

BACCALAUREATE PROGRAMS

Degree BSN
Available Programs Generic Baccalaureate; RN Baccalaureate.
Study Options Full-time.
Program Entrance Requirements Minimum overall college GPA of 2.75, transcript of college record, CPR certification, written essay, health insurance, high school biology, high school chemistry, high school foreign language, 3 years high school math, 2 years high school science, high school transcript, immunizations, minimum GPA in nursing prerequisites of 3.0, professional liability insurance/malpractice insurance, prerequisite course work. *Application deadline:* 2/1 (fall). *Application fee:* $40.
Advanced Placement Credit by examination available. Credit given for nursing courses completed elsewhere dependent upon specific evaluations.
Expenses (2010-11) *Tuition, state resident:* full-time $8541; part-time $237 per quarter hour. *Tuition, nonresident:* full-time $22,725; part-time $631 per quarter hour. *Room and board:* $9930; room only: $6420 per academic year. *Required fees:* full-time $1239; part-time $50 per credit.
Financial Aid 80% of baccalaureate students in nursing programs received some form of financial aid in 2009-10. *Gift aid (need-based):* Federal Pell, FSEOG, state, private, college/university gift aid from institutional funds. *Loans:* Federal Nursing Student Loans, Federal Direct (Subsidized and Unsubsidized Stafford PLUS), Perkins, college/university. *Work-study:* Federal Work-Study, part-time campus jobs. *Financial aid application deadline (priority):* 2/15.
Contact Ms. Georgia Paletta, Counselor and Staff Assistant, College of Nursing, The Ohio State University, Graduate and Professional Admissions, 105 Student Academic Services Building, Columbus, OH 43210. *Telephone:* 614-292-9444. *E-mail:* paletta.4@osu.edu.

GRADUATE PROGRAMS

Expenses (2010-11) *Tuition, state resident:* full-time $10,425; part-time $348 per quarter hour. *Tuition, nonresident:* full-time $25,815; part-time $879 per quarter hour. *Room and board:* $10,305; room only: $6570 per academic year. *Required fees:* full-time $1083; part-time $60 per credit.
Financial Aid 90% of graduate students in nursing programs received some form of financial aid in 2009-10. Fellowships, research assistantships, teaching assistantships, Federal Work-Study, institutionally sponsored loans, and unspecified assistantships available. Aid available to part-time students.
Contact Ms. Jackie Min, Graduate Outreach Coordinator, College of Nursing, The Ohio State University, 1585 Neil Avenue, 212 Newton Hall, Columbus, OH 43210-1289. *Telephone:* 614-688-8145. *Fax:* 614-247-8618. *E-mail:* min.37@osu.edu.

MASTER'S DEGREE PROGRAM

Degrees MS; MS/MPH
Available Programs Accelerated Master's for Non-Nursing College Graduates; Accelerated Master's for Nurses with Non-Nursing Degrees; Master's; Master's for Non-Nursing College Graduates; Master's for Nurses with Non-Nursing Degrees.
Concentrations Available Clinical nurse leader; health-care administration; nurse-midwifery; nursing administration. *Clinical nurse specialist programs in:* adult health, cardiovascular, community health, oncology, psychiatric/mental health, public health. *Nurse practitioner programs in:* acute care, adult health, community health, family health, neonatal health, pediatric, primary care, psychiatric/mental health, women's health.
Study Options Full-time and part-time.
Program Entrance Requirements Minimum overall college GPA of 3.0, transcript of college record, written essay, 3 letters of recommendation, prerequisite course work, resume. *Application deadline:* 5/1 (fall), 11/1 (winter), 2/1 (spring), 2/1 (summer). *Application fee:* $40.
Advanced Placement Credit given for nursing courses completed elsewhere dependent upon specific evaluations.
Degree Requirements 45 total credit hours, thesis or project, comprehensive exam.

POST-MASTER'S PROGRAM

Areas of Study Clinical nurse leader; health-care administration; nurse-midwifery; nursing administration. *Clinical nurse specialist programs in:* adult health, cardiovascular, community health, oncology, psychiatric/mental health, public health. *Nurse practitioner programs in:* acute care, adult health, community health, family health, neonatal health, pediatric, primary care, psychiatric/mental health, women's health.

DOCTORAL DEGREE PROGRAM

Degree DNP

Available Programs Doctorate; Doctorate for Nurses with Non-Nursing Degrees; Post-Baccalaureate Doctorate.

Areas of Study Addiction/substance abuse, advanced practice nursing, aging, bio-behavioral research, biology of health and illness, clinical practice, community health, critical care, ethics, faculty preparation, family health, gerontology, health policy, health promotion/disease prevention, health-care systems, human health and illness, illness and transition, individualized study, information systems, maternity-newborn, neuro-behavior, nurse case management, nursing administration, nursing policy, nursing research, nursing science, oncology, urban health, women's health.

Program Entrance Requirements Clinical experience, minimum overall college GPA of 3.5, interview, 3 letters of recommendation, MSN or equivalent, statistics course, vita, writing sample. Application deadline: 1/15 (fall). Application fee: $40.

Degree Requirements 90 total credit hours, dissertation, oral exam, written exam, residency.

CONTINUING EDUCATION PROGRAM

Contact Ms. Patti Reid, Director of Continuing Education, College of Nursing, The Ohio State University, 1585 Neil Avenue, Columbus, OH 43210-1289. *Telephone:* 614-292-6744. *Fax:* 614-292-7976. *E-mail:* reid.174@osu.edu.

Ohio University

School of Nursing
Athens, Ohio

http://www.ohio.edu/nursing/

Founded in 1804

DEGREES • BSN • MSN

Nursing Program Faculty 9 (89% with doctorates).

Nursing Student Activities Nursing Honor Society, Sigma Theta Tau.

Nursing Student Resources Academic or career counseling; career placement assistance; computer lab; e-mail services; Internet; library services.

Library Facilities 3 million volumes; 46,823 periodical subscriptions.

BACCALAUREATE PROGRAMS

Degree BSN

Available Programs Generic Baccalaureate; RN Baccalaureate.

Online Degree Options Yes.

Program Entrance Requirements Transfer students are accepted.

Contact Dr. Deborah Henderson, Associate Director, School of Nursing, Ohio University, E365 Grover Center, Athens, OH 45701. *Telephone:* 740-593-4494. *Fax:* 740-593-0286. *E-mail:* hendersd@ohio.edu.

GRADUATE PROGRAMS

Contact Dr. Kathy Rose-Grippa, Graduate Coordinator, School of Nursing, Ohio University, E365 Grover Center, Athens, OH 45701-2979. *Telephone:* 740-593-4494. *Fax:* 740-593-0144. *E-mail:* grippa@ohio.edu.

MASTER'S DEGREE PROGRAM

Degree MSN

Available Programs Master's.

Concentrations Available Nursing administration; nursing education. *Nurse practitioner programs in:* family health.

Study Options Full-time and part-time.

Program Entrance Requirements Minimum overall college GPA of 3.0, transcript of college record, written essay, 3 letters of recommendation, resume, statistics course.

Advanced Placement Credit given for nursing courses completed elsewhere dependent upon specific evaluations.

Degree Requirements 55 total credit hours.

Otterbein University

Department of Nursing
Westerville, Ohio

http://www.otterbein.edu/dept/NURS

Founded in 1847

DEGREES • BSN • MSN

Nursing Student Activities Nursing Honor Society, Sigma Theta Tau.

Library Facilities 182,629 volumes; 1,012 periodical subscriptions.

BACCALAUREATE PROGRAMS

Degree BSN

Available Programs Accelerated RN Baccalaureate; Generic Baccalaureate; LPN to Baccalaureate; RN Baccalaureate.

Program Entrance Requirements Transfer students are accepted.

Advanced Placement Credit by examination available. Credit given for nursing courses completed elsewhere dependent upon specific evaluations.

Contact *Telephone:* 614-823-1614. *Fax:* 614-823-3131.

GRADUATE PROGRAMS

Contact *Telephone:* 614-823-1614.

MASTER'S DEGREE PROGRAM

Degree MSN

Available Programs Master's.

Concentrations Available Nursing administration; nursing education. *Clinical nurse specialist programs in:* adult health. *Nurse practitioner programs in:* adult health, family health.

Study Options Part-time.

POST-MASTER'S PROGRAM

Areas of Study Nursing education. *Nurse practitioner programs in:* adult health, family health.

CONTINUING EDUCATION PROGRAM

Contact *Telephone:* 614-823-1614.

Shawnee State University

Department of Nursing
Portsmouth, Ohio

http://www.shawnee.edu/acad/hs/bsn/index.html

Founded in 1986

DEGREE • BSN

Nursing Program Faculty 9.

Nursing Student Activities Student Nurses' Association.

Nursing Student Resources Academic advising; academic or career counseling; assistance for students with disabilities; bookstore; campus computer network; career placement assistance; computer lab; computer-assisted instruction; daycare for children of students; e-mail services; employment services for current students; housing assistance; interactive nursing skills videos; Internet; learning resource lab; library services; nursing audiovisuals; other; placement services for program completers; remedial services; resume preparation assistance; skills, simulation, or other laboratory; tutoring.

Library Facilities 144,595 volumes (8,273 in health, 870 in nursing); 8,148 periodical subscriptions (1,798 health-care related).

BACCALAUREATE PROGRAMS

Degree BSN

Available Programs ADN to Baccalaureate; RN Baccalaureate.

Study Options Full-time and part-time.

Program Entrance Requirements Minimum overall college GPA of 2.5, transcript of college record, CPR certification, health exam, health insurance, high school transcript, immunizations, professional liability insurance/malpractice insurance, prerequisite course work, RN licensure. Transfer students are accepted.

Advanced Placement Credit given for nursing courses completed elsewhere dependent upon specific evaluations.

Contact *Telephone:* 740-351-3378. *Fax:* 740-351-3354.

CONTINUING EDUCATION PROGRAM

Contact *Telephone:* 740-351-3281.

The University of Akron

College of Nursing
Akron, Ohio

http://www.uakron.edu/nursing
Founded in 1870

DEGREES • BSN • MSN • PHD

Nursing Program Faculty 99 (28% with doctorates).
Baccalaureate Enrollment 505 **Women** 81% **Men** 19% **Minority** 10% **Part-time** 6%
Graduate Enrollment 295 **Women** 89% **Men** 11% **Minority** 11% **International** 3% **Part-time** 66%
Distance Learning Courses Available.
Nursing Student Activities Sigma Theta Tau, Student Nurses' Association, nursing club.
Nursing Student Resources Academic advising; academic or career counseling; assistance for students with disabilities; bookstore; campus computer network; career placement assistance; computer lab; computer-assisted instruction; daycare for children of students; e-mail services; employment services for current students; interactive nursing skills videos; Internet; learning resource lab; library services; nursing audiovisuals; remedial services; resume preparation assistance; skills, simulation, or other laboratory; tutoring.
Library Facilities 1.3 million volumes (32,000 in health, 8,920 in nursing); 7,804 periodical subscriptions health-care related.

BACCALAUREATE PROGRAMS

Degree BSN
Available Programs ADN to Baccalaureate; Accelerated Baccalaureate for Second Degree; Generic Baccalaureate; LPN to Baccalaureate; RN Baccalaureate.
Site Options Medina, OH; Orville, OH; Lorain, OH.
Study Options Full-time and part-time.
Program Entrance Requirements Transcript of college record, CPR certification, health exam, immunizations, minimum GPA in nursing prerequisites of 2.75, prerequisite course work. Transfer students are accepted. *Application deadline:* Applications may be processed on a rolling basis for some programs. *Application fee:* $30.
Advanced Placement Credit given for nursing courses completed elsewhere dependent upon specific evaluations.
Expenses (2010-11) *Tuition, state resident:* full-time $7733; part-time $322 per credit hour. *Tuition, nonresident:* full-time $15,389; part-time $641 per credit hour. *Room and board:* $9028; room only: $5830 per academic year. *Required fees:* full-time $2561; part-time $69 per credit; part-time $284 per term.
Financial Aid 80% of baccalaureate students in nursing programs received some form of financial aid in 2009-10. *Gift aid (need-based):* Federal Pell, FSEOG, state, college/university gift aid from institutional funds. *Loans:* Federal Nursing Student Loans, Perkins, college/university. *Work-study:* Federal Work-Study, part-time campus jobs. *Financial aid application deadline (priority):* 2/1.
Contact Dr. Rita A. Klein, Director, Nursing Student Affairs, College of Nursing, The University of Akron, Akron, OH 44325-3701. *Telephone:* 330-972-5103. *Fax:* 330-972-5493. *E-mail:* rklein@uakron.edu.

GRADUATE PROGRAMS

Expenses (2010-11) *Tuition, state resident:* full-time $6800; part-time $378 per credit hour. *Tuition, nonresident:* full-time $11,643; part-time $647 per credit hour. *Room and board:* $9028; room only: $5830 per academic year. *Required fees:* full-time $1265; part-time $52 per credit; part-time $162 per term.
Financial Aid 80% of graduate students in nursing programs received some form of financial aid in 2009-10. 7 research assistantships with full tuition reimbursements available, 8 teaching assistantships with full tuition reimbursements available were awarded; career-related internships or fieldwork and Federal Work-Study also available.
Contact Dr. Marlene S. Huff, Coordinator, Educational Progression and Graduate Programs, College of Nursing, The University of Akron, Akron, OH 44325-3701. *Telephone:* 330-972-5930. *Fax:* 330-972-5737. *E-mail:* mhuff@uakron.edu.

MASTER'S DEGREE PROGRAM

Degree MSN
Available Programs Master's; RN to Master's.
Concentrations Available Nurse anesthesia; nursing administration. *Clinical nurse specialist programs in:* adult health, gerontology, pediatric, psychiatric/mental health. *Nurse practitioner programs in:* adult health, gerontology, pediatric, psychiatric/mental health.
Site Options Orville, OH; Lorain, OH.
Study Options Full-time and part-time.
Program Entrance Requirements Clinical experience, computer literacy, minimum overall college GPA of 3.0, transcript of college record, CPR certification, written essay, immunizations, interview, 3 letters of recommendation, physical assessment course, professional liability insurance/malpractice insurance, prerequisite course work, resume, statistics course, GRE. *Application deadline:* Applications may be processed on a rolling basis for some programs. *Application fee:* $30.
Advanced Placement Credit given for nursing courses completed elsewhere dependent upon specific evaluations.
Degree Requirements 53 total credit hours.

POST-MASTER'S PROGRAM

Areas of Study Nurse anesthesia. *Clinical nurse specialist programs in:* adult health, gerontology, pediatric, psychiatric/mental health. *Nurse practitioner programs in:* adult health, gerontology, pediatric, psychiatric/mental health.

DOCTORAL DEGREE PROGRAM

Degree PhD
Available Programs Doctorate.
Areas of Study Aging, community health, ethics, gerontology, health policy, health promotion/disease prevention, health-care systems, human health and illness, illness and transition, individualized study, maternity-newborn, nursing administration, nursing policy, nursing research, nursing science, women's health.
Program Entrance Requirements Minimum overall college GPA of 3.0, interview by faculty committee, interview, 3 letters of recommendation, MSN or equivalent, vita, writing sample, GRE. Application deadline: Applications may be processed on a rolling basis for some programs. Application fee: $30.
Degree Requirements 72 total credit hours, dissertation, oral exam, written exam, residency.

CONTINUING EDUCATION PROGRAM

Contact Dr. Marlene S. Huff, Coordinator, Educational Progression and Graduate Programs, College of Nursing, The University of Akron, Akron, OH 44325-3701. *Telephone:* 330-972-5930. *Fax:* 330-972-5737. *E-mail:* mhuff@uakron.edu.

See full description on page 494.

University of Cincinnati

College of Nursing
Cincinnati, Ohio

http://www.nursing.uc.edu
Founded in 1819

DEGREES • BSN • MSN • MSN/MBA • MSN/PHD • PHD

Nursing Program Faculty 143 (31% with doctorates).
Baccalaureate Enrollment 631 **Women** 90% **Men** 10% **Minority** 14% **Part-time** 13%
Graduate Enrollment 360 **Women** 86% **Men** 14% **Minority** 14% **International** 2%
Distance Learning Courses Available.
Nursing Student Activities Sigma Theta Tau, Student Nurses' Association.
Nursing Student Resources Academic advising; academic or career counseling; assistance for students with disabilities; bookstore; campus computer network; computer lab; computer-assisted instruction; e-mail services; employment services for current students; externships; housing assistance; interactive nursing skills videos; Internet; learning resource lab; library services; nursing audiovisuals; paid internships; remedial services; resume preparation assistance; skills, simulation, or other laboratory; tutoring; unpaid internships.
Library Facilities 3.7 million volumes (221,630 in health, 21,306 in nursing); 103,066 periodical subscriptions (2,384 health-care related).

BACCALAUREATE PROGRAMS

Degree BSN
Available Programs ADN to Baccalaureate; Accelerated Baccalaureate for Second Degree; Generic Baccalaureate; RN Baccalaureate.
Site Options Cincinnati, OH.
Study Options Full-time.
Program Entrance Requirements Minimum overall college GPA of 2.5, transcript of college record, CPR certification, health insurance, high school biology, high school chemistry, 3 years high school math, high school transcript, immunizations, prerequisite course work. Transfer students are accepted. *Application deadline:* 6/30 (fall).
Advanced Placement Credit by examination available. Credit given for nursing courses completed elsewhere dependent upon specific evaluations.
Contact ***Telephone:*** 513-558-5070. *Fax:* 513-558-7523.

GRADUATE PROGRAMS

Contact ***Telephone:*** 513-558-5072. *Fax:* 513-558-7523.

MASTER'S DEGREE PROGRAM

Degrees MSN; MSN/MBA; MSN/PhD
Available Programs Accelerated Master's for Non-Nursing College Graduates; Master's.
Concentrations Available Nurse anesthesia; nurse-midwifery; nursing administration. *Clinical nurse specialist programs in:* adult health, critical care, gerontology, medical-surgical, occupational health, public health. *Nurse practitioner programs in:* adult health, family health, neonatal health, occupational health, pediatric, women's health.
Site Options Cincinnati, OH.
Study Options Full-time and part-time.
Online Degree Options Yes.
Program Entrance Requirements Clinical experience, computer literacy, transcript of college record, CPR certification, written essay, immunizations, interview, 3 letters of recommendation, physical assessment course, professional liability insurance/malpractice insurance, resume, statistics course, GRE General Test. *Application deadline:* 10/1 (fall), 9/1 (winter), 1/1 (spring), 3/1 (summer). Applications may be processed on a rolling basis for some programs. *Application fee:* $40.
Advanced Placement Credit given for nursing courses completed elsewhere dependent upon specific evaluations.
Degree Requirements 65 total credit hours, thesis or project.

POST-MASTER'S PROGRAM

Areas of Study Nursing education. *Nurse practitioner programs in:* adult health, family health, neonatal health, occupational health, pediatric, psychiatric/mental health, women's health.

DOCTORAL DEGREE PROGRAM

Degree PhD
Available Programs Doctorate; Post-Baccalaureate Doctorate.
Areas of Study Addiction/substance abuse, community health, critical care, ethics, faculty preparation, family health, health promotion/disease prevention, health-care systems, human health and illness, illness and transition, individualized study, maternity-newborn, nursing administration, nursing research, nursing science, oncology, women's health.
Site Options Cincinnati, OH.
Program Entrance Requirements Minimum overall college GPA of 3.0, interview by faculty committee, interview, 3 letters of recommendation, statistics course, vita, writing sample, GRE General Test. Application deadline: 8/15 (fall). Applications may be processed on a rolling basis for some programs. Application fee: $40.
Degree Requirements 135 total credit hours, dissertation, oral exam, written exam, residency.

CONTINUING EDUCATION PROGRAM

Contact ***Telephone:*** 513-558-5311. *Fax:* 513-558-5054.

University of Phoenix–Cleveland Campus

College of Nursing
Independence, Ohio

Founded in 2000

DEGREES • BSN • MSN

Nursing Program Faculty 10 (20% with doctorates).
Baccalaureate Enrollment 17 **Women** 82.4% **Men** 17.6% **Minority** 11.8%
Graduate Enrollment 4 **Women** 100%
Nursing Student Activities Sigma Theta Tau.
Nursing Student Resources Academic advising; academic or career counseling; assistance for students with disabilities; bookstore; campus computer network; computer lab; computer-assisted instruction; e-mail services; interactive nursing skills videos; Internet; learning resource lab; library services; nursing audiovisuals; remedial services; skills, simulation, or other laboratory; tutoring.
Library Facilities 16,781 periodical subscriptions (1,300 health-care related).

BACCALAUREATE PROGRAMS

Degree BSN
Available Programs Accelerated Baccalaureate.
Site Options Beachwood, OH.
Study Options Full-time.
Program Entrance Requirements Transcript of college record, CPR certification, immunizations, 1 letter of recommendation, RN licensure. Transfer students are accepted. *Application deadline:* Applications may be processed on a rolling basis for some programs.
Advanced Placement Credit by examination available. Credit given for nursing courses completed elsewhere dependent upon specific evaluations.
Expenses (2009-10) *Tuition:* full-time $10,560. *Required fees:* full-time $600.
Contact Campus College Chair, Nursing, College of Nursing, University of Phoenix–Cleveland Campus, 5005 Rockside Road, Suite 130, Independence, OH 44131. *Telephone:* 216-447-8807.

GRADUATE PROGRAMS

Expenses (2009-10) *Tuition:* full-time $13,200. *Required fees:* full-time $760.
Financial Aid Institutionally sponsored loans and scholarships available.
Contact Campus College Chair, Nursing, College of Nursing, University of Phoenix–Cleveland Campus, 5005 Rockside Road, Suite 130, Independence, OH 44131. *Telephone:* 216-447-8807.

MASTER'S DEGREE PROGRAM

Degree MSN
Available Programs Master's.
Concentrations Available Nursing administration.
Site Options Beachwood, OH.
Study Options Full-time.
Program Entrance Requirements Clinical experience, computer literacy, minimum overall college GPA of 2.5, transcript of college record. *Application deadline:* Applications may be processed on a rolling basis for some programs. *Application fee:* $45.
Advanced Placement Credit given for nursing courses completed elsewhere dependent upon specific evaluations.
Degree Requirements 39 total credit hours, thesis or project.

University of Rio Grande

Holzer School of Nursing
Rio Grande, Ohio

Founded in 1876

DEGREE • BSN

Nursing Program Faculty 9
Library Facilities 96,731 volumes; 850 periodical subscriptions.

BACCALAUREATE PROGRAMS

Degree BSN
Available Programs RN Baccalaureate.
Study Options Full-time and part-time.
Contact ***Telephone:*** 800-282-7201 Ext. 7308. *Fax:* 740-245-7177.

The University of Toledo
College of Nursing
Toledo, Ohio

http://www.utoledo.edu/nursing
Founded in 1872

DEGREES • BSN • DNP • MSN
Nursing Program Faculty 58 (45% with doctorates).
Baccalaureate Enrollment 474 **Women** 88% **Men** 12% **Minority** 7% **International** 2% **Part-time** 23%
Graduate Enrollment 274 **Women** 88% **Men** 12% **Minority** 7% **Part-time** 77%
Distance Learning Courses Available.
Nursing Student Activities Sigma Theta Tau, Student Nurses' Association, nursing club.
Nursing Student Resources Academic advising; academic or career counseling; assistance for students with disabilities; bookstore; campus computer network; computer lab; computer-assisted instruction; daycare for children of students; e-mail services; interactive nursing skills videos; Internet; learning resource lab; library services; nursing audiovisuals; paid internships; resume preparation assistance; skills, simulation, or other laboratory; tutoring.
Library Facilities 2.1 million volumes (33,000 in health, 4,000 in nursing); 1,841 periodical subscriptions (2,400 health-care related).

BACCALAUREATE PROGRAMS
Degree BSN
Available Programs ADN to Baccalaureate; Generic Baccalaureate.
Study Options Full-time and part-time.
Online Degree Options Yes.
Program Entrance Requirements Minimum overall college GPA of 3.0, transcript of college record, CPR certification, health exam, health insurance, high school biology, high school chemistry, high school foreign language, 3 years high school math, 3 years high school science, high school transcript, immunizations, minimum high school GPA of 3.0, professional liability insurance/malpractice insurance, prerequisite course work. Transfer students are accepted. *Application deadline:* 5/1 (fall), 9/1 (spring), 1/1 (summer).
Advanced Placement Credit given for nursing courses completed elsewhere dependent upon specific evaluations.
Expenses (2010-11) *Tuition, state resident:* full-time $7301; part-time $304 per credit hour. *Tuition, nonresident:* full-time $16,421; part-time $684 per credit hour. *Room and board:* $9746 per academic year. *Required fees:* full-time $5102; part-time $110 per credit; part-time $154 per term.
Financial Aid 60% of baccalaureate students in nursing programs received some form of financial aid in 2009-10. *Gift aid (need-based):* Federal Pell, FSEOG, state, private, college/university gift aid from institutional funds, Academic Competitiveness Grants, National SMART Grants, TEACH Grants. *Loans:* Federal Direct (Subsidized and Unsubsidized Stafford PLUS), Perkins, alternative loans. *Work-study:* Federal Work-Study. *Financial aid application deadline (priority):* 4/1.
Contact Ms. Paula Ballmer, Assistant Dean of Student Services, College of Nursing, The University of Toledo, 3000 Arlington Avenue, Mail Stop 1026, Health Science Campus, Toledo, OH 43614-2598. *Telephone:* 419-383-5839. *Fax:* 419-383-5894. *E-mail:* paula.ballmer@utoledo.edu.

GRADUATE PROGRAMS
Expenses (2010-11) *Tuition, state resident:* full-time $11,426; part-time $476 per credit hour. *Tuition, nonresident:* full-time $21,660; part-time $903 per credit hour. *Required fees:* full-time $5102; part-time $110 per credit; part-time $154 per term.
Financial Aid 60% of graduate students in nursing programs received some form of financial aid in 2009-10. Federal Work-Study, institutionally sponsored loans, and scholarships available.
Contact Ms. Kathleen Mitchell, Graduate Nursing Advisor, College of Nursing, The University of Toledo, Mail Stop #1026, 3000 Arlington Avenue, Toledo, OH 43614-2598. *Telephone:* 419-383-5841. *Fax:* 419-383-5894. *E-mail:* kathleen.mitchell@utoledo.edu.

MASTER'S DEGREE PROGRAM
Degree MSN
Available Programs Master's; Master's for Non-Nursing College Graduates; Master's for Nurses with Non-Nursing Degrees.
Concentrations Available Clinical nurse leader; nursing education. *Clinical nurse specialist programs in:* adult health, psychiatric/mental health. *Nurse practitioner programs in:* adult health, family health, pediatric.
Study Options Full-time and part-time.
Program Entrance Requirements Computer literacy, minimum overall college GPA of 3.0, transcript of college record, written essay, 2 letters of recommendation, prerequisite course work, resume, GRE General Test. *Application deadline:* 1/1 (fall), 8/15 (spring). *Application fee:* $110.
Advanced Placement Credit given for nursing courses completed elsewhere dependent upon specific evaluations.
Degree Requirements 55 total credit hours, thesis or project, comprehensive exam.

POST-MASTER'S PROGRAM
Areas of Study Nursing education. *Clinical nurse specialist programs in:* psychiatric/mental health. *Nurse practitioner programs in:* adult health, family health, pediatric.

DOCTORAL DEGREE PROGRAM
Degree DNP
Available Programs Doctorate.
Areas of Study Advanced practice nursing, nursing administration.
Online Degree Options Yes (online only).
Program Entrance Requirements Clinical experience, minimum overall college GPA of 3.3, interview by faculty committee, interview, 3 letters of recommendation, MSN or equivalent, statistics course, vita, writing sample. Application deadline: 1/1 (fall). Application fee: $110.
Degree Requirements 36 total credit hours.

CONTINUING EDUCATION PROGRAM
Contact Ms. Deborah Mattin, Director, Continuing Nursing Education, College of Nursing, The University of Toledo, Mail Stop #1026, 3000 Arlington Avenue, Toledo, OH 43614-2598. *Telephone:* 419-383-5812. *Fax:* 419-383-5894. *E-mail:* deborah.mattin@utoledo.edu.

Urbana University
BSN Completion Program
Urbana, Ohio

http://www.urbana.edu/index.php/academics/undergraduate_majors/nursing
Founded in 1850

DEGREES • BSN • MSN
Nursing Program Faculty 3 (67% with doctorates).
Baccalaureate Enrollment 120 **Women** 97% **Men** 3% **Minority** 3% **Part-time** 98%
Graduate Enrollment 10
Nursing Student Activities Nursing Honor Society.
Nursing Student Resources Academic advising; academic or career counseling; assistance for students with disabilities; bookstore; campus computer network; career placement assistance; computer lab; e-mail services; Internet; learning resource lab; library services; nursing audiovisuals; placement services for program completers; remedial services; resume preparation assistance; tutoring.
Library Facilities 61,600 volumes; 800 periodical subscriptions.

BACCALAUREATE PROGRAMS
Degree BSN
Available Programs RN Baccalaureate.
Site Options Springfield, OH.
Study Options Full-time and part-time.
Program Entrance Requirements CPR certification, health exam, health insurance, immunizations, professional liability insurance/malpractice insurance, RN licensure. Transfer students are accepted. *Application deadline:* Applications may be processed on a rolling basis for some programs. *Application fee:* $25.
Advanced Placement Credit given for nursing courses completed elsewhere dependent upon specific evaluations.
Expenses (2010-11) *Tuition:* part-time $430 per credit hour. *Required fees:* part-time $150 per term.
Financial Aid 10% of baccalaureate students in nursing programs received some form of financial aid in 2009-10.
Contact Mrs. Judy Donegan, BSN Program Chair, BSN Completion Program, Urbana University, 301 Miller Hall, 330 South Burnett Road, Springfield, OH 45505. *Telephone:* 937-328-9354. *Fax:* 937-328-8668. *E-mail:* jdonegan@urbana.edu.

GRADUATE PROGRAMS

Expenses (2010-11) *Tuition:* part-time $495 per credit hour.
Financial Aid 10% of graduate students in nursing programs received some form of financial aid in 2009-10.
Contact Dr. Nancy Lee Sweeney, Dean, College of Nursing and Allied Health and Professor of Nursing, BSN Completion Program, Urbana University, 579 College Way, Urbana, OH 43078. *Telephone:* 937-328-9610. *Fax:* 937-328-8668. *E-mail:* nsweeney@urbana.edu.

MASTER'S DEGREE PROGRAM

Degree MSN
Available Programs Master's.
Concentrations Available Nursing administration; nursing education.
Site Options Springfield, OH; Dayton, OH.
Study Options Full-time and part-time.
Program Entrance Requirements Minimum overall college GPA of 3.0, transcript of college record, CPR certification, written essay, immunizations, interview, 3 letters of recommendation, professional liability insurance/malpractice insurance, resume. *Application deadline:* 8/15 (fall), 1/5 (spring), 5/15 (summer). Applications may be processed on a rolling basis for some programs. *Application fee:* $25.
Advanced Placement Credit given for nursing courses completed elsewhere dependent upon specific evaluations.
Degree Requirements 46 total credit hours, thesis or project.

Ursuline College

The Breen School of Nursing
Pepper Pike, Ohio

http://www.ursuline.edu/
Founded in 1871

DEGREES • BSN • DNP • MSN
Nursing Program Faculty 25 (28% with doctorates).
Nursing Student Activities Sigma Theta Tau, Student Nurses' Association.
Nursing Student Resources Academic advising; academic or career counseling; assistance for students with disabilities; bookstore; campus computer network; career placement assistance; computer lab; computer-assisted instruction; e-mail services; employment services for current students; externships; housing assistance; interactive nursing skills videos; Internet; learning resource lab; library services; nursing audiovisuals; placement services for program completers; remedial services; resume preparation assistance; skills, simulation, or other laboratory; tutoring.
Library Facilities 136,684 volumes; 7,814 periodical subscriptions.

BACCALAUREATE PROGRAMS

Degree BSN
Available Programs Accelerated Baccalaureate for Second Degree; Accelerated LPN to Baccalaureate; Accelerated RN Baccalaureate; Generic Baccalaureate.
Site Options Cleveland, OH.
Study Options Full-time and part-time.
Program Entrance Requirements Minimum overall college GPA of 2.5, transcript of college record, written essay, health exam, health insurance, high school biology, high school chemistry, 2 years high school math, 2 years high school science, high school transcript, immunizations, 1 letter of recommendation, minimum high school GPA of 2.75, minimum GPA in nursing prerequisites of 2.75. Transfer students are accepted.
Advanced Placement Credit given for nursing courses completed elsewhere dependent upon specific evaluations.
Contact Matthew McCaffrey, Director of Admission, The Breen School of Nursing, Ursuline College, 2550 Lander Road, Pepper Pike, OH 44124-4398. *Telephone:* 440-646-8114. *Fax:* 440-684-6138.

GRADUATE PROGRAMS

Contact Dr. M. Murray Mayo, Director, Graduate Program, The Breen School of Nursing, Ursuline College, 2550 Lander Road, Pepper Pike, OH 44124-4398. *Telephone:* 440-646-8127. *Fax:* 440-684-6053. *E-mail:* mmayo@ursuline.edu.

MASTER'S DEGREE PROGRAM

Degree MSN
Available Programs Accelerated Master's; Master's.

Concentrations Available Nurse case management. *Clinical nurse specialist programs in:* adult health, palliative care. *Nurse practitioner programs in:* adult health, family health.
Study Options Full-time and part-time.
Program Entrance Requirements Clinical experience, minimum overall college GPA of 3.0, transcript of college record, CPR certification, written essay, immunizations, 3 letters of recommendation, resume. *Application deadline:* 6/15 (fall), 12/15 (spring). Applications may be processed on a rolling basis for some programs.
Advanced Placement Credit given for nursing courses completed elsewhere dependent upon specific evaluations.
Degree Requirements 43 total credit hours.

POST-MASTER'S PROGRAM

Areas of Study Nurse case management. *Clinical nurse specialist programs in:* adult health, palliative care. *Nurse practitioner programs in:* adult health, family health.

DOCTORAL DEGREE PROGRAM

Degree DNP
Available Programs Doctorate.
Areas of Study Advanced practice nursing, clinical practice, ethics, faculty preparation, health policy, health promotion/disease prevention, health-care systems, information systems, nursing education, nursing policy, nursing research, nursing science.
Program Entrance Requirements Clinical experience, minimum overall college GPA of 3.0, 2 letters of recommendation, MSN or equivalent, vita, writing sample. Application deadline: 5/15 (fall). Application fee: $25.
Degree Requirements 38 total credit hours, dissertation.

See full description on page 506.

Walsh University

Department of Nursing
North Canton, Ohio

http://www.walsh.edu/
Founded in 1958

DEGREE • BSN

Nursing Program Faculty 16 (40% with doctorates).
Baccalaureate Enrollment 280 **Women** 77% **Men** 23% **Minority** 5% **International** 1% **Part-time** 10%
Distance Learning Courses Available.
Nursing Student Activities Nursing Honor Society, Sigma Theta Tau, Student Nurses' Association.
Nursing Student Resources Academic advising; academic or career counseling; assistance for students with disabilities; bookstore; campus computer network; career placement assistance; computer lab; computer-assisted instruction; e-mail services; employment services for current students; housing assistance; interactive nursing skills videos; Internet; learning resource lab; library services; nursing audiovisuals; placement services for program completers; remedial services; resume preparation assistance; skills, simulation, or other laboratory; tutoring.
Library Facilities 389,094 volumes (4,000 in health, 2,000 in nursing); 21,350 periodical subscriptions (114 health-care related).

BACCALAUREATE PROGRAMS

Degree BSN
Available Programs Accelerated Baccalaureate; Accelerated Baccalaureate for Second Degree; Generic Baccalaureate; RN Baccalaureate.
Site Options Canton, OH; Akron, OH.
Study Options Full-time and part-time.
Program Entrance Requirements Transcript of college record, CPR certification, health exam, health insurance, high school chemistry, high school foreign language, 3 years high school math, 3 years high school science, high school transcript, immunizations, minimum GPA in nursing prerequisites of 2.75, professional liability insurance/malpractice insurance, prerequisite course work. Transfer students are accepted. *Application deadline:* 8/15 (fall), 12/31 (spring), 4/30 (summer). Applications may be processed on a rolling basis for some programs. *Application fee:* $25.
Advanced Placement Credit by examination available. Credit given for nursing courses completed elsewhere dependent upon specific evaluations.
Expenses (2010-11) *Tuition:* full-time $22,000; part-time $710 per credit hour. *Room and board:* $4670; room only: $1950 per academic year.
Financial Aid 94% of baccalaureate students in nursing programs received some form of financial aid in 2009-10.
Contact Dr. Linda G. Linc, Professor and Chair, Department of Nursing, Walsh University, 2020 East Maple Street, North Canton, OH 44720-3336. *Telephone:* 330-490-7251. *Fax:* 330-490-7206. *E-mail:* llinc@walsh.edu.

Wright State University

College of Nursing and Health
Dayton, Ohio

http://www.nursing.wright.edu
Founded in 1964

DEGREES • BSN • DNP • MS • MS/MBA

Nursing Program Faculty 68 (33% with doctorates).
Baccalaureate Enrollment 787 **Women** 84% **Men** 16% **Minority** 16% **International** 1% **Part-time** 35%
Graduate Enrollment 257 **Women** 94% **Men** 6% **Minority** 14% **Part-time** 86%
Distance Learning Courses Available.
Nursing Student Activities Nursing Honor Society, Sigma Theta Tau, Student Nurses' Association, nursing club.
Nursing Student Resources Academic advising; academic or career counseling; assistance for students with disabilities; bookstore; campus computer network; career placement assistance; computer lab; computer-assisted instruction; daycare for children of students; e-mail services; employment services for current students; externships; housing assistance; interactive nursing skills videos; Internet; learning resource lab; library services; nursing audiovisuals; remedial services; resume preparation assistance; skills, simulation, or other laboratory; tutoring.
Library Facilities 703,000 volumes (111,826 in health, 7,646 in nursing); 443,200 periodical subscriptions (1,279 health-care related).

BACCALAUREATE PROGRAMS

Degree BSN
Available Programs Accelerated Baccalaureate for Second Degree; Baccalaureate for Second Degree; Generic Baccalaureate; RN Baccalaureate.
Site Options Dayton, OH; Chillicothe, OH; Celina, OH.
Study Options Full-time and part-time.
Program Entrance Requirements Minimum overall college GPA of 2.5, transcript of college record, written essay, high school transcript, minimum GPA in nursing prerequisites of 2.5, prerequisite course work. Transfer students are accepted. *Application deadline:* 6/30 (fall), 12/30 (spring).
Advanced Placement Credit by examination available. Credit given for nursing courses completed elsewhere dependent upon specific evaluations.
Expenses (2009-10) *Tuition, state resident:* full-time $10,044; part-time $227 per quarter hour. *Tuition, nonresident:* full-time $19,460; part-time $443 per quarter hour. *International tuition:* $19,460 full-time. *Room and board:* $7829 per academic year.
Financial Aid 83% of baccalaureate students in nursing programs received some form of financial aid in 2008-09. *Gift aid (need-based):* Federal Pell, FSEOG, state, private, college/university gift aid from institutional funds, United Negro College Fund, Federal Nursing, Choose Ohio First Scholarships. *Loans:* Federal Nursing Student Loans, Perkins, state, college/university, private loans. *Work-study:* Federal Work-Study. *Financial aid application deadline (priority):* 2/15.
Contact Ms. Theresa A. Haghnazarian, Director, Student and Alumni Affairs, College of Nursing and Health, Wright State University, 3640 Colonel Glenn Highway, Dayton, OH 45435. *Telephone:* 937-775-3132. *Fax:* 937-775-4571. *E-mail:* theresa.haghnazarian@wright.edu.

GRADUATE PROGRAMS

Expenses (2009-10) *Tuition, state resident:* full-time $12,984; part-time $335 per quarter hour. *Tuition, nonresident:* full-time $24,760; part-time $572 per quarter hour. *International tuition:* $24,760 full-time. *Room and board:* $7829 per academic year.
Financial Aid 39% of graduate students in nursing programs received some form of financial aid in 2008-09. 15 fellowships with full tuition reimbursements available were awarded; research assistantships, teaching assistantships, Federal Work-Study, institutionally sponsored

loans, and unspecified assistantships also available. Aid available to part-time students. *Financial aid application deadline:* 6/1.
Contact Dr. Donna Miles Curry, Associate Dean, Graduate Programs, College of Nursing and Health, Wright State University, 3640 Colonel Glenn Highway, Dayton, OH 45435. *Telephone:* 937-775-3577. *Fax:* 937-775-4571. *E-mail:* donna.curry@wright.edu.

MASTER'S DEGREE PROGRAM
Degrees MS; MS/MBA
Available Programs Master's; Master's for Nurses with Non-Nursing Degrees.
Concentrations Available Clinical nurse leader; health-care administration; nursing administration. *Clinical nurse specialist programs in:* adult health, community health, pediatric, public health, school health. *Nurse practitioner programs in:* acute care, family health, pediatric.
Study Options Full-time and part-time.
Online Degree Options Yes.
Program Entrance Requirements Clinical experience, computer literacy, minimum overall college GPA of 3.0, transcript of college record, written essay, interview, physical assessment course, statistics course, GRE General Test. *Application deadline:* Applications may be processed on a rolling basis for some programs. *Application fee:* $30.
Advanced Placement Credit given for nursing courses completed elsewhere dependent upon specific evaluations.
Degree Requirements 48 total credit hours, thesis or project.

POST-MASTER'S PROGRAM
Areas of Study *Clinical nurse specialist programs in:* school health. *Nurse practitioner programs in:* acute care, family health, pediatric.

DOCTORAL DEGREE PROGRAM
Degree DNP
Available Programs Doctorate.
Areas of Study Advanced practice nursing, biology of health and illness, clinical practice, community health, family health, health policy, health promotion/disease prevention, health-care systems, information systems, nursing administration, nursing policy, nursing science.
Online Degree Options Yes (online only).
Program Entrance Requirements Clinical experience, minimum overall college GPA of 3.3, interview by faculty committee, 3 letters of recommendation, MSN or equivalent, statistics course, vita, writing sample.
Degree Requirements 54 total credit hours, dissertation.

CONTINUING EDUCATION PROGRAM
Contact Ms. Teri Houston, Office Assistant, College of Nursing and Health, Wright State University, 3640 Colonel Glenn Highway, Dayton, OH 45435. *Telephone:* 937-775-3577. *Fax:* 937-775-4571. *E-mail:* teresa.houston@wright.edu.

Xavier University
School of Nursing
Cincinnati, Ohio

Founded in 1831

DEGREES • BSN • MSN • MSN/MBA
Nursing Program Faculty 68 (8% with doctorates).
Baccalaureate Enrollment 300 **Women** 92% **Men** 8% **Minority** 12% **Part-time** 1%
Graduate Enrollment 235 **Women** 96% **Men** 4% **Minority** 10% **Part-time** 72%
Nursing Student Activities Sigma Theta Tau, nursing club.
Nursing Student Resources Academic advising; academic or career counseling; assistance for students with disabilities; bookstore; campus computer network; career placement assistance; computer lab; computer-assisted instruction; e-mail services; employment services for current students; externships; housing assistance; interactive nursing skills videos; Internet; learning resource lab; library services; nursing audiovisuals; paid internships; resume preparation assistance; skills, simulation, or other laboratory; tutoring.
Library Facilities 363,140 volumes (8,900 in health, 1,160 in nursing); 54,264 periodical subscriptions (200 health-care related).

BACCALAUREATE PROGRAMS
Degree BSN
Available Programs Generic Baccalaureate.
Study Options Full-time and part-time.
Program Entrance Requirements Minimum overall college GPA of 2.7, transcript of college record, written essay, high school chemistry, high school foreign language, 3 years high school math, 2 years high school science, high school transcript, minimum high school GPA of 2.8. Transfer students are accepted. *Application deadline:* Applications may be processed on a rolling basis for some programs. *Application fee:* $35.
Advanced Placement Credit given for nursing courses completed elsewhere dependent upon specific evaluations.
Expenses (2010-11) *Tuition:* full-time $29,300. *Room and board:* $9900; room only: $5500 per academic year. *Required fees:* full-time $400.
Financial Aid 90% of baccalaureate students in nursing programs received some form of financial aid in 2009-10. *Gift aid (need-based):* Federal Pell, FSEOG, state, private, college/university gift aid from institutional funds. *Loans:* Federal Direct (Subsidized and Unsubsidized Stafford PLUS), Perkins. *Work-study:* Federal Work-Study, part-time campus jobs. *Financial aid application deadline (priority):* 2/15.
Contact Ms. Marilyn Volk Gomez, Director of Nursing Student Services, School of Nursing, Xavier University, 3800 Victory Parkway, Cincinnati, OH 45207-7351. *Telephone:* 513-745-4392. *Fax:* 513-745-1087. *E-mail:* gomez@xavier.edu.

GRADUATE PROGRAMS
Expenses (2010-11) *Tuition:* part-time $566 per credit hour. *Required fees:* part-time $100 per credit.
Financial Aid 30% of graduate students in nursing programs received some form of financial aid in 2009-10.
Contact Ms. Marilyn Volk Gomez, Director of Nursing Student Services, School of Nursing, Xavier University, 3800 Victory Parkway, Cincinnati, OH 45207-7351. *Telephone:* 513-745-4392. *Fax:* 513-745-1087. *E-mail:* gomez@xavier.edu.

MASTER'S DEGREE PROGRAM
Degrees MSN; MSN/MBA
Available Programs Master's; Master's for Nurses with Non-Nursing Degrees; RN to Master's.
Concentrations Available Clinical nurse leader; nursing administration; nursing education; nursing informatics. *Clinical nurse specialist programs in:* forensic nursing, school health.
Study Options Full-time and part-time.
Program Entrance Requirements Minimum overall college GPA of 2.8, transcript of college record, written essay, 3 letters of recommendation, statistics course, GRE. *Application deadline:* Applications may be processed on a rolling basis for some programs. *Application fee:* $35.
Degree Requirements 36 total credit hours, thesis or project.

Youngstown State University
Department of Nursing
Youngstown, Ohio

Founded in 1908

DEGREES • BSN • MSN
Nursing Program Faculty 22 (18% with doctorates).
Baccalaureate Enrollment 22
Graduate Enrollment 24 **Women** 75% **Men** 25% **Minority** 13%
Nursing Student Activities Sigma Theta Tau, Student Nurses' Association.
Nursing Student Resources Academic advising; academic or career counseling; assistance for students with disabilities; bookstore; campus computer network; career placement assistance; computer lab; computer-assisted instruction; e-mail services; housing assistance; interactive nursing skills videos; Internet; learning resource lab; library services; nursing audiovisuals; placement services for program completers; resume preparation assistance; skills, simulation, or other laboratory; tutoring.

BACCALAUREATE PROGRAMS
Degree BSN
Site Options Boardman, OH.
Study Options Full-time.
Program Entrance Requirements Minimum overall college GPA of 2.0, transcript of college record, CPR certification, health exam, health insurance, high school biology, high school chemistry, high school foreign language, 3 years high school math, 3 years high school science, high school transcript, immunizations, minimum high school GPA,

minimum high school rank, minimum GPA in nursing prerequisites of 2.5, prerequisite course work. Transfer students are accepted.
Advanced Placement Credit by examination available. Credit given for nursing courses completed elsewhere dependent upon specific evaluations.
Contact ***Telephone:*** 330-941-2328. *Fax:* 330-941-2309.

GRADUATE PROGRAMS

Contact ***Telephone:*** 330-941-1796. *Fax:* 330-941-2309.

MASTER'S DEGREE PROGRAM

Degree MSN
Concentrations Available Nurse anesthesia; nursing education.
Study Options Full-time and part-time.
Program Entrance Requirements Clinical experience, computer literacy, transcript of college record, CPR certification, written essay, immunizations, nursing research course, physical assessment course, prerequisite course work, resume, GRE General Test.
Advanced Placement Credit given for nursing courses completed elsewhere dependent upon specific evaluations.
Degree Requirements Thesis or project.

OKLAHOMA

Bacone College

Department of Nursing
Muskogee, Oklahoma

Founded in 1880

DEGREE • BSN
Nursing Program Faculty 8
Baccalaureate Enrollment 16 **Women** 100% **Minority** 65%
Nursing Student Activities Student Nurses' Association, nursing club.
Nursing Student Resources Academic advising; bookstore; campus computer network; computer lab; computer-assisted instruction; interactive nursing skills videos; Internet; learning resource lab; library services; nursing audiovisuals; remedial services; skills, simulation, or other laboratory.
Library Facilities 34,564 volumes; 121 periodical subscriptions.

BACCALAUREATE PROGRAMS

Degree BSN
Available Programs Accelerated RN Baccalaureate.
Program Entrance Requirements Transcript of college record, CPR certification, health exam, health insurance, immunizations, 2 letters of recommendation, minimum GPA in nursing prerequisites of 2.5, prerequisite course work, RN licensure.
Contact ***Telephone:*** 888-682-5514.

East Central University

Department of Nursing
Ada, Oklahoma

http://www.ecok.edu/dept/nursing
Founded in 1909

DEGREE • BS
Nursing Program Faculty 17 (31% with doctorates).
Baccalaureate Enrollment 495 **Women** 86% **Men** 14% **Minority** 44% **International** 1% **Part-time** 14%
Distance Learning Courses Available.
Nursing Student Activities Student Nurses' Association.
Nursing Student Resources Academic advising; academic or career counseling; assistance for students with disabilities; bookstore; campus computer network; career placement assistance; computer lab; computer-assisted instruction; daycare for children of students; e-mail services; employment services for current students; externships; housing assistance; interactive nursing skills videos; Internet; learning resource lab; library services; nursing audiovisuals; other; placement services for program completers; resume preparation assistance; skills, simulation, or other laboratory; tutoring.
Library Facilities 251,780 volumes (2,236 in health, 893 in nursing); 16,593 periodical subscriptions (266 health-care related).

BACCALAUREATE PROGRAMS

Degree BS
Available Programs ADN to Baccalaureate; Generic Baccalaureate.
Site Options Ardmore, OK; McAlester, OK; Durant, OK.
Study Options Full-time and part-time.
Program Entrance Requirements Minimum overall college GPA of 2.5, transcript of college record, CPR certification, health exam, immunizations, minimum GPA in nursing prerequisites of 2.5, professional liability insurance/malpractice insurance, prerequisite course work. Transfer students are accepted. *Application deadline:* 9/17 (spring).
Advanced Placement Credit given for nursing courses completed elsewhere dependent upon specific evaluations.
Contact ***Telephone:*** 580-310-5434. *Fax:* 580-310-5785.

Langston University

School of Nursing and Health Professions
Langston, Oklahoma

http://www.lunet.ed/nurs5.html
Founded in 1897

DEGREE • BSN
Nursing Program Faculty 16 (13% with doctorates).
Nursing Student Activities Student Nurses' Association, nursing club.
Nursing Student Resources Academic advising; academic or career counseling; assistance for students with disabilities; bookstore; campus computer network; career placement assistance; computer lab; computer-assisted instruction; daycare for children of students; e-mail services; housing assistance; interactive nursing skills videos; Internet; learning resource lab; library services; nursing audiovisuals; remedial services; resume preparation assistance; skills, simulation, or other laboratory; tutoring.
Library Facilities 97,565 volumes (35,397 in health, 2,664 in nursing); 1,235 periodical subscriptions (978 health-care related).

BACCALAUREATE PROGRAMS

Degree BSN
Available Programs Generic Baccalaureate; LPN to Baccalaureate; RN Baccalaureate.
Site Options Tulsa, OK.
Study Options Full-time and part-time.
Program Entrance Requirements Minimum overall college GPA of 2.5, transcript of college record, written essay, health exam, immunizations, minimum GPA in nursing prerequisites of 2.5, professional liability insurance/malpractice insurance, prerequisite course work. Transfer students are accepted.
Advanced Placement Credit by examination available. Credit given for nursing courses completed elsewhere dependent upon specific evaluations.
Contact ***Telephone:*** 405-466-3411. *Fax:* 405-466-2195.

Northeastern State University

Department of Nursing
Tahlequah, Oklahoma

http://arapaho.nsuok.edu/~nursing
Founded in 1846

DEGREES • BSN • MSN
Nursing Program Faculty 5 (40% with doctorates).
Baccalaureate Enrollment 111 **Women** 93% **Men** 7% **Minority** 27% **Part-time** 100%
Graduate Enrollment 10
Distance Learning Courses Available.
Nursing Student Activities Sigma Theta Tau, Student Nurses' Association.
Nursing Student Resources Academic advising; academic or career counseling; assistance for students with disabilities; bookstore; campus computer network; career placement assistance; computer lab; computer-assisted instruction; e-mail services; employment services for current stu-

dents; housing assistance; Internet; library services; nursing audiovisuals; placement services for program completers; resume preparation assistance; tutoring.
Library Facilities 418,643 volumes (20,000 in health, 15,293 in nursing); 20,141 periodical subscriptions (1,000 health-care related).

BACCALAUREATE PROGRAMS

Degree BSN
Available Programs Accelerated RN Baccalaureate; RN Baccalaureate.
Site Options Muskogee, OK; Broken Arrow, OK; Ponca City, OK.
Online Degree Options Yes (online only).
Program Entrance Requirements Minimum overall college GPA of 2.0, transcript of college record, CPR certification, health exam, immunizations, 3 letters of recommendation, minimum GPA in nursing prerequisites of 2.0, professional liability insurance/malpractice insurance, prerequisite course work, RN licensure. Transfer students are accepted.
Expenses (2010-11) *Tuition, state resident:* full-time $3338; part-time $111 per credit hour. *Tuition, nonresident:* full-time $9675; part-time $323 per credit hour. *Room and board:* $6275; room only: $2590 per academic year. *Required fees:* full-time $3593; part-time $120 per credit; part-time $120 per term.
Financial Aid 70% of baccalaureate students in nursing programs received some form of financial aid in 2009-10. *Gift aid (need-based):* Federal Pell, FSEOG, state, private, college/university gift aid from institutional funds. *Loans:* Federal Direct (Subsidized and Unsubsidized Stafford PLUS), Perkins. *Work-study:* Federal Work-Study, part-time campus jobs. *Financial aid application deadline (priority):* 4/1.
Contact Dr. Joyce A. Van Nostrand, Chair, Nursing Program and Department of Health Professions, Department of Nursing, Northeastern State University, PO Box 549, Muskogee, OK 74402-0549. *Telephone:* 918-781-5410. *Fax:* 918-781-5411. *E-mail:* vannostr@nsuok.edu.

GRADUATE PROGRAMS

Expenses (2010-11) *Tuition, state resident:* full-time $4608; part-time $144 per credit hour. *Tuition, nonresident:* full-time $12,288; part-time $384 per credit hour. *Room and board:* $6275; room only: $2590 per academic year. *Required fees:* full-time $3832; part-time $120 per credit.
Financial Aid 70% of graduate students in nursing programs received some form of financial aid in 2009-10.
Contact Dr. Joyce A. Van Nostrand, Chair, Nursing Program and Department of Health Professions, Department of Nursing, Northeastern State University, PO Box 549, Muskogee, OK 74402-0549. *Telephone:* 918-781-5410. *Fax:* 918-781-5411. *E-mail:* vannostr@nsuok.edu.

MASTER'S DEGREE PROGRAM

Degree MSN
Available Programs Master's.
Concentrations Available Nursing education.
Site Options Muskogee, OK; Broken Arrow, OK; Ponca City, OK.
Study Options Full-time and part-time.
Online Degree Options Yes (online only).
Program Entrance Requirements Minimum overall college GPA of 3, transcript of college record, CPR certification, immunizations, 3 letters of recommendation, nursing research course, professional liability insurance/malpractice insurance, statistics course. *Application deadline:* 8/1 (fall), 1/2 (spring).
Advanced Placement Credit given for nursing courses completed elsewhere dependent upon specific evaluations.
Degree Requirements 32 total credit hours, thesis or project.

Northwestern Oklahoma State University

Division of Nursing
Alva, Oklahoma

http://www.nwosu.edu/nursing
Founded in 1897

DEGREE • BSN

Nursing Program Faculty 12 (.08% with doctorates).
Baccalaureate Enrollment 45 **Women** 99% **Men** 1% **Minority** 2% **International** 2% **Part-time** 1%
Distance Learning Courses Available.
Nursing Student Activities Nursing Honor Society, Student Nurses' Association.
Nursing Student Resources Academic advising; academic or career counseling; assistance for students with disabilities; bookstore; campus computer network; career placement assistance; computer lab; computer-assisted instruction; e-mail services; housing assistance; interactive nursing skills videos; Internet; learning resource lab; library services; nursing audiovisuals; remedial services; skills, simulation, or other laboratory; tutoring.
Library Facilities 266,731 volumes; 12,954 periodical subscriptions (59 health-care related).

BACCALAUREATE PROGRAMS

Degree BSN
Available Programs ADN to Baccalaureate; Accelerated Baccalaureate; Accelerated LPN to Baccalaureate; Accelerated RN Baccalaureate; Baccalaureate for Second Degree; Generic Baccalaureate; LPN to Baccalaureate; LPN to RN Baccalaureate; RN Baccalaureate.
Site Options Enid, OK; Woodward, OK.
Study Options Full-time and part-time.
Program Entrance Requirements Minimum overall college GPA of 2.5, transcript of college record, CPR certification, health exam, high school transcript, immunizations, 3 letters of recommendation, minimum high school GPA of 2.5, minimum GPA in nursing prerequisites of 2.5, professional liability insurance/malpractice insurance, prerequisite course work. Transfer students are accepted. *Application deadline:* 2/2 (spring).
Advanced Placement Credit by examination available. Credit given for nursing courses completed elsewhere dependent upon specific evaluations.
Contact *Telephone:* 580-327-8489. *Fax:* 580-327-8434.

Oklahoma Baptist University

School of Nursing
Shawnee, Oklahoma

http://www.okbu.edu/
Founded in 1910

DEGREES • BSN • MSN

Nursing Program Faculty 24 (28% with doctorates).
Baccalaureate Enrollment 182 **Women** 95% **Men** 5% **Minority** 8% **International** 1% **Part-time** 4%
Graduate Enrollment 34 **Women** 100% **Minority** 8%
Nursing Student Activities Sigma Theta Tau, Student Nurses' Association.
Nursing Student Resources Academic advising; academic or career counseling; assistance for students with disabilities; bookstore; campus computer network; computer lab; computer-assisted instruction; e-mail services; externships; Internet; learning resource lab; library services; nursing audiovisuals; remedial services; resume preparation assistance; skills, simulation, or other laboratory; tutoring; unpaid internships.
Library Facilities 230,000 volumes (10,000 in health, 5,500 in nursing); 1,800 periodical subscriptions (65 health-care related).

BACCALAUREATE PROGRAMS

Degree BSN
Available Programs ADN to Baccalaureate; Baccalaureate for Second Degree; Generic Baccalaureate; LPN to Baccalaureate; RN Baccalaureate.
Study Options Full-time and part-time.
Program Entrance Requirements Minimum overall college GPA of 2.25, transcript of college record, CPR certification, health exam, high school transcript, immunizations, minimum GPA in nursing prerequisites of 2.3, prerequisite course work. Transfer students are accepted. *Application deadline:* 4/1 (fall), 4/1 (winter), 4/1 (spring), 7/15 (summer).
Expenses (2010-11) *Tuition:* full-time $17,220; part-time $474 per credit hour. *International tuition:* $17,260 full-time. *Room and board:* $5630; room only: $3600 per academic year. *Required fees:* full-time $640; part-time $40 per credit; part-time $120 per term.
Financial Aid 93% of baccalaureate students in nursing programs received some form of financial aid in 2009-10. *Gift aid (need-based):* Federal Pell, FSEOG, state, private, college/university gift aid from institutional funds, Academic Competitiveness Grants, National SMART Grants, TEACH Grants. *Loans:* Federal Direct (Subsidized and Unsubsidized Stafford PLUS), Perkins, college/university. *Work-study:* Federal Work-Study. *Financial aid application deadline:* Continuous.
Contact Dr. Lana Bolhouse, Dean, School of Nursing, Oklahoma Baptist University, 500 West University, Shawnee, OK 74804. *Telephone:* 405-878-2081. *Fax:* 405-878-2083. *E-mail:* lana.bolhouse@okbu.edu.

GRADUATE PROGRAMS

Expenses (2010-11) *Tuition:* full-time $11,050; part-time $425 per credit hour. *International tuition:* $11,125 full-time. *Room and board:* $5630; room only: $3600 per academic year.

Financial Aid 100% of graduate students in nursing programs received some form of financial aid in 2009-10.

Contact Dr. Lana Bolhouse, Dean, School of Nursing, Oklahoma Baptist University, 111 North Harrison, Oklahoma City, OK 73104. *Telephone:* 405-878-2081. *Fax:* 405-878-2083. *E-mail:* lana.bolhouse@okbu.edu.

MASTER'S DEGREE PROGRAM

Degree MSN
Available Programs Master's.
Concentrations Available Nursing education.
Site Options Oklahoma City, OK.
Study Options Full-time.
Program Entrance Requirements Clinical experience, minimum overall college GPA of 3.00, transcript of college record, written essay, nursing research course, resume, statistics course. *Application deadline:* 7/30 (fall), 12/20 (winter), 7/30 (spring), 7/30 (summer). Applications may be processed on a rolling basis for some programs.
Degree Requirements 39 total credit hours, thesis or project.

Oklahoma Christian University

Nursing Program
Oklahoma City, Oklahoma

Founded in 1950

DEGREE • BSN

Library Facilities 141,377 volumes; 21,639 periodical subscriptions.

BACCALAUREATE PROGRAMS

Degree BSN
Available Programs Generic Baccalaureate.
Program Entrance Requirements Minimum overall college GPA of 2.75, 3 letters of recommendation.
Contact *Telephone:* 405-425-1921.

Oklahoma City University

Kramer School of Nursing
Oklahoma City, Oklahoma

http://www.okcu.edu/nursing
Founded in 1904

DEGREES • BSN • DNP • MSN • MSN/MBA • PHD

Nursing Program Faculty 30 (30% with doctorates).
Baccalaureate Enrollment 277 **Women** 84% **Men** 16% **Minority** 17% **International** 6% **Part-time** 7%
Graduate Enrollment 26 **Women** 85% **Men** 15% **Minority** 15% **International** 4% **Part-time** 65%
Distance Learning Courses Available.
Nursing Student Activities Sigma Theta Tau, Student Nurses' Association.
Nursing Student Resources Academic advising; academic or career counseling; assistance for students with disabilities; bookstore; campus computer network; career placement assistance; computer lab; computer-assisted instruction; e-mail services; housing assistance; interactive nursing skills videos; Internet; learning resource lab; library services; nursing audiovisuals; placement services for program completers; remedial services; resume preparation assistance; skills, simulation, or other laboratory; tutoring.
Library Facilities 520,953 volumes (2,714 in health, 590 in nursing); 14,000 periodical subscriptions (234 health-care related).

BACCALAUREATE PROGRAMS

Degree BSN
Available Programs ADN to Baccalaureate; Accelerated Baccalaureate for Second Degree; Generic Baccalaureate.
Site Options Catoosa, OK.
Study Options Full-time and part-time.
Program Entrance Requirements Minimum overall college GPA of 3.0, transcript of college record, CPR certification, high school transcript, immunizations, minimum GPA in nursing prerequisites of 3.0, prerequisite course work. Transfer students are accepted. *Application deadline:* 8/1 (fall), 12/1 (spring). Applications may be processed on a rolling basis for some programs. *Application fee:* $40.
Advanced Placement Credit by examination available. Credit given for nursing courses completed elsewhere dependent upon specific evaluations.
Financial Aid 89% of baccalaureate students in nursing programs received some form of financial aid in 2009-10. *Gift aid (need-based):* Federal Pell, FSEOG, state, private, college/university gift aid from institutional funds, United Negro College Fund, Federal Nursing, Native American Grants. *Loans:* Federal Nursing Student Loans, Federal Direct (Subsidized and Unsubsidized Stafford PLUS), Perkins. *Work-study:* Federal Work-Study, part-time campus jobs. *Financial aid application deadline (priority):* 3/1.
Contact Ms. Sherri Christian, Traditional BSN Program Specialist, Kramer School of Nursing, Oklahoma City University, 2501 North Blackwelder Avenue, Oklahoma City, OK 73106-1493. *Telephone:* 405-208-5901. *Fax:* 405-208-5914. *E-mail:* schristian@okcu.edu.

GRADUATE PROGRAMS

Financial Aid 92% of graduate students in nursing programs received some form of financial aid in 2009-10.
Contact Miss Jennifer Clary, Post-Bachelor's Program Specialist, Kramer School of Nursing, Oklahoma City University, 2501 North Blackwelder Avenue, Oklahoma City, OK 73106-1493. *Telephone:* 405-208-5959. *Fax:* 405-208-5914. *E-mail:* jclary@okcu.edu.

MASTER'S DEGREE PROGRAM

Degrees MSN; MSN/MBA
Available Programs Master's.
Concentrations Available Nursing administration; nursing education.
Study Options Full-time and part-time.
Program Entrance Requirements Clinical experience, minimum overall college GPA of 3.0, transcript of college record, physical assessment course, statistics course. *Application deadline:* 8/1 (fall), 12/1 (spring). Applications may be processed on a rolling basis for some programs. *Application fee:* $50.
Advanced Placement Credit given for nursing courses completed elsewhere dependent upon specific evaluations.
Degree Requirements 33 total credit hours, thesis or project.

DOCTORAL DEGREE PROGRAM

Degree DNP
Available Programs Doctorate; Post-Baccalaureate Doctorate; Doctorate for Nurses with Non-Nursing Degrees.
Areas of Study Family health, advanced practice nursing, clinical practice, health-care systems, nursing administration.
Program Entrance Requirements Minimum overall college GPA of 3.0, interview by faculty committee, MSN or equivalent, statistics course, vita, writing sample. *Application deadline*: 4/1 (fall). *Application fee*: $50.
Degree Requirements 30 total credit hours, oral exam, residency.

Degree PhD
Available Programs Doctorate.
Areas of Study Nursing education.
Program Entrance Requirements Minimum overall college GPA of 3.5, interview by faculty committee, MSN or equivalent, statistics course, vita, writing sample. Application deadline: 4/1 (fall). Applications may be processed on a rolling basis for some programs. Application fee: $50.
Degree Requirements 90 total credit hours, dissertation, oral exam, residency.

CONTINUING EDUCATION PROGRAM

Contact Mr. Christopher Black, Director of Communications and Outreach, Kramer School of Nursing, Oklahoma City University, 2501 North Blackwelder Avenue, Oklahoma City, OK 73106-1493. *Telephone:* 405-208-5832. *Fax:* 405-208-5914. *E-mail:* cblack@okcu.edu.

Oklahoma Panhandle State University

Bachelor of Science in Nursing Program
Goodwell, Oklahoma

http://www.opsu.edu
Founded in 1909

DEGREE • BSN
Nursing Program Faculty 4
Baccalaureate Enrollment 57 **Women** 90% **Men** 10% **Minority** 19% **Part-time** 73%
Distance Learning Courses Available.
Nursing Student Activities Student Nurses' Association.
Nursing Student Resources Academic advising; academic or career counseling; assistance for students with disabilities; bookstore; campus computer network; computer-assisted instruction; e-mail services; Internet; library services.
Library Facilities 1,019 volumes in health, 380 volumes in nursing; 2,032 periodical subscriptions health-care related.

BACCALAUREATE PROGRAMS

Degree BSN
Available Programs ADN to Baccalaureate.
Study Options Full-time and part-time.
Online Degree Options Yes (online only).
Program Entrance Requirements Minimum overall college GPA of 2.0, transcript of college record, CPR certification, immunizations, minimum GPA in nursing prerequisites of 2.0, RN licensure. Transfer students are accepted. *Application deadline:* 8/1 (fall), 1/10 (spring), 5/20 (summer).
Advanced Placement Credit given for nursing courses completed elsewhere dependent upon specific evaluations.
Expenses (2009-10) *Tuition, area resident:* part-time $91 per credit. *Required fees:* part-time $111 per credit.
Financial Aid 34% of baccalaureate students in nursing programs received some form of financial aid in 2008-09.
Contact Lynna Brakhage, RN, Director, RN-BSN Program, Bachelor of Science in Nursing Program, Oklahoma Panhandle State University, PO Box 430, Goodwell, OK 73939. *Telephone:* 580-349-1520. *Fax:* 580-349-1529. *E-mail:* nursing@opsu.edu.

Oklahoma Wesleyan University

School of Nursing
Bartlesville, Oklahoma

http://nursing.okwu.edu
Founded in 1909

DEGREE • BSN
Nursing Program Faculty 31 (35% with doctorates).
Baccalaureate Enrollment 140 **Women** 96% **Men** 4% **Minority** 23%
Nursing Student Resources Academic advising; academic or career counseling; assistance for students with disabilities; bookstore; campus computer network; computer lab; computer-assisted instruction; interactive nursing skills videos; Internet; learning resource lab; library services; nursing audiovisuals; skills, simulation, or other laboratory.
Library Facilities 83,859 volumes (946 in health, 483 in nursing); 128 periodical subscriptions (40 health-care related).

BACCALAUREATE PROGRAMS

Degree BSN
Available Programs ADN to Baccalaureate; Accelerated RN Baccalaureate; Baccalaureate for Second Degree; Generic Baccalaureate; International Nurse to Baccalaureate; LPN to Baccalaureate; RN Baccalaureate.
Study Options Full-time.
Program Entrance Requirements Minimum overall college GPA of 2.3, transcript of college record, CPR certification, health exam, health insurance, immunizations, 2 letters of recommendation, minimum GPA in nursing prerequisites of 2.75, professional liability insurance/malpractice insurance, prerequisite course work, RN licensure. Transfer students are accepted.
Advanced Placement Credit by examination available. Credit given for nursing courses completed elsewhere dependent upon specific evaluations.
Contact *Telephone:* 918-335-6254. *Fax:* 918-335-6204.

Oral Roberts University

Anna Vaughn School of Nursing
Tulsa, Oklahoma

http://www.oru.edu/
Founded in 1963

DEGREE • BSN
Nursing Program Faculty 17 (14% with doctorates).
Baccalaureate Enrollment 135 **Women** 89% **Men** 11% **Minority** 25% **International** 9% **Part-time** 4%
Nursing Student Activities Nursing Honor Society, Sigma Theta Tau, Student Nurses' Association.
Nursing Student Resources Academic advising; academic or career counseling; assistance for students with disabilities; bookstore; campus computer network; computer lab; computer-assisted instruction; e-mail services; employment services for current students; housing assistance; interactive nursing skills videos; Internet; learning resource lab; library services; nursing audiovisuals; remedial services; resume preparation assistance; skills, simulation, or other laboratory; tutoring.
Library Facilities 9,809 volumes in health, 2,452 volumes in nursing; 56 periodical subscriptions health-care related.

BACCALAUREATE PROGRAMS

Degree BSN
Available Programs ADN to Baccalaureate; Generic Baccalaureate; RN Baccalaureate.
Study Options Full-time and part-time.
Program Entrance Requirements Minimum overall college GPA of 3.3, transcript of college record, CPR certification, health exam, health insurance, high school chemistry, 2 years high school math, 2 years high school science, high school transcript, immunizations, minimum high school GPA of 2.5, minimum GPA in nursing prerequisites of 2.5. Transfer students are accepted. *Application deadline:* 8/1 (fall), 12/1 (spring). *Application fee:* $35.
Expenses (2010-11) *Tuition:* full-time $19,382; part-time $810 per credit hour. *Room and board:* $8304; room only: $4050 per academic year. *Required fees:* full-time $1112; part-time $1112 per credit.
Financial Aid 98% of baccalaureate students in nursing programs received some form of financial aid in 2009-10.
Contact Dr. Kenda Jezek, Dean, Anna Vaughn School of Nursing, Oral Roberts University, 7777 South Lewis Avenue, Tulsa, OK 74171. *Telephone:* 918-495-6198. *Fax:* 918-495-6020. *E-mail:* kjezek@oru.edu.

Rogers State University

Nursing Program
Claremore, Oklahoma

Founded in 1909

DEGREE • BSN
Baccalaureate Enrollment 18 **Women** 94% **Men** 6% **Minority** 38% **International** 11%
Distance Learning Courses Available.
Nursing Student Activities Student Nurses' Association.
Nursing Student Resources Academic advising; academic or career counseling; assistance for students with disabilities; bookstore; campus computer network; career placement assistance; computer lab; computer-assisted instruction; daycare for children of students; e-mail services; housing assistance; interactive nursing skills videos; Internet; learning resource lab; library services; nursing audiovisuals; placement services for program completers; remedial services; resume preparation assistance; skills, simulation, or other laboratory.
Library Facilities 77,650 volumes; 225 periodical subscriptions.

BACCALAUREATE PROGRAMS

Degree BSN
Available Programs ADN to Baccalaureate.
Site Options Bartlesville, OK.
Program Entrance Requirements Minimum overall college GPA, CPR certification, health exam, health insurance, immunizations, minimum GPA in nursing prerequisites, RN licensure. Transfer students are accepted.

Expenses (2009-10) *Tuition, state resident:* part-time $91 per credit hour. *Room and board:* room only: $4500 per academic year. *Required fees:* part-time $139 per credit.

Financial Aid 60% of baccalaureate students in nursing programs received some form of financial aid in 2008-09. *Gift aid (need-based):* Federal Pell, FSEOG, state, private, college/university gift aid from institutional funds. *Loans:* alternative loans. *Work-study:* Federal Work-Study, part-time campus jobs. *Financial aid application deadline:* Continuous.

Contact Nancy Diede, Department Head, Health Sciences, Nursing Program, Rogers State University, 1701 West Will Rogers Boulevard, Claremore, OK 74017-3252. *Telephone:* 918-343-7885. *Fax:* 918-343-7628. *E-mail:* ndiede@rsu.edu.

Southern Nazarene University

School of Nursing
Bethany, Oklahoma

http://www.snu.edu
Founded in 1899

DEGREES • BS • MS

Nursing Program Faculty 35 (40% with doctorates).

Baccalaureate Enrollment 101 **Women** 90% **Men** 10% **Minority** 35% **International** 2% **Part-time** 10%

Graduate Enrollment 34 **Women** 90% **Men** 10% **Minority** 10%

Distance Learning Courses Available.

Nursing Student Activities Sigma Theta Tau, Student Nurses' Association.

Nursing Student Resources Academic advising; academic or career counseling; assistance for students with disabilities; bookstore; campus computer network; career placement assistance; computer lab; computer-assisted instruction; e-mail services; employment services for current students; externships; housing assistance; interactive nursing skills videos; Internet; learning resource lab; library services; nursing audiovisuals; paid internships; remedial services; skills, simulation, or other laboratory; tutoring.

Library Facilities 95,535 volumes; 225 periodical subscriptions.

BACCALAUREATE PROGRAMS

Degree BS

Available Programs ADN to Baccalaureate; Baccalaureate for Second Degree; Generic Baccalaureate; LPN to Baccalaureate.

Study Options Full-time.

Program Entrance Requirements Minimum overall college GPA of 2.75, transcript of college record, CPR certification, health exam, health insurance, immunizations, minimum GPA in nursing prerequisites of 2.75, professional liability insurance/malpractice insurance, prerequisite course work. Transfer students are accepted. *Application deadline:* 12/5 (fall). Applications may be processed on a rolling basis for some programs.

Advanced Placement Credit by examination available. Credit given for nursing courses completed elsewhere dependent upon specific evaluations.

Financial Aid 90% of baccalaureate students in nursing programs received some form of financial aid in 2008-09. *Gift aid (need-based):* Federal Pell, FSEOG, state, private, college/university gift aid from institutional funds. *Loans:* Federal Direct (Subsidized and Unsubsidized Stafford PLUS), Perkins, alternative loans. *Work-study:* Federal Work-Study, part-time campus jobs. *Financial aid application deadline (priority):* 3/1.

Contact Dr. Carol Jean Dorough, Chair, School of Nursing, Southern Nazarene University, 6729 NW 39th Expressway, Bethany, OK 73008. *Telephone:* 405-717-6217. *Fax:* 405-717-6264. *E-mail:* cdorough@snu.edu.

GRADUATE PROGRAMS

Financial Aid 85% of graduate students in nursing programs received some form of financial aid in 2008-09.

Contact Dr. Carol Jean Dorough, Chair, School of Nursing, Southern Nazarene University, 6729 NW 39th Expressway, Bethany, OK 73008. *Telephone:* 405-717-6217. *Fax:* 405-717-6264. *E-mail:* cdorough@snu.edu.

MASTER'S DEGREE PROGRAM

Degree MS

Available Programs Accelerated Master's; Accelerated Master's for Nurses with Non-Nursing Degrees.

Concentrations Available Nursing administration; nursing education.

Site Options Tulsa, OK.

Study Options Full-time.

Program Entrance Requirements Clinical experience, computer literacy, minimum overall college GPA of 3.0, transcript of college record, immunizations, interview, 3 letters of recommendation, nursing research course, physical assessment course, resume, statistics course. *Application deadline:* Applications may be processed on a rolling basis for some programs.

Advanced Placement Credit given for nursing courses completed elsewhere dependent upon specific evaluations.

Degree Requirements 39 total credit hours, thesis or project.

Southwestern Oklahoma State University

Division of Nursing
Weatherford, Oklahoma

http://www.swosu.edu/academic/nurse
Founded in 1901

DEGREE • BSN

Nursing Program Faculty 8

Baccalaureate Enrollment 82 **Women** 90% **Men** 10% **Minority** 12% **International** 1%

Distance Learning Courses Available.

Nursing Student Activities Sigma Theta Tau, Student Nurses' Association, nursing club.

Nursing Student Resources Academic advising; academic or career counseling; assistance for students with disabilities; bookstore; campus computer network; computer lab; computer-assisted instruction; e-mail services; externships; housing assistance; interactive nursing skills videos; Internet; learning resource lab; library services; nursing audiovisuals; remedial services; skills, simulation, or other laboratory; tutoring.

Library Facilities 284 periodical subscriptions health-care related.

BACCALAUREATE PROGRAMS

Degree BSN

Available Programs ADN to Baccalaureate; Generic Baccalaureate; RN Baccalaureate.

Site Options Oklahoma City, OK; Weatherford, OK; Elk City, OK.

Study Options Full-time.

Online Degree Options Yes.

Program Entrance Requirements Minimum overall college GPA of 2.25, transcript of college record, CPR certification, immunizations, 2 letters of recommendation, minimum GPA in nursing prerequisites of 2.25, professional liability insurance/malpractice insurance, prerequisite course work. Transfer students are accepted. *Application deadline:* 2/1 (fall), 2/1 (spring).

Advanced Placement Credit given for nursing courses completed elsewhere dependent upon specific evaluations.

Expenses (2010-11) *Tuition, state resident:* full-time $6000. *Tuition, nonresident:* full-time $12,000. *Room and board:* $3900 per academic year.

Financial Aid 70% of baccalaureate students in nursing programs received some form of financial aid in 2009-10. *Gift aid (need-based):* Federal Pell, FSEOG, state, private, college/university gift aid from institutional funds. *Loans:* Federal Direct (Subsidized and Unsubsidized Stafford PLUS). *Work-study:* Federal Work-Study. *Financial aid application deadline:* 3/1.

Contact Ms. Debbie Miles, Administrative Assistant, Division of Nursing, Southwestern Oklahoma State University, 100 Campus Drive, Weatherford, OK 73096-3098. *Telephone:* 580-774-3261. *Fax:* 580-774-7075. *E-mail:* debbie.miles@swosu.edu.

University of Central Oklahoma

Department of Nursing
Edmond, Oklahoma

http://nurse.uco.edu/
Founded in 1890

DEGREE • BSN

Nursing Program Faculty 43 (16% with doctorates).
Baccalaureate Enrollment 284 **Women** 90% **Men** 10% **Minority** 16% **International** 3% **Part-time** 1%
Nursing Student Activities Nursing Honor Society, Sigma Theta Tau, Student Nurses' Association.
Nursing Student Resources Academic advising; academic or career counseling; assistance for students with disabilities; bookstore; campus computer network; career placement assistance; computer lab; computer-assisted instruction; e-mail services; externships; interactive nursing skills videos; Internet; library services; nursing audiovisuals; skills, simulation, or other laboratory; tutoring.
Library Facilities 3,000 volumes in health, 1,661 volumes in nursing.

BACCALAUREATE PROGRAMS

Degree BSN
Available Programs Generic Baccalaureate; LPN to Baccalaureate; RN Baccalaureate.
Site Options Midwest City, OK; Oklahoma City, OK.
Study Options Full-time and part-time.
Program Entrance Requirements Minimum overall college GPA of 2.5, transcript of college record, CPR certification, high school math, immunizations, 3 letters of recommendation, professional liability insurance/malpractice insurance, prerequisite course work. Transfer students are accepted. *Application deadline:* 9/10 (fall), 1/28 (spring). *Application fee:* $25.
Advanced Placement Credit given for nursing courses completed elsewhere dependent upon specific evaluations.
Expenses (2010-11) *Tuition, area resident:* full-time $3861; part-time $149 per hour. *International tuition:* $97,452 full-time. *Room and board:* $3895; room only: $2705 per academic year. *Required fees:* full-time $623.
Financial Aid 35% of baccalaureate students in nursing programs received some form of financial aid in 2009-10.
Contact Vicki Addison, Administrative Secretary, Department of Nursing, University of Central Oklahoma, 100 North University Drive, Edmond, OK 73034-5209. *Telephone:* 405-974-5000. *E-mail:* vaddison@ucok.edu.

University of Oklahoma Health Sciences Center

College of Nursing
Oklahoma City, Oklahoma

http://nursing.ouhsc.edu/
Founded in 1890

DEGREES • BSN • MS • PHD

Nursing Program Faculty 185 (16% with doctorates).
Baccalaureate Enrollment 892 **Women** 85% **Men** 15% **Minority** 37% **International** 1% **Part-time** 4%
Graduate Enrollment 256 **Women** 93% **Men** 7% **Minority** 26% **International** 1% **Part-time** 71%
Distance Learning Courses Available.
Nursing Student Activities Sigma Theta Tau, Student Nurses' Association.
Nursing Student Resources Academic advising; academic or career counseling; assistance for students with disabilities; bookstore; campus computer network; computer lab; computer-assisted instruction; e-mail services; employment services for current students; housing assistance; Internet; learning resource lab; library services; nursing audiovisuals; skills, simulation, or other laboratory; tutoring.
Library Facilities 329,056 volumes; 4,850 periodical subscriptions.

BACCALAUREATE PROGRAMS

Degree BSN
Available Programs ADN to Baccalaureate; Accelerated Baccalaureate for Second Degree; Generic Baccalaureate; LPN to RN Baccalaureate.
Site Options Lawton, OK; Tulsa, OK.
Study Options Full-time.
Program Entrance Requirements Minimum overall college GPA of 2.5, transcript of college record, high school transcript, minimum GPA in nursing prerequisites of 2.5, prerequisite course work. Transfer students are accepted. *Application deadline:* 1/15 (fall). *Application fee:* $65.
Advanced Placement Credit by examination available. Credit given for nursing courses completed elsewhere dependent upon specific evaluations.
Expenses (2009-10) *Tuition, state resident:* full-time $3537; part-time $118 per credit hour. *Tuition, nonresident:* full-time $13,518; part-time $451 per credit hour. *Room and board:* room only: $7516 per academic year. *Required fees:* full-time $4923; part-time $164 per credit; part-time $2462 per term.
Financial Aid 87% of baccalaureate students in nursing programs received some form of financial aid in 2008-09. *Loans:* Federal Nursing Student Loans, Perkins, college/university.
Contact Rosalyn Alexander, Admissions Coordinator, College of Nursing, University of Oklahoma Health Sciences Center, PO Box 26901, 1100 North Stonewall Avenue, Oklahoma City, OK 73126-0901. *Telephone:* 405-271-2128. *Fax:* 405-271-7341. *E-mail:* Rosalyn-Alexander@ouhsc.edu.

GRADUATE PROGRAMS

Expenses (2009-10) *Tuition, state resident:* full-time $2808; part-time $156 per credit hour. *Tuition, nonresident:* full-time $10,182; part-time $566 per credit hour. *Room and board:* room only: $7516 per academic year.
Financial Aid 30% of graduate students in nursing programs received some form of financial aid in 2008-09. 6 research assistantships (averaging $6,000 per year) were awarded; teaching assistantships, institutionally sponsored loans, scholarships, and traineeships also available. Aid available to part-time students. *Financial aid application deadline:* 8/1.
Contact Trisha Wilhelm, Admissions Coordinator, College of Nursing, University of Oklahoma Health Sciences Center, PO Box 26901, 1100 North Stonewall Avenue, Oklahoma City, OK 73126-0901. *Telephone:* 405-271-2128. *Fax:* 405-271-7341. *E-mail:* patricia-wilhelm@ouhsc.edu.

MASTER'S DEGREE PROGRAM

Degree MS
Available Programs Master's; Master's for Non-Nursing College Graduates.
Concentrations Available Clinical nurse leader; health-care administration; nursing education. *Clinical nurse specialist programs in:* acute care. *Nurse practitioner programs in:* adult health, family health, neonatal health, pediatric.
Site Options Lawton, OK; Tulsa, OK.
Study Options Full-time and part-time.
Online Degree Options Yes.
Program Entrance Requirements Computer literacy, minimum overall college GPA of 3.0, transcript of college record, 3 letters of recommendation, nursing research course, professional liability insurance/malpractice insurance, prerequisite course work, statistics course. *Application deadline:* 3/1 (fall), 8/1 (spring), 1/15 (summer). *Application fee:* $65.
Advanced Placement Credit given for nursing courses completed elsewhere dependent upon specific evaluations.
Degree Requirements 38 total credit hours, thesis or project, comprehensive exam.

POST-MASTER'S PROGRAM

Areas of Study Clinical nurse leader; health-care administration; nursing education. *Nurse practitioner programs in:* adult health, family health, neonatal health, pediatric.

DOCTORAL DEGREE PROGRAM

Degree PhD
Available Programs Doctorate.
Areas of Study Nursing education.
Program Entrance Requirements Minimum overall college GPA of 3.5, interview by faculty committee, 3 letters of recommendation, scholarly papers, statistics course, vita, writing sample. Application deadline: 4/14 (fall). Application fee: $65.
Degree Requirements 90 total credit hours, dissertation, oral exam, written exam.

CONTINUING EDUCATION PROGRAM

Contact Dr. Beverly Bowers, Assistant Dean for Faculty Development and Professional Continuing Education, College of Nursing, University of Oklahoma Health Sciences Center, PO Box 26901, 1100 North Stonewall Avenue, Oklahoma City, OK 73126-0901. *Telephone:* 405-271-2428. *Fax:* 405-271-7341. *E-mail:* Beverly-Bowers@ouhsc.edu.

University of Phoenix–Oklahoma City Campus
College of Health and Human Services
Oklahoma City, Oklahoma

Founded in 1976
Nursing Program Faculty 1
Nursing Student Activities Sigma Theta Tau.
Nursing Student Resources Academic advising; academic or career counseling; assistance for students with disabilities; bookstore; campus computer network; computer lab; computer-assisted instruction; e-mail services; interactive nursing skills videos; Internet; learning resource lab; library services; nursing audiovisuals; skills, simulation, or other laboratory; tutoring.
Library Facilities 16,781 periodical subscriptions (1,300 health-care related).

University of Phoenix–Tulsa Campus
College of Health and Human Services
Tulsa, Oklahoma

Founded in 1998
Nursing Student Activities Sigma Theta Tau.
Nursing Student Resources Academic advising; academic or career counseling; assistance for students with disabilities; bookstore; campus computer network; computer lab; computer-assisted instruction; e-mail services; interactive nursing skills videos; Internet; learning resource lab; library services; nursing audiovisuals; remedial services; skills, simulation, or other laboratory; tutoring.
Library Facilities 16,781 periodical subscriptions (1,300 health-care related).

University of Tulsa
School of Nursing
Tulsa, Oklahoma

http://www.cba.utulsa.edu/depts/nursing
Founded in 1894

DEGREE • BSN
Nursing Program Faculty 12 (33% with doctorates).
Baccalaureate Enrollment 83 **Women** 93% **Men** 7% **Minority** 25% **Part-time** 2%
Nursing Student Activities Sigma Theta Tau, Student Nurses' Association.
Nursing Student Resources Academic advising; academic or career counseling; assistance for students with disabilities; bookstore; campus computer network; career placement assistance; computer lab; computer-assisted instruction; daycare for children of students; e-mail services; employment services for current students; externships; housing assistance; interactive nursing skills videos; Internet; learning resource lab; library services; nursing audiovisuals; placement services for program completers; remedial services; resume preparation assistance; skills, simulation, or other laboratory; tutoring.
Library Facilities 1.1 million volumes (4,300 in nursing); 27,905 periodical subscriptions (118 health-care related).

BACCALAUREATE PROGRAMS

Degree BSN
Available Programs Generic Baccalaureate; LPN to RN Baccalaureate; RN Baccalaureate.
Study Options Full-time.
Program Entrance Requirements Minimum overall college GPA of 2.5, transcript of college record, CPR certification, written essay, health exam, immunizations, minimum GPA in nursing prerequisites. Transfer students are accepted. *Application deadline:* 2/1 (fall). Applications may be processed on a rolling basis for some programs.
Advanced Placement Credit by examination available. Credit given for nursing courses completed elsewhere dependent upon specific evaluations.
Expenses (2009-10) *Tuition:* full-time $26,722; part-time $899 per credit hour. *International tuition:* $26,722 full-time. *Room and board:* $8544; room only: $4724 per academic year. *Required fees:* full-time $705; part-time $3 per credit.
Financial Aid 90% of baccalaureate students in nursing programs received some form of financial aid in 2008-09.
Contact Dr. Susan Kathleen Gaston, RN, Director, School of Nursing, University of Tulsa, 800 South Tucker Drive, Tulsa, OK 74104-9700. *Telephone:* 918-631-3116. *Fax:* 918-631-2068. *E-mail:* susan-gaston@utulsa.edu.

OREGON

Concordia University
Nursing Program
Portland, Oregon

Founded in 1905

DEGREE • BSN
Nursing Program Faculty 20 (3% with doctorates).
Baccalaureate Enrollment 67
Nursing Student Activities Nursing club.
Nursing Student Resources Academic advising; academic or career counseling; assistance for students with disabilities; bookstore; campus computer network; computer lab; e-mail services; employment services for current students; Internet; learning resource lab; library services; nursing audiovisuals; skills, simulation, or other laboratory; tutoring.
Library Facilities 88,103 volumes; 26,466 periodical subscriptions.

BACCALAUREATE PROGRAMS

Degree BSN
Available Programs Generic Baccalaureate.
Study Options Full-time.
Program Entrance Requirements Transfer students are accepted.
Expenses (2009-10) *Tuition:* full-time $22,900. *International tuition:* $22,900 full-time. *Room and board:* $6700 per academic year.
Financial Aid 100% of baccalaureate students in nursing programs received some form of financial aid in 2008-09.
Contact Mrs. Celeste Krueger, Director of Undergraduate Admissions, Nursing Program, Concordia University, 2811 NE Holman Street, Portland, OR 97211. *Telephone:* 800-321-9371. *E-mail:* admissions@cu-portland.edu.

George Fox University
Nursing Department
Newberg, Oregon

http://www.georgefox.edu/academics/undergrad/departments/nursing/index.html
Founded in 1891

DEGREE • BSN
Nursing Program Faculty 15 (20% with doctorates).
Baccalaureate Enrollment 110 **Women** 91% **Men** 9% **Minority** 8%
Nursing Student Activities Nursing club.
Nursing Student Resources Academic advising; academic or career counseling; assistance for students with disabilities; bookstore; campus computer network; career placement assistance; computer lab; computer-assisted instruction; e-mail services; employment services for current students; housing assistance; interactive nursing skills videos; Internet; learning resource lab; library services; nursing audiovisuals; remedial services; resume preparation assistance; skills, simulation, or other laboratory; tutoring.

Library Facilities 218,240 volumes (490 in health, 100 in nursing); 5,374 periodical subscriptions (5,600 health-care related).

BACCALAUREATE PROGRAMS

Degree BSN

Available Programs Generic Baccalaureate.

Study Options Full-time.

Program Entrance Requirements Minimum overall college GPA of 2.8, transcript of college record, CPR certification, written essay, immunizations, 2 letters of recommendation, minimum GPA in nursing prerequisites of 2.8, prerequisite course work. Transfer students are accepted. *Application deadline:* 10/2 (fall). *Application fee:* $50.

Expenses (2010-11) *Tuition:* full-time $27,640; part-time $840 per credit hour. *Room and board:* $8630; room only: $4880 per academic year. *Required fees:* full-time $930; part-time $180 per credit.

Financial Aid 98% of baccalaureate students in nursing programs received some form of financial aid in 2009-10. *Gift aid (need-based):* Federal Pell, FSEOG, state, private, college/university gift aid from institutional funds, Academic Competitiveness Grants, National SMART Grants, TEACH Grants. *Loans:* Federal Direct (Subsidized and Unsubsidized Stafford PLUS), Perkins, alternative loans. *Work-study:* Federal Work-Study, part-time campus jobs. *Financial aid application deadline (priority):* 2/1.

Contact Elaine Smith, Administrative Assistant, Nursing Department, George Fox University, 414 North Meridian Street, #6273, Newberg, OR 97132. *Telephone:* 503-554-2950. *Fax:* 503-554-3900. *E-mail:* esmith@georgefox.edu.

Linfield College

School of Nursing
McMinnville, Oregon

http://www.linfield.edu/portland

Founded in 1849

DEGREE • BSN

Nursing Program Faculty 64 (22% with doctorates).

Baccalaureate Enrollment 314 **Women** 85.4% **Men** 14.6% **Minority** 17.8% **International** .3% **Part-time** 3.5%

Nursing Student Activities Sigma Theta Tau, Student Nurses' Association, nursing club.

Nursing Student Resources Academic advising; academic or career counseling; bookstore; campus computer network; computer lab; e-mail services; Internet; learning resource lab; library services; nursing audiovisuals; resume preparation assistance; skills, simulation, or other laboratory.

Library Facilities 185,842 volumes (7,201 in health, 1,482 in nursing); 970 periodical subscriptions (249 health-care related).

BACCALAUREATE PROGRAMS

Degree BSN

Available Programs ADN to Baccalaureate; Accelerated Baccalaureate for Second Degree; Baccalaureate for Second Degree; Generic Baccalaureate.

Site Options Portland, OR.

Study Options Full-time.

Program Entrance Requirements Minimum overall college GPA of 2.9, transcript of college record, CPR certification, written essay, health exam, health insurance, immunizations, 1 letter of recommendation, minimum GPA in nursing prerequisites of 2.75, professional liability insurance/malpractice insurance, prerequisite course work. Transfer students are accepted.

Advanced Placement Credit given for nursing courses completed elsewhere dependent upon specific evaluations.

Contact ***Telephone:*** 503-413-8481. *Fax:* 503-413-6283.

CONTINUING EDUCATION PROGRAM

Contact ***Telephone:*** 503-413-7163. *Fax:* 503-413-6846.

Oregon Health & Science University

School of Nursing
Portland, Oregon

http://www.ohsu.edu/son

Founded in 1974

DEGREES • BS • MN/MPH • MS • PHD

Nursing Program Faculty 138 (40% with doctorates).

Baccalaureate Enrollment 573 **Women** 83% **Men** 17% **Minority** 7% **International** 1% **Part-time** 68%

Graduate Enrollment 219 **Women** 74% **Men** 26% **Minority** 4% **International** 2% **Part-time** 56%

Distance Learning Courses Available.

Nursing Student Activities Nursing Honor Society, Sigma Theta Tau, Student Nurses' Association, nursing club.

Nursing Student Resources Academic advising; assistance for students with disabilities; bookstore; campus computer network; computer lab; e-mail services; externships; interactive nursing skills videos; Internet; learning resource lab; library services; nursing audiovisuals; resume preparation assistance; skills, simulation, or other laboratory.

Library Facilities 272,853 volumes (227,344 in health, 7,666 in nursing); 12,888 periodical subscriptions (2,357 health-care related).

BACCALAUREATE PROGRAMS

Degree BS

Available Programs Accelerated Baccalaureate; Generic Baccalaureate; RN Baccalaureate.

Site Options Klamath Falls, OR; Ashland, OR; La Grande, OR.

Study Options Full-time.

Program Entrance Requirements Transcript of college record, written essay, minimum GPA in nursing prerequisites of 3.0, prerequisite course work. Transfer students are accepted. *Application deadline:* 2/15 (fall). *Application fee:* $120.

Advanced Placement Credit given for nursing courses completed elsewhere dependent upon specific evaluations.

Expenses (2010-11) *Tuition, state resident:* full-time $16,538; part-time $289 per credit. *Tuition, nonresident:* full-time $25,824; part-time $836 per credit. *Required fees:* full-time $5325; part-time $547 per term.

Financial Aid 80% of baccalaureate students in nursing programs received some form of financial aid in 2009-10. *Gift aid (need-based):* Federal Pell, FSEOG, state, private, college/university gift aid from institutional funds, Health Profession Scholarships. *Loans:* Federal Nursing Student Loans, Federal Direct (Subsidized and Unsubsidized Stafford PLUS), Perkins, state, college/university, alternative loans. *Work-study:* Federal Work-Study.

Contact Admissions Counselor, School of Nursing, Oregon Health & Science University, Office of Admissions SN-ADM, 3455 SW U.S. Veterans Hospital Road, Portland, OR 97239-2491. *Telephone:* 503-494-7725. *Fax:* 503-494-6433. *E-mail:* proginfo@ohsu.edu.

GRADUATE PROGRAMS

Expenses (2010-11) *Tuition, state resident:* full-time $18,159; part-time $482 per credit. *Tuition, nonresident:* full-time $22,815; part-time $641 per credit. *Required fees:* full-time $5508; part-time $1537 per term.

Financial Aid 45% of graduate students in nursing programs received some form of financial aid in 2009-10. Fellowships, research assistantships, teaching assistantships, career-related internships or fieldwork, Federal Work-Study, institutionally sponsored loans, scholarships, and traineeships available. *Financial aid application deadline:* 3/1.

Contact Admissions Counselor, School of Nursing, Oregon Health & Science University, Office of Admissions SN-ADM, 3455 SW U.S. Veterans Hospital Road, Portland, OR 97239-2491. *Telephone:* 503-494-7725. *Fax:* 503-494-4350. *E-mail:* proginfo@ohsu.edu.

MASTER'S DEGREE PROGRAM

Degrees MN/MPH; MS

Available Programs Accelerated Master's for Non-Nursing College Graduates; Master's.

Concentrations Available Nurse anesthesia; nurse-midwifery; nursing education. *Nurse practitioner programs in:* family health, psychiatric/mental health.

Site Options Klamath Falls, OR; Ashland, OR; La Grande, OR.

Study Options Full-time and part-time.

Program Entrance Requirements Clinical experience, computer literacy, minimum overall college GPA of 3.0, transcript of college record,

CPR certification, written essay, immunizations, interview, 3 letters of recommendation, resume, statistics course, GRE General Test. *Application deadline:* 12/1 (fall). Applications may be processed on a rolling basis for some programs. *Application fee:* $120.
Advanced Placement Credit given for nursing courses completed elsewhere dependent upon specific evaluations.
Degree Requirements 45 total credit hours, comprehensive exam.

POST-MASTER'S PROGRAM

Areas of Study Nurse-midwifery; nursing education. *Nurse practitioner programs in:* family health, gerontology, psychiatric/mental health.

DOCTORAL DEGREE PROGRAM

Degree PhD
Available Programs Doctorate; Post-Baccalaureate Doctorate.
Areas of Study Advanced practice nursing, aging, clinical practice, ethics, faculty preparation, family health, gerontology, health policy, health promotion/disease prevention, health-care systems, human health and illness, illness and transition, nursing policy, nursing research, nursing science, women's health.
Program Entrance Requirements Clinical experience, minimum overall college GPA of 3.0, interview by faculty committee, 3 letters of recommendation, MSN or equivalent, scholarly papers, statistics course, vita, writing sample, GRE General Test. Application deadline: 12/1 (fall). Applications may be processed on a rolling basis for some programs. Application fee: $120.
Degree Requirements 90 total credit hours, dissertation, oral exam, written exam, residency.

POSTDOCTORAL PROGRAM

Areas of Study Adolescent health, aging, chronic illness, family health, gerontology, health promotion/disease prevention, nursing interventions, nursing research, nursing science, outcomes, self-care, vulnerable population, women's health.
Postdoctoral Program Contact Academic Programs Counselor, School of Nursing, Oregon Health & Science University, Office of Admissions SN-ADM, 3455 SW U.S. Veterans Hospital Road, Portland, OR 97239-2491. *Telephone:* 503-494-7725. *Fax:* 503-494-4350. *E-mail:* proginfo@ohsu.edu.

CONTINUING EDUCATION PROGRAM

Contact Paula McNeil, Director of Continuing Education, School of Nursing, Oregon Health & Science University, Office of Continuing Education SN-4N, 3455 SW U.S. Veterans Hospital Road, Portland, OR 97239-2491. *Telephone:* 503-494-6772. *Fax:* 503-494-4350. *E-mail:* snconted@ohsu.edu.

University of Portland
School of Nursing
Portland, Oregon

http://nursing.up.edu/
Founded in 1901

DEGREES • BSN • DNP • MS

Nursing Program Faculty 54 (35% with doctorates).
Baccalaureate Enrollment 650 **Women** 90% **Men** 10% **Minority** 23% **International** 2%
Graduate Enrollment 119 **Women** 83% **Men** 17% **Minority** 12% **International** 1%
Distance Learning Courses Available.
Nursing Student Activities Sigma Theta Tau, Student Nurses' Association, nursing club.
Nursing Student Resources Academic advising; academic or career counseling; assistance for students with disabilities; bookstore; campus computer network; career placement assistance; computer lab; computer-assisted instruction; daycare for children of students; e-mail services; employment services for current students; housing assistance; interactive nursing skills videos; Internet; learning resource lab; library services; nursing audiovisuals; remedial services; resume preparation assistance; skills, simulation, or other laboratory; tutoring.
Library Facilities 350,000 volumes (5,310 in health, 1,226 in nursing); 1,400 periodical subscriptions (496 health-care related).

BACCALAUREATE PROGRAMS

Degree BSN
Available Programs Generic Baccalaureate.
Study Options Full-time.
Program Entrance Requirements Minimum overall college GPA of 2.7, transcript of college record, CPR certification, written essay, health exam, health insurance, high school chemistry, high school transcript, immunizations, 1 letter of recommendation, minimum high school GPA of 2.7, minimum GPA in nursing prerequisites of 2.7, prerequisite course work. Transfer students are accepted. *Application deadline:* 1/15 (fall), 1/15 (spring). *Application fee:* $50.
Advanced Placement Credit by examination available. Credit given for nursing courses completed elsewhere dependent upon specific evaluations.
Expenses (2010-11) *Tuition:* full-time $38,040. *Room and board:* $9320 per academic year. *Required fees:* full-time $1705.
Financial Aid 96% of baccalaureate students in nursing programs received some form of financial aid in 2009-10.
Contact Mr. Jason McDonald, Dean of Admissions, School of Nursing, University of Portland, 5000 North Willamette Boulevard, Portland, OR 97203-5798. *Telephone:* 503-943-7147. *E-mail:* mcdonaja@up.edu.

GRADUATE PROGRAMS

Expenses (2010-11) *Tuition:* part-time $900 per credit hour. *Room and board:* $11,150 per academic year. *Required fees:* part-time $35 per credit.
Financial Aid 91% of graduate students in nursing programs received some form of financial aid in 2009-10. Fellowships, research assistantships, Federal Work-Study and scholarships available. Aid available to part-time students. *Financial aid application deadline:* 3/1.
Contact Mrs. Stacey Boatright, Nursing Program Counselor, School of Nursing, University of Portland, 5000 North Willamette Boulevard, MSC-153, Portland, OR 97203-5798. *Telephone:* 503-943-7423. *Fax:* 503-943-7729. *E-mail:* boatrigh@up.edu.

MASTER'S DEGREE PROGRAM

Degree MS
Available Programs Master's; Master's for Non-Nursing College Graduates; RN to Master's.
Concentrations Available Clinical nurse leader.
Study Options Part-time.
Program Entrance Requirements Computer literacy, minimum overall college GPA of 3.0, transcript of college record, written essay, interview, 2 letters of recommendation, resume, statistics course, GRE General Test or MAT. *Application deadline:* 1/15 (summer). Applications may be processed on a rolling basis for some programs. *Application fee:* $50.
Advanced Placement Credit given for nursing courses completed elsewhere dependent upon specific evaluations.
Degree Requirements 42 total credit hours, thesis or project.

DOCTORAL DEGREE PROGRAM

Degree DNP
Available Programs Doctorate; Post-Baccalaureate Doctorate.
Areas of Study Advanced practice nursing.
Program Entrance Requirements Minimum overall college GPA of 3.0, interview by faculty committee, interview, 3 letters of recommendation, statistics course, vita, writing sample, GRE General Test or MAT. Application deadline: 1/15 (summer). Applications may be processed on a rolling basis for some programs. Application fee: $50.
Degree Requirements 82 total credit hours, residency.

PENNSYLVANIA

Alvernia University
Nursing
Reading, Pennsylvania

http://www.alvernia.edu
Founded in 1958

DEGREE • BSN

Nursing Program Faculty 9 (2% with doctorates).
Baccalaureate Enrollment 203 **Women** 98% **Men** 2% **Minority** 10% **International** 3% **Part-time** 20%
Nursing Student Activities Nursing Honor Society, Sigma Theta Tau, Student Nurses' Association.

Nursing Student Resources Academic advising; academic or career counseling; bookstore; campus computer network; computer lab; computer-assisted instruction; e-mail services; employment services for current students; externships; interactive nursing skills videos; Internet; learning resource lab; library services; nursing audiovisuals; remedial services; skills, simulation, or other laboratory; tutoring.

Library Facilities 85,823 volumes (2,931 in health, 995 in nursing); 362 periodical subscriptions (89 health-care related).

BACCALAUREATE PROGRAMS

Degree BSN

Available Programs Generic Baccalaureate; LPN to Baccalaureate; LPN to RN Baccalaureate; RN Baccalaureate.

Site Options Reading, PA; Pottsville, PA; Ashland, PA.

Study Options Full-time.

Program Entrance Requirements Minimum overall college GPA of 2.7, transcript of college record, CPR certification, written essay, health exam, health insurance, high school biology, high school chemistry, 2 years high school math, 2 years high school science, high school transcript, immunizations, 2 letters of recommendation, minimum high school GPA of 2.7, minimum GPA in nursing prerequisites of 2.7. Transfer students are accepted.

Advanced Placement Credit by examination available. Credit given for nursing courses completed elsewhere dependent upon specific evaluations.

Contact *Telephone:* 610-796-8460. *Fax:* 610-796-8464.

CONTINUING EDUCATION PROGRAM

Contact *Telephone:* 610-796-5611. *Fax:* 610-796-8464.

Bloomsburg University of Pennsylvania

Department of Nursing
Bloomsburg, Pennsylvania

http://www.bloomu.edu/

Founded in 1839

DEGREES • BSN • MSN • MSN/MBA

Nursing Program Faculty 34 (41% with doctorates).

Baccalaureate Enrollment 324 **Women** 89% **Men** 11% **Minority** 8% **Part-time** 5%

Graduate Enrollment 86 **Women** 91% **Men** 9% **Minority** 8% **Part-time** 60%

Distance Learning Courses Available.

Nursing Student Activities Sigma Theta Tau, Student Nurses' Association, nursing club.

Nursing Student Resources Academic advising; academic or career counseling; assistance for students with disabilities; bookstore; campus computer network; career placement assistance; computer lab; computer-assisted instruction; daycare for children of students; e-mail services; employment services for current students; externships; housing assistance; interactive nursing skills videos; Internet; learning resource lab; library services; nursing audiovisuals; paid internships; placement services for program completers; remedial services; resume preparation assistance; skills, simulation, or other laboratory; tutoring; unpaid internships.

Library Facilities 489,636 volumes (8,051 in health, 3,394 in nursing); 1,710 periodical subscriptions (4,392 health-care related).

BACCALAUREATE PROGRAMS

Degree BSN

Available Programs ADN to Baccalaureate; Baccalaureate for Second Degree; Generic Baccalaureate; LPN to RN Baccalaureate; RN Baccalaureate.

Study Options Full-time and part-time.

Program Entrance Requirements Minimum overall college GPA of 2.5, transcript of college record, CPR certification, health exam, health insurance, high school biology, high school chemistry, 2 years high school math, 3 years high school science, high school transcript, immunizations, interview, 3 letters of recommendation, minimum high school GPA of 3.0, minimum high school rank 80%, minimum GPA in nursing prerequisites of 2.5, professional liability insurance/malpractice insurance, prerequisite course work. Transfer students are accepted. *Application deadline:* 11/15 (fall). *Application fee:* $35.

Advanced Placement Credit by examination available. Credit given for nursing courses completed elsewhere dependent upon specific evaluations.

Expenses (2010-11) *Tuition, state resident:* full-time $5804; part-time $242 per credit. *Tuition, nonresident:* full-time $14,510; part-time $605 per credit. *Room and board:* $6890; room only: $4232 per academic year. *Required fees:* full-time $1652; part-time $46 per credit; part-time $123–$230 per term.

Financial Aid 79% of baccalaureate students in nursing programs received some form of financial aid in 2009-10. *Gift aid (need-based):* Federal Pell, FSEOG, state, private, college/university gift aid from institutional funds, Academic Competitiveness Grants, National SMART Grants. *Loans:* Federal Direct (Subsidized and Unsubsidized Stafford PLUS), Perkins, state, alternative loans. *Work-study:* Federal Work-Study, part-time campus jobs. *Financial aid application deadline (priority):* 3/15.

Contact Dr. M. Christine Alichnie, Department Chairperson, Department of Nursing, Bloomsburg University of Pennsylvania, 400 East Second Street, Room 3109, MCHS, Bloomsburg, PA 17815. *Telephone:* 570-389-4426. *Fax:* 570-389-5008. *E-mail:* calichni@bloomu.edu.

GRADUATE PROGRAMS

Expenses (2010-11) *Tuition, state resident:* full-time $6966; part-time $387 per credit. *Tuition, nonresident:* full-time $11,146; part-time $619 per credit. *International tuition:* $11,146 full-time. *Required fees:* full-time $1699; part-time $60 per credit; part-time $123–$230 per term.

Financial Aid 33% of graduate students in nursing programs received some form of financial aid in 2009-10. Unspecified assistantships available.

Contact Dr. Michelle Ficca, Coordinator of Graduate Program, Department of Nursing, Bloomsburg University of Pennsylvania, 400 East Second Street, Room 3136, MCHS, Bloomsburg, PA 17815. *Telephone:* 570-389-4615. *Fax:* 570-389-5008. *E-mail:* mficca@bloomu.edu.

MASTER'S DEGREE PROGRAM

Degrees MSN; MSN/MBA

Available Programs Master's; Master's for Nurses with Non-Nursing Degrees; RN to Master's.

Concentrations Available Nurse anesthesia; nursing administration. *Clinical nurse specialist programs in:* adult health, community health, gerontology, public health, school health. *Nurse practitioner programs in:* adult health, gerontology.

Site Options Danville, PA.

Study Options Full-time and part-time.

Program Entrance Requirements Clinical experience, computer literacy, minimum overall college GPA of 3.0, transcript of college record, CPR certification, immunizations, interview, 3 letters of recommendation, nursing research course, physical assessment course, professional liability insurance/malpractice insurance, prerequisite course work, resume, statistics course. *Application deadline:* Applications may be processed on a rolling basis for some programs. *Application fee:* $35.

Advanced Placement Credit by examination available. Credit given for nursing courses completed elsewhere dependent upon specific evaluations.

Degree Requirements 39–52 total credit hours, comprehensive exam.

POST-MASTER'S PROGRAM

Areas of Study Nurse anesthesia; nursing administration. *Clinical nurse specialist programs in:* school health. *Nurse practitioner programs in:* adult health, family health, gerontology.

CONTINUING EDUCATION PROGRAM

Contact Dr. M. Christine Alichnie, Department Chairperson, Department of Nursing, Bloomsburg University of Pennsylvania, 400 East Second Street, Room 3109, MCHS, Bloomsburg, PA 17815. *Telephone:* 570-389-4426. *Fax:* 570-389-5008. *E-mail:* calichni@bloomu.edu.

California University of Pennsylvania
Department of Nursing
California, Pennsylvania

http://www.cup.edu/eberly/nursing
Founded in 1852

DEGREE • BSN
Nursing Program Faculty 5 (60% with doctorates).
Baccalaureate Enrollment 145 **Women** 83% **Men** 17% **Minority** 3% **Part-time** 92%
Nursing Student Activities Sigma Theta Tau.
Nursing Student Resources Academic advising; academic or career counseling; assistance for students with disabilities; bookstore; campus computer network; career placement assistance; computer lab; computer-assisted instruction; daycare for children of students; e-mail services; employment services for current students; Internet; library services; nursing audiovisuals; placement services for program completers; remedial services; resume preparation assistance; tutoring.
Library Facilities 3,840 volumes in health, 2,010 volumes in nursing; 80 periodical subscriptions health-care related.

BACCALAUREATE PROGRAMS
Degree BSN
Available Programs RN Baccalaureate.
Site Options West Mifflin, PA.
Study Options Full-time and part-time.
Program Entrance Requirements Minimum overall college GPA of 2.0, transcript of college record, CPR certification, health exam, health insurance, immunizations, 2 letters of recommendation, professional liability insurance/malpractice insurance, prerequisite course work, RN licensure. Transfer students are accepted.
Advanced Placement Credit by examination available. Credit given for nursing courses completed elsewhere dependent upon specific evaluations.
Contact ***Telephone:*** 724-938-5739. *Fax:* 724-938-1612.

Carlow University
School of Nursing
Pittsburgh, Pennsylvania

http://www.carlow.edu/academic/nursing.html
Founded in 1929

DEGREES • BSN • MSN
Nursing Program Faculty 31 (23% with doctorates).
Baccalaureate Enrollment 333 **Women** 99% **Men** 1% **Minority** 13% **Part-time** 21%
Graduate Enrollment 54 **Women** 94% **Men** 6% **Minority** 11% **Part-time** 94%
Nursing Student Activities Nursing Honor Society, Sigma Theta Tau, Student Nurses' Association.
Nursing Student Resources Academic advising; academic or career counseling; assistance for students with disabilities; bookstore; campus computer network; career placement assistance; computer lab; computer-assisted instruction; daycare for children of students; e-mail services; employment services for current students; externships; housing assistance; Internet; learning resource lab; library services; nursing audiovisuals; other; paid internships; placement services for program completers; remedial services; resumé preparation assistance; skills, simulation, or other laboratory; tutoring; unpaid internships.
Library Facilities 133,864 volumes (14,100 in health, 5,450 in nursing); 14,784 periodical subscriptions (60 health-care related).

BACCALAUREATE PROGRAMS
Degree BSN
Available Programs Accelerated RN Baccalaureate; Baccalaureate for Second Degree; Generic Baccalaureate.
Site Options Cranberry Township, PA; Greensburg, PA.
Study Options Full-time and part-time.
Program Entrance Requirements Minimum overall college GPA of 3.0, transcript of college record, CPR certification, health exam, health insurance, high school biology, high school chemistry, 2 years high school math, 2 years high school science, high school transcript, immunizations, interview, minimum high school GPA of 3.0, minimum GPA in nursing prerequisites of 2.0, professional liability insurance/malpractice insurance, prerequisite course work. Transfer students are accepted.
Advanced Placement Credit by examination available. Credit given for nursing courses completed elsewhere dependent upon specific evaluations.
Contact ***Telephone:*** 412-578-6059. *Fax:* 412-578-6668.

GRADUATE PROGRAMS
Contact ***Telephone:*** 412-578-8764. *Fax:* 412-578-6321.

MASTER'S DEGREE PROGRAM
Degree MSN
Available Programs Accelerated Master's; Master's; RN to Master's.
Concentrations Available Nurse case management; nursing administration; nursing education. *Clinical nurse specialist programs in:* home health care. *Nurse practitioner programs in:* family health.
Site Options Cranberry Township, PA; Greensburg, PA.
Study Options Full-time and part-time.
Program Entrance Requirements Clinical experience, computer literacy, minimum overall college GPA of 3.0, transcript of college record, CPR certification, written essay, immunizations, interview, 3 letters of recommendation, professional liability insurance/malpractice insurance, prerequisite course work, resume, statistics course.
Advanced Placement Credit by examination available. Credit given for nursing courses completed elsewhere dependent upon specific evaluations.
Degree Requirements 56 total credit hours, thesis or project, comprehensive exam.

POST-MASTER'S PROGRAM
Areas of Study *Clinical nurse specialist programs in:* home health care. *Nurse practitioner programs in:* family health.

CONTINUING EDUCATION PROGRAM
Contact ***Telephone:*** 412-578-8764. *Fax:* 412-578-6321.

Cedar Crest College
Department of Nursing
Allentown, Pennsylvania

http://www.cedarcrest.edu
Founded in 1867

DEGREES • BS • MSN
Nursing Program Faculty 21 (24% with doctorates).
Baccalaureate Enrollment 287 **Women** 96% **Men** 4% **Minority** 23% **International** 8% **Part-time** 68%
Graduate Enrollment 23 **Women** 96% **Men** 4% **Minority** 4% **Part-time** 100%
Nursing Student Activities Nursing Honor Society, Sigma Theta Tau, Student Nurses' Association.
Nursing Student Resources Academic advising; academic or career counseling; assistance for students with disabilities; bookstore; campus computer network; career placement assistance; computer lab; computer-assisted instruction; e-mail services; interactive nursing skills videos; Internet; learning resource lab; library services; nursing audiovisuals; remedial services; skills, simulation, or other laboratory; tutoring.
Library Facilities 144,037 volumes; 15,053 periodical subscriptions.

BACCALAUREATE PROGRAMS
Degree BS
Available Programs Baccalaureate for Second Degree; Generic Baccalaureate; LPN to Baccalaureate; RN Baccalaureate.
Study Options Full-time and part-time.
Program Entrance Requirements Minimum overall college GPA of 2.5, CPR certification, written essay, health exam, health insurance, high school biology, high school chemistry, 3 years high school math, 2 years high school science, high school transcript, immunizations, minimum GPA in nursing prerequisites of 2.7, prerequisite course work. Transfer students are accepted. *Application deadline:* Applications may be processed on a rolling basis for some programs.
Advanced Placement Credit given for nursing courses completed elsewhere dependent upon specific evaluations.
Contact ***Telephone:*** 610-740-3780. *Fax:* 610-606-4647.

GRADUATE PROGRAMS

Contact *Telephone:* 610-606-4666 Ext. 3480.

MASTER'S DEGREE PROGRAM

Degree MSN
Available Programs Master's.
Study Options Part-time.
Program Entrance Requirements Clinical experience, minimum overall college GPA of 3.0, transcript of college record, CPR certification, immunizations, interview, 3 letters of recommendation, nursing research course, physical assessment course, resume, statistics course. *Application deadline:* Applications may be processed on a rolling basis for some programs. *Application fee:* $30.
Advanced Placement Credit given for nursing courses completed elsewhere dependent upon specific evaluations.
Degree Requirements 38 total credit hours, thesis or project.

Chatham University

Program in Nursing
Pittsburgh, Pennsylvania

http://www.chatham.edu/
Founded in 1869

DEGREES • DNP • MSN

Nursing Program Faculty 27 (80% with doctorates).
Graduate Enrollment 117 **Women** 88% **Men** 12% **Minority** 17% **Part-time** 15%
Distance Learning Courses Available.
Nursing Student Resources Academic advising; academic or career counseling; assistance for students with disabilities; bookstore; campus computer network; career placement assistance; computer lab; e-mail services; employment services for current students; housing assistance; Internet; library services; other; placement services for program completers; remedial services; resume preparation assistance; tutoring.
Library Facilities 90,780 volumes (1,747 in health, 1,732 in nursing); 365 periodical subscriptions (967 health-care related).

GRADUATE PROGRAMS

Expenses (2010-11) *Tuition:* part-time $742 per credit. *Required fees:* part-time $18 per credit.
Financial Aid 79% of graduate students in nursing programs received some form of financial aid in 2009-10.
Contact Mr. David Vey, Admission Support Specialist, Program in Nursing, Chatham University, College of Continuing and Professional Studies, Woodland Road, Pittsburgh, PA 15232. *Telephone:* 866-815-2050. *Fax:* 412-365-1720. *E-mail:* dvey@chatham.edu.

MASTER'S DEGREE PROGRAM

Degree MSN
Available Programs Master's.
Concentrations Available Nursing administration; nursing education.
Study Options Full-time and part-time.
Program Entrance Requirements Minimum overall college GPA of 3.0, transcript of college record, resume. *Application deadline:* 8/15 (fall). Applications may be processed on a rolling basis for some programs.
Advanced Placement Credit given for nursing courses completed elsewhere dependent upon specific evaluations.
Degree Requirements 32 total credit hours, thesis or project.

DOCTORAL DEGREE PROGRAM

Degree DNP
Available Programs Doctorate.
Online Degree Options Yes (online only).
Program Entrance Requirements Clinical experience, minimum overall college GPA of 3.0, 2 letters of recommendation, MSN or equivalent, vita, writing sample. Application deadline: 5/1 (fall), 10/1 (spring).
Degree Requirements 27 total credit hours, residency.

Clarion University of Pennsylvania

School of Nursing
Oil City, Pennsylvania

http://www.clarion.edu/
Founded in 1867

DEGREES • BSN • MSN

Nursing Program Faculty 20 (25% with doctorates).
Baccalaureate Enrollment 105 **Women** 90% **Men** 10% **Minority** 2% **International** 1% **Part-time** 88%
Graduate Enrollment 82 **Women** 98% **Men** 2% **Minority** 3% **Part-time** 80%
Distance Learning Courses Available.
Nursing Student Activities Sigma Theta Tau, nursing club.
Nursing Student Resources Academic advising; academic or career counseling; assistance for students with disabilities; bookstore; campus computer network; career placement assistance; computer lab; computer-assisted instruction; daycare for children of students; e-mail services; employment services for current students; externships; housing assistance; interactive nursing skills videos; Internet; learning resource lab; library services; nursing audiovisuals; placement services for program completers; remedial services; resume preparation assistance; skills, simulation, or other laboratory; tutoring.
Library Facilities 442,871 volumes (12,000 in health, 7,000 in nursing); 20,264 periodical subscriptions (300 health-care related).

BACCALAUREATE PROGRAMS

Degree BSN
Available Programs ADN to Baccalaureate; RN Baccalaureate.
Study Options Full-time and part-time.
Online Degree Options Yes (online only).
Program Entrance Requirements Minimum overall college GPA of 2.5, transcript of college record, CPR certification, health exam, health insurance, high school transcript, immunizations, minimum GPA in nursing prerequisites of 2.0, professional liability insurance/malpractice insurance, RN licensure. Transfer students are accepted. *Application deadline:* 8/1 (fall), 12/1 (winter). Applications may be processed on a rolling basis for some programs. *Application fee:* $30.
Financial Aid 70% of baccalaureate students in nursing programs received some form of financial aid in 2009-10.
Contact Dr. Sharon Falkenstern, Director of Nursing and Allied Health, School of Nursing, Clarion University of Pennsylvania, 1801 West First Street, Oil City, PA 16301. *Telephone:* 814-393-1258. *Fax:* 814-676-0251. *E-mail:* sfalkenstern@clarion.edu.

GRADUATE PROGRAMS

Financial Aid 90% of graduate students in nursing programs received some form of financial aid in 2009-10. 2 research assistantships with full tuition reimbursements available (averaging $4,660 per year) were awarded. *Financial aid application deadline:* 3/1.
Contact Dr. Deborah Ciesielka, Coordinator, MSN Family Nurse Practitioner Program, School of Nursing, Clarion University of Pennsylvania, 4900 Friendship Avenue, Pittsburgh, PA 15224. *Telephone:* 412-578-7277. *E-mail:* dciesielka@clarion.edu.

MASTER'S DEGREE PROGRAM

Degree MSN
Available Programs Master's; RN to Master's.
Concentrations Available Nursing education. *Nurse practitioner programs in:* family health.
Site Options Edinboro, PA; Pittsburgh, PA.
Study Options Full-time and part-time.
Program Entrance Requirements Clinical experience, computer literacy, minimum overall college GPA of 3.0, transcript of college record, CPR certification, written essay, immunizations, interview, 3 letters of recommendation, professional liability insurance/malpractice insurance, statistics course. *Application deadline:* 4/1 (fall), 11/1 (winter), 11/1 (spring), 4/1 (summer). *Application fee:* $50.
Advanced Placement Credit given for nursing courses completed elsewhere dependent upon specific evaluations.
Degree Requirements 45 total credit hours, thesis or project, comprehensive exam.

POST-MASTER'S PROGRAM

Areas of Study Nursing education. *Nurse practitioner programs in:* family health.

DeSales University

Department of Nursing and Health
Center Valley, Pennsylvania

http://www.desales.edu
Founded in 1964

DEGREES • BSN • MSN • MSN/MBA

Nursing Program Faculty 74 (23% with doctorates).
Baccalaureate Enrollment 193 **Women** 88% **Men** 12% **Minority** 4% **International** 2% **Part-time** 23%
Graduate Enrollment 85 **Women** 93% **Men** 7% **Minority** 2% **Part-time** 95%
Nursing Student Activities Nursing Honor Society, Sigma Theta Tau, Student Nurses' Association.
Nursing Student Resources Academic advising; academic or career counseling; bookstore; campus computer network; career placement assistance; computer lab; computer-assisted instruction; e-mail services; employment services for current students; externships; interactive nursing skills videos; Internet; learning resource lab; library services; nursing audiovisuals; paid internships; placement services for program completers; remedial services; resume preparation assistance; skills, simulation, or other laboratory; tutoring; unpaid internships.
Library Facilities 154,960 volumes (1,215 in health, 100 in nursing); 8,527 periodical subscriptions (100 health-care related).

BACCALAUREATE PROGRAMS

Degree BSN
Available Programs ADN to Baccalaureate; Accelerated Baccalaureate; Accelerated RN Baccalaureate; Baccalaureate for Second Degree; Generic Baccalaureate; RN Baccalaureate.
Study Options Full-time and part-time.
Program Entrance Requirements Minimum overall college GPA of 2.5, transcript of college record, written essay, high school biology, high school chemistry, high school foreign language, 2 years high school math, 3 years high school science, high school transcript, 2 letters of recommendation, minimum high school GPA of 2.5, minimum high school rank 33%, minimum GPA in nursing prerequisites of 2.0. Transfer students are accepted. *Application deadline:* Applications may be processed on a rolling basis for some programs. *Application fee:* $30.
Advanced Placement Credit by examination available. Credit given for nursing courses completed elsewhere dependent upon specific evaluations.
Expenses (2009-10) *Tuition:* full-time $26,000; part-time $1085 per credit. *International tuition:* $26,000 full-time. *Room and board:* $9200 per academic year.
Financial Aid 47% of baccalaureate students in nursing programs received some form of financial aid in 2008-09. *Gift aid (need-based):* Federal Pell, FSEOG, state, private, college/university gift aid from institutional funds. *Work-study:* Federal Work-Study, part-time campus jobs. *Financial aid application deadline (priority):* 2/1.
Contact Dr. Margaret M. Slusser, Chair, Nursing and Health Department, Department of Nursing and Health, DeSales University, 2755 Station Avenue, Center Valley, PA 18034-9568. *Telephone:* 610-282-1100 Ext. 1285. *Fax:* 610-282-2091. *E-mail:* Margaret.Slusser@desales.edu.

GRADUATE PROGRAMS

Expenses (2009-10) *Tuition:* part-time $665 per credit. *Required fees:* part-time $200 per credit.
Financial Aid 18% of graduate students in nursing programs received some form of financial aid in 2008-09.
Contact Dr. Carol G. Mest, Director of Graduate Program in Nursing, Department of Nursing and Health, DeSales University, 2755 Station Avenue, Center Valley, PA 18034-9568. *Telephone:* 610-282-1100 Ext. 1664. *Fax:* 610-282-2091. *E-mail:* carol.mest@desales.edu.

MASTER'S DEGREE PROGRAM

Degrees MSN; MSN/MBA
Available Programs Accelerated AD/RN to Master's; Master's; RN to Master's.
Concentrations Available Nursing administration; nursing education. *Clinical nurse specialist programs in:* adult health. *Nurse practitioner programs in:* family health.
Study Options Full-time and part-time.
Program Entrance Requirements Minimum overall college GPA of 3.0, transcript of college record, written essay, interview, 3 letters of recommendation, prerequisite course work, statistics course. *Application deadline:* Applications may be processed on a rolling basis for some programs. *Application fee:* $35.
Advanced Placement Credit given for nursing courses completed elsewhere dependent upon specific evaluations.
Degree Requirements 47 total credit hours.

POST-MASTER'S PROGRAM

Areas of Study Nursing education. *Clinical nurse specialist programs in:* adult health. *Nurse practitioner programs in:* family health.

CONTINUING EDUCATION PROGRAM

Contact Dr. Margaret M. Slusser, Chair, Nursing and Health Department, Department of Nursing and Health, DeSales University, 2755 Station Avenue, Center Valley, PA 18034-9568. *Telephone:* 610-282-1100 Ext. 1271. *Fax:* 610-282-2091. *E-mail:* Margaret.Slusser@desales.edu.

Drexel University

College of Nursing and Health Professions
Philadelphia, Pennsylvania

http://www.drexel.edu/
Founded in 1891

DEGREES • BSN • DR NP • MSN

Nursing Program Faculty 73 (52% with doctorates).
Baccalaureate Enrollment 1,350 **Women** 88% **Men** 12% **Minority** 33% **International** 4% **Part-time** 4%
Graduate Enrollment 800 **Women** 88% **Men** 12% **Minority** 15% **Part-time** 80%
Distance Learning Courses Available.
Nursing Student Activities Nursing Honor Society, Sigma Theta Tau, Student Nurses' Association.
Nursing Student Resources Academic advising; academic or career counseling; assistance for students with disabilities; bookstore; campus computer network; career placement assistance; computer lab; computer-assisted instruction; e-mail services; housing assistance; interactive nursing skills videos; Internet; learning resource lab; library services; nursing audiovisuals; paid internships; placement services for program completers; remedial services; resume preparation assistance; skills, simulation, or other laboratory; tutoring.
Library Facilities 643,869 volumes (51,000 in health, 5,015 in nursing); 27,399 periodical subscriptions (63,000 health-care related).

BACCALAUREATE PROGRAMS

Degree BSN
Available Programs ADN to Baccalaureate; Generic Baccalaureate; RN Baccalaureate.
Site Options Philadelphia, PA.
Study Options Full-time.
Program Entrance Requirements CPR certification, written essay, health insurance, high school biology, high school chemistry, 3 years high school math, 2 years high school science, high school transcript, immunizations. Transfer students are accepted. *Application deadline:* Applications may be processed on a rolling basis for some programs. *Application fee:* $75.
Expenses (2010-11) *Tuition:* full-time $38,000. *Room and board:* $13,125; room only: $7875 per academic year. *Required fees:* full-time $2130.
Financial Aid 93% of baccalaureate students in nursing programs received some form of financial aid in 2009-10.
Contact Ms. Margaret Sparzani, Director of Freshman Admissions, College of Nursing and Health Professions, Drexel University, 3141 Chestnut Street, Enrollment Management, Philadelphia, PA 19104. *Telephone:* 215-895-6055. *Fax:* 215-895-5939. *E-mail:* mgts@drexel.edu.

GRADUATE PROGRAMS

Expenses (2010-11) *Tuition:* part-time $960 per credit hour. *Required fees:* part-time $125 per term.

Financial Aid Fellowships, research assistantships, teaching assistantships, career-related internships or fieldwork, Federal Work-Study, institutionally sponsored loans, and tuition waivers (partial) available.
Contact Mr. Redian Furxhui, Academic Advisor, MSN Programs, College of Nursing and Health Professions, Drexel University, 1505 Race Street, Mail Stop 501, Philadelphia, PA 19102-1192. *Telephone:* 215-762-3999. *Fax:* 215-762-1259. *E-mail:* rf53@drexel.edu.

MASTER'S DEGREE PROGRAM

Degree MSN
Available Programs Master's; Master's for Nurses with Non-Nursing Degrees; RN to Master's.
Concentrations Available Nurse anesthesia; nursing administration; nursing education. *Clinical nurse specialist programs in:* women's health. *Nurse practitioner programs in:* acute care, family health, pediatric, psychiatric/mental health, women's health.
Site Options Philadelphia, PA.
Study Options Full-time and part-time.
Online Degree Options Yes.
Program Entrance Requirements Clinical experience, computer literacy, minimum overall college GPA of 3.0, transcript of college record, CPR certification, written essay, immunizations, 2 letters of recommendation, resume. *Application deadline:* Applications may be processed on a rolling basis for some programs. *Application fee:* $75.
Advanced Placement Credit given for nursing courses completed elsewhere dependent upon specific evaluations.
Degree Requirements 55 total credit hours, thesis or project, comprehensive exam.

POST-MASTER'S PROGRAM

Areas of Study Nurse anesthesia; nursing administration; nursing education. *Nurse practitioner programs in:* acute care, family health, pediatric, psychiatric/mental health, women's health.

DOCTORAL DEGREE PROGRAM

Degree Dr NP
Available Programs Doctorate; Post-Baccalaureate Doctorate.
Areas of Study Clinical practice, faculty preparation, nursing administration, nursing education, nursing science.
Site Options Philadelphia, PA.
Program Entrance Requirements Clinical experience, minimum overall college GPA of 3.25, interview by faculty committee, 2 letters of recommendation, MSN or equivalent, vita, writing sample, GRE General Test. Application deadline: 3/1 (fall).
Degree Requirements 48 total credit hours, dissertation, oral exam, written exam, residency.

CONTINUING EDUCATION PROGRAM

Contact Mr. Wayne Miller, Director of Continuing Nursing Education, College of Nursing and Health Professions, Drexel University, 245 North 15th Street, Mail Stop 501, Philadelphia, PA 19102-1192. *Telephone:* 215-762-8521. *Fax:* 215-762-7778. *E-mail:* wdm22@drexel.edu.

Duquesne University
School of Nursing
Pittsburgh, Pennsylvania

http://www.duq.edu/nursing
Founded in 1878

DEGREES • BSN • DNP • MSN • PHD

Nursing Program Faculty 81 (47% with doctorates).
Baccalaureate Enrollment 440 **Women** 87% **Men** 13% **Minority** 7% **International** 2%
Graduate Enrollment 211 **Women** 95% **Men** 5% **Minority** 11% **International** 1% **Part-time** 40%
Distance Learning Courses Available.
Nursing Student Activities Nursing Honor Society, Sigma Theta Tau, Student Nurses' Association, nursing club.
Nursing Student Resources Academic advising; academic or career counseling; assistance for students with disabilities; bookstore; campus computer network; career placement assistance; computer lab; computer-assisted instruction; daycare for children of students; e-mail services; employment services for current students; externships; housing assistance; interactive nursing skills videos; Internet; learning resource lab; library services; nursing audiovisuals; paid internships; placement services for program completers; remedial services; resume preparation assistance; skills, simulation, or other laboratory; tutoring; unpaid internships.
Library Facilities 715,518 volumes (27,613 in health, 1,951 in nursing); 31,060 periodical subscriptions (1,779 health-care related).

BACCALAUREATE PROGRAMS

Degree BSN
Available Programs Accelerated Baccalaureate for Second Degree; Generic Baccalaureate.
Study Options Full-time and part-time.
Program Entrance Requirements Minimum overall college GPA of 3.0, transcript of college record, written essay, high school biology, high school chemistry, high school foreign language, 2 years high school math, 3 years high school science, high school transcript, 2 letters of recommendation, minimum high school GPA of 3.0, minimum high school rank 40%. Transfer students are accepted. *Application deadline:* 5/1 (fall), 11/1 (spring). Applications may be processed on a rolling basis for some programs. *Application fee:* $50.
Advanced Placement Credit by examination available.
Expenses (2010-11) *Tuition:* full-time $25,336; part-time $826 per credit. *Room and board:* $9476 per academic year. *Required fees:* full-time $2166; part-time $84 per credit.
Financial Aid 80% of baccalaureate students in nursing programs received some form of financial aid in 2009-10.
Contact Ms. Susan Hardner, Nursing Recruiter, School of Nursing, Duquesne University, 600 Forbes Avenue, Pittsburgh, PA 15282-1760. *Telephone:* 412-396-4945. *Fax:* 412-396-6346. *E-mail:* hardnersue@duq.edu.

GRADUATE PROGRAMS

Expenses (2010-11) *Tuition:* part-time $907 per credit. *Required fees:* part-time $84 per credit.
Financial Aid 55% of graduate students in nursing programs received some form of financial aid in 2009-10. 14 research assistantships with partial tuition reimbursements available (averaging $2,250 per year), 8 teaching assistantships with partial tuition reimbursements available (averaging $1,075 per year) were awarded; institutionally sponsored loans, scholarships, traineeships, tuition waivers (partial), and unspecified assistantships also available. Aid available to part-time students. *Financial aid application deadline:* 7/1.
Contact Ms. Susan Hardner, Nursing Recruiter, School of Nursing, Duquesne University, 600 Forbes Avenue, Pittsburgh, PA 15282-1760. *Telephone:* 412-396-4945. *Fax:* 412-396-6346. *E-mail:* hardnersue@duq.edu.

MASTER'S DEGREE PROGRAM

Degree MSN
Available Programs Master's.
Concentrations Available Nursing education. *Clinical nurse specialist programs in:* forensic nursing. *Nurse practitioner programs in:* family health.
Study Options Full-time and part-time.
Online Degree Options Yes (online only).
Program Entrance Requirements Clinical experience, computer literacy, minimum overall college GPA of 3.0, transcript of college record, written essay, interview, 2 letters of recommendation, nursing research course, physical assessment course, prerequisite course work, resume, statistics course. *Application deadline:* 3/1 (summer).
Advanced Placement Credit given for nursing courses completed elsewhere dependent upon specific evaluations.
Degree Requirements 47 total credit hours, thesis or project.

POST-MASTER'S PROGRAM

Areas of Study Nursing education. *Clinical nurse specialist programs in:* forensic nursing. *Nurse practitioner programs in:* family health.

DOCTORAL DEGREE PROGRAM

Degree DNP
Available Programs Doctorate.
Areas of Study Nursing practice.
Program Entrance Requirements Minimum overall college GPA of 3.0, 3 letters of recommendation, statistics course, graduate nursing research course, interview by faculty member, current nursing license, current certification if applicable, BSN and MSN or equivalent, vita, personal goal statement, problem statement. *Application deadline:* 2/1 (summer).
Degree Requirements Capstone project, residency.

Degree PhD
Available Programs Doctorate.
Areas of Study Nursing research.
Online Degree Options Yes (online only).
Program Entrance Requirements Minimum overall college GPA of 3.5, interview by faculty committee, 3 letters of recommendation, MSN or equivalent, scholarly papers, statistics course, vita, writing sample, GRE General Test (PhD). Application deadline: 1/15 (summer).
Degree Requirements 58 total credit hours, dissertation, oral exam, written exam, residency.

CONTINUING EDUCATION PROGRAM

Contact Dr. Shirley P. Smith, Assistant Professor, School of Nursing, Duquesne University, 600 Forbes Avenue, Pittsburgh, PA 15282-1760. *Telephone:* 412-396-6535. *Fax:* 412-396-6346. *E-mail:* smithl@duq.edu.

See full description on page 472.

Eastern University
Program in Nursing
St. Davids, Pennsylvania

http://www.eastern.edu/academics/
Founded in 1952

DEGREE • BSN

Nursing Program Faculty 7 (43% with doctorates).
Baccalaureate Enrollment 100 **Women** 92% **Men** 8% **Minority** 25% **International** 32%
Distance Learning Courses Available.
Nursing Student Activities Sigma Theta Tau, Student Nurses' Association.
Nursing Student Resources Academic advising; academic or career counseling; assistance for students with disabilities; bookstore; campus computer network; career placement assistance; computer lab; computer-assisted instruction; e-mail services; employment services for current students; Internet; learning resource lab; library services; nursing audiovisuals; placement services for program completers; remedial services; resume preparation assistance; skills, simulation, or other laboratory; tutoring; unpaid internships.
Library Facilities 5,858 volumes in health, 3,000 volumes in nursing; 821 periodical subscriptions health-care related.

BACCALAUREATE PROGRAMS

Degree BSN
Available Programs Accelerated RN Baccalaureate; Baccalaureate for Second Degree; Generic Baccalaureate; International Nurse to Baccalaureate.
Site Options Wynnewood, PA; West Chester, PA; Harrisburg, PA.
Study Options Full-time.
Program Entrance Requirements Minimum overall college GPA of 3.0, transcript of college record, CPR certification, written essay, health exam, health insurance, high school chemistry, high school transcript, immunizations, interview, 2 letters of recommendation, minimum GPA in nursing prerequisites of 3.0, professional liability insurance/malpractice insurance, prerequisite course work, RN licensure. Transfer students are accepted. *Application deadline:* Applications may be processed on a rolling basis for some programs. *Application fee:* $40.
Expenses (2009-10) *Tuition:* full-time $22,670; part-time $475 per credit hour. *Room and board:* $8870; room only: $4830 per academic year.
Financial Aid 30% of baccalaureate students in nursing programs received some form of financial aid in 2008-09.
Contact Ms. Valerie DiMaio, RN-BSN/BSN TWO Program Advisor, Program in Nursing, Eastern University, 1300 Eagle Road, St. Davids, PA 19087. *Telephone:* 800-732-7669. *Fax:* 610-341-1468. *E-mail:* vdimaio@eastern.edu.

East Stroudsburg University of Pennsylvania
Department of Nursing
East Stroudsburg, Pennsylvania

http://www3.esu/academics/hshp/nurs/home.asp
Founded in 1893

DEGREE • BS

Nursing Program Faculty 14 (77% with doctorates).
Baccalaureate Enrollment 166 **Women** 75% **Men** 25%

Nursing Student Activities Nursing Honor Society, Sigma Theta Tau, Student Nurses' Association, nursing club.
Nursing Student Resources Academic advising; academic or career counseling; assistance for students with disabilities; bookstore; campus computer network; career placement assistance; computer lab; computer-assisted instruction; daycare for children of students; e-mail services; employment services for current students; externships; housing assistance; interactive nursing skills videos; Internet; learning resource lab; library services; nursing audiovisuals; other; placement services for program completers; remedial services; resume preparation assistance; skills, simulation, or other laboratory; tutoring; unpaid internships.
Library Facilities 557,505 volumes (16,810 in health, 2,035 in nursing); 25,747 periodical subscriptions (495 health-care related).

BACCALAUREATE PROGRAMS

Degree BS
Available Programs Generic Baccalaureate; RN Baccalaureate.
Study Options Full-time.
Program Entrance Requirements Minimum overall college GPA of 2.75, transcript of college record, health exam, 2 years high school math, 2 years high school science, high school transcript, immunizations, minimum high school GPA of 3.0, minimum high school rank 75%, minimum GPA in nursing prerequisites of 2.75. Transfer students are accepted. *Application deadline:* 5/1 (fall), 1/1 (winter), 1/1 (spring). Applications may be processed on a rolling basis for some programs. *Application fee:* $100.
Advanced Placement Credit by examination available. Credit given for nursing courses completed elsewhere dependent upon specific evaluations.
Expenses (2010-11) *Tuition, area resident:* full-time $14,436. *Tuition, state resident:* full-time $17,456. *Tuition, nonresident:* full-time $23,260. *Room and board:* $2600; room only: $1400 per academic year. *Required fees:* full-time $2048.
Financial Aid 75% of baccalaureate students in nursing programs received some form of financial aid in 2009-10.
Contact Dr. Laura Waters, Chairperson/Assistant Professor, Department of Nursing, East Stroudsburg University of Pennsylvania, 200 Prospect Street, East Stroudsburg, PA 18301-2999. *Telephone:* 570-422-3569. *Fax:* 570-422-3848. *E-mail:* lwaters@po-box.esu.edu.

Edinboro University of Pennsylvania
Department of Nursing
Edinboro, Pennsylvania

http://www.edinboro.edu/cwis/nursing/nursing.html
Founded in 1857

DEGREE • BS
Nursing Program Faculty 23 (49% with doctorates).
Baccalaureate Enrollment 330 **Women** 83.6% **Men** 16.4% **Minority** 7.5% **International** 3.9% **Part-time** 8.7%
Distance Learning Courses Available.
Nursing Student Activities Sigma Theta Tau, Student Nurses' Association, nursing club.
Nursing Student Resources Academic advising; academic or career counseling; assistance for students with disabilities; bookstore; campus computer network; career placement assistance; computer lab; computer-assisted instruction; e-mail services; employment services for current students; housing assistance; interactive nursing skills videos; Internet; learning resource lab; library services; nursing audiovisuals; remedial services; resume preparation assistance; skills, simulation, or other laboratory; tutoring.
Library Facilities 496,628 volumes (500,000 in health, 100 in nursing); 1,290 periodical subscriptions (105 health-care related).

BACCALAUREATE PROGRAMS

Degree BS
Available Programs ADN to Baccalaureate; Accelerated Baccalaureate; Accelerated Baccalaureate for Second Degree; Baccalaureate for Second Degree; Generic Baccalaureate; International Nurse to Baccalaureate.
Site Options Erie, PA.
Study Options Full-time and part-time.
Program Entrance Requirements Minimum overall college GPA of 2.75, transcript of college record, CPR certification, health exam, high school biology, high school chemistry, 2 years high school math, 2 years high school science, high school transcript, immunizations, minimum high school rank 40%, minimum GPA in nursing prerequisites of 2.75, professional liability insurance/malpractice insurance, prerequisite course work. *Application deadline:* Applications may be processed on a rolling basis for some programs. *Application fee:* $25.
Advanced Placement Credit by examination available.
Expenses (2010-11) *Tuition, state resident:* full-time $5804; part-time $242 per credit. *Tuition, nonresident:* full-time $8706; part-time $363 per credit. *International tuition:* $10,748 full-time. *Room and board:* $9840; room only: $7200 per academic year. *Required fees:* full-time $1925; part-time $101 per credit.
Financial Aid 75% of baccalaureate students in nursing programs received some form of financial aid in 2009-10.
Contact Mrs. Patricia Louise Nosel, Chairperson, Department of Nursing, Edinboro University of Pennsylvania, 215 Scotland Drive, Room 124, Edinboro, PA 16444. *Telephone:* 814-732-1127 Ext. 2900. *Fax:* 814-732-2536. *E-mail:* nosel@edinboro.edu.

Gannon University
Villa Maria School of Nursing
Erie, Pennsylvania

http://www.gannon.edu/
Founded in 1925

DEGREES • BSN • MSN
Nursing Program Faculty 15 (20% with doctorates).
Baccalaureate Enrollment 300 **Women** 88% **Men** 12% **Minority** 4% **International** 3% **Part-time** 5%
Graduate Enrollment 97 **Women** 68% **Men** 32% **Minority** 6% **Part-time** 38%
Distance Learning Courses Available.
Nursing Student Activities Nursing Honor Society, Sigma Theta Tau, nursing club.
Nursing Student Resources Academic advising; academic or career counseling; assistance for students with disabilities; bookstore; campus computer network; career placement assistance; computer lab; computer-assisted instruction; e-mail services; employment services for current students; externships; housing assistance; interactive nursing skills videos; Internet; learning resource lab; library services; nursing audiovisuals; other; paid internships; placement services for program completers; remedial services; resume preparation assistance; skills, simulation, or other laboratory; tutoring; unpaid internships.
Library Facilities 263,600 volumes (14,000 in health, 2,000 in nursing); 39,737 periodical subscriptions (3,000 health-care related).

BACCALAUREATE PROGRAMS

Degree BSN
Available Programs ADN to Baccalaureate; Accelerated Baccalaureate for Second Degree; Baccalaureate for Second Degree; Generic Baccalaureate; International Nurse to Baccalaureate; LPN to RN Baccalaureate; RN Baccalaureate.
Study Options Full-time and part-time.
Program Entrance Requirements Minimum overall college GPA of 2.8, transcript of college record, CPR certification, written essay, health exam, health insurance, high school biology, high school chemistry, 3 years high school math, 3 years high school science, high school transcript, immunizations, 1 letter of recommendation, minimum high school GPA of 2.5, minimum high school rank 40%, minimum GPA in nursing prerequisites of 2.8. Transfer students are accepted. *Application deadline:* Applications may be processed on a rolling basis for some programs. *Application fee:* $25.
Advanced Placement Credit by examination available.
Expenses (2010-11) *Tuition:* full-time $12,475; part-time $750 per credit. *Room and board:* $8000; room only: $6500 per academic year. *Required fees:* full-time $500; part-time $40 per credit.
Financial Aid 40% of baccalaureate students in nursing programs received some form of financial aid in 2009-10. *Gift aid (need-based):* Federal Pell, FSEOG, state, private, college/university gift aid from institutional funds. *Loans:* Federal Nursing Student Loans, Federal Direct (Subsidized and Unsubsidized Stafford PLUS), Perkins. *Work-study:* Federal Work-Study, part-time campus jobs. *Financial aid application deadline (priority):* 3/15.
Contact Ms. Patricia Ann Marshall, Director, Undergraduate Programs in Nursing, Villa Maria School of Nursing, Gannon University, 109 University Square, Morosky Academic Center, Erie, PA 16541-0001. *Tele-*

phone: 814-871-5470. *Fax:* 814-871-5662. *E-mail:* marshall001@gannon.edu.

GRADUATE PROGRAMS

Financial Aid 100% of graduate students in nursing programs received some form of financial aid in 2009-10. Scholarships available. *Financial aid application deadline:* 7/1.
Contact Dr. Kathleen Patterson, School and Graduate Program Director, Villa Maria School of Nursing, Gannon University, 109 University Square, Erie, PA 16541-0001. *Telephone:* 814-871-5547. *Fax:* 814-871-5662. *E-mail:* patterso018@gannon.edu.

MASTER'S DEGREE PROGRAM

Degree MSN
Available Programs Accelerated AD/RN to Master's; Accelerated RN to Master's; Master's; RN to Master's.
Concentrations Available Nurse anesthesia; nursing administration. *Nurse practitioner programs in:* family health.
Study Options Full-time and part-time.
Program Entrance Requirements Clinical experience, computer literacy, minimum overall college GPA of 3.0, transcript of college record, CPR certification, written essay, immunizations, interview, 3 letters of recommendation, nursing research course, professional liability insurance/malpractice insurance, prerequisite course work, statistics course, GRE General Test. *Application deadline:* Applications may be processed on a rolling basis for some programs. *Application fee:* $25.
Advanced Placement Credit given for nursing courses completed elsewhere dependent upon specific evaluations.
Degree Requirements 46 total credit hours, thesis or project.

POST-MASTER'S PROGRAM

Areas of Study Nurse anesthesia; nursing administration. *Nurse practitioner programs in:* family health.

Gwynedd-Mercy College

School of Nursing
Gwynedd Valley, Pennsylvania

Founded in 1948

DEGREES • BSN • MSN

Nursing Program Faculty 21 (43% with doctorates).
Baccalaureate Enrollment 85 **Women** 95% **Men** 5% **Minority** 5% **Part-time** 28%
Graduate Enrollment 40 **Women** 85% **Men** 15% **Minority** 10% **International** 5% **Part-time** 80%
Nursing Student Activities Sigma Theta Tau, Student Nurses' Association.
Nursing Student Resources Academic advising; bookstore; campus computer network; computer lab; computer-assisted instruction; daycare for children of students; e-mail services; interactive nursing skills videos; learning resource lab; library services; nursing audiovisuals; resume preparation assistance; skills, simulation, or other laboratory; tutoring.
Library Facilities 105,070 volumes; 667 periodical subscriptions.

BACCALAUREATE PROGRAMS

Degree BSN
Available Programs ADN to Baccalaureate; Accelerated RN Baccalaureate; RN Baccalaureate.
Site Options Fort Washington, PA.
Study Options Full-time and part-time.
Program Entrance Requirements Minimum overall college GPA of 2.8, transcript of college record, CPR certification, health exam, health insurance, high school biology, high school chemistry, 2 years high school math, high school transcript, immunizations, letters of recommendation, minimum high school rank 33%, minimum GPA in nursing prerequisites, professional liability insurance/malpractice insurance, RN licensure. Transfer students are accepted.
Advanced Placement Credit by examination available. Credit given for nursing courses completed elsewhere dependent upon specific evaluations.
Contact ***Telephone:*** 215-646-7300 Ext. 425. *Fax:* 215-641-5556 Ext. 528.

GRADUATE PROGRAMS

Contact ***Telephone:*** 215-646-7300 Ext. 407. *Fax:* 215-542-5789.

MASTER'S DEGREE PROGRAM

Degree MSN
Available Programs Master's; RN to Master's.
Concentrations Available *Clinical nurse specialist programs in:* gerontology, oncology, pediatric. *Nurse practitioner programs in:* adult health, pediatric.
Study Options Full-time and part-time.
Program Entrance Requirements Clinical experience, minimum overall college GPA of 3.0, transcript of college record, written essay, immunizations, interview, 2 letters of recommendation, physical assessment course, professional liability insurance/malpractice insurance, statistics course, GRE General Test or MAT.
Advanced Placement Credit by examination available. Credit given for nursing courses completed elsewhere dependent upon specific evaluations.
Degree Requirements 43 total credit hours.

POST-MASTER'S PROGRAM

Areas of Study *Nurse practitioner programs in:* adult health, pediatric.

Holy Family University

School of Nursing and Allied Health Professions
Philadelphia, Pennsylvania

http://www.holyfamily.edu/school_nursing/index.html
Founded in 1954

DEGREES • BSN • MSN

Nursing Program Faculty 40 (28% with doctorates).
Baccalaureate Enrollment 183 **Women** 90% **Men** 10% **Minority** 25%
Graduate Enrollment 27 **Women** 97% **Men** 3% **Part-time** 100%
Nursing Student Activities Sigma Theta Tau, Student Nurses' Association.
Nursing Student Resources Academic advising; academic or career counseling; assistance for students with disabilities; bookstore; campus computer network; career placement assistance; computer lab; computer-assisted instruction; daycare for children of students; e-mail services; interactive nursing skills videos; Internet; learning resource lab; library services; nursing audiovisuals; other; resume preparation assistance; skills, simulation, or other laboratory; tutoring.
Library Facilities 142,800 volumes (8,159 in health, 2,177 in nursing); 12,490 periodical subscriptions (279 health-care related).

BACCALAUREATE PROGRAMS

Degree BSN
Available Programs ADN to Baccalaureate; Accelerated Baccalaureate; Generic Baccalaureate; International Nurse to Baccalaureate; LPN to Baccalaureate; LPN to RN Baccalaureate; RN Baccalaureate.
Site Options Bensalem, PA; Newtown, PA.
Study Options Full-time and part-time.
Program Entrance Requirements Transcript of college record, health exam, high school biology, high school chemistry, high school foreign language, 3 years high school math, 3 years high school science, high school transcript, immunizations, letters of recommendation, minimum high school GPA of 2.5, minimum high school rank 60%, minimum GPA in nursing prerequisites of 2.5. Transfer students are accepted.
Contact ***Telephone:*** 215-637-3050. *Fax:* 215-281-1022.

GRADUATE PROGRAMS

Contact ***Telephone:*** 215-637-7203. *Fax:* 215-637-1478.

MASTER'S DEGREE PROGRAM

Degree MSN
Available Programs Master's.
Concentrations Available Health-care administration; nursing education. *Clinical nurse specialist programs in:* community health.
Site Options Newtown, PA.
Study Options Part-time.
Program Entrance Requirements Transcript of college record, written essay, immunizations, 2 letters of recommendation, nursing research course, professional liability insurance/malpractice insurance, prerequisite course work, resume, statistics course.
Advanced Placement Credit by examination available. Credit given for nursing courses completed elsewhere dependent upon specific evaluations.
Degree Requirements 39 total credit hours, comprehensive exam.

CONTINUING EDUCATION PROGRAM

Contact *Telephone:* 215-637-7700 Ext. 5002. *Fax:* 215-633-0558.

See full description on page 478 and display below.

Immaculata University

Department of Nursing
Immaculata, Pennsylvania

http://www.immaculata.edu/nursing/
Founded in 1920

DEGREES • BSN • MSN

Nursing Program Faculty 80 (50% with doctorates).
Baccalaureate Enrollment 1,125 **Women** 92% **Men** 8% **Minority** 13% **International** 2% **Part-time** 90%
Graduate Enrollment 65 **Women** 97% **Men** 3% **Minority** 15% **Part-time** 100%
Nursing Student Activities Sigma Theta Tau, nursing club.
Nursing Student Resources Academic advising; academic or career counseling; assistance for students with disabilities; bookstore; campus computer network; career placement assistance; computer lab; computer-assisted instruction; e-mail services; employment services for current students; externships; interactive nursing skills videos; Internet; learning resource lab; library services; nursing audiovisuals; placement services for program completers; resume preparation assistance; skills, simulation, or other laboratory; tutoring.
Library Facilities 1,500 volumes in health, 1,500 volumes in nursing; 115 periodical subscriptions health-care related.

BACCALAUREATE PROGRAMS

Degree BSN
Available Programs Accelerated RN Baccalaureate; Generic Baccalaureate.
Site Options Christiana, DE; Abington, PA; Immaculata, PA.
Study Options Full-time.
Program Entrance Requirements Transcript of college record, CPR certification, written essay, health exam, high school chemistry, high school foreign language, 2 years high school math, 3 years high school science, high school transcript, immunizations, interview, 2 letters of recommendation, minimum high school GPA of 3.0, prerequisite course work. Transfer students are accepted. *Application deadline:* 1/17 (fall). *Application fee:* $35.
Expenses (2010-11) *Tuition:* full-time $27,870. *Room and board:* $8000; room only: $5220 per academic year.
Financial Aid 50% of baccalaureate students in nursing programs received some form of financial aid in 2009-10.
Contact Ms. Tina Floyd, ACCEL Counselor, Department of Nursing, Immaculata University, 1145 King Road, Immaculata, PA 19345. *Telephone:* 610-647-4400 Ext. 3448. *Fax:* 610-251-1668. *E-mail:* accel@immaculata.edu.

GRADUATE PROGRAMS

Expenses (2010-11) *Tuition:* part-time $585 per credit. *Required fees:* part-time $100 per term.
Financial Aid 25% of graduate students in nursing programs received some form of financial aid in 2009-10.
Contact Dr. Jane Tang, Coordinator, MSN Program, Department of Nursing, Immaculata University, 1145 King Road, Immaculata, PA 19345-0691. *Telephone:* 610-647-4400 Ext. 3309. *Fax:* 610-640-0286. *E-mail:* jtang@immaculata.edu.

MASTER'S DEGREE PROGRAM

Degree MSN
Available Programs Master's; Master's for Non-Nursing College Graduates.
Concentrations Available Nursing administration; nursing education.
Study Options Part-time.
Program Entrance Requirements Minimum overall college GPA of 3.0, transcript of college record, written essay, interview, 3 letters of recommendation, physical assessment course, statistics course. *Application deadline:* Applications may be processed on a rolling basis for some programs. *Application fee:* $50.
Advanced Placement Credit given for nursing courses completed elsewhere dependent upon specific evaluations.
Degree Requirements 39 total credit hours, thesis or project.

Indiana University of Pennsylvania

Department of Nursing and Allied Health
Indiana, Pennsylvania

http://www.hhs.iup.edu/nahp/
Founded in 1875

DEGREES • BSN • MS • PHD

Nursing Program Faculty 40 (40% with doctorates).
Baccalaureate Enrollment 580 **Women** 89% **Men** 11% **Minority** 9% **International** 7%
Graduate Enrollment 56 **Women** 97% **Men** 3% **Minority** 5% **Part-time** 100%
Nursing Student Activities Nursing Honor Society, Sigma Theta Tau, Student Nurses' Association, nursing club.
Nursing Student Resources Academic advising; academic or career counseling; assistance for students with disabilities; bookstore; campus computer network; career placement assistance; computer lab; computer-assisted instruction; e-mail services; employment services for current students; housing assistance; interactive nursing skills videos; Internet; learning resource lab; library services; nursing audiovisuals; remedial services; resume preparation assistance; skills, simulation, or other laboratory; tutoring.
Library Facilities 875,888 volumes (5,758 in health, 3,395 in nursing); 23,425 periodical subscriptions (225 health-care related).

BACCALAUREATE PROGRAMS

Degree BSN
Available Programs Baccalaureate for Second Degree; Generic Baccalaureate; LPN to Baccalaureate; RN Baccalaureate.
Site Options Slate Lick, PA.
Study Options Full-time and part-time.
Program Entrance Requirements Minimum overall college GPA of 2.5, transcript of college record, CPR certification, health exam, 2 years high school math, high school transcript, immunizations, minimum high school GPA of 3.0, professional liability insurance/malpractice insurance, prerequisite course work. Transfer students are accepted. *Application deadline:* Applications may be processed on a rolling basis for some programs. *Application fee:* $40.
Expenses (2010-11) *Tuition, state resident:* full-time $5804; part-time $242 per credit. *Tuition, nonresident:* full-time $14,510; part-time $605 per credit. *Room and board:* $6450 per academic year. *Required fees:* full-time $1767; part-time $286 per term.
Financial Aid 92% of baccalaureate students in nursing programs received some form of financial aid in 2009-10.
Contact Mr. Mike Husenits, Director of Admissions, Department of Nursing and Allied Health, Indiana University of Pennsylvania, 117 Sutton Hall, Indiana, PA 15705. *E-mail:* admissions-inquiry@iup.edu.

GRADUATE PROGRAMS

Expenses (2010-11) *Tuition, state resident:* full-time $6966; part-time $387 per credit. *Tuition, nonresident:* full-time $11,146; part-time $619 per credit. *International tuition:* $11,146 full-time. *Required fees:* full-time $1118; part-time $58 per credit; part-time $153 per term.
Financial Aid 29% of graduate students in nursing programs received some form of financial aid in 2009-10. 4 fellowships (averaging $875 per year), 5 research assistantships with full and partial tuition reimbursements available (averaging $2,190 per year), 2 teaching assistantships (averaging $16,153 per year) were awarded; Federal Work-Study also available. Aid available to part-time students. *Financial aid application deadline:* 3/15.
Contact Dr. Elizabeth A. Palmer, Department Chair, Department of Nursing and Allied Health, Indiana University of Pennsylvania, 1010 Oakland Avenue, Indiana, PA 15705-1087. *Telephone:* 724-357-2557. *Fax:* 724-357-3267. *E-mail:* lpalmer@iup.edu.

MASTER'S DEGREE PROGRAM

Degree MS
Available Programs Master's; Master's for Nurses with Non-Nursing Degrees.
Concentrations Available Nursing administration; nursing education.
Site Options Monroeville, PA; Slate Lick, PA; Johnstown, PA.
Study Options Part-time.
Program Entrance Requirements Clinical experience, computer literacy, minimum overall college GPA of 3.0, transcript of college record, written essay, 2 letters of recommendation, nursing research course, professional liability insurance/malpractice insurance, resume, statistics course. *Application deadline:* Applications may be processed on a rolling basis for some programs. *Application fee:* $40.
Advanced Placement Credit given for nursing courses completed elsewhere dependent upon specific evaluations.
Degree Requirements 36 total credit hours, thesis or project.

DOCTORAL DEGREE PROGRAM

Degree PhD
Available Programs Doctorate.
Areas of Study Nursing education.
Program Entrance Requirements Minimum overall college GPA of 3.5, interview by faculty committee, 2 letters of recommendation, MSN or equivalent, statistics course, vita, writing sample. Application deadline: Applications may be processed on a rolling basis for some programs. Application fee: $40.
Degree Requirements 60 total credit hours, dissertation, oral exam, written exam, residency.

La Roche College

Department of Nursing and Nursing Management
Pittsburgh, Pennsylvania

http://www.laroche.edu
Founded in 1963

DEGREES • BSN • MSN

Nursing Program Faculty 11 (45% with doctorates).
Baccalaureate Enrollment 46 **Women** 89% **Men** 11% **International** 17% **Part-time** 74%
Graduate Enrollment 18 **Women** 83% **Men** 17% **International** 5% **Part-time** 94%
Distance Learning Courses Available.
Nursing Student Activities Sigma Theta Tau.
Nursing Student Resources Academic advising; academic or career counseling; assistance for students with disabilities; bookstore; campus computer network; computer lab; e-mail services; externships; Internet; library services; resume preparation assistance; tutoring.
Library Facilities 122,642 volumes; 582 periodical subscriptions (713 health-care related).

BACCALAUREATE PROGRAMS

Degree BSN
Available Programs Accelerated RN Baccalaureate; RN Baccalaureate.
Site Options Pittsburgh, PA.
Study Options Full-time and part-time.
Program Entrance Requirements Minimum overall college GPA of 2.5, transcript of college record, high school transcript, 2 letters of recommendation, professional liability insurance/malpractice insurance, prerequisite course work, RN licensure. Transfer students are accepted. *Application deadline:* Applications may be processed on a rolling basis for some programs. *Application fee:* $50.
Advanced Placement Credit by examination available. Credit given for nursing courses completed elsewhere dependent upon specific evaluations.
Expenses (2009-10) *Tuition:* full-time $10,370; part-time $525 per credit. *International tuition:* $10,370 full-time. *Room and board:* $4000; room only: $2742 per academic year. *Required fees:* full-time $400; part-time $9 per credit.
Financial Aid 87% of baccalaureate students in nursing programs received some form of financial aid in 2008-09. *Gift aid (need-based):* Federal Pell, FSEOG, state, private, college/university gift aid from institutional funds. *Loans:* Federal Direct (Subsidized and Unsubsidized Stafford PLUS), Perkins, state. *Work-study:* Federal Work-Study. *Financial aid application deadline (priority):* 5/1.
Contact Ms. Hope A. Schiffgens, Director, Graduate Studies and Adult Education, Department of Nursing and Nursing Management, La Roche College, 9000 Babcock Boulevard, Pittsburgh, PA 15237. *Telephone:* 412-536-1266. *Fax:* 412-536-1283. *E-mail:* hope.schiffgens@laroche.edu.

GRADUATE PROGRAMS

Expenses (2009-10) *Tuition:* part-time $525 per credit hour. *International tuition:* $525 full-time. *Room and board:* $4000; room only:

$2742 per academic year. *Required fees:* full-time $200; part-time $9 per credit; part-time $9 per term.
Financial Aid 85% of graduate students in nursing programs received some form of financial aid in 2008-09.
Contact Ms. Hope A. Schiffgens, Director, Graduate Studies and Adult Education, Department of Nursing and Nursing Management, La Roche College, 9000 Babcock Boulevard, Pittsburgh, PA 15237. *Telephone:* 412-536-1262. *Fax:* 412-536-1283. *E-mail:* hope.schiffgens@laroche.edu.

MASTER'S DEGREE PROGRAM

Degree MSN
Available Programs Master's; RN to Master's.
Concentrations Available Health-care administration; nursing administration; nursing education. *Clinical nurse specialist programs in:* community health. *Nurse practitioner programs in:* school health.
Study Options Full-time and part-time.
Online Degree Options Yes (online only).
Program Entrance Requirements Clinical experience, minimum overall college GPA of 3.0, transcript of college record, immunizations, interview, 2 letters of recommendation, professional liability insurance/malpractice insurance, resume. *Application deadline:* Applications may be processed on a rolling basis for some programs. *Application fee:* $50.
Advanced Placement Credit given for nursing courses completed elsewhere dependent upon specific evaluations.
Degree Requirements 41 total credit hours.

CONTINUING EDUCATION PROGRAM

Contact Ms. Hope A. Schiffgens, Director, Graduate Studies and Adult Education, Department of Nursing and Nursing Management, La Roche College, 9000 Babcock Boulevard, Pittsburgh, PA 15237. *Telephone:* 412-536-1262. *Fax:* 412-536-1283. *E-mail:* hope.schiffgens@laroche.edu.

La Salle University

School of Nursing and Health Sciences
Philadelphia, Pennsylvania

http://www.lasalle.edu/academ/nursing
Founded in 1863

DEGREES • BSN • MSN • MSN/MBA

Nursing Program Faculty 45 (32% with doctorates).
Nursing Student Activities Sigma Theta Tau, Student Nurses' Association, nursing club.
Nursing Student Resources Academic advising; academic or career counseling; assistance for students with disabilities; bookstore; campus computer network; career placement assistance; computer lab; computer-assisted instruction; e-mail services; employment services for current students; externships; housing assistance; interactive nursing skills videos; Internet; learning resource lab; library services; nursing audiovisuals; placement services for program completers; remedial services; resume preparation assistance; skills, simulation, or other laboratory; tutoring.
Library Facilities 400,000 volumes (8,350 in nursing); 9,250 periodical subscriptions (310 health-care related).

BACCALAUREATE PROGRAMS

Degree BSN
Available Programs Baccalaureate for Second Degree; Generic Baccalaureate; LPN to Baccalaureate; RN Baccalaureate.
Site Options Newtown, PA.
Study Options Full-time and part-time.
Program Entrance Requirements Minimum overall college GPA of 2.75, transcript of college record, CPR certification, written essay, health exam, health insurance, high school biology, high school chemistry, 3 years high school math, 3 years high school science, high school transcript, immunizations, interview, 2 letters of recommendation, minimum high school GPA of 3.0, minimum high school rank 25%, minimum GPA in nursing prerequisites of 2.75, professional liability insurance/malpractice insurance, prerequisite course work. Transfer students are accepted.
Advanced Placement Credit by examination available. Credit given for nursing courses completed elsewhere dependent upon specific evaluations.
Contact *Telephone:* 215-951-1430. *Fax:* 215-951-1896.

GRADUATE PROGRAMS

Contact *Telephone:* 215-951-1413. *Fax:* 215-951-1896.

MASTER'S DEGREE PROGRAM

Degrees MSN; MSN/MBA
Available Programs Master's; RN to Master's.
Concentrations Available Nurse anesthesia; nursing administration. *Clinical nurse specialist programs in:* adult health, public health. *Nurse practitioner programs in:* adult health, family health.
Site Options Newtown, PA.
Study Options Full-time and part-time.
Program Entrance Requirements Clinical experience, minimum overall college GPA of 3.0, transcript of college record, CPR certification, written essay, immunizations, interview, 2 letters of recommendation, nursing research course, physical assessment course, professional liability insurance/malpractice insurance, resume, statistics course.
Advanced Placement Credit given for nursing courses completed elsewhere dependent upon specific evaluations.
Degree Requirements 41 total credit hours.

POST-MASTER'S PROGRAM

Areas of Study Nurse anesthesia; nursing administration; nursing education. *Clinical nurse specialist programs in:* adult health, public health. *Nurse practitioner programs in:* adult health, family health.

CONTINUING EDUCATION PROGRAM

Contact *Telephone:* 215-951-1432. *Fax:* 215-951-1896.

Mansfield University of Pennsylvania

Department of Health Sciences–Nursing
Mansfield, Pennsylvania

http://www.mansfield.edu/
Founded in 1857

DEGREES • BSN • MSN

Nursing Program Faculty 12 (50% with doctorates).
Baccalaureate Enrollment 186 **Women** 95% **Men** 5% **Minority** 4% **International** 1% **Part-time** 5%
Graduate Enrollment 52 **Women** 98% **Men** 2% **Minority** 1% **Part-time** 100%
Distance Learning Courses Available.
Nursing Student Activities Nursing Honor Society, Student Nurses' Association, nursing club.
Nursing Student Resources Academic advising; academic or career counseling; assistance for students with disabilities; bookstore; campus computer network; career placement assistance; computer lab; daycare for children of students; e-mail services; employment services for current students; housing assistance; Internet; learning resource lab; library services; nursing audiovisuals; remedial services; resume preparation assistance; skills, simulation, or other laboratory; tutoring.
Library Facilities 249,874 volumes (1,300 in health, 500 in nursing); 631 periodical subscriptions (550 health-care related).

BACCALAUREATE PROGRAMS

Degree BSN
Available Programs Generic Baccalaureate; RN Baccalaureate.
Site Options Sayre, PA.
Study Options Full-time and part-time.
Program Entrance Requirements Minimum overall college GPA of 2.7, transcript of college record, CPR certification, health exam, health insurance, high school biology, high school chemistry, 2 years high school math, 2 years high school science, high school transcript, immunizations, minimum high school GPA of 2.7, minimum high school rank 60%, professional liability insurance/malpractice insurance. Transfer students are accepted. *Application deadline:* Applications may be processed on a rolling basis for some programs. *Application fee:* $25.
Advanced Placement Credit by examination available. Credit given for nursing courses completed elsewhere dependent upon specific evaluations.
Expenses (2010-11) *Room and board:* $7276; room only: $2906 per academic year. *Required fees:* full-time $5804; part-time $233 per credit; part-time $2902 per term.

Financial Aid 90% of baccalaureate students in nursing programs received some form of financial aid in 2009-10.

Contact Admissions Office, Department of Health Sciences–Nursing, Mansfield University of Pennsylvania, Alumni Hall, Mansfield, PA 16933. *Telephone:* 570-662-4243. *Fax:* 570-662-4121. *E-mail:* admissions@mansfield.edu.

GRADUATE PROGRAMS

Expenses (2010-11) *Tuition, state resident:* full-time $3483; part-time $387 per credit. *Tuition, nonresident:* full-time $5573; part-time $619 per credit. *Required fees:* full-time $1206; part-time $54 per credit.

Financial Aid 50% of graduate students in nursing programs received some form of financial aid in 2009-10.

Contact Dr. Janeen Bartlett Sheehe, Department Chair and Nursing Program Director, Department of Health Sciences–Nursing, Mansfield University of Pennsylvania, 212C Elliott Hall, Mansfield, PA 16933. *Telephone:* 570-662-4522. *Fax:* 570-662-4137. *E-mail:* jsheehe@mansfield.edu.

MASTER'S DEGREE PROGRAM

Degree MSN

Available Programs Master's.

Concentrations Available Nursing administration; nursing education.

Study Options Part-time.

Online Degree Options Yes (online only).

Program Entrance Requirements Minimum overall college GPA of 3.0, transcript of college record, 1 letter of recommendation, nursing research course, prerequisite course work. *Application deadline:* Applications may be processed on a rolling basis for some programs. *Application fee:* $25.

Advanced Placement Credit given for nursing courses completed elsewhere dependent upon specific evaluations.

Degree Requirements 33 total credit hours, thesis or project.

Marywood University

Department of Nursing
Scranton, Pennsylvania

http://www.marywood.edu/uscat/nurs.htm

Founded in 1915

DEGREES • BSN • MSN • MSN/MPH

Nursing Program Faculty 16 (50% with doctorates).

Baccalaureate Enrollment 117 **Women** 90% **Men** 10% **Minority** 5% **International** 3% **Part-time** 5%

Graduate Enrollment 17 **Women** 100% **Part-time** 90%

Distance Learning Courses Available.

Nursing Student Activities Sigma Theta Tau, Student Nurses' Association.

Nursing Student Resources Academic advising; academic or career counseling; assistance for students with disabilities; bookstore; campus computer network; computer lab; daycare for children of students; e-mail services; employment services for current students; interactive nursing skills videos; Internet; learning resource lab; library services; nursing audiovisuals; skills, simulation, or other laboratory; tutoring.

Library Facilities 220,998 volumes (7,400 in health, 3,006 in nursing); 17,923 periodical subscriptions (750 health-care related).

BACCALAUREATE PROGRAMS

Degree BSN

Available Programs ADN to Baccalaureate; Generic Baccalaureate; International Nurse to Baccalaureate; LPN to Baccalaureate; RN Baccalaureate.

Study Options Full-time and part-time.

Program Entrance Requirements Transcript of college record, high school biology, high school chemistry, 1 year of high school math, high school transcript, 1 letter of recommendation. Transfer students are accepted.

Advanced Placement Credit given for nursing courses completed elsewhere dependent upon specific evaluations.

Contact ***Telephone:*** 570-348-6211 Ext. 2374. *Fax:* 570-961-4761.

GRADUATE PROGRAMS

Contact ***Telephone:*** 570-348-6211 Ext. 2475. *Fax:* 570-961-4761.

MASTER'S DEGREE PROGRAM

Degrees MSN; MSN/MPH

Available Programs Master's.

Concentrations Available Nursing administration.

Study Options Full-time and part-time.

Program Entrance Requirements Clinical experience, minimum overall college GPA of 3.0, transcript of college record, written essay, 2 letters of recommendation, nursing research course, physical assessment course, statistics course.

Degree Requirements 39 total credit hours, thesis or project.

CONTINUING EDUCATION PROGRAM

Contact ***Telephone:*** 570-340-6060. *Fax:* 570-961-4776.

Messiah College

Department of Nursing
Grantham, Pennsylvania

http://www.messiah.edu/

Founded in 1909

DEGREE • BSN

Nursing Program Faculty 23 (26% with doctorates).

Baccalaureate Enrollment 241 **Women** 95% **Men** 5% **Minority** 13% **International** 1% **Part-time** 1%

Distance Learning Courses Available.

Nursing Student Activities Nursing Honor Society, Sigma Theta Tau, Student Nurses' Association.

Nursing Student Resources Academic advising; academic or career counseling; assistance for students with disabilities; bookstore; campus computer network; career placement assistance; computer lab; computer-assisted instruction; e-mail services; employment services for current students; interactive nursing skills videos; Internet; learning resource lab; library services; nursing audiovisuals; remedial services; resume preparation assistance; skills, simulation, or other laboratory; tutoring.

Library Facilities 289,053 volumes (7,589 in health, 549 in nursing); 48,840 periodical subscriptions (4,530 health-care related).

BACCALAUREATE PROGRAMS

Degree BSN

Available Programs Generic Baccalaureate.

Study Options Full-time and part-time.

Program Entrance Requirements Minimum overall college GPA of 2.8, transcript of college record, CPR certification, health exam, health insurance, high school foreign language, 2 years high school math, 2 years high school science, high school transcript, immunizations, minimum GPA in nursing prerequisites of 2.5, prerequisite course work. Transfer students are accepted. *Application deadline:* Applications may be processed on a rolling basis for some programs. *Application fee:* $30.

Advanced Placement Credit given for nursing courses completed elsewhere dependent upon specific evaluations.

Expenses (2010-11) *Tuition:* full-time $26,680; part-time $1115 per credit hour. *Room and board:* $8160; room only: $4320 per academic year. *Required fees:* full-time $440.

Financial Aid 100% of baccalaureate students in nursing programs received some form of financial aid in 2009-10. *Gift aid (need-based):* Federal Pell, FSEOG, state, private, college/university gift aid from institutional funds. *Loans:* Federal Nursing Student Loans, Federal Direct (Subsidized and Unsubsidized Stafford PLUS), Perkins. *Work-study:* Federal Work-Study, part-time campus jobs. *Financial aid application deadline (priority):* 4/1.

Contact Dana Britton, Director of Admissions, Department of Nursing, Messiah College, PO Box 3005, One College Avenue, Grantham, PA 17027. *Telephone:* 800-233-4220. *Fax:* 717-796-5374. *E-mail:* admiss@messiah.edu.

Millersville University of Pennsylvania

Department of Nursing
Millersville, Pennsylvania

http://muweb.millersville.edu/~nursing/
Founded in 1855

DEGREES • BSN • MSN

Nursing Program Faculty 5 (100% with doctorates).
Baccalaureate Enrollment 40 **Women** 95% **Men** 5% **Minority** 18% **Part-time** 80%
Graduate Enrollment 45 **Women** 86% **Men** 14% **Minority** 3% **Part-time** 100%
Nursing Student Activities Sigma Theta Tau.
Nursing Student Resources Academic advising; academic or career counseling; assistance for students with disabilities; bookstore; computer lab; e-mail services; interactive nursing skills videos; Internet; library services; nursing audiovisuals.
Library Facilities 603,224 volumes; 16,712 periodical subscriptions (82 health-care related).

BACCALAUREATE PROGRAMS

Degree BSN
Available Programs RN Baccalaureate.
Study Options Full-time and part-time.
Program Entrance Requirements Transcript of college record, CPR certification, health exam, immunizations, professional liability insurance/malpractice insurance, RN licensure. Transfer students are accepted.
Financial Aid 50% of baccalaureate students in nursing programs received some form of financial aid in 2009-10. *Gift aid (need-based):* Federal Pell, FSEOG, state, private, college/university gift aid from institutional funds, Schock Scholarships. *Loans:* Perkins. *Work-study:* Federal Work-Study, part-time campus jobs. *Financial aid application deadline (priority):* 3/15.
Contact Dr. Barbara Zimmerman, Chairperson, Department of Nursing, Millersville University of Pennsylvania, Caputo Hall, PO Box 1002, Millersville, PA 17551-0302. *Telephone:* 717-872-3376. *Fax:* 717-871-4877. *E-mail:* barbara.zimmerman@millersville.edu.

GRADUATE PROGRAMS

Financial Aid 5% of graduate students in nursing programs received some form of financial aid in 2009-10. 3 research assistantships with partial tuition reimbursements available (averaging $1,578 per year) were awarded; institutionally sponsored loans and unspecified assistantships also available. Aid available to part-time students. *Financial aid application deadline:* 3/15.
Contact Dr. Deborah Castellucci, Graduate Program Coordinator, Department of Nursing, Millersville University of Pennsylvania, Caputo Hall, PO Box 1002, Millersville, PA 17551-0302. *Telephone:* 717-871-5341. *Fax:* 717-871-4887. *E-mail:* deborah.castellucci@millersville.edu.

MASTER'S DEGREE PROGRAM

Degree MSN
Available Programs Master's.
Concentrations Available Nursing education. *Nurse practitioner programs in:* family health.
Program Entrance Requirements Clinical experience, minimum overall college GPA of 3.0, transcript of college record, interview, 3 letters of recommendation, nursing research course, physical assessment course, resume, statistics course.
Degree Requirements 42 total credit hours, thesis or project.

POST-MASTER'S PROGRAM

Areas of Study Nursing education. *Nurse practitioner programs in:* family health.

CONTINUING EDUCATION PROGRAM

Contact Ms. Bili Mattes, Director, Professional Training and Education, Department of Nursing, Millersville University of Pennsylvania, Office of Professional Training and Education, PO Box 1002, Millersville, PA 17551-0302. *Telephone:* 717-872-3030. *Fax:* 717-871-2022. *E-mail:* bili.mattes@millersville.edu.

Misericordia University

Department of Nursing
Dallas, Pennsylvania

http://www.misericordia.edu/nursing
Founded in 1924

DEGREES • BSN • MSN

Nursing Program Faculty 35 (4% with doctorates).
Baccalaureate Enrollment 273 **Women** 85% **Men** 15% **Minority** 3% **Part-time** 30%
Graduate Enrollment 65 **Women** 94% **Men** 6% **Minority** 1% **Part-time** 100%
Distance Learning Courses Available.
Nursing Student Activities Nursing Honor Society, Sigma Theta Tau, Student Nurses' Association, nursing club.
Nursing Student Resources Academic advising; academic or career counseling; assistance for students with disabilities; bookstore; campus computer network; career placement assistance; computer lab; computer-assisted instruction; e-mail services; employment services for current students; externships; housing assistance; interactive nursing skills videos; Internet; learning resource lab; library services; nursing audiovisuals; placement services for program completers; remedial services; resume preparation assistance; skills, simulation, or other laboratory; tutoring.
Library Facilities 79,503 volumes (5 in health, 5 in nursing); 355 periodical subscriptions (15 health-care related).

BACCALAUREATE PROGRAMS

Degree BSN
Available Programs Accelerated RN Baccalaureate; Baccalaureate for Second Degree; Generic Baccalaureate; RN Baccalaureate.
Site Options Nanticoke , PA; Shamokin, PA.
Study Options Full-time and part-time.
Program Entrance Requirements Minimum overall college GPA of 3.0, transcript of college record, CPR certification, health exam, health insurance, high school biology, high school chemistry, 1 year of high school math, high school transcript, immunizations, letters of recommendation, minimum high school GPA of 2.5, minimum high school rank, minimum GPA in nursing prerequisites of 3.0, professional liability insurance/malpractice insurance. Transfer students are accepted. *Application deadline:* Applications may be processed on a rolling basis for some programs. *Application fee:* $200.
Advanced Placement Credit by examination available. Credit given for nursing courses completed elsewhere dependent upon specific evaluations.
Expenses (2010-11) *Tuition:* full-time $11,875; part-time $450 per credit. *Room and board:* $5145; room only: $3020 per academic year. *Required fees:* full-time $620; part-time $200 per credit.
Financial Aid 75% of baccalaureate students in nursing programs received some form of financial aid in 2009-10. *Gift aid (need-based):* Federal Pell, FSEOG, state, private, college/university gift aid from institutional funds, Federal Nursing. *Loans:* Federal Nursing Student Loans, Perkins, state. *Work-study:* Federal Work-Study. *Financial aid application deadline (priority):* 3/1.
Contact Mr. Glenn Bozinski, Admissions, Department of Nursing, Misericordia University, 301 Lake Street, Dallas, PA 18612. *Telephone:* 570-674-6434. *E-mail:* gbozinsk@misericordia.edu.

GRADUATE PROGRAMS

Financial Aid 90% of graduate students in nursing programs received some form of financial aid in 2009-10. Teaching assistantships, career-related internships or fieldwork, scholarships, traineeships, tuition waivers (partial), and unspecified assistantships available. Aid available to part-time students. *Financial aid application deadline:* 6/30.
Contact Miss Larree Brown, Adult Education Counselor, Graduate Programs, Department of Nursing, Misericordia University, 301 Lake Street, Dallas, PA 18612. *Telephone:* 570-674-6451. *Fax:* 570-674-8902. *E-mail:* lbrown@misericordia.edu.

MASTER'S DEGREE PROGRAM

Degree MSN
Available Programs Master's; RN to Master's.
Concentrations Available Nursing education. *Nurse practitioner programs in:* family health.
Study Options Part-time.
Program Entrance Requirements Clinical experience, computer literacy, minimum overall college GPA of 3.0, transcript of college record, written essay, 3 letters of recommendation, nursing research course,

physical assessment course, professional liability insurance/malpractice insurance, statistics course, GRE General Test or MAT (minimum 35th percentile). *Application deadline:* Applications may be processed on a rolling basis for some programs. *Application fee:* $200.
Advanced Placement Credit given for nursing courses completed elsewhere dependent upon specific evaluations.
Degree Requirements 45 total credit hours, thesis or project.

POST-MASTER'S PROGRAM

Areas of Study Nursing education. *Nurse practitioner programs in:* family health.

Moravian College

St. Luke's School of Nursing
Bethlehem, Pennsylvania

http://www.moravian.edu/academics/departments/nursing
Founded in 1742

DEGREES • BS • MS

Nursing Program Faculty 29 (34% with doctorates).
Baccalaureate Enrollment 238 **Women** 95% **Men** 5% **Minority** 3% **International** 1% **Part-time** 40%
Graduate Enrollment 49 **Women** 97% **Men** 3% **Minority** 4% **Part-time** 100%
Nursing Student Activities Sigma Theta Tau, Student Nurses' Association.
Nursing Student Resources Academic advising; academic or career counseling; assistance for students with disabilities; bookstore; campus computer network; career placement assistance; computer lab; computer-assisted instruction; e-mail services; employment services for current students; externships; housing assistance; interactive nursing skills videos; Internet; learning resource lab; library services; nursing audiovisuals; placement services for program completers; remedial services; resume preparation assistance; skills, simulation, or other laboratory; tutoring.
Library Facilities 249,308 volumes (4,600 in health, 1,900 in nursing); 22,946 periodical subscriptions (275 health-care related).

BACCALAUREATE PROGRAMS

Degree BS
Available Programs Generic Baccalaureate; RN Baccalaureate.
Study Options Full-time.
Program Entrance Requirements CPR certification, written essay, health exam, health insurance, high school biology, high school foreign language, 3 years high school math, 3 years high school science, high school transcript, immunizations, minimum GPA in nursing prerequisites of 2.7, prerequisite course work. Transfer students are accepted. *Application deadline:* 3/1 (fall).
Advanced Placement Credit by examination available. Credit given for nursing courses completed elsewhere dependent upon specific evaluations.
Expenses (2010-11) *Tuition:* full-time $31,662. *Room and board:* $5314 per academic year. *Required fees:* full-time $515.
Financial Aid 90% of baccalaureate students in nursing programs received some form of financial aid in 2009-10. *Gift aid (need-based):* Federal Pell, FSEOG, state, private, college/university gift aid from institutional funds. *Loans:* Perkins. *Work-study:* Federal Work-Study, part-time campus jobs. *Financial aid application deadline (priority):* 2/14.
Contact Mr. Bernard J. Story, Dean of Admissions, St. Luke's School of Nursing, Moravian College, 1200 Main Street, Bethlehem, PA 18018. *Telephone:* 800-441-3191. *E-mail:* storyb@moravian.edu.

GRADUATE PROGRAMS

Expenses (2010-11) *Tuition:* part-time $647 per credit hour. *Required fees:* part-time $40 per term.
Contact Dr. Lori Hoffman, MS Program Coordinator, St. Luke's School of Nursing, Moravian College, 1200 Main Street, Bethlehem, PA 18018. *Telephone:* 610-625-7769. *Fax:* 610-625-7861. *E-mail:* lorihoffman@moravian.edu.

MASTER'S DEGREE PROGRAM

Degree MS
Available Programs Master's.
Concentrations Available Clinical nurse leader; nursing administration; nursing education.
Study Options Part-time.
Program Entrance Requirements Computer literacy, minimum overall college GPA of 3.0, transcript of college record, written essay, 2 letters of recommendation, prerequisite course work, resume, statistics course. *Application deadline:* Applications may be processed on a rolling basis for some programs. *Application fee:* $35.
Advanced Placement Credit given for nursing courses completed elsewhere dependent upon specific evaluations.
Degree Requirements 36 total credit hours.

CONTINUING EDUCATION PROGRAM

Contact Mrs. Dawn Goodolf, RN-to-BS Program Coordinator, St. Luke's School of Nursing, Moravian College, 1200 Main Street, Bethlehem, PA 18018. *Telephone:* 610-625-7764. *Fax:* 610-625-7861. *E-mail:* medmg01@moravian.edu.

Mount Aloysius College

Division of Nursing
Cresson, Pennsylvania

http://www.mtaloy.edu/
Founded in 1939

DEGREE • BSN

Nursing Program Faculty 7 (14% with doctorates).
Baccalaureate Enrollment 72 **Women** 88% **Men** 12% **Minority** 1% **Part-time** 89%
Distance Learning Courses Available.
Nursing Student Activities Student Nurses' Association.
Nursing Student Resources Academic advising; academic or career counseling; assistance for students with disabilities; bookstore; campus computer network; computer lab; computer-assisted instruction; daycare for children of students; e-mail services; interactive nursing skills videos; Internet; learning resource lab; library services; nursing audiovisuals; remedial services; resume preparation assistance; skills, simulation, or other laboratory; tutoring.
Library Facilities 7,000 volumes in health, 900 volumes in nursing; 41 periodical subscriptions health-care related.

BACCALAUREATE PROGRAMS

Degree BSN
Available Programs ADN to Baccalaureate; Accelerated RN Baccalaureate.
Site Options Johnstown, PA; Altoona, PA.
Study Options Full-time and part-time.
Online Degree Options Yes.
Program Entrance Requirements Transcript of college record, health exam, high school transcript, immunizations, RN licensure. Transfer students are accepted. *Application deadline:* Applications may be processed on a rolling basis for some programs. *Application fee:* $30.
Advanced Placement Credit by examination available. Credit given for nursing courses completed elsewhere dependent upon specific evaluations.
Expenses (2010-11) *Tuition:* full-time $19,400; part-time $520 per credit. *Room and board:* $8460; room only: $4740 per academic year. *Required fees:* part-time $30 per term.
Financial Aid 90% of baccalaureate students in nursing programs received some form of financial aid in 2009-10. *Gift aid (need-based):* Federal Pell, FSEOG, state, private, college/university gift aid from institutional funds. *Loans:* Federal Nursing Student Loans, Federal Direct (Subsidized and Unsubsidized Stafford PLUS), Perkins, alternative loans. *Work-study:* Federal Work-Study. *Financial aid application deadline (priority):* 2/15.
Contact Dr. Nickole M. Tickerhoof George, Chairperson, RN-BSN Department, Division of Nursing, Mount Aloysius College, 7373 Admiral Peary Highway, Cresson, PA 16630. *Telephone:* 814-886-6401. *Fax:* 814-886-6374. *E-mail:* ngeorge@mtaloy.edu.

CONTINUING EDUCATION PROGRAM

Contact Director of Graduate and Continuing Education, Division of Nursing, Mount Aloysius College, 7373 Admiral Peary Highway, Cresson, PA 16630. *Telephone:* 814-886-6537. *Fax:* 814-886-2978.

Neumann University
Program in Nursing and Health Sciences
Aston, Pennsylvania

http://www.neumann.edu/
Founded in 1965

DEGREES • BS • MS

Nursing Program Faculty 31 (20% with doctorates).
Baccalaureate Enrollment 526 **Women** 93% **Men** 7% **Minority** 15% **International** 2% **Part-time** 22%
Graduate Enrollment 24 **Women** 100% **Minority** 5% **Part-time** 100%
Nursing Student Activities Nursing Honor Society, Sigma Theta Tau, Student Nurses' Association.
Nursing Student Resources Academic advising; academic or career counseling; assistance for students with disabilities; bookstore; campus computer network; career placement assistance; computer lab; computer-assisted instruction; e-mail services; employment services for current students; externships; housing assistance; interactive nursing skills videos; Internet; learning resource lab; library services; nursing audiovisuals; paid internships; remedial services; resume preparation assistance; skills, simulation, or other laboratory; tutoring; unpaid internships.
Library Facilities 75,000 volumes (3,956 in health, 1,170 in nursing); 400 periodical subscriptions (155 health-care related).

BACCALAUREATE PROGRAMS

Degree BS
Available Programs ADN to Baccalaureate; Baccalaureate for Second Degree; Generic Baccalaureate; International Nurse to Baccalaureate; LPN to RN Baccalaureate; RN Baccalaureate.
Study Options Full-time and part-time.
Program Entrance Requirements Minimum overall college GPA of 2.5, transcript of college record, CPR certification, health exam, health insurance, high school biology, high school chemistry, high school foreign language, 2 years high school math, 4 years high school science, high school transcript, immunizations, minimum high school GPA of 2.5, minimum GPA in nursing prerequisites of 2.5, prerequisite course work, RN licensure. Transfer students are accepted. *Application deadline:* Applications may be processed on a rolling basis for some programs. *Application fee:* $25.
Advanced Placement Credit by examination available. Credit given for nursing courses completed elsewhere dependent upon specific evaluations.
Expenses (2010-11) *Tuition:* full-time $10,728; part-time $490 per credit hour. *Room and board:* $10,162; room only: $5976 per academic year. *Required fees:* full-time $1800; part-time $900 per term.
Financial Aid 95% of baccalaureate students in nursing programs received some form of financial aid in 2009-10. *Gift aid (need-based):* Federal Pell, FSEOG, state, private, college/university gift aid from institutional funds. *Loans:* Federal Nursing Student Loans, Federal Direct (Subsidized and Unsubsidized Stafford PLUS), Perkins. *Work-study:* Federal Work-Study, part-time campus jobs. *Financial aid application deadline:* Continuous.
Contact Mr. Justin Wright, Admissions Counselor, Program in Nursing and Health Sciences, Neumann University, One Neumann Drive, Aston, PA 19014-1298. *Telephone:* 800-963-8626 Ext. 5531. *Fax:* 610-558-5652. *E-mail:* nursediv@neumann.edu.

GRADUATE PROGRAMS

Expenses (2010-11) *Tuition:* part-time $594 per credit hour.
Financial Aid 50% of graduate students in nursing programs received some form of financial aid in 2009-10. Available to part-time students. *Application deadline:* 3/15.
Contact Ms. Kittie Pain, Admissions Counselor, Program in Nursing and Health Sciences, Neumann University, One Neumann Drive, Aston, PA 19014-1298. *Telephone:* 800-963-8626 Ext. 5613. *Fax:* 610-558-5652. *E-mail:* nursediv@neumann.edu.

MASTER'S DEGREE PROGRAM

Degree MS
Available Programs Master's; RN to Master's.
Concentrations Available Nursing education. *Clinical nurse specialist programs in:* gerontology. *Nurse practitioner programs in:* adult health, gerontology.
Study Options Full-time and part-time.
Program Entrance Requirements Computer literacy, minimum overall college GPA of 3.0, transcript of college record, CPR certification, immunizations, interview, 2 letters of recommendation, nursing research course, physical assessment course, professional liability insurance/malpractice insurance, prerequisite course work, statistics course, GRE or MAT. *Application deadline:* Applications may be processed on a rolling basis for some programs. *Application fee:* $25.
Advanced Placement Credit by examination available. Credit given for nursing courses completed elsewhere dependent upon specific evaluations.
Degree Requirements 43 total credit hours, thesis or project.

POST-MASTER'S PROGRAM

Areas of Study Nursing education. *Clinical nurse specialist programs in:* gerontology. *Nurse practitioner programs in:* adult health, gerontology.

Penn State University Park
School of Nursing
State College, University Park, Pennsylvania

http://www.hhdev.psu.edu/nurs
Founded in 1855

DEGREES • BS • MS • MSN/PHD • PHD

Nursing Program Faculty 110 (20% with doctorates).
Baccalaureate Enrollment 824 **Women** 95% **Men** 5% **Minority** 7% **Part-time** 43%
Graduate Enrollment 61 **Women** 92% **Men** 8% **Minority** 10% **Part-time** 59%
Distance Learning Courses Available.
Nursing Student Activities Sigma Theta Tau, Student Nurses' Association.
Nursing Student Resources Academic advising; academic or career counseling; assistance for students with disabilities; bookstore; campus computer network; career placement assistance; computer lab; computer-assisted instruction; daycare for children of students; e-mail services; employment services for current students; externships; housing assistance; interactive nursing skills videos; Internet; learning resource lab; library services; nursing audiovisuals; paid internships; remedial services; resume preparation assistance; skills, simulation, or other laboratory; tutoring.
Library Facilities 5.4 million volumes (244,000 in health); 88,668 periodical subscriptions (3,500 health-care related).

BACCALAUREATE PROGRAMS

Degree BS
Available Programs ADN to Baccalaureate; Generic Baccalaureate; RN Baccalaureate.
Site Options Uniontown, PA; New Kensington, PA; Harrisburg, PA; Hershey, PA; University Park, PA; Altoona, PA; Mont Alto, PA; Sharon, PA: Scranton, PA.
Study Options Full-time.
Online Degree Options Yes.
Program Entrance Requirements Transcript of college record, 3 years high school math, 3 years high school science, high school transcript. Transfer students are accepted. *Application deadline:* 11/30 (fall). *Application fee:* $50.
Advanced Placement Credit given for nursing courses completed elsewhere dependent upon specific evaluations.
Contact ***Telephone:*** 814-863-8185. *Fax:* 814-863-2925.

GRADUATE PROGRAMS

Contact ***Telephone:*** 814-863-2211. *Fax:* 814-865-2925.

MASTER'S DEGREE PROGRAM

Degrees MS; MSN/PhD
Available Programs Master's.
Concentrations Available Nursing administration. *Clinical nurse specialist programs in:* adult health, community health, gerontology. *Nurse practitioner programs in:* adult health, family health.
Site Options Hershey, PA; University Park, PA.
Study Options Full-time and part-time.
Online Degree Options Yes.
Program Entrance Requirements Computer literacy, minimum overall college GPA of 3.0, transcript of college record, CPR certification, written essay, immunizations, 2 letters of recommendation, professional liability insurance/malpractice insurance. *Application deadline:* Applications may be processed on a rolling basis for some programs. *Application fee:* $65.

Advanced Placement Credit given for nursing courses completed elsewhere dependent upon specific evaluations.
Degree Requirements 43 total credit hours, thesis or project.

POST-MASTER'S PROGRAM
Areas of Study *Nurse practitioner programs in:* family health.

DOCTORAL DEGREE PROGRAM
Degree PhD
Available Programs Doctorate.
Areas of Study Bio-behavioral research, faculty preparation, gerontology, human health and illness, illness and transition, individualized study, nursing research, nursing science.
Site Options Hershey, PA; University Park, PA.
Program Entrance Requirements Minimum overall college GPA of 3.5, interview, 3 letters of recommendation, MSN or equivalent, writing sample. Application deadline: Applications may be processed on a rolling basis for some programs. Application fee: $65.
Degree Requirements 58 total credit hours, dissertation, oral exam, written exam, residency.

POSTDOCTORAL PROGRAM
Areas of Study Gerontology.
Postdoctoral Program Contact ***Telephone:*** 814-865-9337. *Fax:* 814-865-2925.

CONTINUING EDUCATION PROGRAM
Contact ***Telephone:*** 814-865-8469. *Fax:* 814-865-3779.

Pennsylvania College of Technology
School of Health Sciences
Williamsport, Pennsylvania

Founded in 1965
DEGREE • BSN
Nursing Program Faculty 37 (5% with doctorates).
Baccalaureate Enrollment 12 **Women** 100% **International** 1% **Part-time** 92%
Nursing Student Activities Student Nurses' Association.
Nursing Student Resources Academic advising; academic or career counseling; assistance for students with disabilities; bookstore; campus computer network; career placement assistance; computer lab; computer-assisted instruction; daycare for children of students; e-mail services; employment services for current students; externships; housing assistance; interactive nursing skills videos; Internet; learning resource lab; library services; nursing audiovisuals; placement services for program completers; remedial services; resume preparation assistance; skills, simulation, or other laboratory; tutoring.
Library Facilities 127,995 volumes; 30,883 periodical subscriptions.

BACCALAUREATE PROGRAMS
Degree BSN
Available Programs RN Baccalaureate.
Program Entrance Requirements Transfer students are accepted.
Contact ***Telephone:*** 800-367-9222 Ext. 4525.

Robert Morris University
School of Nursing and Health Sciences
Moon Township, Pennsylvania

http://www.rmu.edu/
Founded in 1921
DEGREES • BSN • DNP • MSN
Nursing Program Faculty 21 (57% with doctorates).
Baccalaureate Enrollment 223 **Women** 78% **Men** 22% **Minority** 5% **International** 1% **Part-time** 3%
Graduate Enrollment 177 **Women** 88% **Men** 12% **Minority** 9% **International** 1% **Part-time** 100%
Distance Learning Courses Available.
Nursing Student Activities Nursing Honor Society, Sigma Theta Tau, Student Nurses' Association.
Nursing Student Resources Academic advising; academic or career counseling; assistance for students with disabilities; bookstore; campus computer network; career placement assistance; computer lab; computer-assisted instruction; e-mail services; employment services for current students; externships; housing assistance; interactive nursing skills videos; Internet; learning resource lab; library services; nursing audiovisuals; paid internships; placement services for program completers; remedial services; resume preparation assistance; skills, simulation, or other laboratory; tutoring; unpaid internships.
Library Facilities 125,121 volumes (4,548 in health, 2,784 in nursing); 766 periodical subscriptions (2,280 health-care related).

BACCALAUREATE PROGRAMS
Degree BSN
Available Programs Baccalaureate for Second Degree; Generic Baccalaureate.
Study Options Full-time.
Program Entrance Requirements Minimum overall college GPA of 3.0, transcript of college record, written essay, health exam, health insurance, high school biology, high school chemistry, 2 years high school math, 2 years high school science, high school transcript, immunizations, 2 letters of recommendation, minimum high school GPA of 3.0, minimum GPA in nursing prerequisites of 2.0, prerequisite course work. Transfer students are accepted. *Application deadline:* 5/1 (fall), 11/1 (spring). Applications may be processed on a rolling basis for some programs. *Application fee:* $30.
Advanced Placement Credit given for nursing courses completed elsewhere dependent upon specific evaluations.
Expenses (2010-11) *Tuition:* full-time $21,860; part-time $775 per credit. *Room and board:* $10,660; room only: $5110 per academic year. *Required fees:* full-time $1090.
Financial Aid 90% of baccalaureate students in nursing programs received some form of financial aid in 2009-10. *Gift aid (need-based):* Federal Pell, FSEOG, state, private, college/university gift aid from institutional funds. *Loans:* Perkins, alternative private loans. *Work-study:* Federal Work-Study, part-time campus jobs. *Financial aid application deadline:* Continuous.
Contact Enrollment Services, School of Nursing and Health Sciences, Robert Morris University, 6001 University Boulevard, Moon Township, PA 15108-1189. *Telephone:* 412-397-5200. *Fax:* 412-397-2425. *E-mail:* admissionsoffice@rmu.edu.

GRADUATE PROGRAMS
Expenses (2010-11) *Tuition:* part-time $775 per credit. *Required fees:* part-time $40 per credit.
Financial Aid 80% of graduate students in nursing programs received some form of financial aid in 2009-10. Federal Work-Study, institutionally sponsored loans, and unspecified assistantships available. *Financial aid application deadline:* 5/1.
Contact Enrollment Services, School of Nursing and Health Sciences, Robert Morris University, 6001 University Boulevard, Moon Township, PA 15108-1189. *Telephone:* 412-397-5200. *Fax:* 412-397-2425. *E-mail:* GraduateAdmissions@rmu.edu.

MASTER'S DEGREE PROGRAM
Degree MSN
Available Programs Master's.
Concentrations Available Nursing education.
Site Options Cranberry, PA.
Study Options Part-time.
Program Entrance Requirements Clinical experience, minimum overall college GPA of 3.25, transcript of college record, CPR certification, written essay, 2 letters of recommendation, statistics course. *Application deadline:* Applications may be processed on a rolling basis for some programs. *Application fee:* $35.
Degree Requirements 36 total credit hours, comprehensive exam.

DOCTORAL DEGREE PROGRAM
Degree DNP
Available Programs Doctorate; Post-Baccalaureate Doctorate.
Areas of Study Advanced practice nursing, family health.
Program Entrance Requirements Clinical experience, minimum overall college GPA of 3.25, interview by faculty committee, 2 letters of recommendation, vita, writing sample. Application deadline: Applications may be processed on a rolling basis for some programs. Application fee: $35.

Saint Francis University

Department of Nursing
Loretto, Pennsylvania

http://www.francis.edu/academic/Undergraduate/Nursing/Nursinghome.shtml

Founded in 1847

DEGREE • BSN

Nursing Program Faculty 7 (2% with doctorates).

Baccalaureate Enrollment 81 **Women** 90% **Men** 10% **Minority** 2%

Nursing Student Activities Student Nurses' Association, nursing club.

Nursing Student Resources Academic advising; academic or career counseling; assistance for students with disabilities; bookstore; campus computer network; career placement assistance; computer lab; computer-assisted instruction; e-mail services; employment services for current students; externships; interactive nursing skills videos; Internet; learning resource lab; library services; nursing audiovisuals; resume preparation assistance; skills, simulation, or other laboratory; tutoring.

Library Facilities 126,167 volumes (120,000 in nursing); 23,038 periodical subscriptions.

BACCALAUREATE PROGRAMS

Degree BSN

Available Programs Generic Baccalaureate; RN Baccalaureate.

Study Options Full-time and part-time.

Program Entrance Requirements Transcript of college record, high school biology, high school chemistry, 2 years high school math, 2 years high school science, high school transcript, minimum high school GPA of 3.0, minimum high school rank 50%, minimum GPA in nursing prerequisites of 2.0, prerequisite course work. Transfer students are accepted. *Application deadline:* Applications may be processed on a rolling basis for some programs. *Application fee:* $30.

Advanced Placement Credit by examination available. Credit given for nursing courses completed elsewhere dependent upon specific evaluations.

Expenses (2009-10) *Room and board:* $4654; room only: $2190 per academic year.

Financial Aid 100% of baccalaureate students in nursing programs received some form of financial aid in 2008-09. *Gift aid (need-based):* Federal Pell, FSEOG, state, private, college/university gift aid from institutional funds. *Loans:* Federal Direct (Subsidized and Unsubsidized Stafford PLUS), Perkins, private alternative loans. *Work-study:* Federal Work-Study, part-time campus jobs. *Financial aid application deadline (priority):* 5/1.

Contact Dr. Lisa J. Devineni, PhD, Chairperson, Department of Nursing, Saint Francis University, PO Box 600, 117 Evergreen Drive, 103 Schwab Hall, Loretto, PA 15940-0600. *Telephone:* 814-472-3027. *Fax:* 814-472-3849. *E-mail:* ldevineni@francis.edu.

Slippery Rock University of Pennsylvania

Department of Nursing
Slippery Rock, Pennsylvania

http://www.sru.edu/pages/1791.asp

Founded in 1889

DEGREE • BSN

Nursing Program Faculty 7 (100% with doctorates).

Baccalaureate Enrollment 230 **Women** 95% **Men** 5% **Minority** 1% **Part-time** 97%

Distance Learning Courses Available.

Nursing Student Activities Sigma Theta Tau.

Nursing Student Resources Academic advising; academic or career counseling; assistance for students with disabilities; bookstore; campus computer network; career placement assistance; computer lab; computer-assisted instruction; daycare for children of students; e-mail services; employment services for current students; housing assistance; Internet; library services; nursing audiovisuals; placement services for program completers; resume preparation assistance; tutoring.

Library Facilities 515,095 volumes (7,214 in health, 925 in nursing); 436 periodical subscriptions (1,299 health-care related).

BACCALAUREATE PROGRAMS

Degree BSN

Available Programs ADN to Baccalaureate; RN Baccalaureate.

Study Options Full-time and part-time.

Online Degree Options Yes (online only).

Program Entrance Requirements Minimum overall college GPA of 2.5, transcript of college record, minimum GPA in nursing prerequisites of 2.5, professional liability insurance/malpractice insurance, RN licensure. Transfer students are accepted. *Application deadline:* Applications may be processed on a rolling basis for some programs. *Application fee:* $30.

Advanced Placement Credit by examination available. Credit given for nursing courses completed elsewhere dependent upon specific evaluations.

Expenses (2010-11) *Tuition, state resident:* part-time $242 per credit. *Tuition, nonresident:* part-time $247 per credit. *Required fees:* part-time $122 per credit.

Financial Aid 45% of baccalaureate students in nursing programs received some form of financial aid in 2009-10. *Gift aid (need-based):* Federal Pell, FSEOG, state, private, college/university gift aid from institutional funds. *Loans:* Federal Direct (Subsidized and Unsubsidized Stafford PLUS), Perkins. *Work-study:* Federal Work-Study, part-time campus jobs. *Financial aid application deadline (priority):* 3/15.

Contact Dr. Judith A. DePalma, Professor and Chair, Department of Nursing, Slippery Rock University of Pennsylvania, 119 Behavioral Science Building, Slippery Rock, PA 16057. *Telephone:* 724-738-4921. *Fax:* 724-738-2509. *E-mail:* judith.depalma@sru.edu.

Temple University

Department of Nursing
Philadelphia, Pennsylvania

http://www.temple.edu/nursing

Founded in 1884

DEGREES • BSN • DNP • MSN

Nursing Program Faculty 37 (50% with doctorates).

Baccalaureate Enrollment 400 **Women** 85% **Men** 15% **Minority** 49% **Part-time** 62%

Graduate Enrollment 120 **Women** 95% **Men** 5% **Minority** 16% **Part-time** 100%

Distance Learning Courses Available.

Nursing Student Activities Nursing Honor Society, Sigma Theta Tau, Student Nurses' Association, nursing club.

Nursing Student Resources Academic advising; academic or career counseling; assistance for students with disabilities; bookstore; campus computer network; career placement assistance; computer lab; computer-assisted instruction; e-mail services; externships; housing assistance; interactive nursing skills videos; Internet; learning resource lab; library services; nursing audiovisuals; remedial services; resume preparation assistance; skills, simulation, or other laboratory; tutoring.

Library Facilities 60,374 volumes in health, 1,350 volumes in nursing; 60,586 periodical subscriptions (1,350 health-care related).

BACCALAUREATE PROGRAMS

Degree BSN

Available Programs Generic Baccalaureate; RN Baccalaureate.

Study Options Full-time.

Program Entrance Requirements Minimum overall college GPA of 3.0, transcript of college record, CPR certification, written essay, health exam, health insurance, high school biology, high school chemistry, high school foreign language, 3 years high school math, 3 years high school science, high school transcript, immunizations, interview, minimum high school GPA of 3.0, minimum GPA in nursing prerequisites of 3.0, prerequisite course work. Transfer students are accepted. *Application deadline:* 2/15 (fall). *Application fee:* $50.

Advanced Placement Credit given for nursing courses completed elsewhere dependent upon specific evaluations.

Financial Aid 70% of baccalaureate students in nursing programs received some form of financial aid in 2009-10.

Contact Ms. Sylvia Kaikai, Student Services Coordinator, Department of Nursing, Temple University, 3307 North Broad Street, Philadelphia, PA 19140. *Telephone:* 215-707-4618. *Fax:* 215-707-1599.

GRADUATE PROGRAMS

Financial Aid 100% of graduate students in nursing programs received some form of financial aid in 2009-10. Teaching assistantships with full tuition reimbursements available, career-related internships or fieldwork, institutionally sponsored loans, and traineeships available. Aid available to part-time students. *Financial aid application deadline:* 1/15.
Contact Dr. Delores Zygmont, Interim Director of Graduate Studies, Department of Nursing, Temple University, 3307 North Broad Street, Philadelphia, PA 19140. *Telephone:* 215-707-3789. *Fax:* 215-707-1599. *E-mail:* zygmont@temple.edu.

MASTER'S DEGREE PROGRAM

Degree MSN
Available Programs Master's.
Concentrations Available Nursing education. *Clinical nurse specialist programs in:* psychiatric/mental health. *Nurse practitioner programs in:* adult health, family health, pediatric.
Study Options Full-time and part-time.
Program Entrance Requirements Clinical experience, minimum overall college GPA of 3.0, transcript of college record, CPR certification, written essay, immunizations, interview, 2 letters of recommendation, nursing research course, physical assessment course, professional liability insurance/malpractice insurance, statistics course, GRE General Test.
Advanced Placement Credit given for nursing courses completed elsewhere dependent upon specific evaluations.
Degree Requirements 36 total credit hours.

POST-MASTER'S PROGRAM

Areas of Study Nursing education. *Clinical nurse specialist programs in:* psychiatric/mental health. *Nurse practitioner programs in:* adult health, family health, pediatric.

DOCTORAL DEGREE PROGRAM

Degree DNP
Available Programs Doctorate.

Thomas Jefferson University

Department of Nursing
Philadelphia, Pennsylvania

http://www.tju.edu
Founded in 1824

DEGREES • BSN • DNP • MSN

Nursing Program Faculty 38 (42% with doctorates).
Nursing Student Activities Nursing Honor Society, Sigma Theta Tau, Student Nurses' Association.
Nursing Student Resources Academic advising; academic or career counseling; assistance for students with disabilities; bookstore; campus computer network; career placement assistance; computer lab; computer-assisted instruction; e-mail services; interactive nursing skills videos; Internet; learning resource lab; library services; nursing audiovisuals; paid internships; placement services for program completers; remedial services; resume preparation assistance; skills, simulation, or other laboratory; tutoring.
Library Facilities 146,000 volumes in health, 4,700 volumes in nursing; 2,100 periodical subscriptions health-care related.

BACCALAUREATE PROGRAMS

Degree BSN
Available Programs ADN to Baccalaureate; Accelerated Baccalaureate; Accelerated Baccalaureate for Second Degree; Accelerated RN Baccalaureate; Baccalaureate for Second Degree; Generic Baccalaureate; RN Baccalaureate.
Site Options Atlantic City, NJ; Philadelphia, PA.
Study Options Full-time and part-time.
Program Entrance Requirements Minimum overall college GPA of 2.9, transcript of college record, CPR certification, written essay, health exam, health insurance, high school transcript, immunizations, 2 letters of recommendation, prerequisite course work. Transfer students are accepted.
Advanced Placement Credit by examination available. Credit given for nursing courses completed elsewhere dependent upon specific evaluations.
Contact *Telephone:* 215-503-8104. *Fax:* 215-503-0376.

GRADUATE PROGRAMS

Contact *Telephone:* 215-503-8057. *Fax:* 215-932-1468.

MASTER'S DEGREE PROGRAM

Degree MSN
Available Programs Accelerated Master's; Accelerated RN to Master's; Master's; Master's for Non-Nursing College Graduates; Master's for Nurses with Non-Nursing Degrees; RN to Master's.
Concentrations Available Nurse anesthesia; nursing education; nursing informatics. *Clinical nurse specialist programs in:* acute care, adult health, community health, critical care, home health care, medical-surgical, oncology, pediatric, public health. *Nurse practitioner programs in:* acute care, adult health, family health, neonatal health, oncology, pediatric.
Site Options Philadelphia, PA.
Study Options Full-time and part-time.
Program Entrance Requirements Clinical experience, computer literacy, minimum overall college GPA of 3.0, transcript of college record, CPR certification, written essay, interview, 3 letters of recommendation, nursing research course, physical assessment course, professional liability insurance/malpractice insurance, resume, statistics course.
Advanced Placement Credit given for nursing courses completed elsewhere dependent upon specific evaluations.
Degree Requirements 36 total credit hours.

POST-MASTER'S PROGRAM

Areas of Study Nursing education; nursing informatics. *Nurse practitioner programs in:* acute care, adult health, family health, neonatal health, oncology, pediatric.

DOCTORAL DEGREE PROGRAM

Degree DNP
Available Programs Doctorate.
Areas of Study Advanced practice nursing, clinical practice, individualized study.
Program Entrance Requirements Clinical experience, minimum overall college GPA of 3.2, interview by faculty committee, interview, 3 letters of recommendation, MSN or equivalent, scholarly papers, statistics course, vita, writing sample.
Degree Requirements 36 total credit hours, written exam, residency.

CONTINUING EDUCATION PROGRAM

Contact *Telephone:* 215-503-8057. *Fax:* 215-503-0376.

University of Pennsylvania

School of Nursing
Philadelphia, Pennsylvania

http://www.nursing.upenn.edu/
Founded in 1740

DEGREES • BSN • MSN • MSN/MPH • MSN/PHD • PHD

Nursing Program Faculty 338 (17% with doctorates).
Baccalaureate Enrollment 544 **Women** 91% **Men** 9% **Minority** 28% **International** 2% **Part-time** 2%
Graduate Enrollment 498 **Women** 92% **Men** 8% **Minority** 17% **International** 10% **Part-time** 59%
Nursing Student Activities Nursing Honor Society, Sigma Theta Tau, Student Nurses' Association.
Nursing Student Resources Academic advising; academic or career counseling; assistance for students with disabilities; bookstore; campus computer network; career placement assistance; computer lab; computer-assisted instruction; daycare for children of students; e-mail services; employment services for current students; externships; housing assistance; interactive nursing skills videos; Internet; learning resource lab; library services; nursing audiovisuals; other; paid internships; placement services for program completers; remedial services; resume preparation assistance; skills, simulation, or other laboratory; tutoring; unpaid internships.
Library Facilities 5.8 million volumes; 72,688 periodical subscriptions.

BACCALAUREATE PROGRAMS

Degree BSN
Available Programs ADN to Baccalaureate; Accelerated Baccalaureate; Accelerated Baccalaureate for Second Degree; Accelerated RN Bacca-

laureate; Baccalaureate for Second Degree; Generic Baccalaureate; RN Baccalaureate.
Study Options Full-time and part-time.
Program Entrance Requirements Minimum overall college GPA of 3.0, transcript of college record, written essay, health exam, health insurance, high school biology, high school chemistry, high school foreign language, 4 years high school math, 4 years high school science, high school transcript, immunizations, interview, 2 letters of recommendation, minimum high school GPA of 3.0, minimum high school rank 10%. Transfer students are accepted. *Application deadline:* 1/1 (fall). *Application fee:* $70.
Advanced Placement Credit by examination available. Credit given for nursing courses completed elsewhere dependent upon specific evaluations.
Financial Aid 96% of baccalaureate students in nursing programs received some form of financial aid in 2009-10.
Contact Office of Enrollment Management, School of Nursing, University of Pennsylvania, 418 Curie Boulevard, Philadelphia, PA 19104-4217. *Telephone:* 215-898-4271. *Fax:* 215-573-8439. *E-mail:* admissions@nursing.upenn.edu.

GRADUATE PROGRAMS

Financial Aid 94% of graduate students in nursing programs received some form of financial aid in 2009-10. Fellowships, research assistantships, teaching assistantships, institutionally sponsored loans, scholarships, traineeships, and unspecified assistantships available. *Financial aid application deadline:* 12/15.
Contact Office of Enrollment Management, School of Nursing, University of Pennsylvania, 418 Curie Boulevard, Philadelphia, PA 19104-4217. *Telephone:* 215-898-4271. *Fax:* 215-573-8439. *E-mail:* admissions@nursing.upenn.edu.

MASTER'S DEGREE PROGRAM

Degrees MSN; MSN/MPH; MSN/PhD
Available Programs Accelerated AD/RN to Master's; Accelerated Master's for Non-Nursing College Graduates; Accelerated RN to Master's; Master's.
Concentrations Available Health-care administration; nurse anesthesia; nurse-midwifery; nursing administration. *Clinical nurse specialist programs in:* adult health, pediatric, psychiatric/mental health. *Nurse practitioner programs in:* acute care, adult health, family health, gerontology, neonatal health, pediatric, primary care, psychiatric/mental health, women's health.
Study Options Full-time and part-time.
Program Entrance Requirements Clinical experience, computer literacy, minimum overall college GPA of 3.0, transcript of college record, CPR certification, written essay, immunizations, interview, 3 letters of recommendation, prerequisite course work, resume, statistics course, GRE General Test. *Application deadline:* 7/1 (fall), 11/1 (winter), 11/1 (spring), 3/1 (summer). Applications may be processed on a rolling basis for some programs. *Application fee:* $70.
Advanced Placement Credit given for nursing courses completed elsewhere dependent upon specific evaluations.
Degree Requirements 36 total credit hours.

POST-MASTER'S PROGRAM

Areas of Study Health-care administration; nurse anesthesia; nurse-midwifery; nursing administration; nursing education. *Clinical nurse specialist programs in:* acute care, adult health, critical care, family health, gerontology, home health care, maternity-newborn, medical-surgical, oncology, pediatric, psychiatric/mental health. *Nurse practitioner programs in:* acute care, adult health, family health, gerontology, neonatal health, oncology, pediatric, primary care, psychiatric/mental health, women's health.

DOCTORAL DEGREE PROGRAM

Degree PhD
Available Programs Doctorate; Post-Baccalaureate Doctorate.
Areas of Study Addiction/substance abuse, aging, bio-behavioral research, biology of health and illness, clinical practice, community health, critical care, ethics, faculty preparation, family health, gerontology, health policy, health promotion/disease prevention, health-care systems, human health and illness, illness and transition, individualized study, information systems, maternity-newborn, neuro-behavior, nursing administration, nursing policy, nursing research, nursing science, oncology, urban health, women's health.
Program Entrance Requirements Minimum overall college GPA of 3.5, interview by faculty committee, interview, 3 letters of recommendation, MSN or equivalent, statistics course, vita, writing sample, GRE General Test. Application deadline: 12/1 (fall). Application fee: $70.
Degree Requirements 39 total credit hours, dissertation, oral exam, written exam, residency.

POSTDOCTORAL PROGRAM

Areas of Study Adolescent health, aging, cancer care, chronic illness, community health, family health, gerontology, health promotion/disease prevention, individualized study, nursing informatics, nursing interventions, nursing research, nursing science, outcomes, self-care, vulnerable population, women's health.
Postdoctoral Program Contact Dr. Yvonne Paterson, Associate Dean for Nursing Research, School of Nursing, University of Pennsylvania, 418 Curie Boulevard, Claire M. Fagin Hall, 4th Floor, Philadelphia, PA 19104-4271. *Telephone:* 215-898-3151. *E-mail:* research@nursing.upenn.edu.

CONTINUING EDUCATION PROGRAM

Contact Janet L. Tomcavage, Program Management, School of Nursing, University of Pennsylvania, 418 Curie Boulevard, Philadelphia, PA 19104-4271. *Telephone:* 215-898-5422. *E-mail:* tomcavag@nursing.upenn.edu.

University of Pittsburgh

School of Nursing
Pittsburgh, Pennsylvania

http://www.nursing.pitt.edu/
Founded in 1787

DEGREES • BSN • MSN • PHD

Nursing Program Faculty 112 (58% with doctorates).
Baccalaureate Enrollment 644 **Women** 86% **Men** 14% **Minority** 9% **International** .5% **Part-time** 3%
Graduate Enrollment 386 **Women** 87% **Men** 13% **Minority** 9% **International** 4% **Part-time** 54%
Distance Learning Courses Available.
Nursing Student Activities Nursing Honor Society, Sigma Theta Tau, Student Nurses' Association.
Nursing Student Resources Academic advising; academic or career counseling; assistance for students with disabilities; bookstore; campus computer network; career placement assistance; computer lab; computer-assisted instruction; daycare for children of students; e-mail services; employment services for current students; externships; housing assistance; interactive nursing skills videos; Internet; learning resource lab; library services; nursing audiovisuals; other; paid internships; placement services for program completers; remedial services; resume preparation assistance; skills, simulation, or other laboratory; tutoring.
Library Facilities 5.5 million volumes (386,000 in health, 7,000 in nursing); 59,141 periodical subscriptions (4,775 health-care related).

BACCALAUREATE PROGRAMS

Degree BSN
Available Programs Accelerated Baccalaureate for Second Degree; Generic Baccalaureate; RN Baccalaureate.
Study Options Full-time.
Program Entrance Requirements Minimum overall college GPA of 3.0, transcript of college record, written essay, health exam, health insurance, high school biology, high school chemistry, 4 years high school math, 3 years high school science, high school transcript, immunizations, 1 letter of recommendation, minimum high school GPA of 3.3, minimum GPA in nursing prerequisites of 3.0. Transfer students are accepted. *Application deadline:* Applications may be processed on a rolling basis for some programs. *Application fee:* $45.
Advanced Placement Credit by examination available.
Expenses (2010-11) *Tuition, state resident:* full-time $17,720; part-time $738 per credit. *Tuition, nonresident:* full-time $30,162; part-time $1256 per credit. *Room and board:* $5700; room only: $2950 per academic year. *Required fees:* full-time $884; part-time $226 per term.
Financial Aid 71% of baccalaureate students in nursing programs received some form of financial aid in 2009-10. *Gift aid (need-based):* Federal Pell, FSEOG, state, private, college/university gift aid from institutional funds, Federal Nursing. *Loans:* Federal Nursing Student Loans, Federal Direct (Subsidized and Unsubsidized Stafford PLUS), Perkins, state, college/university. *Work-study:* Federal Work-Study. *Financial aid application deadline (priority):* 3/1.

Contact Mrs. Suzanne Brody, Associate Director of Student Services Recruitment, School of Nursing, University of Pittsburgh, 239 Victoria Building, 3500 Victoria Street, Pittsburgh, PA 15261. *Telephone:* 412-624-1291. *Fax:* 412-624-2409. *E-mail:* brodys@pitt.edu.

GRADUATE PROGRAMS

Expenses (2010-11) *Tuition, state resident:* full-time $20,288; part-time $829 per credit. *Tuition, nonresident:* full-time $24,412; part-time $999 per credit. *International tuition:* $24,412 full-time. *Required fees:* full-time $764; part-time $212 per term.

Financial Aid 68% of graduate students in nursing programs received some form of financial aid in 2009-10. 12 fellowships with partial tuition reimbursements available (averaging $21,000 per year), 12 research assistantships with full tuition reimbursements available (averaging $19,000 per year), 22 teaching assistantships with full tuition reimbursements available (averaging $12,000 per year) were awarded; scholarships, traineeships, and unspecified assistantships also available. Aid available to part-time students. *Financial aid application deadline:* 7/1.

Contact Mrs. Suzanne Brody, Associate Director of Student Services Recruitment, School of Nursing, University of Pittsburgh, 239 Victoria Building, 3500 Victoria Street, Pittsburgh, PA 15261. *Telephone:* 412-624-1291. *Fax:* 412-624-2409. *E-mail:* brodys@pitt.edu.

MASTER'S DEGREE PROGRAM

Degree MSN

Available Programs Master's; RN to Master's.

Concentrations Available Clinical nurse leader; nurse anesthesia; nursing administration; nursing education; nursing informatics. *Clinical nurse specialist programs in:* medical-surgical, psychiatric/mental health. *Nurse practitioner programs in:* acute care, adult health, family health, neonatal health, pediatric, psychiatric/mental health.

Site Options Bradford, PA; Greensburg, PA; Johnstown, PA.

Study Options Full-time and part-time.

Online Degree Options Yes.

Program Entrance Requirements Clinical experience, minimum overall college GPA of 3.0, transcript of college record, CPR certification, written essay, immunizations, interview, 3 letters of recommendation, professional liability insurance/malpractice insurance, resume, statistics course, GRE or MAT. *Application deadline:* Applications may be processed on a rolling basis for some programs. *Application fee:* $50.

Advanced Placement Credit by examination available. Credit given for nursing courses completed elsewhere dependent upon specific evaluations.

Degree Requirements 52 total credit hours, comprehensive exam.

POST-MASTER'S PROGRAM

Areas of Study Nursing education; nursing informatics. *Nurse practitioner programs in:* acute care, neonatal health, psychiatric/mental health.

DOCTORAL DEGREE PROGRAM

Degree PhD

Available Programs Doctorate; Post-Baccalaureate Doctorate.

Areas of Study Nursing research, nursing science.

Program Entrance Requirements Minimum overall college GPA of 3.5, interview by faculty committee, interview, 3 letters of recommendation, MSN or equivalent, statistics course, vita, writing sample, GRE. Application deadline: Applications may be processed on a rolling basis for some programs. Application fee: $50.

Degree Requirements 64 total credit hours, dissertation.

POSTDOCTORAL PROGRAM

Areas of Study Nursing research, nursing science.

Postdoctoral Program Contact Dr. Judith A. Erlen, PhD Program Coordinator/Associate Director of Center for Research in Chronic Disorders, School of Nursing, University of Pittsburgh, 3500 Victoria Street, Pittsburgh, PA 15261. *Telephone:* 412-624-1905. *Fax:* 412-624-8521. *E-mail:* jae001@pitt.edu.

CONTINUING EDUCATION PROGRAM

Contact Mrs. Mary Rodgers Schubert, Interim Director of Continuing Education Program, School of Nursing, University of Pittsburgh, 226 Victoria Building, 3500 Victoria Street, Pittsburgh, PA 15261. *Telephone:* 412-624-3156. *E-mail:* mschuber@pitt.edu.

University of Pittsburgh at Bradford

Department of Nursing
Bradford, Pennsylvania

http://www.upb.pitt.edu/academics/nursing.aspx
Founded in 1963

DEGREE • BSN

Nursing Program Faculty 12 (17% with doctorates).

Baccalaureate Enrollment 15 **Women** 80% **Men** 20% **Part-time** 60%

Distance Learning Courses Available.

Nursing Student Activities Nursing club.

Nursing Student Resources Academic advising; academic or career counseling; assistance for students with disabilities; bookstore; campus computer network; career placement assistance; computer lab; computer-assisted instruction; e-mail services; employment services for current students; externships; housing assistance; Internet; learning resource lab; library services; nursing audiovisuals; remedial services; resume preparation assistance; skills, simulation, or other laboratory; tutoring; unpaid internships.

Library Facilities 97,963 volumes (219 in health, 196 in nursing); 245 periodical subscriptions (13 health-care related).

BACCALAUREATE PROGRAMS

Degree BSN

Available Programs Generic Baccalaureate; RN Baccalaureate.

Site Options St. Marys, PA.

Study Options Full-time and part-time.

Program Entrance Requirements Transcript of college record, CPR certification, health exam, health insurance, high school transcript, immunizations, minimum high school GPA of 2.50, minimum GPA in nursing prerequisites of 2.5, professional liability insurance/malpractice insurance, prerequisite course work, RN licensure. Transfer students are accepted. *Application deadline:* Applications may be processed on a rolling basis for some programs. *Application fee:* $45.

Advanced Placement Credit by examination available. Credit given for nursing courses completed elsewhere dependent upon specific evaluations.

Expenses (2010-11) *Tuition, state resident:* full-time $14,456; part-time $602 per credit. *Tuition, nonresident:* full-time $26,890; part-time $1120 per credit. *Room and board:* $7650; room only: $4680 per academic year. *Required fees:* full-time $772; part-time $142 per credit.

Financial Aid 80% of baccalaureate students in nursing programs received some form of financial aid in 2009-10. *Gift aid (need-based):* Federal Pell, FSEOG, state, private, college/university gift aid from institutional funds, Academic Competitiveness Grants, National SMART Grants. *Loans:* Perkins. *Work-study:* Federal Work-Study, part-time campus jobs. *Financial aid application deadline (priority):* 3/1.

Contact Nursing Admissions, Department of Nursing, University of Pittsburgh at Bradford, 300 Campus Drive, Bradford, PA 16701. *Telephone:* 800-872-1787.

The University of Scranton

Department of Nursing
Scranton, Pennsylvania

Founded in 1888

DEGREES • BS • MSN

Nursing Program Faculty 40 (85% with doctorates).

Baccalaureate Enrollment 270 **Women** 92% **Men** 8% **Minority** 7% **Part-time** 8%

Graduate Enrollment 95 **Women** 70% **Men** 30% **Minority** 6% **Part-time** 50%

Nursing Student Activities Nursing Honor Society, Sigma Theta Tau, Student Nurses' Association, nursing club.

Nursing Student Resources Academic advising; academic or career counseling; bookstore; campus computer network; career placement assistance; computer lab; computer-assisted instruction; e-mail services; employment services for current students; interactive nursing skills videos; Internet; learning resource lab; library services; nursing audiovisuals; placement services for program completers; remedial services; resume preparation assistance; skills, simulation, or other laboratory; tutoring.

Library Facilities 389,832 volumes (28,400 in health, 8,484 in nursing); 35,296 periodical subscriptions (106 health-care related).

BACCALAUREATE PROGRAMS

Degree BS

Available Programs Baccalaureate for Second Degree; Generic Baccalaureate; LPN to RN Baccalaureate; RN Baccalaureate.

Study Options Full-time and part-time.

Program Entrance Requirements Minimum overall college GPA of 2.5, transcript of college record, written essay, health exam, health insurance, high school biology, high school chemistry, high school foreign language, 3 years high school math, 3 years high school science, high school transcript, immunizations, minimum high school rank 30%, minimum GPA in nursing prerequisites. Transfer students are accepted. *Application deadline:* 3/1 (fall). Applications may be processed on a rolling basis for some programs.

Advanced Placement Credit by examination available. Credit given for nursing courses completed elsewhere dependent upon specific evaluations.

Expenses (2010-11) *Tuition:* full-time $35,000; part-time $713 per credit. *Room and board:* $13,000; room only: $10,000 per academic year. *Required fees:* full-time $400; part-time $75 per term.

Financial Aid 80% of baccalaureate students in nursing programs received some form of financial aid in 2009-10. *Gift aid (need-based):* Federal Pell, FSEOG, state, private, college/university gift aid from institutional funds, TEACH Grants. *Loans:* Federal Nursing Student Loans, Federal Direct (Subsidized and Unsubsidized Stafford PLUS), Perkins. *Work-study:* Federal Work-Study, part-time campus jobs. *Financial aid application deadline (priority):* 2/15.

Contact Dr. Patricia Harrington, Chairperson, Department of Nursing, The University of Scranton, 800 Linden Street, McGurrin Hall, Scranton, PA 18510-4595. *Telephone:* 570-941-7673. *Fax:* 570-941-7903. *E-mail:* harringtonp1@scranton.edu.

GRADUATE PROGRAMS

Expenses (2010-11) *Tuition:* part-time $813 per credit. *Required fees:* full-time $50.

Financial Aid 90% of graduate students in nursing programs received some form of financial aid in 2009-10. 8 teaching assistantships with full and partial tuition reimbursements available (averaging $6,600 per year) were awarded; career-related internships or fieldwork, Federal Work-Study, and unspecified assistantships also available. Aid available to part-time students. *Financial aid application deadline:* 3/1.

Contact Dr. Mary Jane Hanson, Director, Graduate Nursing Program, Department of Nursing, The University of Scranton, 800 Linden Street, McGurrin Hall, Scranton, PA 18510-4595. *Telephone:* 570-941-4060. *Fax:* 570-941-7903. *E-mail:* hansonm2@scranton.edu.

MASTER'S DEGREE PROGRAM

Degree MSN

Available Programs Accelerated AD/RN to Master's; Accelerated RN to Master's; Master's; RN to Master's.

Concentrations Available Nurse anesthesia; nursing education. *Clinical nurse specialist programs in:* adult health. *Nurse practitioner programs in:* family health.

Study Options Full-time and part-time.

Program Entrance Requirements Clinical experience, minimum overall college GPA of 3.0, transcript of college record, CPR certification, written essay, immunizations, interview, 3 letters of recommendation, nursing research course, physical assessment course, professional liability insurance/malpractice insurance, prerequisite course work, statistics course. *Application deadline:* Applications may be processed on a rolling basis for some programs. *Application fee:* $50.

Advanced Placement Credit given for nursing courses completed elsewhere dependent upon specific evaluations.

Degree Requirements 46 total credit hours, comprehensive exam.

POST-MASTER'S PROGRAM

Areas of Study Nurse anesthesia; nursing education. *Clinical nurse specialist programs in:* adult health. *Nurse practitioner programs in:* family health.

Villanova University
College of Nursing
Villanova, Pennsylvania

http://www.nursing.villanova.edu/
Founded in 1842

DEGREES • BSN • MSN • PHD

Nursing Program Faculty 86 (44% with doctorates).
Baccalaureate Enrollment 567 **Women** 95% **Men** 5% **Minority** 24% **International** 3.5% **Part-time** 6%
Graduate Enrollment 215 **Women** 88% **Men** 12% **Minority** 24% **International** 2% **Part-time** 86%
Distance Learning Courses Available.
Nursing Student Activities Nursing Honor Society, Sigma Theta Tau, Student Nurses' Association, nursing club.
Nursing Student Resources Academic advising; academic or career counseling; assistance for students with disabilities; bookstore; campus computer network; career placement assistance; computer lab; computer-assisted instruction; e-mail services; employment services for current students; externships; housing assistance; interactive nursing skills videos; Internet; learning resource lab; library services; nursing audiovisuals; remedial services; resume preparation assistance; skills, simulation, or other laboratory; tutoring.
Library Facilities 730,000 volumes (27,980 in health, 15,580 in nursing); 12,000 periodical subscriptions (1,900 health-care related).

BACCALAUREATE PROGRAMS

Degree BSN
Available Programs ADN to Baccalaureate; Accelerated Baccalaureate for Second Degree; Baccalaureate for Second Degree; Generic Baccalaureate; International Nurse to Baccalaureate; RN Baccalaureate.
Site Options Philadelphia, PA.
Study Options Full-time and part-time.
Program Entrance Requirements Minimum overall college GPA of 2.75, transcript of college record, CPR certification, written essay, health exam, health insurance, high school biology, high school chemistry, high school foreign language, 3 years high school math, 3 years high school science, high school transcript, immunizations, 2 letters of recommendation, minimum high school GPA of 3.0. Transfer students are accepted. *Application deadline:* 11/1 (fall), 1/7 (winter). *Application fee:* $75.
Advanced Placement Credit by examination available. Credit given for nursing courses completed elsewhere dependent upon specific evaluations.
Expenses (2010-11) *Tuition:* full-time $39,350; part-time $1640 per credit. *Room and board:* $11,000; room only: $5640 per academic year. *Required fees:* full-time $580; part-time $475 per credit; part-time $30 per term.
Financial Aid 76% of baccalaureate students in nursing programs received some form of financial aid in 2009-10. *Gift aid (need-based):* Federal Pell, FSEOG, state, private, college/university gift aid from institutional funds, endowed and restricted grants. *Loans:* Federal Nursing Student Loans, Perkins, Villanova Loan. *Work-study:* Federal Work-Study, part-time campus jobs. *Financial aid application deadline (priority):* 2/1.
Contact Dr. M. Frances Keen, Assistant Dean and Director, Undergraduate Program, College of Nursing, Villanova University, Driscoll Hall, 800 Lancaster Avenue, Villanova, PA 19085-1690. *Telephone:* 610-519-4926. *Fax:* 610-519-7650. *E-mail:* frances.keen@villanova.edu.

GRADUATE PROGRAMS

Expenses (2010-11) *Tuition:* full-time $4200; part-time $700 per credit. *Required fees:* part-time $60 per credit.
Financial Aid 58% of graduate students in nursing programs received some form of financial aid in 2009-10. 5 teaching assistantships with full tuition reimbursements available (averaging $13,100 per year) were awarded; institutionally sponsored loans, scholarships, traineeships, tuition waivers (full), and unspecified assistantships also available. *Financial aid application deadline:* 3/1.
Contact Dr. Marguerite K. Schlag, Assistant Dean and Director, Graduate Program, College of Nursing, Villanova University, Driscoll Hall, 800 Lancaster Avenue, Villanova, PA 19085-1690. *Telephone:* 610-519-4934. *Fax:* 610-519-7997. *E-mail:* marguerite.schlag@villanova.edu.

MASTER'S DEGREE PROGRAM

Degree MSN
Available Programs Accelerated Master's; Master's; RN to Master's.

Concentrations Available Health-care administration; nurse anesthesia; nursing education. *Nurse practitioner programs in:* adult health, family health, gerontology, pediatric.
Study Options Full-time and part-time.
Program Entrance Requirements Clinical experience, computer literacy, minimum overall college GPA of 3.0, transcript of college record, CPR certification, written essay, immunizations, 3 letters of recommendation, physical assessment course, professional liability insurance/malpractice insurance, prerequisite course work, resume, statistics course, GRE or MAT. *Application deadline:* 11/1 (fall), 4/1 (spring), 7/1 (summer). Applications may be processed on a rolling basis for some programs. *Application fee:* $50.
Advanced Placement Credit given for nursing courses completed elsewhere dependent upon specific evaluations.
Degree Requirements 45 total credit hours, thesis or project.

POST-MASTER'S PROGRAM

Areas of Study Nurse anesthesia; nursing education. *Nurse practitioner programs in:* adult health, gerontology, pediatric.

DOCTORAL DEGREE PROGRAM

Degree PhD
Available Programs Doctorate.
Areas of Study Faculty preparation, nursing education, nursing research.
Program Entrance Requirements Clinical experience, minimum overall college GPA of 3.5, interview, 3 letters of recommendation, MSN or equivalent, scholarly papers, vita, writing sample, GRE. Application deadline: 1/15 (fall), 1/15 (summer). Application fee: $50.
Degree Requirements 51 total credit hours, dissertation, oral exam, written exam.

CONTINUING EDUCATION PROGRAM

Contact Dr. Lynore DeSilets, Assistant Dean and Director, Continuing Education, College of Nursing, Villanova University, Driscoll Hall, 800 Lancaster Avenue, Villanova, PA 19085-1690. *Telephone:* 610-519-4931. *Fax:* 610-519-6780. *E-mail:* lyn.desilets@villanova.edu.

Waynesburg University

Department of Nursing
Waynesburg, Pennsylvania

http://www.waynesburg.edu/
Founded in 1849

DEGREES • BSN • DNP • MSN • MSN/MBA

Nursing Program Faculty 48 (39% with doctorates).
Baccalaureate Enrollment 337 **Women** 91% **Men** 9% **Minority** 1%
Graduate Enrollment 240 **Women** 95% **Men** 5% **Minority** 1% **Part-time** 95%
Nursing Student Activities Sigma Theta Tau, Student Nurses' Association.
Nursing Student Resources Academic advising; academic or career counseling; assistance for students with disabilities; bookstore; campus computer network; career placement assistance; computer lab; computer-assisted instruction; e-mail services; employment services for current students; externships; Internet; learning resource lab; library services; nursing audiovisuals; paid internships; placement services for program completers; remedial services; resume preparation assistance; skills, simulation, or other laboratory; tutoring.
Library Facilities 100,000 volumes (4,500 in nursing); 1,206 periodical subscriptions (46 health-care related).

BACCALAUREATE PROGRAMS

Degree BSN
Available Programs Accelerated Baccalaureate; Accelerated Baccalaureate for Second Degree; Generic Baccalaureate; LPN to Baccalaureate.
Site Options Monroeville, PA; Canonsburg, PA; Wexford, PA.
Study Options Full-time.
Program Entrance Requirements Minimum overall college GPA of 3.0, transcript of college record, CPR certification, health exam, high school biology, high school chemistry, 2 years high school math, 2 years high school science, high school transcript, immunizations, minimum high school GPA of 3.0, minimum GPA in nursing prerequisites of 3.0, professional liability insurance/malpractice insurance, prerequisite course work. Transfer students are accepted. *Application deadline:* Applications may be processed on a rolling basis for some programs. *Application fee:* $75.
Advanced Placement Credit by examination available.
Expenses (2010-11) *Tuition:* full-time $18,050; part-time $760 per credit. *Room and board:* $7580; room only: $3850 per academic year. *Required fees:* full-time $360.
Financial Aid 90% of baccalaureate students in nursing programs received some form of financial aid in 2009-10. *Gift aid (need-based):* Federal Pell, FSEOG, state, private, college/university gift aid from institutional funds, United Negro College Fund. *Loans:* Federal Nursing Student Loans, Federal Direct (Subsidized and Unsubsidized Stafford PLUS), Perkins. *Work-study:* Federal Work-Study. *Financial aid application deadline:* Continuous.
Contact Dr. Nancy R. Mosser, Director/Chairperson, Department of Nursing, Waynesburg University, 51 West College Street, Waynesburg, PA 15370-1222. *Telephone:* 724-852-3356. *Fax:* 724-852-3220. *E-mail:* nmosser@waynesburg.edu.

GRADUATE PROGRAMS

Expenses (2010-11) *Tuition:* part-time $500 per credit.
Financial Aid 50% of graduate students in nursing programs received some form of financial aid in 2009-10.
Contact Dr. Lynette Jack, Director of Graduate and Professional Studies Program, Department of Nursing, Waynesburg University, 1001 Corporate Drive, Canonsburg, PA 15317. *Telephone:* 724-743-2256. *Fax:* 724-743-4425. *E-mail:* ljack@waynesburg.edu.

MASTER'S DEGREE PROGRAM

Degrees MSN; MSN/MBA
Available Programs Accelerated Master's; Accelerated Master's for Nurses with Non-Nursing Degrees; Accelerated RN to Master's.
Concentrations Available Nursing administration; nursing education.
Site Options Monroeville, PA; Canonsburg, PA; Wexford, PA.
Study Options Part-time.
Program Entrance Requirements Clinical experience, computer literacy, minimum overall college GPA of 3.0, transcript of college record, 2 letters of recommendation, resume. *Application deadline:* Applications may be processed on a rolling basis for some programs. *Application fee:* $75.
Degree Requirements 36 total credit hours, thesis or project.

DOCTORAL DEGREE PROGRAM

Degree DNP
Available Programs Doctorate; Post-Baccalaureate Doctorate.
Areas of Study Advanced practice nursing, health-care systems, nursing administration.
Site Options Monroeville, PA.
Program Entrance Requirements Minimum overall college GPA of 3.0, interview by faculty committee, interview, letters of recommendation, MSN or equivalent, statistics course, vita, writing sample. Application deadline: Applications may be processed on a rolling basis for some programs.
Degree Requirements 80 total credit hours, oral exam, written exam, residency.

West Chester University of Pennsylvania

Department of Nursing
West Chester, Pennsylvania

http://health-sciences.wcupa.edu/nursing
Founded in 1871

DEGREES • BSN • MSN

Nursing Program Faculty 34 (30% with doctorates).
Baccalaureate Enrollment 364 **Women** 91.9% **Men** 8.1% **Minority** 12% **International** .3% **Part-time** 20.1%
Graduate Enrollment 55 **Women** 97.83% **Men** 2.17% **International** 1% **Part-time** 84.6%
Nursing Student Activities Nursing Honor Society, Sigma Theta Tau, Student Nurses' Association.
Nursing Student Resources Academic advising; academic or career counseling; assistance for students with disabilities; bookstore; campus computer network; career placement assistance; computer lab; computer-assisted instruction; daycare for children of students; e-mail services; employment services for current students; externships; housing assistance; interactive nursing skills videos; Internet; learning resource lab;

library services; nursing audiovisuals; remedial services; resume preparation assistance; skills, simulation, or other laboratory; tutoring.
Library Facilities 1.3 million volumes (88 in nursing); 9,661 periodical subscriptions (173 health-care related).

BACCALAUREATE PROGRAMS

Degree BSN
Available Programs Accelerated Baccalaureate for Second Degree; Accelerated RN Baccalaureate; Generic Baccalaureate.
Study Options Full-time and part-time.
Program Entrance Requirements Minimum overall college GPA, transcript of college record, written essay, health exam, health insurance, high school biology, high school chemistry, 2 years high school math, 2 years high school science, high school transcript, immunizations, minimum high school GPA, minimum high school rank, minimum GPA in nursing prerequisites of 2.75. *Application deadline:* Applications may be processed on a rolling basis for some programs. *Application fee:* $35.
Advanced Placement Credit given for nursing courses completed elsewhere dependent upon specific evaluations.
Expenses (2010-11) *Tuition, state resident:* full-time $2902; part-time $242 per credit. *Tuition, nonresident:* full-time $7255; part-time $645 per credit. *Room and board:* $5307; room only: $2405 per academic year. *Required fees:* full-time $858; part-time $130 per credit.
Financial Aid 85% of baccalaureate students in nursing programs received some form of financial aid in 2009-10.
Contact Dr. Charlotte H. Mackey, Chairperson, Department of Nursing, West Chester University of Pennsylvania, 855 South New Street, West Chester, PA 19383. *Telephone:* 610-436-2219. *Fax:* 610-436-3083. *E-mail:* cmackey@wcupa.edu.

GRADUATE PROGRAMS

Expenses (2010-11) *Tuition, state resident:* full-time $3483; part-time $387 per credit. *Tuition, nonresident:* full-time $5573; part-time $619 per credit. *Required fees:* full-time $866; part-time $158 per credit.
Financial Aid 60% of graduate students in nursing programs received some form of financial aid in 2009-10. 1 research assistantship with full and partial tuition reimbursement available (averaging $5,000 per year) was awarded; unspecified assistantships also available. Aid available to part-time students. *Financial aid application deadline:* 2/15.
Contact Janet S. Hickman, Graduate Program Coordinator, Department of Nursing, West Chester University of Pennsylvania, Sturzebecker Health Sciences Center, South New Street, West Chester, PA 19383. *Telephone:* 610-436-2258. *Fax:* 610-436-3083. *E-mail:* jhickman@wcupa.edu.

MASTER'S DEGREE PROGRAM

Degree MSN
Available Programs Master's.
Concentrations Available *Clinical nurse specialist programs in:* public health.
Study Options Full-time and part-time.
Program Entrance Requirements Clinical experience, minimum overall college GPA of 2.5, transcript of college record, interview, 3 letters of recommendation, physical assessment course, professional liability insurance/malpractice insurance, resume, statistics course. *Application deadline:* Applications may be processed on a rolling basis for some programs. *Application fee:* $35.
Advanced Placement Credit given for nursing courses completed elsewhere dependent upon specific evaluations.
Degree Requirements 39 total credit hours, comprehensive exam.

Widener University

School of Nursing
Chester, Pennsylvania

http://www.widener.edu/
Founded in 1821

DEGREES • BSN • DNP • MSN • MSN/PHD • PHD

Nursing Program Faculty 64 (33% with doctorates).
Baccalaureate Enrollment 546 **Women** 90% **Men** 10% **Minority** 26% **International** 1% **Part-time** 4%
Graduate Enrollment 156 **Women** 88% **Men** 12% **Minority** 24% **International** 1% **Part-time** 84%
Distance Learning Courses Available.
Nursing Student Activities Nursing Honor Society, Sigma Theta Tau, Student Nurses' Association.
Nursing Student Resources Academic advising; academic or career counseling; assistance for students with disabilities; bookstore; campus computer network; career placement assistance; computer lab; computer-assisted instruction; e-mail services; employment services for current students; housing assistance; interactive nursing skills videos; Internet; learning resource lab; library services; nursing audiovisuals; placement services for program completers; remedial services; resume preparation assistance; skills, simulation, or other laboratory; tutoring.
Library Facilities 218,284 volumes (18,175 in health, 12,225 in nursing); 2,335 periodical subscriptions (275 health-care related).

BACCALAUREATE PROGRAMS

Degree BSN
Available Programs ADN to Baccalaureate; Generic Baccalaureate; RN Baccalaureate.
Study Options Full-time.
Program Entrance Requirements Transcript of college record, CPR certification, health exam, health insurance, high school biology, high school chemistry, high school foreign language, 3 years high school math, 3 years high school science, high school transcript, immunizations, 1 letter of recommendation, minimum high school GPA of 2.85, minimum GPA in nursing prerequisites of 3.0, professional liability insurance/malpractice insurance, prerequisite course work. Transfer students are accepted. *Application deadline:* Applications may be processed on a rolling basis for some programs.
Advanced Placement Credit by examination available. Credit given for nursing courses completed elsewhere dependent upon specific evaluations.
Expenses (2010-11) *Tuition:* full-time $32,750; part-time $1090 per credit. *Room and board:* $5860; room only: $3026 per academic year. *Required fees:* full-time $760; part-time $155 per term.
Financial Aid 97% of baccalaureate students in nursing programs received some form of financial aid in 2009-10. *Gift aid (need-based):* Federal Pell, FSEOG, state, private, college/university gift aid from institutional funds, Federal Nursing. *Loans:* Perkins. *Work-study:* Federal Work-Study, part-time campus jobs. *Financial aid application deadline (priority):* 2/15.
Contact Dr. Kathleen Black, Associate Dean, Undergraduate Program, School of Nursing, Widener University, One University Place, Chester, PA 19013-5892. *Telephone:* 610-499-4211. *Fax:* 610-499-4216. *E-mail:* kblack@widener.edu.

GRADUATE PROGRAMS

Expenses (2010-11) *Tuition:* full-time $13,860; part-time $770 per credit hour. *Required fees:* full-time $155; part-time $67 per term.
Financial Aid 63% of graduate students in nursing programs received some form of financial aid in 2009-10. Career-related internships or fieldwork, Federal Work-Study, and traineeships available. Aid available to part-time students. *Financial aid application deadline:* 4/1.
Contact Dr. Mary B. Walker, Associate Dean for Graduate Studies, School of Nursing, Widener University, One University Place, Chester, PA 19013-5892. *Telephone:* 610-499-4208. *Fax:* 610-499-4216. *E-mail:* mbwalker@widener.edu.

MASTER'S DEGREE PROGRAM

Degrees MSN; MSN/PhD
Available Programs Master's; Master's for Nurses with Non-Nursing Degrees.
Concentrations Available Nursing education. *Clinical nurse specialist programs in:* adult health, critical care, psychiatric/mental health. *Nurse practitioner programs in:* family health.
Site Options Harrisburg, PA.
Study Options Full-time and part-time.
Program Entrance Requirements Clinical experience, computer literacy, minimum overall college GPA of 3.0, transcript of college record, CPR certification, immunizations, interview, 2 letters of recommendation, nursing research course, physical assessment course, professional liability insurance/malpractice insurance, prerequisite course work, resume, statistics course, GRE General Test. *Application deadline:* 7/15 (fall), 11/15 (spring), 3/16 (summer). Applications may be processed on a rolling basis for some programs.
Advanced Placement Credit given for nursing courses completed elsewhere dependent upon specific evaluations.
Degree Requirements 42 total credit hours.

POST-MASTER'S PROGRAM

Areas of Study Nursing education. *Clinical nurse specialist programs in:* adult health, critical care, psychiatric/mental health. *Nurse practitioner programs in:* family health.

DOCTORAL DEGREE PROGRAM

Degree DNP
Available Programs Doctorate.
Areas of Study Primary care (family nurse practitioners), adult health, community health, emergency/critical care, psychiatric/mental health.
Program Entrance Requirements Minimum overall college GPA of 3.2, interview, 2 letters of recommendation, statistics course, MSN, vita. *Application deadline:* 7/15 (fall), 11/15 (spring), 3/17 (summer). Applications are processed on a rolling basis.
Degree Requirements 37 total credit hours, Capstone project.

Degree PhD
Available Programs Doctorate.
Areas of Study Faculty preparation, nursing education, nursing research, nursing science.
Program Entrance Requirements Minimum overall college GPA of 3.5, interview, 2 letters of recommendation, MSN or equivalent, statistics course, vita, writing sample, GRE General Test. Application deadline: 7/15 (fall), 11/15 (spring), 3/17 (summer). Applications may be processed on a rolling basis for some programs.
Degree Requirements 63 total credit hours, dissertation, written exam.

CONTINUING EDUCATION PROGRAM

Contact Ms. Marcia Bowers, Director for Community Relations and Continuing Education, School of Nursing, Widener University, One University Place, Chester, PA 19013. *Telephone:* 610-499-1327. *Fax:* 601-499-4216. *E-mail:* mdbowers@widener.edu.

Wilkes University

Department of Nursing
Wilkes-Barre, Pennsylvania

http://www.wilkes.edu
Founded in 1933

DEGREES • BS • MS

Nursing Program Faculty 25 (20% with doctorates).
Baccalaureate Enrollment 300 **Women** 90% **Men** 10% **Minority** 5% **Part-time** 15%
Graduate Enrollment 65 **Women** 85% **Men** 15% **Minority** 5% **Part-time** 75%
Distance Learning Courses Available.
Nursing Student Activities Sigma Theta Tau, Student Nurses' Association, nursing club.
Nursing Student Resources Academic advising; academic or career counseling; assistance for students with disabilities; bookstore; campus computer network; career placement assistance; computer lab; computer-assisted instruction; daycare for children of students; e-mail services; employment services for current students; externships; housing assistance; interactive nursing skills videos; Internet; learning resource lab; library services; nursing audiovisuals; paid internships; placement services for program completers; remedial services; resume preparation assistance; skills, simulation, or other laboratory; tutoring; unpaid internships.
Library Facilities 13,450 volumes in health, 13,000 volumes in nursing; 70 periodical subscriptions health-care related.

BACCALAUREATE PROGRAMS

Degree BS
Available Programs ADN to Baccalaureate; Accelerated Baccalaureate for Second Degree; Accelerated LPN to Baccalaureate; Accelerated RN Baccalaureate; Generic Baccalaureate; LPN to RN Baccalaureate; RN Baccalaureate.
Study Options Full-time and part-time.
Program Entrance Requirements Minimum overall college GPA of 2.0, transcript of college record, CPR certification, health exam, health insurance, high school biology, high school chemistry, 2 years high school math, 3 years high school science, high school transcript, immunizations, minimum high school GPA, professional liability insurance/malpractice insurance. Transfer students are accepted.
Advanced Placement Credit by examination available. Credit given for nursing courses completed elsewhere dependent upon specific evaluations.
Contact *Telephone:* 570-408-4074. *Fax:* 570-408-7807.

GRADUATE PROGRAMS

Contact *Telephone:* 570-408-4078. *Fax:* 570-408-7807.

MASTER'S DEGREE PROGRAM

Degree MS
Available Programs Accelerated AD/RN to Master's; Accelerated RN to Master's; Master's; Master's for Non-Nursing College Graduates; RN to Master's.
Concentrations Available Nursing administration; nursing education. *Clinical nurse specialist programs in:* gerontology, psychiatric/mental health.
Study Options Full-time and part-time.
Program Entrance Requirements Clinical experience, minimum overall college GPA of 3.0, transcript of college record, CPR certification, immunizations, interview, 3 letters of recommendation, nursing research course, physical assessment course, professional liability insurance/malpractice insurance, statistics course.
Advanced Placement Credit given for nursing courses completed elsewhere dependent upon specific evaluations.
Degree Requirements 37 total credit hours, thesis or project.

POST-MASTER'S PROGRAM

Areas of Study Nursing administration; nursing education. *Clinical nurse specialist programs in:* gerontology, psychiatric/mental health.

CONTINUING EDUCATION PROGRAM

Contact *Telephone:* 570-408-4462.

York College of Pennsylvania

Department of Nursing
York, Pennsylvania

http://www.ycp.edu/nursing/index.html
Founded in 1787

DEGREES • BS • MS

Nursing Program Faculty 63 (11% with doctorates).
Baccalaureate Enrollment 588 **Women** 94% **Men** 6% **Minority** 4% **Part-time** 6%
Graduate Enrollment 65 **Women** 98% **Men** 2% **Minority** 1% **International** 1% **Part-time** 47%
Distance Learning Courses Available.
Nursing Student Activities Nursing Honor Society, Sigma Theta Tau, Student Nurses' Association, nursing club.
Nursing Student Resources Academic advising; academic or career counseling; assistance for students with disabilities; bookstore; campus computer network; career placement assistance; computer lab; computer-assisted instruction; e-mail services; employment services for current students; externships; housing assistance; interactive nursing skills videos; Internet; learning resource lab; library services; nursing audiovisuals; paid internships; placement services for program completers; remedial services; resume preparation assistance; skills, simulation, or other laboratory; tutoring.
Library Facilities 159,273 volumes (6,681 in health, 1,226 in nursing); 138,319 periodical subscriptions (83 health-care related).

BACCALAUREATE PROGRAMS

Degree BS
Available Programs Generic Baccalaureate; LPN to RN Baccalaureate; RN Baccalaureate.
Site Options Chambersburg, PA; Hanover, PA; Harrisburg, PA.
Study Options Full-time and part-time.
Program Entrance Requirements Minimum overall college GPA of 2.8, transcript of college record, CPR certification, written essay, health exam, health insurance, high school biology, high school chemistry, 1 year of high school math, high school science, high school transcript, immunizations, 2 letters of recommendation, minimum high school rank 40%, minimum GPA in nursing prerequisites of 2.8, professional liability insurance/malpractice insurance, prerequisite course work. *Application deadline:* Applications may be processed on a rolling basis for some programs.
Advanced Placement Credit by examination available. Credit given for nursing courses completed elsewhere dependent upon specific evaluations.
Expenses (2009-10) *Tuition:* full-time $14,460; part-time $385 per credit. *International tuition:* $14,460 full-time. *Room and board:*

$8080 per academic year. *Required fees:* full-time $1080; part-time $90 per credit.

Financial Aid 90% of baccalaureate students in nursing programs received some form of financial aid in 2008-09. *Gift aid (need-based):* Federal Pell, FSEOG, state, private, college/university gift aid from institutional funds. *Loans:* Federal Nursing Student Loans, Federal Direct (Subsidized and Unsubsidized Stafford PLUS), Perkins, college/university. *Work-study:* Federal Work-Study, part-time campus jobs. *Financial aid application deadline (priority):* 3/1.

Contact Dr. Jacquelin H. Harrington, RN, Chairperson, Department of Nursing, York College of Pennsylvania, York, PA 17405-7199. *Telephone:* 717-815-1420. *Fax:* 717-849-1651. *E-mail:* jharring@ycp.edu.

GRADUATE PROGRAMS

Expenses (2009-10) *Tuition:* part-time $578 per credit. *Room and board:* $8080 per academic year. *Required fees:* part-time $298 per credit.

Financial Aid 8% of graduate students in nursing programs received some form of financial aid in 2008-09.

Contact Dr. Lynn Warner, RN, Coordinator, Department of Nursing, York College of Pennsylvania, York, PA 17405-7199. *Telephone:* 717-815-1212. *Fax:* 717-849-1651.

MASTER'S DEGREE PROGRAM

Degree MS

Available Programs Master's; RN to Master's.

Concentrations Available Nurse anesthesia; nursing administration; nursing education. *Clinical nurse specialist programs in:* adult health. *Nurse practitioner programs in:* adult health.

Site Options Chambersburg, PA; Hanover, PA; Harrisburg, PA.

Study Options Part-time.

Program Entrance Requirements Clinical experience, computer literacy, minimum overall college GPA of 3.0, transcript of college record, CPR certification, written essay, immunizations, 2 letters of recommendation, nursing research course, physical assessment course, professional liability insurance/malpractice insurance, resume, statistics course. *Application deadline:* 5/30 (fall). Applications may be processed on a rolling basis for some programs. *Application fee:* $75.

Advanced Placement Credit given for nursing courses completed elsewhere dependent upon specific evaluations.

Degree Requirements 41 total credit hours, thesis or project.

POST-MASTER'S PROGRAM

Areas of Study *Clinical nurse specialist programs in:* adult health. *Nurse practitioner programs in:* adult health.

PUERTO RICO

Inter American University of Puerto Rico, Arecibo Campus

Nursing Program
Arecibo, Puerto Rico

Founded in 1957

DEGREE • BS

Library Facilities 73,642 volumes; 640 periodical subscriptions.

BACCALAUREATE PROGRAMS

Degree BS

Available Programs Generic Baccalaureate.

Contact Undergraduate Program, Nursing Program, Inter American University of Puerto Rico, Arecibo Campus, Arecibo, PR 00614-4050. *Telephone:* 787-878-5475.

Inter American University of Puerto Rico, Metropolitan Campus

Carmen Torres de Tiburcio School of Nursing
San Juan, Puerto Rico

http://www.metro.inter.edu/progacad/enfe/nursing/index.html

Founded in 1960

DEGREE • BSN

Nursing Program Faculty 26 (27% with doctorates).

Baccalaureate Enrollment 312 **Women** 57% **Men** 43%

Nursing Student Activities Student Nurses' Association.

Nursing Student Resources Academic advising; academic or career counseling; assistance for students with disabilities; bookstore; campus computer network; career placement assistance; computer lab; computer-assisted instruction; daycare for children of students; e-mail services; employment services for current students; externships; interactive nursing skills videos; Internet; learning resource lab; library services; nursing audiovisuals; paid internships; placement services for program completers; remedial services; skills, simulation, or other laboratory; tutoring.

Library Facilities 171,173 volumes (36,000 in health, 21,759 in nursing); 41,660 periodical subscriptions (2,090 health-care related).

BACCALAUREATE PROGRAMS

Degree BSN

Available Programs ADN to Baccalaureate; Accelerated Baccalaureate; Generic Baccalaureate.

Study Options Full-time and part-time.

Program Entrance Requirements Minimum overall college GPA of 2.0, transcript of college record, CPR certification, health exam, health insurance, high school transcript, immunizations, 2 letters of recommendation, minimum high school rank 4%, minimum GPA in nursing prerequisites of 2. Transfer students are accepted.

Advanced Placement Credit by examination available. Credit given for nursing courses completed elsewhere dependent upon specific evaluations.

Contact ***Telephone:*** 787-763-3066. *Fax:* 787-250-1242 Ext. 2159.

Pontifical Catholic University of Puerto Rico

Department of Nursing
Ponce, Puerto Rico

http://www.pucpr.edu/catalogo/espanol/ciencias/dep_enf.htm

Founded in 1948

DEGREE • BSN

Library Facilities 1,499 volumes in nursing.

BACCALAUREATE PROGRAMS

Degree BSN

Available Programs Generic Baccalaureate.

Program Entrance Requirements Minimum overall college GPA of 2.0, CPR certification, health exam, health insurance, immunizations, interview, letters of recommendation, minimum high school GPA of 2.5, prerequisite course work.

Contact ***Telephone:*** 787-841-2000 Ext. 1604.

Universidad Adventista de las Antillas

Department of Nursing
Mayagüez, Puerto Rico

Founded in 1957

DEGREE • BSN

Nursing Program Faculty 11 (18% with doctorates).

Baccalaureate Enrollment 257 **Women** 69% **Men** 31% **Minority** 100% **International** 13% **Part-time** 1%
Nursing Student Activities Nursing club.
Nursing Student Resources Academic advising; academic or career counseling; assistance for students with disabilities; campus computer network; computer lab; computer-assisted instruction; e-mail services; employment services for current students; housing assistance; interactive nursing skills videos; Internet; learning resource lab; library services; nursing audiovisuals; remedial services; resume preparation assistance; skills, simulation, or other laboratory; tutoring; unpaid internships.
Library Facilities 2,488 volumes in health, 1,556 volumes in nursing; 29 periodical subscriptions health-care related.

BACCALAUREATE PROGRAMS

Degree BSN
Available Programs Generic Baccalaureate; RN Baccalaureate.
Study Options Full-time.
Program Entrance Requirements Minimum overall college GPA of 2.3, transcript of college record, health exam, health insurance, high school transcript, immunizations, interview, 2 letters of recommendation, minimum high school GPA of 2.5. Transfer students are accepted.
Advanced Placement Credit given for nursing courses completed elsewhere dependent upon specific evaluations.
Contact ***Telephone:*** 787-834-9595 Ext. 2209. *Fax:* 787-834-9597.

CONTINUING EDUCATION PROGRAM

Contact ***Telephone:*** 787-834-9595 Ext. 2284. *Fax:* 787-834-9597.

Universidad del Turabo

Nursing Program
Gurabo, Puerto Rico

Founded in 1972

DEGREE • BS

BACCALAUREATE PROGRAMS

Degree BS
Available Programs Generic Baccalaureate.
Contact ***Telephone:*** 787-743-7979.

Universidad Metropolitana

Department of Nursing
San Juan, Puerto Rico

http://www.suagm.edu/umet/umet_new_web/escuelas/ciencias_tecnologia/ciencias_tecnologia.htm
Founded in 1980

DEGREE • BSN

Library Facilities 5,438 volumes in health; 110 periodical subscriptions health-care related.

BACCALAUREATE PROGRAMS

Degree BSN
Contact ***Telephone:*** 787-766-1717 Ext. 6422. *Fax:* 787-769-7663.

University of Puerto Rico at Arecibo

Department of Nursing
Arecibo, Puerto Rico

http://upra.edu/asuntosacademicos/enfermeria/menu_enfe.htm
Founded in 1967

DEGREE • BSN

Nursing Program Faculty 21
Library Facilities 65,000 volumes; 3,660 periodical subscriptions.

BACCALAUREATE PROGRAMS

Degree BSN
Available Programs Generic Baccalaureate.
Contact ***Telephone:*** 787-878-2830. *Fax:* 787-880-4972.

University of Puerto Rico at Humacao

Department of Nursing
Humacao, Puerto Rico

http://cuhwww.upr.clu.edu/~enfe/
Founded in 1962

DEGREE • BS

Nursing Program Faculty 16 (12% with doctorates).
Nursing Student Activities Student Nurses' Association.
Nursing Student Resources Skills, simulation, or other laboratory.
Library Facilities 74,732 volumes; 53,598 periodical subscriptions.

BACCALAUREATE PROGRAMS

Degree BS
Available Programs Generic Baccalaureate.
Study Options Full-time and part-time.
Program Entrance Requirements Minimum overall college GPA, transcript of college record, health exam, health insurance, high school transcript, immunizations, minimum high school GPA of 2.0, minimum GPA in nursing prerequisites of 2.5. Transfer students are accepted.
Advanced Placement Credit by examination available. Credit given for nursing courses completed elsewhere dependent upon specific evaluations.
Contact ***Telephone:*** 787-850-9346. *Fax:* 787-850-9411.

University of Puerto Rico, Mayagüez Campus

Department of Nursing
Mayagüez, Puerto Rico

http://www.uprm.edu/enfe/
Founded in 1911

DEGREE • BSN

Nursing Program Faculty 21 (10% with doctorates).
Nursing Student Activities Nursing Honor Society, Sigma Theta Tau, Student Nurses' Association.
Nursing Student Resources Academic advising; academic or career counseling; assistance for students with disabilities; bookstore; campus computer network; career placement assistance; computer lab; computer-assisted instruction; e-mail services; employment services for current students; interactive nursing skills videos; Internet; learning resource lab; library services; nursing audiovisuals; paid internships; placement services for program completers; remedial services; resume preparation assistance; skills, simulation, or other laboratory; tutoring.
Library Facilities 68 periodical subscriptions health-care related.

BACCALAUREATE PROGRAMS

Degree BSN
Available Programs Generic Baccalaureate.
Study Options Full-time.
Program Entrance Requirements High school transcript, immunizations. Transfer students are accepted.
Advanced Placement Credit by examination available.
Contact ***Telephone:*** 787-263-3482. *Fax:* 787-832-3875.

CONTINUING EDUCATION PROGRAM

Contact ***Telephone:*** 787-265-3842. *Fax:* 787-832-3875.

University of Puerto Rico, Medical Sciences Campus

School of Nursing
San Juan, Puerto Rico

Founded in 1950

DEGREES • BSN • MSN

Nursing Program Faculty 37 (25% with doctorates).
Baccalaureate Enrollment 241 **Women** 85% **Men** 15% **Part-time** 12%
Graduate Enrollment 158 **Women** 79% **Men** 21% **Part-time** 6%
Nursing Student Activities Sigma Theta Tau, Student Nurses' Association.
Nursing Student Resources Academic advising; academic or career counseling; assistance for students with disabilities; computer lab; computer-assisted instruction; e-mail services; employment services for current students; interactive nursing skills videos; Internet; library services; nursing audiovisuals; skills, simulation, or other laboratory; tutoring.
Library Facilities 7,830 volumes in health, 1,143 volumes in nursing; 1,215 periodical subscriptions health-care related.

BACCALAUREATE PROGRAMS

Degree BSN
Available Programs ADN to Baccalaureate; Generic Baccalaureate.
Study Options Full-time and part-time.
Program Entrance Requirements Minimum overall college GPA of 2.0, transcript of college record, health exam, immunizations, interview, minimum high school GPA of 2.0, prerequisite course work. Transfer students are accepted.
Contact *Telephone:* 787-758-2525 Ext. 1984. *Fax:* 787-281-0721.

GRADUATE PROGRAMS

Contact *Telephone:* 787-758-2525 Ext. 3105. *Fax:* 787-281-0721.

MASTER'S DEGREE PROGRAM

Degree MSN
Available Programs Master's.
Concentrations Available Nurse anesthesia; nursing administration; nursing education. *Clinical nurse specialist programs in:* adult health, community health, critical care, gerontology, maternity-newborn, pediatric, psychiatric/mental health.
Site Options Mayaguez, PR.
Study Options Full-time and part-time.
Program Entrance Requirements Clinical experience, minimum overall college GPA of 2.5, transcript of college record, immunizations, interview, resume, statistics course, GRE or EXADEP.
Degree Requirements 48 total credit hours, thesis or project.

CONTINUING EDUCATION PROGRAM

Contact *Telephone:* 787-758-2525 Ext. 2102. *Fax:* 787-281-0721.

University of the Sacred Heart

Program in Nursing
San Juan, Puerto Rico

Founded in 1935

DEGREES • BSN • MSN

Nursing Student Resources Skills, simulation, or other laboratory.

BACCALAUREATE PROGRAMS

Degree BSN
Available Programs Generic Baccalaureate.
Contact *Telephone:* 787-728-1515. *Fax:* 787-727-1250.

GRADUATE PROGRAMS

Contact *Telephone:* 787-728-1515 Ext. 2427. *Fax:* 787-727-1250.

MASTER'S DEGREE PROGRAM

Degree MSN
Available Programs Master's.
Concentrations Available *Nurse practitioner programs in:* occupational health.
Degree Requirements 37 total credit hours.

RHODE ISLAND

Rhode Island College

Department of Nursing
Providence, Rhode Island

http://www.ric.edu/nursing
Founded in 1854

DEGREES • BSN • MSN

Nursing Program Faculty 49 (39% with doctorates).
Baccalaureate Enrollment 415 **Women** 89% **Men** 11% **Minority** 36% **Part-time** 38%
Graduate Enrollment 43 **Women** 98% **Men** 2% **Minority** 19% **Part-time** 98%
Distance Learning Courses Available.
Nursing Student Activities Sigma Theta Tau, Student Nurses' Association, nursing club.
Nursing Student Resources Academic advising; academic or career counseling; assistance for students with disabilities; bookstore; campus computer network; career placement assistance; computer lab; computer-assisted instruction; daycare for children of students; e-mail services; employment services for current students; housing assistance; interactive nursing skills videos; Internet; learning resource lab; library services; nursing audiovisuals; paid internships; placement services for program completers; remedial services; resume preparation assistance; skills, simulation, or other laboratory; tutoring.
Library Facilities 694,541 volumes (574 in nursing); 1.3 million periodical subscriptions (63 health-care related).

BACCALAUREATE PROGRAMS

Degree BSN
Available Programs Baccalaureate for Second Degree; Generic Baccalaureate; RN Baccalaureate.
Site Options Providence, RI.
Study Options Full-time and part-time.
Program Entrance Requirements Minimum overall college GPA of 2.7, CPR certification, health exam, health insurance, high school biology, high school chemistry, high school foreign language, 4 years high school math, 2 years high school science, high school transcript, immunizations, letters of recommendation, minimum GPA in nursing prerequisites of 3.0, prerequisite course work. Transfer students are accepted. *Application deadline:* 10/15 (fall), 4/15 (spring).
Advanced Placement Credit given for nursing courses completed elsewhere dependent upon specific evaluations.
Expenses (2010-11) *Tuition, state resident:* full-time $5420; part-time $226 per credit hour. *Tuition, nonresident:* full-time $14,500; part-time $604 per credit hour. *Room and board:* $8618; room only: $4968 per academic year. *Required fees:* full-time $898; part-time $24 per credit.
Financial Aid 62% of baccalaureate students in nursing programs received some form of financial aid in 2009-10. *Gift aid (need-based):* Federal Pell, FSEOG, state, private, college/university gift aid from institutional funds. *Loans:* Perkins, state, private loans. *Work-study:* Federal Work-Study. *Financial aid application deadline (priority):* 3/1.
Contact Dr. Jane Williams, Dean, Department of Nursing, Rhode Island College, 600 Mount Pleasant Avenue, Providence, RI 02908-1991. *Telephone:* 401-456-8014. *Fax:* 401-456-8206. *E-mail:* jwilliams@ric.edu.

GRADUATE PROGRAMS

Expenses (2010-11) *Tuition, state resident:* full-time $5580; part-time $310 per credit hour. *Tuition, nonresident:* full-time $11,088; part-time $616 per credit hour. *Required fees:* full-time $288; part-time $16 per credit.
Financial Aid 60% of graduate students in nursing programs received some form of financial aid in 2009-10.
Contact Dr. Cynthia Padula, Masters Program Director, Department of Nursing, Rhode Island College, 600 Mount Pleasant Avenue, Providence, RI 02908-1991. *Telephone:* 401-456-9720. *Fax:* 401-456-8206. *E-mail:* cpadula@ric.edu.

MASTER'S DEGREE PROGRAM

Degree MSN
Available Programs Master's.
Concentrations Available *Clinical nurse specialist programs in:* acute care, adult health, community health. *Nurse practitioner programs in:* acute care, adult health.
Site Options Providence, RI.
Study Options Full-time and part-time.
Program Entrance Requirements Minimum overall college GPA of 3.0, transcript of college record, written essay, letters of recommendation, resume, statistics course. *Application deadline:* 2/15 (fall). *Application fee:* $50.
Advanced Placement Credit given for nursing courses completed elsewhere dependent upon specific evaluations.
Degree Requirements 45 total credit hours, thesis or project.

Salve Regina University

Department of Nursing
Newport, Rhode Island

http://www.salve.edu/departments/nur/index.cfm
Founded in 1934

DEGREE • BS

Nursing Program Faculty 22 (18% with doctorates).
Baccalaureate Enrollment 200 **Women** 93% **Men** 7% **Minority** 7% **Part-time** 20%
Nursing Student Activities Sigma Theta Tau, Student Nurses' Association, nursing club.
Nursing Student Resources Academic advising; academic or career counseling; assistance for students with disabilities; bookstore; campus computer network; career placement assistance; computer lab; computer-assisted instruction; e-mail services; housing assistance; interactive nursing skills videos; Internet; learning resource lab; library services; nursing audiovisuals; paid internships; resume preparation assistance; skills, simulation, or other laboratory; tutoring; unpaid internships.
Library Facilities 6,882 volumes in health, 1,081 volumes in nursing; 76 periodical subscriptions health-care related.

BACCALAUREATE PROGRAMS

Degree BS
Available Programs Generic Baccalaureate; RN Baccalaureate.
Site Options Pawtucket, RI; Warwick, RI.
Study Options Full-time and part-time.
Program Entrance Requirements Minimum overall college GPA of 2.7, transcript of college record, written essay, high school biology, high school chemistry, high school foreign language, 3 years high school math, 3 years high school science, high school transcript, 2 letters of recommendation, minimum GPA in nursing prerequisites of 2.0, prerequisite course work. Transfer students are accepted. *Application deadline:* 2/1 (fall). Applications may be processed on a rolling basis for some programs. *Application fee:* $50.
Advanced Placement Credit by examination available. Credit given for nursing courses completed elsewhere dependent upon specific evaluations.
Expenses (2010-11) *Tuition:* full-time $31,250; part-time $1042 per credit. *Room and board:* $11,300 per academic year. *Required fees:* full-time $200; part-time $40 per term.
Financial Aid 78% of baccalaureate students in nursing programs received some form of financial aid in 2009-10. *Gift aid (need-based):* Federal Pell, FSEOG, state, private, college/university gift aid from institutional funds. *Loans:* Federal Nursing Student Loans, Perkins, college/university, alternative loans. *Work-study:* Federal Work-Study, part-time campus jobs. *Financial aid application deadline (priority):* 3/1.
Contact Mrs. Colleen Emerson, Dean of Undergraduate Admissions, Department of Nursing, Salve Regina University, 100 Ochre Point Avenue, Newport, RI 02840-4192. *Telephone:* 888-467-2583. *Fax:* 401-848-2823. *E-mail:* sruadmis@salve.edu.

CONTINUING EDUCATION PROGRAM

Contact Ms. Kelly Alverson, Continuing Education and Graduate Enrollment, Department of Nursing, Salve Regina University, Graduate Studies and Continuing Education Office, Newport, RI 02840-4192. *Telephone:* 800-637-0002. *Fax:* 401-341-2973. *E-mail:* kelly.alverson@salve.edu.

University of Rhode Island

College of Nursing
Kingston, Rhode Island

http://www.uri.edu/nursing
Founded in 1892

DEGREES • BS • MS • PHD

Nursing Program Faculty 47 (50% with doctorates).
Baccalaureate Enrollment 851 **Women** 87% **Men** 13% **Minority** 24% **International** 1% **Part-time** 10%
Graduate Enrollment 110 **Women** 95% **Men** 5% **Minority** 5% **International** 6% **Part-time** 75%
Nursing Student Activities Sigma Theta Tau, Student Nurses' Association.
Nursing Student Resources Academic advising; academic or career counseling; assistance for students with disabilities; bookstore; campus computer network; career placement assistance; computer lab; computer-assisted instruction; e-mail services; externships; housing assistance; interactive nursing skills videos; Internet; learning resource lab; library services; nursing audiovisuals; remedial services; resume preparation assistance; skills, simulation, or other laboratory; tutoring.
Library Facilities 1.4 million volumes; 18,742 periodical subscriptions.

BACCALAUREATE PROGRAMS

Degree BS
Available Programs ADN to Baccalaureate; Generic Baccalaureate; RN Baccalaureate.
Site Options Providence, RI.
Study Options Full-time and part-time.
Program Entrance Requirements Minimum overall college GPA of 2.5, transcript of college record, CPR certification, written essay, health exam, health insurance, high school foreign language, 3 years high school math, 2 years high school science, high school transcript, immunizations, 2 letters of recommendation, minimum high school rank 30%, minimum GPA in nursing prerequisites of 2.2. Transfer students are accepted.
Advanced Placement Credit given for nursing courses completed elsewhere dependent upon specific evaluations.
Expenses (2009-10) *Tuition, state resident:* full-time $9528. *Tuition, nonresident:* full-time $26,026. *Room and board:* $10,638 per academic year.
Financial Aid 70% of baccalaureate students in nursing programs received some form of financial aid in 2008-09. *Gift aid (need-based):* Federal Pell, FSEOG, state, private, college/university gift aid from institutional funds. *Loans:* Federal Nursing Student Loans, Federal Direct (Subsidized and Unsubsidized Stafford PLUS), Perkins, college/university. *Work-study:* Federal Work-Study. *Financial aid application deadline (priority):* 3/1.
Contact Undergraduate Admissions Office, College of Nursing, University of Rhode Island, Newman Hall, 14 Upper College Road, Kingston, RI 02881. *Telephone:* 401-874-7100.

GRADUATE PROGRAMS

Financial Aid 50% of graduate students in nursing programs received some form of financial aid in 2008-09. 3 teaching assistantships with full and partial tuition reimbursements available (averaging $8,428 per year) were awarded. *Financial aid application deadline:* 4/15.
Contact Dr. Mary Sullivan, Director of Graduate Programs, College of Nursing, University of Rhode Island, White Hall, Kingston, RI 02881. *Telephone:* 401-874-2766. *Fax:* 401-874-2061. *E-mail:* mcsullivan@uri.edu.

MASTER'S DEGREE PROGRAM

Degree MS
Available Programs Master's; RN to Master's.
Concentrations Available Clinical nurse leader; nursing administration; nursing education. *Clinical nurse specialist programs in:* gerontology, psychiatric/mental health. *Nurse practitioner programs in:* family health, gerontology.
Site Options Providence, RI.
Study Options Full-time and part-time.
Program Entrance Requirements Clinical experience, minimum overall college GPA of 3.0, transcript of college record, written essay, immunizations, 3 letters of recommendation, nursing research course, professional liability insurance/malpractice insurance, resume, statistics course, GRE or MAT.

Degree Requirements 41 total credit hours, thesis or project, comprehensive exam.

POST-MASTER'S PROGRAM

Areas of Study Nursing administration; nursing education. *Clinical nurse specialist programs in:* gerontology, psychiatric/mental health. *Nurse practitioner programs in:* family health, gerontology.

DOCTORAL DEGREE PROGRAM

Degree PhD
Available Programs Doctorate.
Areas of Study Nursing research, nursing science.
Program Entrance Requirements Clinical experience, minimum overall college GPA of 3.0, interview by faculty committee, 3 letters of recommendation, MSN or equivalent, scholarly papers, statistics course, vita, writing sample, GRE.
Degree Requirements 61 total credit hours, dissertation, oral exam, written exam, residency.

SOUTH CAROLINA

Charleston Southern University

Wingo School of Nursing
Charleston, South Carolina

http://www.csuniv.edu/
Founded in 1964

DEGREES • BSN • MSN

Nursing Program Faculty 18 (39% with doctorates).
Baccalaureate Enrollment 95 **Women** 90% **Men** 10% **Minority** 25%
Graduate Enrollment 27 **Women** 96% **Men** 4% **Minority** 22%
Distance Learning Courses Available.
Nursing Student Activities Sigma Theta Tau, Student Nurses' Association.
Nursing Student Resources Academic advising; academic or career counseling; assistance for students with disabilities; bookstore; campus computer network; career placement assistance; computer lab; computer-assisted instruction; e-mail services; externships; interactive nursing skills videos; Internet; learning resource lab; library services; nursing audiovisuals; remedial services; resume preparation assistance; skills, simulation, or other laboratory; tutoring.
Library Facilities 192,600 volumes (2,400 in health, 250 in nursing); 1,111 periodical subscriptions (55 health-care related).

BACCALAUREATE PROGRAMS

Degree BSN
Available Programs ADN to Baccalaureate; Generic Baccalaureate; RN Baccalaureate.
Study Options Full-time.
Program Entrance Requirements Minimum overall college GPA of 2.5, transcript of college record, CPR certification, written essay, health exam, health insurance, immunizations, minimum GPA in nursing prerequisites of 2.75, professional liability insurance/malpractice insurance, prerequisite course work. Transfer students are accepted. *Application deadline:* 3/15 (fall).
Advanced Placement Credit given for nursing courses completed elsewhere dependent upon specific evaluations.
Expenses (2010-11) *Tuition:* full-time $9000. *Required fees:* full-time $1000.
Financial Aid 90% of baccalaureate students in nursing programs received some form of financial aid in 2009-10.
Contact Dr. Tara Hulsey, Dean of Nursing, Wingo School of Nursing, Charleston Southern University, 9200 University Boulevard, PO Box 118087, Charleston, SC 29423-8087. *Telephone:* 843-863-7075. *Fax:* 843-863-7540. *E-mail:* thulsey@csuniv.edu.

GRADUATE PROGRAMS

Expenses (2010-11) *Tuition:* full-time $3000; part-time $420 per credit hour. *Required fees:* full-time $1000.
Financial Aid 95% of graduate students in nursing programs received some form of financial aid in 2009-10.
Contact Dr. Tara Hulsey, Dean, Wingo School of Nursing, Charleston Southern University, 9200 University Boulevard, PO Box 118087, Charleston, SC 29423. *Telephone:* 843-863-7075. *Fax:* 843-863-7540. *E-mail:* thulsey@csuniv.edu.

MASTER'S DEGREE PROGRAM

Degree MSN
Available Programs Master's; RN to Master's.
Concentrations Available Nursing education.
Study Options Full-time and part-time.
Online Degree Options Yes (online only).
Program Entrance Requirements Clinical experience, minimum overall college GPA of 3.0, transcript of college record, written essay, 3 letters of recommendation, resume. *Application deadline:* 6/31 (fall). *Application fee:* $20.
Advanced Placement Credit given for nursing courses completed elsewhere dependent upon specific evaluations.
Degree Requirements 39 total credit hours, thesis or project.

Clemson University

School of Nursing
Clemson, South Carolina

http://www.hehd.clemson.edu/nursing
Founded in 1889

DEGREES • BS • MS

Nursing Program Faculty 24 (71% with doctorates).
Baccalaureate Enrollment 402 **Women** 99% **Men** 1% **Minority** 11%
Graduate Enrollment 82 **Women** 96.3% **Men** 3.7% **Minority** 9.8%
Part-time 65.9%
Nursing Student Activities Nursing Honor Society, Sigma Theta Tau, Student Nurses' Association.
Nursing Student Resources Academic advising; academic or career counseling; assistance for students with disabilities; bookstore; campus computer network; career placement assistance; computer lab; computer-assisted instruction; e-mail services; employment services for current students; externships; housing assistance; interactive nursing skills videos; Internet; learning resource lab; library services; nursing audiovisuals; other; remedial services; resume preparation assistance; skills, simulation, or other laboratory; tutoring; unpaid internships.
Library Facilities 1.2 million volumes (29,800 in health, 5,548 in nursing); 5,587 periodical subscriptions (877 health-care related).

BACCALAUREATE PROGRAMS

Degree BS
Available Programs Generic Baccalaureate; RN Baccalaureate.
Study Options Full-time and part-time.
Program Entrance Requirements Minimum overall college GPA of 2.5, transcript of college record, CPR certification, health insurance, high school biology, high school chemistry, 3 years high school math, 3 years high school science, high school transcript, immunizations, minimum high school GPA of 2.5, professional liability insurance/malpractice insurance, prerequisite course work. Transfer students are accepted.
Advanced Placement Credit by examination available. Credit given for nursing courses completed elsewhere dependent upon specific evaluations.
Contact *Telephone:* 864-656-5463. *Fax:* 864-656-2464.

GRADUATE PROGRAMS

Contact *Telephone:* 864-250-8881. *Fax:* 864-250-6711.

MASTER'S DEGREE PROGRAM

Degree MS
Available Programs Master's; RN to Master's.
Concentrations Available Nursing administration; nursing education. *Clinical nurse specialist programs in:* adult health, gerontology, maternity-newborn, parent-child, pediatric. *Nurse practitioner programs in:* adult health, family health, gerontology.
Study Options Full-time and part-time.
Program Entrance Requirements Clinical experience, computer literacy, minimum overall college GPA of 3.0, transcript of college record, CPR certification, 2 letters of recommendation, nursing research course, physical assessment course, professional liability insurance/malpractice insurance, prerequisite course work, resume, statistics course, GRE General Test.

Advanced Placement Credit by examination available. Credit given for nursing courses completed elsewhere dependent upon specific evaluations.

Degree Requirements 45 total credit hours, thesis or project, comprehensive exam.

POST-MASTER'S PROGRAM

Areas of Study Nursing administration; nursing education. *Clinical nurse specialist programs in:* adult health, gerontology, maternity-newborn, parent-child, pediatric. *Nurse practitioner programs in:* adult health, family health, gerontology.

DOCTORAL DEGREE PROGRAM

Program Entrance Requirements GRE General Test.

CONTINUING EDUCATION PROGRAM

Contact *Telephone:* 864-656-3078. *Fax:* 864-656-1877.

Francis Marion University

Department of Nursing
Florence, South Carolina

http://www.fmarion.edu/
Founded in 1970

DEGREE • BSN

Nursing Program Faculty 23 (5% with doctorates).

Baccalaureate Enrollment 159 **Women** 90% **Men** 10% **Minority** 26% **Part-time** 7%

Nursing Student Activities Nursing Honor Society, Sigma Theta Tau, Student Nurses' Association.

Nursing Student Resources Academic advising; academic or career counseling; assistance for students with disabilities; bookstore; campus computer network; career placement assistance; computer lab; computer-assisted instruction; daycare for children of students; e-mail services; externships; housing assistance; interactive nursing skills videos; Internet; learning resource lab; library services; nursing audiovisuals; paid internships; placement services for program completers; remedial services; resume preparation assistance; skills, simulation, or other laboratory; tutoring; unpaid internships.

Library Facilities 343,220 volumes; 1,338 periodical subscriptions.

BACCALAUREATE PROGRAMS

Degree BSN

Available Programs ADN to Baccalaureate; Generic Baccalaureate.

Site Options Lake City, SC; Marion, SC.

Study Options Full-time.

Program Entrance Requirements Transcript of college record, CPR certification, written essay, health insurance, immunizations, 3 letters of recommendation, minimum GPA in nursing prerequisites of 3.0, prerequisite course work. Transfer students are accepted. *Application deadline:* 3/1 (fall), 10/1 (spring). *Application fee:* $75.

Expenses (2010-11) *Tuition, state resident:* full-time $6368; part-time $6368 per semester. *Tuition, nonresident:* full-time $12,737; part-time $12,737 per semester. *Room and board:* $2045 per academic year. *Required fees:* full-time $1300.

Financial Aid 90% of baccalaureate students in nursing programs received some form of financial aid in 2009-10. *Gift aid (need-based):* Federal Pell, FSEOG, state, private, Academic Competitiveness Grants, National SMART Grants. *Loans:* Federal Direct (Subsidized and Unsubsidized Stafford PLUS), Perkins, state. *Work-study:* Federal Work-Study, part-time campus jobs. *Financial aid application deadline (priority):* 3/1.

Contact Mrs. Lauren K. Vause, Coordinator of Student Services, Department of Nursing, Francis Marion University, PO Box 100547, Florence, SC 29502-0547. *Telephone:* 843-661-1226. *Fax:* 843-661-1696. *E-mail:* kpadgett@fmarion.edu.

Lander University

School of Nursing
Greenwood, South Carolina

http://www.lander.edu/nursing/
Founded in 1872

DEGREE • BSN

Nursing Program Faculty 21 (10% with doctorates).
Baccalaureate Enrollment 273 **Women** 92% **Men** 8% **Minority** 21% **Part-time** 16%
Distance Learning Courses Available.
Nursing Student Activities Sigma Theta Tau, Student Nurses' Association.
Nursing Student Resources Academic advising; academic or career counseling; assistance for students with disabilities; bookstore; campus computer network; career placement assistance; computer lab; computer-assisted instruction; e-mail services; externships; housing assistance; interactive nursing skills videos; Internet; learning resource lab; library services; nursing audiovisuals; resume preparation assistance; skills, simulation, or other laboratory.
Library Facilities 186,690 volumes (6,209 in health, 1,145 in nursing); 657 periodical subscriptions (36 health-care related).

BACCALAUREATE PROGRAMS

Degree BSN
Available Programs Accelerated Baccalaureate; Accelerated Baccalaureate for Second Degree; Accelerated RN Baccalaureate; Baccalaureate for Second Degree; Generic Baccalaureate; RN Baccalaureate.
Site Options Greenwood, SC.
Study Options Full-time and part-time.
Online Degree Options Yes.
Program Entrance Requirements Minimum overall college GPA of 2.6, transcript of college record, CPR certification, health exam, health insurance, immunizations, professional liability insurance/malpractice insurance, prerequisite course work. Transfer students are accepted. *Application deadline:* Applications may be processed on a rolling basis for some programs. *Application fee:* $35.
Advanced Placement Credit given for nursing courses completed elsewhere dependent upon specific evaluations.
Expenses (2009-10) *Tuition, state resident:* full-time $8760; part-time $365 per credit hour. *Tuition, nonresident:* full-time $16,560; part-time $690 per credit hour. *Room and board:* $6400; room only: $4000 per academic year.
Financial Aid 60% of baccalaureate students in nursing programs received some form of financial aid in 2008-09.
Contact Mrs. Jennifer M. Mathis, Director of Admissions, School of Nursing, Lander University, 320 Stanley Avenue, Greenwood, SC 29649-2099. *Telephone:* 864-388-8307. *Fax:* 864-388-8125. *E-mail:* jmathis@lander.edu.

Medical University of South Carolina

College of Nursing
Charleston, South Carolina

http://www.musc.edu/nursing
Founded in 1824

DEGREES • BSN • BSN • DNP • PHD

Nursing Program Faculty 37 (76% with doctorates).
Baccalaureate Enrollment 173 **Women** 81% **Men** 19% **Minority** 21% **Part-time** 1%
Graduate Enrollment 156 **Women** 94% **Men** 6% **Minority** 17% **Part-time** 42%
Distance Learning Courses Available.
Nursing Student Activities Sigma Theta Tau, Student Nurses' Association.
Nursing Student Resources Academic advising; bookstore; campus computer network; computer lab; computer-assisted instruction; e-mail services; housing assistance; interactive nursing skills videos; Internet; learning resource lab; library services; nursing audiovisuals; other; resume preparation assistance; skills, simulation, or other laboratory; tutoring.

Library Facilities 193,599 volumes (48,000 in health, 1,500 in nursing); 17,532 periodical subscriptions (19,000 health-care related).

BACCALAUREATE PROGRAMS

Degree BSN
Available Programs Accelerated Baccalaureate; Accelerated Baccalaureate for Second Degree.
Study Options Full-time.
Program Entrance Requirements Transcript of college record, CPR certification, written essay, health exam, health insurance, immunizations, 3 letters of recommendation, minimum GPA in nursing prerequisites of 3.0, prerequisite course work. Transfer students are accepted. *Application deadline:* 1/15 (fall), 9/15 (spring). *Application fee:* $95.
Advanced Placement Credit by examination available. Credit given for nursing courses completed elsewhere dependent upon specific evaluations.
Expenses (2010-11) *Tuition, state resident:* full-time $20,886; part-time $630 per credit hour. *Tuition, nonresident:* full-time $33,399; part-time $1030 per credit hour. *Required fees:* full-time $930; part-time $805 per term.
Financial Aid 85% of baccalaureate students in nursing programs received some form of financial aid in 2009-10.
Contact Mrs. Mardi Long, Program Coordinator, College of Nursing, Medical University of South Carolina, 99 Jonathan Lucas Street, MSC 160, Charleston, SC 29425-1600. *Telephone:* 843-792-6683. *Fax:* 843-792-9258. *E-mail:* longm@musc.edu.

GRADUATE PROGRAMS

Expenses (2010-11) *Tuition, state resident:* full-time $22,065; part-time $758 per credit hour. *Tuition, nonresident:* full-time $26,055; part-time $895 per credit hour. *Required fees:* full-time $1050; part-time $750 per term.
Financial Aid 74% of graduate students in nursing programs received some form of financial aid in 2009-10. Federal Work-Study, scholarships, and traineeships available. Aid available to part-time students. *Financial aid application deadline:* 3/10.
Contact Dr. Robin L. Bissinger, Director of Graduate Programs, College of Nursing, Medical University of South Carolina, 99 Jonathan Lucas Street, Room 209, MSC 160, Charleston, SC 29425-1600. *Telephone:* 843-792-0531. *Fax:* 843-792-1741. *E-mail:* bissinrl@musc.edu.

MASTER'S DEGREE PROGRAM

Degree MSN
Available Programs Master's.
Concentrations Available Nursing administration; nursing education. *Nurse practitioner programs in:* adult health, family health, pediatric.
Study Options Full-time and part-time.
Online Degree Options Yes (online only).
Program Entrance Requirements Minimum overall college GPA of 3.0, transcript of college record, CPR certification, written essay, immunizations, 3 letters of recommendation, prerequisite course work, resume, statistics course. *Application deadline:* 2/1 (fall). *Application fee:* $95.
Advanced Placement Credit given for nursing courses completed elsewhere dependent upon specific evaluations.
Degree Requirements 58 total credit hours.

POST-MASTER'S PROGRAM

Areas of Study Nursing administration; nursing education.

DOCTORAL DEGREE PROGRAM

Degree DNP
Available Programs Doctorate; Post-Baccalaureate Doctorate; Doctorate for Nurses with Non-Nursing Degrees.
Areas of Study Advanced practice nursing, health-care systems.
Online Degree Options Yes.
Program Entrance Requirements Minimum overall college GPA of 3.0, 3 letters of recommendation, vita, writing sample, interview by faculty committee. *Application deadline*: 5/1 (fall), 1/1 (winter), 1/1 (spring), 1/1 (summer). *Application fee*: $50.
Degree Requirements 61 total credit hours, oral exam, residency.

Degree PhD
Available Programs Doctorate; Post-Baccalaureate Doctorate.
Areas of Study Community health, family health, nursing administration, nursing education, nursing policy, nursing research.
Online Degree Options Yes (online only).
Program Entrance Requirements Minimum overall college GPA of 3.5, interview by faculty committee, interview, 3 letters of recommendation, MSN or equivalent, statistics course, vita, writing sample, GRE General Test (PhD). Application deadline: 2/1 (fall). Applications may be processed on a rolling basis for some programs. Application fee: $95.
Degree Requirements 62 total credit hours, dissertation, oral exam, written exam.

POSTDOCTORAL PROGRAM

Areas of Study Gerontology, nursing interventions, nursing research, vulnerable population.
Postdoctoral Program Contact Dr. William Basco, Program Director, College of Nursing, Medical University of South Carolina, Rutledge Towers, MSC 106, Charleston, SC 29425. *Telephone:* 843-876-6512. *Fax:* 843-876-8709. *E-mail:* bascob@musc.edu.

CONTINUING EDUCATION PROGRAM

Contact Ms. Carol Whelan, Administrative Assistant, College of Nursing, Medical University of South Carolina, 99 Jonathan Lucas Street, MSC 160, Charleston, SC 29425-1600. *Telephone:* 843-792-2651. *Fax:* 843-792-2104. *E-mail:* whelanc@musc.edu.

South Carolina State University

Department of Nursing
Orangeburg, South Carolina

Founded in 1896

DEGREE • BSN

Library Facilities 313,329 volumes; 3,031 periodical subscriptions.

BACCALAUREATE PROGRAMS

Degree BSN
Available Programs Generic Baccalaureate; RN Baccalaureate.
Program Entrance Requirements Minimum overall college GPA of 2.8, immunizations, minimum high school GPA of 2.8.
Contact ***Telephone:*** 803-536-7063. *Fax:* 803-536-8593.

University of South Carolina

College of Nursing
Columbia, South Carolina

http://www.sc.edu/nursing
Founded in 1801

DEGREES • BSN • DNP • MSN • PHD

Nursing Program Faculty 92 (27% with doctorates).
Baccalaureate Enrollment 1,002 **Women** 92% **Men** 8% **Minority** 17% **International** .4% **Part-time** 4%
Graduate Enrollment 210 **Women** 89% **Men** 11% **Minority** 16% **Part-time** 59%
Distance Learning Courses Available.
Nursing Student Activities Nursing Honor Society, Sigma Theta Tau, Student Nurses' Association.
Nursing Student Resources Academic advising; academic or career counseling; assistance for students with disabilities; bookstore; campus computer network; career placement assistance; computer lab; computer-assisted instruction; daycare for children of students; e-mail services; housing assistance; interactive nursing skills videos; Internet; learning resource lab; library services; nursing audiovisuals; remedial services; resume preparation assistance; skills, simulation, or other laboratory; tutoring.
Library Facilities 3.3 million volumes (98,901 in health, 10,716 in nursing); 66,309 periodical subscriptions (285 health-care related).

BACCALAUREATE PROGRAMS

Degree BSN
Available Programs Generic Baccalaureate.
Site Options Walterboro, SC; Lancaster, SC; Allendale, SC.
Study Options Full-time and part-time.
Program Entrance Requirements Minimum overall college GPA of 3.0, transcript of college record, high school biology, high school chemistry, high school foreign language, 1.5 years high school math, 1.5 years high school science, high school transcript, immunizations, minimum GPA in nursing prerequisites of 3.0. Transfer students are accepted. *Application deadline:* 12/1 (fall), 11/1 (spring), 5/1 (summer). *Application fee:* $50.

Advanced Placement Credit by examination available. Credit given for nursing courses completed elsewhere dependent upon specific evaluations.
Expenses (2010-11) *Tuition, state resident:* full-time $10,686; part-time $485 per credit hour. *Tuition, nonresident:* full-time $27,362; part-time $1200 per credit hour. *Room and board:* $7440; room only: $4957 per academic year. *Required fees:* full-time $2350; part-time $17 per credit; part-time $113 per term.
Financial Aid 60% of baccalaureate students in nursing programs received some form of financial aid in 2009-10. *Gift aid (need-based):* Federal Pell, FSEOG, state, private, college/university gift aid from institutional funds, United Negro College Fund, Federal Nursing. *Loans:* Federal Nursing Student Loans, Federal Direct (Subsidized and Unsubsidized Stafford PLUS), Perkins. *Work-study:* Federal Work-Study, part-time campus jobs. *Financial aid application deadline (priority):* 4/1.
Contact Mrs. Gail S. Vereen, Director of Recruitment and Undergraduate Advisement, College of Nursing, University of South Carolina, 1601 Greene Street, Columbia, SC 29208. *Telephone:* 803-777-2526. *Fax:* 803-777-0616. *E-mail:* gsveree@mailbox.sc.edu.

GRADUATE PROGRAMS

Expenses (2010-11) *Tuition, state resident:* full-time $11,990; part-time $540 per credit hour. *Tuition, nonresident:* full-time $24,550; part-time $1045 per credit hour. *Room and board:* room only: $835 per academic year. *Required fees:* full-time $2150; part-time $204 per credit; part-time $169 per term.
Financial Aid 39% of graduate students in nursing programs received some form of financial aid in 2009-10. 1 fellowship (averaging $1,200 per year), 3 research assistantships with partial tuition reimbursements available (averaging $2,790 per year), 11 teaching assistantships (averaging $5,533 per year) were awarded; scholarships, traineeships, and unspecified assistantships also available. *Financial aid application deadline:* 4/1.
Contact Ms. Cheryl Nelson, Student Services Coordinator, Graduate Programs, College of Nursing, University of South Carolina, 1601 Greene Street, Columbia, SC 29208. *Telephone:* 803-777-3754. *Fax:* 803-777-9080. *E-mail:* cyjackso@mailbox.sc.edu.

MASTER'S DEGREE PROGRAM

Degree MSN
Available Programs Master's.
Concentrations Available *Nurse practitioner programs in:* acute care, family health.
Study Options Full-time and part-time.
Program Entrance Requirements Minimum overall college GPA of 3.0, transcript of college record, written essay, immunizations, 2 letters of recommendation, resume, GRE General Test, MAT. *Application deadline:* 5/1 (fall). *Application fee:* $50.
Advanced Placement Credit given for nursing courses completed elsewhere dependent upon specific evaluations.
Degree Requirements 45 total credit hours.

POST-MASTER'S PROGRAM

Areas of Study *Nurse practitioner programs in:* acute care, family health.

DOCTORAL DEGREE PROGRAM

Degree DNP
Available Programs Doctorate; Post-Baccalaureate Doctorate; Doctorate for Nurses with Non-Nursing Degrees.
Areas of Study Advanced practice nursing, health-care systems.
Online Degree Options Yes.
Program Entrance Requirements Minimum overall college GPA of 3.0, 3 letters of recommendation, vita, writing sample, interview by faculty committee. *Application deadline*: 5/1 (fall), 1/1 (winter), 1/1 (spring), 1/1 (summer). *Application fee*: $50.
Degree Requirements 61 total credit hours, oral exam, residency.

Degree PhD
Available Programs Doctorate; Post-Baccalaureate Doctorate.
Areas of Study Health-care systems, individualized study, nursing science.
Program Entrance Requirements Minimum overall college GPA of 3.0, interview by faculty committee, 3 letters of recommendation, scholarly papers, vita, writing sample, GRE General Test. Application deadline: 5/1 (fall). Application fee: $50.
Degree Requirements 61 total credit hours, dissertation, written exam, residency.

CONTINUING EDUCATION PROGRAM

Contact Dr. Eileen Shake, Director, Center for Nursing Leadership, College of Nursing, University of South Carolina, 1601 Greene Street, Columbia, SC 29208. *Telephone:* 803-777-5881. *Fax:* 803-777-6800. *E-mail:* shakee@mailbox.sc.edu.

University of South Carolina Aiken

School of Nursing
Aiken, South Carolina

http://www.usca.edu/nursing/
Founded in 1961

DEGREE • BSN

Nursing Program Faculty 16 (50% with doctorates).
Baccalaureate Enrollment 250 **Women** 90% **Men** 10% **Minority** 30% **International** 1% **Part-time** 3%
Distance Learning Courses Available.
Nursing Student Activities Sigma Theta Tau, Student Nurses' Association.
Nursing Student Resources Academic advising; academic or career counseling; assistance for students with disabilities; bookstore; campus computer network; career placement assistance; computer lab; computer-assisted instruction; daycare for children of students; e-mail services; employment services for current students; housing assistance; interactive nursing skills videos; Internet; learning resource lab; library services; nursing audiovisuals; placement services for program completers; resume preparation assistance; skills, simulation, or other laboratory; tutoring.
Library Facilities 200 volumes in health, 100 volumes in nursing; 100 periodical subscriptions health-care related.

BACCALAUREATE PROGRAMS

Degree BSN
Available Programs ADN to Baccalaureate; Generic Baccalaureate; International Nurse to Baccalaureate; LPN to Baccalaureate; RN Baccalaureate.
Study Options Full-time and part-time.
Online Degree Options Yes.
Program Entrance Requirements CPR certification, written essay, health exam, immunizations, 2 letters of recommendation, minimum GPA in nursing prerequisites of 2.75, prerequisite course work. Transfer students are accepted. *Application deadline:* 3/15 (fall), 10/15 (spring).
Advanced Placement Credit by examination available. Credit given for nursing courses completed elsewhere dependent upon specific evaluations.
Financial Aid 50% of baccalaureate students in nursing programs received some form of financial aid in 2009-10.
Contact Ms. Kathy Simmons, Administrative Assistant, School of Nursing, University of South Carolina Aiken, 471 University Parkway, Aiken, SC 29801. *Telephone:* 803-648-3392. *Fax:* 803-641-3725. *E-mail:* kathers@usca.edu.

University of South Carolina Beaufort

Nursing Program
Bluffton, South Carolina

Founded in 1959

DEGREE • BSN

Nursing Program Faculty 9 (43% with doctorates).
Baccalaureate Enrollment 80
Nursing Student Activities Student Nurses' Association.
Nursing Student Resources Academic advising; academic or career counseling; assistance for students with disabilities; bookstore; campus computer network; career placement assistance; computer lab; computer-assisted instruction; e-mail services; employment services for current students; externships; housing assistance; interactive nursing skills videos; Internet; learning resource lab; library services; nursing audiovisuals; paid internships; remedial services; resume preparation assistance; skills, simulation, or other laboratory; tutoring; unpaid internships.
Library Facilities 84,865 volumes; 146 periodical subscriptions.

BACCALAUREATE PROGRAMS

Degree BSN
Available Programs Generic Baccalaureate; RN Baccalaureate.
Contact *Telephone:* 843-208-8124. *E-mail:* Nursing@uscb.edu.

University of South Carolina Upstate

Mary Black School of Nursing
Spartanburg, South Carolina

http://www.uscs.edu/academics/mbsn/
Founded in 1967

DEGREE • BSN

Nursing Program Faculty 61 (18% with doctorates).
Baccalaureate Enrollment 450 **Women** 88% **Men** 12% **Minority** 25% **International** 2% **Part-time** 5%
Distance Learning Courses Available.
Nursing Student Activities Nursing Honor Society, Sigma Theta Tau, Student Nurses' Association.
Nursing Student Resources Academic advising; academic or career counseling; assistance for students with disabilities; bookstore; campus computer network; career placement assistance; computer lab; computer-assisted instruction; daycare for children of students; e-mail services; employment services for current students; externships; housing assistance; interactive nursing skills videos; Internet; learning resource lab; library services; nursing audiovisuals; paid internships; resume preparation assistance; skills, simulation, or other laboratory; tutoring; unpaid internships.
Library Facilities 201,237 volumes (214,998 in health, 23,359 in nursing); 27,405 periodical subscriptions.

BACCALAUREATE PROGRAMS

Degree BSN
Available Programs Generic Baccalaureate; RN Baccalaureate.
Site Options Greenville, SC.
Study Options Full-time and part-time.
Online Degree Options Yes.
Program Entrance Requirements Transcript of college record, CPR certification, health exam, immunizations, minimum GPA in nursing prerequisites of 2.75, professional liability insurance/malpractice insurance, prerequisite course work. Transfer students are accepted. *Application deadline:* 1/15 (fall), 5/1 (spring).
Advanced Placement Credit by examination available. Credit given for nursing courses completed elsewhere dependent upon specific evaluations.
Expenses (2010-11) *Tuition, state resident:* full-time $8792; part-time $357 per credit hour. *Tuition, nonresident:* full-time $17,864; part-time $759 per credit hour. *Room and board:* $7400; room only: $5200 per academic year. *Required fees:* full-time $1810; part-time $89 per credit.
Financial Aid 85% of baccalaureate students in nursing programs received some form of financial aid in 2009-10.
Contact Dr. Katharine M. Gibb, Associate Dean, Mary Black School of Nursing, University of South Carolina Upstate, 800 University Way, Spartanburg, SC 29303. *Telephone:* 864-503-5447. *Fax:* 864-503-5405. *E-mail:* kgibb@uscupstate.edu.

SOUTH DAKOTA

Augustana College

Department of Nursing
Sioux Falls, South Dakota

http://www.augie.edu/
Founded in 1860

DEGREE • BA

Nursing Program Faculty 15 (20% with doctorates).
Baccalaureate Enrollment 255 **Women** 90% **Men** 10% **Minority** 4% **Part-time** 2%
Distance Learning Courses Available.
Nursing Student Activities Sigma Theta Tau, Student Nurses' Association.
Nursing Student Resources Academic advising; academic or career counseling; assistance for students with disabilities; bookstore; campus computer network; career placement assistance; computer lab; computer-assisted instruction; daycare for children of students; e-mail services; employment services for current students; housing assistance; interactive nursing skills videos; Internet; learning resource lab; library services; nursing audiovisuals; remedial services; resume preparation assistance; skills, simulation, or other laboratory; tutoring; unpaid internships.
Library Facilities 258,451 volumes; 6,341 periodical subscriptions.

BACCALAUREATE PROGRAMS

Degree BA
Available Programs Generic Baccalaureate.
Study Options Full-time.
Program Entrance Requirements Minimum overall college GPA of 2.7, transcript of college record, CPR certification, written essay, health exam, health insurance, high school transcript, immunizations, 2 letters of recommendation, minimum high school GPA of 3.5, minimum GPA in nursing prerequisites of 2.7, prerequisite course work. Transfer students are accepted. *Application deadline:* 2/15 (fall). Applications may be processed on a rolling basis for some programs.
Advanced Placement Credit given for nursing courses completed elsewhere dependent upon specific evaluations.
Expenses (2010-11) *Tuition:* full-time $24,790. *Room and board:* $6486 per academic year. *Required fees:* full-time $334.
Financial Aid 98% of baccalaureate students in nursing programs received some form of financial aid in 2009-10. *Gift aid (need-based):* Federal Pell, FSEOG, state, private, college/university gift aid from institutional funds, need-linked special talent scholarships, minority scholarships. *Loans:* Federal Nursing Student Loans, Federal Direct (Subsidized and Unsubsidized Stafford PLUS), Perkins, college/university, Minnesota SELF Loans, private alternative loans. *Work-study:* Federal Work-Study, part-time campus jobs. *Financial aid application deadline (priority):* 3/1.
Contact Debbie Anderson, Office Assistant, Department of Nursing, Augustana College, 2001 South Summit Avenue, Sioux Falls, SD 57197. *Telephone:* 605-274-4721. *Fax:* 605-274-4723. *E-mail:* debbie.anderson@augie.edu.

Dakota Wesleyan University

Nursing Department
Mitchell, South Dakota

Founded in 1885

DEGREE • BA

Library Facilities 78,928 volumes; 1,100 periodical subscriptions.

BACCALAUREATE PROGRAMS

Degree BA
Available Programs RN Baccalaureate.
Program Entrance Requirements CPR certification, immunizations, RN licensure. Transfer students are accepted.
Contact Adele Jacobson, RN-BAN Completion Program Director. *Telephone:* 605-352-2662. *E-mail:* adjacobs@dwu.edu.

Mount Marty College

Nursing Program
Yankton, South Dakota

http://www.mtmc.edu
Founded in 1936

DEGREE • BSN

Nursing Program Faculty 13 (15% with doctorates).
Baccalaureate Enrollment 89 **Women** 89% **Men** 11% **Minority** 7% **Part-time** 2%
Nursing Student Activities Sigma Theta Tau, Student Nurses' Association, nursing club.
Nursing Student Resources Academic advising; academic or career counseling; assistance for students with disabilities; bookstore; campus computer network; career placement assistance; computer lab; computer-

assisted instruction; daycare for children of students; e-mail services; employment services for current students; externships; housing assistance; interactive nursing skills videos; Internet; learning resource lab; library services; nursing audiovisuals; paid internships; placement services for program completers; remedial services; resume preparation assistance; skills, simulation, or other laboratory; tutoring; unpaid internships.
Library Facilities 76,571 volumes (8,750 in health, 5,350 in nursing); 424 periodical subscriptions (85 health-care related).

BACCALAUREATE PROGRAMS

Degree BSN
Available Programs ADN to Baccalaureate; Accelerated LPN to Baccalaureate; Generic Baccalaureate; International Nurse to Baccalaureate; LPN to Baccalaureate; LPN to RN Baccalaureate; RN Baccalaureate.
Site Options Watertown, SD.
Study Options Full-time and part-time.
Program Entrance Requirements Minimum overall college GPA of 2.7, transcript of college record, CPR certification, health exam, health insurance, high school transcript, immunizations, minimum GPA in nursing prerequisites of 2.0, prerequisite course work. Transfer students are accepted. *Application deadline:* Applications may be processed on a rolling basis for some programs.
Advanced Placement Credit given for nursing courses completed elsewhere dependent upon specific evaluations.
Contact ***Telephone:*** 605-668-1594. *Fax:* 605-668-1607.

National American University
School of Nursing
Rapid City, South Dakota

Founded in 1941

DEGREE • BSN

Library Facilities 31,018 volumes; 268 periodical subscriptions.

BACCALAUREATE PROGRAMS

Degree BSN
Available Programs Generic Baccalaureate.
Contact Dodie Serafini, RN, Nursing Program Chair, School of Nursing, National American University, Denver, CO 80222. *Telephone:* 303-876-7181. *Fax:* 303-876-7105. *E-mail:* dserafini@national.edu.

Presentation College
Department of Nursing
Aberdeen, South Dakota

http://www.presentation.edu
Founded in 1951

DEGREE • BSN

Nursing Program Faculty 21 (9% with doctorates).
Baccalaureate Enrollment 185 **Women** 95% **Men** 5% **Minority** 4% **Part-time** 24%
Distance Learning Courses Available.
Nursing Student Activities Nursing Honor Society, Sigma Theta Tau, Student Nurses' Association, nursing club.
Nursing Student Resources Academic advising; academic or career counseling; assistance for students with disabilities; bookstore; campus computer network; career placement assistance; computer lab; computer-assisted instruction; e-mail services; employment services for current students; externships; interactive nursing skills videos; Internet; learning resource lab; library services; nursing audiovisuals; placement services for program completers; remedial services; resume preparation assistance; skills, simulation, or other laboratory; tutoring; unpaid internships.
Library Facilities 40,000 volumes (378 in health, 353 in nursing); 44,215 periodical subscriptions (2,172 health-care related).

BACCALAUREATE PROGRAMS

Degree BSN
Available Programs ADN to Baccalaureate; Baccalaureate for Second Degree; Generic Baccalaureate; LPN to RN Baccalaureate; RN Baccalaureate.
Site Options Fargo , ND; Fairmont, MN.
Study Options Full-time and part-time.
Online Degree Options Yes.
Program Entrance Requirements Minimum overall college GPA of 2.5, transcript of college record, CPR certification, written essay, health exam, high school biology, high school chemistry, 2 years high school math, high school transcript, immunizations, 2 letters of recommendation, minimum high school GPA of 2.7, minimum GPA in nursing prerequisites of 2.5, prerequisite course work. Transfer students are accepted. *Application deadline:* 3/1 (fall).
Advanced Placement Credit by examination available. Credit given for nursing courses completed elsewhere dependent upon specific evaluations.
Expenses (2009-10) *Tuition:* full-time $14,250; part-time $525 per credit hour. *Room and board:* $5500; room only: $4100 per academic year. *Required fees:* full-time $1331; part-time $333 per term.
Financial Aid 91% of baccalaureate students in nursing programs received some form of financial aid in 2008-09.
Contact Ms. JoEllen Lindner, Dean of Admissions, Department of Nursing, Presentation College, 1500 North Main Street, Aberdeen, SD 57401. *Telephone:* 605-229-8492. *Fax:* 605-229-8489. *E-mail:* lindnerjo@presentation.edu.

South Dakota State University
College of Nursing
Brookings, South Dakota

http://www.sdstate.org/Academics/CollegeOfNursing/
Founded in 1881

DEGREES • BS • MS • PHD

Nursing Program Faculty 127 (22% with doctorates).
Baccalaureate Enrollment 553 **Women** 82% **Men** 18% **Minority** 4%
Graduate Enrollment 166 **Women** 96% **Men** 4% **Minority** 2% **Part-time** 100%
Distance Learning Courses Available.
Nursing Student Activities Sigma Theta Tau, Student Nurses' Association, nursing club.
Nursing Student Resources Academic advising; academic or career counseling; assistance for students with disabilities; bookstore; campus computer network; career placement assistance; computer lab; computer-assisted instruction; e-mail services; employment services for current students; externships; interactive nursing skills videos; Internet; learning resource lab; library services; nursing audiovisuals; paid internships; placement services for program completers; remedial services; resume preparation assistance; skills, simulation, or other laboratory; tutoring.
Library Facilities 926,000 volumes (20,000 in health, 5,700 in nursing); 44,579 periodical subscriptions (4,402 health-care related).

BACCALAUREATE PROGRAMS

Degree BS
Available Programs Accelerated Baccalaureate; Generic Baccalaureate; RN Baccalaureate.
Site Options Rapid City, SD; Sioux Falls, SD.
Study Options Full-time.
Online Degree Options Yes.
Program Entrance Requirements Minimum overall college GPA of 2.7, transcript of college record, CPR certification, health exam, health insurance, immunizations, interview, minimum GPA in nursing prerequisites of 2.7, professional liability insurance/malpractice insurance, prerequisite course work. Transfer students are accepted. *Application deadline:* 1/25 (fall), 9/25 (spring).
Advanced Placement Credit given for nursing courses completed elsewhere dependent upon specific evaluations.
Expenses (2009-10) *Tuition, state resident:* part-time $92 per credit. *Tuition, nonresident:* part-time $291 per credit. *Room and board:* $5668; room only: $2540 per academic year. *Required fees:* part-time $236 per credit; part-time $460 per term.
Financial Aid 86% of baccalaureate students in nursing programs received some form of financial aid in 2008-09. *Gift aid (need-based):* Federal Pell, FSEOG, state, private, college/university gift aid from institutional funds, United Negro College Fund, Federal Nursing, Academic Competitiveness Grants, National SMART Grants, TEACH Grants, TRiO Scholarships. *Loans:* Federal Nursing Student Loans, Federal Direct (Subsidized and Unsubsidized Stafford PLUS), Perkins, college/university, Health Professions Loans, private alternative loans. *Work-study:* Federal Work-Study, part-time campus jobs. *Financial aid application deadline (priority):* 3/11.

Contact Dr. Janet Lord, Undergraduate Department Head, College of Nursing, South Dakota State University, Box 2275, SNF 327, Brookings, SD 57007-0098. *Telephone:* 605-688-6153. *Fax:* 605-688-6523. *E-mail:* Janet.Lord@sdstate.edu.

GRADUATE PROGRAMS

Expenses (2009-10) *Tuition, state resident:* part-time $139 per credit. *Tuition, nonresident:* part-time $294 per credit. *Required fees:* part-time $123 per credit; part-time $185 per term.
Financial Aid 86% of graduate students in nursing programs received some form of financial aid in 2008-09. 2 fellowships, 1 research assistantship, 3 teaching assistantships were awarded; career-related internships or fieldwork, Federal Work-Study, scholarships, and unspecified assistantships also available.
Contact Dr. Sandra Bunkers, Department Head, College of Nursing, South Dakota State University, Box 2275, Rotunda Lane, NFA 217, Brookings, SD 57007-0098. *Telephone:* 605-688-4114. *Fax:* 605-688-5827. *E-mail:* sandra.bunkers@sdstate.edu.

MASTER'S DEGREE PROGRAM

Degree MS
Available Programs Master's; RN to Master's.
Concentrations Available Clinical nurse leader; nursing administration; nursing education. *Nurse practitioner programs in:* family health, neonatal health, psychiatric/mental health.
Site Options Rapid City, SD; Sioux Falls, SD.
Study Options Full-time and part-time.
Online Degree Options Yes.
Program Entrance Requirements Clinical experience, minimum overall college GPA of 3.0, transcript of college record, CPR certification, written essay, immunizations, 3 letters of recommendation, professional liability insurance/malpractice insurance, statistics course. *Application deadline:* 3/1 (fall). *Application fee:* $200.
Advanced Placement Credit given for nursing courses completed elsewhere dependent upon specific evaluations.
Degree Requirements 48 total credit hours, thesis or project, comprehensive exam.

POST-MASTER'S PROGRAM

Areas of Study Nursing education. *Nurse practitioner programs in:* family health.

DOCTORAL DEGREE PROGRAM

Degree PhD
Available Programs Doctorate.
Areas of Study Nursing research.
Site Options Sioux Falls, SD.
Program Entrance Requirements Minimum overall college GPA of 3.3, interview by faculty committee, 4 letters of recommendation, MSN or equivalent, scholarly papers, vita, writing sample. Application deadline: 3/1 (fall).
Degree Requirements 60 total credit hours, dissertation, oral exam, written exam.

CONTINUING EDUCATION PROGRAM

Contact Dr. Roberta K. Olson, Dean, College of Nursing, South Dakota State University, Box 2275, SNF 255, Brookings, SD 57007-0098. *Telephone:* 605-688-5178. *Fax:* 605-688-5745. *E-mail:* Roberta.Olson@sdstate.edu.

TENNESSEE

Aquinas College
Department of Nursing
Nashville, Tennessee

http://www.aquinas-tn.edu/nursing/index.htm
Founded in 1961

DEGREE • BSN
Nursing Student Resources Library services.
Library Facilities 71,339 volumes; 13,602 periodical subscriptions.

BACCALAUREATE PROGRAMS

Degree BSN
Available Programs RN Baccalaureate.
Program Entrance Requirements Interview, 2 letters of recommendation, RN licensure.
Advanced Placement Credit given for nursing courses completed elsewhere dependent upon specific evaluations.
Contact *Telephone:* 615-222-4038.

Austin Peay State University
School of Nursing
Clarksville, Tennessee

http://www.apsu.edu/nursing01
Founded in 1927

DEGREE • BSN
Nursing Program Faculty 20 (20% with doctorates).
Baccalaureate Enrollment 250
Nursing Student Activities Nursing Honor Society, Sigma Theta Tau, Student Nurses' Association.
Nursing Student Resources Academic advising; computer lab; computer-assisted instruction; interactive nursing skills videos; Internet; nursing audiovisuals; skills, simulation, or other laboratory.
Library Facilities 416,874 volumes (8,249 in health, 1,111 in nursing); 29,666 periodical subscriptions (146 health-care related).

BACCALAUREATE PROGRAMS

Degree BSN
Available Programs Generic Baccalaureate; RN Baccalaureate.
Study Options Full-time.
Program Entrance Requirements Minimum overall college GPA of 3.0, transcript of college record, CPR certification, health insurance, immunizations, minimum GPA in nursing prerequisites of 3.0, prerequisite course work. Transfer students are accepted. *Application deadline:* 5/1 (fall), 9/1 (spring).
Contact *Telephone:* 931-221-7708. *Fax:* 931-221-7595.

Baptist College of Health Sciences
Nursing Division
Memphis, Tennessee

Founded in 1994

DEGREE • BSN
Nursing Program Faculty 40 (20% with doctorates).
Baccalaureate Enrollment 731 **Women** 89% **Men** 11% **Minority** 43% **Part-time** 45%
Distance Learning Courses Available.
Nursing Student Activities Sigma Theta Tau, Student Nurses' Association.
Nursing Student Resources Academic advising; academic or career counseling; assistance for students with disabilities; bookstore; campus computer network; computer lab; computer-assisted instruction; e-mail services; employment services for current students; externships; housing assistance; interactive nursing skills videos; Internet; learning resource lab; library services; nursing audiovisuals; paid internships; placement services for program completers; resume preparation assistance; skills, simulation, or other laboratory; tutoring.
Library Facilities 14,547 volumes (2,573 in health, 1,790 in nursing); 260 periodical subscriptions (213 health-care related).

BACCALAUREATE PROGRAMS

Degree BSN
Available Programs Generic Baccalaureate; LPN to Baccalaureate; RN Baccalaureate.
Study Options Full-time and part-time.
Program Entrance Requirements Minimum overall college GPA of 2.5, CPR certification, health exam, health insurance, 2 years high school math, 2 years high school science, high school transcript, immunizations, 3 letters of recommendation, minimum high school GPA of 2.75. Transfer students are accepted. *Application deadline:* 6/1 (fall), 11/1 (spring). *Application fee:* $25.

Contact *Telephone:* 901-572-2441. *Fax:* 901-572-2461.

Belmont University
School of Nursing
Nashville, Tennessee

http://www.belmont.edu/nursing
Founded in 1951

DEGREES • BSN • MSN
Nursing Program Faculty 65 (19% with doctorates).
Baccalaureate Enrollment 406 **Women** 84% **Men** 16% **Minority** 6% **International** 3% **Part-time** 8%
Graduate Enrollment 43 **Women** 98% **Men** 2% **Minority** 12% **International** 2% **Part-time** 63%
Nursing Student Activities Nursing Honor Society, Sigma Theta Tau, Student Nurses' Association.
Nursing Student Resources Academic advising; academic or career counseling; assistance for students with disabilities; bookstore; campus computer network; career placement assistance; computer lab; computer-assisted instruction; e-mail services; employment services for current students; externships; housing assistance; interactive nursing skills videos; Internet; learning resource lab; library services; nursing audiovisuals; placement services for program completers; remedial services; resume preparation assistance; skills, simulation, or other laboratory; tutoring.
Library Facilities 220,637 volumes (6,000 in health, 800 in nursing); 1,072 periodical subscriptions (7,500 health-care related).

BACCALAUREATE PROGRAMS

Degree BSN
Available Programs ADN to Baccalaureate; Accelerated Baccalaureate; Accelerated Baccalaureate for Second Degree; Baccalaureate for Second Degree; Generic Baccalaureate; LPN to RN Baccalaureate; RN Baccalaureate.
Study Options Full-time and part-time.
Program Entrance Requirements Minimum overall college GPA of 2.5, transcript of college record, CPR certification, written essay, health exam, health insurance, high school biology, high school chemistry, 3 years high school math, 3 years high school science, high school transcript, immunizations, 1 letter of recommendation, minimum high school GPA of 2.5, minimum GPA in nursing prerequisites of 3.0. Transfer students are accepted. *Application deadline:* Applications may be processed on a rolling basis for some programs. *Application fee:* $50.
Advanced Placement Credit by examination available. Credit given for nursing courses completed elsewhere dependent upon specific evaluations.
Expenses (2009-10) *Tuition:* full-time $21,270; part-time $820 per credit hour. *International tuition:* $21,270 full-time. *Room and board:* $8470; room only: $4600 per academic year. *Required fees:* full-time $1090; part-time $545 per term.
Financial Aid 85% of baccalaureate students in nursing programs received some form of financial aid in 2008-09. *Gift aid (need-based):* Federal Pell, FSEOG, state, private, college/university gift aid from institutional funds. *Loans:* Federal Direct PLUS), Perkins, college/university. *Work-study:* Federal Work-Study. *Financial aid application deadline (priority):* 3/1.
Contact Mrs. Maren Bishop, Admissions Assistant, School of Nursing, Belmont University, 1900 Belmont Boulevard, Nashville, TN 37212-3757. *Telephone:* 615-460-6120. *Fax:* 615-460-6125. *E-mail:* maren.bishop@mail.belmont.edu.

GRADUATE PROGRAMS

Expenses (2009-10) *Tuition:* part-time $860 per credit hour. *Room and board:* $8470; room only: $4600 per academic year.
Financial Aid 95% of graduate students in nursing programs received some form of financial aid in 2008-09. Scholarships and traineeships available. *Financial aid application deadline:* 3/1.
Contact Dr. Leslie Higgins, Director, Graduate Program, School of Nursing, Belmont University, 1900 Belmont Boulevard, Nashville, TN 37212-3757. *Telephone:* 615-460-6027. *Fax:* 615-460-6125. *E-mail:* leslie.higgins@mail.belmont.edu.

MASTER'S DEGREE PROGRAM

Degree MSN
Available Programs Master's.
Concentrations Available Nursing education. *Nurse practitioner programs in:* family health.
Study Options Full-time and part-time.
Program Entrance Requirements Clinical experience, minimum overall college GPA of 3.0, transcript of college record, CPR certification, written essay, immunizations, interview, 2 letters of recommendation, resume, GRE. *Application fee:* $50.
Advanced Placement Credit given for nursing courses completed elsewhere dependent upon specific evaluations.
Degree Requirements 41 total credit hours, comprehensive exam.

POST-MASTER'S PROGRAM

Areas of Study Nursing education. *Nurse practitioner programs in:* family health.

Bethel University
Nursing Program
McKenzie, Tennessee

http://www.bethelu.edu/
Founded in 1842

DEGREE • BSN
Nursing Program Faculty 7
Baccalaureate Enrollment 25 **Women** 70% **Men** 30% **Minority** .8% **International** .4%
Nursing Student Activities Student Nurses' Association.
Nursing Student Resources Academic advising; academic or career counseling; assistance for students with disabilities; bookstore; campus computer network; career placement assistance; computer lab; computer-assisted instruction; e-mail services; housing assistance; interactive nursing skills videos; Internet; learning resource lab; library services; nursing audiovisuals; remedial services; resume preparation assistance; skills, simulation, or other laboratory; tutoring.
Library Facilities 45,000 volumes (1,146 in nursing); 111,700 periodical subscriptions (99 health-care related).

BACCALAUREATE PROGRAMS

Degree BSN
Available Programs Generic Baccalaureate.
Study Options Full-time.
Program Entrance Requirements Minimum overall college GPA of 2.75, transcript of college record, CPR certification, health exam, health insurance, immunizations, minimum GPA in nursing prerequisites of 2.0, professional liability insurance/malpractice insurance, prerequisite course work. Transfer students are accepted. *Application deadline:* 3/1 (spring). *Application fee:* $25.
Advanced Placement Credit given for nursing courses completed elsewhere dependent upon specific evaluations.
Expenses (2010-11) *Tuition:* full-time $11,592. *Room and board:* $3463 per academic year. *Required fees:* full-time $500.
Financial Aid 80% of baccalaureate students in nursing programs received some form of financial aid in 2009-10.
Contact Ms. Mary Bess Griffith, Director, Nursing Program, Bethel University, 325 Cherry Avenue, McKenzie, TN 38201. *Telephone:* 731-352-6768. *Fax:* 731-352-6772. *E-mail:* griffithmb@bethelu.edu.

Carson-Newman College
Department of Nursing
Jefferson City, Tennessee

http://www.cn.edu/
Founded in 1851

DEGREES • BSN • MSN
Nursing Program Faculty 15 (47% with doctorates).
Baccalaureate Enrollment 114 **Women** 89% **Men** 11% **Minority** 16% **International** 1%
Graduate Enrollment 50 **Women** 80% **Men** 20% **Minority** 6% **Part-time** 58%
Distance Learning Courses Available.
Nursing Student Activities Sigma Theta Tau, Student Nurses' Association.
Nursing Student Resources Academic advising; academic or career counseling; assistance for students with disabilities; bookstore; campus computer network; career placement assistance; computer lab; computer-assisted instruction; e-mail services; employment services for current stu-

dents; externships; housing assistance; interactive nursing skills videos; Internet; learning resource lab; library services; nursing audiovisuals; placement services for program completers; remedial services; resume preparation assistance; skills, simulation, or other laboratory; tutoring; unpaid internships.
Library Facilities 218,371 volumes (6,497 in health, 5,419 in nursing); 3,966 periodical subscriptions (3,481 health-care related).

BACCALAUREATE PROGRAMS

Degree BSN
Available Programs Accelerated Baccalaureate; Accelerated Baccalaureate for Second Degree; Generic Baccalaureate; LPN to RN Baccalaureate; RN Baccalaureate.
Study Options Full-time.
Online Degree Options Yes.
Program Entrance Requirements Minimum overall college GPA of 2.75, transcript of college record, health exam, high school transcript, immunizations, minimum GPA in nursing prerequisites of 2.75, prerequisite course work. Transfer students are accepted. *Application deadline:* 3/1 (fall), 9/1 (spring), 3/1 (summer). Applications may be processed on a rolling basis for some programs.
Advanced Placement Credit given for nursing courses completed elsewhere dependent upon specific evaluations.
Expenses (2010-11) *Tuition:* full-time $19,628; part-time $818 per credit hour. *Room and board:* $7680; room only: $4208 per academic year. *Required fees:* full-time $2064; part-time $824 per term.
Financial Aid 95% of baccalaureate students in nursing programs received some form of financial aid in 2009-10. *Gift aid (need-based):* Federal Pell, FSEOG, state, private, college/university gift aid from institutional funds. *Loans:* Perkins, state, college/university, alternative loans. *Work-study:* Federal Work-Study, part-time campus jobs. *Financial aid application deadline (priority):* 4/1.
Contact Dr. Gregory A. Casalenuovo, Chair, Undergraduate Studies in Nursing, Department of Nursing, Carson-Newman College, 1646 Russell Avenue, C-N Box 71883, Jefferson City, TN 37760. *Telephone:* 865-471-3236. *Fax:* 865-471-4574. *E-mail:* gcasalenuovo@cn.edu.

GRADUATE PROGRAMS

Expenses (2010-11) *Tuition:* full-time $8730; part-time $485 per credit hour. *Room and board:* $7700; room only: $4200 per academic year. *Required fees:* full-time $264; part-time $154 per term.
Financial Aid 100% of graduate students in nursing programs received some form of financial aid in 2009-10.
Contact Dr. Kimberly S. Bolton, Chair, Graduate Studies in Nursing, Department of Nursing, Carson-Newman College, 1646 Russell Avenue, C-N Box 71883, Jefferson City, TN 37760. *Telephone:* 865-471-4056. *Fax:* 865-471-4574. *E-mail:* kbolton@cn.edu.

MASTER'S DEGREE PROGRAM

Degree MSN
Available Programs Master's; RN to Master's.
Concentrations Available Nursing education. *Nurse practitioner programs in:* family health.
Study Options Full-time and part-time.
Program Entrance Requirements Minimum overall college GPA of 3.0, transcript of college record, written essay, interview, 3 letters of recommendation. *Application deadline:* 4/15 (fall), 10/15 (spring), 3/15 (summer). Applications may be processed on a rolling basis for some programs. *Application fee:* $50.
Advanced Placement Credit given for nursing courses completed elsewhere dependent upon specific evaluations.
Degree Requirements 45 total credit hours, thesis or project, comprehensive exam.

POST-MASTER'S PROGRAM

Areas of Study Nursing education. *Nurse practitioner programs in:* family health.

Cumberland University
Rudy School of Nursing and Health Professions
Lebanon, Tennessee

http://www.cumberland.edu/academics/nursing/index.html
Founded in 1842

DEGREE • BSN

Nursing Program Faculty 12 (25% with doctorates).
Baccalaureate Enrollment 276 **Women** 90% **Men** 10% **Minority** 3% **International** .5% **Part-time** .5%
Nursing Student Activities Sigma Theta Tau, Student Nurses' Association.
Nursing Student Resources Academic advising; academic or career counseling; assistance for students with disabilities; bookstore; campus computer network; career placement assistance; computer lab; computer-assisted instruction; e-mail services; housing assistance; interactive nursing skills videos; Internet; learning resource lab; library services; nursing audiovisuals; remedial services; resume preparation assistance; skills, simulation, or other laboratory; tutoring.
Library Facilities 75,000 volumes (125 in health, 66 in nursing); 335 periodical subscriptions (25 health-care related).

BACCALAUREATE PROGRAMS

Degree BSN
Available Programs ADN to Baccalaureate; Accelerated Baccalaureate; Accelerated Baccalaureate for Second Degree; Baccalaureate for Second Degree; Generic Baccalaureate; LPN to Baccalaureate; LPN to RN Baccalaureate; RN Baccalaureate.
Site Options Mt. Juliet, TN.
Study Options Full-time and part-time.
Program Entrance Requirements Minimum overall college GPA of 3.0, transcript of college record, CPR certification, health exam, health insurance, high school transcript, immunizations, minimum high school GPA of 2.75, minimum GPA in nursing prerequisites of 3.0, professional liability insurance/malpractice insurance, prerequisite course work. Transfer students are accepted. *Application deadline:* 6/1 (fall), 10/1 (winter), 2/1 (summer). Applications may be processed on a rolling basis for some programs. *Application fee:* $25.
Advanced Placement Credit by examination available. Credit given for nursing courses completed elsewhere dependent upon specific evaluations.
Expenses (2010-11) *Tuition:* full-time $17,356; part-time $723 per credit hour. *Room and board:* $6160; room only: $5630 per academic year. *Required fees:* full-time $1800; part-time $275 per credit; part-time $125 per term.
Financial Aid 95% of baccalaureate students in nursing programs received some form of financial aid in 2009-10.
Contact Dr. Carole Ann Bach, Professor and Dean, Rudy School of Nursing and Health Professions, Cumberland University, One Cumberland Square, McFarland Campus, Lebanon, TN 37087-3554. *Telephone:* 615-547-1200. *Fax:* 615-449-1368. *E-mail:* cbach@cumberland.edu.

East Tennessee State University
College of Nursing
Johnson City, Tennessee

http://www.etsu.edu/nursing
Founded in 1911

DEGREES • BSN • MSN • PHD

Nursing Program Faculty 70 (36% with doctorates).
Baccalaureate Enrollment 630 **Women** 83% **Men** 17% **Minority** 7% **Part-time** 11%
Graduate Enrollment 217 **Women** 94% **Men** 6% **Minority** 2% **International** 1% **Part-time** 57%
Distance Learning Courses Available.
Nursing Student Activities Sigma Theta Tau, Student Nurses' Association.
Nursing Student Resources Academic advising; academic or career counseling; assistance for students with disabilities; bookstore; campus computer network; career placement assistance; computer lab; computer-assisted instruction; daycare for children of students; e-mail services; employment services for current students; externships; housing assistance; interactive nursing skills videos; Internet; learning resource lab; library services; nursing audiovisuals; remedial services; resume preparation assistance; skills, simulation, or other laboratory; tutoring.
Library Facilities 1.1 million volumes; 3,714 periodical subscriptions.

BACCALAUREATE PROGRAMS

Degree BSN
Available Programs ADN to Baccalaureate; Accelerated Baccalaureate for Second Degree; Accelerated RN Baccalaureate; Generic Baccalaureate; LPN to Baccalaureate; RN Baccalaureate.

Site Options Pellissippi, TN; Sevierville, TN; Cleveland and Kingsport, TN.
Study Options Full-time and part-time.
Online Degree Options Yes.
Program Entrance Requirements Minimum overall college GPA of 2.6, transcript of college record, minimum GPA in nursing prerequisites of 2.6, prerequisite course work. Transfer students are accepted. *Application deadline:* 10/1 (fall), 2/1 (spring).
Advanced Placement Credit given for nursing courses completed elsewhere dependent upon specific evaluations.
Expenses (2010-11) *Tuition, state resident:* full-time $3001; part-time $1500 per semester. *Tuition, nonresident:* full-time $9800; part-time $4700 per semester. *Room and board:* $2964; room only: $1825 per academic year. *Required fees:* full-time $700.
Financial Aid 95% of baccalaureate students in nursing programs received some form of financial aid in 2009-10.
Contact Mr. Scott Vaughn, Director, Student Services, College of Nursing, East Tennessee State University, PO Box 70664, Office of Student Services, Johnson City, TN 37614. *Telephone:* 423-439-4578. *Fax:* 423-439-4522. *E-mail:* nursing@etsu.edu.

GRADUATE PROGRAMS

Expenses (2010-11) *Tuition, state resident:* full-time $3850; part-time $1920 per semester. *Tuition, nonresident:* full-time $9750; part-time $4875 per semester. *Room and board:* $2740; room only: $1650 per academic year. *Required fees:* full-time $700; part-time $100 per credit; part-time $350 per term.
Financial Aid 90% of graduate students in nursing programs received some form of financial aid in 2009-10. 6 research assistantships with full tuition reimbursements available (averaging $5,500 per year), 4 teaching assistantships with full tuition reimbursements available (averaging $5,500 per year) were awarded; career-related internships or fieldwork, traineeships, and unspecified assistantships also available. Aid available to part-time students. *Financial aid application deadline:* 7/1.
Contact Ms. Amy Bower, Coordinator, College of Nursing, East Tennessee State University, PO Box 70664, Office of Student Services, Johnson City, TN 37614. *Telephone:* 423-439-4531. *Fax:* 423-439-4522. *E-mail:* bowera@etsu.edu.

MASTER'S DEGREE PROGRAM

Degree MSN
Available Programs Master's; Master's for Nurses with Non-Nursing Degrees.
Concentrations Available Clinical nurse leader; nursing administration; nursing education; nursing informatics. *Nurse practitioner programs in:* adult health, family health, gerontology, psychiatric/mental health.
Study Options Full-time and part-time.
Online Degree Options Yes.
Program Entrance Requirements Minimum overall college GPA of 3.0, transcript of college record, written essay, 3 letters of recommendation, prerequisite course work, resume, GRE General Test. *Application deadline:* 2/1 (fall), 7/1 (spring), 12/1 (summer). *Application fee:* $25.
Advanced Placement Credit given for nursing courses completed elsewhere dependent upon specific evaluations.
Degree Requirements 48 total credit hours, comprehensive exam.

POST-MASTER'S PROGRAM

Areas of Study Health-care administration. *Nurse practitioner programs in:* adult health, family health, gerontology, psychiatric/mental health.

DOCTORAL DEGREE PROGRAM

Degree PhD
Available Programs Doctorate.
Areas of Study Individualized study.
Program Entrance Requirements Clinical experience, minimum overall college GPA of 3.0, interview by faculty committee, 3 letters of recommendation, MSN or equivalent, statistics course, vita, writing sample. Application deadline: 2/1 (spring). Application fee: $35.
Degree Requirements 62 total credit hours, dissertation, written exam, residency.

CONTINUING EDUCATION PROGRAM

Contact Dr. Joy Wachs, Professor and Coordinator, Continuing Education, College of Nursing, East Tennessee State University, 807 University Parkway, Box 70629, Johnson City, TN 37614-1709. *Telephone:* 423-439-4549. *Fax:* 423-439-4100. *E-mail:* wadhs@etsu.edu.

King College

School of Nursing
Bristol, Tennessee

Founded in 1867

DEGREES • BSN • MSN • MSN/MBA

Nursing Program Faculty 31 (26% with doctorates).
Baccalaureate Enrollment 366 **Women** 96% **Men** 4% **Minority** 1% **International** 1%
Graduate Enrollment 35 **Women** 99% **Men** 1% **Minority** 1%
Distance Learning Courses Available.
Nursing Student Activities Student Nurses' Association.
Nursing Student Resources Academic advising; academic or career counseling; assistance for students with disabilities; bookstore; campus computer network; career placement assistance; computer lab; computer-assisted instruction; e-mail services; employment services for current students; externships; interactive nursing skills videos; Internet; learning resource lab; library services; nursing audiovisuals; paid internships; remedial services; resume preparation assistance; skills, simulation, or other laboratory; tutoring.
Library Facilities 97,836 volumes (929 in health, 158 in nursing); 352 periodical subscriptions (87 health-care related).

BACCALAUREATE PROGRAMS

Degree BSN
Available Programs Accelerated RN Baccalaureate; Generic Baccalaureate.
Site Options Kingsport, TN.
Study Options Full-time.
Program Entrance Requirements Minimum overall college GPA of 2.0, transcript of college record, CPR certification, written essay, health exam, health insurance, high school biology, high school chemistry, high school foreign language, 2 years high school math, 2 years high school science, high school transcript, immunizations, minimum high school GPA of 2.6, minimum high school rank 25%, minimum GPA in nursing prerequisites of 2.75. Transfer students are accepted. *Application deadline:* 6/1 (fall). *Application fee:* $100.
Expenses (2009-10) *Tuition:* full-time $21,880. *Room and board:* $7418; room only: $3726 per academic year. *Required fees:* full-time $600.
Financial Aid 90% of baccalaureate students in nursing programs received some form of financial aid in 2008-09. *Gift aid (need-based):* Federal Pell, FSEOG, state, private, college/university gift aid from institutional funds. *Loans:* Perkins, college/university. *Work-study:* Federal Work-Study, part-time campus jobs. *Financial aid application deadline (priority):* 3/1.
Contact Dr. Jane E. Castle, Interim Dean and Professor, School of Nursing, King College, 1350 King College Road, Bristol, TN 37620. *Telephone:* 423-652-4841. *Fax:* 423-652-4833. *E-mail:* jecastle@king.edu.

GRADUATE PROGRAMS

Expenses (2009-10) *Tuition:* part-time $3300 per semester.
Financial Aid 100% of graduate students in nursing programs received some form of financial aid in 2008-09.
Contact Dr. Jane E. Castle, Interim Dean and Professor, School of Nursing, King College, 1350 King College Road, Bristol, TN 37620. *Telephone:* 423-652-4841. *Fax:* 423-652-4833. *E-mail:* jecastle@king.edu.

MASTER'S DEGREE PROGRAM

Degrees MSN; MSN/MBA
Available Programs Accelerated RN to Master's; Master's.
Concentrations Available *Clinical nurse specialist programs in:* acute care, adult health, oncology.
Study Options Full-time.
Program Entrance Requirements Clinical experience, computer literacy, minimum overall college GPA of 3.0, transcript of college record, CPR certification, written essay, immunizations, 2 letters of recommendation, nursing research course, physical assessment course, resume, statistics course. *Application deadline:* 4/15 (fall). *Application fee:* $100.
Degree Requirements 39 total credit hours, thesis or project.

Lincoln Memorial University
Caylor School of Nursing
Harrogate, Tennessee

http://www.lmunet.edu/academics/undergrad/nursing/
Founded in 1897

DEGREE • BSN
Nursing Program Faculty 7 (57% with doctorates).
Nursing Student Activities Student Nurses' Association.
Nursing Student Resources Academic advising; academic or career counseling; bookstore; campus computer network; career placement assistance; computer lab; e-mail services; externships; interactive nursing skills videos; Internet; learning resource lab; library services; nursing audiovisuals; other; placement services for program completers; skills, simulation, or other laboratory; tutoring.
Library Facilities 199,892 volumes (1,230 in health, 630 in nursing); 334 periodical subscriptions (36 health-care related).

BACCALAUREATE PROGRAMS
Degree BSN
Available Programs RN Baccalaureate.
Site Options Knoxville, TN.
Program Entrance Requirements Minimum overall college GPA of 2.25, transcript of college record, CPR certification, immunizations, 3 letters of recommendation, professional liability insurance/malpractice insurance, prerequisite course work, RN licensure. Transfer students are accepted.
Advanced Placement Credit given for nursing courses completed elsewhere dependent upon specific evaluations.
Contact *Telephone:* 423-869-3611. *Fax:* 423-869-6444.

Lipscomb University
Department of Nursing
Nashville, Tennessee

Founded in 1891

DEGREE • BSN
Library Facilities 253,398 volumes; 850 periodical subscriptions.

BACCALAUREATE PROGRAMS
Degree BSN
Available Programs Generic Baccalaureate.
Contact Sonya Colvert, Department of Nursing, Lipscomb University, One University Park Drive, Nashville, TN 37204-3951. *Telephone:* 615-996-6650. *E-mail:* sonya.colvert@lipscomb.edu.

Martin Methodist College
Division of Nursing
Pulaski, Tennessee

http://martinmethodist.edu/
Founded in 1870

DEGREE • BSN
Nursing Program Faculty 7 (60% with doctorates).
Baccalaureate Enrollment 33 **Women** 96% **Men** 4% **Minority** 11.5%
Nursing Student Activities Student Nurses' Association.
Nursing Student Resources Academic advising; academic or career counseling; bookstore; campus computer network; career placement assistance; computer lab; computer-assisted instruction; e-mail services; employment services for current students; housing assistance; interactive nursing skills videos; Internet; learning resource lab; library services; nursing audiovisuals; placement services for program completers; remedial services; resume preparation assistance; skills, simulation, or other laboratory; tutoring; unpaid internships.
Library Facilities 84,000 volumes (875 in nursing); 664 periodical subscriptions (400 health-care related).

BACCALAUREATE PROGRAMS
Degree BSN
Available Programs Generic Baccalaureate.
Study Options Full-time.
Program Entrance Requirements CPR certification, health insurance, immunizations, prerequisite course work. Transfer students are accepted. *Application deadline:* 2/1 (fall), 2/1 (winter). *Application fee:* $30.
Expenses (2010-11) *Tuition:* full-time $18,998; part-time $790 per credit. *Room and board:* $6700 per academic year. *Required fees:* full-time $750.
Contact Dr. Kenneth R. Burns, Professor and Chair, Division of Nursing, Martin Methodist College, 433 West Madison Street, Pulaski, TN 38478. *Telephone:* 931-424-7395. *Fax:* 931-363-9891. *E-mail:* kburns@martinmethodist.edu.

Middle Tennessee State University
School of Nursing
Murfreesboro, Tennessee

http://www.mtsu.edu/~nursing/
Founded in 1911

DEGREES • BSN • MSN
Nursing Program Faculty 45 (60% with doctorates).
Baccalaureate Enrollment 300 **Women** 85% **Men** 15% **Minority** 15%
Graduate Enrollment 100 **Women** 80% **Men** 20% **Minority** 15% **Part-time** 50%
Distance Learning Courses Available.
Nursing Student Activities Sigma Theta Tau, Student Nurses' Association.
Nursing Student Resources Academic advising; academic or career counseling; assistance for students with disabilities; bookstore; campus computer network; career placement assistance; computer lab; computer-assisted instruction; e-mail services; interactive nursing skills videos; Internet; learning resource lab; library services; nursing audiovisuals; remedial services; resume preparation assistance; skills, simulation, or other laboratory; tutoring.
Library Facilities 100 volumes in health, 45 volumes in nursing; 100 periodical subscriptions health-care related.

BACCALAUREATE PROGRAMS
Degree BSN
Available Programs Generic Baccalaureate; LPN to RN Baccalaureate; RN Baccalaureate.
Study Options Full-time.
Online Degree Options Yes.
Program Entrance Requirements Minimum overall college GPA of 2.80, transcript of college record, CPR certification, health insurance, immunizations, interview, minimum GPA in nursing prerequisites of 2.0, professional liability insurance/malpractice insurance, prerequisite course work. Transfer students are accepted. *Application deadline:* 2/1 (fall), 10/1 (spring).
Advanced Placement Credit by examination available. Credit given for nursing courses completed elsewhere dependent upon specific evaluations.
Contact Dr. Lynn C. Parsons, RN, Professor and Director, School of Nursing, Middle Tennessee State University, PO Box 81, 1301 East Main Street, Murfreesboro, TN 37132-0001. *Telephone:* 615-898-2437. *Fax:* 615-898-5441. *E-mail:* lparsons@mtsu.edu.

GRADUATE PROGRAMS
Contact Lynn C. Parsons, RN, Professor and Director, School of Nursing, Middle Tennessee State University, PO Box 81, 1301 East Main Street, Murfreesboro, TN 37132-0001. *Telephone:* 615-898-2437. *Fax:* 615-898-5441. *E-mail:* lparsons@mtsu.edu.

MASTER'S DEGREE PROGRAM
Degree MSN
Available Programs Accelerated AD/RN to Master's; Master's.
Concentrations Available Nursing administration; nursing education; nursing informatics. *Nurse practitioner programs in:* family health.
Site Options multiple cities.
Study Options Full-time and part-time.
Online Degree Options Yes.
Program Entrance Requirements Minimum overall college GPA of 3.0, transcript of college record, 3 letters of recommendation, prerequisite course work, resume. *Application deadline:* Applications may be processed on a rolling basis for some programs.
Degree Requirements 43 total credit hours, thesis or project.

POST-MASTER'S PROGRAM

Areas of Study *Nurse practitioner programs in:* family health.

Milligan College

Department of Nursing
Milligan College, Tennessee

http://www.milligan.edu/BSN/
Founded in 1866

DEGREE • BSN

Nursing Program Faculty 10 (25% with doctorates).
Baccalaureate Enrollment 195 **Women** 90% **Men** 10% **Minority** 2%
Nursing Student Activities Nursing Honor Society, Student Nurses' Association.
Nursing Student Resources Academic advising; academic or career counseling; assistance for students with disabilities; bookstore; campus computer network; career placement assistance; computer lab; computer-assisted instruction; e-mail services; employment services for current students; externships; interactive nursing skills videos; Internet; learning resource lab; library services; nursing audiovisuals; placement services for program completers; remedial services; resume preparation assistance; skills, simulation, or other laboratory; tutoring; unpaid internships.
Library Facilities 145,605 volumes (2,430 in health, 184 in nursing); 11,097 periodical subscriptions (340 health-care related).

BACCALAUREATE PROGRAMS

Degree BSN
Available Programs ADN to Baccalaureate; Baccalaureate for Second Degree; Generic Baccalaureate; LPN to Baccalaureate; LPN to RN Baccalaureate; RN Baccalaureate.
Study Options Full-time and part-time.
Program Entrance Requirements Minimum overall college GPA of 2.5, transcript of college record, CPR certification, written essay, health exam, immunizations, letters of recommendation, minimum GPA in nursing prerequisites of 2.5, professional liability insurance/malpractice insurance, prerequisite course work. Transfer students are accepted. *Application deadline:* Applications may be processed on a rolling basis for some programs. *Application fee:* $30.
Advanced Placement Credit given for nursing courses completed elsewhere dependent upon specific evaluations.
Expenses (2010-11) *Tuition:* full-time $22,666; part-time $360 per semester. *Room and board:* $2825; room only: $1325 per academic year. *Required fees:* full-time $200.
Financial Aid 94% of baccalaureate students in nursing programs received some form of financial aid in 2009-10. *Gift aid (need-based):* Federal Pell, FSEOG, state, private, college/university gift aid from institutional funds. *Loans:* Federal Direct (Subsidized and Unsubsidized Stafford PLUS), Perkins, alternative loans. *Work-study:* Federal Work-Study, part-time campus jobs. *Financial aid application deadline (priority):* 3/1.
Contact Dr. Melinda K. Collins, Area Chair and Director of Nursing, Department of Nursing, Milligan College, Wilson Way, Suite 302, Milligan College, TN 37682. *Telephone:* 423-461-8655. *Fax:* 423-461-8982. *E-mail:* mcollins@milligan.edu.

South College

Department of Nursing
Knoxville, Tennessee

Founded in 1882

DEGREE • BSN

BACCALAUREATE PROGRAMS

Degree BSN
Available Programs Generic Baccalaureate.
Program Entrance Requirements Immunizations, minimum high school GPA of 2.5. Transfer students are accepted.
Contact ***Telephone:*** 865-251-1800.

Southern Adventist University

School of Nursing
Collegedale, Tennessee

http://nursing.southern.edu/
Founded in 1892

DEGREES • BS • MSN • MSN/MBA

Nursing Program Faculty 18 (22% with doctorates).
Baccalaureate Enrollment 114 **Women** 80% **Men** 20% **Minority** 29% **International** 15% **Part-time** 37%
Graduate Enrollment 72 **Women** 85% **Men** 15% **Minority** 7% **Part-time** 45%
Nursing Student Activities Sigma Theta Tau, nursing club.
Nursing Student Resources Academic advising; academic or career counseling; assistance for students with disabilities; bookstore; campus computer network; computer lab; computer-assisted instruction; e-mail services; employment services for current students; housing assistance; interactive nursing skills videos; Internet; learning resource lab; library services; nursing audiovisuals; remedial services; resume preparation assistance; skills, simulation, or other laboratory; tutoring.
Library Facilities 166,905 volumes (7,795 in health, 974 in nursing); 40,304 periodical subscriptions (86 health-care related).

BACCALAUREATE PROGRAMS

Degree BS
Available Programs ADN to Baccalaureate.
Site Options Chattanooga, TN.
Study Options Full-time and part-time.
Program Entrance Requirements Minimum overall college GPA of 2.5, transcript of college record, CPR certification, health exam, high school transcript, immunizations, 2 letters of recommendation, minimum GPA in nursing prerequisites of 2.0, prerequisite course work, RN licensure. Transfer students are accepted. *Application deadline:* 2/1 (fall), 9/1 (winter). Applications may be processed on a rolling basis for some programs.
Advanced Placement Credit given for nursing courses completed elsewhere dependent upon specific evaluations.
Expenses (2010-11) *Tuition:* full-time $17,534; part-time $740 per credit hour. *Room and board:* $5356; room only: $3286 per academic year. *Required fees:* full-time $790; part-time $15 per credit.
Financial Aid 80% of baccalaureate students in nursing programs received some form of financial aid in 2009-10. *Gift aid (need-based):* Federal Pell, FSEOG, state, private, college/university gift aid from institutional funds. *Loans:* Federal Nursing Student Loans, Federal Direct (Subsidized and Unsubsidized Stafford PLUS), Perkins, college/university. *Work-study:* Federal Work-Study, part-time campus jobs. *Financial aid application deadline (priority):* 3/1.
Contact Mrs. Linda Marlowe, Admissions and Progression Coordinator, School of Nursing, Southern Adventist University, PO Box 370, Collegedale, TN 37315-0370. *Telephone:* 423-236-2941. *Fax:* 423-236-1940. *E-mail:* lmarlowe@southern.edu.

GRADUATE PROGRAMS

Expenses (2010-11) *Tuition:* full-time $9072; part-time $504 per credit hour.
Financial Aid 50% of graduate students in nursing programs received some form of financial aid in 2009-10.
Contact Mrs. Diane Proffitt, Applications Manager, School of Nursing, Southern Adventist University, PO Box 370, Collegedale, TN 37315-0370. *Telephone:* 423-236-2957. *Fax:* 423-236-1940. *E-mail:* dproffit@southern.edu.

MASTER'S DEGREE PROGRAM

Degrees MSN; MSN/MBA
Available Programs Accelerated RN to Master's; Master's.
Concentrations Available Nursing education. *Nurse practitioner programs in:* acute care, adult health, family health.
Study Options Full-time and part-time.
Program Entrance Requirements Clinical experience, minimum overall college GPA of 3.0, transcript of college record, CPR certification, written essay, immunizations, interview, 2 letters of recommendation, prerequisite course work, statistics course. *Application deadline:* 7/1 (fall), 11/1 (winter). *Application fee:* $25.
Advanced Placement Credit given for nursing courses completed elsewhere dependent upon specific evaluations.
Degree Requirements 46 total credit hours, thesis or project.

CONTINUING EDUCATION PROGRAM

Contact Mrs. Linda Marlowe, Admissions and Progression Coordinator, School of Nursing, Southern Adventist University, PO Box 370, Collegedale, TN 37315-0370. *Telephone:* 423-236-2941. *Fax:* 423-236-1940. *E-mail:* lmarlowe@southern.edu.

Tennessee State University

School of Nursing
Nashville, Tennessee

http://www.tnstate.edu/nurs
Founded in 1912

DEGREES • BSN • MSN

Nursing Program Faculty 41 (39% with doctorates).
Baccalaureate Enrollment 103 **Women** 85% **Men** 15% **Minority** 78% **Part-time** 3%
Graduate Enrollment 189 **Women** 94% **Men** 6% **Minority** 36% **International** 4% **Part-time** 88%
Distance Learning Courses Available.
Nursing Student Activities Nursing Honor Society, Sigma Theta Tau, Student Nurses' Association.
Nursing Student Resources Academic advising; academic or career counseling; assistance for students with disabilities; bookstore; campus computer network; computer lab; e-mail services; interactive nursing skills videos; Internet; learning resource lab; library services; nursing audiovisuals; skills, simulation, or other laboratory; tutoring.
Library Facilities 630,890 volumes (50,000 in health, 25,000 in nursing); 300 periodical subscriptions health-care related.

BACCALAUREATE PROGRAMS

Degree BSN
Available Programs Generic Baccalaureate; LPN to Baccalaureate; RN Baccalaureate.
Site Options Nashville, TN.
Study Options Full-time and part-time.
Program Entrance Requirements Minimum overall college GPA of 2.8, transcript of college record, CPR certification, health exam, immunizations, minimum GPA in nursing prerequisites of 2.8, professional liability insurance/malpractice insurance, prerequisite course work. Transfer students are accepted. *Application deadline:* 3/15 (fall).
Expenses (2010-11) *Tuition, state resident:* full-time $5824; part-time $254 per credit hour. *Tuition, nonresident:* full-time $18,880; part-time $776 per credit hour. *Room and board:* $5760; room only: $3160 per academic year. *Required fees:* full-time $1076; part-time $25 per credit.
Financial Aid 80% of baccalaureate students in nursing programs received some form of financial aid in 2009-10.
Contact Dr. Pamela D. Ark, BSN Program Director, School of Nursing, Tennessee State University, 3500 John A. Merritt Boulevard, Box 9590, Nashville, TN 37209-1561. *Telephone:* 615-963-7615. *Fax:* 615-963-5593. *E-mail:* park@tnstate.edu.

GRADUATE PROGRAMS

Expenses (2010-11) *Tuition, state resident:* full-time $7360; part-time $377 per credit hour. *Tuition, nonresident:* full-time $18,840; part-time $951 per credit hour. *Room and board:* $7750; room only: $5150 per academic year. *Required fees:* full-time $450; part-time $25 per credit.
Financial Aid 75% of graduate students in nursing programs received some form of financial aid in 2009-10. Research assistantships (averaging $6,500 per year), 3 teaching assistantships (averaging $6,500 per year) were awarded.
Contact Dr. Jane C. Norman, MSN Program Director, School of Nursing, Tennessee State University, 3500 John A. Merritt Boulevard, Box 9590, Nashville, TN 37209-1561. *Telephone:* 615-963-5255. *Fax:* 615-963-7614. *E-mail:* jnorman@tnstate.edu.

MASTER'S DEGREE PROGRAM

Degree MSN
Available Programs RN to Master's.
Concentrations Available Nursing education. *Clinical nurse specialist programs in:* family health. *Nurse practitioner programs in:* family health.
Site Options Nashville, TN.
Study Options Full-time and part-time.
Online Degree Options Yes.
Program Entrance Requirements Clinical experience, computer literacy, minimum overall college GPA of 3.0, transcript of college record, CPR certification, written essay, immunizations, interview, 3 letters of recommendation, physical assessment course, professional liability insurance/malpractice insurance, resume, statistics course, GRE General Test or MAT. *Application deadline:* 7/15 (fall), 11/15 (spring), 3/15 (summer).
Advanced Placement Credit given for nursing courses completed elsewhere dependent upon specific evaluations.
Degree Requirements 43 total credit hours, thesis or project, comprehensive exam.

POST-MASTER'S PROGRAM

Areas of Study *Clinical nurse specialist programs in:* family health. *Nurse practitioner programs in:* family health.

CONTINUING EDUCATION PROGRAM

Contact Dr. Kathy L. Martin, Dean, School of Nursing, Tennessee State University, 3500 John A. Merritt Boulevard, Box 9590, Nashville, TN 37209-1561. *Telephone:* 615-963-5251. *Fax:* 615-963-5049. *E-mail:* kmartin3@tnstate.edu.

Tennessee Technological University

Whitson-Hester School of Nursing
Cookeville, Tennessee

http://www.tntech.edu/nursing
Founded in 1915

DEGREES • BSN • M SC N • MSN

Nursing Program Faculty 21 (14% with doctorates).
Baccalaureate Enrollment 189 **Women** 89% **Men** 11% **Minority** 2% **Part-time** 1%
Graduate Enrollment 41 **Women** 90% **Men** 10% **Minority** 2% **Part-time** 76%
Distance Learning Courses Available.
Nursing Student Activities Sigma Theta Tau, Student Nurses' Association.
Nursing Student Resources Academic advising; academic or career counseling; assistance for students with disabilities; bookstore; campus computer network; career placement assistance; computer lab; computer-assisted instruction; daycare for children of students; e-mail services; employment services for current students; externships; housing assistance; Internet; learning resource lab; library services; nursing audiovisuals; paid internships; placement services for program completers; remedial services; resume preparation assistance; skills, simulation, or other laboratory; tutoring; unpaid internships.
Library Facilities 693,169 volumes (312,892 in health, 11,893 in nursing); 1,636 periodical subscriptions (96 health-care related).

BACCALAUREATE PROGRAMS

Degree BSN
Available Programs ADN to Baccalaureate; Baccalaureate for Second Degree; Generic Baccalaureate; RN Baccalaureate.
Study Options Full-time.
Program Entrance Requirements Minimum overall college GPA of 2.5, transcript of college record, CPR certification, health exam, high school biology, high school foreign language, 4 years high school math, 2 years high school science, high school transcript, immunizations, minimum high school GPA of 3.0, minimum GPA in nursing prerequisites of 2.5, professional liability insurance/malpractice insurance, prerequisite course work. Transfer students are accepted. *Application deadline:* 2/1 (fall), 6/1 (spring).
Advanced Placement Credit given for nursing courses completed elsewhere dependent upon specific evaluations.
Expenses (2010-11) *Tuition, state resident:* full-time $6038; part-time $268 per credit hour. *Tuition, nonresident:* full-time $19,034; part-time $790 per credit hour. *Room and board:* $7158; room only: $3700 per academic year. *Required fees:* full-time $735; part-time $25 per credit.
Financial Aid 85% of baccalaureate students in nursing programs received some form of financial aid in 2009-10. *Gift aid (need-based):* Federal Pell, FSEOG, state, private, college/university gift aid from institutional funds, United Negro College Fund. *Loans:* Federal Direct (Subsidized and Unsubsidized Stafford PLUS), Perkins, college/university.

Work-study: Federal Work-Study, part-time campus jobs. *Financial aid application deadline (priority):* 3/15.

Contact Ms. Kristi L. Burris, Academic Advisor, Whitson-Hester School of Nursing, Tennessee Technological University, Box 5001, Cookeville, TN 38505-0001. *Telephone:* 931-372-3203. *Fax:* 931-372-6244. *E-mail:* nursing@tntech.edu.

GRADUATE PROGRAMS

Expenses (2010-11) *Tuition, state resident:* part-time $404 per credit hour. *Tuition, nonresident:* part-time $978 per credit hour.

Financial Aid 5% of graduate students in nursing programs received some form of financial aid in 2009-10.

Contact Ms. Kristi L. Burris, Academic Advisor, Whitson-Hester School of Nursing, Tennessee Technological University, Box 5001, Cookeville, TN 38505-0001. *Telephone:* 931-372-3203. *Fax:* 931-372-6244. *E-mail:* nursing@tntech.edu.

MASTER'S DEGREE PROGRAM

Degrees M Sc N; MSN

Available Programs Master's; Master's for Nurses with Non-Nursing Degrees.

Concentrations Available Health-care administration; nursing education; nursing informatics. *Nurse practitioner programs in:* family health.

Study Options Full-time and part-time.

Online Degree Options Yes (online only).

Program Entrance Requirements Computer literacy, minimum overall college GPA of 3.0, transcript of college record, CPR certification, immunizations, 3 letters of recommendation, professional liability insurance/malpractice insurance, resume. *Application deadline:* 8/1 (fall), 12/1 (spring), 5/1 (summer). Applications may be processed on a rolling basis for some programs. *Application fee:* $25.

Advanced Placement Credit given for nursing courses completed elsewhere dependent upon specific evaluations.

Degree Requirements 46 total credit hours, thesis or project.

Tennessee Wesleyan College
Fort Sanders Nursing Department
Knoxville, Tennessee

http://www.twcnet.edu/academics/nursing

Founded in 1857

DEGREE • BSN

Nursing Program Faculty 15 (20% with doctorates).

Baccalaureate Enrollment 101 **Women** 92% **Men** 8% **Minority** 3% **International** 2% **Part-time** 4%

Distance Learning Courses Available.

Nursing Student Activities Nursing Honor Society, Sigma Theta Tau, Student Nurses' Association.

Nursing Student Resources Academic advising; assistance for students with disabilities; bookstore; computer lab; Internet; library services; nursing audiovisuals; other; skills, simulation, or other laboratory.

Library Facilities 5,000 volumes in health, 4,000 volumes in nursing; 135 periodical subscriptions health-care related.

BACCALAUREATE PROGRAMS

Degree BSN

Available Programs ADN to Baccalaureate; Generic Baccalaureate; RN Baccalaureate.

Site Options Knoxville, TN.

Study Options Full-time and part-time.

Program Entrance Requirements Minimum overall college GPA of 2.7, transcript of college record, CPR certification, written essay, health exam, high school transcript, immunizations, interview, prerequisite course work. Transfer students are accepted. *Application deadline:* 1/15 (fall). *Application fee:* $25.

Advanced Placement Credit given for nursing courses completed elsewhere dependent upon specific evaluations.

Contact ***Telephone:*** 865-777-5100. *Fax:* 865-777-5114.

Union University
School of Nursing
Jackson, Tennessee

http://www.uu.edu/academics/son/

Founded in 1823

DEGREES • BSN • MSN

Nursing Program Faculty 28 (36% with doctorates).

Baccalaureate Enrollment 285 **Women** 93% **Men** 7% **Minority** 27% **International** 2% **Part-time** 56%

Graduate Enrollment 55 **Women** 80% **Men** 20% **Minority** 25% **Part-time** 4%

Nursing Student Activities Nursing Honor Society, Sigma Theta Tau, Student Nurses' Association.

Nursing Student Resources Academic advising; academic or career counseling; assistance for students with disabilities; bookstore; campus computer network; career placement assistance; computer lab; computer-assisted instruction; e-mail services; employment services for current students; housing assistance; Internet; learning resource lab; library services; nursing audiovisuals; resume preparation assistance; skills, simulation, or other laboratory; tutoring.

Library Facilities 155,500 volumes (6,005 in nursing); 20,324 periodical subscriptions (1,284 health-care related).

BACCALAUREATE PROGRAMS

Degree BSN

Available Programs Accelerated Baccalaureate for Second Degree; Generic Baccalaureate; LPN to Baccalaureate; RN Baccalaureate.

Site Options Germantown, TN.

Study Options Full-time.

Program Entrance Requirements Minimum overall college GPA of 2.8, transcript of college record, CPR certification, health exam, immunizations, minimum GPA in nursing prerequisites of 2.8, prerequisite course work. Transfer students are accepted.

Advanced Placement Credit by examination available. Credit given for nursing courses completed elsewhere dependent upon specific evaluations.

Contact ***Telephone:*** 731-661-5538. *Fax:* 731-661-5504.

GRADUATE PROGRAMS

Contact ***Telephone:*** 731-661-5538. *Fax:* 901-661-5504.

MASTER'S DEGREE PROGRAM

Degree MSN

Available Programs Master's.

Concentrations Available Nurse anesthesia; nursing administration; nursing education. *Clinical nurse specialist programs in:* adult health, pediatric. *Nurse practitioner programs in:* family health.

Site Options Germantown, TN.

Study Options Full-time and part-time.

Program Entrance Requirements Minimum overall college GPA of 3.0, transcript of college record, CPR certification, written essay, immunizations, interview, 3 letters of recommendation, professional liability insurance/malpractice insurance, GRE.

Advanced Placement Credit given for nursing courses completed elsewhere dependent upon specific evaluations.

Degree Requirements 46 total credit hours.

POST-MASTER'S PROGRAM

Areas of Study Nursing administration; nursing education. *Clinical nurse specialist programs in:* adult health, pediatric. *Nurse practitioner programs in:* family health.

CONTINUING EDUCATION PROGRAM

Contact ***Telephone:*** 731-661-5152. *Fax:* 731-661-5504.

University of Memphis
Loewenberg School of Nursing
Memphis, Tennessee

http://nursing.memphis.edu

Founded in 1912

DEGREES • BSN • MSN

Nursing Program Faculty 65 (22% with doctorates).

Baccalaureate Enrollment 441 **Women** 91% **Men** 9% **Minority** 23% **Part-time** 15%
Graduate Enrollment 124 **Women** 92% **Men** 8% **Minority** 30% **Part-time** 75%
Distance Learning Courses Available.
Nursing Student Activities Sigma Theta Tau, Student Nurses' Association.
Nursing Student Resources Academic advising; academic or career counseling; assistance for students with disabilities; bookstore; campus computer network; career placement assistance; computer lab; computer-assisted instruction; daycare for children of students; e-mail services; externships; housing assistance; interactive nursing skills videos; Internet; learning resource lab; library services; nursing audiovisuals; paid internships; remedial services; resume preparation assistance; skills, simulation, or other laboratory; tutoring.
Library Facilities 1.8 million volumes (74,513 in health); 7,065 periodical subscriptions (878 health-care related).

BACCALAUREATE PROGRAMS

Degree BSN
Available Programs ADN to Baccalaureate; Accelerated Baccalaureate; Accelerated Baccalaureate for Second Degree; Accelerated RN Baccalaureate; Baccalaureate for Second Degree; Generic Baccalaureate; RN Baccalaureate.
Site Options Jackson, TN.
Study Options Full-time.
Program Entrance Requirements Minimum overall college GPA of 2.7, transcript of college record, CPR certification, health exam, high school biology, high school chemistry, high school foreign language, 3 years high school math, 2 years high school science, high school transcript, immunizations, minimum high school GPA of 3.0, minimum GPA in nursing prerequisites of 2.4, prerequisite course work. Transfer students are accepted.
Advanced Placement Credit by examination available. Credit given for nursing courses completed elsewhere dependent upon specific evaluations.
Contact *Telephone:* 901-678-2003. *Fax:* 901-678-4906.

GRADUATE PROGRAMS

Contact *Telephone:* 901-678-2003. *Fax:* 901-678-4906.

MASTER'S DEGREE PROGRAM

Degree MSN
Available Programs Accelerated Master's for Nurses with Non-Nursing Degrees; Master's; Master's for Non-Nursing College Graduates; Master's for Nurses with Non-Nursing Degrees.
Concentrations Available Nursing administration; nursing education. *Nurse practitioner programs in:* family health.
Site Options Jackson, TN.
Study Options Full-time and part-time.
Online Degree Options Yes.
Program Entrance Requirements Minimum overall college GPA of 2.8, CPR certification, immunizations, 3 letters of recommendation, professional liability insurance/malpractice insurance.
Advanced Placement Credit given for nursing courses completed elsewhere dependent upon specific evaluations.
Degree Requirements 45 total credit hours, comprehensive exam.

POST-MASTER'S PROGRAM

Areas of Study *Nurse practitioner programs in:* family health.

The University of Tennessee

College of Nursing
Knoxville, Tennessee

http://www.nightingale.con.utk.edu/
Founded in 1794

DEGREES • BSN • MSN • PHD

Nursing Program Faculty 54 (54% with doctorates).
Baccalaureate Enrollment 215 **Women** 91% **Men** 9% **Minority** 5.6% **International** 3.3% **Part-time** 7.4%
Graduate Enrollment 139 **Women** 89.3% **Men** 10.7% **Minority** 3.5% **International** 1.4% **Part-time** 32%
Distance Learning Courses Available.
Nursing Student Activities Sigma Theta Tau, Student Nurses' Association.
Nursing Student Resources Academic advising; academic or career counseling; assistance for students with disabilities; bookstore; campus computer network; computer lab; computer-assisted instruction; e-mail services; employment services for current students; externships; interactive nursing skills videos; Internet; learning resource lab; library services; nursing audiovisuals; remedial services; skills, simulation, or other laboratory; tutoring.
Library Facilities 3 million volumes (59,214 in health, 3,711 in nursing); 38,965 periodical subscriptions (572 health-care related).

BACCALAUREATE PROGRAMS

Degree BSN
Available Programs Accelerated Baccalaureate; Accelerated RN Baccalaureate; Generic Baccalaureate.
Study Options Full-time and part-time.
Program Entrance Requirements Transcript of college record, CPR certification, written essay, health exam, health insurance, high school biology, high school chemistry, 3 years high school math, 2 years high school science, high school transcript, immunizations, interview, minimum high school GPA of 3.2, minimum GPA in nursing prerequisites of 3.2, professional liability insurance/malpractice insurance, prerequisite course work. Transfer students are accepted. *Application deadline:* 12/1 (fall), 12/1 (summer). *Application fee:* $30.
Advanced Placement Credit given for nursing courses completed elsewhere dependent upon specific evaluations.
Expenses (2010-11) *Tuition, state resident:* full-time $6450; part-time $270 per credit. *Tuition, nonresident:* full-time $15,038; part-time $627 per credit. *Room and board:* $10,000; room only: $6800 per academic year. *Required fees:* full-time $3166; part-time $266 per credit; part-time $266 per term.
Financial Aid 90% of baccalaureate students in nursing programs received some form of financial aid in 2009-10. *Gift aid (need-based):* Federal Pell, FSEOG, state, private, college/university gift aid from institutional funds, Federal Nursing. *Loans:* Perkins, college/university. *Work-study:* Federal Work-Study. *Financial aid application deadline (priority):* 3/1.
Contact Director, Student Services, College of Nursing, The University of Tennessee, 1200 Volunteer Boulevard, Knoxville, TN 37996-4180. *Telephone:* 865-974-7606. *Fax:* 865-974-3569. *E-mail:* bbarret@utk.edu.

GRADUATE PROGRAMS

Expenses (2010-11) *Tuition, state resident:* full-time $7440; part-time $414 per credit. *Tuition, nonresident:* full-time $15,038; part-time $836 per credit. *Room and board:* $10,000; room only: $6800 per academic year. *Required fees:* full-time $922; part-time $43 per credit.
Financial Aid 75% of graduate students in nursing programs received some form of financial aid in 2009-10. 3 fellowships, 1 research assistantship were awarded; teaching assistantships, Federal Work-Study, institutionally sponsored loans, and unspecified assistantships also available. *Financial aid application deadline:* 2/1.
Contact Dr. Mary Gunther, Chair, Masters Program and Director, Graduate Studies, College of Nursing, The University of Tennessee, 1200 Volunteer Boulevard, Knoxville, TN 37996-4180. *Telephone:* 865-974-4151. *Fax:* 865-974-3569. *E-mail:* mgunther@utk.edu.

MASTER'S DEGREE PROGRAM

Degree MSN
Available Programs Accelerated Master's for Nurses with Non-Nursing Degrees; Accelerated RN to Master's; Master's; Master's for Non-Nursing College Graduates; Master's for Nurses with Non-Nursing Degrees; RN to Master's.
Concentrations Available Nurse anesthesia; nursing administration. *Clinical nurse specialist programs in:* adult health, pediatric, psychiatric/mental health. *Nurse practitioner programs in:* adult health, family health, pediatric, psychiatric/mental health.
Study Options Full-time.
Program Entrance Requirements Minimum overall college GPA of 3.0, transcript of college record, CPR certification, written essay, immunizations, 3 letters of recommendation, physical assessment course, professional liability insurance/malpractice insurance, prerequisite course work, statistics course, GRE General Test. *Application deadline:* 2/1 (fall), 10/1 (spring), 10/1 (summer). *Application fee:* $30.
Advanced Placement Credit by examination available. Credit given for nursing courses completed elsewhere dependent upon specific evaluations.
Degree Requirements 41 total credit hours, comprehensive exam.

POST-MASTER'S PROGRAM

Areas of Study Nurse anesthesia; nursing administration; nursing education. *Clinical nurse specialist programs in:* adult health, pediatric, psychiatric/mental health. *Nurse practitioner programs in:* adult health, family health, pediatric, psychiatric/mental health.

DOCTORAL DEGREE PROGRAM

Degree PhD
Available Programs Doctorate; Post-Baccalaureate Doctorate.
Areas of Study Bio-behavioral research, biology of health and illness, faculty preparation, family health, gerontology, health policy, health promotion/disease prevention, human health and illness, individualized study, neuro-behavior, nursing administration, nursing education, nursing research, nursing science, women's health.
Online Degree Options Yes (online only).
Program Entrance Requirements Minimum overall college GPA of 3.0, interview by faculty committee, interview, 3 letters of recommendation, writing sample, GRE General Test. Application deadline: 10/1 (summer). Application fee: $30.
Degree Requirements 67 total credit hours, dissertation, oral exam, written exam, residency.

CONTINUING EDUCATION PROGRAM

Contact Dr. Maureen Nalle, Coordinator, Continuing Education, College of Nursing, The University of Tennessee, 1200 Volunteer Boulevard, Knoxville, TN 37996-4180. *Telephone:* 865-974-7598. *Fax:* 865-974-3569. *E-mail:* mnalle@utk.edu.

The University of Tennessee at Chattanooga

School of Nursing
Chattanooga, Tennessee

http://www.utc.edu/Academic/Nursing
Founded in 1886

DEGREES • BSN • DNP • MSN

Nursing Program Faculty 27 (48% with doctorates).
Baccalaureate Enrollment 126 **Women** 90% **Men** 10% **Minority** 8%
Graduate Enrollment 107 **Women** 70% **Men** 30% **Minority** 15% **Part-time** 32%
Distance Learning Courses Available.
Nursing Student Activities Sigma Theta Tau, Student Nurses' Association.
Nursing Student Resources Academic advising; academic or career counseling; assistance for students with disabilities; bookstore; campus computer network; computer lab; computer-assisted instruction; e-mail services; interactive nursing skills videos; Internet; learning resource lab; library services; nursing audiovisuals; skills, simulation, or other laboratory; tutoring.
Library Facilities 596,000 volumes (19,370 in health, 3,100 in nursing); 2,718 periodical subscriptions (200 health-care related).

BACCALAUREATE PROGRAMS

Degree BSN
Available Programs ADN to Baccalaureate; Baccalaureate for Second Degree; Generic Baccalaureate.
Study Options Full-time.
Program Entrance Requirements Minimum overall college GPA of 2.75, transcript of college record, CPR certification, health exam, health insurance, high school foreign language, 3 years high school math, high school transcript, immunizations, 2 letters of recommendation, minimum high school GPA of 2.0, minimum GPA in nursing prerequisites of 2.75, professional liability insurance/malpractice insurance, prerequisite course work. Transfer students are accepted. *Application deadline:* 3/1 (fall), 9/1 (spring).
Advanced Placement Credit by examination available. Credit given for nursing courses completed elsewhere dependent upon specific evaluations.
Financial Aid 60% of baccalaureate students in nursing programs received some form of financial aid in 2009-10. *Gift aid (need-based):* Federal Pell, FSEOG, state, private, college/university gift aid from institutional funds, United Negro College Fund, Federal Nursing. *Loans:* Perkins, college/university. *Work-study:* Federal Work-Study, part-time campus jobs. *Financial aid application deadline (priority):* 4/1.
Contact Dr. Katherine S. Lindgren, Director, School of Nursing, The University of Tennessee at Chattanooga, 615 McCallie Avenue, Department 1051, Chattanooga, TN 37403-2598. *Telephone:* 423-425-4750. *Fax:* 423-425-4668. *E-mail:* kay-lindgren@utc.edu.

GRADUATE PROGRAMS

Financial Aid 70% of graduate students in nursing programs received some form of financial aid in 2009-10. Career-related internships or fieldwork and scholarships available. Aid available to part-time students.
Contact Dr. Katherine S. Lindgren, Director, School of Nursing, The University of Tennessee at Chattanooga, 615 McCallie Avenue, Department 1051, Chattanooga, TN 37403-2598. *Telephone:* 423-425-4750. *Fax:* 423-425-4668. *E-mail:* kay-lindgren@utc.edu.

MASTER'S DEGREE PROGRAM

Degree MSN
Available Programs Master's.
Concentrations Available Nurse anesthesia. *Nurse practitioner programs in:* family health.
Site Options Tupelo, MS.
Study Options Full-time and part-time.
Program Entrance Requirements Clinical experience, computer literacy, minimum overall college GPA of 3.0, transcript of college record, CPR certification, written essay, immunizations, interview, 3 letters of recommendation, nursing research course, physical assessment course, professional liability insurance/malpractice insurance, resume, statistics course, GRE General Test, MAT. *Application deadline:* 2/1 (winter), 8/1 (summer).
Advanced Placement Credit given for nursing courses completed elsewhere dependent upon specific evaluations.
Degree Requirements 48 total credit hours, comprehensive exam.

POST-MASTER'S PROGRAM

Areas of Study Nurse anesthesia. *Nurse practitioner programs in:* family health.

DOCTORAL DEGREE PROGRAM

Degree DNP
Available Programs Doctorate.
Online Degree Options Yes (online only).
Program Entrance Requirements Clinical experience, minimum overall college GPA of 3.0, interview by faculty committee, 3.0 letters of recommendation, MSN or equivalent, vita. Application deadline: 11/1 (winter).
Degree Requirements 36 total credit hours.

CONTINUING EDUCATION PROGRAM

Contact Dr. Katherine S. Lindgren, Director, School of Nursing, The University of Tennessee at Chattanooga, 615 McCallie Avenue, Department 1051, Chattanooga, TN 37403-2598. *Telephone:* 423-425-4750. *Fax:* 423-425-4668. *E-mail:* kay-lindgren@utc.edu.

The University of Tennessee at Martin

Department of Nursing
Martin, Tennessee

http://www.utm.edu
Founded in 1900

DEGREE • BSN

Nursing Program Faculty 15 (20% with doctorates).
Baccalaureate Enrollment 198 **Women** 88% **Men** 12% **Minority** 5% **International** 1% **Part-time** 18%
Distance Learning Courses Available.
Nursing Student Activities Nursing Honor Society, Sigma Theta Tau, Student Nurses' Association, nursing club.
Nursing Student Resources Academic advising; academic or career counseling; assistance for students with disabilities; bookstore; campus computer network; career placement assistance; computer lab; computer-assisted instruction; daycare for children of students; e-mail services; employment services for current students; housing assistance; interactive nursing skills videos; Internet; learning resource lab; library services; nursing audiovisuals; remedial services; resume preparation assistance; skills, simulation, or other laboratory; tutoring.

Library Facilities 534,802 volumes (1,772 in health, 1,645 in nursing); 1,132 periodical subscriptions (10,803 health-care related).

BACCALAUREATE PROGRAMS

Degree BSN
Available Programs ADN to Baccalaureate; Generic Baccalaureate; LPN to RN Baccalaureate.
Site Options Selmer, TN; Parsons, TN; Ripley, TN.
Study Options Full-time.
Program Entrance Requirements Minimum overall college GPA of 2.0, transcript of college record, CPR certification, health exam, health insurance, high school biology, high school chemistry, high school foreign language, 3 years high school math, 2 years high school science, high school transcript, immunizations, interview, minimum high school GPA of 3.0, minimum GPA in nursing prerequisites of 2.0, professional liability insurance/malpractice insurance, prerequisite course work. Transfer students are accepted. *Application deadline:* 2/1 (fall).
Advanced Placement Credit by examination available. Credit given for nursing courses completed elsewhere dependent upon specific evaluations.
Expenses (2009-10) *Tuition, state resident:* full-time $5675; part-time $238 per credit hour. *Tuition, nonresident:* full-time $17,169; part-time $715 per credit hour. *International tuition:* $17,169 full-time. *Room and board:* room only: $2300 per academic year. *Required fees:* full-time $1200; part-time $238 per credit; part-time $500 per term.
Financial Aid 95% of baccalaureate students in nursing programs received some form of financial aid in 2008-09. *Gift aid (need-based):* Federal Pell, FSEOG, state, private, college/university gift aid from institutional funds. *Loans:* Perkins. *Work-study:* Federal Work-Study. *Financial aid application deadline (priority):* 3/1.
Contact Mrs. Brenda W. Campbell, Program Resource Specialist, Department of Nursing, The University of Tennessee at Martin, Gooch Hall 136J, Martin, TN 38238. *Telephone:* 731-881-7138. *Fax:* 731-881-7939. *E-mail:* brendac@utm.edu.

CONTINUING EDUCATION PROGRAM

Contact Dr. Victoria S. Seng, PhD, Interim Chair, Department of Nursing, The University of Tennessee at Martin, Gooch Hall 136H, 538 University Street, Martin, TN 38238. *Telephone:* 731-881-7140. *Fax:* 731-881-7939. *E-mail:* vseng@utm.edu.

The University of Tennessee Health Science Center

College of Nursing
Memphis, Tennessee

http://www.utmem.edu/nursing
Founded in 1911

DEGREES • DNP • MSN
Nursing Program Faculty 51 (87% with doctorates).
Graduate Enrollment 227 **Women** 85% **Men** 15% **Minority** 22%
Distance Learning Courses Available.
Nursing Student Activities Sigma Theta Tau, Student Nurses' Association.
Nursing Student Resources Academic advising; academic or career counseling; assistance for students with disabilities; bookstore; campus computer network; computer lab; computer-assisted instruction; e-mail services; housing assistance; interactive nursing skills videos; Internet; learning resource lab; library services; nursing audiovisuals; paid internships; remedial services; skills, simulation, or other laboratory; tutoring.
Library Facilities 165,200 volumes (198,936 in health, 8,061 in nursing); 1,784 periodical subscriptions (3,800 health-care related).

GRADUATE PROGRAMS

Expenses (2009-10) *Tuition, state resident:* full-time $9376; part-time $521 per credit hour. *Tuition, nonresident:* full-time $22,585; part-time $1254 per credit hour. *Required fees:* full-time $684.
Financial Aid 65% of graduate students in nursing programs received some form of financial aid in 2008-09. Fellowships with partial tuition reimbursements available, teaching assistantships, Federal Work-Study, institutionally sponsored loans, scholarships, and traineeships available. Aid available to part-time students. *Financial aid application deadline:* 2/28.
Contact Mr. Justin Casey, Assistant Director, Student Affairs, College of Nursing, The University of Tennessee Health Science Center, 877 Madison Avenue, Suite 637, Memphis, TN 38163. *Telephone:* 901-448-6139. *Fax:* 901-448-4121. *E-mail:* jcasey4@uthsc.edu.

MASTER'S DEGREE PROGRAM

Degree MSN
Available Programs Accelerated Master's for Non-Nursing College Graduates.
Concentrations Available Clinical nurse leader.
Study Options Full-time.
Program Entrance Requirements Computer literacy, minimum overall college GPA of 3.0, transcript of college record, CPR certification, written essay, immunizations, interview, 3 letters of recommendation, prerequisite course work, statistics course, GRE General Test. *Application deadline:* 1/15 (summer).
Degree Requirements 80 total credit hours.

POST-MASTER'S PROGRAM

Areas of Study Nurse anesthesia. *Clinical nurse specialist programs in:* acute care, critical care, family health, psychiatric/mental health, public health. *Nurse practitioner programs in:* acute care, family health, neonatal health, pediatric, primary care, psychiatric/mental health.

DOCTORAL DEGREE PROGRAM

Degree DNP
Available Programs Doctorate; Post-Baccalaureate Doctorate.
Areas of Study Addiction/substance abuse, advanced practice nursing, clinical practice, community health, critical care, family health, forensic nursing, gerontology, women's health.
Online Degree Options Yes (online only).
Program Entrance Requirements Minimum overall college GPA of 3.0, interview by faculty committee, interview, 3 letters of recommendation, writing sample. Application deadline: 2/1 (fall).
Degree Requirements Residency.

Vanderbilt University

School of Nursing
Nashville, Tennessee

http://www.nursing.vanderbilt.edu/
Founded in 1873

DEGREES • DNP • MSN • MSN/MDIV • MSN/MTS • PHD
Nursing Program Faculty 133 (44% with doctorates).
Graduate Enrollment 776 **Women** 91% **Men** 9% **Minority** 13% **International** 2% **Part-time** 48%
Distance Learning Courses Available.
Nursing Student Activities Nursing Honor Society, Sigma Theta Tau.
Nursing Student Resources Academic advising; academic or career counseling; assistance for students with disabilities; bookstore; campus computer network; career placement assistance; computer lab; computer-assisted instruction; daycare for children of students; e-mail services; housing assistance; interactive nursing skills videos; Internet; learning resource lab; library services; nursing audiovisuals; remedial services; resume preparation assistance; skills, simulation, or other laboratory; tutoring.
Library Facilities 1.8 million volumes (195,900 in health); 26,885 periodical subscriptions (3,113 health-care related).

GRADUATE PROGRAMS

Expenses (2010-11) *Tuition:* full-time $40,989; part-time $1051 per credit hour. *Required fees:* full-time $3257; part-time $1597 per term.
Financial Aid 89% of graduate students in nursing programs received some form of financial aid in 2009-10. 1 research assistantship (averaging $5,000 per year) was awarded; teaching assistantships, scholarships and tuition waivers also available. Aid available to part-time students. *Financial aid application deadline:* 3/15.
Contact Patricia Peerman, Assistant Dean of Enrollment Management, School of Nursing, Vanderbilt University, 207 Godchaux Hall, Nashville, TN 37240. *Telephone:* 615-322-3800. *Fax:* 615-343-0333. *E-mail:* paddy.peerman@vanderbilt.edu.

MASTER'S DEGREE PROGRAM

Degrees MSN; MSN/MDIV; MSN/MTS
Available Programs Accelerated AD/RN to Master's; Accelerated Master's; Accelerated Master's for Non-Nursing College Graduates;

Accelerated RN to Master's; Master's; Master's for Non-Nursing College Graduates; RN to Master's.

Concentrations Available Health-care administration; nurse-midwifery; nursing administration; nursing informatics. *Nurse practitioner programs in:* acute care, adult health, family health, gerontology, neonatal health, pediatric, psychiatric/mental health, women's health.

Study Options Full-time and part-time.

Online Degree Options Yes.

Program Entrance Requirements Computer literacy, minimum overall college GPA of 3.0, transcript of college record, CPR certification, written essay, immunizations, 3 letters of recommendation, physical assessment course, prerequisite course work, statistics course, GRE General Test. *Application deadline:* 12/1 (fall). Applications may be processed on a rolling basis for some programs. *Application fee:* $50.

Advanced Placement Credit by examination available. Credit given for nursing courses completed elsewhere dependent upon specific evaluations.

Degree Requirements 39 total credit hours.

POST-MASTER'S PROGRAM

Areas of Study Health-care administration; nurse-midwifery; nursing administration; nursing informatics. *Nurse practitioner programs in:* acute care, adult health, family health, gerontology, neonatal health, pediatric, psychiatric/mental health, women's health.

DOCTORAL DEGREE PROGRAM

Degree DNP

Available Programs Doctorate.

Areas of Study Aging, biology of health and illness, clinical practice, community health, critical care, family health, gerontology, health policy, health promotion/disease prevention, health-care systems, human health and illness, information systems, maternity-newborn, nursing administration, nursing policy, women's health.

Program Entrance Requirements Clinical experience, minimum overall college GPA of 3.5, interview by faculty committee, interview, 3 letters of recommendation, MSN or equivalent, statistics course, vita, writing sample, GRE General Test. Application deadline: 1/15 (fall). Applications may be processed on a rolling basis for some programs. Application fee: $50.

Degree Requirements 74 total credit hours, oral exam.

Degree PhD

Available Programs Doctorate.

Areas of Study health services research, clinical research.

Program Entrance Requirements Minimum overall college GPA of 3.5, 3 letters of recommendation, MSN or equivalent, clinical experience, interview by faculty committee, interview, statistics course, vita, writing sample. *Application deadline*: 1/15 (fall).

Degree Requirements 72 total credit hours, dissertation, oral exam.

POSTDOCTORAL PROGRAM

Areas of Study Individualized study.

Postdoctoral Program Contact Dr. Ann Minnick, Director, School of Nursing, Vanderbilt University, 415 Godchaux Hall, Nashville, TN 37240. *Telephone:* 615-343-2998. *Fax:* 615-343-5898. *E-mail:* ann.minnick@vanderbilt.edu.

See full description on page 508.

TEXAS

Abilene Christian University

Patty Hanks Shelton School of Nursing
Abilene, Texas

See description of programs under
Patty Hanks Shelton School of Nursing (Abilene, Texas)

Angelo State University
Department of Nursing
San Angelo, Texas

http://www.angelo.edu/dept/nursing
Founded in 1928

DEGREES • BSN • MSN

Nursing Program Faculty 36 (27% with doctorates).
Baccalaureate Enrollment 99 **Women** 83% **Men** 17% **Minority** 29% **Part-time** 87%
Graduate Enrollment 98 **Women** 89% **Men** 11% **Minority** 25% **International** 1% **Part-time** 81%
Distance Learning Courses Available.
Nursing Student Activities Student Nurses' Association.
Nursing Student Resources Academic advising; academic or career counseling; bookstore; campus computer network; computer lab; computer-assisted instruction; e-mail services; housing assistance; interactive nursing skills videos; Internet; learning resource lab; library services; nursing audiovisuals; skills, simulation, or other laboratory; tutoring.
Library Facilities 650,000 volumes (3,352 in health, 837 in nursing); 34,916 periodical subscriptions (173 health-care related).

BACCALAUREATE PROGRAMS

Degree BSN
Available Programs Accelerated Baccalaureate for Second Degree; RN Baccalaureate.
Online Degree Options Yes (online only).
Program Entrance Requirements Minimum overall college GPA of 2.5, transcript of college record, CPR certification, health insurance, immunizations, 2 letters of recommendation, RN licensure. Transfer students are accepted. *Application deadline:* 2/15 (fall), 10/15 (spring).
Expenses (2010-11) *Tuition, state resident:* full-time $8444; part-time $587 per credit hour. *Tuition, nonresident:* full-time $19,208; part-time $897 per credit hour. *Room and board:* $6815; room only: $4215 per academic year. *Required fees:* full-time $1800; part-time $50 per credit; part-time $25 per term.
Financial Aid 30% of baccalaureate students in nursing programs received some form of financial aid in 2009-10. *Gift aid (need-based):* Federal Pell, FSEOG, state, private, college/university gift aid from institutional funds, Federal Nursing. *Loans:* Federal Nursing Student Loans, Perkins, state, college/university, alternative loans. *Work-study:* Federal Work-Study, part-time campus jobs. *Financial aid application deadline (priority):* 4/1.
Contact Ms. Joanna Rabourn, Office Coordinator, Department of Nursing, Angelo State University, ASU Station #10911, San Angelo, TX 76909. *Telephone:* 325-942-2630. *Fax:* 325-942-2631. *E-mail:* joanna.rabourn@angelo.edu.

GRADUATE PROGRAMS

Expenses (2010-11) *Tuition, state resident:* full-time $9682; part-time $607 per credit hour. *Tuition, nonresident:* full-time $20,446; part-time $917 per credit hour. *Room and board:* $6815; room only: $4215 per academic year. *Required fees:* full-time $1800; part-time $50 per credit; part-time $25 per term.
Financial Aid 75% of graduate students in nursing programs received some form of financial aid in 2009-10. Career-related internships or fieldwork, Federal Work-Study, and scholarships available. Aid available to part-time students. *Financial aid application deadline:* 3/1.
Contact Dr. Molly Walker, Graduate Adviser, MSN Program, Department of Nursing, Angelo State University, ASU Station #10902, San Angelo, TX 76909. *Telephone:* 325-942-2224. *Fax:* 325-942-2236. *E-mail:* molly.walker@angelo.edu.

MASTER'S DEGREE PROGRAM

Degree MSN
Available Programs Master's; Master's for Non-Nursing College Graduates; RN to Master's.
Concentrations Available Nursing education. *Clinical nurse specialist programs in:* adult health, medical-surgical. *Nurse practitioner programs in:* family health.
Study Options Full-time and part-time.
Online Degree Options Yes (online only).
Program Entrance Requirements Computer literacy, minimum overall college GPA of 3.0, transcript of college record, CPR certification, written essay, immunizations, 2 letters of recommendation, physical assessment course, prerequisite course work, statistics course, GRE General Test. *Application deadline:* 7/1 (fall), 10/1 (spring).
Advanced Placement Credit given for nursing courses completed elsewhere dependent upon specific evaluations.
Degree Requirements 43 total credit hours, comprehensive exam.

Baylor University
Louise Herrington School of Nursing
Dallas, Texas

http://www.baylor.edu/nursing
Founded in 1845

DEGREES • BSN • DNP • MSN

Nursing Program Faculty 55 (24% with doctorates).
Baccalaureate Enrollment 288 **Women** 93% **Men** 7% **Minority** 32% **International** 4% **Part-time** 4%
Graduate Enrollment 76 **Women** 93.3% **Men** 6.7% **Minority** 25.3% **International** 1.3% **Part-time** 52%
Nursing Student Activities Sigma Theta Tau, Student Nurses' Association.
Nursing Student Resources Academic advising; campus computer network; computer lab; e-mail services; housing assistance; interactive nursing skills videos; Internet; learning resource lab; library services; nursing audiovisuals; skills, simulation, or other laboratory.
Library Facilities 2.3 million volumes (6,000 in health, 5,000 in nursing); 8,429 periodical subscriptions (147 health-care related).

BACCALAUREATE PROGRAMS

Degree BSN
Available Programs Accelerated Baccalaureate for Second Degree; Generic Baccalaureate.
Study Options Full-time.
Program Entrance Requirements Minimum overall college GPA of 3.0, transcript of college record, CPR certification, written essay, health exam, health insurance, immunizations, 3 letters of recommendation, minimum GPA in nursing prerequisites of 3.0, prerequisite course work. Transfer students are accepted. *Application deadline:* 1/15 (fall), 5/1 (spring).
Expenses (2010-11) *Tuition:* full-time $26,966; part-time $1124 per credit hour. *Required fees:* full-time $4208; part-time $50 per credit.
Financial Aid 94% of baccalaureate students in nursing programs received some form of financial aid in 2009-10. *Gift aid (need-based):* Federal Pell, FSEOG, state, college/university gift aid from institutional funds. *Loans:* Federal Nursing Student Loans, Federal Direct (Subsidized and Unsubsidized Stafford PLUS), Perkins, state, private loans. *Work-study:* Federal Work-Study, part-time campus jobs. *Financial aid application deadline (priority):* 3/1.
Contact Academic Advisor, Louise Herrington School of Nursing, Baylor University, 3700 Worth Street, Dallas, TX 75246. *Telephone:* 214-820-3361. *Fax:* 214-820-3835. *E-mail:* BU_Nursing@baylor.edu.

GRADUATE PROGRAMS

Expenses (2010-11) *Tuition:* full-time $26,966; part-time $1124 per credit hour. *Required fees:* full-time $4208; part-time $115 per credit.
Financial Aid 100% of graduate students in nursing programs received some form of financial aid in 2009-10.
Contact Dr. Mary C. Brucker, Director, Graduate Program, Louise Herrington School of Nursing, Baylor University, 3700 Worth Street, Dallas, TX 75246. *Telephone:* 214-820-3361. *Fax:* 214-820-4770. *E-mail:* mary_brucker@baylor.edu.

MASTER'S DEGREE PROGRAM

Degree MSN
Available Programs Master's.
Concentrations Available *Nurse practitioner programs in:* family health, neonatal health.
Site Options Waco, TX.
Study Options Full-time and part-time.
Program Entrance Requirements Clinical experience, minimum overall college GPA of 3.0, transcript of college record, CPR certification, written essay, immunizations, 3 letters of recommendation, prerequisite course work, statistics course, GRE General Test. *Application deadline:* 6/1 (fall). *Application fee:* $40.
Advanced Placement Credit given for nursing courses completed elsewhere dependent upon specific evaluations.
Degree Requirements 39 total credit hours.

POST-MASTER'S PROGRAM

Areas of Study *Nurse practitioner programs in:* family health, neonatal health.

DOCTORAL DEGREE PROGRAM

Degree DNP.

Available Programs Doctorate.

Areas of Study Maternity-newborn.

Site Options Waco, TX.

Program Entrance Requirements Clinical experience, minimum overall college GPA of 3, interview, 3 letters of recommendation, MSN or equivalent, vita, writing sample. Application deadline: 6/1 (fall). Application fee: $40.

Degree Requirements 75 total credit hours.

See full description on page 464.

East Texas Baptist University

Department of Nursing
Marshall, Texas

http://www.etbu.edu/academicSchools/School_of_Nursing

Founded in 1912

DEGREE • BSN

Nursing Program Faculty 8 (25% with doctorates).

Baccalaureate Enrollment 42 **Women** 81% **Men** 19% **Minority** 19%

Nursing Student Activities Student Nurses' Association.

Nursing Student Resources Academic advising; academic or career counseling; assistance for students with disabilities; bookstore; campus computer network; computer lab; computer-assisted instruction; e-mail services; employment services for current students; housing assistance; interactive nursing skills videos; Internet; learning resource lab; library services; nursing audiovisuals; remedial services; resume preparation assistance; skills, simulation, or other laboratory; tutoring.

Library Facilities 245,374 volumes (568 in health, 291 in nursing); 22,000 periodical subscriptions (2,100 health-care related).

BACCALAUREATE PROGRAMS

Degree BSN

Available Programs Generic Baccalaureate.

Study Options Full-time.

Program Entrance Requirements Transcript of college record, CPR certification, written essay, health insurance, immunizations, 2 letters of recommendation, minimum GPA in nursing prerequisites of 2.8, prerequisite course work. Transfer students are accepted. *Application deadline:* 3/1 (fall).

Advanced Placement Credit given for nursing courses completed elsewhere dependent upon specific evaluations.

Expenses (2010-11) *Tuition:* full-time $19,000; part-time $625 per credit hour. *Room and board:* $4920; room only: $2800 per academic year. *Required fees:* full-time $2050.

Financial Aid 99% of baccalaureate students in nursing programs received some form of financial aid in 2009-10.

Contact Susan Fratangelo, Admissions Coordinator, Department of Nursing, East Texas Baptist University, 1209 North Grove Street, Marshall, TX 75670-1498. *Telephone:* 903-923-2214. *Fax:* 903-938-9225. *E-mail:* sfratangelo@etbu.edu.

Hardin-Simmons University

Patty Hanks Shelton School of Nursing
Abilene, Texas

See description of programs under

Patty Hanks Shelton School of Nursing (Abilene, Texas).

Houston Baptist University
School of Nursing and Allied Health
Houston, Texas

Founded in 1960

DEGREE • BSN

Nursing Program Faculty 23 (6% with doctorates).
Baccalaureate Enrollment 60 **Women** 90% **Men** 10% **Minority** 20% **International** 10%
Nursing Student Activities Nursing Honor Society, Sigma Theta Tau, Student Nurses' Association.
Nursing Student Resources Academic advising; academic or career counseling; assistance for students with disabilities; bookstore; career placement assistance; computer lab; e-mail services; employment services for current students; externships; housing assistance; interactive nursing skills videos; Internet; learning resource lab; library services; nursing audiovisuals; paid internships; placement services for program completers; remedial services; resume preparation assistance; skills, simulation, or other laboratory; tutoring; unpaid internships.
Library Facilities 235,973 volumes (4,276 in health, 1,200 in nursing); 59,855 periodical subscriptions (117 health-care related).

BACCALAUREATE PROGRAMS

Degree BSN
Site Options Houston, TX.
Study Options Full-time.
Program Entrance Requirements Minimum overall college GPA of 2.5, minimum GPA in nursing prerequisites of 2.5. Transfer students are accepted.
Advanced Placement Credit by examination available.
Contact ***Telephone:*** 281-649-3300. *Fax:* 281-649-3340.

Lamar University
Department of Nursing
Beaumont, Texas

http://dept.lamar.edu/nursing/
Founded in 1923

DEGREES • BSN • MSN • MSN/MBA

Nursing Program Faculty 39 (31% with doctorates).
Baccalaureate Enrollment 271 **Women** 85% **Men** 15% **Minority** 31% **Part-time** 3.5%
Graduate Enrollment 32 **Women** 91% **Men** 9% **Minority** 17% **Part-time** 88%
Distance Learning Courses Available.
Nursing Student Activities Sigma Theta Tau, Student Nurses' Association.
Nursing Student Resources Academic advising; academic or career counseling; assistance for students with disabilities; bookstore; campus computer network; career placement assistance; computer lab; computer-assisted instruction; daycare for children of students; e-mail services; employment services for current students; housing assistance; interactive nursing skills videos; Internet; learning resource lab; library services; nursing audiovisuals; placement services for program completers; remedial services; resume preparation assistance; skills, simulation, or other laboratory; tutoring.
Library Facilities 526,180 volumes (6,825 in health, 3,160 in nursing); 26,618 periodical subscriptions (166 health-care related).

BACCALAUREATE PROGRAMS

Degree BSN
Available Programs ADN to Baccalaureate; Generic Baccalaureate; RN Baccalaureate.
Study Options Full-time.
Online Degree Options Yes.
Program Entrance Requirements Minimum overall college GPA of 2.5, transcript of college record, CPR certification, health exam, immunizations, minimum GPA in nursing prerequisites of 2.5, professional liability insurance/malpractice insurance, prerequisite course work. Transfer students are accepted. *Application deadline:* 3/1 (fall), 10/1 (spring). *Application fee:* $25.
Advanced Placement Credit given for nursing courses completed elsewhere dependent upon specific evaluations.
Expenses (2010-11) *Tuition, state resident:* full-time $8223. *Tuition, nonresident:* full-time $18,762. *Room and board:* $5742; room only: $4500 per academic year. *Required fees:* full-time $300; part-time $150 per term.
Financial Aid 71% of baccalaureate students in nursing programs received some form of financial aid in 2009-10. *Gift aid (need-based):* Federal Pell, FSEOG, state, college/university gift aid from institutional funds. *Loans:* Perkins, state, college/university. *Work-study:* Federal Work-Study, part-time campus jobs. *Financial aid application deadline (priority):* 4/1.
Contact Ms. Melissa I. Chandler, Academic Advisor, Department of Nursing, Lamar University, PO Box 10081, Beaumont, TX 77710. *Telephone:* 409-880-8868. *Fax:* 409-880-7736. *E-mail:* nursing@lamar.edu.

GRADUATE PROGRAMS

Expenses (2010-11) *Tuition, state resident:* full-time $5750; part-time $423 per credit hour. *Tuition, nonresident:* full-time $11,486; part-time $773 per credit hour. *Room and board:* $5742; room only: $4500 per academic year. *Required fees:* full-time $300; part-time $150 per term.
Financial Aid 71% of graduate students in nursing programs received some form of financial aid in 2009-10.
Contact Dr. Nancy Bume, Director of Graduate Nursing Studies, Department of Nursing, Lamar University, PO Box 10081, Beaumont, TX 77710. *Telephone:* 409-880-7720. *Fax:* 409-880-8698. *E-mail:* nancy.blume@lamar.edu.

MASTER'S DEGREE PROGRAM

Degrees MSN; MSN/MBA
Available Programs Master's.
Concentrations Available Nursing administration; nursing education.
Study Options Full-time and part-time.
Online Degree Options Yes (online only).
Program Entrance Requirements Computer literacy, minimum overall college GPA of 3.0, transcript of college record, immunizations, professional liability insurance/malpractice insurance, prerequisite course work, statistics course. *Application deadline:* Applications may be processed on a rolling basis for some programs. *Application fee:* $25.
Advanced Placement Credit given for nursing courses completed elsewhere dependent upon specific evaluations.
Degree Requirements 37 total credit hours, thesis or project, comprehensive exam.

POST-MASTER'S PROGRAM

Areas of Study Nursing administration; nursing education.

CONTINUING EDUCATION PROGRAM

Contact Dr. Cindy Stinson, Coordinator of Continuing Education, Department of Nursing, Lamar University, PO Box 10081, Beaumont, TX 77710. *Telephone:* 409-880-8833. *Fax:* 409-880-1865. *E-mail:* cynthia.stinson@lamar.edu.

Lubbock Christian University
Department of Nursing
Lubbock, Texas

Founded in 1957

DEGREE • BSN

Nursing Program Faculty 5 (40% with doctorates).
Library Facilities 172,464 volumes; 580 periodical subscriptions.

BACCALAUREATE PROGRAMS

Degree BSN
Available Programs RN Baccalaureate.
Study Options Part-time.
Program Entrance Requirements Minimum overall college GPA of 2.5, transcript of college record, CPR certification, health exam, immunizations, interview, 2 letters of recommendation, minimum high school GPA, minimum GPA in nursing prerequisites of 2.5, professional liability insurance/malpractice insurance, prerequisite course work, RN licensure. Transfer students are accepted.

McMurry University
Patty Hanks Shelton School of Nursing
Abilene, Texas

See description of programs under
Patty Hanks Shelton School of Nursing (Abilene, Texas).

Midwestern State University
Nursing Program
Wichita Falls, Texas

Founded in 1922

DEGREES • BSN • MN/MHSA • MSN • MSN/MHA

Nursing Program Faculty 22 (4.4% with doctorates).
Baccalaureate Enrollment 271 **Women** 82% **Men** 18% **Minority** 54% **International** 4% **Part-time** 1%
Graduate Enrollment 65 **Women** 86% **Men** 14% **Minority** 46% **International** 6% **Part-time** 70%
Nursing Student Activities Nursing Honor Society, Sigma Theta Tau, Student Nurses' Association.
Nursing Student Resources Academic advising; academic or career counseling; assistance for students with disabilities; bookstore; campus computer network; career placement assistance; computer lab; computer-assisted instruction; e-mail services; employment services for current students; externships; housing assistance; interactive nursing skills videos; Internet; learning resource lab; library services; nursing audiovisuals; other; paid internships; placement services for program completers; remedial services; resume preparation assistance; skills, simulation, or other laboratory; tutoring; unpaid internships.
Library Facilities 515,252 volumes (10,000 in health, 5,000 in nursing); 889 periodical subscriptions (200 health-care related).

BACCALAUREATE PROGRAMS

Degree BSN
Available Programs ADN to Baccalaureate; Generic Baccalaureate; RN Baccalaureate.
Study Options Full-time and part-time.
Program Entrance Requirements Transcript of college record, CPR certification, health exam, health insurance, high school transcript, immunizations, minimum GPA in nursing prerequisites of 3.0, professional liability insurance/malpractice insurance, prerequisite course work. Transfer students are accepted.
Advanced Placement Credit by examination available. Credit given for nursing courses completed elsewhere dependent upon specific evaluations.
Contact *Telephone:* 940-397-4601. *Fax:* 940-397-4911.

GRADUATE PROGRAMS

Contact *Telephone:* 940-397-4601. *Fax:* 940-397-4911.

MASTER'S DEGREE PROGRAM

Degrees MN/MHSA; MSN; MSN/MHA
Available Programs Master's; RN to Master's.
Concentrations Available Health-care administration; nursing administration; nursing education. *Nurse practitioner programs in:* family health.
Study Options Full-time and part-time.
Program Entrance Requirements Clinical experience, computer literacy, minimum overall college GPA of 3.0, transcript of college record, CPR certification, immunizations, interview, nursing research course, physical assessment course, professional liability insurance/malpractice insurance, prerequisite course work, statistics course, GRE General Test or MAT.
Degree Requirements 36 total credit hours, thesis or project.

POST-MASTER'S PROGRAM

Areas of Study Nursing education. *Nurse practitioner programs in:* family health.

CONTINUING EDUCATION PROGRAM

Contact *Telephone:* 940-397-4048. *Fax:* 940-397-4513.

Patty Hanks Shelton School of Nursing
Patty Hanks Shelton School of Nursing
Abilene, Texas

http://www.aisn.edu/

DEGREES • BSN • MSN

Nursing Program Faculty 17 (33% with doctorates).
Baccalaureate Enrollment 130 **Women** 90% **Men** 10% **Minority** 15% **International** 4%
Graduate Enrollment 23 **Women** 75% **Men** 25% **Minority** 10%
Distance Learning Courses Available.
Nursing Student Activities Nursing Honor Society, Sigma Theta Tau, Student Nurses' Association.
Nursing Student Resources Academic advising; academic or career counseling; assistance for students with disabilities; bookstore; campus computer network; career placement assistance; computer lab; computer-assisted instruction; e-mail services; employment services for current students; externships; interactive nursing skills videos; Internet; learning resource lab; library services; nursing audiovisuals; remedial services; resume preparation assistance; skills, simulation, or other laboratory; tutoring.
Library Facilities 9,200 volumes in health, 1,300 volumes in nursing; 140 periodical subscriptions health-care related.

BACCALAUREATE PROGRAMS

Degree BSN
Available Programs Generic Baccalaureate; RN Baccalaureate.
Study Options Full-time.
Program Entrance Requirements Minimum overall college GPA of 3.0, transcript of college record, CPR certification, health exam, health insurance, immunizations, interview, 2 letters of recommendation, minimum GPA in nursing prerequisites of 3.0, professional liability insurance/malpractice insurance, prerequisite course work. Transfer students are accepted. *Application deadline:* 2/12 (fall). *Application fee:* $80.
Advanced Placement Credit by examination available. Credit given for nursing courses completed elsewhere dependent upon specific evaluations.
Financial Aid 80% of baccalaureate students in nursing programs received some form of financial aid in 2008-09.
Contact Mrs. Rachel King, Director, Learning and Student Development, Patty Hanks Shelton School of Nursing, 2149 Hickory Street, Abilene, TX 79601. *Telephone:* 325-671-2353. *Fax:* 325-671-2386. *E-mail:* rking@phssn.edu.

GRADUATE PROGRAMS

Financial Aid 50% of graduate students in nursing programs received some form of financial aid in 2008-09.
Contact Dr. Amy Roberts Toone, Director of the Graduate Program, Patty Hanks Shelton School of Nursing, 2149 Hickory Street, Abilene, TX 79601. *Telephone:* 325-671-2361. *Fax:* 325-671-2386. *E-mail:* atoone@phssn.edu.

MASTER'S DEGREE PROGRAM

Degree MSN
Available Programs Master's.
Concentrations Available Nursing administration; nursing education. *Nurse practitioner programs in:* family health.
Study Options Full-time and part-time.
Program Entrance Requirements Clinical experience, minimum overall college GPA of 3.5, transcript of college record, CPR certification, written essay, immunizations, interview, 3 letters of recommendation, physical assessment course, professional liability insurance/malpractice insurance, resume, statistics course.
Advanced Placement Credit given for nursing courses completed elsewhere dependent upon specific evaluations.
Degree Requirements 49 total credit hours.

POST-MASTER'S PROGRAM

Areas of Study *Nurse practitioner programs in:* family health.

CONTINUING EDUCATION PROGRAM

Contact Dr. Nina Ouimette, Dean and Associate Professor, Patty Hanks Shelton School of Nursing, 2149 Hickory Street, Abilene, TX 79601.

Telephone: 325-671-2399. *Fax:* 325-671-2386. *E-mail:* nouimette@phssn.edu.

Prairie View A&M University
College of Nursing
Houston, Texas

http://www.pvamu.edu/nursing
Founded in 1878

DEGREES • BSN • MSN
Nursing Program Faculty 66 (26% with doctorates).
Baccalaureate Enrollment 447 **Women** 85% **Men** 15% **Minority** 38% **International** 2% **Part-time** 19%
Graduate Enrollment 103 **Women** 95% **Men** 5% **Minority** 25% **International** 2% **Part-time** 78%
Distance Learning Courses Available.
Nursing Student Activities Nursing Honor Society, Sigma Theta Tau, Student Nurses' Association, nursing club.
Nursing Student Resources Academic advising; academic or career counseling; assistance for students with disabilities; bookstore; campus computer network; career placement assistance; computer lab; computer-assisted instruction; e-mail services; employment services for current students; interactive nursing skills videos; Internet; learning resource lab; library services; nursing audiovisuals; placement services for program completers; resume preparation assistance; skills, simulation, or other laboratory; tutoring.
Library Facilities 1.2 million volumes (355,707 in health, 7,899 in nursing); 42,660 periodical subscriptions (9,283 health-care related).

BACCALAUREATE PROGRAMS

Degree BSN
Available Programs Generic Baccalaureate; LPN to Baccalaureate; RN Baccalaureate.
Site Options Woodlands, TX; College Station, TX.
Study Options Full-time and part-time.
Program Entrance Requirements Minimum overall college GPA of 2.5, transcript of college record, CPR certification, health exam, immunizations, minimum GPA in nursing prerequisites of 2.0, professional liability insurance/malpractice insurance, prerequisite course work. Transfer students are accepted. *Application deadline:* 3/1 (fall), 10/1 (spring). *Application fee:* $25.
Advanced Placement Credit given for nursing courses completed elsewhere dependent upon specific evaluations.
Expenses (2009-10) *Tuition, area resident:* full-time $4232; part-time $163 per credit hour. *Tuition, nonresident:* full-time $11,435; part-time $440 per credit hour. *International tuition:* $11,435 full-time. *Required fees:* full-time $2181; part-time $272 per credit; part-time $864 per term.
Financial Aid 95% of baccalaureate students in nursing programs received some form of financial aid in 2008-09.
Contact Dr. Forest Smith, Director, Admissions and Student Services, College of Nursing, Prairie View A&M University, 6436 Fannin Street, Suite 109, Houston, TX 77030. *Telephone:* 713-797-7031. *Fax:* 713-797-7092. *E-mail:* fdsmith@pvamu.edu.

GRADUATE PROGRAMS

Expenses (2009-10) *Tuition, area resident:* full-time $6170; part-time $213 per credit hour. *Tuition, nonresident:* full-time $15,738; part-time $492 per credit hour. *International tuition:* $15,738 full-time. *Required fees:* full-time $3257; part-time $633 per credit; part-time $1086 per term.
Financial Aid 38% of graduate students in nursing programs received some form of financial aid in 2008-09. Career-related internships or fieldwork, Federal Work-Study, institutionally sponsored loans, scholarships, and traineeships available. Aid available to part-time students. *Financial aid application deadline:* 4/1.
Contact Dr. Jennifer Goodman, Director, College of Nursing, Prairie View A&M University, 6436 Fannin Street, Suite 1254, Houston, TX 77030. *Telephone:* 713-797-7015. *Fax:* 713-797-7011. *E-mail:* jjgoodman@pvamu.edu.

MASTER'S DEGREE PROGRAM

Degree MSN
Available Programs Master's.
Concentrations Available Nursing administration; nursing education. *Nurse practitioner programs in:* family health.
Study Options Full-time and part-time.
Program Entrance Requirements Clinical experience, minimum overall college GPA of 2.75, transcript of college record, CPR certification, immunizations, interview, 3 letters of recommendation, physical assessment course, prerequisite course work, resume, statistics course, MAT or GRE. *Application deadline:* 6/1 (fall), 10/1 (spring), 4/1 (summer). *Application fee:* $25.
Advanced Placement Credit by examination available. Credit given for nursing courses completed elsewhere dependent upon specific evaluations.
Degree Requirements 53 total credit hours, thesis or project.

POST-MASTER'S PROGRAM

Areas of Study Nursing administration; nursing education. *Nurse practitioner programs in:* family health.

Southwestern Adventist University
Department of Nursing
Keene, Texas

http://www.swau.edu/
Founded in 1894

DEGREE • BS
Nursing Program Faculty 17 (24% with doctorates).
Baccalaureate Enrollment 115 **Women** 80% **Men** 20% **Minority** 63% **International** 13%
Nursing Student Activities Student Nurses' Association.
Nursing Student Resources Academic advising; academic or career counseling; assistance for students with disabilities; bookstore; campus computer network; computer lab; computer-assisted instruction; e-mail services; externships; interactive nursing skills videos; Internet; learning resource lab; library services; nursing audiovisuals; remedial services; resume preparation assistance; skills, simulation, or other laboratory; tutoring.
Library Facilities 135,774 volumes (6,575 in nursing); 4,500 periodical subscriptions (60 health-care related).

BACCALAUREATE PROGRAMS

Degree BS
Available Programs ADN to Baccalaureate; Generic Baccalaureate; LPN to Baccalaureate.
Study Options Full-time and part-time.
Program Entrance Requirements Transcript of college record, CPR certification, health exam, health insurance, immunizations, 3 letters of recommendation, minimum GPA in nursing prerequisites of 2.75, prerequisite course work. Transfer students are accepted. *Application deadline:* 11/30 (spring). *Application fee:* $100.
Advanced Placement Credit by examination available.
Expenses (2010-11) *Tuition:* full-time $16,456; part-time $669 per credit. *Room and board:* $7242; room only: $3222 per academic year. *Required fees:* full-time $400.
Financial Aid 65% of baccalaureate students in nursing programs received some form of financial aid in 2009-10.
Contact Dr. Ronald Mitchell, Chair, Department of Nursing, Southwestern Adventist University, 100 West Hillcrest Street, Keene, TX 76059. *Telephone:* 817-202-6230. *Fax:* 817-202-6713. *E-mail:* rmitchell@swau.edu.

Stephen F. Austin State University
Richard and Lucille Dewitt School of Nursing
Nacogdoches, Texas

http://www.fp.sfasu.edu/nursing/
Founded in 1923

DEGREE • BSN
Nursing Program Faculty 19 (16% with doctorates).
Baccalaureate Enrollment 128 **Women** 96% **Men** 4% **Minority** 1%
Nursing Student Activities Sigma Theta Tau, Student Nurses' Association.

Nursing Student Resources Academic advising; academic or career counseling; bookstore; computer lab; computer-assisted instruction; e-mail services; interactive nursing skills videos; Internet; library services; nursing audiovisuals; skills, simulation, or other laboratory; tutoring.
Library Facilities 735,445 volumes; 1,378 periodical subscriptions.

BACCALAUREATE PROGRAMS

Degree BSN
Available Programs RN Baccalaureate.
Site Options Lufkin, TX.
Study Options Full-time.
Program Entrance Requirements Minimum overall college GPA of 2.75, transcript of college record, CPR certification, health insurance, high school transcript, immunizations, minimum GPA in nursing prerequisites of 2.5, professional liability insurance/malpractice insurance, prerequisite course work. Transfer students are accepted.
Advanced Placement Credit given for nursing courses completed elsewhere dependent upon specific evaluations.
Contact *Telephone:* 936-468-3604. *Fax:* 936-468-1696.

Tarleton State University

Department of Nursing
Stephenville, Texas

http://www.tarleton.edu/~nursing
Founded in 1899

DEGREE • BSN

Nursing Program Faculty 19 (14% with doctorates).
Baccalaureate Enrollment 230 **Women** 95% **Men** 5% **Minority** 15% **International** 2% **Part-time** 25%
Nursing Student Activities Sigma Theta Tau, Student Nurses' Association.
Nursing Student Resources Academic advising; academic or career counseling; assistance for students with disabilities; bookstore; computer lab; computer-assisted instruction; daycare for children of students; e-mail services; employment services for current students; externships; learning resource lab; library services; nursing audiovisuals; remedial services; resume preparation assistance; skills, simulation, or other laboratory; tutoring; unpaid internships.
Library Facilities 400,000 volumes; 25,800 periodical subscriptions.

BACCALAUREATE PROGRAMS

Degree BSN
Available Programs ADN to Baccalaureate; Generic Baccalaureate; LPN to Baccalaureate.
Study Options Full-time and part-time.
Program Entrance Requirements Transcript of college record, CPR certification, written essay, health exam, high school transcript, immunizations, 3 letters of recommendation, minimum GPA in nursing prerequisites of 2.75, professional liability insurance/malpractice insurance, prerequisite course work. Transfer students are accepted.
Advanced Placement Credit by examination available. Credit given for nursing courses completed elsewhere dependent upon specific evaluations.
Contact *Telephone:* 254-968-9139. *Fax:* 254-968-9716.

CONTINUING EDUCATION PROGRAM

Contact *Telephone:* 325-649-8058. *Fax:* 325-649-8959.

Texas A&M Health Science Center

College of Nursing
College Station, Texas

Founded in 1999

DEGREE • BSN

BACCALAUREATE PROGRAMS

Degree BSN
Available Programs Accelerated Baccalaureate for Second Degree; Generic Baccalaureate; RN Baccalaureate.
Online Degree Options Yes.
Program Entrance Requirements Minimum overall college GPA of 3.0, transcript of college record, CPR certification, written essay, health exam, immunizations, 3 letters of recommendation, minimum GPA in nursing prerequisites of 3.25, professional liability insurance/malpractice insurance. Transfer students are accepted. *Application deadline:* 2/1 (fall). *Application fee:* $50.
Contact Dean, College of Nursing, Texas A&M Health Science Center, 8447 State Highway 47, Bryan, TX 77807-3260. *Telephone:* 979-436-0110. *Fax:* 979-436-0098. *E-mail:* wilkerson@tamhsc.edu.

Texas A&M International University

Canseco School of Nursing
Laredo, Texas

Founded in 1969

DEGREES • BSN • MSN

Nursing Program Faculty 18 (20% with doctorates).
Baccalaureate Enrollment 175 **Women** 70% **Men** 30% **Minority** 98% **International** 1% **Part-time** 25%
Graduate Enrollment 12 **Women** 75% **Men** 25% **Minority** 75% **Part-time** 100%
Nursing Student Activities Nursing Honor Society, Student Nurses' Association.
Nursing Student Resources Academic advising; academic or career counseling; assistance for students with disabilities; bookstore; campus computer network; career placement assistance; computer lab; computer-assisted instruction; daycare for children of students; e-mail services; employment services for current students; externships; housing assistance; interactive nursing skills videos; Internet; learning resource lab; library services; nursing audiovisuals; paid internships; placement services for program completers; remedial services; resume preparation assistance; skills, simulation, or other laboratory; tutoring.
Library Facilities 368,166 volumes (8,500 in nursing); 32,689 periodical subscriptions (80 health-care related).

BACCALAUREATE PROGRAMS

Degree BSN
Available Programs Generic Baccalaureate; RN Baccalaureate.
Study Options Full-time.
Program Entrance Requirements Minimum overall college GPA of 2.5, transcript of college record, written essay, health exam, immunizations, 2 letters of recommendation, minimum GPA in nursing prerequisites of 2.5, prerequisite course work. Transfer students are accepted. *Application deadline:* 9/1 (fall).
Advanced Placement Credit given for nursing courses completed elsewhere dependent upon specific evaluations.
Expenses (2009-10) *Tuition, state resident:* full-time $4740; part-time $288 per credit hour. *Tuition, nonresident:* full-time $11,386; part-time $564 per credit hour.
Financial Aid 85% of baccalaureate students in nursing programs received some form of financial aid in 2008-09.
Contact Dr. Regina C. Aune, RN, Dean, Canseco School of Nursing, Texas A&M International University, 5201 University Boulevard, Laredo, TX 78041-1900. *Telephone:* 956-326-2450. *Fax:* 956-326-2449. *E-mail:* regina.aune@tamiu.edu.

GRADUATE PROGRAMS

Expenses (2009-10) *Tuition, state resident:* full-time $4980; part-time $307 per credit hour. *Tuition, nonresident:* full-time $8634; part-time $558 per credit hour.
Financial Aid 85% of graduate students in nursing programs received some form of financial aid in 2008-09.
Contact Dr. Regina C. Aune, RN, Dean, Canseco School of Nursing, Texas A&M International University, 5201 University Boulevard, Laredo, TX 78041-1900. *Telephone:* 956-326-2450. *Fax:* 956-326-2449. *E-mail:* sbaker@tamiu.edu.

MASTER'S DEGREE PROGRAM

Degree MSN
Available Programs Master's; Master's for Nurses with Non-Nursing Degrees.
Concentrations Available *Nurse practitioner programs in:* family health.

Study Options Full-time and part-time.
Program Entrance Requirements Clinical experience, minimum overall college GPA of 3.0, transcript of college record, CPR certification, written essay, immunizations, interview, 2 letters of recommendation.
Advanced Placement Credit given for nursing courses completed elsewhere dependent upon specific evaluations.
Degree Requirements 45 total credit hours.

Texas A&M University–Corpus Christi

School of Nursing and Health Sciences
Corpus Christi, Texas

http://conhs.tamucc.edu/
Founded in 1947

DEGREES • BSN • MSN

Nursing Program Faculty 55 (45% with doctorates).
Baccalaureate Enrollment 425 **Women** 72% **Men** 28% **Minority** 52% **International** 1% **Part-time** 20%
Graduate Enrollment 345 **Women** 87% **Men** 13% **Minority** 38% **International** 1% **Part-time** 99%
Distance Learning Courses Available.
Nursing Student Activities Nursing Honor Society, Sigma Theta Tau, Student Nurses' Association.
Nursing Student Resources Academic advising; academic or career counseling; assistance for students with disabilities; bookstore; campus computer network; career placement assistance; computer lab; computer-assisted instruction; e-mail services; employment services for current students; housing assistance; interactive nursing skills videos; Internet; learning resource lab; library services; nursing audiovisuals; placement services for program completers; remedial services; resume preparation assistance; skills, simulation, or other laboratory; tutoring.
Library Facilities 731,586 volumes (500 in health, 350 in nursing); 1,901 periodical subscriptions (100 health-care related).

BACCALAUREATE PROGRAMS

Degree BSN
Available Programs ADN to Baccalaureate; Accelerated Baccalaureate for Second Degree; Baccalaureate for Second Degree; Generic Baccalaureate; RN Baccalaureate.
Study Options Full-time and part-time.
Online Degree Options Yes.
Program Entrance Requirements Minimum overall college GPA of 3.0, transcript of college record, CPR certification, immunizations, professional liability insurance/malpractice insurance, prerequisite course work. Transfer students are accepted. *Application deadline:* 2/16 (fall), 8/3 (spring), 12/1 (summer). *Application fee:* $25.
Advanced Placement Credit by examination available. Credit given for nursing courses completed elsewhere dependent upon specific evaluations.
Expenses (2009-10) *Tuition, area resident:* full-time $5317; part-time $141 per credit. *Tuition, state resident:* full-time $5317; part-time $144 per credit. *Tuition, nonresident:* full-time $16,276; part-time $422 per credit. *International tuition:* $16,276 full-time. *Room and board:* $1900; room only: $900 per academic year. *Required fees:* full-time $4376; part-time $150 per credit; part-time $1044 per term.
Financial Aid 70% of baccalaureate students in nursing programs received some form of financial aid in 2008-09. *Gift aid (need-based):* Federal Pell, FSEOG, state, college/university gift aid from institutional funds. *Loans:* Perkins, state, college/university. *Work-study:* Federal Work-Study, part-time campus jobs. *Financial aid application deadline (priority):* 3/31.
Contact Ms. Angelica M. Santillan, Academic Advisor, School of Nursing and Health Sciences, Texas A&M University–Corpus Christi, 6300 Ocean Drive, Unit 5805, Corpus Christi, TX 78412. *Telephone:* 361-825-2461. *E-mail:* angelica.santillan@tamucc.edu.

GRADUATE PROGRAMS

Expenses (2009-10) *Tuition, area resident:* full-time $4103; part-time $70 per credit hour. *Tuition, state resident:* full-time $10,751; part-time $70 per credit hour. *Tuition, nonresident:* full-time $10,751; part-time $448 per credit hour. *International tuition:* $10,751 full-time. *Required fees:* full-time $1081; part-time $155 per credit; part-time $455 per term.
Financial Aid 20% of graduate students in nursing programs received some form of financial aid in 2008-09.
Contact Dr. Eve Layman, RN, Graduate Department Chair, School of Nursing and Health Sciences, Texas A&M University–Corpus Christi, 6300 Ocean Drive, Unit 5805, Corpus Christi, TX 78412. *Telephone:* 361-825-3781. *Fax:* 361-825-5853. *E-mail:* eve.layman@tamucc.edu.

MASTER'S DEGREE PROGRAM

Degree MSN
Available Programs Accelerated AD/RN to Master's; Accelerated RN to Master's; Master's.
Concentrations Available Nursing administration. *Clinical nurse specialist programs in:* adult health. *Nurse practitioner programs in:* family health.
Site Options Temple, TX.
Study Options Part-time.
Online Degree Options Yes (online only).
Program Entrance Requirements Computer literacy, minimum overall college GPA of 3.0, transcript of college record, CPR certification, written essay, immunizations, 3 letters of recommendation, nursing research course, resume, statistics course. *Application deadline:* 7/14 (fall), 11/15 (spring), 4/15 (summer). *Application fee:* $40.
Advanced Placement Credit given for nursing courses completed elsewhere dependent upon specific evaluations.
Degree Requirements 49 total credit hours.

POST-MASTER'S PROGRAM

Areas of Study Nursing administration; nursing education. *Clinical nurse specialist programs in:* adult health. *Nurse practitioner programs in:* family health.

CONTINUING EDUCATION PROGRAM

Contact Ms. Petra Martinez, Chair of Continuing Education Committee, School of Nursing and Health Sciences, Texas A&M University–Corpus Christi, 6300 Ocean Drive, ST 316, Corpus Christi, TX 78412. *Telephone:* 361-825-2353. *Fax:* 361-825-3491. *E-mail:* petra.martinez@tamucc.edu.

Texas A&M University–Texarkana

Nursing Department
Texarkana, Texas

http://www.tamut.edu/nursing/index.php?pageid=13
Founded in 1971

DEGREES • BSN • MSN

Nursing Program Faculty 5 (60% with doctorates).
Baccalaureate Enrollment 31 **Women** 87% **Men** 13% **Minority** 23% **Part-time** 94%
Graduate Enrollment 26 **Women** 96% **Men** 4% **Minority** 15% **Part-time** 100%
Nursing Student Activities Nursing club.
Nursing Student Resources Academic advising; academic or career counseling; assistance for students with disabilities; bookstore; campus computer network; career placement assistance; computer lab; computer-assisted instruction; e-mail services; Internet; library services; nursing audiovisuals; resume preparation assistance.
Library Facilities 8,743 volumes in health, 2,558 volumes in nursing; 80 periodical subscriptions health-care related.

BACCALAUREATE PROGRAMS

Degree BSN
Available Programs ADN to Baccalaureate.
Study Options Full-time and part-time.
Program Entrance Requirements Minimum overall college GPA of 2.0, transcript of college record, CPR certification, health exam, health insurance, immunizations, letters of recommendation, professional liability insurance/malpractice insurance, prerequisite course work, RN licensure. Transfer students are accepted. *Application deadline:* 7/15 (fall), 12/1 (spring), 4/1 (summer).
Advanced Placement Credit given for nursing courses completed elsewhere dependent upon specific evaluations.
Expenses (2009-10) *Tuition, state resident:* full-time $3900; part-time $130 per credit hour. *Tuition, nonresident:* full-time $12,210; part-time $407 per credit hour. *International tuition:* $12,210 full-time. *Required fees:* full-time $656; part-time $21 per credit.

Financial Aid 12% of baccalaureate students in nursing programs received some form of financial aid in 2008-09. *Gift aid (need-based):* Federal Pell, FSEOG, state, private, college/university gift aid from institutional funds. *Loans:* college/university. *Work-study:* Federal Work-Study. *Financial aid application deadline (priority):* 5/1.
Contact Jo Kahler, EdD, Dean of the College of Health and Behavioral Sciences, Nursing Department, Texas A&M University–Texarkana, PO Box 5518, 2600 North Robison Road, Texarkana, TX 75501. *Telephone:* 903-223-3175. *Fax:* 903-223-3107. *E-mail:* Jo.Kahler@tamut.edu.

GRADUATE PROGRAMS

Expenses (2009-10) *Tuition, state resident:* full-time $3600; part-time $150 per credit hour. *Tuition, nonresident:* full-time $10,248; part-time $427 per credit hour. *International tuition:* $10,248 full-time. *Required fees:* full-time $532; part-time $20 per credit; part-time $9 per term.
Contact Dr. Jo Kahler, Dean, College of Health and Behavioral Sciences, Nursing Department, Texas A&M University–Texarkana, PO Box 5518, 2600 North Robison Road, Texarkana, TX 75505. *Telephone:* 903-223-3175. *E-mail:* jo.kahler@tamut.edu.

MASTER'S DEGREE PROGRAM

Degree MSN
Available Programs Master's.
Concentrations Available Nursing administration; nursing education.
Study Options Full-time and part-time.
Program Entrance Requirements Minimum overall college GPA of 3.0, transcript of college record, written essay, 3 letters of recommendation, resume. *Application deadline:* 7/15 (fall), 12/1 (spring), 4/1 (summer).
Degree Requirements 36 total credit hours.

Texas Christian University
Harris College of Nursing
Fort Worth, Texas

http://www.nursing.tcu.edu/
Founded in 1873

DEGREES • BSN • DNP • MSN

Nursing Program Faculty 50 (62% with doctorates).
Baccalaureate Enrollment 653 **Women** 92.5% **Men** 7.5% **Minority** 20% **International** 1%
Graduate Enrollment 282 **Women** 61% **Men** 39% **Minority** 79% **Part-time** 11%
Distance Learning Courses Available.
Nursing Student Activities Sigma Theta Tau, Student Nurses' Association.
Nursing Student Resources Academic advising; academic or career counseling; assistance for students with disabilities; bookstore; campus computer network; career placement assistance; computer lab; computer-assisted instruction; e-mail services; externships; interactive nursing skills videos; Internet; learning resource lab; library services; nursing audiovisuals; other; remedial services; resume preparation assistance; skills, simulation, or other laboratory; tutoring; unpaid internships.
Library Facilities 1.4 million volumes (17,565 in health, 1,525 in nursing); 56,856 periodical subscriptions (180 health-care related).

BACCALAUREATE PROGRAMS

Degree BSN
Available Programs Accelerated Baccalaureate for Second Degree; Generic Baccalaureate.
Site Options Fort Worth, TX.
Study Options Full-time and part-time.
Program Entrance Requirements Minimum overall college GPA of 2.5, transcript of college record, CPR certification, written essay, high school foreign language, 2 years high school math, 4 years high school science, high school transcript, immunizations, minimum high school GPA of 3.0, minimum GPA in nursing prerequisites of 2.5, prerequisite course work. Transfer students are accepted. *Application deadline:* 2/1 (fall), 10/1 (spring), 11/15 (summer). *Application fee:* $40.
Advanced Placement Credit by examination available. Credit given for nursing courses completed elsewhere dependent upon specific evaluations.
Expenses (2010-11) *Tuition:* full-time $30,090; part-time $980 per credit hour. *Room and board:* $6300; room only: $3710 per academic year. *Required fees:* full-time $680.
Financial Aid 80% of baccalaureate students in nursing programs received some form of financial aid in 2009-10. *Gift aid (need-based):* Federal Pell, FSEOG, state, private, college/university gift aid from institutional funds. *Loans:* Federal Nursing Student Loans, Perkins, state. *Work-study:* Federal Work-Study, part-time campus jobs. *Financial aid application deadline:* 5/1.
Contact Ms. Zoranna Jones, Assistant Director of Nursing Recruitment and Retention, Harris College of Nursing, Texas Christian University, TCU Box 298620, Fort Worth, TX 76129. *Telephone:* 817-257-7650. *Fax:* 817-257-7944. *E-mail:* z.jones@tcu.edu.

GRADUATE PROGRAMS

Expenses (2010-11) *Tuition:* full-time $34,000; part-time $1040 per credit hour. *Required fees:* full-time $702.
Financial Aid 100% of graduate students in nursing programs received some form of financial aid in 2009-10.
Contact Ms. Sybil White, Assistant to Dean of Graduate Studies, Harris College of Nursing, Texas Christian University, TCU Box 298625, Fort Worth, TX 76129. *Telephone:* 817-257-6750. *Fax:* 817-257-6751. *E-mail:* s.white@tcu.edu.

MASTER'S DEGREE PROGRAM

Degree MSN
Available Programs Master's.
Concentrations Available Clinical nurse leader; nurse anesthesia; nursing education. *Clinical nurse specialist programs in:* adult health, medical-surgical, pediatric.
Site Options Fort Worth, TX.
Study Options Full-time and part-time.
Online Degree Options Yes (online only).
Program Entrance Requirements Clinical experience, computer literacy, minimum overall college GPA of 3.0, transcript of college record, CPR certification, written essay, immunizations, 3 letters of recommendation, professional liability insurance/malpractice insurance, prerequisite course work, resume. *Application deadline:* 2/1 (spring). *Application fee:* $50.
Advanced Placement Credit given for nursing courses completed elsewhere dependent upon specific evaluations.
Degree Requirements 40 total credit hours, thesis or project.

POST-MASTER'S PROGRAM

Areas of Study Clinical nurse leader; nursing education. *Clinical nurse specialist programs in:* adult health, medical-surgical, pediatric.

DOCTORAL DEGREE PROGRAM

Degree DNP
Available Programs Doctorate; Post-Baccalaureate Doctorate.
Areas of Study Advanced practice nursing, nursing administration.
Site Options Fort Worth, TX.
Online Degree Options Yes (online only).
Program Entrance Requirements Clinical experience, minimum overall college GPA of 3.0, interview, 3 letters of recommendation, MSN or equivalent, vita, writing sample. Application deadline: 12/15 (fall). Application fee: $50.
Degree Requirements 30 total credit hours, oral exam, written exam.

CONTINUING EDUCATION PROGRAM

Contact Ms. Barbara Patten, Program Planning and Continuing Nursing Education Coordinator, Harris College of Nursing, Texas Christian University, TCU Box 298620, Fort Worth, TX 76129. *Telephone:* 817-257-7368. *Fax:* 817-257-7944. *E-mail:* bapatten@tcu.edu.

Texas Tech University Health Sciences Center
School of Nursing
Lubbock, Texas

http://www.ttuhsc.edu/son
Founded in 1969

DEGREES • BSC PN • DNP • MSN

Nursing Program Faculty 101 (53% with doctorates).
Baccalaureate Enrollment 1,020 **Women** 85% **Men** 15% **Minority** 40% **International** 32% **Part-time** 2%
Graduate Enrollment 473 **Women** 85% **Men** 15% **Minority** 34% **Part-time** 86%

Distance Learning Courses Available.
Nursing Student Activities Sigma Theta Tau, Student Nurses' Association.
Nursing Student Resources Academic advising; academic or career counseling; assistance for students with disabilities; bookstore; campus computer network; computer lab; e-mail services; Internet; learning resource lab; library services; nursing audiovisuals; other; skills, simulation, or other laboratory; tutoring.
Library Facilities 305,436 volumes in health, 11,000 volumes in nursing; 14,020 periodical subscriptions health-care related.

BACCALAUREATE PROGRAMS

Degree BSc PN
Available Programs Accelerated Baccalaureate for Second Degree; Accelerated RN Baccalaureate; Generic Baccalaureate.
Site Options El Paso, TX; Abilene, TX; Odessa, TX.
Study Options Full-time.
Online Degree Options Yes (online only).
Program Entrance Requirements Transcript of college record, written essay, immunizations, minimum GPA in nursing prerequisites of 2.5, prerequisite course work, RN licensure. *Application deadline:* 12/15 (fall). *Application fee:* $40.
Advanced Placement Credit given for nursing courses completed elsewhere dependent upon specific evaluations.
Expenses (2010-11) *Tuition, state resident:* full-time $2325. *Tuition, nonresident:* full-time $6975. *Required fees:* full-time $4524.
Financial Aid 85% of baccalaureate students in nursing programs received some form of financial aid in 2009-10.
Contact Dr. Cynthia O'Neal, Department Chair of Traditional Undergraduate Studies, School of Nursing, Texas Tech University Health Sciences Center, 3601 4th Street, MS 6264, Lubbock, TX 79430. *Telephone:* 806-743-2730. *Fax:* 806-743-1648. *E-mail:* cynthia.oneal@ttuhsc.edu.

GRADUATE PROGRAMS

Expenses (2010-11) *Tuition, state resident:* full-time $1845. *Tuition, nonresident:* full-time $4293. *Required fees:* full-time $3468.
Financial Aid 80% of graduate students in nursing programs received some form of financial aid in 2009-10. Institutionally sponsored loans, scholarships, and traineeships available. Aid available to part-time students. *Financial aid application deadline:* 12/1.
Contact Ms. Georgina Barrera, Graduate Program Coordinator, School of Nursing, Texas Tech University Health Sciences Center, 3601 4th Street, MS 6264, Lubbock, TX 79430. *Telephone:* 806-743-2762. *Fax:* 806-743-2324. *E-mail:* georgina.barrera@ttuhsc.edu.

MASTER'S DEGREE PROGRAM

Degree MSN
Available Programs Master's; RN to Master's.
Concentrations Available Nurse-midwifery; nursing administration; nursing education. *Nurse practitioner programs in:* acute care, family health, gerontology, pediatric.
Study Options Full-time and part-time.
Online Degree Options Yes (online only).
Program Entrance Requirements Clinical experience, computer literacy, minimum overall college GPA of 3.0, transcript of college record, CPR certification, written essay, immunizations, 3 letters of recommendation, nursing research course, statistics course. *Application deadline:* 5/1 (fall), 9/1 (spring). *Application fee:* $40.
Advanced Placement Credit given for nursing courses completed elsewhere dependent upon specific evaluations.
Degree Requirements 48 total credit hours, thesis or project, comprehensive exam.

POST-MASTER'S PROGRAM

Areas of Study *Nurse practitioner programs in:* acute care, family health, gerontology, pediatric.

DOCTORAL DEGREE PROGRAM

Degree DNP
Available Programs Doctorate.
Areas of Study Nursing administration, nursing education.
Program Entrance Requirements Clinical experience, minimum overall college GPA of 3.0, interview by faculty committee, interview, 3 letters of recommendation, MSN or equivalent, statistics course, vita, writing sample. Application deadline: 1/15 (summer). Application fee: $40.
Degree Requirements 48 total credit hours.

CONTINUING EDUCATION PROGRAM

Contact Dr. Susan Anderson, Director of Continuing Nursing Education, School of Nursing, Texas Tech University Health Sciences Center, 3601 4th Street, MS 6264, Lubbock, TX 79430. *Telephone:* 806-743-2732. *Fax:* 806-743-1198. *E-mail:* susan.anderson@ttuhsc.edu.

Texas Woman's University

College of Nursing
Denton, Texas

Founded in 1901

DEGREES • BS • MS • MSN/MHA • PHD
Nursing Program Faculty 175 (33% with doctorates).
Baccalaureate Enrollment 983 **Women** 90% **Men** 10% **Minority** 51% **International** 4% **Part-time** 14%
Graduate Enrollment 545 **Women** 94% **Men** 6% **Minority** 40% **International** 1% **Part-time** 85%
Distance Learning Courses Available.
Nursing Student Activities Sigma Theta Tau, Student Nurses' Association.
Nursing Student Resources Academic advising; academic or career counseling; assistance for students with disabilities; bookstore; campus computer network; career placement assistance; computer lab; computer-assisted instruction; e-mail services; employment services for current students; Internet; learning resource lab; library services; nursing audiovisuals; placement services for program completers; remedial services; skills, simulation, or other laboratory.
Library Facilities 643,323 volumes (250,000 in health, 26,463 in nursing); 35,625 periodical subscriptions (2,644 health-care related).

BACCALAUREATE PROGRAMS

Degree BS
Available Programs Accelerated Baccalaureate for Second Degree; Baccalaureate for Second Degree; Generic Baccalaureate; RN Baccalaureate.
Site Options Dallas, TX; Houston, TX.
Study Options Full-time and part-time.
Online Degree Options Yes.
Program Entrance Requirements Transcript of college record, CPR certification, high school transcript, immunizations, minimum GPA in nursing prerequisites of 3.0, professional liability insurance/malpractice insurance, prerequisite course work. Transfer students are accepted. *Application deadline:* 2/1 (fall), 9/1 (spring). *Application fee:* $30.
Advanced Placement Credit given for nursing courses completed elsewhere dependent upon specific evaluations.
Contact ***Telephone:*** 940-898-2412. *Fax:* 940-898-2437.

GRADUATE PROGRAMS

Contact ***Telephone:*** 940-898-3415.

MASTER'S DEGREE PROGRAM

Degrees MS; MSN/MHA
Available Programs Master's; RN to Master's.
Concentrations Available Nursing administration; nursing education. *Clinical nurse specialist programs in:* adult health, pediatric, women's health. *Nurse practitioner programs in:* acute care, adult health, family health, pediatric, women's health.
Site Options Dallas, TX; Houston, TX.
Study Options Full-time and part-time.
Online Degree Options Yes.
Program Entrance Requirements Clinical experience, minimum overall college GPA of 3.0, transcript of college record, CPR certification, immunizations, professional liability insurance/malpractice insurance, statistics course, GRE or MAT.
Advanced Placement Credit given for nursing courses completed elsewhere dependent upon specific evaluations.
Degree Requirements 48 total credit hours, thesis or project.

POST-MASTER'S PROGRAM

Areas of Study *Nurse practitioner programs in:* acute care, adult health, family health, pediatric, women's health.

DOCTORAL DEGREE PROGRAM

Degree PhD
Available Programs Doctorate.
Areas of Study Nursing research, nursing science, women's health.
Site Options Dallas, TX; Houston, TX.

Program Entrance Requirements Minimum overall college GPA of 3.5, 2 letters of recommendation, MSN or equivalent, statistics course, vita, GRE (Verbal 460, Quantitative 500) or MAT (50).
Degree Requirements 60 total credit hours, dissertation, oral exam, written exam.

University of Houston–Victoria
School of Nursing
Victoria, Texas

Founded in 1973

DEGREES • BSN • MSN

Library Facilities 50,000 volumes; 70,000 periodical subscriptions.

BACCALAUREATE PROGRAMS

Degree BSN
Available Programs Accelerated Baccalaureate for Second Degree; RN Baccalaureate.
Contact Baccalaureate programs, School of Nursing, University of Houston–Victoria, 3007 North Ben Wilson, Victoria, TX 77901. *Telephone:* 361-570-4848. *E-mail:* nursing@uhv.edu.

GRADUATE PROGRAMS

Contact Masters Programs, School of Nursing, University of Houston–Victoria, 3007 North Ben Wilson, Victoria, TX 77901. *Telephone:* 361-570-4848. *E-mail:* nursing@uhv.edu.

MASTER'S DEGREE PROGRAM

Degree MSN
Available Programs Master's; RN to Master's.
Concentrations Available Nursing administration; nursing education.
Program Entrance Requirements GRE or MAT.

University of Mary Hardin-Baylor
College of Nursing
Belton, Texas

http://www.umhb.edu/
Founded in 1845

DEGREES • BSN • MSN

Nursing Program Faculty 22 (36% with doctorates).
Baccalaureate Enrollment 290 **Women** 92% **Men** 8% **Minority** 25% **Part-time** 1%
Graduate Enrollment 15 **Women** 90% **Men** 10% **Minority** 40% **Part-time** 20%
Nursing Student Activities Sigma Theta Tau, Student Nurses' Association.
Nursing Student Resources Academic advising; academic or career counseling; assistance for students with disabilities; bookstore; campus computer network; career placement assistance; computer lab; e-mail services; employment services for current students; housing assistance; Internet; learning resource lab; library services; nursing audiovisuals; placement services for program completers; remedial services; resume preparation assistance; skills, simulation, or other laboratory; tutoring.
Library Facilities 7,769 volumes in health, 6,771 volumes in nursing; 120 periodical subscriptions health-care related.

BACCALAUREATE PROGRAMS

Degree BSN
Available Programs ADN to Baccalaureate; Generic Baccalaureate.
Study Options Full-time and part-time.
Program Entrance Requirements Minimum overall college GPA of 2.75, transcript of college record, CPR certification, written essay, health exam, health insurance, high school transcript, immunizations, minimum high school rank 50%, minimum GPA in nursing prerequisites of 2.75, professional liability insurance/malpractice insurance, prerequisite course work. Transfer students are accepted. *Application deadline:* 3/1 (fall), 10/1 (spring). Applications may be processed on a rolling basis for some programs.
Advanced Placement Credit given for nursing courses completed elsewhere dependent upon specific evaluations.
Expenses (2010-11) *Tuition:* full-time $26,064; part-time $645 per credit hour. *Room and board:* $3020 per academic year. *Required fees:* full-time $640; part-time $90 per credit.
Financial Aid 95% of baccalaureate students in nursing programs received some form of financial aid in 2009-10. *Gift aid (need-based):* Federal Pell, FSEOG, state, private, college/university gift aid from institutional funds. *Loans:* Federal Direct (Subsidized and Unsubsidized Stafford PLUS), Perkins, state. *Work-study:* Federal Work-Study, part-time campus jobs. *Financial aid application deadline (priority):* 3/1.
Contact Dr. Sharon Souter, Dean and Professor, College of Nursing, University of Mary Hardin-Baylor, Box 8015, 900 College Street, Belton, TX 76513-2599. *Telephone:* 254-295-4665. *Fax:* 254-295-4141. *E-mail:* lpehl@umhb.edu.

GRADUATE PROGRAMS

Expenses (2010-11) *Tuition:* full-time $5995; part-time $665 per credit hour. *Required fees:* full-time $690; part-time $90 per credit.
Financial Aid 10% of graduate students in nursing programs received some form of financial aid in 2009-10.
Contact Dr. Margaret Prydun, Director and Associate Professor, College of Nursing, University of Mary Hardin-Baylor, Box 8015, 900 College Street, Belton, TX 76513-2599. *Telephone:* 254-295-4674. *Fax:* 254-295-4141. *E-mail:* m.prydun@umhb.edu.

MASTER'S DEGREE PROGRAM

Degree MSN
Available Programs Master's.
Concentrations Available Clinical nurse leader; nursing education. *Clinical nurse specialist programs in:* adult health.
Study Options Full-time and part-time.
Program Entrance Requirements Clinical experience, computer literacy, minimum overall college GPA of 3.0, transcript of college record, CPR certification, written essay, immunizations, interview, 2 letters of recommendation, nursing research course, physical assessment course, professional liability insurance/malpractice insurance, prerequisite course work, resume, statistics course. *Application deadline:* 10/1 (fall).
Degree Requirements 36 total credit hours, comprehensive exam.

CONTINUING EDUCATION PROGRAM

Contact Dr. Ann Crawford, Program Administrator, College of Nursing, University of Mary Hardin-Baylor, Box 8015, 900 College Street, Belton, TX 76513-2599. *Telephone:* 254-295-4671. *Fax:* 254-295-4141. *E-mail:* acrawford@umhb.edu.

The University of Texas at Arlington
College of Nursing
Arlington, Texas

http://www.uta.edu/nursing
Founded in 1895

DEGREES • BSN • DNP • MSN • MSN/MBA • MSN/MHA • MSN/MPH • PHD

Nursing Program Faculty 126 (34% with doctorates).
Baccalaureate Enrollment 2,243 **Women** 89% **Men** 11% **Minority** 40% **International** 10% **Part-time** 8%
Graduate Enrollment 542 **Women** 91% **Men** 9% **Minority** 22% **Part-time** 70%
Distance Learning Courses Available.
Nursing Student Activities Nursing Honor Society, Sigma Theta Tau, Student Nurses' Association, nursing club.
Nursing Student Resources Academic advising; campus computer network; computer lab; e-mail services; externships; interactive nursing skills videos; Internet; learning resource lab; nursing audiovisuals; skills, simulation, or other laboratory; tutoring.
Library Facilities 1.4 million volumes (36,000 in health, 23,300 in nursing); 54,149 periodical subscriptions (530 health-care related).

BACCALAUREATE PROGRAMS

Degree BSN
Available Programs Accelerated Baccalaureate; Accelerated Baccalaureate for Second Degree; Accelerated RN Baccalaureate; Baccalaureate for Second Degree; Generic Baccalaureate; RN Baccalaureate.

Site Options Fort Worth, TX; Dallas, TX; Waco, Grayson, Paris, Kaufman, TX.
Study Options Full-time and part-time.
Program Entrance Requirements Minimum overall college GPA of 2.5, transcript of college record, CPR certification, health insurance, immunizations, minimum high school GPA of 2.5, minimum GPA in nursing prerequisites of 2.5, professional liability insurance/malpractice insurance, prerequisite course work. Transfer students are accepted. *Application deadline:* 1/5 (fall), 6/1 (spring).
Advanced Placement Credit given for nursing courses completed elsewhere dependent upon specific evaluations.
Expenses (2010-11) *Room and board:* $6097 per academic year.
Financial Aid 90% of baccalaureate students in nursing programs received some form of financial aid in 2009-10. *Gift aid (need-based):* Federal Pell, FSEOG, state, private, college/university gift aid from institutional funds, United Negro College Fund. *Loans:* Federal Direct (Subsidized and Unsubsidized Stafford PLUS), Perkins, state. *Work-study:* Federal Work-Study, part-time campus jobs. *Financial aid application deadline (priority):* 4/1.
Contact Ms. Jean Ashwill, Assistant Dean, Undergraduate Student Services, School of Nursing, The University of Texas at Arlington, 411 South Nedderman Drive, Box 19407, Arlington, TX 76019-0407. *Telephone:* 817-272-2776. *Fax:* 817-272-5006. *E-mail:* nursing@uta.edu.

GRADUATE PROGRAMS

Expenses (2010-11) *Tuition, state resident:* full-time $12,262; part-time $1500 per course. *Tuition, nonresident:* full-time $19,504; part-time $2465 per course. *International tuition:* $21,966 full-time. *Required fees:* full-time $500; part-time $150 per term.
Financial Aid 50% of graduate students in nursing programs received some form of financial aid in 2009-10. 24 fellowships with partial tuition reimbursements available (averaging $3,000 per year), 6 research assistantships (averaging $7,992 per year), 7 teaching assistantships (averaging $10,080 per year) were awarded; career-related internships or fieldwork and traineeships also available. *Financial aid application deadline:* 6/1.
Contact Dr. Mary Schira, Associate Dean and Associate Professor, School of Nursing, The University of Texas at Arlington, 411 South Nedderman Drive, Box 19407, Arlington, TX 76019-0407. *Telephone:* 817-272-2776. *Fax:* 817-272-5006. *E-mail:* schira@uta.edu.

MASTER'S DEGREE PROGRAM

Degrees MSN; MSN/MBA; MSN/MHA; MSN/MPH
Available Programs Master's.
Concentrations Available Health-care administration; nursing administration; nursing education. *Nurse practitioner programs in:* acute care, adult health, family health, gerontology, neonatal health, pediatric, psychiatric/mental health.
Site Options Fort Worth, TX; Dallas, TX.
Study Options Full-time and part-time.
Online Degree Options Yes (Nursing Administration only).
Program Entrance Requirements Clinical experience, computer literacy, minimum overall college GPA of 3.0, transcript of college record, CPR certification, written essay, immunizations, physical assessment course, statistics course, GRE General Test. *Application deadline:* 6/1 (fall), 10/15 (spring). *Application fee:* $70.
Advanced Placement Credit given for nursing courses completed elsewhere dependent upon specific evaluations.
Degree Requirements 36–51total credit hours.

POST-MASTER'S PROGRAM

Areas of Study *Nurse practitioner programs in:* acute care, adult health, family health, gerontology, neonatal health, pediatric, psychiatric/mental health.

DOCTORAL DEGREE PROGRAM

Degree DNP
Available Programs Doctorate.
Areas of Study Advanced practice nursing, clinical practice, faculty preparation, nursing education, nursing research.
Program Entrance Requirements Minimum overall college GPA of 3.0, clinical experience, statistics course, statement of goals. *Application deadline*: 6/1 (fall), 10/1 (spring). *Application fee*: $70.
Degree Requirements 45 total credit hours, dissertation, residency, clinical project.

Degree PhD
Available Programs Doctorate; Post-Baccalaureate Doctorate.
Areas of Study Faculty preparation, nursing education, nursing research.
Program Entrance Requirements Clinical experience, minimum overall college GPA of 3.0, interview by faculty committee, interview, 3 letters of recommendation, statistics course, statement of goals, GRE General Test. Application deadline: 4/2 (fall). Application fee: $70.
Degree Requirements 54 total credit hours, dissertation, residency.

CONTINUING EDUCATION PROGRAM

Contact Dr. Toni McKenna, Director, School of Nursing, The University of Texas at Arlington, 411 South Nedderman Drive, Box 19197, Arlington, TX 76019-0419. *Telephone:* 817-272-0720. *Fax:* 817-272-5371. *E-mail:* tmckenna@uta.edu.

The University of Texas at Austin
School of Nursing
Austin, Texas

http://www.utexas.edu/nursing
Founded in 1883

DEGREES • BSN • MSN • MSN/MBA • PHD
Nursing Program Faculty 73 (62% with doctorates).
Baccalaureate Enrollment 701 **Women** 90.5% **Men** 9.5% **Minority** 33% **International** 1% **Part-time** 13%
Graduate Enrollment 222 **Women** 88% **Men** 12% **Minority** 27% **International** 9% **Part-time** 24%
Nursing Student Activities Nursing Honor Society, Sigma Theta Tau, Student Nurses' Association, nursing club.
Nursing Student Resources Academic advising; academic or career counseling; assistance for students with disabilities; bookstore; campus computer network; career placement assistance; computer lab; computer-assisted instruction; daycare for children of students; e-mail services; employment services for current students; externships; housing assistance; interactive nursing skills videos; Internet; learning resource lab; library services; nursing audiovisuals; other; paid internships; placement services for program completers; remedial services; resume preparation assistance; skills, simulation, or other laboratory; tutoring; unpaid internships.
Library Facilities 9.9 million volumes (100,000 in health, 80,000 in nursing); 504 periodical subscriptions health-care related.

BACCALAUREATE PROGRAMS

Degree BSN
Available Programs Generic Baccalaureate; RN Baccalaureate.
Study Options Full-time.
Program Entrance Requirements Minimum overall college GPA of 2.5, transcript of college record, CPR certification, written essay, 3 years high school math, 2 years high school science, high school transcript, immunizations, 3 letters of recommendation, minimum GPA in nursing prerequisites of 2.5, professional liability insurance/malpractice insurance, prerequisite course work. Transfer students are accepted.
Advanced Placement Credit by examination available. Credit given for nursing courses completed elsewhere dependent upon specific evaluations.
Contact ***Telephone:*** 512-232-4780. *Fax:* 512-232-4777.

GRADUATE PROGRAMS

Contact ***Telephone:*** 512-471-7927. *Fax:* 512-232-4777.

MASTER'S DEGREE PROGRAM

Degrees MSN; MSN/MBA
Available Programs Master's; Master's for Non-Nursing College Graduates; Master's for Nurses with Non-Nursing Degrees.
Concentrations Available Nursing administration. *Clinical nurse specialist programs in:* adult health, community health, medical-surgical, public health. *Nurse practitioner programs in:* family health, pediatric.
Study Options Full-time and part-time.
Program Entrance Requirements Clinical experience, minimum overall college GPA of 3.0, transcript of college record, CPR certification, written essay, immunizations, interview, 3 letters of recommendation, physical assessment course, professional liability insurance/malpractice insurance, prerequisite course work, resume, statistics course, GRE General Test.
Advanced Placement Credit given for nursing courses completed elsewhere dependent upon specific evaluations.
Degree Requirements 48 total credit hours.

POST-MASTER'S PROGRAM

Areas of Study *Nurse practitioner programs in:* family health, pediatric.

DOCTORAL DEGREE PROGRAM

Degree PhD
Available Programs Doctorate.
Areas of Study Aging, community health, faculty preparation, gerontology, health promotion/disease prevention, health-care systems, human health and illness, illness and transition, maternity-newborn, nursing administration, nursing research, women's health.
Program Entrance Requirements Minimum overall college GPA of 3.0, interview, 3 letters of recommendation, MSN or equivalent, statistics course, vita, GRE General Test.
Degree Requirements 64 total credit hours, dissertation, oral exam, written exam, residency.

POSTDOCTORAL PROGRAM

Areas of Study Women's health.
Postdoctoral Program Contact ***Telephone:*** 512-232-4751. *Fax:* 512-232-4777.

The University of Texas at Brownsville

Department of Nursing
Brownsville, Texas

http://www.ntmain.utb.edu/shs/nursing_dept.html
Founded in 1973

DEGREES • BSN • MSN

Nursing Program Faculty 25 (12% with doctorates).
Baccalaureate Enrollment 21 **Women** 90% **Men** 10% **Part-time** 70%
Graduate Enrollment 11 **Women** 90% **Men** 10% **Part-time** 80%
Nursing Student Resources Academic advising; academic or career counseling; assistance for students with disabilities; bookstore; campus computer network; career placement assistance; computer lab; computer-assisted instruction; daycare for children of students; e-mail services; employment services for current students; housing assistance; interactive nursing skills videos; Internet; learning resource lab; library services; nursing audiovisuals; remedial services; skills, simulation, or other laboratory; tutoring.
Library Facilities 174,660 volumes; 4,447 periodical subscriptions.

BACCALAUREATE PROGRAMS

Degree BSN
Available Programs ADN to Baccalaureate.
Study Options Full-time and part-time.
Program Entrance Requirements Minimum overall college GPA of 2.5, transcript of college record, CPR certification, immunizations, minimum GPA in nursing prerequisites of 2.5, professional liability insurance/malpractice insurance, prerequisite course work, RN licensure. Transfer students are accepted.
Advanced Placement Credit by examination available.
Contact ***Telephone:*** 956-882-5071. *Fax:* 956-882-5100.

GRADUATE PROGRAMS

Contact ***Telephone:*** 956-882-5079. *Fax:* 956-882-5100.

MASTER'S DEGREE PROGRAM

Degree MSN
Available Programs Master's.
Concentrations Available Nursing administration; nursing education. *Clinical nurse specialist programs in:* public health.
Study Options Full-time and part-time.
Program Entrance Requirements Minimum overall college GPA of 3.0, transcript of college record, immunizations, 2 letters of recommendation, professional liability insurance/malpractice insurance, statistics course.
Degree Requirements 37 total credit hours, thesis or project.

The University of Texas at El Paso

School of Nursing
El Paso, Texas

http://www.utep.edu/nursing
Founded in 1913

DEGREES • BSN • MSN

Nursing Program Faculty 64 (27% with doctorates).
Baccalaureate Enrollment 514 **Women** 76.5% **Men** 23.5% **Minority** 80.4% **International** 2.7% **Part-time** 58.8%
Graduate Enrollment 153 **Women** 81% **Men** 19% **Minority** 61.4% **International** 3.3% **Part-time** 78.4%
Distance Learning Courses Available.
Nursing Student Activities Nursing Honor Society, Sigma Theta Tau, Student Nurses' Association.
Nursing Student Resources Academic advising; academic or career counseling; assistance for students with disabilities; bookstore; campus computer network; career placement assistance; computer lab; computer-assisted instruction; e-mail services; employment services for current students; interactive nursing skills videos; Internet; learning resource lab; library services; nursing audiovisuals; remedial services; skills, simulation, or other laboratory; tutoring.
Library Facilities 1.3 million volumes (71,389 in health, 13,043 in nursing); 3,065 periodical subscriptions (314 health-care related).

BACCALAUREATE PROGRAMS

Degree BSN
Available Programs Accelerated Baccalaureate; Generic Baccalaureate; RN Baccalaureate.
Site Options El Paso, TX.
Study Options Full-time and part-time.
Program Entrance Requirements Minimum overall college GPA of 2.0, transcript of college record, CPR certification, health exam, high school biology, high school math, high school science, high school transcript, immunizations, minimum GPA in nursing prerequisites of 2.5, professional liability insurance/malpractice insurance, prerequisite course work. Transfer students are accepted. *Application deadline:* 2/28 (fall), 9/30 (spring), 2/28 (summer).
Advanced Placement Credit by examination available. Credit given for nursing courses completed elsewhere dependent upon specific evaluations.
Expenses (2010-11) *Tuition, state resident:* full-time $4806; part-time $160 per credit hour. *Tuition, nonresident:* full-time $13,116; part-time $437 per credit hour. *Room and board:* room only: $4500 per academic year. *Required fees:* full-time $1631; part-time $46 per credit; part-time $178 per term.
Financial Aid 67% of baccalaureate students in nursing programs received some form of financial aid in 2009-10.
Contact Ms. Patricia Fowler, Assistant Dean, Undergraduate Education, School of Nursing, The University of Texas at El Paso, 1101 North Campbell Street, El Paso, TX 79902. *Telephone:* 915-747-7267. *Fax:* 915-747-8266. *E-mail:* pfowler@utep.edu.

GRADUATE PROGRAMS

Expenses (2010-11) *Tuition, state resident:* full-time $3928; part-time $218 per credit hour. *Tuition, nonresident:* full-time $8914; part-time $495 per credit hour. *Room and board:* room only: $4500 per academic year. *Required fees:* full-time $1193; part-time $47 per credit; part-time $178 per term.
Financial Aid 34% of graduate students in nursing programs received some form of financial aid in 2009-10. Research assistantships with partial tuition reimbursements available (averaging $18,825 per year), teaching assistantships with partial tuition reimbursements available (averaging $18,000 per year) were awarded; fellowships with partial tuition reimbursements available, institutionally sponsored loans, scholarships, tuition waivers (partial), and unspecified assistantships also available. Aid available to part-time students. *Financial aid application deadline:* 3/15.
Contact Dr. Kristynia Robinson, Assistant Dean, Graduate Education, School of Nursing, The University of Texas at El Paso, 1101 North Campbell Street, El Paso, TX 79902. *Telephone:* 915-747-7226. *Fax:* 915-747-8266. *E-mail:* krobinson@utep.edu.

MASTER'S DEGREE PROGRAM

Degree MSN
Available Programs Master's; RN to Master's.

Concentrations Available Nursing administration; nursing education. *Nurse practitioner programs in:* family health.
Site Options El Paso, TX.
Study Options Full-time and part-time.
Online Degree Options Yes (online only).
Program Entrance Requirements Clinical experience, minimum overall college GPA of 3.0, transcript of college record, CPR certification, written essay, immunizations, interview, nursing research course, professional liability insurance/malpractice insurance, resume, statistics course, GRE. *Application deadline:* 9/1 (fall), 2/1 (spring). Applications may be processed on a rolling basis for some programs. *Application fee:* $45.
Advanced Placement Credit given for nursing courses completed elsewhere dependent upon specific evaluations.
Degree Requirements 33 total credit hours, thesis or project, comprehensive exam.

POST-MASTER'S PROGRAM
Areas of Study Nursing administration; nursing education. *Nurse practitioner programs in:* family health.

DOCTORAL DEGREE PROGRAM
Program Entrance Requirements GRE.

The University of Texas at Tyler
Program in Nursing
Tyler, Texas

http://www.uttyler.edu/nursing
Founded in 1971

DEGREES • BSN • DNS • MSN • MSN/MBA
Nursing Program Faculty 65 (25% with doctorates).
Baccalaureate Enrollment 500 **Women** 70% **Men** 30% **Minority** 10% **International** 1% **Part-time** 15%
Graduate Enrollment 175 **Women** 88% **Men** 12% **Minority** 11% **Part-time** 88%
Nursing Student Activities Nursing Honor Society, Sigma Theta Tau, Student Nurses' Association, nursing club.
Nursing Student Resources Academic advising; academic or career counseling; assistance for students with disabilities; bookstore; campus computer network; career placement assistance; computer lab; computer-assisted instruction; e-mail services; employment services for current students; externships; interactive nursing skills videos; Internet; learning resource lab; library services; nursing audiovisuals; remedial services; resume preparation assistance; skills, simulation, or other laboratory; tutoring.
Library Facilities 486,895 volumes (11,000 in health, 5,500 in nursing); 525 periodical subscriptions (150 health-care related).

BACCALAUREATE PROGRAMS
Degree BSN
Available Programs ADN to Baccalaureate; Accelerated RN Baccalaureate; Generic Baccalaureate; International Nurse to Baccalaureate; LPN to Baccalaureate; LPN to RN Baccalaureate; RN Baccalaureate.
Site Options Longview, TX; Palestine, TX.
Study Options Full-time and part-time.
Online Degree Options Yes (online only).
Program Entrance Requirements Minimum overall college GPA of 2.75, transcript of college record, CPR certification, health exam, immunizations, minimum GPA in nursing prerequisites of 2.75, professional liability insurance/malpractice insurance, prerequisite course work. Transfer students are accepted. *Application deadline:* 2/15 (fall), 9/15 (spring).
Advanced Placement Credit given for nursing courses completed elsewhere dependent upon specific evaluations.
Financial Aid 70% of baccalaureate students in nursing programs received some form of financial aid in 2009-10.
Contact Ms. Renee Lampkin, Director of Marketing/Advising, Program in Nursing, The University of Texas at Tyler, 3900 University Boulevard, Tyler, TX 75799. *Telephone:* 903-565-5534. *Fax:* 903-565-5533. *E-mail:* rlampkin@uttyler.edu.

GRADUATE PROGRAMS
Financial Aid 60% of graduate students in nursing programs received some form of financial aid in 2009-10. 1 fellowship (averaging $10,000 per year), 3 research assistantships (averaging $2,200 per year) were awarded; institutionally sponsored loans and scholarships also available. *Financial aid application deadline:* 7/1.
Contact Ms. Renee Lampkin, Director of Marketing/Advising, Program in Nursing, The University of Texas at Tyler, 3900 University Boulevard, Tyler, TX 75799. *Telephone:* 903-565-5534. *Fax:* 903-565-5901. *E-mail:* rlampkin@uttyler.edu.

MASTER'S DEGREE PROGRAM
Degrees MSN; MSN/MBA
Available Programs Accelerated AD/RN to Master's; Accelerated RN to Master's; Master's; RN to Master's.
Concentrations Available Nursing administration; nursing education. *Nurse practitioner programs in:* acute care, adult health, family health, gerontology, pediatric, women's health.
Study Options Full-time and part-time.
Program Entrance Requirements Computer literacy, minimum overall college GPA of 3.0, transcript of college record, CPR certification, immunizations, 4 letters of recommendation, nursing research course, professional liability insurance/malpractice insurance, prerequisite course work, resume, statistics course, GRE General Test or MAT, GMAT.
Advanced Placement Credit given for nursing courses completed elsewhere dependent upon specific evaluations.
Degree Requirements 36 total credit hours, thesis or project, comprehensive exam.

POST-MASTER'S PROGRAM
Areas of Study Nursing administration; nursing education. *Nurse practitioner programs in:* acute care, adult health, family health, gerontology, pediatric, women's health.

DOCTORAL DEGREE PROGRAM
Degree DNS
Available Programs Doctorate.
Areas of Study Nursing science.
Program Entrance Requirements Minimum overall college GPA of 3.0, interview by faculty committee, 3 letters of recommendation, MSN or equivalent, scholarly papers, statistics course, vita, writing sample.
Degree Requirements 65 total credit hours, dissertation, written exam.

CONTINUING EDUCATION PROGRAM
Contact Dr. Pamela Martin, Assistant Dean of Undergraduate Studies, Program in Nursing, The University of Texas at Tyler, 3900 University Boulevard, Tyler, TX 75799. *Telephone:* 903-566-7320. *Fax:* 903-565-5533. *E-mail:* pmartin@uttyler.edu.

The University of Texas Health Science Center at Houston
School of Nursing
Houston, Texas

http://son.uth.tmc.edu/
Founded in 1972

DEGREES • BSN • MSN • MSN/MPH • PHD
Nursing Program Faculty 112 (54% with doctorates).
Baccalaureate Enrollment 497 **Women** 86% **Men** 14% **Minority** 45% **International** 1% **Part-time** 20%
Graduate Enrollment 350 **Women** 87% **Men** 13% **Minority** 35% **International** 12% **Part-time** 60%
Distance Learning Courses Available.
Nursing Student Activities Sigma Theta Tau, Student Nurses' Association.
Nursing Student Resources Academic advising; academic or career counseling; assistance for students with disabilities; bookstore; campus computer network; computer lab; computer-assisted instruction; e-mail services; employment services for current students; housing assistance; interactive nursing skills videos; Internet; learning resource lab; library services; nursing audiovisuals; paid internships; remedial services; skills, simulation, or other laboratory; tutoring.
Library Facilities 364,744 volumes; 12,106 periodical subscriptions.

BACCALAUREATE PROGRAMS
Degree BSN
Available Programs ADN to Baccalaureate; Accelerated Baccalaureate for Second Degree; Generic Baccalaureate.
Site Options Houston, TX.

Study Options Full-time.
Program Entrance Requirements Transcript of college record, CPR certification, written essay, health exam, immunizations, interview, minimum GPA in nursing prerequisites of 2.75, prerequisite course work. Transfer students are accepted. *Application deadline:* 1/15 (fall), 9/1 (spring), 12/1 (summer). *Application fee:* $30.
Advanced Placement Credit given for nursing courses completed elsewhere dependent upon specific evaluations.
Expenses (2010-11) *Tuition, state resident:* full-time $7238. *Tuition, nonresident:* full-time $31,537. *Required fees:* full-time $1270.
Financial Aid 83% of baccalaureate students in nursing programs received some form of financial aid in 2009-10.
Contact Ms. Laurie G. Rutherford, Director of Student Affairs, School of Nursing, The University of Texas Health Science Center at Houston, 6901 Bertner Avenue, Suite 220, Houston, TX 77030. *Telephone:* 713-500-2101. *Fax:* 713-500-2107. *E-mail:* soninfo@uth.tmc.edu.

GRADUATE PROGRAMS

Expenses (2010-11) *Tuition, state resident:* full-time $4172. *Tuition, nonresident:* full-time $18,732. *International tuition:* $18,732 full-time. *Required fees:* full-time $1126.
Financial Aid 37% of graduate students in nursing programs received some form of financial aid in 2009-10. Research assistantships with tuition reimbursements available, teaching assistantships with tuition reimbursements available, institutionally sponsored loans, scholarships, traineeships, and tuition waivers (full) available. Aid available to part-time students.
Contact Ms. Laurie G. Rutherford, Director of Student Affairs, School of Nursing, The University of Texas Health Science Center at Houston, 6901 Bertner Avenue, Suite 220, Houston, TX 77030. *Telephone:* 713-500-2101. *Fax:* 713-500-2107. *E-mail:* soninfo@uth.tmc.edu.

MASTER'S DEGREE PROGRAM

Degrees MSN; MSN/MPH
Available Programs Master's.
Concentrations Available Nurse anesthesia; nursing administration; nursing education. *Clinical nurse specialist programs in:* acute care, adult health, critical care, gerontology. *Nurse practitioner programs in:* acute care, adult health, family health, gerontology, pediatric, psychiatric/mental health, women's health.
Study Options Full-time and part-time.
Program Entrance Requirements Clinical experience, minimum overall college GPA of 3.0, transcript of college record, CPR certification, immunizations, interview, 3 letters of recommendation, prerequisite course work, resume, statistics course, GRE or MAT. *Application deadline:* 4/15 (fall), 2/15 (summer). *Application fee:* $30.
Advanced Placement Credit given for nursing courses completed elsewhere dependent upon specific evaluations.
Degree Requirements 48 total credit hours, thesis or project.

POST-MASTER'S PROGRAM

Areas of Study Nursing administration; nursing education. *Clinical nurse specialist programs in:* acute care, adult health, critical care, gerontology, oncology. *Nurse practitioner programs in:* acute care, adult health, family health, gerontology, oncology, pediatric, psychiatric/mental health, women's health.

DOCTORAL DEGREE PROGRAM

Degree PhD
Available Programs Doctorate.
Areas of Study Addiction/substance abuse, advanced practice nursing, aging, bio-behavioral research, biology of health and illness, clinical practice, community health, critical care, ethics, faculty preparation, family health, gerontology, health policy, health promotion/disease prevention, health-care systems, human health and illness, illness and transition, individualized study, information systems, maternity-newborn, neuro-behavior, nurse case management, nursing administration, nursing education, nursing policy, nursing research, nursing science, oncology, urban health, women's health.
Program Entrance Requirements Minimum overall college GPA of 3.0, interview by faculty committee, 3 letters of recommendation, MSN or equivalent, vita, writing sample, GRE. Application deadline: 4/1 (fall). Application fee: $30.
Degree Requirements 66 total credit hours, dissertation.

CONTINUING EDUCATION PROGRAM

Contact Dr. Vaunette P. Fay, Associate Professor of Clinical Nursing, School of Nursing, The University of Texas Health Science Center at Houston, 6901 Bertner Avenue, Suite 846, Houston, TX 77030. *Telephone:* 713-500-2116. *Fax:* 713-500-2026. *E-mail:* vaunette.p.fay@uth.tmc.edu.

The University of Texas Health Science Center at San Antonio

School of Nursing
San Antonio, Texas

http://www.nursing.uthscsa.edu
Founded in 1976

DEGREES • BSN • MSN • MSN/MPH • PHD
Nursing Program Faculty 109 (39% with doctorates).
Baccalaureate Enrollment 508 **Women** 81% **Men** 19% **Minority** 52% **International** 1% **Part-time** 10%
Graduate Enrollment 212 **Women** 85% **Men** 15% **Minority** 47% **International** 1% **Part-time** 75%
Distance Learning Courses Available.
Nursing Student Activities Nursing Honor Society, Sigma Theta Tau, Student Nurses' Association, nursing club.
Nursing Student Resources Academic advising; academic or career counseling; assistance for students with disabilities; bookstore; campus computer network; career placement assistance; computer lab; computer-assisted instruction; e-mail services; housing assistance; interactive nursing skills videos; Internet; learning resource lab; library services; nursing audiovisuals; remedial services; resume preparation assistance; skills, simulation, or other laboratory; tutoring.
Library Facilities 205,641 volumes in health, 2,056 volumes in nursing; 250 periodical subscriptions health-care related.

BACCALAUREATE PROGRAMS

Degree BSN
Available Programs ADN to Baccalaureate; Accelerated Baccalaureate for Second Degree; Generic Baccalaureate.
Study Options Full-time and part-time.
Program Entrance Requirements Minimum overall college GPA of 2.5, transcript of college record, CPR certification, written essay, health insurance, immunizations, minimum GPA in nursing prerequisites of 2.5, professional liability insurance/malpractice insurance, prerequisite course work. Transfer students are accepted. *Application deadline:* 1/1 (fall), 7/1 (spring). *Application fee:* $45.
Advanced Placement Credit given for nursing courses completed elsewhere dependent upon specific evaluations.
Expenses (2009-10) *Tuition, state resident:* full-time $5000; part-time $165 per credit hour. *Tuition, nonresident:* full-time $15,000; part-time $500 per credit hour. *International tuition:* $15,000 full-time. *Required fees:* full-time $2110; part-time $120 per credit; part-time $916 per term.
Financial Aid 80% of baccalaureate students in nursing programs received some form of financial aid in 2008-09.
Contact Dr. Suzanne Yarbrough, RN, Associate Dean for Undergraduate Studies, School of Nursing, The University of Texas Health Science Center at San Antonio, 7703 Floyd Curl Drive, MC 7945, San Antonio, TX 78229-3900. *Telephone:* 210-567-5810. *Fax:* 210-567-3813. *E-mail:* yarbrough@uthscsa.edu.

GRADUATE PROGRAMS

Expenses (2009-10) *Tuition, state resident:* full-time $2400; part-time $50 per credit hour. *Tuition, nonresident:* full-time $7848; part-time $327 per credit hour. *International tuition:* $7848 full-time. *Required fees:* part-time $1818 per term.
Financial Aid 50% of graduate students in nursing programs received some form of financial aid in 2008-09. 2 fellowships with full tuition reimbursements available (averaging $30,000 per year) were awarded; research assistantships, teaching assistantships, institutionally sponsored loans and scholarships also available. *Financial aid application deadline:* 4/1.
Contact Dr. Beverly Robinson, PhD, Associate Dean for Graduate Nursing Program, School of Nursing, The University of Texas Health Science Center at San Antonio, 7703 Floyd Curl Drive, MC 7945, San Antonio, TX 78229-3900. *Telephone:* 210-567-5815. *Fax:* 210-567-3813. *E-mail:* robinsonb@uthscsa.edu.

MASTER'S DEGREE PROGRAM

Degrees MSN; MSN/MPH
Available Programs Master's; RN to Master's.

Concentrations Available Nursing administration; nursing education; nursing informatics. *Clinical nurse specialist programs in:* critical care, medical-surgical. *Nurse practitioner programs in:* acute care, family health, pediatric, psychiatric/mental health.
Study Options Full-time and part-time.
Program Entrance Requirements Clinical experience, computer literacy, minimum overall college GPA of 3.0, transcript of college record, CPR certification, immunizations, interview, 3 letters of recommendation, physical assessment course, professional liability insurance/malpractice insurance, statistics course. *Application deadline:* 2/1 (fall), 9/1 (spring). *Application fee:* $45.
Advanced Placement Credit given for nursing courses completed elsewhere dependent upon specific evaluations.
Degree Requirements 47 total credit hours.

POST-MASTER'S PROGRAM
Areas of Study *Nurse practitioner programs in:* acute care, family health, pediatric, psychiatric/mental health.

DOCTORAL DEGREE PROGRAM
Degree PhD
Available Programs Doctorate; Post-Baccalaureate Doctorate.
Areas of Study Nursing education, nursing research, nursing science.
Program Entrance Requirements Clinical experience, minimum overall college GPA of 3.0, interview by faculty committee, interview, 3 letters of recommendation, statistics course, GRE, MAT. Application deadline: 2/1 (fall). Application fee: $45.
Degree Requirements 55 total credit hours, dissertation, oral exam, written exam.

CONTINUING EDUCATION PROGRAM
Contact Ms. Rosalie Tierney-Gumaer, Director of Nursing Continuing Education, School of Nursing, The University of Texas Health Science Center at San Antonio, 7703 Floyd Curl Drive, San Antonio, TX 78229-3900. *Telephone:* 210-567-5850. *Fax:* 210-567-5909. *E-mail:* tierneyguma@uthsca.edu.

The University of Texas Medical Branch
School of Nursing
Galveston, Texas

http://www.son.utmb.edu/
Founded in 1891

DEGREES • BSN • MSN • PHD
Nursing Program Faculty 52 (60% with doctorates).
Baccalaureate Enrollment 390 **Women** 85% **Men** 15% **Minority** 33% **International** 1% **Part-time** 23%
Graduate Enrollment 325 **Women** 88% **Men** 12% **Minority** 29% **International** .1% **Part-time** 74%
Distance Learning Courses Available.
Nursing Student Activities Nursing Honor Society, Sigma Theta Tau, Student Nurses' Association, nursing club.
Nursing Student Resources Academic advising; academic or career counseling; assistance for students with disabilities; bookstore; campus computer network; career placement assistance; computer lab; computer-assisted instruction; e-mail services; employment services for current students; housing assistance; interactive nursing skills videos; Internet; learning resource lab; library services; nursing audiovisuals; resume preparation assistance; skills, simulation, or other laboratory; tutoring.
Library Facilities 248,763 volumes in health, 6,105 volumes in nursing; 9,078 periodical subscriptions health-care related.

BACCALAUREATE PROGRAMS
Degree BSN
Available Programs Accelerated Baccalaureate for Second Degree; Generic Baccalaureate; RN Baccalaureate.
Study Options Full-time.
Online Degree Options Yes (online only).
Program Entrance Requirements Minimum overall college GPA of 3.0, transcript of college record, CPR certification, written essay, health exam, health insurance, immunizations, interview, minimum GPA in nursing prerequisites of 3.0, professional liability insurance/malpractice insurance, prerequisite course work. Transfer students are accepted. *Application deadline:* 2/15 (fall), 7/15 (spring). *Application fee:* $50.
Advanced Placement Credit by examination available. Credit given for nursing courses completed elsewhere dependent upon specific evaluations.
Expenses (2010-11) *Tuition, state resident:* full-time $8424; part-time $176 per credit hour. *Tuition, nonresident:* full-time $23,304; part-time $486 per credit hour. *Room and board:* $3110; room only: $2109 per academic year. *Required fees:* full-time $4703; part-time $289 per credit; part-time $1526 per term.
Financial Aid 95% of baccalaureate students in nursing programs received some form of financial aid in 2009-10.
Contact Dr. Linda Rath, Associate Professor and Director of Baccalaureate Programs, School of Nursing, The University of Texas Medical Branch, 301 University Boulevard, 3.630 SON/SAHS Building, Galveston, TX 77555-1029. *Telephone:* 409-772-8247. *Fax:* 409-772-3770. *E-mail:* lrath@utmb.edu.

GRADUATE PROGRAMS
Expenses (2010-11) *Tuition, state resident:* full-time $7860; part-time $262 per credit hour. *Tuition, nonresident:* full-time $17,160; part-time $572 per credit hour. *Room and board:* $3110; room only: $2109 per academic year. *Required fees:* full-time $2885; part-time $289 per credit; part-time $910 per term.
Financial Aid 30% of graduate students in nursing programs received some form of financial aid in 2009-10.
Contact Dr. Bruce Leonard, Associate Professor and Masters Program Director, School of Nursing, The University of Texas Medical Branch, 301 University Boulevard, Galveston, TX 77555-1029. *Telephone:* 409-772-8225. *Fax:* 409-772-8323. *E-mail:* brleonard@utmb.edu.

MASTER'S DEGREE PROGRAM
Degree MSN
Available Programs Master's.
Concentrations Available Nursing administration; nursing education. *Nurse practitioner programs in:* family health, gerontology, neonatal health.
Study Options Full-time and part-time.
Online Degree Options Yes (online only).
Program Entrance Requirements Clinical experience, computer literacy, minimum overall college GPA of 3.0, transcript of college record, CPR certification, immunizations, interview, 3 letters of recommendation, professional liability insurance/malpractice insurance, prerequisite course work, statistics course. *Application deadline:* 3/15 (fall), 9/15 (spring). *Application fee:* $50.
Advanced Placement Credit given for nursing courses completed elsewhere dependent upon specific evaluations.
Degree Requirements 48 total credit hours, thesis or project.

POST-MASTER'S PROGRAM
Areas of Study Nursing administration; nursing education. *Nurse practitioner programs in:* family health, gerontology, neonatal health.

DOCTORAL DEGREE PROGRAM
Degree PhD
Available Programs Doctorate; Post-Baccalaureate Doctorate.
Areas of Study Health promotion/disease prevention.
Online Degree Options Yes (online only).
Program Entrance Requirements Clinical experience, minimum overall college GPA of 3.5, interview by faculty committee, interview, 3 letters of recommendation, MSN or equivalent, statistics course, vita, writing sample. Application deadline: 3/1 (fall). Application fee: $50.
Degree Requirements 63 total credit hours, dissertation, oral exam, written exam, residency.

The University of Texas–Pan American
Department of Nursing
Edinburg, Texas

http://www.panam.edu
Founded in 1927

DEGREES • BSN • MSN
Nursing Program Faculty 23 (45% with doctorates).
Baccalaureate Enrollment 170 **Women** 78% **Men** 22% **Minority** 90%
Graduate Enrollment 65 **Women** 88% **Men** 12% **Minority** 88% **Part-time** 75%

Nursing Student Activities Sigma Theta Tau, Student Nurses' Association.

Nursing Student Resources Academic advising; academic or career counseling; assistance for students with disabilities; bookstore; campus computer network; career placement assistance; computer lab; computer-assisted instruction; daycare for children of students; e-mail services; employment services for current students; housing assistance; interactive nursing skills videos; Internet; learning resource lab; library services; nursing audiovisuals; remedial services; skills, simulation, or other laboratory; tutoring.

Library Facilities 230 volumes in health, 200 volumes in nursing; 300 periodical subscriptions health-care related.

BACCALAUREATE PROGRAMS

Degree BSN

Available Programs ADN to Baccalaureate; Generic Baccalaureate; RN Baccalaureate.

Study Options Full-time.

Program Entrance Requirements Transcript of college record, CPR certification, immunizations, minimum GPA in nursing prerequisites of 2.5, professional liability insurance/malpractice insurance, prerequisite course work. Transfer students are accepted. *Application deadline:* 10/1 (fall), 10/1 (spring).

Expenses (2009-10) *Tuition, state resident:* full-time $5425; part-time $50 per credit hour. *Tuition, nonresident:* full-time $13,735; part-time $327 per credit hour. *International tuition:* $13,735 full-time. *Room and board:* $6456; room only: $4456 per academic year. *Required fees:* full-time $1033; part-time $15 per credit; part-time $162 per term.

Financial Aid 92% of baccalaureate students in nursing programs received some form of financial aid in 2008-09.

Contact Dr. Sandy M. Snchez, BSN Program Coordinator, Department of Nursing, The University of Texas–Pan American, 1201 West University Drive, Edinburg, TX 78539. *Telephone:* 956-381-3491. *Fax:* 956-381-2875. *E-mail:* sandy@utpa.edu.

GRADUATE PROGRAMS

Expenses (2009-10) *Tuition, state resident:* full-time $4437; part-time $100 per credit hour. *Tuition, nonresident:* full-time $9423; part-time $377 per credit hour. *International tuition:* $9423 full-time. *Room and board:* $6984; room only: $4984 per academic year. *Required fees:* full-time $404; part-time $30 per credit; part-time $140 per term.

Financial Aid 50% of graduate students in nursing programs received some form of financial aid in 2008-09. Scholarships and traineeships available.

Contact Dr. Janice A. Maville, MSN Coordinator, Department of Nursing, The University of Texas–Pan American, 1201 West University Drive, Edinburg, TX 78539. *Telephone:* 956-381-3491. *Fax:* 956-381-2875. *E-mail:* jmaville@utpa.edu.

MASTER'S DEGREE PROGRAM

Degree MSN

Available Programs Master's.

Concentrations Available *Clinical nurse specialist programs in:* adult health. *Nurse practitioner programs in:* family health, pediatric.

Study Options Full-time and part-time.

Program Entrance Requirements Minimum overall college GPA of 2.75, transcript of college record, written essay, immunizations, 3 letters of recommendation, resume, statistics course. *Application deadline:* 7/1 (fall), 10/1 (winter), 4/1 (spring), 4/1 (summer).

Advanced Placement Credit given for nursing courses completed elsewhere dependent upon specific evaluations.

Degree Requirements 48 total credit hours, thesis or project.

POST-MASTER'S PROGRAM

Areas of Study *Clinical nurse specialist programs in:* adult health. *Nurse practitioner programs in:* family health, pediatric.

University of the Incarnate Word

Program in Nursing
San Antonio, Texas

http://www.uiw.edu/snhp

Founded in 1881

DEGREES • BSN • MSN

Nursing Program Faculty 35 (57% with doctorates).

Baccalaureate Enrollment 238 **Women** 88% **Men** 12% **Minority** 57%

Graduate Enrollment 60 **Women** 83% **Men** 17% **Minority** 59% **International** 10% **Part-time** 76%

Distance Learning Courses Available.

Nursing Student Activities Sigma Theta Tau, Student Nurses' Association.

Nursing Student Resources Academic advising; academic or career counseling; assistance for students with disabilities; bookstore; campus computer network; career placement assistance; computer lab; computer-assisted instruction; e-mail services; employment services for current students; externships; housing assistance; interactive nursing skills videos; Internet; learning resource lab; library services; nursing audiovisuals; paid internships; placement services for program completers; remedial services; resume preparation assistance; skills, simulation, or other laboratory; tutoring; unpaid internships.

Library Facilities 271,657 volumes (6,000 in health, 6,000 in nursing); 46,637 periodical subscriptions (3,048 health-care related).

BACCALAUREATE PROGRAMS

Degree BSN

Available Programs ADN to Baccalaureate; Baccalaureate for Second Degree; Generic Baccalaureate.

Study Options Full-time.

Online Degree Options Yes.

Program Entrance Requirements Minimum overall college GPA of 2.5, transcript of college record, CPR certification, health exam, health insurance, immunizations, minimum GPA in nursing prerequisites of 2.5, professional liability insurance/malpractice insurance, prerequisite course work. Transfer students are accepted. *Application deadline:* 2/1 (fall), 9/1 (spring). *Application fee:* $20.

Advanced Placement Credit given for nursing courses completed elsewhere dependent upon specific evaluations.

Expenses (2010-11) *Tuition:* full-time $21,000; part-time $695 per credit hour. *Room and board:* $8000; room only: $4500 per academic year. *Required fees:* full-time $2400; part-time $1200 per term.

Financial Aid 90% of baccalaureate students in nursing programs received some form of financial aid in 2009-10.

Contact Office of Admissions, Program in Nursing, University of the Incarnate Word, 4301 Broadway, San Antonio, TX 78209. *Telephone:* 210-829-6005.

GRADUATE PROGRAMS

Expenses (2010-11) *Tuition:* part-time $695 per credit hour. *Room and board:* $8000; room only: $6000 per academic year. *Required fees:* part-time $100 per credit.

Financial Aid 75% of graduate students in nursing programs received some form of financial aid in 2009-10. Federal Work-Study, scholarships, and traineeships available. Aid available to part-time students.

Contact Dr. Holly Cassells, Chair of Graduate Program, Program in Nursing, University of the Incarnate Word, 4301 Broadway, San Antonio, TX 78209. *Telephone:* 210-283-5093. *Fax:* 210-829-3174. *E-mail:* cassells@uiwtx.edu.

MASTER'S DEGREE PROGRAM

Degree MSN

Available Programs Accelerated AD/RN to Master's; Master's.

Concentrations Available Clinical nurse leader. *Clinical nurse specialist programs in:* adult health.

Study Options Full-time and part-time.

Program Entrance Requirements Clinical experience, minimum overall college GPA of 3.0, transcript of college record, immunizations, 3 letters of recommendation, physical assessment course, professional liability insurance/malpractice insurance, statistics course. *Application deadline:* Applications may be processed on a rolling basis for some programs. *Application fee:* $20.

Advanced Placement Credit given for nursing courses completed elsewhere dependent upon specific evaluations.

Degree Requirements 40 total credit hours, thesis or project.

POST-MASTER'S PROGRAM

Areas of Study Clinical nurse leader. *Clinical nurse specialist programs in:* adult health.

Wayland Baptist University

Bachelor of Science in Nursing Program
Plainview, Texas

Founded in 1908

DEGREE • BSN

Library Facilities 129,082 volumes; 466 periodical subscriptions.

BACCALAUREATE PROGRAMS

Degree BSN
Available Programs RN Baccalaureate.
Contact Diane Frazor, Dean, Bachelor of Science in Nursing Program, Wayland Baptist University, 11550 IH 35 North, San Antonio, TX 78233. *Telephone:* 210-826-7595 Ext. 228. *E-mail:* frazord@wbu.edu.

West Texas A&M University

Division of Nursing
Canyon, Texas

http://www.wtamu.edu/nursing
Founded in 1909

DEGREES • BSN • MSN

Nursing Program Faculty 30 (23% with doctorates).
Baccalaureate Enrollment 380 **Women** 84% **Men** 16% **Minority** 27% **International** 1% **Part-time** 35%
Graduate Enrollment 54 **Women** 85% **Men** 15% **Minority** 9% **Part-time** 52%
Nursing Student Activities Sigma Theta Tau, Student Nurses' Association.
Nursing Student Resources Academic advising; academic or career counseling; assistance for students with disabilities; bookstore; campus computer network; career placement assistance; computer lab; computer-assisted instruction; daycare for children of students; e-mail services; employment services for current students; housing assistance; interactive nursing skills videos; Internet; learning resource lab; library services; nursing audiovisuals; placement services for program completers; remedial services; resume preparation assistance; skills, simulation, or other laboratory; tutoring.
Library Facilities 1.1 million volumes (17,000 in health, 10,000 in nursing); 19,022 periodical subscriptions (75 health-care related).

BACCALAUREATE PROGRAMS

Degree BSN
Available Programs ADN to Baccalaureate; Generic Baccalaureate; LPN to Baccalaureate.
Study Options Full-time and part-time.
Program Entrance Requirements Minimum overall college GPA of 2.5, transcript of college record, CPR certification, immunizations, minimum GPA in nursing prerequisites of 2.0, prerequisite course work. Transfer students are accepted.
Advanced Placement Credit given for nursing courses completed elsewhere dependent upon specific evaluations.
Contact ***Telephone:*** 806-651-2661. *Fax:* 806-651-2632.

GRADUATE PROGRAMS

Contact ***Telephone:*** 806-651-2637. *Fax:* 806-651-2632.

MASTER'S DEGREE PROGRAM

Degree MSN
Available Programs Master's; RN to Master's.
Concentrations Available Nursing administration; nursing education. *Nurse practitioner programs in:* family health.
Study Options Full-time and part-time.
Program Entrance Requirements Clinical experience, computer literacy, minimum overall college GPA of 3.0, transcript of college record, CPR certification, immunizations, nursing research course, prerequisite course work, statistics course, GRE General Test.
Advanced Placement Credit given for nursing courses completed elsewhere dependent upon specific evaluations.
Degree Requirements 39 total credit hours, thesis or project.

POST-MASTER'S PROGRAM

Areas of Study *Nurse practitioner programs in:* family health.

UTAH

Brigham Young University

College of Nursing
Provo, Utah

http://nursing.byu.edu/
Founded in 1875

DEGREES • BS • MS

Nursing Program Faculty 46 (43% with doctorates).
Baccalaureate Enrollment 329 **Women** 91.5% **Men** 8.5% **Minority** 5.5% **International** 3%
Graduate Enrollment 31 **Women** 68% **Men** 32% **Minority** 9% **International** 3% **Part-time** 9.6%
Nursing Student Activities Nursing Honor Society, Sigma Theta Tau, Student Nurses' Association.
Nursing Student Resources Academic advising; academic or career counseling; assistance for students with disabilities; bookstore; campus computer network; career placement assistance; computer lab; computer-assisted instruction; e-mail services; employment services for current students; housing assistance; interactive nursing skills videos; Internet; learning resource lab; library services; nursing audiovisuals; other; paid internships; resume preparation assistance; skills, simulation, or other laboratory; tutoring.
Library Facilities 3.5 million volumes (72,332 in health, 5,217 in nursing); 27,161 periodical subscriptions (10,500 health-care related).

BACCALAUREATE PROGRAMS

Degree BS
Available Programs RN Baccalaureate.
Study Options Full-time.
Program Entrance Requirements Minimum overall college GPA, transcript of college record, CPR certification, written essay, 2 letters of recommendation, minimum GPA in nursing prerequisites of 3.0, prerequisite course work. Transfer students are accepted. *Application deadline:* 5/31 (fall), 9/30 (winter).
Advanced Placement Credit given for nursing courses completed elsewhere dependent upon specific evaluations.
Expenses (2010-11) *Tuition:* full-time $2210; part-time $227 per credit hour.
Financial Aid 33% of baccalaureate students in nursing programs received some form of financial aid in 2009-10.
Contact Dr. Mark E. White, Advisement Center Supervisor, College of Nursing, Brigham Young University, 550 SWKT, Provo, UT 84602-5532. *Telephone:* 801-422-7211. *Fax:* 801-422-0536. *E-mail:* mark_white@byu.edu.

GRADUATE PROGRAMS

Expenses (2010-11) *Tuition:* full-time $2790; part-time $310 per credit hour.
Financial Aid 100% of graduate students in nursing programs received some form of financial aid in 2009-10. 2 research assistantships with full and partial tuition reimbursements available (averaging $10,000 per year), 3 teaching assistantships with full and partial tuition reimbursements available (averaging $10,000 per year) were awarded; institutionally sponsored loans, scholarships, tuition waivers (full), and unspecified assistantships also available. Aid available to part-time students. *Financial aid application deadline:* 2/1.
Contact Ms. Stephanie Wilson, Research Center and Graduate Program Secretary, College of Nursing, Brigham Young University, 400 SWKT, Provo, UT 84602-5532. *Telephone:* 801-422-4142. *Fax:* 801-422-0536. *E-mail:* stephanie-wilson@byu.edu.

MASTER'S DEGREE PROGRAM

Degree MS
Available Programs Master's.
Concentrations Available *Nurse practitioner programs in:* family health.
Study Options Full-time and part-time.
Program Entrance Requirements Clinical experience, minimum overall college GPA of 3.0, transcript of college record, CPR certification, written essay, immunizations, interview, 3 letters of recommendation, prerequisite course work, resume, statistics course, GRE. *Application deadline:* 12/1 (spring). *Application fee:* $50.

Advanced Placement Credit given for nursing courses completed elsewhere dependent upon specific evaluations.
Degree Requirements 56 total credit hours, thesis or project.

POST-MASTER'S PROGRAM

Areas of Study *Nurse practitioner programs in:* family health.

Dixie State College of Utah

Nursing Department
St. George, Utah

Founded in 1911

DEGREE • BSN

Library Facilities 153,051 volumes; 203 periodical subscriptions.

BACCALAUREATE PROGRAMS

Degree BSN
Available Programs RN Baccalaureate.
Program Entrance Requirements Written essay, immunizations, RN licensure. *Application deadline:* 3/15 (fall), 9/15 (spring).
Contact Dr. Carole Grady, Associate Dean of Nursing and Allied Health. *Telephone:* 435-879-4802. *E-mail:* grady@dixie.edu.

Southern Utah University

Department of Nursing
Cedar City, Utah

http://www.suu.edu/sci/nursing
Founded in 1897

DEGREE • BSN

Nursing Program Faculty 9
Baccalaureate Enrollment 126 **Women** 70% **Men** 30% **Minority** 5% **International** 1%
Nursing Student Activities Student Nurses' Association, nursing club.
Nursing Student Resources Academic advising; academic or career counseling; assistance for students with disabilities; bookstore; campus computer network; career placement assistance; computer lab; computer-assisted instruction; e-mail services; employment services for current students; externships; housing assistance; interactive nursing skills videos; Internet; learning resource lab; library services; nursing audiovisuals; remedial services; resume preparation assistance; skills, simulation, or other laboratory; tutoring.
Library Facilities 1,000 volumes in health, 1,000 volumes in nursing; 5,000 periodical subscriptions health-care related.

BACCALAUREATE PROGRAMS

Degree BSN
Available Programs Generic Baccalaureate; LPN to Baccalaureate; RN Baccalaureate.
Study Options Full-time.
Program Entrance Requirements Minimum overall college GPA of 3.0, transcript of college record, CPR certification, written essay, health insurance, high school transcript, immunizations, 3 letters of recommendation, minimum GPA in nursing prerequisites of 3.0, prerequisite course work. Transfer students are accepted. *Application deadline:* 2/11 (fall), 9/9 (spring). *Application fee:* $20.
Advanced Placement Credit given for nursing courses completed elsewhere dependent upon specific evaluations.
Expenses (2010-11) *Tuition, state resident:* full-time $4200. *Tuition, nonresident:* full-time $13,500. *Room and board:* room only: $1043 per academic year. *Required fees:* full-time $540.
Financial Aid 90% of baccalaureate students in nursing programs received some form of financial aid in 2009-10.
Contact Vikki Robertson, Department Secretary, Department of Nursing, Southern Utah University, 351 West University Boulevard, GC 005, Cedar City, UT 84720. *Telephone:* 435-586-1906. *Fax:* 435-586-1984. *E-mail:* robertsonv@suu.edu.

University of Phoenix–Utah Campus

College of Health and Human Services
Salt Lake City, Utah

Founded in 1984
Nursing Program Faculty 2
Nursing Student Activities Sigma Theta Tau.
Nursing Student Resources Academic advising; academic or career counseling; assistance for students with disabilities; bookstore; campus computer network; computer lab; computer-assisted instruction; e-mail services; interactive nursing skills videos; Internet; learning resource lab; library services; nursing audiovisuals; remedial services; skills, simulation, or other laboratory; tutoring.
Library Facilities 16,871 periodical subscriptions (1,300 health-care related).

University of Utah

College of Nursing
Salt Lake City, Utah

http://www.nursing.utah.edu/
Founded in 1850

DEGREES • BS • DNP • MS • MSN/MPH • PHD

Nursing Program Faculty 97 (52% with doctorates).
Baccalaureate Enrollment 322 **Women** 75% **Men** 25% **Minority** 6% **International** 5% **Part-time** 37%
Graduate Enrollment 319 **Women** 84% **Men** 16% **Minority** 17% **International** 3% **Part-time** 23%
Distance Learning Courses Available.
Nursing Student Activities Sigma Theta Tau, Student Nurses' Association.
Nursing Student Resources Academic advising; academic or career counseling; assistance for students with disabilities; bookstore; campus computer network; career placement assistance; computer lab; computer-assisted instruction; e-mail services; externships; interactive nursing skills videos; Internet; learning resource lab; library services; nursing audiovisuals; paid internships; remedial services; resume preparation assistance; skills, simulation, or other laboratory; unpaid internships.
Library Facilities 4.1 million volumes (212,579 in health, 6,603 in nursing); 64,843 periodical subscriptions (5,201 health-care related).

BACCALAUREATE PROGRAMS

Degree BS
Available Programs Accelerated Baccalaureate; Generic Baccalaureate; RN Baccalaureate.
Study Options Full-time.
Program Entrance Requirements Minimum overall college GPA of 2.8, transcript of college record, CPR certification, written essay, health exam, immunizations, 3 letters of recommendation, minimum GPA in nursing prerequisites of 3.0, prerequisite course work. Transfer students are accepted. *Application deadline:* 1/15 (fall).
Advanced Placement Credit by examination available. Credit given for nursing courses completed elsewhere dependent upon specific evaluations.
Financial Aid 62% of baccalaureate students in nursing programs received some form of financial aid in 2009-10.
Contact Ms. Cynthia Weatbrook, Undergraduate Academic Advisor, College of Nursing, University of Utah, 10 South 2000 East, Salt Lake City, UT 84112-5880. *Telephone:* 801-581-3414. *Fax:* 801-585-9705. *E-mail:* cynthia.weatbrook@nurs.utah.edu.

GRADUATE PROGRAMS

Financial Aid 41% of graduate students in nursing programs received some form of financial aid in 2009-10. Fellowships with partial tuition reimbursements available, research assistantships with partial tuition reimbursements available, teaching assistantships with partial tuition reimbursements available, scholarships available. *Financial aid application deadline:* 2/1.
Contact Ms. Liz Leckie, Co Director, Academic Programs and Student Services, College of Nursing, University of Utah, 10 South 2000 East, Salt Lake City, UT 84112-5880. *Telephone:* 801-585-6658. *Fax:* 801-585-9705. *E-mail:* liz.leckie@nurs.utah.edu.

MASTER'S DEGREE PROGRAM

Degrees MS; MSN/MPH
Available Programs Master's.
Concentrations Available Clinical nurse leader; nurse-midwifery; nursing education; nursing informatics. *Clinical nurse specialist programs in:* psychiatric/mental health. *Nurse practitioner programs in:* gerontology, psychiatric/mental health.
Site Options St. George, UT.
Study Options Full-time and part-time.
Program Entrance Requirements Clinical experience, computer literacy, minimum overall college GPA of 3.0, transcript of college record, CPR certification, written essay, immunizations, interview, 3 letters of recommendation, professional liability insurance/malpractice insurance, resume, statistics course, GRE General Test (if undergraduate GPA less than 3.2). *Application deadline:* 1/15 (fall).
Advanced Placement Credit given for nursing courses completed elsewhere dependent upon specific evaluations.
Degree Requirements 40 total credit hours, thesis or project, comprehensive exam.

POST-MASTER'S PROGRAM

Areas of Study Nurse-midwifery; nursing education; nursing informatics. *Clinical nurse specialist programs in:* acute care, family health, pediatric, psychiatric/mental health, women's health. *Nurse practitioner programs in:* acute care, adult health, community health, family health, neonatal health, pediatric, primary care, psychiatric/mental health, women's health.

DOCTORAL DEGREE PROGRAM

Degree DNP, DNP/MPH.
Available Programs Doctorate; Post-Baccalaureate Doctorate.
Areas of Study Acute care, adult health, community health, neonatal health, pediatric, primary care.
Program Entrance Requirements Minimum overall college GPA of 3.0, 3 letters of recommendation, interview, vita.
Degree Requirements Dissertation, residency.

Degree PhD
Available Programs Doctorate; Doctorate for Nurses with Non-Nursing Degrees; Post-Baccalaureate Doctorate.
Areas of Study Aging, bio-behavioral research, community health, ethics, faculty preparation, family health, gerontology, health policy, health promotion/disease prevention, health-care systems, human health and illness, illness and transition, individualized study, information systems, maternity-newborn, nursing administration, nursing education, nursing policy, nursing research, nursing science, oncology, women's health.
Program Entrance Requirements Clinical experience, minimum overall college GPA of 3.3, interview by faculty committee, interview, 3 letters of recommendation, vita, writing sample, GRE General Test. Application deadline: 1/15 (fall).
Degree Requirements 62 total credit hours, dissertation, oral exam, written exam, residency.

POSTDOCTORAL PROGRAM

Areas of Study Aging, cancer care, gerontology, nursing informatics, nursing interventions, nursing research, nursing science.
Postdoctoral Program Contact Dr. Ginette A. Pepper, Associate Dean for Research and PhD Programs, College of Nursing, University of Utah, 10 South 2000 East, Salt Lake City, UT 84112-5880. *Telephone:* 801-585-7872. *Fax:* 801-581-4642. *E-mail:* ginny.pepper@nurs.utah.edu.

Utah Valley University
Department of Nursing
Orem, Utah

http://www.uvsc.edu/nurs/
Founded in 1941

DEGREE • BSN
Nursing Program Faculty 22 (25% with doctorates).
Baccalaureate Enrollment 100 **Women** 60% **Men** 40% **Part-time** 99%
Nursing Student Activities Student Nurses' Association.
Nursing Student Resources Academic advising; academic or career counseling; assistance for students with disabilities; bookstore; campus computer network; career placement assistance; computer lab; computer-assisted instruction; daycare for children of students; e-mail services; employment services for current students; interactive nursing skills videos; Internet; learning resource lab; library services; nursing audiovisuals; resume preparation assistance; skills, simulation, or other laboratory; tutoring; unpaid internships.
Library Facilities 228,000 volumes (4,640 in health, 361 in nursing); 568 periodical subscriptions (200 health-care related).

BACCALAUREATE PROGRAMS

Degree BSN
Available Programs ADN to Baccalaureate.
Study Options Part-time.
Program Entrance Requirements CPR certification, health exam, health insurance, immunizations, minimum GPA in nursing prerequisites of 2.5, prerequisite course work, RN licensure. Transfer students are accepted.
Advanced Placement Credit by examination available.
Contact *Telephone:* 801-863-8199. *Fax:* 801-863-6093.

Weber State University
Program in Nursing
Ogden, Utah

http://weber.edu/nursing
Founded in 1889

DEGREES • BSN • MSN
Nursing Program Faculty 42 (5% with doctorates).
Baccalaureate Enrollment 280 **Women** 88% **Men** 12% **Minority** 3% **International** 1% **Part-time** 5%
Graduate Enrollment 45 **Women** 85% **Men** 15% **Minority** 1%
Distance Learning Courses Available.
Nursing Student Activities Sigma Theta Tau, Student Nurses' Association.
Nursing Student Resources Academic advising; academic or career counseling; assistance for students with disabilities; bookstore; campus computer network; career placement assistance; computer lab; computer-assisted instruction; daycare for children of students; e-mail services; employment services for current students; housing assistance; interactive nursing skills videos; Internet; learning resource lab; library services; nursing audiovisuals; placement services for program completers; resume preparation assistance; skills, simulation, or other laboratory; tutoring; unpaid internships.
Library Facilities 646,666 volumes (800 in health, 800 in nursing); 120 periodical subscriptions health-care related.

BACCALAUREATE PROGRAMS

Degree BSN
Available Programs ADN to Baccalaureate; Accelerated Baccalaureate.
Study Options Full-time and part-time.
Online Degree Options Yes.
Program Entrance Requirements Minimum overall college GPA of 3.0, transcript of college record, CPR certification, health insurance, immunizations, minimum GPA in nursing prerequisites of 3.0, prerequisite course work, RN licensure. Transfer students are accepted. *Application deadline:* 3/10 (fall), 10/10 (spring). *Application fee:* $25.
Advanced Placement Credit by examination available. Credit given for nursing courses completed elsewhere dependent upon specific evaluations.
Financial Aid 15% of baccalaureate students in nursing programs received some form of financial aid in 2009-10.
Contact Mr. Doug Watson, Academic Admissions Advisor, Program in Nursing, Weber State University, 3907 University Circle, Ogden, UT 84408-3907. *Telephone:* 801-626-6128. *Fax:* 801-626-6382. *E-mail:* dwatson@weber.edu.

GRADUATE PROGRAMS

Contact Mr. Robert W. Holt, Enrollment Director, Program in Nursing, Weber State University, 3903 University Circle, Ogden, UT 84408-3903. *Telephone:* 801-626-7774. *Fax:* 801-626-6397. *E-mail:* rholt@weber.edu.

MASTER'S DEGREE PROGRAM

Degree MSN
Available Programs Master's.
Concentrations Available Nursing administration; nursing education.
Study Options Full-time.

Program Entrance Requirements Clinical experience, minimum overall college GPA of 3.0, transcript of college record, CPR certification, written essay, immunizations, interview, 2 letters of recommendation, nursing research course, professional liability insurance/malpractice insurance, prerequisite course work, resume, statistics course. *Application deadline:* 3/1 (fall). *Application fee:* $100.
Degree Requirements 40 total credit hours, thesis or project.

Western Governors University
Online College of Health Professions
Salt Lake City, Utah

Founded in 1998
DEGREES • BS • MS

BACCALAUREATE PROGRAMS

Degree BS
Available Programs RN Baccalaureate.
Online Degree Options Yes.
Contact Admissions, Online College of Health Professions, Western Governors University, 4001 South 700 East, Suite 700, Salt Lake City, UT 84107-2533. *Telephone:* 801-274-3280. *Fax:* 801-274-3305.

GRADUATE PROGRAMS

Contact Admissions, Online College of Health Professions, Western Governors University, 4001 South 700 East, Suite 700, Salt Lake City, UT 84107-2533. *Telephone:* 801-274-3280. *Fax:* 801-274-3305.

MASTER'S DEGREE PROGRAM

Degree MS
Available Programs RN to Master's.
Concentrations Available Clinical nurse leader; nursing education.
Online Degree Options Yes.

Westminster College
School of Nursing and Health Sciences
Salt Lake City, Utah

http://www.westminstercollege.edu
Founded in 1875
DEGREES • BSN • MSN
Nursing Student Activities Sigma Theta Tau, Student Nurses' Association, nursing club.
Nursing Student Resources Academic advising; academic or career counseling; assistance for students with disabilities; bookstore; campus computer network; career placement assistance; computer lab; computer-assisted instruction; e-mail services; employment services for current students; housing assistance; interactive nursing skills videos; Internet; learning resource lab; library services; nursing audiovisuals; placement services for program completers; remedial services; resume preparation assistance; skills, simulation, or other laboratory; tutoring.
Library Facilities 168,573 volumes; 9,857 periodical subscriptions.

BACCALAUREATE PROGRAMS

Degree BSN
Available Programs Baccalaureate for Second Degree; Generic Baccalaureate; RN Baccalaureate.
Study Options Full-time.
Program Entrance Requirements Transcript of college record, written essay, 3 letters of recommendation, minimum GPA in nursing prerequisites of 2.5, prerequisite course work. Transfer students are accepted.
Contact ***Telephone:*** 801-832-2150. *Fax:* 801-832-3110.

GRADUATE PROGRAMS

Contact ***Telephone:*** 801-832-2150. *Fax:* 801-832-3110.

MASTER'S DEGREE PROGRAM

Degree MSN
Available Programs Master's.
Concentrations Available Nursing education. *Nurse practitioner programs in:* family health.
Program Entrance Requirements Transcript of college record, written essay, 3 letters of recommendation, resume, GRE.
Advanced Placement Credit given for nursing courses completed elsewhere dependent upon specific evaluations.
Degree Requirements 42 total credit hours, thesis or project.

POST-MASTER'S PROGRAM

Areas of Study *Nurse practitioner programs in:* family health.

VERMONT

Norwich University
Department of Nursing
Northfield, Vermont

http://www.norwich.edu/acad/nursing
Founded in 1819
DEGREE • BSN
Nursing Program Faculty 8 (10% with doctorates).
Baccalaureate Enrollment 90 **Women** 90% **Men** 10% **Minority** 10%
Part-time 20%
Nursing Student Activities Student Nurses' Association, nursing club.
Nursing Student Resources Academic advising; academic or career counseling; assistance for students with disabilities; bookstore; campus computer network; career placement assistance; computer lab; e-mail services; employment services for current students; externships; housing assistance; interactive nursing skills videos; Internet; learning resource lab; library services; nursing audiovisuals; placement services for program completers; remedial services; resume preparation assistance; skills, simulation, or other laboratory; tutoring; unpaid internships.
Library Facilities 280,000 volumes; 904 periodical subscriptions.

BACCALAUREATE PROGRAMS

Degree BSN
Available Programs ADN to Baccalaureate; Generic Baccalaureate; RN Baccalaureate.
Site Options Rutland, VT.
Study Options Full-time and part-time.
Program Entrance Requirements Minimum overall college GPA of 2.5, transcript of college record, CPR certification, written essay, health exam, health insurance, high school biology, high school chemistry, 2 years high school math, 2 years high school science, high school transcript, immunizations, interview, 2 letters of recommendation, minimum GPA in nursing prerequisites of 2.5. Transfer students are accepted.
Advanced Placement Credit given for nursing courses completed elsewhere dependent upon specific evaluations.
Contact ***Telephone:*** 802-485-2008. *Fax:* 802-485-2032.

Southern Vermont College
Department of Nursing
Bennington, Vermont

http://www.svc.edu/academics/divisions/nursing.html
Founded in 1926
DEGREE • BSN
Nursing Program Faculty 7
Distance Learning Courses Available.
Nursing Student Resources Academic advising; academic or career counseling; assistance for students with disabilities; bookstore; computer lab; e-mail services; Internet; library services; resume preparation assistance; tutoring.
Library Facilities 26,000 volumes; 250 periodical subscriptions.

BACCALAUREATE PROGRAMS

Degree BSN
Available Programs ADN to Baccalaureate; RN Baccalaureate.
Advanced Placement Credit by examination available.
Contact ***Telephone:*** 802-447-6335. *Fax:* 802-447-4652.

University of Vermont

Department of Nursing
Burlington, Vermont

http://www.uvm.edu/~cnhs/nursing

Founded in 1791

DEGREES • BS • MS

Nursing Program Faculty 37 (14% with doctorates).

Baccalaureate Enrollment 282 **Women** 95% **Men** 5% **Minority** 9%

Graduate Enrollment 78 **Women** 90% **Men** 10% **Minority** 9% **Part-time** 23%

Distance Learning Courses Available.

Nursing Student Activities Nursing Honor Society, Sigma Theta Tau, Student Nurses' Association.

Nursing Student Resources Academic advising; academic or career counseling; assistance for students with disabilities; bookstore; campus computer network; career placement assistance; computer lab; computer-assisted instruction; e-mail services; employment services for current students; interactive nursing skills videos; Internet; learning resource lab; library services; nursing audiovisuals; remedial services; resume preparation assistance; skills, simulation, or other laboratory; tutoring.

Library Facilities 2.6 million volumes (126,689 in health, 1,437 in nursing); 23,642 periodical subscriptions (5,084 health-care related).

BACCALAUREATE PROGRAMS

Degree BS

Available Programs ADN to Baccalaureate; Generic Baccalaureate.

Study Options Full-time and part-time.

Program Entrance Requirements Minimum overall college GPA of 3.0, transcript of college record, written essay, health insurance, high school biology, high school chemistry, high school foreign language, 3 years high school math, 2 years high school science, high school transcript, immunizations, letters of recommendation, minimum GPA in nursing prerequisites of 2.0. Transfer students are accepted. *Application deadline:* 1/15 (fall). *Application fee:* $55.

Advanced Placement Credit by examination available. Credit given for nursing courses completed elsewhere dependent upon specific evaluations.

Expenses (2009-10) *Tuition, state resident:* full-time $11,712; part-time $488 per credit hour. *Tuition, nonresident:* full-time $29,568; part-time $1232 per credit hour. *Room and board:* $9026 per academic year. *Required fees:* full-time $1812.

Financial Aid 87% of baccalaureate students in nursing programs received some form of financial aid in 2008-09. *Gift aid (need-based):* Federal Pell, FSEOG, state, private, college/university gift aid from institutional funds, Federal Nursing. *Loans:* Federal Nursing Student Loans, Perkins, state, college/university. *Work-study:* Federal Work-Study. *Financial aid application deadline (priority):* 2/10.

Contact Ms. Erica S. Caloiero, Director of Student Services, Department of Nursing, University of Vermont, Rowell Building, Room 106, Burlington, VT 05405-0068. *Telephone:* 802-656-0968. *E-mail:* Erica.Caloiero@uvm.edu.

GRADUATE PROGRAMS

Expenses (2009-10) *Tuition, state resident:* full-time $8784; part-time $488 per credit hour. *Tuition, nonresident:* full-time $22,176; part-time $1232 per credit hour.

Financial Aid 36% of graduate students in nursing programs received some form of financial aid in 2008-09. *Application deadline:* 3/1.

Contact Ms. Miriam Harms, Graduate Program Assistant, Department of Nursing, University of Vermont, 216 Rowell Building, 106 Carrigan Drive, Burlington, VT 05405. *Telephone:* 802-656-2018. *Fax:* 802-656-8306. *E-mail:* Miriam.Harms@uvm.edu.

MASTER'S DEGREE PROGRAM

Degree MS

Available Programs Master's; Master's for Non-Nursing College Graduates; Master's for Nurses with Non-Nursing Degrees; RN to Master's.

Concentrations Available Nursing administration. *Nurse practitioner programs in:* adult health, family health, psychiatric/mental health.

Study Options Full-time and part-time.

Program Entrance Requirements Minimum overall college GPA of 3.0, transcript of college record, written essay, 3 letters of recommendation, physical assessment course, statistics course, GRE General Test. *Application deadline:* Applications may be processed on a rolling basis for some programs. *Application fee:* $40.

Advanced Placement Credit by examination available. Credit given for nursing courses completed elsewhere dependent upon specific evaluations.

Degree Requirements 57 total credit hours, thesis or project, comprehensive exam.

POST-MASTER'S PROGRAM

Areas of Study *Nurse practitioner programs in:* adult health, family health, psychiatric/mental health.

VIRGIN ISLANDS

University of the Virgin Islands

Division of Nursing
Saint Thomas, Virgin Islands

http://www.uvi.edu/

Founded in 1962

DEGREE • BSN

Nursing Program Faculty 6 (33% with doctorates).

Baccalaureate Enrollment 165 **Women** 97.58% **Men** 2.42% **Minority** 97% **International** 3% **Part-time** 20%

Nursing Student Activities Student Nurses' Association.

Nursing Student Resources Academic advising; academic or career counseling; assistance for students with disabilities; bookstore; campus computer network; computer lab; computer-assisted instruction; e-mail services; employment services for current students; externships; housing assistance; interactive nursing skills videos; Internet; learning resource lab; library services; nursing audiovisuals; paid internships; skills, simulation, or other laboratory; tutoring.

Library Facilities 106,361 volumes (95,000 in health, 600 in nursing); 113,623 periodical subscriptions (15 health-care related).

BACCALAUREATE PROGRAMS

Degree BSN

Available Programs ADN to Baccalaureate; Generic Baccalaureate; LPN to Baccalaureate; RN Baccalaureate.

Site Options St. Croix, VI.

Study Options Full-time and part-time.

Program Entrance Requirements Minimum overall college GPA of 2.5, CPR certification, health exam, 2 years high school math, high school transcript, immunizations, minimum GPA in nursing prerequisites of 2.5, professional liability insurance/malpractice insurance, prerequisite course work. Transfer students are accepted. *Application deadline:* 10/15 (fall), 4/15 (spring). Applications may be processed on a rolling basis for some programs. *Application fee:* $25.

Advanced Placement Credit by examination available. Credit given for nursing courses completed elsewhere dependent upon specific evaluations.

Expenses (2010-11) *Tuition, state resident:* full-time $3750; part-time $125 per credit. *Tuition, nonresident:* full-time $11,240; part-time $375 per credit. *Room and board:* $4050; room only: $1610 per academic year. *Required fees:* full-time $523.

Financial Aid 99% of baccalaureate students in nursing programs received some form of financial aid in 2009-10.

Contact Dr. Cheryl P. Franklin, Dean, Division of Nursing, University of the Virgin Islands, RR1 Box 10000, Kingshill, St. Croix, VI 00850-9781. *Telephone:* 340-778-1620 Ext. 4117. *Fax:* 340-693-1285. *E-mail:* cfrankl@uvi.edu.

VIRGINIA

Eastern Mennonite University

Department of Nursing
Harrisonburg, Virginia

Founded in 1917

DEGREES • BSN • MSN

Nursing Program Faculty 12 (25% with doctorates).

Baccalaureate Enrollment 146 **Women** 92.5% **Men** 7.5% **Minority** 8.2%

Graduate Enrollment 13 **Women** 84.6% **Men** 15.4% **Minority** 8% **Part-time** 8%

Distance Learning Courses Available.

Nursing Student Activities Sigma Theta Tau, Student Nurses' Association.

Nursing Student Resources Academic advising; academic or career counseling; assistance for students with disabilities; bookstore; campus computer network; career placement assistance; computer lab; computer-assisted instruction; e-mail services; employment services for current students; externships; housing assistance; interactive nursing skills videos; Internet; learning resource lab; library services; nursing audiovisuals; placement services for program completers; remedial services; resume preparation assistance; skills, simulation, or other laboratory; tutoring.

Library Facilities 166,154 volumes (1,256 in health, 926 in nursing); 861 periodical subscriptions (33 health-care related).

BACCALAUREATE PROGRAMS

Degree BSN

Available Programs ADN to Baccalaureate; Baccalaureate for Second Degree; Generic Baccalaureate; LPN to Baccalaureate; RN Baccalaureate.

Site Options Lancaster , PA.

Study Options Full-time and part-time.

Program Entrance Requirements Minimum overall college GPA of 2.8, transcript of college record, CPR certification, written essay, health exam, health insurance, high school chemistry, high school transcript, immunizations, 3 letters of recommendation, minimum high school GPA of 2.0, minimum GPA in nursing prerequisites of 2.8, professional liability insurance/malpractice insurance, prerequisite course work. Transfer students are accepted. *Application deadline:* 2/2 (fall), 6/1 (spring). Applications may be processed on a rolling basis for some programs.

Advanced Placement Credit by examination available. Credit given for nursing courses completed elsewhere dependent upon specific evaluations.

Expenses (2010-11) *Tuition:* full-time $25,200; part-time $350 per credit hour. *Room and board:* $8040 per academic year. *Required fees:* full-time $1400; part-time $700 per term.

Financial Aid 98% of baccalaureate students in nursing programs received some form of financial aid in 2009-10.

Contact Mrs. Stephanie C. Shafer, Director of Admissions, Department of Nursing, Eastern Mennonite University, 1200 Park Road, Harrisonburg, VA 22802. *Telephone:* 800-368-2665. *Fax:* 540-432-4118. *E-mail:* stephanie.schafer@emu.edu.

GRADUATE PROGRAMS

Expenses (2010-11) *Tuition:* full-time $9000; part-time $500 per credit hour.

Financial Aid 58% of graduate students in nursing programs received some form of financial aid in 2009-10.

Contact Dr. Ann G. Hershberger, Coordinator, Department of Nursing, Eastern Mennonite University, 1200 Park Road, Harrisonburg, VA 22802. *Telephone:* 540-432-4000 Ext. 4192. *Fax:* 540-432-4000 Ext. 4444. *E-mail:* hershbea@emu.edu.

MASTER'S DEGREE PROGRAM

Degree MSN

Available Programs Master's; Master's for Nurses with Non-Nursing Degrees.

Concentrations Available Nursing administration.

Online Degree Options Yes (online only).

Program Entrance Requirements Clinical experience, computer literacy, minimum overall college GPA of 3.0, transcript of college record, written essay, 2 letters of recommendation, nursing research course. *Application deadline:* 4/1 (fall). Applications may be processed on a rolling basis for some programs. *Application fee:* $25.

Degree Requirements 37 total credit hours, thesis or project.

ECPI College of Technology

BSN Program
Virginia Beach, Virginia

Founded in 1966

DEGREE • BSN

Distance Learning Courses Available.

Library Facilities 107,640 volumes; 293 periodical subscriptions.

BACCALAUREATE PROGRAMS

Degree BSN

Available Programs RN Baccalaureate.

Online Degree Options Yes.

Contact Bachelors Degree Program, BSN Program, ECPI College of Technology, 5501 Greenwich Road, Suite 100, Virginia Beach, VA 23462. *Telephone:* 757-497-8400.

George Mason University

College of Health and Human Services
Fairfax, Virginia

http://chhs.gmu.edu/

Founded in 1957

DEGREES • BSN • MSN • PHD

Nursing Program Faculty 39 (69% with doctorates).

Baccalaureate Enrollment 360 **Women** 89% **Men** 11% **Minority** 51% **International** 3% **Part-time** 4%

Graduate Enrollment 345 **Women** 95% **Men** 5% **Minority** 33% **International** 2% **Part-time** 86%

Distance Learning Courses Available.

Nursing Student Activities Nursing Honor Society, Sigma Theta Tau, Student Nurses' Association.

Nursing Student Resources Academic advising; academic or career counseling; assistance for students with disabilities; bookstore; campus computer network; career placement assistance; computer lab; computer-assisted instruction; e-mail services; employment services for current students; housing assistance; interactive nursing skills videos; Internet; library services; nursing audiovisuals; remedial services; resume preparation assistance; skills, simulation, or other laboratory; tutoring.

Library Facilities 1.9 million volumes (16,172 in nursing); 56,433 periodical subscriptions (200 health-care related).

BACCALAUREATE PROGRAMS

Degree BSN

Available Programs Accelerated Baccalaureate for Second Degree; Generic Baccalaureate; RN Baccalaureate.

Study Options Full-time.

Online Degree Options Yes.

Program Entrance Requirements Minimum overall college GPA of 2.0, CPR certification, written essay, health exam, health insurance, immunizations, minimum GPA in nursing prerequisites of 3.0, professional liability insurance/malpractice insurance, prerequisite course work. Transfer students are accepted. *Application deadline:* 1/15 (fall).

Expenses (2010-11) *Tuition, state resident:* full-time $8484; part-time $354 per credit. *Tuition, nonresident:* full-time $25,248; part-time $1052 per credit. *Room and board:* $8150; room only: $6350 per academic year. *Required fees:* full-time $1388.

Financial Aid 65% of baccalaureate students in nursing programs received some form of financial aid in 2009-10. *Gift aid (need-based):* Federal Pell, FSEOG, state, private, college/university gift aid from institutional funds. *Loans:* Federal Nursing Student Loans, Federal Direct (Subsidized and Unsubsidized Stafford PLUS), Perkins. *Work-study:* Federal Work-Study. *Financial aid application deadline (priority):* 3/1.

Contact Dr. Carol Urban, Assistant Dean, Division of Undergraduate Studies, School of Nursing, College of Health and Human Services, George Mason University, Mailstop 3C4, 4400 University Drive, Fairfax, VA 22030-4444. *Telephone:* 703-993-2991. *Fax:* 703-993-1949. *E-mail:* curban@gmu.edu.

GRADUATE PROGRAMS

Expenses (2010-11) *Tuition, state resident:* full-time $5778; part-time $482 per credit. *Tuition, nonresident:* full-time $13,158; part-time $1096 per credit. *Required fees:* full-time $160; part-time $60 per credit.
Financial Aid 10 research assistantships (averaging $3,654 per year), 2 teaching assistantships (averaging $2,790 per year) were awarded; fellowships, Federal Work-Study, scholarships, tuition waivers (partial), unspecified assistantships, and health care benefits (full-time research or teaching assistantship recipients) also available.
Contact Dr. Margaret Rodan, Assistant Dean for Graduate Programs, College of Health and Human Services, George Mason University, Mailstop 3C4, 4400 University Drive, Fairfax, VA 22030-4444. *Telephone:* 703-993-1727. *Fax:* 703-993-1949. *E-mail:* mrodan@gmu.edu.

MASTER'S DEGREE PROGRAM

Degree MSN
Available Programs Master's; RN to Master's.
Concentrations Available Nursing administration; nursing education. *Clinical nurse specialist programs in:* acute care, adult health, cardiovascular, critical care, medical-surgical, oncology. *Nurse practitioner programs in:* adult health, family health, primary care.
Site Options Loudoun County, VA; Prince William County, VA.
Study Options Full-time and part-time.
Online Degree Options Yes (online only).
Program Entrance Requirements Clinical experience, minimum overall college GPA of 3.0, CPR certification, written essay, immunizations, 2 letters of recommendation, physical assessment course, statistics course. *Application deadline:* 4/1 (fall), 11/1 (spring). *Application fee:* $50.
Degree Requirements 44 total credit hours, thesis or project.

POST-MASTER'S PROGRAM

Areas of Study Nursing administration; nursing education.

DOCTORAL DEGREE PROGRAM

Degree PhD
Available Programs Doctorate.
Areas of Study Individualized study.
Online Degree Options Yes (online only).
Program Entrance Requirements Clinical experience, minimum overall college GPA of 3.5, interview, 3 letters of recommendation, MSN or equivalent, statistics course, writing sample, MAT. Application deadline: 3/1 (spring). Application fee: $60.
Degree Requirements 48 total credit hours, dissertation, written exam.

POSTDOCTORAL PROGRAM

Postdoctoral Program Contact Jean Sorrell, Coordinator, College of Health and Human Services, George Mason University, Mailstop 3C4, 4400 University Drive, Fairfax, VA 22030-4444. *Telephone:* 703-993-1944. *Fax:* 703-993-1942. *E-mail:* jsorrell@gmu.edu.

CONTINUING EDUCATION PROGRAM

Contact Dr. Mona Ternus, Director, Academic Outreach, College of Health and Human Services, George Mason University, Mailstop 3C4, 4400 University Drive, Fairfax, VA 22030-4444. *Telephone:* 703-993-1910. *Fax:* 703-993-1622. *E-mail:* mternus@gmu.edu.

Hampton University

School of Nursing
Hampton, Virginia

http://www.hamptonu.edu/nursing/Index.htm
Founded in 1868

DEGREES • BS • MS • PHD

Nursing Program Faculty 26 (51% with doctorates).
Baccalaureate Enrollment 470 **Women** 93% **Men** 7% **Minority** 90% **International** 4% **Part-time** 4%
Graduate Enrollment 66 **Women** 100% **Minority** 80% **Part-time** 25%
Distance Learning Courses Available.
Nursing Student Activities Sigma Theta Tau, Student Nurses' Association.
Nursing Student Resources Academic advising; bookstore; computer lab; e-mail services; interactive nursing skills videos; Internet; library services; skills, simulation, or other laboratory; tutoring.
Library Facilities 526,154 volumes (4,000 in health, 2,000 in nursing); 32,187 periodical subscriptions (500 health-care related).

BACCALAUREATE PROGRAMS

Degree BS
Available Programs Accelerated Baccalaureate; Generic Baccalaureate; LPN to Baccalaureate; LPN to RN Baccalaureate; RN Baccalaureate.
Site Options Virginia Beach, VA.
Study Options Full-time and part-time.
Program Entrance Requirements Minimum overall college GPA of 2.3, transcript of college record, CPR certification, written essay, health exam, health insurance, high school biology, high school chemistry, 3 years high school math, 2 years high school science, high school transcript, immunizations, 2 letters of recommendation, minimum high school GPA of 2.0, minimum high school rank 50%, minimum GPA in nursing prerequisites of 2.0, professional liability insurance/malpractice insurance. Transfer students are accepted. *Application deadline:* 3/1 (fall), 12/1 (spring).
Advanced Placement Credit by examination available. Credit given for nursing courses completed elsewhere dependent upon specific evaluations.
Expenses (2010-11) *Tuition:* full-time $16,238; part-time $410 per semester. *Room and board:* $8048; room only: $4186 per academic year.
Financial Aid 93% of baccalaureate students in nursing programs received some form of financial aid in 2009-10. *Gift aid (need-based):* Federal Pell, FSEOG, state, private, college/university gift aid from institutional funds, Federal Nursing. *Loans:* Federal Nursing Student Loans, Perkins, college/university, private loans. *Work-study:* Federal Work-Study, part-time campus jobs. *Financial aid application deadline:* 4/15(priority: 3/1).
Contact Dr. Barbara Wright, Chairperson, Department of Undergraduate Nursing Education, School of Nursing, Hampton University, William Freeman Hall, 100 East Queen Street, Hampton, VA 23668. *Telephone:* 757-727-5251. *E-mail:* nursing@hamptonu.edu.

GRADUATE PROGRAMS

Expenses (2010-11) *Tuition:* full-time $8119; part-time $410 per semester. *International tuition:* $8119 full-time.
Financial Aid 90% of graduate students in nursing programs received some form of financial aid in 2009-10. Fellowships, research assistantships, teaching assistantships, career-related internships or fieldwork, Federal Work-Study, institutionally sponsored loans, and scholarships available. Aid available to part-time students. *Financial aid application deadline:* 5/1.
Contact Dr. Arlene J. Montgomery, Chairperson, Department of Graduate Nursing Education, School of Nursing, Hampton University, Freeman Hall, Hampton, VA 23668. *Telephone:* 757-727-5251. *Fax:* 757-727-5423.

MASTER'S DEGREE PROGRAM

Degree MS
Available Programs Master's; RN to Master's.
Concentrations Available Health-care administration; nursing administration; nursing education. *Nurse practitioner programs in:* family health, gerontology, pediatric, primary care, women's health.
Study Options Full-time and part-time.
Online Degree Options Yes.
Program Entrance Requirements Clinical experience, computer literacy, minimum overall college GPA of 2.5, transcript of college record, written essay, interview, 2 letters of recommendation, nursing research course, physical assessment course, resume, statistics course, GRE General Test. *Application deadline:* 3/30 (fall), 11/1 (spring).
Advanced Placement Credit given for nursing courses completed elsewhere dependent upon specific evaluations.
Degree Requirements 46 total credit hours, thesis or project, comprehensive exam.

DOCTORAL DEGREE PROGRAM

Degree PhD
Available Programs Doctorate.
Areas of Study Family health.
Online Degree Options Yes (online only).
Program Entrance Requirements Minimum overall college GPA of 3.5, interview by faculty committee, interview, 3 letters of recommendation, MSN or equivalent, statistics course, vita, writing sample. Application deadline: 3/30 (fall).
Degree Requirements 44 total credit hours, dissertation, oral exam, written exam, residency.

James Madison University
Department of Nursing
Harrisonburg, Virginia

http://www.nursing.jmu.edu
Founded in 1908

DEGREES • BSN • MSN

Nursing Program Faculty 35 (40% with doctorates).
Baccalaureate Enrollment 808 **Women** 95% **Men** 5% **Minority** 7%
Graduate Enrollment 47 **Women** 93% **Men** 7% **Minority** 5% **Part-time** 45%
Distance Learning Courses Available.
Nursing Student Activities Nursing Honor Society, Sigma Theta Tau, Student Nurses' Association.
Nursing Student Resources Academic advising; academic or career counseling; assistance for students with disabilities; bookstore; campus computer network; career placement assistance; computer lab; computer-assisted instruction; e-mail services; employment services for current students; externships; housing assistance; interactive nursing skills videos; Internet; learning resource lab; library services; nursing audiovisuals; paid internships; remedial services; resume preparation assistance; skills, simulation, or other laboratory; unpaid internships.
Library Facilities 1.3 million volumes (67,716 in health, 12,054 in nursing); 12,830 periodical subscriptions.

BACCALAUREATE PROGRAMS

Degree BSN
Available Programs Accelerated RN Baccalaureate; Generic Baccalaureate.
Study Options Full-time and part-time.
Program Entrance Requirements Minimum overall college GPA of 2.8, transcript of college record, CPR certification, written essay, health exam, health insurance, immunizations, minimum GPA in nursing prerequisites of 2.0, prerequisite course work. Transfer students are accepted. *Application deadline:* Applications may be processed on a rolling basis for some programs.
Advanced Placement Credit given for nursing courses completed elsewhere dependent upon specific evaluations.
Expenses (2009-10) *Tuition, state resident:* full-time $7244. *Tuition, nonresident:* full-time $19,366. *Room and board:* $7386 per academic year. *Required fees:* full-time $532.
Financial Aid 37% of baccalaureate students in nursing programs received some form of financial aid in 2008-09. *Gift aid (need-based):* Federal Pell, FSEOG, state, private, college/university gift aid from institutional funds. *Loans:* Federal Nursing Student Loans, Federal Direct (Subsidized and Unsubsidized Stafford PLUS), Perkins. *Work-study:* Federal Work-Study, part-time campus jobs. *Financial aid application deadline (priority):* 3/1.
Contact Ms. Kelly Brown, Administrative Assistant, Department of Nursing, James Madison University, 701 Carrier Drive, Health and Human Services Building, MSC 4305, Harrisonburg, VA 22807. *Telephone:* 540-568-6314. *Fax:* 540-568-7896. *E-mail:* brownkd@jmu.edu.

GRADUATE PROGRAMS

Expenses (2009-10) *Tuition, state resident:* part-time $305 per credit hour. *Tuition, nonresident:* part-time $890 per credit hour.
Financial Aid 95% of graduate students in nursing programs received some form of financial aid in 2008-09.
Contact Christy Comer, Administrative Assistant, Department of Nursing, James Madison University, 701 Carrier Drive, Health and Human Services Building, MSC 4305, Harrisonburg, VA 22807. *Telephone:* 540-568-6314. *Fax:* 540-568-7896. *E-mail:* comerca@jmu.edu.

MASTER'S DEGREE PROGRAM

Degree MSN
Available Programs Master's.
Concentrations Available Clinical nurse leader; nurse-midwifery; nursing administration. *Nurse practitioner programs in:* adult health, family health, gerontology.
Study Options Full-time and part-time.
Program Entrance Requirements Clinical experience, computer literacy, minimum overall college GPA of 2.8, transcript of college record, CPR certification, written essay, immunizations, 2 letters of recommendation, physical assessment course, prerequisite course work, resume, statistics course. *Application deadline:* Applications may be processed on a rolling basis for some programs.
Advanced Placement Credit given for nursing courses completed elsewhere dependent upon specific evaluations.
Degree Requirements 43 total credit hours.

POST-MASTER'S PROGRAM

Areas of Study Clinical nurse leader; nurse-midwifery; nursing administration. *Nurse practitioner programs in:* adult health, family health, gerontology.

Jefferson College of Health Sciences
Nursing Education Program
Roanoke, Virginia

http://www.jchs.edu
Founded in 1982

DEGREES • BSN • MSN

Nursing Program Faculty 24 (17% with doctorates).
Baccalaureate Enrollment 260 **Women** 93% **Men** 7% **Minority** 15% **Part-time** 47%
Graduate Enrollment 32 **Women** 91% **Men** 9% **Minority** 9% **Part-time** 3%
Distance Learning Courses Available.
Nursing Student Activities Nursing Honor Society, Sigma Theta Tau, Student Nurses' Association.
Nursing Student Resources Academic advising; academic or career counseling; assistance for students with disabilities; bookstore; campus computer network; computer lab; computer-assisted instruction; e-mail services; externships; housing assistance; interactive nursing skills videos; Internet; learning resource lab; library services; nursing audiovisuals; skills, simulation, or other laboratory; tutoring.
Library Facilities 10,533 volumes (4,403 in health, 1,422 in nursing); 376 periodical subscriptions (277 health-care related).

BACCALAUREATE PROGRAMS

Degree BSN
Available Programs ADN to Baccalaureate; Generic Baccalaureate; RN Baccalaureate.
Site Options Roanoke, VA.
Study Options Full-time and part-time.
Program Entrance Requirements Minimum overall college GPA of 2.0, transcript of college record, CPR certification, health exam, health insurance, high school biology, high school chemistry, 2 years high school math, 2 years high school science, high school transcript, immunizations, minimum high school GPA of 2.0, prerequisite course work. Transfer students are accepted.
Advanced Placement Credit by examination available. Credit given for nursing courses completed elsewhere dependent upon specific evaluations.
Contact *Telephone:* 540-985-9083. *Fax:* 540-224-6703.

GRADUATE PROGRAMS

Contact *Telephone:* 540-985-9083. *Fax:* 540-224-6703.

MASTER'S DEGREE PROGRAM

Degree MSN
Available Programs Master's; Master's for Nurses with Non-Nursing Degrees.
Concentrations Available Nursing administration; nursing education.
Site Options Roanoke, VA.
Study Options Full-time.
Program Entrance Requirements Clinical experience, computer literacy, transcript of college record, 2 letters of recommendation, nursing research course, resume, statistics course.
Degree Requirements 37 total credit hours, thesis or project.

CONTINUING EDUCATION PROGRAM

Contact *Telephone:* 540-767-6072.

Liberty University
Department of Nursing
Lynchburg, Virginia

http://www.liberty.edu
Founded in 1971

DEGREES • BSN • MSN

Nursing Program Faculty 25 (25% with doctorates).
Baccalaureate Enrollment 358 **Women** 93% **Men** 7% **Minority** 7% **International** 8%
Graduate Enrollment 280 **Women** 89% **Men** 11% **Minority** 29% **International** 3% **Part-time** 99%
Distance Learning Courses Available.
Nursing Student Activities Student Nurses' Association.
Nursing Student Resources Academic advising; academic or career counseling; assistance for students with disabilities; bookstore; campus computer network; career placement assistance; computer lab; e-mail services; externships; interactive nursing skills videos; Internet; learning resource lab; library services; nursing audiovisuals; resume preparation assistance; skills, simulation, or other laboratory; tutoring.
Library Facilities 495,255 volumes (3,632 in health, 3,000 in nursing); 72,245 periodical subscriptions (46 health-care related).

BACCALAUREATE PROGRAMS

Degree BSN
Available Programs Generic Baccalaureate; RN Baccalaureate.
Site Options Lynchburg, VA.
Study Options Full-time and part-time.
Program Entrance Requirements Minimum overall college GPA of 3.0, transcript of college record, CPR certification, written essay, immunizations, 2 letters of recommendation, minimum GPA in nursing prerequisites of 3.0, professional liability insurance/malpractice insurance, prerequisite course work. Transfer students are accepted. *Application deadline:* 2/11 (spring).
Advanced Placement Credit given for nursing courses completed elsewhere dependent upon specific evaluations.
Contact ***Telephone:*** 804-582-2519. *Fax:* 804-582-7035.

GRADUATE PROGRAMS

Contact ***Telephone:*** 804-582-2519.

MASTER'S DEGREE PROGRAM

Degree MSN
Available Programs Master's.
Concentrations Available Nursing education. *Clinical nurse specialist programs in:* acute care.
Site Options Lynchburg, VA.
Study Options Full-time and part-time.
Online Degree Options Yes (online only).
Program Entrance Requirements Clinical experience, computer literacy, minimum overall college GPA of 3.0, transcript of college record, CPR certification, written essay, immunizations, interview, 3 letters of recommendation, nursing research course, physical assessment course, prerequisite course work, resume, statistics course. *Application deadline:* Applications may be processed on a rolling basis for some programs. *Application fee:* $50.
Degree Requirements 36 total credit hours, thesis or project.

Lynchburg College
School of Health Sciences and Human Performance
Lynchburg, Virginia

http://www.lynchburg.edu/nursing.xml
Founded in 1903

DEGREES • BS • MSN • MSN/MBA

Nursing Program Faculty 15 (33% with doctorates).
Baccalaureate Enrollment 206 **Women** 85% **Men** 15% **Minority** 10% **International** 1% **Part-time** 5%
Graduate Enrollment 12
Nursing Student Activities Sigma Theta Tau, Student Nurses' Association.
Nursing Student Resources Academic advising; academic or career counseling; assistance for students with disabilities; bookstore; campus computer network; career placement assistance; computer lab; computer-assisted instruction; e-mail services; employment services for current students; externships; Internet; learning resource lab; library services; nursing audiovisuals; resume preparation assistance; skills, simulation, or other laboratory; tutoring; unpaid internships.
Library Facilities 234,000 volumes (6,259 in health, 1,881 in nursing); 254 periodical subscriptions (65 health-care related).

BACCALAUREATE PROGRAMS

Degree BS
Available Programs Accelerated Baccalaureate; Generic Baccalaureate.
Study Options Full-time and part-time.
Program Entrance Requirements Transcript of college record, 3 years high school math, minimum GPA in nursing prerequisites of 3.0, prerequisite course work. Transfer students are accepted. *Application deadline:* 4/1 (fall), 4/1 (summer).
Advanced Placement Credit given for nursing courses completed elsewhere dependent upon specific evaluations.
Expenses (2010-11) *Tuition:* full-time $14,480; part-time $800 per credit hour. *Room and board:* $3600; room only: $2000 per academic year. *Required fees:* full-time $500; part-time $100 per credit.
Financial Aid 97% of baccalaureate students in nursing programs received some form of financial aid in 2009-10. *Gift aid (need-based):* Federal Pell, FSEOG, state, private, college/university gift aid from institutional funds. *Loans:* Federal Direct (Subsidized and Unsubsidized Stafford PLUS), Perkins. *Work-study:* Federal Work-Study, part-time campus jobs. *Financial aid application deadline (priority):* 3/5.
Contact Dr. Angela S. Taylor, Director of Nursing Program and Associate Professor, School of Health Sciences and Human Performance, Lynchburg College, 1501 Lakeside Drive, McMillan Nursing Building, Lynchburg, VA 24501-3199. *Telephone:* 434-544-8901. *Fax:* 434-544-8323. *E-mail:* taylor.a@lynchburg.edu.

GRADUATE PROGRAMS

Expenses (2010-11) *Tuition:* part-time $400 per credit hour.
Financial Aid 75% of graduate students in nursing programs received some form of financial aid in 2009-10.
Contact Dr. Angela S. Taylor, Director of Nursing Program, School of Health Sciences and Human Performance, Lynchburg College, 1501 Lakeside Drive, Lynchburg, VA 24501. *Telephone:* 434-544-8901. *Fax:* 434-544-8323. *E-mail:* taylor.a@lynchburg.edu.

MASTER'S DEGREE PROGRAM

Degrees MSN; MSN/MBA
Available Programs Master's.
Concentrations Available Clinical nurse leader; nursing education.
Study Options Full-time and part-time.
Program Entrance Requirements Clinical experience, minimum overall college GPA of 2.5, transcript of college record, 3 letters of recommendation, physical assessment course, statistics course. *Application deadline:* Applications may be processed on a rolling basis for some programs.
Advanced Placement Credit given for nursing courses completed elsewhere dependent upon specific evaluations.
Degree Requirements 37 total credit hours, thesis or project.

Marymount University
School of Health Professions
Arlington, Virginia

http://www.marymount.edu/academic/healthprof/index.html
Founded in 1950

DEGREES • BSN • DNP • MSN

Nursing Program Faculty 18 (61% with doctorates).
Baccalaureate Enrollment 350 **Women** 90% **Men** 10% **Minority** 32% **International** 4% **Part-time** 17%
Graduate Enrollment 479 **Women** 91% **Men** 9% **Minority** 48% **International** 5% **Part-time** 84%
Distance Learning Courses Available.
Nursing Student Activities Sigma Theta Tau, Student Nurses' Association.
Nursing Student Resources Academic advising; academic or career counseling; assistance for students with disabilities; bookstore; campus computer network; career placement assistance; computer lab; computer-

assisted instruction; e-mail services; externships; housing assistance; interactive nursing skills videos; Internet; learning resource lab; library services; nursing audiovisuals; paid internships; remedial services; resume preparation assistance; skills, simulation, or other laboratory; tutoring; unpaid internships.
Library Facilities 236,315 volumes (10,657 in health, 1,500 in nursing); 955 periodical subscriptions (100 health-care related).

BACCALAUREATE PROGRAMS

Degree BSN
Available Programs ADN to Baccalaureate; Accelerated Baccalaureate for Second Degree; Accelerated RN Baccalaureate; Baccalaureate for Second Degree; Generic Baccalaureate; RN Baccalaureate.
Site Options Arlington, VA.
Study Options Full-time and part-time.
Online Degree Options Yes.
Program Entrance Requirements Minimum overall college GPA of 2.5, health exam, health insurance, high school transcript, 2 letters of recommendation, minimum high school GPA of 2.5. Transfer students are accepted. *Application deadline:* Applications may be processed on a rolling basis for some programs. *Application fee:* $40.
Advanced Placement Credit by examination available. Credit given for nursing courses completed elsewhere dependent upon specific evaluations.
Expenses (2009-10) *Tuition:* full-time $22,370; part-time $725 per credit hour. *Room and board:* $9745 per academic year.
Financial Aid 84% of baccalaureate students in nursing programs received some form of financial aid in 2008-09. *Gift did (need-based):* Federal Pell, FSEOG, state, private, college/university gift aid from institutional funds. *Loans:* Federal Direct (Subsidized and Unsubsidized Stafford PLUS), Perkins. *Work-study:* Federal Work-Study. *Financial aid application deadline (priority):* 3/1.
Contact Dr. Rosemarie Berman, Chair, School of Health Professions, Marymount University, 2807 North Glebe Road, Arlington, VA 22207-4299. *Telephone:* 703-284-1627. *Fax:* 703-284-3819. *E-mail:* rosemarie.berman@marymount.edu.

GRADUATE PROGRAMS

Expenses (2009-10) *Tuition:* part-time $725 per credit hour.
Financial Aid 57% of graduate students in nursing programs received some form of financial aid in 2008-09. Research assistantships with full and partial tuition reimbursements available, career-related internships or fieldwork, Federal Work-Study, scholarships, and unspecified assistantships available. Aid available to part-time students.
Contact Ms. Francesca Reed, Coordinator, Graduate Admissions, School of Health Professions, Marymount University, 2807 North Glebe Road, Arlington, VA 22207-4299. *Telephone:* 703-284-5906. *E-mail:* francesca.reed@marymount.edu.

MASTER'S DEGREE PROGRAM

Degree MSN
Available Programs Master's.
Concentrations Available Nursing education. *Nurse practitioner programs in:* family health.
Site Options Arlington, VA.
Study Options Full-time and part-time.
Program Entrance Requirements Minimum overall college GPA of 3.0, transcript of college record, CPR certification, immunizations, interview, 2 letters of recommendation, professional liability insurance/malpractice insurance, resume, statistics course, GRE, MAT. *Application deadline:* Applications may be processed on a rolling basis for some programs. *Application fee:* $40.
Advanced Placement Credit given for nursing courses completed elsewhere dependent upon specific evaluations.
Degree Requirements 40 total credit hours, comprehensive exam.

POST-MASTER'S PROGRAM

Areas of Study Nursing education. *Nurse practitioner programs in:* family health.

DOCTORAL DEGREE PROGRAM

Degree DNP
Available Programs Doctorate; Post-Baccalaureate Doctorate.
Areas of Study Advanced practice nursing.
Site Options Arlington, VA.
Program Entrance Requirements Clinical experience, minimum overall college GPA of 3.0, interview by faculty committee, interview, 2 letters of recommendation, MSN or equivalent, vita, GRE. Application deadline: 4/1 (fall). Application fee: $40.
Degree Requirements 32 total credit hours, residency.

Norfolk State University
Department of Nursing
Norfolk, Virginia

http://www.nsu.edu/schools/sciencetech/nursing/
Founded in 1935

DEGREE • BSN

Nursing Program Faculty 26 (40% with doctorates).
Baccalaureate Enrollment 133 **Women** 90% **Men** 10% **Minority** 85% **International** 15% **Part-time** 45%
Distance Learning Courses Available.
Nursing Student Activities Nursing Honor Society, Student Nurses' Association, nursing club.
Nursing Student Resources Academic advising; academic or career counseling; assistance for students with disabilities; bookstore; campus computer network; career placement assistance; computer lab; computer-assisted instruction; daycare for children of students; e-mail services; employment services for current students; externships; housing assistance; interactive nursing skills videos; Internet; learning resource lab; library services; nursing audiovisuals; paid internships; remedial services; resume preparation assistance; skills, simulation, or other laboratory; tutoring; unpaid internships.
Library Facilities 348,953 volumes (600 in health, 300 in nursing); 127,601 periodical subscriptions (125 health-care related).

BACCALAUREATE PROGRAMS

Degree BSN
Available Programs Accelerated Baccalaureate for Second Degree; Accelerated LPN to Baccalaureate; RN Baccalaureate.
Site Options Virginia Beach , VA.
Study Options Full-time and part-time.
Program Entrance Requirements Minimum overall college GPA of 2.5, transcript of college record, CPR certification, health exam, health insurance, high school biology, high school chemistry, 2 years high school math, high school transcript, immunizations, minimum high school GPA of 2.5, minimum GPA in nursing prerequisites of 2.5, professional liability insurance/malpractice insurance, prerequisite course work. Transfer students are accepted. *Application deadline:* 8/1 (fall), 12/1 (winter), 2/1 (spring), 8/1 (summer).
Advanced Placement Credit by examination available. Credit given for nursing courses completed elsewhere dependent upon specific evaluations.
Expenses (2009-10) *Tuition, state resident:* full-time $2986; part-time $260 per credit hour. *Tuition, nonresident:* full-time $9016; part-time $662 per credit hour. *International tuition:* $9016 full-time. *Room and board:* $3665; room only: $2335 per academic year. *Required fees:* full-time $205.
Financial Aid 87% of baccalaureate students in nursing programs received some form of financial aid in 2008-09.
Contact Dr. Bennie L. Marshall, Department Head, Department of Nursing, Norfolk State University, 700 Park Avenue, Norfolk, VA 23504. *Telephone:* 757-823-9015. *Fax:* 757-823-2131. *E-mail:* blmarshall@nsu.edu.

Old Dominion University
Department of Nursing
Norfolk, Virginia

http://www.odu.edu/nursson
Founded in 1930

DEGREES • BSN • DNP • MSN

Nursing Program Faculty 27 (33% with doctorates).
Baccalaureate Enrollment 399 **Women** 91% **Men** 9% **Minority** 40% **Part-time** 46%
Graduate Enrollment 219 **Women** 92% **Men** 8% **Minority** 23% **Part-time** 47%
Distance Learning Courses Available.
Nursing Student Activities Sigma Theta Tau, Student Nurses' Association.
Nursing Student Resources Academic advising; academic or career counseling; assistance for students with disabilities; bookstore; campus

computer network; career placement assistance; computer lab; computer-assisted instruction; e-mail services; externships; interactive nursing skills videos; Internet; learning resource lab; library services; nursing audiovisuals; paid internships; remedial services; resume preparation assistance; skills, simulation, or other laboratory; tutoring; unpaid internships.

Library Facilities 1.2 million volumes (44,144 in health, 3,622 in nursing); 10,495 periodical subscriptions (3,035 health-care related).

BACCALAUREATE PROGRAMS

Degree BSN

Available Programs Accelerated Baccalaureate; Generic Baccalaureate; RN Baccalaureate.

Site Options Olympia, WA; Yavapai, AZ.

Study Options Full-time.

Program Entrance Requirements Transcript of college record, CPR certification, immunizations, minimum GPA in nursing prerequisites of 2.5, prerequisite course work. Transfer students are accepted. *Application deadline:* 2/1 (fall). *Application fee:* $40.

Contact ***Telephone:*** 757-683-5245. *Fax:* 757-683-5253.

GRADUATE PROGRAMS

Contact ***Telephone:*** 757-683-4298. *Fax:* 757-683-5253.

MASTER'S DEGREE PROGRAM

Degree MSN

Available Programs Master's; RN to Master's.

Concentrations Available Nurse anesthesia; nurse-midwifery; nursing administration; nursing education. *Nurse practitioner programs in:* family health, women's health.

Site Options Athens, GA; Olympia, WA; Yavapai, AZ.

Study Options Full-time and part-time.

Online Degree Options Yes (online only).

Program Entrance Requirements Clinical experience, computer literacy, minimum overall college GPA of 3.0, transcript of college record, CPR certification, written essay, immunizations, interview, 3 letters of recommendation, physical assessment course, statistics course. *Application deadline:* 6/1 (fall), 12/1 (winter). *Application fee:* $40.

Advanced Placement Credit given for nursing courses completed elsewhere dependent upon specific evaluations.

Degree Requirements 47 total credit hours, comprehensive exam.

POST-MASTER'S PROGRAM

Areas of Study Nurse anesthesia; nurse-midwifery; nursing administration; nursing education. *Nurse practitioner programs in:* family health, women's health.

DOCTORAL DEGREE PROGRAM

Degree DNP

Available Programs Doctorate.

Areas of Study Advanced practice nursing.

Online Degree Options Yes (online only).

Program Entrance Requirements Clinical experience, minimum overall college GPA of 3.0, 3 letters of recommendation, MSN or equivalent, statistics course, vita, writing sample. Application deadline: 11/15 (fall), 11/15 (winter), 11/15 (spring).

Degree Requirements 36 total credit hours.

CONTINUING EDUCATION PROGRAM

Contact ***Telephone:*** 757-683-5261. *Fax:* 757-683-5253.

Radford University

School of Nursing
Radford, Virginia

http://www.radford.edu/nurs-web

Founded in 1910

DEGREES • BSN • DNP

Nursing Program Faculty 42 (8% with doctorates).

Baccalaureate Enrollment 264 **Women** 93% **Men** 7% **Minority** 9% **International** 3%

Graduate Enrollment 18 **Women** 100% **Minority** 5% **Part-time** 30%

Distance Learning Courses Available.

Nursing Student Activities Nursing Honor Society, Sigma Theta Tau, Student Nurses' Association.

Nursing Student Resources Academic advising; academic or career counseling; assistance for students with disabilities; bookstore; campus computer network; career placement assistance; computer lab; computer-assisted instruction; e-mail services; employment services for current students; externships; housing assistance; interactive nursing skills videos; Internet; learning resource lab; library services; nursing audiovisuals; resume preparation assistance; skills, simulation, or other laboratory; unpaid internships.

Library Facilities 383,664 volumes; 9,935 periodical subscriptions.

BACCALAUREATE PROGRAMS

Degree BSN

Available Programs Baccalaureate for Second Degree; Generic Baccalaureate; RN Baccalaureate.

Site Options Roanoke, VA.

Study Options Full-time.

Online Degree Options Yes.

Program Entrance Requirements Minimum overall college GPA of 2.5, transcript of college record, CPR certification, written essay, health exam, health insurance, immunizations, minimum GPA in nursing prerequisites of 2.5, prerequisite course work. Transfer students are accepted. *Application deadline:* 11/15 (fall), 8/1 (spring).

Advanced Placement Credit given for nursing courses completed elsewhere dependent upon specific evaluations.

Expenses (2010-11) *Tuition, state resident:* full-time $7694; part-time $321 per credit hour. *Tuition, nonresident:* full-time $18,428; part-time $768 per credit hour. *Room and board:* $7198; room only: $3828 per academic year.

Financial Aid 50% of baccalaureate students in nursing programs received some form of financial aid in 2009-10. *Gift aid (need-based):* Federal Pell, FSEOG, state, private, college/university gift aid from institutional funds. *Loans:* Federal Nursing Student Loans, Federal Direct (Subsidized and Unsubsidized Stafford PLUS), Perkins, state, college/university. *Work-study:* Federal Work-Study, part-time campus jobs. *Financial aid application deadline (priority):* 2/15.

Contact Prof. Anthony Ray Ramsey, Undergraduate Program Coordinator, School of Nursing, Radford University, PO Box 6964, Radford, VA 24142. *Telephone:* 540-831-7700. *Fax:* 540-831-7716. *E-mail:* nurs-web@radford.edu.

GRADUATE PROGRAMS

Expenses (2010-11) *Tuition, state resident:* full-time $8380; part-time $350 per credit hour. *Tuition, nonresident:* full-time $16,808; part-time $702 per credit hour. *International tuition:* $16,808 full-time. *Room and board:* $7198; room only: $3828 per academic year.

Financial Aid 90% of graduate students in nursing programs received some form of financial aid in 2009-10. 4 teaching assistantships with partial tuition reimbursements available (averaging $8,700 per year) were awarded; career-related internships or fieldwork, Federal Work-Study, institutionally sponsored loans, scholarships, and unspecified assistantships also available. *Financial aid application deadline:* 3/1.

Contact Dr. Virginia Burggraf, Graduate Program Coordinator, School of Nursing, Radford University, PO Box 6964, Radford, VA 24142. *Telephone:* 540-831-7714. *Fax:* 540-831-7716. *E-mail:* nurs-web@radford.edu.

MASTER'S DEGREE PROGRAM

Program Entrance Requirements GRE.

DOCTORAL DEGREE PROGRAM

Degree DNP

Available Programs Doctorate; Post-Baccalaureate Doctorate.

Areas of Study Advanced practice nursing, aging, clinical practice, faculty preparation, family health, gerontology, individualized study, maternity-newborn.

Online Degree Options Yes (online only).

Program Entrance Requirements Clinical experience, minimum overall college GPA of 3.0, interview by faculty committee, 3 letters of recommendation, vita, writing sample. Application deadline: 4/1 (fall). Application fee: $50.

Degree Requirements Residency.

Shenandoah University

Division of Nursing
Winchester, Virginia

http://www.su.edu/nursing/index.html
Founded in 1875

DEGREES • BSN • MSN

Nursing Program Faculty 44 (30% with doctorates).

Baccalaureate Enrollment 239 **Women** 97% **Men** 3% **Minority** 10% **International** 3% **Part-time** 15%

Graduate Enrollment 28 **Women** 97% **Men** 3% **Minority** 10% **Part-time** 25%

Nursing Student Activities Nursing Honor Society, Sigma Theta Tau, Student Nurses' Association.

Nursing Student Resources Academic advising; academic or career counseling; assistance for students with disabilities; bookstore; campus computer network; computer lab; daycare for children of students; e-mail services; interactive nursing skills videos; Internet; learning resource lab; library services; nursing audiovisuals; resume preparation assistance; skills, simulation, or other laboratory; tutoring.

Library Facilities 202,815 volumes (500 in health, 200 in nursing); 54,215 periodical subscriptions (250 health-care related).

BACCALAUREATE PROGRAMS

Degree BSN

Available Programs ADN to Baccalaureate; Accelerated Baccalaureate for Second Degree; Generic Baccalaureate; LPN to Baccalaureate; LPN to RN Baccalaureate; RN Baccalaureate.

Site Options Leesburg, VA.

Study Options Full-time and part-time.

Program Entrance Requirements Minimum overall college GPA of 2.5, transcript of college record, CPR certification, health exam, health insurance, high school biology, high school chemistry, 2 years high school math, high school transcript, immunizations, minimum high school GPA of 2.5, minimum GPA in nursing prerequisites of 2.0, prerequisite course work. Transfer students are accepted.

Advanced Placement Credit by examination available. Credit given for nursing courses completed elsewhere dependent upon specific evaluations.

Contact ***Telephone:*** 540-678-4381. *Fax:* 540-665-5519.

GRADUATE PROGRAMS

Contact ***Telephone:*** 540-665-5512. *Fax:* 540-665-5519.

MASTER'S DEGREE PROGRAM

Degree MSN

Available Programs Master's; RN to Master's.

Concentrations Available Nurse case management; nurse-midwifery. *Clinical nurse specialist programs in:* psychiatric/mental health. *Nurse practitioner programs in:* family health, psychiatric/mental health.

Study Options Full-time and part-time.

Program Entrance Requirements Clinical experience, computer literacy, minimum overall college GPA of 2.8, transcript of college record, CPR certification, immunizations, interview, 3 letters of recommendation, nursing research course, physical assessment course, professional liability insurance/malpractice insurance, prerequisite course work, resume, statistics course, GRE General Test.

Advanced Placement Credit given for nursing courses completed elsewhere dependent upon specific evaluations.

Degree Requirements 37 total credit hours, thesis or project.

POST-MASTER'S PROGRAM

Areas of Study Nurse-midwifery. *Nurse practitioner programs in:* family health, psychiatric/mental health.

CONTINUING EDUCATION PROGRAM

Contact ***Telephone:*** 540-665-4584.

University of Virginia

School of Nursing
Charlottesville, Virginia

http://www.nursing.virginia.edu/
Founded in 1819

DEGREES • BSN • MSN • MSN/MBA • MSN/PHD • PHD

Nursing Program Faculty 99 (65% with doctorates).

Baccalaureate Enrollment 350 **Women** 95% **Men** 5% **Minority** 20% **International** 2% **Part-time** 5%

Graduate Enrollment 300 **Women** 90% **Men** 10% **Minority** 20% **International** 2% **Part-time** 40%

Distance Learning Courses Available.

Nursing Student Activities Nursing Honor Society, Sigma Theta Tau, Student Nurses' Association, nursing club.

Nursing Student Resources Academic advising; academic or career counseling; assistance for students with disabilities; bookstore; campus computer network; career placement assistance; computer-assisted instruction; e-mail services; employment services for current students; housing assistance; interactive nursing skills videos; Internet; learning resource lab; library services; nursing audiovisuals; placement services for program completers; remedial services; resume preparation assistance; skills, simulation, or other laboratory; tutoring.

Library Facilities 5.6 million volumes (200,000 in health); 172,057 periodical subscriptions (1,000 health-care related).

BACCALAUREATE PROGRAMS

Degree BSN

Available Programs ADN to Baccalaureate; Generic Baccalaureate; RN Baccalaureate.

Study Options Full-time.

Program Entrance Requirements Transcript of college record, written essay, health insurance, high school biology, 2 years high school math, 2 years high school science, high school transcript, 1 letter of recommendation, minimum GPA in nursing prerequisites of 2.0. Transfer students are accepted. *Application deadline:* 1/1 (fall). *Application fee:* $60.

Advanced Placement Credit by examination available.

Expenses (2010-11) *Tuition, state resident:* full-time $10,836. *Tuition, nonresident:* full-time $33,992. *International tuition:* $34,092 full-time. *Room and board:* $8590; room only: $4660 per academic year. *Required fees:* full-time $18; part-time $18 per term.

Financial Aid 60% of baccalaureate students in nursing programs received some form of financial aid in 2009-10. *Gift aid (need-based):* Federal Pell, FSEOG, state, private, college/university gift aid from institutional funds, Federal Nursing. *Loans:* Federal Nursing Student Loans, Perkins, college/university, alternative private loans. *Work-study:* Federal Work-Study. *Financial aid application deadline (priority):* 3/1.

Contact Mr. Clay Hysell, Assistant Dean for Admissions and Financial Aid, School of Nursing, University of Virginia, Claude Moore Nursing Education Building, PO Box 800826, Charlottesville, VA 22908. *Telephone:* 888-283-8703. *Fax:* 434-924-0528. *E-mail:* nur-osa@virginia.edu.

GRADUATE PROGRAMS

Financial Aid 80% of graduate students in nursing programs received some form of financial aid in 2009-10. Fellowships, research assistantships, teaching assistantships, Federal Work-Study and scholarships available.

Contact Mr. Clay D. Hysell, Assistant Dean for Graduate Student Services, School of Nursing, University of Virginia, Claude Moore Nursing Education Building, PO Box 800826, Charlottesville, VA 22908. *Telephone:* 888-283-8703. *Fax:* 434-924-0528. *E-mail:* nur-osa@virginia.edu.

MASTER'S DEGREE PROGRAM

Degrees MSN; MSN/MBA; MSN/PhD

Available Programs Master's; Master's for Non-Nursing College Graduates; Master's for Nurses with Non-Nursing Degrees.

Concentrations Available Clinical nurse leader; nursing administration. *Clinical nurse specialist programs in:* acute care, adult health, community health, critical care, medical-surgical, oncology, palliative care, psychiatric/mental health, public health. *Nurse practitioner programs in:* acute care, community health, family health, oncology, pediatric, primary care, psychiatric/mental health.

Study Options Full-time and part-time.

Program Entrance Requirements Clinical experience, minimum overall college GPA of 3.0, transcript of college record, written essay, 3

letters of recommendation, physical assessment course, prerequisite course work, resume, statistics course, GRE General Test, MAT. *Application deadline:* 4/1 (fall), 11/1 (spring). Applications may be processed on a rolling basis for some programs. *Application fee:* $60.
Advanced Placement Credit given for nursing courses completed elsewhere dependent upon specific evaluations.
Degree Requirements 34 total credit hours.

POST-MASTER'S PROGRAM

Areas of Study Nursing administration. *Clinical nurse specialist programs in:* acute care, adult health, community health, critical care, medical-surgical, oncology, psychiatric/mental health, public health. *Nurse practitioner programs in:* acute care, family health, oncology, pediatric, primary care, psychiatric/mental health.

DOCTORAL DEGREE PROGRAM

Degree PhD
Available Programs Doctorate; Post-Baccalaureate Doctorate.
Areas of Study Advanced practice nursing, aging, bio-behavioral research, clinical practice, community health, critical care, ethics, faculty preparation, family health, forensic nursing, gerontology, health policy, health promotion/disease prevention, health-care systems, information systems, maternity-newborn, nursing administration, nursing education, nursing policy, nursing research, nursing science, oncology, women's health.
Program Entrance Requirements Minimum overall college GPA of 3.0, interview by faculty committee, interview, 3 letters of recommendation, statistics course, vita, writing sample, GRE General Test. Application deadline: 2/1 (fall). Applications may be processed on a rolling basis for some programs. Application fee: $60.
Degree Requirements 46 total credit hours, dissertation, written exam, residency.

POSTDOCTORAL PROGRAM

Areas of Study Nursing research, nursing science.
Postdoctoral Program Contact Mr. Clay D. Hysell, Assistant Dean for Admissions and Financial Aid, School of Nursing, University of Virginia, McLeod Hall, PO Box 800826, Charlottesville, VA 22908. *Telephone:* 434-924-0141. *Fax:* 434-924-0528. *E-mail:* cdh6n@virginia.edu.

The University of Virginia's College at Wise

Department of Nursing
Wise, Virginia

http://www.uvawise.edu
Founded in 1954

DEGREE • BSN

Nursing Program Faculty 10 (20% with doctorates).
Baccalaureate Enrollment 47 **Women** 79% **Men** 21% **Minority** 15% **Part-time** 5%
Nursing Student Activities Sigma Theta Tau, Student Nurses' Association.
Nursing Student Resources Academic advising; academic or career counseling; assistance for students with disabilities; bookstore; campus computer network; computer lab; computer-assisted instruction; e-mail services; employment services for current students; externships; housing assistance; interactive nursing skills videos; Internet; learning resource lab; library services; nursing audiovisuals; resume preparation assistance; skills, simulation, or other laboratory; tutoring.
Library Facilities 157,706 volumes (4,654 in health, 2,761 in nursing); 3,155 periodical subscriptions (40 health-care related).

BACCALAUREATE PROGRAMS

Degree BSN
Available Programs ADN to Baccalaureate; Generic Baccalaureate; RN Baccalaureate.
Site Options Abingdon, VA.
Study Options Full-time.
Program Entrance Requirements Minimum overall college GPA of 2.7, transcript of college record, CPR certification, health exam, health insurance, immunizations, letters of recommendation, minimum GPA in nursing prerequisites of 2.5, professional liability insurance/malpractice insurance, prerequisite course work. Transfer students are accepted. *Application deadline:* 2/1 (fall). Applications may be processed on a rolling basis for some programs. *Application fee:* $25.
Advanced Placement Credit given for nursing courses completed elsewhere dependent upon specific evaluations.
Contact *Telephone:* 276-376-1030. *Fax:* 276-376-4589.

Virginia Commonwealth University

School of Nursing
Richmond, Virginia

http://www.nursing.vcu.edu
Founded in 1838

DEGREES • BS • MS • PHD

Nursing Program Faculty 137 (30% with doctorates).
Baccalaureate Enrollment 653 **Women** 91% **Men** 9% **Minority** 27% **International** 1% **Part-time** 44%
Graduate Enrollment 315 **Women** 92% **Men** 8% **Minority** 30% **International** 1% **Part-time** 55%
Distance Learning Courses Available.
Nursing Student Activities Sigma Theta Tau, Student Nurses' Association.
Nursing Student Resources Academic advising; academic or career counseling; assistance for students with disabilities; bookstore; campus computer network; career placement assistance; computer lab; computer-assisted instruction; daycare for children of students; e-mail services; employment services for current students; externships; housing assistance; interactive nursing skills videos; Internet; learning resource lab; library services; nursing audiovisuals; paid internships; placement services for program completers; remedial services; resume preparation assistance; skills, simulation, or other laboratory; tutoring.
Library Facilities 1.9 million volumes (476,122 in health, 15,562 in nursing); 50,461 periodical subscriptions (9,969 health-care related).

BACCALAUREATE PROGRAMS

Degree BS
Available Programs ADN to Baccalaureate; Accelerated Baccalaureate for Second Degree; Generic Baccalaureate.
Site Options Danville, VA; Fredericksburg, VA; Portsmouth, VA.
Study Options Full-time.
Program Entrance Requirements Minimum overall college GPA of 2.5, transcript of college record, CPR certification, written essay, health exam, immunizations, 3 letters of recommendation, minimum GPA in nursing prerequisites of 2.5, prerequisite course work. Transfer students are accepted. *Application deadline:* 1/15 (fall). *Application fee:* $40.
Advanced Placement Credit by examination available. Credit given for nursing courses completed elsewhere dependent upon specific evaluations.
Expenses (2009-10) *Tuition, state resident:* full-time $5185; part-time $217 per credit. *Tuition, nonresident:* full-time $18,409; part-time $768 per credit. *International tuition:* $18,409 full-time. *Room and board:* $9517; room only: $6267 per academic year. *Required fees:* full-time $1878; part-time $71 per credit.
Contact Mrs. Susan L. Lipp, RN, Assistant Dean of Enrollment and Student Services, School of Nursing, Virginia Commonwealth University, 1100 East Leigh Street, PO Box 980567, Richmond, VA 23298-0567. *Telephone:* 804-828-5171. *Fax:* 804-828-7743. *E-mail:* slipp@vcu.edu.

GRADUATE PROGRAMS

Expenses (2009-10) *Tuition, state resident:* full-time $8116; part-time $451 per credit. *Tuition, nonresident:* full-time $16,871; part-time $938 per credit. *International tuition:* $16,871 full-time. *Room and board:* $9517; room only: $6267 per academic year. *Required fees:* full-time $1878; part-time $71 per credit; part-time $7 per term.
Financial Aid Fellowships, research assistantships, teaching assistantships, career-related internships or fieldwork and institutionally sponsored loans available.
Contact Mrs. Susan L. Lipp, RN, Assistant Dean of Enrollment and Student Services, School of Nursing, Virginia Commonwealth University, 1100 East Leigh Street, PO Box 980567, Richmond, VA 23298-0567. *Telephone:* 804-828-5171. *Fax:* 804-828-7743. *E-mail:* slipp@vcu.edu.

MASTER'S DEGREE PROGRAM

Degree MS

Available Programs Accelerated Master's for Non-Nursing College Graduates; Master's; Master's for Nurses with Non-Nursing Degrees; RN to Master's.
Concentrations Available Clinical nurse leader; nursing administration; nursing education. *Clinical nurse specialist programs in:* acute care. *Nurse practitioner programs in:* acute care, adult health, family health, pediatric, primary care, women's health.
Study Options Full-time and part-time.
Program Entrance Requirements Computer literacy, minimum overall college GPA of 3.0, transcript of college record, CPR certification, written essay, immunizations, 3 letters of recommendation, prerequisite course work, resume, statistics course, GRE General Test. *Application deadline:* 2/1 (fall), 10/1 (spring). *Application fee:* $50.
Advanced Placement Credit given for nursing courses completed elsewhere dependent upon specific evaluations.
Degree Requirements 55 total credit hours.

POST-MASTER'S PROGRAM
Areas of Study Clinical nurse leader; nursing administration; nursing education. *Clinical nurse specialist programs in:* acute care. *Nurse practitioner programs in:* acute care, adult health, family health, pediatric, primary care, women's health.

DOCTORAL DEGREE PROGRAM
Degree PhD
Available Programs Doctorate; Post-Baccalaureate Doctorate.
Areas of Study Bio-behavioral research.
Program Entrance Requirements Minimum overall college GPA of 3.0, interview by faculty committee, interview, 3 letters of recommendation, MSN or equivalent, statistics course, vita, writing sample, GRE General Test. Application deadline: 2/1 (fall). Application fee: $50.
Degree Requirements 61 total credit hours, dissertation, written exam, residency.

POSTDOCTORAL PROGRAM
Postdoctoral Program Contact Ms. Susan L. Lipp, RN, Assistant Dean of Enrollment and Student Services, School of Nursing, Virginia Commonwealth University, 1100 East Leigh Street, PO Box 980567, Richmond, VA 23298-0567. *Telephone:* 804-828-5171. *Fax:* 804-828-7743. *E-mail:* slipp@vcu.edu.

WASHINGTON

Eastern Washington University
Intercollegiate College of Nursing/Washington State University
Cheney, Washington

See description of programs under
Intercollegiate College of Nursing/Washington State University (Spokane, Washington).

Gonzaga University
Department of Nursing
Spokane, Washington

http://www.gonzaga.edu/nursing
Founded in 1887

DEGREES • BSN • MSN
Nursing Program Faculty 15 (73% with doctorates).
Baccalaureate Enrollment 233 **Women** 93% **Men** 7%
Graduate Enrollment 337 **Women** 94% **Men** 6% **Part-time** 14%
Distance Learning Courses Available.
Nursing Student Activities Sigma Theta Tau, Student Nurses' Association.
Nursing Student Resources Academic advising; academic or career counseling; assistance for students with disabilities; bookstore; campus computer network; computer lab; computer-assisted instruction; e-mail services; housing assistance; interactive nursing skills videos; Internet; learning resource lab; library services; nursing audiovisuals; resume preparation assistance; skills, simulation, or other laboratory; tutoring.
Library Facilities 305,517 volumes (35,000 in health, 950 in nursing); 32,106 periodical subscriptions (206 health-care related).

BACCALAUREATE PROGRAMS
Degree BSN
Available Programs Generic Baccalaureate.
Study Options Full-time and part-time.
Program Entrance Requirements Minimum overall college GPA of 2.9, transcript of college record, written essay, high school biology, high school chemistry, 4 years high school math, 4 years high school science, high school transcript, 2 letters of recommendation, minimum high school GPA of 2.9, minimum GPA in nursing prerequisites of 2.0, prerequisite course work. Transfer students are accepted. *Application deadline:* 1/15 (fall), 9/15 (spring). *Application fee:* $50.
Advanced Placement Credit given for nursing courses completed elsewhere dependent upon specific evaluations.
Expenses (2010-11) *Tuition:* full-time $30,440; part-time $850 per credit.
Financial Aid 90% of baccalaureate students in nursing programs received some form of financial aid in 2009-10. *Gift aid (need-based):* Federal Pell, FSEOG, state, private, college/university gift aid from institutional funds, United Negro College Fund, Federal Nursing, Academic Competitiveness Grants, National SMART Grants, TEACH Grants. *Loans:* Federal Nursing Student Loans, Perkins, state, college/university. *Work-study:* Federal Work-Study, part-time campus jobs. *Financial aid application deadline (priority):* 2/1.
Contact Marcy Heldt, Program Assistant, Department of Nursing, Gonzaga University, 502 East Boone Avenue, Spokane, WA 99258-0038. *Telephone:* 509-313-3580. *Fax:* 509-313-5827. *E-mail:* heldt@gonzaga.edu.

GRADUATE PROGRAMS
Expenses (2010-11) *Tuition:* full-time $9300; part-time $775 per credit.
Financial Aid 78% of graduate students in nursing programs received some form of financial aid in 2009-10. *Application deadline:* 3/1.
Contact Mrs. Molly Woof, Program Assistant, Department of Nursing, Gonzaga University, 502 East Boone Avenue, Spokane, WA 99258-0038. *Telephone:* 509-313-6640. *Fax:* 509-323-5827. *E-mail:* woodm@gonzaga.edu.

MASTER'S DEGREE PROGRAM
Degree MSN
Available Programs Accelerated RN to Master's; Master's; Master's for Nurses with Non-Nursing Degrees.
Concentrations Available Health-care administration; nursing administration; nursing education. *Clinical nurse specialist programs in:* psychiatric/mental health. *Nurse practitioner programs in:* family health, primary care, psychiatric/mental health.
Study Options Full-time and part-time.
Online Degree Options Yes (online only).
Program Entrance Requirements Computer literacy, minimum overall college GPA of 3.0, transcript of college record, written essay, 2 letters of recommendation, resume, statistics course, MAT. *Application deadline:* Applications may be processed on a rolling basis for some programs.
Advanced Placement Credit given for nursing courses completed elsewhere dependent upon specific evaluations.
Degree Requirements 36 total credit hours.

POST-MASTER'S PROGRAM
Areas of Study Health-care administration; nursing administration; nursing education. *Clinical nurse specialist programs in:* psychiatric/mental health. *Nurse practitioner programs in:* family health, primary care, psychiatric/mental health.

Northwest University
The Mark and Huldah Buntain School of Nursing
Kirkland, Washington

http://www.northwestu.edu/
Founded in 1934

DEGREE • BS
Nursing Program Faculty 24 (16% with doctorates).
Baccalaureate Enrollment 50 **Women** 87% **Men** 13% **Minority** 11%

Nursing Student Resources Academic advising; academic or career counseling; assistance for students with disabilities; bookstore; campus computer network; computer lab; computer-assisted instruction; e-mail services; employment services for current students; housing assistance; interactive nursing skills videos; Internet; learning resource lab; library services; nursing audiovisuals; other; remedial services; resume preparation assistance; skills, simulation, or other laboratory; tutoring; unpaid internships.
Library Facilities 100,356 volumes (1,922 in health, 387 in nursing); 13,443 periodical subscriptions (815 health-care related).

BACCALAUREATE PROGRAMS

Degree BS
Available Programs Generic Baccalaureate.
Study Options Full-time.
Program Entrance Requirements Minimum overall college GPA of 3.0, transcript of college record, CPR certification, written essay, health exam, health insurance, high school transcript, immunizations, 2 letters of recommendation, minimum GPA in nursing prerequisites of 3.0, prerequisite course work. Transfer students are accepted. *Application deadline:* 1/30 (fall). *Application fee:* $35.
Contact *Telephone:* 800-669-3781 Ext. 7822. *Fax:* 425-889-7822.

Olympic College
Nursing Programs
Bremerton, Washington

Founded in 1946

DEGREE • BSN

Library Facilities 60,000 volumes; 541 periodical subscriptions.

BACCALAUREATE PROGRAMS

Degree BSN
Available Programs RN Baccalaureate.
Study Options Full-time and part-time.
Program Entrance Requirements Minimum overall college GPA of 2.5, minimum GPA in nursing prerequisites of 2.0, RN licensure.
Contact Administrative Office, Nursing Programs, Olympic College, 1600 Chester Avenue, Bremerton, WA 98337-1699. *Telephone:* 360-475-7748. *Fax:* 360-475-7628. *E-mail:* nursing@olympic.edu.

Pacific Lutheran University
School of Nursing
Tacoma, Washington

http://www.plu.edu/~nurs/
Founded in 1890

DEGREES • BSN • MSN • MSN/MBA

Nursing Program Faculty 30 (40% with doctorates).
Baccalaureate Enrollment 236 **Women** 92% **Men** 8% **Minority** 14% **International** 2% **Part-time** 1%
Graduate Enrollment 70 **Women** 96% **Men** 4% **Minority** 15% **International** 1% **Part-time** 5%
Nursing Student Activities Nursing Honor Society, Sigma Theta Tau, Student Nurses' Association, nursing club.
Nursing Student Resources Academic advising; academic or career counseling; assistance for students with disabilities; bookstore; campus computer network; career placement assistance; computer lab; computer-assisted instruction; e-mail services; employment services for current students; housing assistance; interactive nursing skills videos; Internet; learning resource lab; library services; nursing audiovisuals; resume preparation assistance; skills, simulation, or other laboratory; tutoring; unpaid internships.
Library Facilities 15,000 volumes in health, 6,500 volumes in nursing; 150 periodical subscriptions health-care related.

BACCALAUREATE PROGRAMS

Degree BSN
Available Programs ADN to Baccalaureate; Generic Baccalaureate; LPN to Baccalaureate.
Study Options Full-time.
Program Entrance Requirements Minimum overall college GPA of 3.0, transcript of college record, CPR certification, written essay, health exam, health insurance, 2 years high school math, high school transcript, immunizations, 2 letters of recommendation, minimum GPA in nursing prerequisites of 2.75, professional liability insurance/malpractice insurance, prerequisite course work. Transfer students are accepted. *Application deadline:* 2/1 (fall), 2/1 (spring), 2/1 (summer). Applications may be processed on a rolling basis for some programs. *Application fee:* $15.
Advanced Placement Credit by examination available. Credit given for nursing courses completed elsewhere dependent upon specific evaluations.
Financial Aid 95% of baccalaureate students in nursing programs received some form of financial aid in 2009-10. *Gift aid (need-based):* Federal Pell, FSEOG, state, private, college/university gift aid from institutional funds, Federal Nursing. *Loans:* Federal Nursing Student Loans, Federal Direct (Subsidized and Unsubsidized Stafford PLUS), Perkins, state. *Work-study:* Federal Work-Study, part-time campus jobs. *Financial aid application deadline (priority):* 1/31.
Contact Dr. Amy S. Manoso, Admission/Retention/Recruitment Coordinator, School of Nursing, Pacific Lutheran University, 12180 Park Avenue South, Tacoma, WA 98447-0029. *Telephone:* 253-535-7672. *Fax:* 253-535-7590. *E-mail:* manosoas@plu,edu.

GRADUATE PROGRAMS

Financial Aid 90% of graduate students in nursing programs received some form of financial aid in 2009-10. Fellowships, Federal Work-Study, scholarships, and unspecified assistantships available. *Financial aid application deadline:* 3/1.
Contact Dr. Amy S. Manoso, Admissions Coordinator, School of Nursing, Pacific Lutheran University, 12180 Park Avenue South, Tacoma, WA 98447-0029. *Telephone:* 253-535-7672. *Fax:* 253-535-7590. *E-mail:* gradnurs@plu.edu.

MASTER'S DEGREE PROGRAM

Degrees MSN; MSN/MBA
Available Programs Accelerated Master's; Master's; Master's for Non-Nursing College Graduates; Master's for Nurses with Non-Nursing Degrees.
Concentrations Available Clinical nurse leader; health-care administration; nurse case management; nursing administration; nursing education. *Nurse practitioner programs in:* family health.
Study Options Full-time and part-time.
Program Entrance Requirements Clinical experience, computer literacy, minimum overall college GPA of 3.0, transcript of college record, CPR certification, written essay, immunizations, interview, 2 letters of recommendation, nursing research course, professional liability insurance/malpractice insurance, prerequisite course work, resume, statistics course, GRE General Test. *Application deadline:* 3/1 (fall), 11/15 (summer). Applications may be processed on a rolling basis for some programs. *Application fee:* $40.
Advanced Placement Credit given for nursing courses completed elsewhere dependent upon specific evaluations.
Degree Requirements 37 total credit hours, thesis or project.

CONTINUING EDUCATION PROGRAM

Contact Ms. Terry L. Bennett, Coordinator, Continuing Nursing Education and Clinical Placements, School of Nursing, Pacific Lutheran University, 12180 Park Avenue South, Tacoma, WA 98447-0029. *Telephone:* 253-535-7683. *Fax:* 253-535-7590. *E-mail:* bennettl@plu.edu.

Seattle Pacific University
School of Health Sciences
Seattle, Washington

http://www.spu.edu/depts/hsc
Founded in 1891

DEGREES • BS • MSN

Nursing Program Faculty 23 (39% with doctorates).
Baccalaureate Enrollment 98 **Women** 91% **Men** 9% **Minority** 21% **International** 2%
Graduate Enrollment 61 **Women** 89% **Men** 11% **Minority** 39% **Part-time** 49%
Nursing Student Activities Nursing Honor Society, Sigma Theta Tau, Student Nurses' Association, nursing club.
Nursing Student Resources Academic advising; academic or career counseling; assistance for students with disabilities; bookstore; campus

computer network; career placement assistance; computer lab; computer-assisted instruction; e-mail services; employment services for current students; housing assistance; Internet; learning resource lab; library services; nursing audiovisuals; placement services for program completers; remedial services; resume preparation assistance; skills, simulation, or other laboratory; tutoring; unpaid internships.

Library Facilities 212,247 volumes (11,539 in health, 1,791 in nursing); 2,241 periodical subscriptions (274 health-care related).

BACCALAUREATE PROGRAMS

Degree BS

Available Programs Generic Baccalaureate; RN Baccalaureate.

Study Options Full-time.

Program Entrance Requirements Minimum overall college GPA of 2.75, transcript of college record, CPR certification, written essay, health exam, health insurance, high school transcript, immunizations, 1 letter of recommendation, minimum GPA in nursing prerequisites of 2.75, prerequisite course work. Transfer students are accepted. *Application deadline:* 1/15 (fall).

Advanced Placement Credit given for nursing courses completed elsewhere dependent upon specific evaluations.

Expenses (2010-11) *Tuition:* full-time $28,602. *Room and board:* $9500; room only: $5500 per academic year. *Required fees:* full-time $1800.

Financial Aid 94% of baccalaureate students in nursing programs received some form of financial aid in 2009-10. *Gift aid (need-based):* Federal Pell, FSEOG, state, private, college/university gift aid from institutional funds. *Loans:* Federal Nursing Student Loans, Federal Direct (Subsidized and Unsubsidized Stafford PLUS), Perkins, college/university. *Work-study:* Federal Work-Study, part-time campus jobs. *Financial aid application deadline (priority):* 2/1.

Contact Dr. Chris Henshaw, Associate Dean, School of Health Sciences, Seattle Pacific University, 3307 Third Avenue West, Marson Hall, Suite 106, Seattle, WA 98119-1922. *Telephone:* 206-281-2612. *Fax:* 206-281-2767. *E-mail:* chenshaw@spu.edu.

GRADUATE PROGRAMS

Financial Aid 60% of graduate students in nursing programs received some form of financial aid in 2009-10. 2 teaching assistantships were awarded; career-related internships or fieldwork and traineeships also available.

Contact Beth Van Camp, MSN Admission Counselor, School of Health Sciences, Seattle Pacific University, 3307 Third Avenue West, Suite 111, Seattle, WA 98119-1922. *Telephone:* 206-281-2888. *Fax:* 206-378-5480. *E-mail:* beth.vancamp@spu.edu.

MASTER'S DEGREE PROGRAM

Degree MSN

Available Programs Master's; Master's for Nurses with Non-Nursing Degrees.

Concentrations Available Nursing administration; nursing education. *Clinical nurse specialist programs in:* acute care, adult health, community health, critical care, gerontology, medical-surgical, oncology, palliative care, parent-child, pediatric, women's health. *Nurse practitioner programs in:* adult health, family health.

Study Options Full-time and part-time.

Program Entrance Requirements Clinical experience, computer literacy, minimum overall college GPA of 3.0, transcript of college record, CPR certification, written essay, immunizations, interview, 3 letters of recommendation, nursing research course, professional liability insurance/malpractice insurance, prerequisite course work, resume, statistics course, GRE General Test. *Application deadline:* 5/1 (fall). *Application fee:* $50.

Advanced Placement Credit given for nursing courses completed elsewhere dependent upon specific evaluations.

Degree Requirements 59 total credit hours, thesis or project, comprehensive exam.

POST-MASTER'S PROGRAM

Areas of Study Nursing education. *Nurse practitioner programs in:* adult health, family health.

Seattle University

College of Nursing
Seattle, Washington

http://www.seattleu.edu/nurs
Founded in 1891

DEGREES • BSN • MSN

Nursing Program Faculty 81 (42% with doctorates).
Baccalaureate Enrollment 418 **Women** 90% **Men** 10% **Minority** 37% **International** 1%
Graduate Enrollment 110 **Women** 89% **Men** 11% **Minority** 18% **International** 1%
Distance Learning Courses Available.
Nursing Student Activities Sigma Theta Tau, Student Nurses' Association.
Nursing Student Resources Academic advising; academic or career counseling; assistance for students with disabilities; bookstore; campus computer network; career placement assistance; computer lab; computer-assisted instruction; e-mail services; employment services for current students; housing assistance; interactive nursing skills videos; Internet; learning resource lab; library services; nursing audiovisuals; paid internships; remedial services; resume preparation assistance; skills, simulation, or other laboratory; tutoring.
Library Facilities 258,540 volumes; 1,802 periodical subscriptions.

BACCALAUREATE PROGRAMS

Degree BSN
Available Programs Baccalaureate for Second Degree; Generic Baccalaureate.
Study Options Full-time.
Program Entrance Requirements Minimum overall college GPA of 2.75, transcript of college record, CPR certification, written essay, health insurance, high school biology, high school chemistry, high school foreign language, 3 years high school math, 2 years high school science, high school transcript, immunizations, minimum GPA in nursing prerequisites of 3.0, professional liability insurance/malpractice insurance, prerequisite course work. Transfer students are accepted. *Application deadline:* 1/5 (winter). *Application fee:* $50.
Expenses (2009-10) *Tuition:* full-time $29,340. *International tuition:* $29,340 full-time. *Room and board:* $8805 per academic year. *Required fees:* full-time $800.
Financial Aid 80% of baccalaureate students in nursing programs received some form of financial aid in 2008-09. *Gift aid (need-based):* Federal Pell, FSEOG, state, private, college/university gift aid from institutional funds, Federal Nursing. *Loans:* Federal Nursing Student Loans, Federal Direct (Subsidized and Unsubsidized Stafford PLUS), Perkins. *Work-study:* Federal Work-Study, part-time campus jobs. *Financial aid application deadline (priority):* 2/1.
Contact Rita Tower, Pre-Major Advisor, College of Nursing, Seattle University, 901 12th Avenue, PO Box 222000, Seattle, WA 98122-1090. *Telephone:* 206-296-2242. *Fax:* 206-296-5544. *E-mail:* rstower@seattleu.edu.

GRADUATE PROGRAMS

Financial Aid 81% of graduate students in nursing programs received some form of financial aid in 2008-09. Fellowships, research assistantships, career-related internships or fieldwork and Federal Work-Study available. Aid available to part-time students.
Contact Dr. Katherine Camacho Carr, Assistant Dean for Graduate Program, College of Nursing, Seattle University, 901 12th Avenue, PO Box 222000, Seattle, WA 98122-1090. *Telephone:* 206-296-5666. *Fax:* 206-296-5544. *E-mail:* kcarr@seattleu.edu.

MASTER'S DEGREE PROGRAM

Degree MSN
Available Programs Accelerated Master's for Nurses with Non-Nursing Degrees; Master's.
Concentrations Available *Clinical nurse specialist programs in:* community health. *Nurse practitioner programs in:* adult health, family health, psychiatric/mental health.
Study Options Full-time and part-time.
Program Entrance Requirements Clinical experience, computer literacy, minimum overall college GPA of 3.0, transcript of college record, CPR certification, written essay, immunizations, interview, 2 letters of recommendation, professional liability insurance/malpractice insurance, prerequisite course work, resume, statistics course, GRE General Test. *Application deadline:* 12/1 (fall), 4/1 (spring). *Application fee:* $55.

Advanced Placement Credit given for nursing courses completed elsewhere dependent upon specific evaluations.
Degree Requirements 108 total credit hours, thesis or project.

POST-MASTER'S PROGRAM

Areas of Study *Clinical nurse specialist programs in:* community health. *Nurse practitioner programs in:* adult health, family health, psychiatric/mental health.

University of Washington
School of Nursing
Seattle, Washington

http://nursing.uw.edu/
Founded in 1861

DEGREES • BSN • DNP • MN • MN/MPH • MS • PHD

Nursing Program Faculty 246 (78% with doctorates).
Baccalaureate Enrollment 587 **Women** 85% **Men** 15% **Minority** 33% **International** .5% **Part-time** 55%
Graduate Enrollment 581 **Women** 89.5% **Men** 10.5% **Minority** 23% **International** 4% **Part-time** 54%
Distance Learning Courses Available.
Nursing Student Activities Sigma Theta Tau, Student Nurses' Association.
Nursing Student Resources Academic advising; academic or career counseling; assistance for students with disabilities; bookstore; campus computer network; computer lab; computer-assisted instruction; e-mail services; employment services for current students; interactive nursing skills videos; Internet; learning resource lab; library services; nursing audiovisuals; skills, simulation, or other laboratory.
Library Facilities 5.8 million volumes (350,000 in health); 50,245 periodical subscriptions (2,400 health-care related).

BACCALAUREATE PROGRAMS

Degree BSN
Available Programs ADN to Baccalaureate; Accelerated Baccalaureate; Generic Baccalaureate.
Site Options Bothell, WA; Tacoma, WA.
Study Options Full-time.
Program Entrance Requirements Minimum overall college GPA of 2.0, transcript of college record, CPR certification, written essay, immunizations, 1 letter of recommendation, minimum GPA in nursing prerequisites of 2.8, prerequisite course work. *Application deadline:* 1/15 (fall).
Expenses (2010-11) *Tuition, state resident:* full-time $8703; part-time $291 per credit. *Tuition, nonresident:* full-time $25,328; part-time $845 per credit. *Room and board:* $10,215; room only: $4905 per academic year. *Required fees:* full-time $2083.
Contact Academic Services, School of Nursing, University of Washington, Box 357260, Health Sciences Building, Room T310, Seattle, WA 98195. *Telephone:* 206-543-8736. *Fax:* 206-543-3624. *E-mail:* sonas@u.washington.edu.

GRADUATE PROGRAMS

Expenses (2010-11) *Tuition, state resident:* full-time $18,000; part-time $856 per credit. *Tuition, nonresident:* full-time $35,000; part-time $1667 per credit. *International tuition:* $35,000 full-time. *Room and board:* $10,215; room only: $4905 per academic year. *Required fees:* full-time $2880.
Financial Aid 16% of graduate students in nursing programs received some form of financial aid in 2009-10. Fellowships with full tuition reimbursements available, research assistantships with partial tuition reimbursements available, teaching assistantships with partial tuition reimbursements available, Federal Work-Study, institutionally sponsored loans, scholarships, and traineeships available. *Financial aid application deadline:* 2/28.
Contact Academic Services, School of Nursing, University of Washington, Box 357260, Health Sciences Building, Room T310, Seattle, WA 98195. *Telephone:* 206-543-8736. *Fax:* 206-543-3624. *E-mail:* sonas@u.washington.edu.

MASTER'S DEGREE PROGRAM

Degrees MN; MN/MPH; MS
Available Programs Master's; Master's for Nurses with Non-Nursing Degrees.
Concentrations Available Nurse-midwifery; nursing informatics; individualized study. *Clinical nurse specialist programs in:* acute care, adult health, cardiovascular, community health, critical care, gerontology, maternity-newborn, medical-surgical, occupational health, oncology, parent-child, perinatal. *Nurse practitioner programs in:* acute care, adult health, family health, neonatal health, pediatric, primary care, psychiatric/mental health.
Site Options Bothell, WA; Tacoma, WA.
Study Options Full-time and part-time.
Program Entrance Requirements Minimum overall college GPA of 3.0, transcript of college record, CPR certification, written essay, immunizations, 3 letters of recommendation, resume, statistics course, GRE. *Application deadline:* 1/15 (fall).
Advanced Placement Credit given for nursing courses completed elsewhere dependent upon specific evaluations.
Degree Requirements 40–49 total credit hours, thesis or project.

POST-MASTER'S PROGRAM

Areas of Study Nurse-midwifery; nursing education. *Clinical nurse specialist programs in:* occupational health. *Nurse practitioner programs in:* acute care, adult health, psychiatric/mental health.

DOCTORAL DEGREE PROGRAM

Degree DNP
Available Programs Doctorate.
Areas of Study Advanced practice nursing, bio-behavioral research, health policy, health-care systems, nursing policy, nursing research.
Program Entrance Requirements Minimum overall college GPA of 3.0, 3 letters of recommendation, clinical experience, statistics course, vita, writing sample. *Application deadline*: 1/15 (fall).
Degree Requirements 90 total credit hours, Capstone project, oral exam, written exam.

Degree PhD
Available Programs Doctorate; Doctorate for Nurses with Non-Nursing Degrees; Post-Baccalaureate Doctorate.
Areas of Study Faculty preparation, individualized study, nursing research.
Program Entrance Requirements Minimum overall college GPA of 3.0, 3 letters of recommendation, scholarly papers, vita, GRE. Application deadline: 1/15 (fall).
Degree Requirements 93 total credit hours, dissertation, oral exam, written exam.

POSTDOCTORAL PROGRAM

Areas of Study Aging, cancer care, chronic illness, gerontology, health promotion/disease prevention, infection prevention/skin care, neurobehavior, nursing interventions, nursing research, self-care, women's health.
Postdoctoral Program Contact Academic Services, School of Nursing, University of Washington, Box 357260, Health Sciences Building, Room T310, Seattle, WA 98195. *Telephone:* 206-543-8736. *Fax:* 206-685-1613. *E-mail:* sonas@u.washington.edu.

CONTINUING EDUCATION PROGRAM

Contact Martha Duhamel, Assistant Dean for Continuing Nursing Education, School of Nursing, University of Washington, Box 359440, Seattle, WA 98195-9440. *Telephone:* 206-543-1047. *Fax:* 206-543-6953. *E-mail:* marthadu@u.washington.edu.

Walla Walla University
School of Nursing
College Place, Washington

http://www.wallawalla.edu/nursing
Founded in 1892

DEGREE • BS

Nursing Program Faculty 25 (12% with doctorates).
Baccalaureate Enrollment 175 **Women** 79% **Men** 21% **Minority** 14% **International** 1% **Part-time** 1%
Nursing Student Activities Nursing Honor Society, nursing club.
Nursing Student Resources Academic advising; assistance for students with disabilities; bookstore; campus computer network; computer lab; e-mail services; Internet; learning resource lab; library services; nursing audiovisuals; resume preparation assistance; skills, simulation, or other laboratory; tutoring.
Library Facilities 273,266 volumes (10,000 in health, 7,000 in nursing); 3,727 periodical subscriptions (450 health-care related).

BACCALAUREATE PROGRAMS

Degree BS

Available Programs ADN to Baccalaureate; Generic Baccalaureate; LPN to Baccalaureate; RN Baccalaureate.

Site Options Portland, OR.

Study Options Full-time.

Program Entrance Requirements Minimum overall college GPA of 2.75, transcript of college record, CPR certification, written essay, health exam, health insurance, high school biology, 3 years high school math, 2 years high school science, high school transcript, immunizations, 3 letters of recommendation, minimum high school GPA of 2.75, minimum GPA in nursing prerequisites of 2.75, prerequisite course work. Transfer students are accepted. *Application deadline:* 4/15 (fall), 2/1 (summer). *Application fee:* $40.

Advanced Placement Credit given for nursing courses completed elsewhere dependent upon specific evaluations.

Expenses (2010-11) *Tuition:* full-time $23,229; part-time $607 per quarter hour. *Room and board:* $5180; room only: $2841 per academic year. *Required fees:* full-time $700; part-time $20 per credit; part-time $75 per term.

Financial Aid 95% of baccalaureate students in nursing programs received some form of financial aid in 2009-10.

Contact Jan Thurnhofer, Student Program Advisor, School of Nursing, Walla Walla University, 10345 SE Market Street, Portland, OR 97216. *Telephone:* 503-251-6115 Ext. 7304. *Fax:* 503-251-6249. *E-mail:* jant@wallawalla.edu.

Washington State University

Intercollegiate College of Nursing/Washington State University
Pullman, Washington

See description of programs under
Intercollegiate College of Nursing/Washington State University (Spokane, Washington).

Washington State University College of Nursing and Consortium

Washington State University College of Nursing and Consortium
Spokane, Washington

http://www.nursing.wsu.edu/

DEGREES • BSN • MN • PHD

Nursing Program Faculty 114 (39% with doctorates).

Baccalaureate Enrollment 737 **Women** 85% **Men** 15% **Minority** 17% **International** 1% **Part-time** 29%

Graduate Enrollment 271 **Women** 88% **Men** 12% **Minority** 12% **Part-time** 81%

Distance Learning Courses Available.

Nursing Student Activities Nursing Honor Society, Sigma Theta Tau, Student Nurses' Association, nursing club.

Nursing Student Resources Academic advising; academic or career counseling; assistance for students with disabilities; bookstore; campus computer network; computer lab; computer-assisted instruction; e-mail services; interactive nursing skills videos; Internet; learning resource lab; library services; nursing audiovisuals; other; remedial services; resume preparation assistance; skills, simulation, or other laboratory; tutoring; unpaid internships.

Library Facilities 15,000 volumes in health, 7,000 volumes in nursing; 2,000 periodical subscriptions health-care related.

BACCALAUREATE PROGRAMS

Degree BSN

Available Programs Generic Baccalaureate; RN Baccalaureate.

Site Options Richland, WA; Yakima, WA; Vancouver, WA.

Study Options Full-time.

Program Entrance Requirements Minimum overall college GPA of 2.8, transcript of college record, CPR certification, health insurance, immunizations, interview, minimum GPA in nursing prerequisites of 2.8, professional liability insurance/malpractice insurance, prerequisite course work. Transfer students are accepted. *Application deadline:* 1/15 (fall), 8/5 (spring).

Advanced Placement Credit given for nursing courses completed elsewhere dependent upon specific evaluations.

Expenses (2010-11) *Tuition, state resident:* full-time $8592; part-time $430 per credit. *Tuition, nonresident:* full-time $19,634; part-time $982 per credit. *Required fees:* full-time $1124.

Financial Aid 68% of baccalaureate students in nursing programs received some form of financial aid in 2009-10.

Contact Ms. Renae J. Richter, Academic Coordinator, Washington State University College of Nursing and Consortium, PO Box 1495, Spokane, WA 99210-1495. *Telephone:* 509-324-7337. *Fax:* 509-324-7336. *E-mail:* richre@wsu.edu.

GRADUATE PROGRAMS

Expenses (2010-11) *Tuition, state resident:* full-time $15,288; part-time $764 per credit. *Tuition, nonresident:* full-time $29,768; part-time $1488 per course. *Required fees:* full-time $420.

Financial Aid 53% of graduate students in nursing programs received some form of financial aid in 2009-10.

Contact Ms. Tamara Kelley, Principal Assistant, Washington State University College of Nursing and Consortium, PO Box 1495, Spokane, WA 99210-1495. *Telephone:* 509-324-7334. *Fax:* 509-324-7336. *E-mail:* kelleyt@wsu.edu.

MASTER'S DEGREE PROGRAM

Degree MN

Available Programs Accelerated Master's for Nurses with Non-Nursing Degrees; Accelerated RN to Master's; Master's.

Concentrations Available Nurse case management; nursing administration; nursing education. *Clinical nurse specialist programs in:* community health. *Nurse practitioner programs in:* family health, psychiatric/mental health.

Site Options Richland, WA; Yakima, WA; Vancouver, WA.

Study Options Full-time and part-time.

Program Entrance Requirements Computer literacy, minimum overall college GPA of 3.0, transcript of college record, CPR certification, written essay, immunizations, interview, 3 letters of recommendation, physical assessment course, professional liability insurance/malpractice insurance, prerequisite course work, statistics course. *Application deadline:* 2/1 (fall), 10/1 (spring).

Advanced Placement Credit given for nursing courses completed elsewhere dependent upon specific evaluations.

Degree Requirements 45 total credit hours, thesis or project.

POST-MASTER'S PROGRAM

Areas of Study *Nurse practitioner programs in:* family health, psychiatric/mental health.

DOCTORAL DEGREE PROGRAM

Degree PhD

Available Programs Doctorate.

Areas of Study Nursing education, nursing research.

Program Entrance Requirements Minimum overall college GPA of 3.5, interview by faculty committee, 3 letters of recommendation, MSN or equivalent, scholarly papers, statistics course, vita. Application deadline: 1/10 (summer).

Degree Requirements 72 total credit hours, dissertation.

CONTINUING EDUCATION PROGRAM

Contact Ms. Carol Johns, Director of Professional Development, Washington State University College of Nursing and Consortium, PO Box 1495, Spokane, WA 99210-1495. *Telephone:* 509-324-7354. *Fax:* 509-324-7341. *E-mail:* cjohns@wsu.edu.

Whitworth College

Intercollegiate College of Nursing/Washington State University
Spokane, Washington

See description of programs under
Intercollegiate College of Nursing/Washington State University (Spokane, Washington).

WEST VIRGINIA

Alderson-Broaddus College

Department of Nursing
Philippi, West Virginia

http://www.ab.edu/
Founded in 1871

DEGREE • BSN

Nursing Program Faculty 13 (1% with doctorates).

Baccalaureate Enrollment 96 **Women** 94% **Men** 6% **Minority** 2% **International** 1% **Part-time** 2%

Nursing Student Activities Student Nurses' Association.

Nursing Student Resources Academic advising; academic or career counseling; assistance for students with disabilities; bookstore; campus computer network; career placement assistance; computer lab; computer-assisted instruction; e-mail services; employment services for current students; Internet; learning resource lab; library services; nursing audiovisuals; remedial services; resume preparation assistance; skills, simulation, or other laboratory; tutoring.

Library Facilities 60,000 volumes (6,000 in health, 1,000 in nursing); 11,000 periodical subscriptions (172 health-care related).

BACCALAUREATE PROGRAMS

Degree BSN

Available Programs Generic Baccalaureate; LPN to RN Baccalaureate; RN Baccalaureate.

Study Options Full-time.

Program Entrance Requirements Minimum overall college GPA of 2.0, transcript of college record, CPR certification, health exam, high school chemistry, high school transcript, immunizations, minimum GPA in nursing prerequisites of 2.25, professional liability insurance/malpractice insurance, prerequisite course work. Transfer students are accepted. *Application deadline:* 7/30 (fall), 1/5 (winter). Applications may be processed on a rolling basis for some programs. *Application fee:* $25.

Advanced Placement Credit by examination available. Credit given for nursing courses completed elsewhere dependent upon specific evaluations.

Expenses (2010-11) *Tuition:* full-time $21,444. *Room and board:* $7002 per academic year. *Required fees:* full-time $210.

Financial Aid 98% of baccalaureate students in nursing programs received some form of financial aid in 2009-10. *Gift aid (need-based):* Federal Pell, FSEOG, state, private, college/university gift aid from institutional funds, Federal Nursing, National Health Service Corps Scholarships, Scholarships for Disadvantaged Students. *Loans:* Federal Nursing Student Loans, Federal Direct (Subsidized and Unsubsidized Stafford PLUS), Perkins. *Work-study:* Federal Work-Study, part-time campus jobs. *Financial aid application deadline (priority):* 3/1.

Contact Dr. Dawn Margaret Scheick, Chairperson, Department of Nursing, Alderson-Broaddus College, 101 College Hill Drive, Philippi, WV 26416. *Telephone:* 304-457-6384. *Fax:* 304-457-6293. *E-mail:* scheickdm@ab.edu.

Bluefield State College

Program in Nursing
Bluefield, West Virginia

http://www.bluefieldstate.edu/
Founded in 1895

DEGREE • BSN

Nursing Program Faculty 3 (30% with doctorates).
Baccalaureate Enrollment 33 **Women** 87% **Men** 13% **Part-time** 12%
Distance Learning Courses Available.
Nursing Student Activities Sigma Theta Tau, Student Nurses' Association.
Nursing Student Resources Academic advising; academic or career counseling; assistance for students with disabilities; bookstore; campus computer network; career placement assistance; computer lab; computer-assisted instruction; e-mail services; housing assistance; interactive nursing skills videos; Internet; learning resource lab; library services; nursing audiovisuals; resume preparation assistance; skills, simulation, or other laboratory; tutoring.
Library Facilities 5,649 volumes in health, 1,250 volumes in nursing; 200 periodical subscriptions health-care related.

BACCALAUREATE PROGRAMS

Degree BSN
Available Programs ADN to Baccalaureate; RN Baccalaureate.
Site Options Beckley, WV.
Study Options Full-time and part-time.
Program Entrance Requirements Minimum overall college GPA of 2.5, transcript of college record, CPR certification, health exam, immunizations, letters of recommendation, minimum GPA in nursing prerequisites of 2.0, prerequisite course work, RN licensure. Transfer students are accepted. *Application deadline:* 4/15 (spring).
Expenses (2010-11) *Tuition, state resident:* full-time $2298; part-time $192 per credit hour. *Tuition, nonresident:* full-time $4644; part-time $387 per credit hour. *Room and board:* $3600 per academic year. *Required fees:* full-time $280; part-time $35 per credit.
Financial Aid 52% of baccalaureate students in nursing programs received some form of financial aid in 2009-10. *Gift aid (need-based):* Federal Pell, FSEOG, state. *Loans:* Federal Direct (Subsidized and Unsubsidized Stafford PLUS), Perkins. *Work-study:* Federal Work-Study, part-time campus jobs. *Financial aid application deadline (priority):* 3/1.
Contact Ms. Beth Pritchett, Director, Program in Nursing, Bluefield State College, 219 Rock Street, Bluefield, WV 24701. *Telephone:* 304-327-4139. *Fax:* 304-327-4219. *E-mail:* bpritchett@bluefieldstate.edu.

Fairmont State University

School of Nursing and Allied Health Administration
Fairmont, West Virginia

http://www.fairmontstate.edu/
Founded in 1865

DEGREE • BSN

Nursing Program Faculty 4 (50% with doctorates).
Baccalaureate Enrollment 120 **Women** 96% **Men** 4% **International** 1% **Part-time** 40%
Nursing Student Activities Sigma Theta Tau, Student Nurses' Association.
Nursing Student Resources Academic advising; academic or career counseling; assistance for students with disabilities; bookstore; campus computer network; career placement assistance; computer lab; computer-assisted instruction; e-mail services; housing assistance; interactive nursing skills videos; Internet; learning resource lab; library services; nursing audiovisuals; placement services for program completers; remedial services; resume preparation assistance; skills, simulation, or other laboratory; tutoring.
Library Facilities 280,000 volumes (9,000 in health, 1,100 in nursing); 895 periodical subscriptions (50 health-care related).

BACCALAUREATE PROGRAMS

Degree BSN
Available Programs ADN to Baccalaureate; Accelerated RN Baccalaureate; LPN to RN Baccalaureate; RN Baccalaureate.

Study Options Full-time and part-time.
Program Entrance Requirements Minimum overall college GPA of 2.5, transcript of college record, CPR certification, health exam, high school chemistry, immunizations, letters of recommendation, minimum GPA in nursing prerequisites of 3.0, prerequisite course work, RN licensure. Transfer students are accepted. *Application deadline:* 8/15 (fall), 8/15 (winter), 1/2 (spring), 5/15 (summer). Applications may be processed on a rolling basis for some programs.
Advanced Placement Credit by examination available. Credit given for nursing courses completed elsewhere dependent upon specific evaluations.
Expenses (2010-11) *Tuition, state resident:* full-time $2586; part-time $216 per credit. *Tuition, nonresident:* full-time $5452; part-time $454 per credit. *Room and board:* $3383; room only: $1689 per academic year. *Required fees:* full-time $50; part-time $50 per credit; part-time $50 per term.
Financial Aid 80% of baccalaureate students in nursing programs received some form of financial aid in 2009-10.
Contact Dr. Mary M. Meighen, Professor, School of Nursing and Allied Health Administration, Fairmont State University, 1201 Locust Avenue, Fairmont, WV 26554. *Telephone:* 304-367-4761. *Fax:* 304-367-4268. *E-mail:* mmeighen@fairmontstate.edu.

CONTINUING EDUCATION PROGRAM

Contact Dr. Tanya Rogers, Associate Professor, School of Nursing and Allied Health Administration, Fairmont State University, 1201 Locust Avenue, Fairmont, WV 26554. *Telephone:* 304-367-4074. *Fax:* 304-367-4268. *E-mail:* tanya.rogers@fairmontstate.edu.

Marshall University

College of Health Professions
Huntington, West Virginia

http://www.marshall.edu/conhp
Founded in 1837

DEGREES • BSN • MSN
Nursing Program Faculty 35 (23% with doctorates).
Baccalaureate Enrollment 345 **Women** 80% **Men** 20% **Minority** 5% **Part-time** 35%
Graduate Enrollment 100 **Women** 90% **Men** 10% **Part-time** 60%
Nursing Student Activities Sigma Theta Tau, Student Nurses' Association, nursing club.
Nursing Student Resources Academic advising; academic or career counseling; assistance for students with disabilities; bookstore; campus computer network; career placement assistance; computer lab; computer-assisted instruction; daycare for children of students; e-mail services; employment services for current students; externships; housing assistance; interactive nursing skills videos; Internet; learning resource lab; library services; nursing audiovisuals; placement services for program completers; remedial services; resume preparation assistance; skills, simulation, or other laboratory; tutoring.
Library Facilities 1.5 million volumes (20,200 in health, 6,400 in nursing); 41,118 periodical subscriptions (500 health-care related).

BACCALAUREATE PROGRAMS

Degree BSN
Available Programs Accelerated RN Baccalaureate; Generic Baccalaureate.
Study Options Full-time and part-time.
Program Entrance Requirements Minimum overall college GPA of 2.5, transcript of college record, high school transcript, minimum high school GPA of 2.5. Transfer students are accepted.
Advanced Placement Credit given for nursing courses completed elsewhere dependent upon specific evaluations.
Contact ***Telephone:*** 304-696-2639. *Fax:* 304-696-6739.

GRADUATE PROGRAMS

Contact ***Telephone:*** 304-696-2639. *Fax:* 304-696-6739.

MASTER'S DEGREE PROGRAM

Degree MSN
Available Programs Master's.
Concentrations Available Nursing administration; nursing education. *Nurse practitioner programs in:* family health.
Study Options Full-time and part-time.
Program Entrance Requirements Minimum overall college GPA of 3.0, transcript of college record, nursing research course, resume, statistics course, GRE General Test.
Advanced Placement Credit given for nursing courses completed elsewhere dependent upon specific evaluations.
Degree Requirements 36 total credit hours, thesis or project.

POST-MASTER'S PROGRAM

Areas of Study Nursing administration; nursing education. *Nurse practitioner programs in:* family health.

Mountain State University

College of Nursing
Beckley, West Virginia

http://www.mountainstate.edu/majors/onlinecatalogs/undergrad/programs/NursingBSN.aspx
Founded in 1933

DEGREES • BSN • MSN
Nursing Program Faculty 92 (4% with doctorates).
Baccalaureate Enrollment 493 **Women** 86% **Men** 14% **Minority** 14% **International** 8% **Part-time** 19%
Graduate Enrollment 97 **Women** 93% **Men** 7% **Minority** 6% **International** 3% **Part-time** 22%
Distance Learning Courses Available.
Nursing Student Activities Nursing Honor Society, Student Nurses' Association.
Nursing Student Resources Academic advising; academic or career counseling; assistance for students with disabilities; bookstore; campus computer network; career placement assistance; computer lab; computer-assisted instruction; e-mail services; employment services for current students; externships; interactive nursing skills videos; Internet; learning resource lab; library services; nursing audiovisuals; placement services for program completers; remedial services; resume preparation assistance; skills, simulation, or other laboratory; tutoring.
Library Facilities 121,378 volumes (10,936 in health, 610 in nursing); 157 periodical subscriptions (2,632 health-care related).

BACCALAUREATE PROGRAMS

Degree BSN
Available Programs Generic Baccalaureate; RN Baccalaureate.
Site Options Martinsburg, WV; Orlando, FL.
Study Options Full-time.
Program Entrance Requirements Minimum overall college GPA of 2.5, transcript of college record, CPR certification, health exam, health insurance, high school biology, 2 years high school science, high school transcript, immunizations, minimum high school GPA of 2.75. Transfer students are accepted. *Application deadline:* 4/1 (fall), 11/1 (spring), 3/1 (summer). Applications may be processed on a rolling basis for some programs. *Application fee:* $25.
Advanced Placement Credit by examination available. Credit given for nursing courses completed elsewhere dependent upon specific evaluations.
Expenses (2010-11) *Tuition:* full-time $8640; part-time $360 per credit hour. *Room and board:* $7990; room only: $4750 per academic year.
Financial Aid 84% of baccalaureate students in nursing programs received some form of financial aid in 2009-10. *Gift aid (need-based):* Federal Pell, FSEOG, state, private, college/university gift aid from institutional funds, Federal Nursing. *Loans:* private educational loans. *Work-study:* Federal Work-Study. *Financial aid application deadline:* Continuous.
Contact Dr. Nancey France, Dean of the School of Nursing, College of Nursing, Mountain State University, PO Box 9003, Beckley, WV 25802-9003. *Telephone:* 304-929-1516. *Fax:* 304-929-1600. *E-mail:* nfrance@mountainstate.edu.

GRADUATE PROGRAMS

Expenses (2010-11) *Tuition:* full-time $4500; part-time $375 per credit hour. *Room and board:* $7990; room only: $4750 per academic year.
Financial Aid 68% of graduate students in nursing programs received some form of financial aid in 2009-10.
Contact Dr. Jessica Sharp, Senior Academic Officer for Graduate Nursing, College of Nursing, Mountain State University, PO Box 9003, Beckley, WV 25802-9003. *Telephone:* 304-929-1425. *Fax:* 304-253-0789. *E-mail:* jsharp@mountainstate.edu.

MASTER'S DEGREE PROGRAM

Degree MSN
Available Programs Master's.
Concentrations Available Nurse anesthesia; nursing administration; nursing education. *Nurse practitioner programs in:* family health.
Site Options Martinsburg, WV; Orlando, FL.
Study Options Full-time and part-time.
Program Entrance Requirements Clinical experience, computer literacy, minimum overall college GPA of 3.0, transcript of college record, CPR certification, written essay, immunizations, 3 letters of recommendation, nursing research course, physical assessment course, prerequisite course work, resume, statistics course. *Application deadline:* Applications may be processed on a rolling basis for some programs. *Application fee:* $25.
Advanced Placement Credit given for nursing courses completed elsewhere dependent upon specific evaluations.
Degree Requirements 35 total credit hours, thesis or project, comprehensive exam.

POST-MASTER'S PROGRAM

Areas of Study Nurse anesthesia; nursing administration; nursing education. *Nurse practitioner programs in:* family health.

Shepherd University

Department of Nursing Education
Shepherdstown, West Virginia

http://www.shepherd.edu/nurseweb/
Founded in 1871

DEGREE • BSN

Nursing Program Faculty 8 (50% with doctorates).
Baccalaureate Enrollment 144 **Women** 92% **Men** 8% **Minority** 18% **International** 4%
Nursing Student Activities Nursing Honor Society, Student Nurses' Association.
Nursing Student Resources Academic advising; academic or career counseling; assistance for students with disabilities; bookstore; campus computer network; career placement assistance; computer lab; computer-assisted instruction; e-mail services; interactive nursing skills videos; Internet; learning resource lab; library services; nursing audiovisuals; remedial services; resume preparation assistance; skills, simulation, or other laboratory; tutoring.
Library Facilities 169,899 volumes (4,997 in health, 462 in nursing); 19,361 periodical subscriptions (1,956 health-care related).

BACCALAUREATE PROGRAMS

Degree BSN
Available Programs ADN to Baccalaureate; Generic Baccalaureate; RN Baccalaureate.
Study Options Full-time.
Program Entrance Requirements Minimum overall college GPA of 2.5, transcript of college record, CPR certification, written essay, health exam, health insurance, immunizations, interview, minimum GPA in nursing prerequisites of 2.0, professional liability insurance/malpractice insurance, prerequisite course work. Transfer students are accepted. *Application deadline:* 3/1 (fall), 10/1 (spring).
Advanced Placement Credit by examination available. Credit given for nursing courses completed elsewhere dependent upon specific evaluations.
Expenses (2009-10) *Tuition, state resident:* full-time $2617; part-time $214 per credit. *Tuition, nonresident:* full-time $6787; part-time $561 per credit. *Room and board:* $3908 per academic year. *Required fees:* full-time $3000.
Financial Aid 86% of baccalaureate students in nursing programs received some form of financial aid in 2008-09.
Contact Dr. Sharon K. Mailey, Professor and Chair, Department of Nursing Education, Department of Nursing Education, Shepherd University, 301 North King Street, PO Box 5000, Shepherdstown, WV 25443. *Telephone:* 304-876-5341. *Fax:* 304-876-5169. *E-mail:* smailey@shepherd.edu.

CONTINUING EDUCATION PROGRAM

Contact Dr. Sharon K. Mailey, Professor and Chair, Department of Nursing Education, Department of Nursing Education, Shepherd University, 301 North King Street, PO Box 5000, Shepherdstown, WV 25443. *Telephone:* 304-876-5341. *Fax:* 304-876-5169. *E-mail:* smailey@shepherd.edu.

University of Charleston

Department of Nursing
Charleston, West Virginia

http://www.ucwv.edu/dhs/bsn
Founded in 1888

DEGREE • BSN

Nursing Program Faculty 7 (42% with doctorates).
Baccalaureate Enrollment 65 **Women** 97% **Men** 3% **Minority** 3% **International** 1% **Part-time** 1%
Nursing Student Activities Nursing Honor Society, Sigma Theta Tau, Student Nurses' Association, nursing club.
Nursing Student Resources Academic advising; academic or career counseling; assistance for students with disabilities; bookstore; campus computer network; career placement assistance; computer lab; computer-assisted instruction; e-mail services; employment services for current students; externships; housing assistance; interactive nursing skills videos; Internet; learning resource lab; library services; nursing audiovisuals; paid internships; placement services for program completers; remedial services; resume preparation assistance; skills, simulation, or other laboratory; tutoring; unpaid internships.
Library Facilities 164,457 volumes (3,900 in health, 1,550 in nursing); 14,192 periodical subscriptions (75 health-care related).

BACCALAUREATE PROGRAMS

Degree BSN
Available Programs Generic Baccalaureate.
Study Options Full-time and part-time.
Program Entrance Requirements Minimum overall college GPA of 2.75, transcript of college record, CPR certification, health exam, high school biology, 1 year of high school math, high school transcript, immunizations, minimum high school GPA of 2.25, minimum GPA in nursing prerequisites of 2.75, professional liability insurance/malpractice insurance, prerequisite course work. Transfer students are accepted. *Application deadline:* Applications may be processed on a rolling basis for some programs.
Advanced Placement Credit given for nursing courses completed elsewhere dependent upon specific evaluations.
Expenses (2010-11) *Tuition:* full-time $12,350; part-time $410 per credit. *Room and board:* $8700; room only: $4750 per academic year. *Required fees:* full-time $460; part-time $180 per term.
Financial Aid 100% of baccalaureate students in nursing programs received some form of financial aid in 2009-10.
Contact Amanda Pritt, Office of Undergraduate Admissions, Department of Nursing, University of Charleston, 2300 MacCorkle Avenue SE, Charleston, WV 25304. *Telephone:* 304-357-4750. *Fax:* 304-357-4781. *E-mail:* admissions@ucwv.edu.

West Liberty University

Department of Health Sciences
West Liberty, West Virginia

http://www.westliberty.edu/nursing/index.htm
Founded in 1837

DEGREE • BSN

Nursing Program Faculty 8
Baccalaureate Enrollment 100 **Women** 88% **Men** 12% **Minority** 3%
Distance Learning Courses Available.
Nursing Student Activities Student Nurses' Association.
Nursing Student Resources Academic advising; academic or career counseling; assistance for students with disabilities; bookstore; campus computer network; career placement assistance; computer lab; computer-assisted instruction; e-mail services; externships; housing assistance; interactive nursing skills videos; Internet; learning resource lab; library services; nursing audiovisuals; placement services for program completers; remedial services; resume preparation assistance; skills, simulation, or other laboratory; tutoring; unpaid internships.
Library Facilities 194,715 volumes (2,500 in health, 750 in nursing); 485 periodical subscriptions (350 health-care related).

BACCALAUREATE PROGRAMS

Degree BSN
Available Programs Accelerated RN Baccalaureate; Generic Baccalaureate.
Site Options Tridelphia, WV; Wheeling, WV.
Study Options Full-time and part-time.
Program Entrance Requirements Minimum overall college GPA of 2.8, transcript of college record, health exam, minimum high school GPA of 3.0, prerequisite course work. Transfer students are accepted. *Application deadline:* 3/31 (fall), 3/31 (spring).
Advanced Placement Credit by examination available. Credit given for nursing courses completed elsewhere dependent upon specific evaluations.
Expenses (2009-10) *Tuition, area resident:* full-time $4880; part-time $203 per contact hour. *Tuition, state resident:* full-time $9560; part-time $398 per contact hour. *Tuition, nonresident:* full-time $11,950; part-time $498 per contact hour. *International tuition:* $11,950 full-time. *Room and board:* $6870; room only: $6870 per academic year.
Financial Aid 90% of baccalaureate students in nursing programs received some form of financial aid in 2008-09. *Gift aid (need-based):* Federal Pell, FSEOG, state, private, college/university gift aid from institutional funds. *Loans:* Federal Nursing Student Loans, Federal Direct (Subsidized and Unsubsidized Stafford PLUS), Perkins, alternative loans. *Work-study:* Federal Work-Study, part-time campus jobs. *Financial aid application deadline (priority):* 3/1.
Contact Ms. Sara E. Smith, RN, Nursing Program Director, Interim, Department of Health Sciences, West Liberty University, PO Box 295, CMC #140, West Liberty, WV 26074. *Telephone:* 304-336-8630. *Fax:* 304-336-5104. *E-mail:* ssmith1@westliberty.edu.

West Virginia University
School of Nursing
Morgantown, West Virginia

http://www.hsc.wvu.edu/son/
Founded in 1867

DEGREES • BSN • DNP • MSN • PHD
Nursing Program Faculty 85 (42% with doctorates).
Baccalaureate Enrollment 610 **Women** 88% **Men** 12% **Minority** 3.8% **International** .1% **Part-time** 22%
Graduate Enrollment 181 **Women** 94% **Men** 6% **Minority** 9% **Part-time** 75%
Distance Learning Courses Available.
Nursing Student Activities Nursing Honor Society, Sigma Theta Tau, Student Nurses' Association.
Nursing Student Resources Academic advising; academic or career counseling; assistance for students with disabilities; bookstore; campus computer network; career placement assistance; computer lab; computer-assisted instruction; e-mail services; employment services for current students; externships; housing assistance; interactive nursing skills videos; Internet; learning resource lab; library services; nursing audiovisuals; other; paid internships; remedial services; resume preparation assistance; skills, simulation, or other laboratory; tutoring.
Library Facilities 1.6 million volumes (211,803 in health, 2,663 in nursing); 44,866 periodical subscriptions (1,662 health-care related).

BACCALAUREATE PROGRAMS

Degree BSN
Available Programs ADN to Baccalaureate; Accelerated Baccalaureate; Accelerated Baccalaureate for Second Degree; Generic Baccalaureate; RN Baccalaureate.
Site Options Charleston, WV; Montgomery, WV; Glenville/Keyser, WV.
Study Options Full-time.
Program Entrance Requirements Minimum overall college GPA of 3.0, transcript of college record, CPR certification, high school biology, high school chemistry, 3 years high school math, 3 years high school science, high school transcript, immunizations, interview, minimum high school GPA of 3.2, minimum GPA in nursing prerequisites of 3.0, prerequisite course work. Transfer students are accepted. *Application deadline:* 2/1 (fall). *Application fee:* $25.
Advanced Placement Credit by examination available. Credit given for nursing courses completed elsewhere dependent upon specific evaluations.
Expenses (2010-11) *Tuition, state resident:* full-time $5174; part-time $217 per credit hour. *Tuition, nonresident:* full-time $18,698; part-time $781 per credit hour. *Room and board:* $8610; room only: $5392 per academic year. *Required fees:* full-time $1586; part-time $54 per credit; part-time $156 per term.
Financial Aid 67% of baccalaureate students in nursing programs received some form of financial aid in 2009-10. *Gift aid (need-based):* Federal Pell, FSEOG, state, private, college/university gift aid from institutional funds. *Loans:* Federal Direct (Subsidized and Unsubsidized Stafford PLUS), Perkins, college/university. *Work-study:* Federal Work-Study, part-time campus jobs. *Financial aid application deadline:* 3/1.
Contact Mr. Stuart R. Wells, Director of Admission and Enrollment, School of Nursing, West Virginia University, PO Box 9600, Morgantown, WV 26506-9600. *Telephone:* 304-293-1386. *Fax:* 304-293-2784. *E-mail:* swells@hsc.wvu.edu.

GRADUATE PROGRAMS

Expenses (2010-11) *Tuition, state resident:* full-time $6028; part-time $337 per credit hour. *Tuition, nonresident:* full-time $20,356; part-time $1133 per credit hour. *International tuition:* $20,356 full-time. *Room and board:* $8610; room only: $5392 per academic year. *Required fees:* full-time $1274; part-time $73 per credit.
Financial Aid 49% of graduate students in nursing programs received some form of financial aid in 2009-10. 1 teaching assistantship with tuition reimbursement available (averaging $10,000 per year) was awarded; institutionally sponsored loans, tuition waivers (partial), and graduate administrative assistantships also available. *Financial aid application deadline:* 2/1.
Contact Mr. Stuart R. Wells, Director of Admission and Enrollment, School of Nursing, West Virginia University, 6406 Health Sciences Center South, PO Box 9600, Morgantown, WV 26506-9600. *Telephone:* 304-293-1386. *Fax:* 304-293-2784. *E-mail:* swells@hsc.wvu.edu.

MASTER'S DEGREE PROGRAM

Degree MSN
Available Programs Accelerated AD/RN to Master's; Accelerated Master's; Accelerated RN to Master's; Master's; RN to Master's.
Concentrations Available Nursing administration. *Nurse practitioner programs in:* family health, gerontology, neonatal health, pediatric, women's health.
Site Options Charleston, WV.
Study Options Full-time and part-time.
Online Degree Options Yes (online only).
Program Entrance Requirements Computer literacy, minimum overall college GPA of 3.0, transcript of college record, CPR certification, written essay, immunizations, 3 letters of recommendation, nursing research course, physical assessment course, resume, statistics course. *Application deadline:* 3/1 (fall). *Application fee:* $50.
Advanced Placement Credit by examination available. Credit given for nursing courses completed elsewhere dependent upon specific evaluations.
Degree Requirements 44 total credit hours.

POST-MASTER'S PROGRAM

Areas of Study Nursing administration. *Nurse practitioner programs in:* family health, gerontology, neonatal health, pediatric, women's health.

DOCTORAL DEGREE PROGRAM

Degree DNP
Available Programs Doctorate.
Areas of Study Advanced practice nursing, clinical practice, individualized study, nursing administration.
Site Options Charleston, WV.
Online Degree Options Yes (online only).
Program Entrance Requirements Minimum overall college GPA of 3.0, interview, 3 letters of recommendation, MSN or equivalent, statistics course, vita, writing sample, GRE General Test (PhD). Application deadline: 3/1 (fall). Application fee: $50.
Degree Requirements 44 total credit hours, oral exam, written exam.

Degree PhD
Available Programs Doctorate.
Areas of Study Nursing research.
Program Entrance Requirements Minimum overall college GPA of 3.0, interview, 3 letters of recommendation, statistics course, MSN or equivalent, vita, writing sample. *Application deadline*: 2/1 (fall). *Application fee:* $50.
Degree Requirements 54 total credit hours, dissertation, oral exam, written exam.

CONTINUING EDUCATION PROGRAM

Contact Office of Extended Learning, School of Nursing, West Virginia University, PO Box 6800, Morgantown, WV 26506-6800. *Telephone:* 800-253-2762. *Fax:* 304-293-4233.

West Virginia Wesleyan College

School of Nursing
Buckhannon, West Virginia

http://www.wvwc.edu/
Founded in 1890

DEGREES • BSN • MSN

Nursing Program Faculty 7 (60% with doctorates).
Baccalaureate Enrollment 141 **Women** 93% **Men** 7% **Minority** 3%
Graduate Enrollment 20 **Women** 97% **Men** 3% **Minority** 3%
Nursing Student Activities Sigma Theta Tau, Student Nurses' Association.
Nursing Student Resources Academic advising; academic or career counseling; assistance for students with disabilities; bookstore; campus computer network; career placement assistance; computer-assisted instruction; e-mail services; employment services for current students; externships; interactive nursing skills videos; Internet; learning resource lab; library services; nursing audiovisuals; placement services for program completers; remedial services; resume preparation assistance; skills, simulation, or other laboratory; tutoring.
Library Facilities 130,000 volumes (4,000 in health, 600 in nursing); 14,500 periodical subscriptions (90 health-care related).

BACCALAUREATE PROGRAMS

Degree BSN
Available Programs Generic Baccalaureate.
Study Options Full-time and part-time.
Program Entrance Requirements Minimum overall college GPA of 2.75, transcript of college record, CPR certification, health exam, health insurance, high school transcript, immunizations, interview, minimum high school GPA of 2.5, minimum GPA in nursing prerequisites of 2.0, prerequisite course work. Transfer students are accepted. *Application deadline:* 6/15 (fall), 12/15 (spring). Applications may be processed on a rolling basis for some programs.
Advanced Placement Credit by examination available. Credit given for nursing courses completed elsewhere dependent upon specific evaluations.
Expenses (2010-11) *Tuition:* full-time $11,565; part-time $340 per credit. *Room and board:* $3570; room only: $1855 per academic year. *Required fees:* full-time $900; part-time $425 per term.
Financial Aid 95% of baccalaureate students in nursing programs received some form of financial aid in 2009-10. *Gift aid (need-based):* Federal Pell, FSEOG, state, private, college/university gift aid from institutional funds, Federal Nursing. *Loans:* Federal Nursing Student Loans, Federal Direct (Subsidized and Unsubsidized Stafford PLUS), Perkins, college/university. *Work-study:* Federal Work-Study, part-time campus jobs. *Financial aid application deadline (priority):* 2/15.
Contact Dr. Judith McKinney, Professor and Director, School of Nursing, West Virginia Wesleyan College, 59 College Avenue, Buckhannon, WV 26201-2995. *Telephone:* 304-473-8224. *Fax:* 304-473-8435. *E-mail:* mckinney@wvwc.edu.

GRADUATE PROGRAMS

Expenses (2010-11) *Tuition:* part-time $360 per credit hour. *Room and board:* $3570; room only: $1855 per academic year. *Required fees:* full-time $400; part-time $200 per term.
Financial Aid 50% of graduate students in nursing programs received some form of financial aid in 2009-10.
Contact Dr. Sue Leight, Associate Professor and Director of MSN Program, School of Nursing, West Virginia Wesleyan College, 59 College Avenue, Buckhannon, WV 26201. *Telephone:* 304-473-8228. *E-mail:* leight@wvwc.edu.

MASTER'S DEGREE PROGRAM

Degree MSN
Available Programs Master's.
Concentrations Available Nursing administration; nursing education.
Study Options Full-time and part-time.
Program Entrance Requirements Transcript of college record, interview, letters of recommendation, resume. *Application deadline:* 8/1 (fall), 12/10 (spring), 5/1 (summer). Applications may be processed on a rolling basis for some programs.
Degree Requirements 36 total credit hours, thesis or project.

Wheeling Jesuit University

Department of Nursing
Wheeling, West Virginia

http://www.wju.edu/academics/nursing/welcome.asp
Founded in 1954

DEGREES • BSN • MSN

Nursing Program Faculty 24 (33% with doctorates).
Baccalaureate Enrollment 178 **Women** 95% **Men** 5% **Minority** 1% **International** 1% **Part-time** 26%
Graduate Enrollment 130 **Women** 96% **Men** 4% **Part-time** 88%
Nursing Student Activities Sigma Theta Tau, Student Nurses' Association.
Nursing Student Resources Academic advising; academic or career counseling; bookstore; campus computer network; career placement assistance; computer lab; computer-assisted instruction; e-mail services; employment services for current students; externships; housing assistance; Internet; library services; nursing audiovisuals; placement services for program completers; remedial services; resume preparation assistance; skills, simulation, or other laboratory; tutoring.
Library Facilities 148,117 volumes (5,065 in nursing); 432 periodical subscriptions (90 health-care related).

BACCALAUREATE PROGRAMS

Degree BSN
Available Programs Accelerated Baccalaureate for Second Degree; Generic Baccalaureate; RN Baccalaureate.
Study Options Full-time and part-time.
Program Entrance Requirements Health exam, health insurance, 2 years high school math, 1 year of high school science, high school transcript, immunizations, minimum high school rank 50%. Transfer students are accepted.
Advanced Placement Credit by examination available. Credit given for nursing courses completed elsewhere dependent upon specific evaluations.
Expenses (2010-11) *Tuition:* full-time $23,950; part-time $655 per credit. *Room and board:* $6720; room only: $1930 per academic year. *Required fees:* full-time $2002.
Financial Aid ***Gift aid (need-based):*** Federal Pell, FSEOG, state, private, college/university gift aid from institutional funds, Federal Nursing. *Loans:* Federal Nursing Student Loans, Federal Direct (Subsidized and Unsubsidized Stafford PLUS), Perkins, alternative loans. *Work-study:* Federal Work-Study, part-time campus jobs. *Financial aid application deadline (priority):* 3/1.
Contact Admissions Office, Department of Nursing, Wheeling Jesuit University, 316 Washington Avenue, Wheeling, WV 26003-6233. *Telephone:* 304-243-2359. *Fax:* 304-243-2397.

GRADUATE PROGRAMS

Expenses (2010-11) *Tuition:* part-time $525 per credit. *Required fees:* full-time $460.
Financial Aid Scholarships and unspecified assistantships available.
Contact Mrs. Carol Carroll, Program Contact, Department of Nursing, Wheeling Jesuit University, 316 Washington Avenue, Wheeling, WV 26003-6233. *Telephone:* 304-243-2344. *Fax:* 304-243-2608.

MASTER'S DEGREE PROGRAM

Degree MSN
Available Programs Master's; RN to Master's.
Concentrations Available Nursing administration; nursing education. *Nurse practitioner programs in:* family health.
Study Options Full-time and part-time.
Program Entrance Requirements Computer literacy, minimum overall college GPA of 3.0, 3 letters of recommendation, statistics course, GRE General Test.
Advanced Placement Credit given for nursing courses completed elsewhere dependent upon specific evaluations.
Degree Requirements 42 total credit hours, thesis or project, comprehensive exam.

POST-MASTER'S PROGRAM

Areas of Study Nursing administration; nursing education. *Nurse practitioner programs in:* family health.

WISCONSIN

Alverno College
Division of Nursing
Milwaukee, Wisconsin

http://www.alverno.edu
Founded in 1887

DEGREES • BSN • MSN

Nursing Program Faculty 39 (5% with doctorates).

Baccalaureate Enrollment 763 **Women** 100% **Minority** 24% **Part-time** 22%

Graduate Enrollment 43 **Women** 96% **Men** 4% **Minority** 9% **Part-time** 62%

Nursing Student Activities Student Nurses' Association.

Nursing Student Resources Academic advising; academic or career counseling; assistance for students with disabilities; bookstore; campus computer network; career placement assistance; computer lab; computer-assisted instruction; daycare for children of students; e-mail services; employment services for current students; externships; housing assistance; interactive nursing skills videos; Internet; learning resource lab; library services; nursing audiovisuals; remedial services; resume preparation assistance; skills, simulation, or other laboratory; tutoring; unpaid internships.

Library Facilities 106,372 volumes; 26,768 periodical subscriptions.

BACCALAUREATE PROGRAMS

Degree BSN

Available Programs ADN to Baccalaureate; Baccalaureate for Second Degree; Generic Baccalaureate; LPN to Baccalaureate; RN Baccalaureate.

Study Options Full-time and part-time.

Program Entrance Requirements Minimum overall college GPA of 2.5, transcript of college record, written essay, high school biology, high school chemistry, 3 years high school math, 2 years high school science, high school transcript, minimum high school GPA of 2.0, prerequisite course work. Transfer students are accepted.

Advanced Placement Credit by examination available. Credit given for nursing courses completed elsewhere dependent upon specific evaluations.

Contact ***Telephone:*** 414-382-6276. *Fax:* 414-382-6279.

GRADUATE PROGRAMS

Contact ***Telephone:*** 414-382-6278. *Fax:* 414-382-6279.

MASTER'S DEGREE PROGRAM

Degree MSN

Available Programs Master's.

Concentrations Available Nursing education. *Clinical nurse specialist programs in:* adult health, gerontology, medical-surgical.

Study Options Full-time and part-time.

Program Entrance Requirements Clinical experience, transcript of college record, CPR certification, written essay, immunizations, 3 letters of recommendation, physical assessment course, statistics course.

Advanced Placement Credit given for nursing courses completed elsewhere dependent upon specific evaluations.

Degree Requirements 39 total credit hours, thesis or project.

CONTINUING EDUCATION PROGRAM

Contact ***Telephone:*** 414-382-6177. *Fax:* 414-382-6354.

Bellin College
Nursing Program
Green Bay, Wisconsin

http://www.bcon.edu
Founded in 1909

DEGREES • BSN • MSN

Nursing Program Faculty 20 (21% with doctorates).

Baccalaureate Enrollment 274 **Women** 92% **Men** 8% **Minority** 5% **International** 1% **Part-time** 9%

Graduate Enrollment 32 **Women** 93% **Men** 7% **Minority** 2% **Part-time** 81%

Distance Learning Courses Available.

Nursing Student Activities Sigma Theta Tau, Student Nurses' Association.

Nursing Student Resources Academic advising; academic or career counseling; assistance for students with disabilities; career placement assistance; computer lab; computer-assisted instruction; e-mail services; interactive nursing skills videos; Internet; learning resource lab; library services; nursing audiovisuals; resume preparation assistance; skills, simulation, or other laboratory; tutoring.

Library Facilities 7,000 volumes (7,000 in health, 4,000 in nursing); 225 periodical subscriptions (190 health-care related).

BACCALAUREATE PROGRAMS

Degree BSN

Available Programs Accelerated Baccalaureate; Accelerated Baccalaureate for Second Degree; Baccalaureate for Second Degree; Generic Baccalaureate.

Study Options Full-time and part-time.

Program Entrance Requirements Minimum overall college GPA of 2.7, transcript of college record, CPR certification, health exam, health insurance, high school biology, high school chemistry, 3 years high school math, 3 years high school science, high school transcript, immunizations, interview, 3 letters of recommendation, minimum high school GPA of 3.25, minimum GPA in nursing prerequisites of 2.7. Transfer students are accepted. *Application deadline:* Applications may be processed on a rolling basis for some programs. *Application fee:* $30.

Advanced Placement Credit by examination available. Credit given for nursing courses completed elsewhere dependent upon specific evaluations.

Expenses (2009-10) *Tuition:* full-time $18,500; part-time $884 per credit. *International tuition:* $18,500 full-time. *Required fees:* full-time $339; part-time $339 per credit.

Financial Aid 92% of baccalaureate students in nursing programs received some form of financial aid in 2008-09.

Contact Ms. Katie Klaus, Director of Admission, Nursing Program, Bellin College, 3201 Eaton Road, Green Bay, WI 54311. *Telephone:* 920-433-6651. *Fax:* 920-433-1922. *E-mail:* katie.klaus@bellincollege.edu.

GRADUATE PROGRAMS

Expenses (2009-10) *Tuition:* full-time $19,500; part-time $650 per credit. *International tuition:* $19,500 full-time. *Required fees:* full-time $500.

Financial Aid 63% of graduate students in nursing programs received some form of financial aid in 2008-09.

Contact Dr. Vera Dauffenbach, Director of Graduate Program, Nursing Program, Bellin College, 3201 Eaton Road, Green Bay, WI 54311. *Telephone:* 920-433-3624. *Fax:* 920-433-1922. *E-mail:* vera.dauffenbach@bellincollege.edu.

MASTER'S DEGREE PROGRAM

Degree MSN

Available Programs Master's.

Concentrations Available Nursing administration; nursing education.

Study Options Full-time and part-time.

Online Degree Options Yes.

Program Entrance Requirements Computer literacy, minimum overall college GPA of 3.0, transcript of college record, written essay, interview, 3 letters of recommendation, nursing research course, resume, statistics course. *Application deadline:* Applications may be processed on a rolling basis for some programs. *Application fee:* $50.

Advanced Placement Credit given for nursing courses completed elsewhere dependent upon specific evaluations.

Degree Requirements 38 total credit hours, thesis or project.

Cardinal Stritch University

Ruth S. Coleman College of Nursing
Milwaukee, Wisconsin

http://www.stritch.edu/nursing
Founded in 1937

DEGREES • BSN • MSN

Nursing Program Faculty 36 (11% with doctorates).

Baccalaureate Enrollment 98 **Women** 90% **Men** 10% **Minority** 17% **International** 6%

Graduate Enrollment 15 **Women** 100% **Minority** 13%

Nursing Student Activities Student Nurses' Association.

Nursing Student Resources Academic advising; academic or career counseling; assistance for students with disabilities; bookstore; campus computer network; career placement assistance; computer lab; e-mail services; employment services for current students; interactive nursing skills videos; Internet; learning resource lab; library services; nursing audiovisuals; remedial services; resume preparation assistance; skills, simulation, or other laboratory; tutoring.

Library Facilities 124,897 volumes (4,500 in health, 600 in nursing); 667 periodical subscriptions (1,500 health-care related).

BACCALAUREATE PROGRAMS

Degree BSN

Available Programs ADN to Baccalaureate.

Site Options Menomonee Falls, WI; Milwaukee, WI.

Study Options Full-time and part-time.

Program Entrance Requirements Minimum overall college GPA of 2.33, transcript of college record, RN licensure. Transfer students are accepted. *Application deadline:* Applications may be processed on a rolling basis for some programs.

Advanced Placement Credit by examination available. Credit given for nursing courses completed elsewhere dependent upon specific evaluations.

Expenses (2010-11) *Tuition:* full-time $23,520; part-time $580 per credit. *Required fees:* part-time $255 per credit.

Financial Aid 75% of baccalaureate students in nursing programs received some form of financial aid in 2009-10.

Contact Ms. Stacey Wegener, Nursing Admissions Counselor, Ruth S. Coleman College of Nursing, Cardinal Stritch University, 6801 North Yates Road, Milwaukee, WI 53217-3985. *Telephone:* 414-410-4966. *Fax:* 414-410-4049. *E-mail:* slwegener@stritch.edu.

GRADUATE PROGRAMS

Expenses (2010-11) *Tuition:* full-time $23,520; part-time $660 per credit. *Required fees:* part-time $160 per credit.

Financial Aid 53% of graduate students in nursing programs received some form of financial aid in 2009-10.

Contact Ms. Stacey Wegener, Nursing Admissions Counselor, Ruth S. Coleman College of Nursing, Cardinal Stritch University, 6801 North Yates Road, Milwaukee, WI 53217-3985. *Telephone:* 414-410-4966. *Fax:* 414-410-4049. *E-mail:* slwegener@stritch.edu.

MASTER'S DEGREE PROGRAM

Degree MSN

Available Programs Accelerated Master's.

Concentrations Available Nursing education.

Study Options Full-time.

Program Entrance Requirements Computer literacy, minimum overall college GPA of 3.0, transcript of college record, CPR certification, written essay, immunizations, interview, 3 letters of recommendation, nursing research course, resume. *Application deadline:* Applications may be processed on a rolling basis for some programs.

Advanced Placement Credit given for nursing courses completed elsewhere dependent upon specific evaluations.

Degree Requirements 36 total credit hours, thesis or project.

Carroll University

Nursing Program
Waukesha, Wisconsin

http://www.carrollu.edu/programs/nursing/
Founded in 1846

DEGREE • BSN

Nursing Program Faculty 15 (6.6% with doctorates).

Baccalaureate Enrollment 290 **Women** 90% **Men** 10% **Minority** 15% **Part-time** 5%

Nursing Student Activities Sigma Theta Tau, Student Nurses' Association.

Nursing Student Resources Academic advising; academic or career counseling; assistance for students with disabilities; bookstore; campus computer network; computer lab; computer-assisted instruction; e-mail services; housing assistance; interactive nursing skills videos; Internet; learning resource lab; library services; nursing audiovisuals; skills, simulation, or other laboratory; tutoring.

Library Facilities 150,000 volumes; 65,200 periodical subscriptions.

BACCALAUREATE PROGRAMS

Degree BSN

Available Programs ADN to Baccalaureate; Generic Baccalaureate.

Study Options Full-time.

Program Entrance Requirements Minimum overall college GPA of 2.75, transcript of college record, written essay, health exam, health insurance, high school biology, high school chemistry, 3 years high school math, high school transcript, minimum high school GPA of 2.75. Transfer students are accepted. *Application deadline:* Applications may be processed on a rolling basis for some programs.

Expenses (2010-11) *Tuition:* full-time $23,582; part-time $377 per credit. *Room and board:* $7371; room only: $4023 per academic year. *Required fees:* full-time $915; part-time $425 per term.

Financial Aid 98% of baccalaureate students in nursing programs received some form of financial aid in 2009-10. *Gift aid (need-based):* Federal Pell, FSEOG, state, private, college/university gift aid from institutional funds. *Loans:* Federal Direct (Subsidized and Unsubsidized Stafford PLUS), Perkins, state, college/university. *Work-study:* Federal Work-Study, part-time campus jobs. *Financial aid application deadline:* Continuous.

Contact Ms. Angela Rose Brindowski, Chair, Department of Nursing, Nursing Program, Carroll University, 100 North East Avenue, Waukesha, WI 53186. *Telephone:* 262-524-4927. *E-mail:* abrindow@carrollu.edu.

Columbia College of Nursing

Columbia College of Nursing/Mount Mary College Nursing Program
Milwaukee, Wisconsin

See description of programs under
Columbia College of Nursing/Mount Mary College Nursing Program (Milwaukee, Wisconsin).

Columbia College of Nursing/Mount Mary College Nursing Program

Columbia College of Nursing/Mount Mary College Nursing Program
Milwaukee, Wisconsin

http://www.mtmary.edu/nursing.htm
Founded in 2002

DEGREE • BSN

Nursing Program Faculty 20 (7% with doctorates).

Baccalaureate Enrollment 250 **Women** 95% **Men** 5% **Minority** 15% **Part-time** 20%

Nursing Student Activities Sigma Theta Tau, Student Nurses' Association.

Nursing Student Resources Academic advising; academic or career counseling; bookstore; campus computer network; career placement assistance; computer lab; computer-assisted instruction; daycare for children of students; e-mail services; employment services for current students; housing assistance; interactive nursing skills videos; Internet; learning resource lab; library services; nursing audiovisuals; resume preparation assistance; skills, simulation, or other laboratory; tutoring.

BACCALAUREATE PROGRAMS

Degree BSN

Available Programs Baccalaureate for Second Degree; Generic Baccalaureate; RN Baccalaureate.

Site Options Milwaukee, WI.

Study Options Full-time and part-time.

Program Entrance Requirements Minimum overall college GPA of 2.8, transcript of college record, health exam, health insurance, high school biology, high school chemistry, 2 years high school math, 2 years high school science, high school transcript, minimum high school GPA of 2.5, minimum high school rank 40%, minimum GPA in nursing prerequisites of 2.8, prerequisite course work. Transfer students are accepted.

Advanced Placement Credit by examination available. Credit given for nursing courses completed elsewhere dependent upon specific evaluations.

Contact ***Telephone:*** 414-256-1219 Ext. 193. *Fax:* 414-256-0180.

See full description on page 466.

Concordia University Wisconsin

Program in Nursing
Mequon, Wisconsin

http://www.cuw.edu/

Founded in 1881

DEGREES • BSN • DNP • MSN

Nursing Program Faculty 12 (3% with doctorates).

Baccalaureate Enrollment 423 **Women** 92% **Men** 8% **Minority** 10% **International** 1% **Part-time** 32%

Graduate Enrollment 510 **Women** 95% **Men** 5% **Minority** 8% **International** 1% **Part-time** 44%

Distance Learning Courses Available.

Nursing Student Activities Nursing Honor Society, Sigma Theta Tau, Student Nurses' Association.

Nursing Student Resources Academic advising; academic or career counseling; assistance for students with disabilities; bookstore; campus computer network; career placement assistance; computer lab; computer-assisted instruction; e-mail services; employment services for current students; externships; interactive nursing skills videos; Internet; learning resource lab; library services; nursing audiovisuals; paid internships; placement services for program completers; resume preparation assistance; skills, simulation, or other laboratory; tutoring.

Library Facilities 3,893 volumes in health, 878 volumes in nursing; 922 periodical subscriptions health-care related.

BACCALAUREATE PROGRAMS

Degree BSN

Available Programs ADN to Baccalaureate; Generic Baccalaureate; LPN to RN Baccalaureate; RN Baccalaureate.

Site Options Mequon, WI; Milwaukee, WI.

Study Options Full-time.

Program Entrance Requirements Transcript of college record, CPR certification, health exam, health insurance, high school transcript, immunizations, minimum high school GPA of 2.75, minimum GPA in nursing prerequisites of 2.75, RN licensure. Transfer students are accepted. *Application deadline:* 7/15 (fall), 7/15 (winter), 10/15 (spring), 3/15 (summer). *Application fee:* $50.

Advanced Placement Credit given for nursing courses completed elsewhere dependent upon specific evaluations.

Expenses (2010-11) *Tuition:* full-time $21,940. *Room and board:* $8310 per academic year. *Required fees:* full-time $210.

Financial Aid 98% of baccalaureate students in nursing programs received some form of financial aid in 2009-10. *Gift aid (need-based):* Federal Pell, FSEOG, state, private, college/university gift aid from institutional funds. *Loans:* Federal Direct (Subsidized and Unsubsidized Stafford PLUS), state. *Work-study:* Federal Work-Study. *Financial aid application deadline (priority):* 3/15.

Contact Mrs. Sandra Hannemann, Administrative Assistant, Nursing Department, Program in Nursing, Concordia University Wisconsin, 12800 North Lake Shore Drive, Mequon, WI 53097. *Telephone:* 262-243-4374. *Fax:* 262-243-4466. *E-mail:* sandy.hannemann@cuw.edu.

GRADUATE PROGRAMS

Expenses (2010-11) *Tuition:* full-time $8175; part-time $545 per credit. *Required fees:* full-time $105; part-time $35 per term.

Financial Aid 57% of graduate students in nursing programs received some form of financial aid in 2009-10. *Application deadline:* 8/1.

Contact Dr. Teri Kaul, Director, Masters Program in Nursing and DNP, Program in Nursing, Concordia University Wisconsin, 12800 North Lake Shore Drive, Mequon, WI 53097. *Telephone:* 262-243-4538. *Fax:* 262-243-4506. *E-mail:* teri.kaul@cuw.edu.

MASTER'S DEGREE PROGRAM

Degree MSN

Available Programs Master's.

Concentrations Available Nursing education. *Nurse practitioner programs in:* family health, gerontology.

Site Options Mequon, WI; Milwaukee, WI; multiple cities and states.

Study Options Full-time and part-time.

Program Entrance Requirements Clinical experience, computer literacy, minimum overall college GPA of 3.0, transcript of college record, CPR certification, written essay, immunizations, interview, 2 letters of recommendation, physical assessment course, professional liability insurance/malpractice insurance, resume, statistics course. *Application deadline:* 6/15 (fall), 6/15 (winter), 10/15 (spring). *Application fee:* $35.

Advanced Placement Credit given for nursing courses completed elsewhere dependent upon specific evaluations.

Degree Requirements 44 total credit hours, thesis or project.

POST-MASTER'S PROGRAM

Areas of Study *Nurse practitioner programs in:* family health.

DOCTORAL DEGREE PROGRAM

Degree DNP

Available Programs Doctorate.

Areas of Study Family health, gerontology.

Site Options Mequon, WI; Milwaukee, WI; multiple cities and states.

Online Degree Options Yes (online only).

Program Entrance Requirements Clinical experience, minimum overall college GPA of 3.0, 2 letters of recommendation, MSN or equivalent, vita, writing sample. Application deadline: 4/1 (spring). Application fee: $35.

Degree Requirements 35 total credit hours, dissertation.

Edgewood College

Program in Nursing
Madison, Wisconsin

http://nursing.edgewood.edu

Founded in 1927

DEGREES • BS • MS • MSN/MBA

Nursing Program Faculty 36 (25% with doctorates).

Baccalaureate Enrollment 220 **Women** 90% **Men** 10% **Minority** 2% **International** 1% **Part-time** 35%

Graduate Enrollment 45 **Women** 86% **Men** 14% **Minority** 2% **Part-time** 100%

Distance Learning Courses Available.

Nursing Student Activities Sigma Theta Tau, Student Nurses' Association.

Nursing Student Resources Academic advising; academic or career counseling; assistance for students with disabilities; bookstore; campus computer network; career placement assistance; computer lab; computer-assisted instruction; e-mail services; employment services for current students; externships; housing assistance; interactive nursing skills videos; Internet; learning resource lab; library services; nursing audiovisuals; paid internships; remedial services; resume preparation assistance; skills, simulation, or other laboratory; tutoring; unpaid internships.

Library Facilities 107,873 volumes (4,500 in health, 1,000 in nursing); 164 periodical subscriptions (45 health-care related).

BACCALAUREATE PROGRAMS

Degree BS
Available Programs Accelerated Baccalaureate for Second Degree; Baccalaureate for Second Degree; Generic Baccalaureate.
Site Options Madison, WI.
Study Options Full-time and part-time.
Program Entrance Requirements Minimum overall college GPA of 2.75, transcript of college record, CPR certification, written essay, health exam, high school biology, high school chemistry, high school foreign language, high school math, high school transcript, immunizations, interview, minimum high school GPA of 2.75, minimum GPA in nursing prerequisites of 2.75, prerequisite course work. Transfer students are accepted. *Application deadline:* 1/15 (fall), 9/15 (spring). *Application fee:* $40.
Advanced Placement Credit given for nursing courses completed elsewhere dependent upon specific evaluations.
Expenses (2009-10) *Tuition:* full-time $21,042; part-time $662 per credit. *Room and board:* $6866 per academic year. *Required fees:* full-time $662.
Financial Aid 85% of baccalaureate students in nursing programs received some form of financial aid in 2008-09. *Gift aid (need-based):* Federal Pell, FSEOG, state, private, college/university gift aid from institutional funds. *Loans:* Perkins, state, college/university. *Work-study:* Federal Work-Study, part-time campus jobs. *Financial aid application deadline (priority):* 3/1.
Contact Dr. Margaret C. Noreuil, Dean, School of Nursing, Program in Nursing, Edgewood College, 1000 Edgewood College Drive, Madison, WI 53711. *Telephone:* 608-663-2280. *Fax:* 608-663-2863. *E-mail:* mnoreuil@edgewood.edu.

GRADUATE PROGRAMS

Expenses (2009-10) *Tuition:* part-time $688 per credit.
Financial Aid 10% of graduate students in nursing programs received some form of financial aid in 2008-09.
Contact Dr. Margaret C. Noreuil, Dean, School of Nursing, Program in Nursing, Edgewood College, 1000 Edgewood College Drive, Madison, WI 53711. *Telephone:* 608-663-2280. *Fax:* 608-663-2863. *E-mail:* mnoreuil@edgewood.edu.

MASTER'S DEGREE PROGRAM

Degrees MS; MSN/MBA
Available Programs Master's.
Concentrations Available Nursing administration; nursing education.
Site Options Madison, WI.
Study Options Full-time and part-time.
Program Entrance Requirements Clinical experience, computer literacy, minimum overall college GPA of 3.0, transcript of college record, CPR certification, written essay, immunizations, interview, 2 letters of recommendation, nursing research course, prerequisite course work, resume, statistics course. *Application deadline:* Applications may be processed on a rolling basis for some programs.
Advanced Placement Credit given for nursing courses completed elsewhere dependent upon specific evaluations.
Degree Requirements 36 total credit hours, thesis or project.

Maranatha Baptist Bible College

Nursing Department
Watertown, Wisconsin

Founded in 1968

DEGREE • BSN

Baccalaureate Enrollment 58
Nursing Student Activities Student Nurses' Association.
Nursing Student Resources Academic advising; academic or career counseling; assistance for students with disabilities; bookstore; campus computer network; career placement assistance; computer lab; computer-assisted instruction; e-mail services; employment services for current students; housing assistance; interactive nursing skills videos; Internet; learning resource lab; library services; nursing audiovisuals; skills, simulation, or other laboratory; tutoring.
Library Facilities 122,251 volumes; 502 periodical subscriptions.

BACCALAUREATE PROGRAMS

Degree BSN
Available Programs RN Baccalaureate.
Program Entrance Requirements Minimum overall college GPA of 2.5, CPR certification, written essay, health exam, immunizations, interview, minimum high school GPA, minimum GPA in nursing prerequisites of 2.5, prerequisite course work. Transfer students are accepted. *Application deadline:* Applications may be processed on a rolling basis for some programs.
Contact Mrs. Kelly Ann Crum, RN, Chair, Department of Nursing, Nursing Department, Maranatha Baptist Bible College, 745 West Main Street, Watertown, WI 53094. *Telephone:* 920-206-4050. *E-mail:* kelly.crum@mbbc.edu.

Marian University

School of Nursing
Fond du Lac, Wisconsin

http://www.mariancollege.edu
Founded in 1936

DEGREES • BSN • MSN

Baccalaureate Enrollment 221 **Women** 95% **Men** 5% **Minority** 1% **Part-time** 7%
Graduate Enrollment 39 **Women** 97% **Men** 3% **Part-time** 15%
Nursing Student Activities Student Nurses' Association.
Nursing Student Resources Academic advising; academic or career counseling; assistance for students with disabilities; bookstore; career placement assistance; computer lab; daycare for children of students; e-mail services; externships; interactive nursing skills videos; Internet; learning resource lab; library services; nursing audiovisuals.
Library Facilities 116,270 volumes (3,000 in health, 2,500 in nursing); 1,464 periodical subscriptions (91 health-care related).

BACCALAUREATE PROGRAMS

Degree BSN
Available Programs ADN to Baccalaureate; Generic Baccalaureate.
Site Options Appleton, WI; Beaver Dam, WI.
Study Options Full-time and part-time.
Program Entrance Requirements Transcript of college record, high school biology, high school chemistry, 3 years high school math, high school science, high school transcript, minimum high school GPA of 2.5. Transfer students are accepted.
Advanced Placement Credit given for nursing courses completed elsewhere dependent upon specific evaluations.
Contact ***Telephone:*** 920-923-8732. *Fax:* 920-923-8770.

GRADUATE PROGRAMS

Contact ***Telephone:*** 920-923-8094. *Fax:* 920-923-8094.

MASTER'S DEGREE PROGRAM

Degree MSN
Available Programs Master's.
Concentrations Available Nursing education. *Nurse practitioner programs in:* adult health.
Study Options Full-time and part-time.
Program Entrance Requirements Clinical experience, minimum overall college GPA of 3.0, transcript of college record, CPR certification, written essay, immunizations, 3 letters of recommendation, nursing research course, professional liability insurance/malpractice insurance, resume, statistics course.
Advanced Placement Credit given for nursing courses completed elsewhere dependent upon specific evaluations.
Degree Requirements 39 total credit hours, thesis or project.

POST-MASTER'S PROGRAM

Areas of Study Nursing education.

Marquette University

College of Nursing
Milwaukee, Wisconsin

http://www.marquette.edu/nursing
Founded in 1881

DEGREES • BSN • DNP • MSN • MSN/MBA • PHD

Nursing Program Faculty 50 (60% with doctorates).

Baccalaureate Enrollment 413 **Women** 94% **Men** 6% **Minority** 15% **Part-time** 1%
Graduate Enrollment 337 **Women** 94% **Men** 6% **Minority** 11% **Part-time** 62%
Distance Learning Courses Available.
Nursing Student Activities Nursing Honor Society, Sigma Theta Tau, Student Nurses' Association.
Nursing Student Resources Academic advising; academic or career counseling; assistance for students with disabilities; bookstore; campus computer network; career placement assistance; computer lab; computer-assisted instruction; daycare for children of students; e-mail services; employment services for current students; externships; housing assistance; interactive nursing skills videos; Internet; learning resource lab; library services; nursing audiovisuals; placement services for program completers; remedial services; resume preparation assistance; skills, simulation, or other laboratory; tutoring.
Library Facilities 54,388 volumes in health, 9,322 volumes in nursing; 27,425 periodical subscriptions (3,255 health-care related).

BACCALAUREATE PROGRAMS

Degree BSN
Available Programs Generic Baccalaureate.
Study Options Full-time and part-time.
Program Entrance Requirements Minimum overall college GPA of 2.5, transcript of college record, written essay, high school biology, high school chemistry, 3 years high school math, high school transcript, 1 letter of recommendation, minimum high school GPA of 2.5, minimum high school rank 25%. *Application deadline:* 12/1 (fall).
Advanced Placement Credit given for nursing courses completed elsewhere dependent upon specific evaluations.
Expenses (2010-11) *Tuition:* full-time $30,040; part-time $875 per credit. *Room and board:* $9890 per academic year. *Required fees:* full-time $422; part-time $211 per term.
Financial Aid 87% of baccalaureate students in nursing programs received some form of financial aid in 2009-10. *Gift aid (need-based):* Federal Pell, FSEOG, state, private, college/university gift aid from institutional funds. *Loans:* Federal Nursing Student Loans, Federal Direct (Subsidized and Unsubsidized Stafford PLUS), Perkins, state, college/university. *Work-study:* Federal Work-Study, part-time campus jobs. *Financial aid application deadline:* Continuous.
Contact Dr. Kerry Kosmoski-Goepfert, Associate Dean for Undergraduate Programs, College of Nursing, Marquette University, Clark Hall, PO Box 1881, Milwaukee, WI 53201-1881. *Telephone:* 414-288-3809. *Fax:* 414-288-1597. *E-mail:* kerry.goepfert@marquette.edu.

GRADUATE PROGRAMS

Expenses (2010-11) *Tuition:* part-time $905 per credit. *Required fees:* part-time $75 per term.
Financial Aid 72% of graduate students in nursing programs received some form of financial aid in 2009-10. 6 research assistantships, 1 teaching assistantship were awarded; career-related internships or fieldwork, Federal Work-Study, institutionally sponsored loans, scholarships, and tuition waivers (full and partial) also available. Aid available to part-time students. *Financial aid application deadline:* 2/15.
Contact Dr. Maureen O'Brien, Associate Dean for Graduate Programs, College of Nursing, Marquette University, Clark Hall, PO Box 1881, Milwaukee, WI 53201-1881. *Telephone:* 414-288-3869. *Fax:* 414-288-1597. *E-mail:* maureen.obrien@marquette.edu.

MASTER'S DEGREE PROGRAM

Degrees MSN; MSN/MBA
Available Programs Master's; Master's for Non-Nursing College Graduates; Master's for Nurses with Non-Nursing Degrees; RN to Master's.
Concentrations Available Clinical nurse leader; nurse-midwifery; nursing administration. *Clinical nurse specialist programs in:* adult health, gerontology, pediatric. *Nurse practitioner programs in:* acute care, adult health, gerontology, pediatric.
Study Options Full-time and part-time.
Program Entrance Requirements Minimum overall college GPA of 3.0, transcript of college record, CPR certification, written essay, immunizations, 3 letters of recommendation, nursing research course, physical assessment course, resume, statistics course, GRE General Test. *Application deadline:* 2/15 (fall), 11/15 (spring). Applications may be processed on a rolling basis for some programs. *Application fee:* $50.
Advanced Placement Credit given for nursing courses completed elsewhere dependent upon specific evaluations.
Degree Requirements 42 total credit hours, comprehensive exam.

POST-MASTER'S PROGRAM

Areas of Study Nurse-midwifery; nursing administration. *Clinical nurse specialist programs in:* adult health, gerontology, pediatric. *Nurse practitioner programs in:* acute care, adult health, gerontology, pediatric.

DOCTORAL DEGREE PROGRAM

Degree DNP
Available Programs Doctorate; Post-Baccalaureate Doctorate.
Areas of Study Advanced nursing practice, nursing administration.
Program Entrance Requirements Minimum overall college GPA of 3.2, 3 letters of recommendation, statistics course, MSN or equivalent, vita. Applications are processed on a rolling basis.
Degree Requirements 24 total credit hours (post-master's), 66 total credit hours (post-baccalaureate), residency, written exam.

Degree PhD
Available Programs Doctorate; Post-Baccalaureate Doctorate.
Areas of Study Aging, ethics, faculty preparation, health promotion/disease prevention, health-care systems, human health and illness, illness and transition, nursing administration, nursing education, nursing research, nursing science.
Program Entrance Requirements Minimum overall college GPA of 3.3, interview by faculty committee, interview, 3 letters of recommendation, MSN or equivalent, statistics course, vita, writing sample. Application deadline: 2/15 (fall), 11/15 (spring). Applications may be processed on a rolling basis for some programs. Application fee: $50.
Degree Requirements 51 total credit hours, dissertation, oral exam, written exam, residency.

See full description on page 486.

Milwaukee School of Engineering

School of Nursing
Milwaukee, Wisconsin

http://www.msoe.edu/nursing
Founded in 1903

DEGREE • BSN

Nursing Program Faculty 26 (23% with doctorates).
Baccalaureate Enrollment 185 **Women** 85% **Men** 15% **Minority** 20% **Part-time** 3%
Nursing Student Activities Nursing Honor Society, Student Nurses' Association.
Nursing Student Resources Academic advising; academic or career counseling; assistance for students with disabilities; bookstore; campus computer network; career placement assistance; computer lab; computer-assisted instruction; e-mail services; externships; housing assistance; interactive nursing skills videos; Internet; learning resource lab; library services; nursing audiovisuals; placement services for program completers; remedial services; resume preparation assistance; skills, simulation, or other laboratory; tutoring.
Library Facilities 84,325 volumes (1,956 in health, 1,126 in nursing); 389 periodical subscriptions (116 health-care related).

BACCALAUREATE PROGRAMS

Degree BSN
Available Programs Generic Baccalaureate; RN Baccalaureate.
Study Options Full-time and part-time.
Program Entrance Requirements Minimum overall college GPA of 2.75, transcript of college record, CPR certification, health exam, health insurance, high school biology, high school chemistry, 3 years high school math, 3 years high school science, high school transcript, immunizations, minimum high school GPA of 2.8, professional liability insurance/malpractice insurance. Transfer students are accepted. *Application deadline:* 9/1 (fall), 12/1 (winter), 3/1 (spring). Applications may be processed on a rolling basis for some programs. *Application fee:* $25.
Advanced Placement Credit by examination available. Credit given for nursing courses completed elsewhere dependent upon specific evaluations.
Expenses (2010-11) *Tuition:* full-time $9840; part-time $513 per credit. *Room and board:* $7557; room only: $4737 per academic year.
Financial Aid 95% of baccalaureate students in nursing programs received some form of financial aid in 2009-10.
Contact Dr. Debra L. Jenks, Chair, School of Nursing, Milwaukee School of Engineering, 1025 North Broadway Street, Milwaukee, WI 53202-3109. *Telephone:* 414-277-4516. *Fax:* 414-277-4540. *E-mail:* jenks@msoe.edu.

Mount Mary College

Columbia College of Nursing/Mount Mary College Nursing Program
Milwaukee, Wisconsin

See description of programs under
Columbia College of Nursing/Mount Mary College Nursing Program (Milwaukee, Wisconsin).

Silver Lake College

Nursing Program
Manitowoc, Wisconsin

Founded in 1869

DEGREE • BSN

Nursing Program Faculty 11 (1% with doctorates).
Baccalaureate Enrollment 19 **Women** 90% **Men** 10% **Minority** 5% **Part-time** 100%
Distance Learning Courses Available.
Nursing Student Resources Academic advising; academic or career counseling; assistance for students with disabilities; bookstore; campus computer network; computer lab; computer-assisted instruction; e-mail services; Internet; library services; nursing audiovisuals; tutoring.
Library Facilities 62,531 volumes; 251 periodical subscriptions.

BACCALAUREATE PROGRAMS

Degree BSN
Available Programs ADN to Baccalaureate.
Site Options Wausau, WI; Green Bay, WI.
Study Options Part-time.
Online Degree Options Yes.
Program Entrance Requirements Transcript of college record, health exam, immunizations, 1 letter of recommendation, RN licensure. Transfer students are accepted. *Application deadline:* Applications may be processed on a rolling basis for some programs. *Application fee:* $50.
Advanced Placement Credit given for nursing courses completed elsewhere dependent upon specific evaluations.
Expenses (2010-11) *Tuition:* part-time $410 per credit.
Financial Aid ***Gift aid (need-based):*** Federal Pell, FSEOG, state, private, college/university gift aid from institutional funds. *Loans:* Federal Direct (Subsidized and Unsubsidized Stafford PLUS), state. *Work-study:* Federal Work-Study, part-time campus jobs. *Financial aid application deadline (priority):* 3/15.
Contact Brianna Neuser, BSN Completion Program Director, Nursing Program, Silver Lake College, 2406 South Alverno Road, Manitowoc, WI 54220. *Telephone:* 920-686-6213. *Fax:* 920-684-7082. *E-mail:* bneuser@silver.sl.edu.

University of Phoenix–Milwaukee Campus

College of Health and Human Services
Milwaukee, Wisconsin

http://www.phoenix.edu/campus-locations/wi/milwaukee-campus/milwaukee-campus.html

DEGREES • BSN • MSN • PHD

BACCALAUREATE PROGRAMS

Degree BSN
Available Programs RN Baccalaureate.

Contact Campus College Chair, Nursing, College of Health and Human Services, University of Phoenix–Milwaukee Campus, Brookfield, WI 53045-3573. *Telephone:* 262-785-0608.

GRADUATE PROGRAMS

Contact Campus College Chair, Nursing, College of Health and Human Services, University of Phoenix–Milwaukee Campus, Brookfield, WI 53045-3573. *Telephone:* 262-785-0608.

MASTER'S DEGREE PROGRAM

Degree MSN
Available Programs Master's.

DOCTORAL DEGREE PROGRAM

Degree PhD
Available Programs Doctorate.

University of Wisconsin–Eau Claire

College of Nursing and Health Sciences
Eau Claire, Wisconsin

http://www.uwec.edu/conhs/index.htm
Founded in 1916

DEGREES • BSN • DNP • MSN
Nursing Program Faculty 47 (28% with doctorates).
Baccalaureate Enrollment 401 **Women** 91% **Men** 9% **Minority** 4% **Part-time** 20%
Graduate Enrollment 102 **Women** 96% **Men** 4% **Minority** 1% **Part-time** 61%
Distance Learning Courses Available.
Nursing Student Activities Sigma Theta Tau, Student Nurses' Association.
Nursing Student Resources Academic advising; academic or career counseling; assistance for students with disabilities; bookstore; campus computer network; career placement assistance; computer lab; computer-assisted instruction; daycare for children of students; e-mail services; employment services for current students; housing assistance; interactive nursing skills videos; Internet; learning resource lab; library services; nursing audiovisuals; other; placement services for program completers; remedial services; resume preparation assistance; skills, simulation, or other laboratory; tutoring.
Library Facilities 944,303 volumes (17,256 in health, 1,984 in nursing); 18,382 periodical subscriptions (3,893 health-care related).

BACCALAUREATE PROGRAMS

Degree BSN
Available Programs ADN to Baccalaureate; Accelerated Baccalaureate for Second Degree; Generic Baccalaureate; RN Baccalaureate.
Site Options Marshfield, WI.
Study Options Full-time.
Program Entrance Requirements Minimum overall college GPA of 3.0, transcript of college record, CPR certification, written essay, health exam, high school biology, high school chemistry, high school foreign language, 3 years high school math, 3 years high school science, high school transcript, immunizations, minimum GPA in nursing prerequisites of 2.5, prerequisite course work. Transfer students are accepted. *Application deadline:* 5/1 (fall), 12/1 (spring). *Application fee:* $86.
Advanced Placement Credit given for nursing courses completed elsewhere dependent upon specific evaluations.
Expenses (2010-11) *Tuition, state resident:* full-time $6122; part-time $255 per credit. *Tuition, nonresident:* full-time $13,695; part-time $571 per credit. *Room and board:* $5830; room only: $2920 per academic year. *Required fees:* full-time $1242; part-time $52 per credit; part-time $621 per term.
Financial Aid 69% of baccalaureate students in nursing programs received some form of financial aid in 2009-10.
Contact Dr. Mary Zwygart-Stauffacher, Interim Dean, College of Nursing and Health Sciences, University of Wisconsin–Eau Claire, 105 Garfield Avenue, Eau Claire, WI 54702-4004. *Telephone:* 715-836-5287. *Fax:* 715-836-5925. *E-mail:* zwygarmc@uwec.edu.

GRADUATE PROGRAMS

Expenses (2010-11) *Tuition, state resident:* full-time $7001; part-time $389 per credit. *Tuition, nonresident:* full-time $16,771; part-time $932 per credit. *Room and board:* $5830; room only: $2920 per academic year. *Required fees:* full-time $1057; part-time $58 per credit; part-time $528 per term.
Financial Aid 58% of graduate students in nursing programs received some form of financial aid in 2009-10. Federal Work-Study and unspecified assistantships available. *Financial aid application deadline:* 3/1.
Contact Dr. Mary Zwygart-Stauffacher, Interim Dean, College of Nursing and Health Sciences, University of Wisconsin–Eau Claire, 105 Garfield Avenue, Eau Claire, WI 54702-4004. *Telephone:* 715-836-5287. *Fax:* 715-836-5925. *E-mail:* zwygarmc@uwec.edu.

MASTER'S DEGREE PROGRAM

Degree MSN
Available Programs Master's; RN to Master's.
Concentrations Available Nursing administration; nursing education. *Clinical nurse specialist programs in:* adult health. *Nurse practitioner programs in:* adult health, family health, gerontology.
Site Options Marshfield, WI.
Study Options Full-time and part-time.
Program Entrance Requirements Clinical experience, minimum overall college GPA of 3.0, transcript of college record, CPR certification, written essay, immunizations, 3 letters of recommendation, physical assessment course, professional liability insurance/malpractice insurance, statistics course. *Application deadline:* 1/15 (summer). Applications may be processed on a rolling basis for some programs. *Application fee:* $86.
Advanced Placement Credit given for nursing courses completed elsewhere dependent upon specific evaluations.
Degree Requirements 42 total credit hours, thesis or project.

POST-MASTER'S PROGRAM

Areas of Study Nursing administration; nursing education. *Clinical nurse specialist programs in:* adult health. *Nurse practitioner programs in:* adult health, family health, gerontology.

DOCTORAL DEGREE PROGRAM

Degree DNP
Available Programs Doctorate; Post-Baccalaureate Doctorate.
Areas of Study Family health, gerontology, nursing administration.
Program Entrance Requirements Clinical experience, minimum overall college GPA of 3.00, 3 letters of recommendation, statistics course, vita, writing sample. Application deadline: 1/4 (summer). Applications may be processed on a rolling basis for some programs. Application fee: $86.
Degree Requirements 72 total credit hours.

CONTINUING EDUCATION PROGRAM

Contact Ms. Peggy Ore, Program Manager, College of Nursing and Health Sciences, University of Wisconsin–Eau Claire, Continuing Education Department, Eau Claire, WI 54702-4004. *Telephone:* 715-836-5645. *Fax:* 715-836-5263. *E-mail:* orepd@uwec.edu.

University of Wisconsin–Green Bay

BSN–LINC Online RN–BSN Program
Green Bay, Wisconsin

http://www.uwgb.edu/nursing/
Founded in 1968

DEGREE • BSN
Nursing Program Faculty 7 (86% with doctorates).
Baccalaureate Enrollment 296 **Women** 91% **Men** 9% **Minority** 11% **International** 1% **Part-time** 91%
Distance Learning Courses Available.
Nursing Student Activities Sigma Theta Tau, Student Nurses' Association.
Nursing Student Resources Academic advising; academic or career counseling; assistance for students with disabilities; bookstore; campus computer network; career placement assistance; computer lab; computer-assisted instruction; e-mail services; employment services for current students; Internet; learning resource lab; library services; nursing audiovi-

suals; resume preparation assistance; skills, simulation, or other laboratory.
Library Facilities 360,795 volumes (1,000 in health, 675 in nursing); 4,452 periodical subscriptions (100 health-care related).

BACCALAUREATE PROGRAMS

Degree BSN
Available Programs RN Baccalaureate.
Site Options Marinette, WI; Rhinelander, WI.
Study Options Full-time and part-time.
Online Degree Options Yes.
Program Entrance Requirements Minimum overall college GPA of 2.5, transcript of college record, RN licensure. Transfer students are accepted. *Application fee:* $44.
Expenses (2010-11) *Tuition, state resident:* part-time $291 per credit. *Tuition, nonresident:* part-time $385 per credit.
Financial Aid 25% of baccalaureate students in nursing programs received some form of financial aid in 2009-10. *Gift aid (need-based):* Federal Pell, FSEOG, state, private, college/university gift aid from institutional funds. *Loans:* Perkins. *Work-study:* Federal Work-Study, part-time campus jobs. *Financial aid application deadline (priority):* 4/15.
Contact Ms. Sharon Gajeski, Advisor, BSN–LINC Online RN–BSN Program, University of Wisconsin–Green Bay, 2420 Nicolet Drive, Green Bay, WI 54311-7001. *Telephone:* 920-465-2570. *Fax:* 920-465-2854. *E-mail:* gajeskis@uwgb.edu.

University of Wisconsin–Madison

School of Nursing
Madison, Wisconsin

http://www.son.wisc.edu/
Founded in 1848

DEGREES • BS • PHD

Nursing Program Faculty 52 (35% with doctorates).
Baccalaureate Enrollment 384 **Women** 86% **Men** 14% **Minority** 11% **International** 2% **Part-time** 25%
Graduate Enrollment 164 **Women** 95% **Men** 5% **Minority** 7% **International** 4% **Part-time** 60%
Distance Learning Courses Available.
Nursing Student Activities Nursing Honor Society, Sigma Theta Tau, Student Nurses' Association, nursing club.
Nursing Student Resources Academic advising; academic or career counseling; assistance for students with disabilities; bookstore; campus computer network; computer lab; computer-assisted instruction; e-mail services; externships; interactive nursing skills videos; Internet; learning resource lab; library services; nursing audiovisuals; resume preparation assistance; skills, simulation, or other laboratory; tutoring.
Library Facilities 334,000 volumes in health, 8,300 volumes in nursing; 1,500 periodical subscriptions health-care related.

BACCALAUREATE PROGRAMS

Degree BS
Available Programs Generic Baccalaureate; RN Baccalaureate.
Site Options La Crosse, WI.
Study Options Full-time.
Program Entrance Requirements Minimum overall college GPA of 2.75, transcript of college record, CPR certification, written essay, high school chemistry, high school foreign language, 3 years high school math, 3 years high school science, high school transcript, immunizations, minimum GPA in nursing prerequisites of 2.75, prerequisite course work. Transfer students are accepted. *Application deadline:* 2/1 (fall). *Application fee:* $50.
Advanced Placement Credit by examination available. Credit given for nursing courses completed elsewhere dependent upon specific evaluations.
Expenses (2010-11) *Tuition, state resident:* full-time $8986; part-time $376 per credit. *Tuition, nonresident:* full-time $24,237; part-time $1011 per credit. *Room and board:* $7900; room only: $6000 per academic year. *Required fees:* full-time $1054; part-time $45 per credit; part-time $527 per term.
Financial Aid 65% of baccalaureate students in nursing programs received some form of financial aid in 2009-10. *Gift aid (need-based):* Federal Pell, FSEOG, state, private, college/university gift aid from institutional funds. *Loans:* Federal Nursing Student Loans, Federal Direct (Subsidized and Unsubsidized Stafford PLUS), Perkins, state. *Work-study:* Federal Work-Study. *Financial aid application deadline:* Continuous.
Contact Nursing Admissions, School of Nursing, University of Wisconsin–Madison, 600 Highland Avenue, Room K6/146, Madison, WI 53792-2455. *Telephone:* 608-263-5202. *Fax:* 608-263-5296. *E-mail:* ugadmit@son.wisc.edu.

GRADUATE PROGRAMS

Expenses (2010-11) *Tuition, state resident:* full-time $10,940; part-time $685 per credit. *Tuition, nonresident:* full-time $25,108; part-time $1571 per credit. *Required fees:* full-time $1054; part-time $67 per credit; part-time $527 per term.
Financial Aid 55% of graduate students in nursing programs received some form of financial aid in 2009-10. 12 fellowships with full tuition reimbursements available (averaging $22,000 per year), 6 research assistantships with full tuition reimbursements available (averaging $21,000 per year), 7 teaching assistantships with full tuition reimbursements available (averaging $14,000 per year) were awarded; career-related internships or fieldwork, Federal Work-Study, institutionally sponsored loans, scholarships, traineeships, and unspecified assistantships also available. Aid available to part-time students. *Financial aid application deadline:* 3/1.
Contact Ms. Marcia Voss, Graduate Program Coordinator, School of Nursing, University of Wisconsin–Madison, 600 Highland Avenue, K6/140, Clinical Science Center, Madison, WI 53792-2455. *Telephone:* 608-263-5258. *Fax:* 608-263-5296. *E-mail:* mlvoss@wisc.edu.

DOCTORAL DEGREE PROGRAM

Degree PhD
Available Programs Doctorate; Post-Baccalaureate Doctorate.
Areas of Study Aging, bio-behavioral research, biology of health and illness, community health, faculty preparation, family health, gerontology, health policy, health promotion/disease prevention, human health and illness, information systems, nursing education, nursing research, oncology, women's health.
Program Entrance Requirements Minimum overall college GPA of 3.0, interview, 3 letters of recommendation, scholarly papers, vita, writing sample, GRE General Test. Application deadline: 1/15 (fall), 9/15 (spring). Application fee: $56.
Degree Requirements 60 total credit hours, dissertation, written exam, residency.

POSTDOCTORAL PROGRAM

Areas of Study Adolescent health, aging, cancer care, chronic illness, community health, family health, gerontology, health promotion/disease prevention, individualized study, nursing informatics, nursing interventions, nursing research, vulnerable population, women's health.
Postdoctoral Program Contact Carol Aspinwall,

CONTINUING EDUCATION PROGRAM

Contact Ms. LeaRae Galarowicz, Clinical Professor, School of Nursing, University of Wisconsin–Madison, 600 Highland Avenue, H6/158, Clinical Science Center, Madison, WI 53792-2455. *Telephone:* 608-263-5336. *Fax:* 608-263-5332. *E-mail:* lbgalaro@facstaff.wisc.edu.

See full description on page 502.

University of Wisconsin–Milwaukee

College of Nursing
Milwaukee, Wisconsin

http://www.nursing.uwm.edu/
Founded in 1956

DEGREES • BSN • DNP • MN • MSN/MBA • PHD

Nursing Program Faculty 34 (100% with doctorates).
Baccalaureate Enrollment 1,166 **Women** 88% **Men** 12% **Minority** 19% **International** 1% **Part-time** 27%
Graduate Enrollment 279 **Women** 89% **Men** 11% **Minority** 13% **International** 1% **Part-time** 75%
Distance Learning Courses Available.
Nursing Student Activities Sigma Theta Tau, Student Nurses' Association.

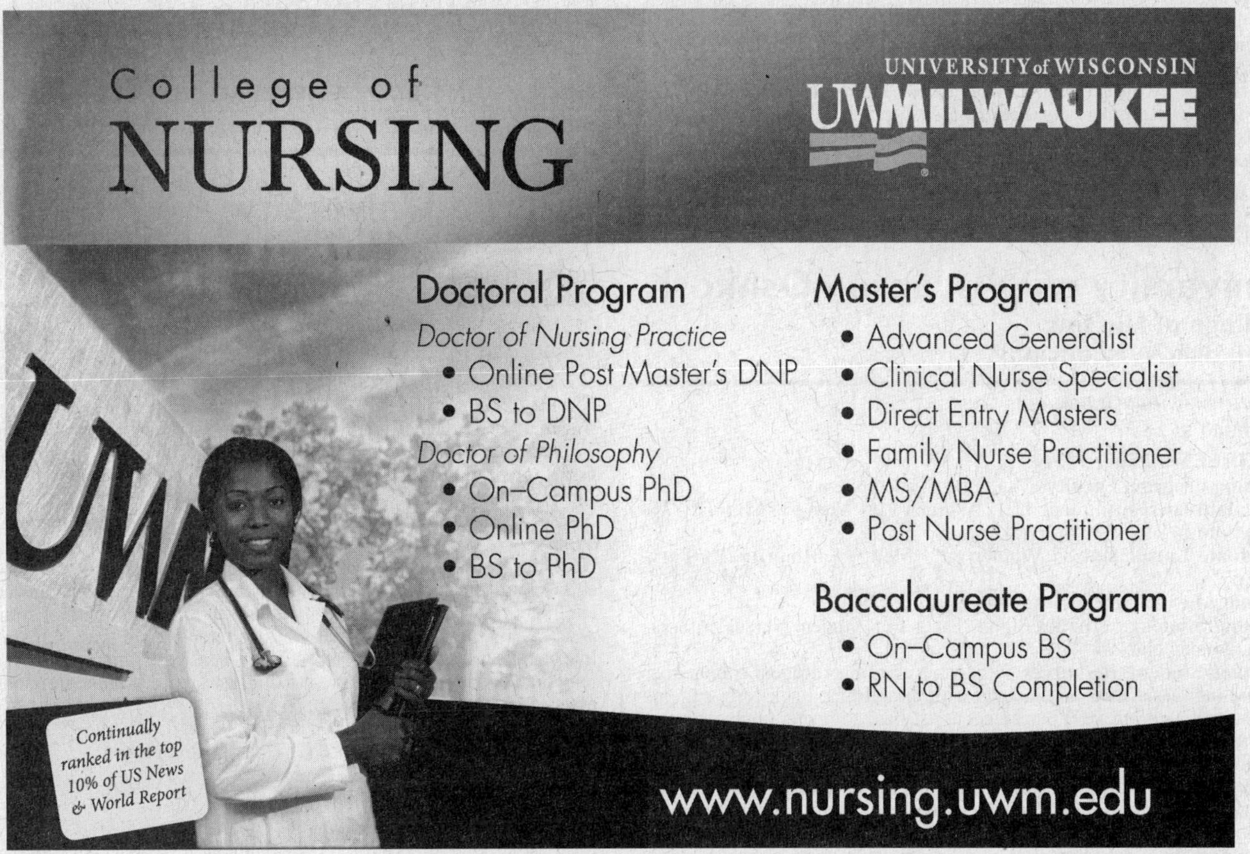

Nursing Student Resources Academic advising; academic or career counseling; campus computer network; computer lab; computer-assisted instruction; e-mail services; interactive nursing skills videos; Internet; learning resource lab; library services; nursing audiovisuals; remedial services; skills, simulation, or other laboratory; tutoring.
Library Facilities 1.4 million volumes (330,089 in health, 179,089 in nursing); 8,240 periodical subscriptions (926 health-care related).

BACCALAUREATE PROGRAMS

Degree BSN
Available Programs Generic Baccalaureate; RN Baccalaureate.
Site Options West Bend, WI; Kenosha, WI.
Study Options Full-time and part-time.
Program Entrance Requirements Minimum overall college GPA of 2.5, transcript of college record, written essay, high school biology, high school chemistry, high school foreign language, 3 years high school math, 3 years high school science, high school transcript, minimum high school GPA of 2.0, minimum GPA in nursing prerequisites of 2.5, prerequisite course work. Transfer students are accepted. *Application deadline:* 1/15 (fall), 8/15 (spring).
Advanced Placement Credit given for nursing courses completed elsewhere dependent upon specific evaluations.
Expenses (2010-11) *Tuition, state resident:* full-time $7270; part-time $303 per credit. *Tuition, nonresident:* full-time $16,998; part-time $708 per credit. *Room and board:* $17,800; room only: $10,400 per academic year. *Required fees:* full-time $882; part-time $441 per term.
Financial Aid 70% of baccalaureate students in nursing programs received some form of financial aid in 2009-10.
Contact Ms. Donna Wier, Senior Advisor, College of Nursing, University of Wisconsin–Milwaukee, PO Box 413, Student Affairs, Milwaukee, WI 53201. *Telephone:* 414-229-5481. *Fax:* 414-229-5554. *E-mail:* ddw@uwm.edu.

GRADUATE PROGRAMS

Expenses (2010-11) *Tuition, state resident:* full-time $9564; part-time $598 per credit. *Tuition, nonresident:* full-time $22,852; part-time $1428 per credit. *International tuition:* $22,852 full-time. *Room and board:* $9420; room only: $2020 per academic year. *Required fees:* full-time $882; part-time $441 per term.
Financial Aid 69% of graduate students in nursing programs received some form of financial aid in 2009-10. 8 teaching assistantships were awarded; career-related internships or fieldwork, Federal Work-Study, and unspecified assistantships also available. Aid available to part-time students. *Financial aid application deadline:* 4/15.
Contact Ms. Robin Jens, Director, Student Services, College of Nursing, University of Wisconsin–Milwaukee, PO Box 413, Student Affairs, Milwaukee, WI 53201. *Telephone:* 414-229-2494. *Fax:* 414-229-5554. *E-mail:* rjens@uwm.edu.

MASTER'S DEGREE PROGRAM

Degrees MN; MSN/MBA
Available Programs Master's; Master's for Non-Nursing College Graduates.
Concentrations Available Clinical nurse leader.
Site Options Kenosha, WI.
Study Options Full-time and part-time.
Program Entrance Requirements Minimum overall college GPA of 2.75, transcript of college record, written essay, interview, 3 letters of recommendation, prerequisite course work, resume, statistics course, GRE General Test or MAT. *Application deadline:* 1/1 (fall), 9/1 (spring). *Application fee:* $56.
Advanced Placement Credit given for nursing courses completed elsewhere dependent upon specific evaluations.
Degree Requirements 33 total credit hours, thesis or project.

DOCTORAL DEGREE PROGRAM

Degree DNP
Available Programs Doctorate; Post-Baccalaureate Doctorate.
Areas of Study Advanced practice nursing, clinical practice, community health, family health, health-care systems, human health and illness, individualized study, maternity-newborn.
Online Degree Options Yes.
Program Entrance Requirements Minimum overall college GPA of 2.75, interview, 3 letters of recommendation, statistics course, vita, writing sample, GRE. Application deadline: 1/1 (fall), 9/1 (spring), 11/1 (summer). Application fee: $56.
Degree Requirements 64 total credit hours, residency.

Degree PhD
Available Programs Doctorate; Post-Baccalaureate Doctorate.

Areas of Study Individualized study, nursing research.
Online Degree Options Yes.
Program Entrance Requirements Minimum overall college GPA of 3.2, interview, 3 letters of recommendation, MSN or equivalent, scholarly papers, vita, writing sample. *Application deadline*: 1/1 (fall), 9/1 (spring), 11/1 (summer). *Application fee*: $56.
Degree Requirements 49 total credit hours, dissertation, oral exam, written exam.

See full description on page 504.

University of Wisconsin–Oshkosh

College of Nursing
Oshkosh, Wisconsin

http://www.uwosh.edu/con
Founded in 1871

DEGREES • BSN • MSN
Nursing Program Faculty 69 (17% with doctorates).
Baccalaureate Enrollment 1,212 **Women** 91% **Men** 9% **Minority** 7% **Part-time** 14%
Graduate Enrollment 85 **Women** 91% **Men** 9% **Minority** 2% **Part-time** 81%
Distance Learning Courses Available.
Nursing Student Activities Sigma Theta Tau, Student Nurses' Association, nursing club.
Nursing Student Resources Academic advising; academic or career counseling; assistance for students with disabilities; bookstore; campus computer network; career placement assistance; computer lab; computer-assisted instruction; daycare for children of students; e-mail services; employment services for current students; externships; housing assistance; interactive nursing skills videos; Internet; learning resource lab; library services; nursing audiovisuals; other; paid internships; placement services for program completers; remedial services; resume preparation assistance; skills, simulation, or other laboratory; tutoring; unpaid internships.
Library Facilities 446,774 volumes; 5,219 periodical subscriptions.

BACCALAUREATE PROGRAMS

Degree BSN
Available Programs Accelerated Baccalaureate; Accelerated Baccalaureate for Second Degree; Accelerated RN Baccalaureate; Baccalaureate for Second Degree; Generic Baccalaureate; RN Baccalaureate.
Site Options Sheboygan, WI; Manitowoc, WI; Wausau, WI.
Study Options Full-time and part-time.
Online Degree Options Yes.
Program Entrance Requirements Minimum overall college GPA of 2.75, transcript of college record, CPR certification, written essay, health exam, 3 years high school math, 3 years high school science, immunizations, interview, minimum high school rank 50%, minimum GPA in nursing prerequisites of 2.75, prerequisite course work. Transfer students are accepted. *Application deadline:* 1/30 (fall), 8/30 (spring).
Advanced Placement Credit by examination available. Credit given for nursing courses completed elsewhere dependent upon specific evaluations.
Contact ***Telephone:*** 920-424-1028. *Fax:* 920-424-0123.

GRADUATE PROGRAMS

Contact ***Telephone:*** 920-424-2106. *Fax:* 920-424-0123.

MASTER'S DEGREE PROGRAM

Degree MSN
Available Programs Master's.
Concentrations Available Clinical nurse leader; nursing education. *Nurse practitioner programs in:* adult health, family health.
Study Options Full-time and part-time.
Program Entrance Requirements Computer literacy, minimum overall college GPA of 3.0, transcript of college record, CPR certification, written essay, immunizations, interview, 3 letters of recommendation, physical assessment course, prerequisite course work, resume, statistics course. *Application deadline:* 4/1 (fall). *Application fee:* $56.
Advanced Placement Credit given for nursing courses completed elsewhere dependent upon specific evaluations.
Degree Requirements 48 total credit hours, thesis or project.

POST-MASTER'S PROGRAM

Areas of Study Nursing education. *Nurse practitioner programs in:* adult health, family health.

CONTINUING EDUCATION PROGRAM

Contact ***Telephone:*** 920-424-1129. *Fax:* 920-424-1803.

Viterbo University

School of Nursing
La Crosse, Wisconsin

http://www.viterbo.edu/
Founded in 1890

DEGREES • BSN • MSN
Nursing Program Faculty 32 (8% with doctorates).
Baccalaureate Enrollment 674 **Women** 94% **Men** 6% **Minority** 3% **International** 1% **Part-time** 5%
Graduate Enrollment 60 **Women** 99% **Men** 1% **Minority** 1% **Part-time** 15%
Nursing Student Activities Sigma Theta Tau, Student Nurses' Association.
Nursing Student Resources Academic advising; academic or career counseling; assistance for students with disabilities; bookstore; campus computer network; career placement assistance; computer lab; computer-assisted instruction; e-mail services; interactive nursing skills videos; Internet; learning resource lab; library services; nursing audiovisuals; remedial services; resume preparation assistance; skills, simulation, or other laboratory; tutoring.
Library Facilities 89,072 volumes (5,200 in health, 3,398 in nursing); 30,094 periodical subscriptions (312 health-care related).

BACCALAUREATE PROGRAMS

Degree BSN
Available Programs Generic Baccalaureate; RN Baccalaureate.
Site Options Rochester, MN; Madison, WI; Janesville, WI.
Study Options Full-time and part-time.
Program Entrance Requirements Minimum overall college GPA of 2.75, transcript of college record, CPR certification, health exam, high school chemistry, 2 years high school math, 2 years high school science, high school transcript, immunizations, minimum high school GPA of 3.0, minimum high school rank 55%, minimum GPA in nursing prerequisites of 2.75, prerequisite course work. Transfer students are accepted. *Application deadline:* Applications may be processed on a rolling basis for some programs. *Application fee:* $25.
Advanced Placement Credit given for nursing courses completed elsewhere dependent upon specific evaluations.
Expenses (2010-11) *Tuition:* full-time $21,280; part-time $625 per credit. *Room and board:* $3830; room only: $2035 per academic year. *Required fees:* full-time $800.
Financial Aid 90% of baccalaureate students in nursing programs received some form of financial aid in 2009-10.
Contact Mr. Robert Forget, Dean of Admission, School of Nursing, Viterbo University, 900 Viterbo Drive, La Crosse, WI 54601. *Telephone:* 608-796-3012. *Fax:* 608-796-3050. *E-mail:* rlforget@viterbo.edu.

GRADUATE PROGRAMS

Expenses (2010-11) *Tuition:* part-time $655 per credit.
Financial Aid 33% of graduate students in nursing programs received some form of financial aid in 2009-10.
Contact Dr. Bonnie Nesbitt, Director, School of Nursing, Viterbo University, 900 Viterbo Drive, La Crosse, WI 54601. *Telephone:* 608-796-3688. *Fax:* 608-796-3668. *E-mail:* bjnesbitt@viterbo.edu.

MASTER'S DEGREE PROGRAM

Degree MSN
Available Programs Master's.
Concentrations Available Clinical nurse leader; nursing education. *Nurse practitioner programs in:* adult health, family health.
Study Options Full-time and part-time.
Program Entrance Requirements Clinical experience, computer literacy, minimum overall college GPA of 3.0, transcript of college record, CPR certification, written essay, immunizations, interview, 3 letters of recommendation, nursing research course, physical assessment course,

resume, statistics course. *Application deadline:* 2/15 (fall). *Application fee:* $50.

Advanced Placement Credit given for nursing courses completed elsewhere dependent upon specific evaluations.

Degree Requirements 40 total credit hours, thesis or project.

POST-MASTER'S PROGRAM

Areas of Study Nursing education. *Nurse practitioner programs in:* adult health, family health.

CONTINUING EDUCATION PROGRAM

Contact Ms. Delayne Vogel, Continuing Education Coordinator, School of Nursing, Viterbo University, 900 Viterbo Drive, La Crosse, WI 54601. *Telephone:* 608-796-3692. *Fax:* 608-796-3668. *E-mail:* dgvogel@viterbo.edu.

Wisconsin Lutheran College

Nursing Program
Milwaukee, Wisconsin

Founded in 1973

DEGREE • BSN

Nursing Program Faculty 2

Baccalaureate Enrollment 14

Nursing Student Activities Student Nurses' Association.

Nursing Student Resources Academic advising; academic or career counseling; assistance for students with disabilities; bookstore; campus computer network; career placement assistance; computer lab; computer-assisted instruction; e-mail services; externships; housing assistance; interactive nursing skills videos; Internet; learning resource lab; library services; nursing audiovisuals; skills, simulation, or other laboratory; tutoring.

Library Facilities 78,107 volumes; 310 periodical subscriptions.

BACCALAUREATE PROGRAMS

Degree BSN

Available Programs Generic Baccalaureate.

Study Options Full-time.

Program Entrance Requirements Minimum overall college GPA of 2.75, transcript of college record, written essay, high school foreign language, interview, 3 letters of recommendation, minimum GPA in nursing prerequisites of 2.0, prerequisite course work. Transfer students are accepted. *Application deadline:* 3/15 (spring).

Expenses (2009-10) *Tuition:* full-time $27,000. *Room and board:* $10,000 per academic year.

Financial Aid 90% of baccalaureate students in nursing programs received some form of financial aid in 2008-09.

Contact Admissions Office, Nursing Program, Wisconsin Lutheran College, 8800 West Bluemound Road, Milwaukee, WI 53226. *Telephone:* 414-443-8800.

CONTINUING EDUCATION PROGRAM

Contact School of Nursing, Nursing Program, Wisconsin Lutheran College, 8800 West Bluemound Road, Milwaukee, WI 53226. *Telephone:* 414-443-8800.

WYOMING

University of Wyoming

Fay W. Whitney School of Nursing
Laramie, Wyoming

http://www.uwyo.edu/nursing
Founded in 1886

DEGREES • BSN • MS

Nursing Program Faculty 38 (29% with doctorates).
Baccalaureate Enrollment 418 **Women** 89% **Men** 11% **Minority** 8% **International** 1% **Part-time** 65%
Graduate Enrollment 69 **Women** 88% **Men** 12% **Minority** 7% **Part-time** 62%
Distance Learning Courses Available.
Nursing Student Activities Sigma Theta Tau, Student Nurses' Association.
Nursing Student Resources Academic advising; academic or career counseling; assistance for students with disabilities; bookstore; campus computer network; career placement assistance; computer lab; computer-assisted instruction; e-mail services; employment services for current students; externships; housing assistance; interactive nursing skills videos; Internet; learning resource lab; library services; nursing audiovisuals; paid internships; remedial services; resume preparation assistance; skills, simulation, or other laboratory; tutoring; unpaid internships.
Library Facilities 3 million volumes (56,231 in health); 75,864 periodical subscriptions (1,689 health-care related).

BACCALAUREATE PROGRAMS

Degree BSN
Available Programs ADN to Baccalaureate; Accelerated Baccalaureate for Second Degree; Generic Baccalaureate.
Study Options Full-time.
Online Degree Options Yes.
Program Entrance Requirements Transcript of college record, CPR certification, written essay, immunizations, 2 letters of recommendation, minimum GPA in nursing prerequisites of 2.75, professional liability insurance/malpractice insurance, prerequisite course work. Transfer students are accepted. *Application deadline:* 2/1 (fall). *Application fee:* $30.
Advanced Placement Credit given for nursing courses completed elsewhere dependent upon specific evaluations.
Expenses (2010-11) *Tuition, state resident:* part-time $94 per credit hour. *Tuition, nonresident:* part-time $358 per credit hour. *Required fees:* full-time $906; part-time $30 per credit; part-time $20 per term.
Financial Aid ***Gift aid (need-based):*** Federal Pell, FSEOG, state, private, college/university gift aid from institutional funds. *Loans:* Perkins, alternative loans. *Work-study:* Federal Work-Study. *Financial aid application deadline (priority):* 2/1.
Contact Ms. Debbie A. Shoefelt, Credentials Analyst/Academic Advisor, Fay W. Whitney School of Nursing, University of Wyoming, Department 3065, 1000 East University Avenue, Laramie, WY 82071. *Telephone:* 307-766-4292. *Fax:* 307-766-4294. *E-mail:* basicbsn@uwyo.edu.

GRADUATE PROGRAMS

Expenses (2010-11) *Tuition, state resident:* part-time $183 per credit hour. *Tuition, nonresident:* part-time $523 per credit hour. *Required fees:* full-time $906; part-time $30 per credit; part-time $20 per term.
Financial Aid Research assistantships (averaging $10,062 per year), teaching assistantships (averaging $10,062 per year) were awarded; career-related internships or fieldwork, institutionally sponsored loans, scholarships, traineeships, and unspecified assistantships also available.
Contact Ms. Crystal McFadden, Office Associate, Fay W. Whitney School of Nursing, University of Wyoming, Department 3065, 1000 East University Avenue, Laramie, WY 82071. *Telephone:* 307-766-6568. *Fax:* 307-766-4294. *E-mail:* gradnurse@uwyo.edu.

MASTER'S DEGREE PROGRAM

Degree MS
Available Programs Master's; Master's for Nurses with Non-Nursing Degrees.
Concentrations Available Nursing education. *Nurse practitioner programs in:* family health, psychiatric/mental health.
Study Options Full-time and part-time.
Online Degree Options Yes.
Program Entrance Requirements Minimum overall college GPA of 3.0, transcript of college record, CPR certification, written essay, immu-

nizations, interview, 3 letters of recommendation, professional liability insurance/malpractice insurance, resume, statistics course, GRE General Test. *Application deadline:* 2/1 (fall). *Application fee:* $30.

Advanced Placement Credit given for nursing courses completed elsewhere dependent upon specific evaluations.

Degree Requirements 53 total credit hours, thesis or project.

POST-MASTER'S PROGRAM
Areas of Study Nursing education. *Nurse practitioner programs in:* family health, psychiatric/mental health.

CANADA

ALBERTA

Athabasca University
Centre for Nursing and Health Studies
Athabasca, Alberta

http://www.athabascau.ca/cnhs/
Founded in 1970

DEGREES • BN • MN • MN/MBA • MN/MHSA
Nursing Program Faculty 112 (49% with doctorates).
Baccalaureate Enrollment 2,984
Graduate Enrollment 1,214
Distance Learning Courses Available.
Nursing Student Activities Student Nurses' Association.
Nursing Student Resources Academic advising; academic or career counseling; assistance for students with disabilities; bookstore; campus computer network; computer lab; computer-assisted instruction; e-mail services; interactive nursing skills videos; Internet; library services; nursing audiovisuals; remedial services; skills, simulation, or other laboratory; tutoring.
Library Facilities 178,808 volumes; 32,619 periodical subscriptions.

BACCALAUREATE PROGRAMS
Degree BN
Available Programs Generic Baccalaureate; LPN to RN Baccalaureate; RN Baccalaureate.
Site Options Calgary, AB.
Study Options Full-time and part-time.
Program Entrance Requirements Minimum overall college GPA of 2.5, transcript of college record, CPR certification, high school biology, 3 years high school math, 3 years high school science, high school transcript, immunizations, minimum high school GPA of 2.0, minimum GPA in nursing prerequisites of 2.0, RN licensure. Transfer students are accepted. *Application deadline:* Applications may be processed on a rolling basis for some programs.
Advanced Placement Credit by examination available. Credit given for nursing courses completed elsewhere dependent upon specific evaluations.
Expenses (2010-11) *Tuition, state resident:* part-time CAN$646 per course. *Tuition, nonresident:* part-time CAN$751 per course. *International tuition:* CAN$1216 full-time.
Contact Gayle Deren-Purdy, Undergraduate Student Advisor, Centre for Nursing and Health Studies, Athabasca University, 1 University Drive, Athabasca, AB T9S 3A3. *Telephone:* 800-788-9041 Ext. 6446. *Fax:* 780-675-6468. *E-mail:* gayled@athabascau.ca.

GRADUATE PROGRAMS
Expenses (2010-11) *Tuition, state resident:* part-time CAN$1145 per course. *Tuition, nonresident:* part-time CAN$1145 per course. *International tuition:* CAN$1345 full-time.
Contact Ms. Donna Dunn Hart, Graduate Student Advisor, Centre for Nursing and Health Studies, Athabasca University, 1 University Drive, Athabasca, AB T9S 3A3. *Telephone:* 800-788-9041 Ext. 6300. *Fax:* 780-675-6468. *E-mail:* donnad@athabascau.ca.

MASTER'S DEGREE PROGRAM
Degrees MN; MN/MBA; MN/MHSA
Available Programs Master's; Master's for Nurses with Non-Nursing Degrees.
Concentrations Available Nursing administration; nursing education. *Nurse practitioner programs in:* community health, family health, primary care.
Study Options Full-time and part-time.
Online Degree Options Yes.
Program Entrance Requirements Clinical experience, computer literacy, minimum overall college GPA of 3.0, transcript of college record, written essay, 3 letters of recommendation, resume. *Application deadline:* 3/1 (fall), 12/1 (spring). *Application fee:* CAN$80.
Advanced Placement Credit given for nursing courses completed elsewhere dependent upon specific evaluations.
Degree Requirements 33 total credit hours, thesis or project, comprehensive exam.

POST-MASTER'S PROGRAM
Areas of Study *Nurse practitioner programs in:* community health, family health.

University of Alberta
Faculty of Nursing
Edmonton, Alberta

http://www.nursing.ualberta.ca/
Founded in 1906

DEGREES • BSCN • MN • PHD
Nursing Program Faculty 110 (50% with doctorates).
Baccalaureate Enrollment 1,600 **Women** 93% **Men** 7% **International** 1% **Part-time** 7%
Graduate Enrollment 200 **Women** 92% **Men** 8% **International** 7% **Part-time** 60%
Distance Learning Courses Available.
Nursing Student Activities Nursing Honor Society, Sigma Theta Tau, Student Nurses' Association.
Nursing Student Resources Academic advising; academic or career counseling; assistance for students with disabilities; bookstore; campus computer network; career placement assistance; computer lab; computer-assisted instruction; daycare for children of students; e-mail services; employment services for current students; housing assistance; interactive nursing skills videos; Internet; learning resource lab; library services; nursing audiovisuals; other; paid internships; remedial services; resume preparation assistance; skills, simulation, or other laboratory; tutoring; unpaid internships.
Library Facilities 9.7 million volumes (115,000 in health, 19,000 in nursing); 2,400 periodical subscriptions health-care related.

BACCALAUREATE PROGRAMS
Degree BScN
Available Programs Accelerated Baccalaureate for Second Degree; Baccalaureate for Second Degree; Generic Baccalaureate; RN Baccalaureate; RPN to Baccalaureate.
Site Options Fort McMurray, AB; Red Deer, AB; Grande Prairie, AB.
Study Options Full-time.
Program Entrance Requirements Minimum overall college GPA of 3.0, transcript of college record, CPR certification, health exam, high school biology, high school chemistry, 3 years high school math, 3 years high school science, high school transcript, immunizations, minimum

high school GPA of 3.0, minimum high school rank 78%. Transfer students are accepted. *Application deadline:* 2/1 (fall). *Application fee:* CAN$115.

Advanced Placement Credit by examination available.

Financial Aid 50% of baccalaureate students in nursing programs received some form of financial aid in 2009-10.

Contact Ms. Kristan Morin, Student Recruiter, Faculty of Nursing, University of Alberta, 2-143 Clinical Sciences Building, Edmonton, AB T6G 2G3. *Telephone:* 780-492-1242. *Fax:* 780-492-2551. *E-mail:* kristan.morin@ualberta.ca.

GRADUATE PROGRAMS

Expenses (2010-11) *Tuition, area resident:* full-time CAN$6000. *International tuition:* CAN$8750 full-time.

Financial Aid 47% of graduate students in nursing programs received some form of financial aid in 2009-10. 12 fellowships with partial tuition reimbursements available (averaging $23,868 per year), 27 research assistantships with partial tuition reimbursements available (averaging $6,186 per year), 12 teaching assistantships with partial tuition reimbursements available (averaging $2,365 per year) were awarded; institutionally sponsored loans and scholarships also available.

Contact Yvette Labiuk, Graduate Services Administrator, Faculty of Nursing, University of Alberta, Clinical Sciences Building, 5-111, Edmonton, AB T6G 2G3. *Telephone:* 780-492-8055. *Fax:* 780-492-2551. *E-mail:* yvette.labiuk@ualberta.ca.

MASTER'S DEGREE PROGRAM

Degree MN

Available Programs Master's.

Concentrations Available *Nurse practitioner programs in:* adult health, gerontology.

Study Options Full-time and part-time.

Program Entrance Requirements Clinical experience, computer literacy, minimum overall college GPA of 3.0, transcript of college record, CPR certification, 3 letters of recommendation, nursing research course, physical assessment course, resume, statistics course. *Application deadline:* 10/1 (fall). *Application fee:* CAN$100.

Advanced Placement Credit given for nursing courses completed elsewhere dependent upon specific evaluations.

Degree Requirements 39 total credit hours, thesis or project.

POST-MASTER'S PROGRAM

Areas of Study *Nurse practitioner programs in:* adult health, gerontology.

DOCTORAL DEGREE PROGRAM

Degree PhD

Available Programs Doctorate.

Areas of Study Aging, community health, ethics, family health, gerontology, health policy, health promotion/disease prevention, health-care systems, nursing education, nursing policy, nursing research.

Program Entrance Requirements Clinical experience, minimum overall college GPA of 3.0, 3 letters of recommendation, MSN or equivalent, scholarly papers, statistics course, vita, writing sample. Application deadline: 10/1 (fall). Application fee: $100.

Degree Requirements 36 total credit hours, dissertation, oral exam, written exam, residency.

POSTDOCTORAL PROGRAM

Postdoctoral Program Contact Dr. Phyllis Giovannetti, Associate Dean, Graduate Education, Faculty of Nursing, University of Alberta, Clinical Sciences Building, 3rd Floor, Edmonton, AB T6G 2G3. *Telephone:* 780-492-6764. *Fax:* 780-492-2551. *E-mail:* phyllis.giovannetti@ualberta.ca.

University of Calgary

Faculty of Nursing
Calgary, Alberta

http://www.ucalgary.ca/nu
Founded in 1945

DEGREES • BN • MN • PHD

Nursing Program Faculty 50 (85% with doctorates).

Baccalaureate Enrollment 930 **Women** 90% **Men** 10% **Minority** 5% **International** 1%

Graduate Enrollment 110 **Women** 95% **Men** 5% **Minority** 1% **International** 1% **Part-time** 21%

Nursing Student Activities Student Nurses' Association.

Nursing Student Resources Academic advising; academic or career counseling; assistance for students with disabilities; bookstore; campus computer network; career placement assistance; computer lab; computer-assisted instruction; daycare for children of students; e-mail services; externships; housing assistance; interactive nursing skills videos; Internet; learning resource lab; library services; nursing audiovisuals; remedial services; resume preparation assistance; skills, simulation, or other laboratory; tutoring.

Library Facilities 3.3 million volumes; 37,285 periodical subscriptions.

BACCALAUREATE PROGRAMS

Degree BN

Available Programs Accelerated Baccalaureate; Accelerated Baccalaureate for Second Degree; Baccalaureate for Second Degree; Generic Baccalaureate; RN Baccalaureate.

Site Options Medicine Hat, AB.

Study Options Full-time.

Program Entrance Requirements Minimum overall college GPA of 3.3, transcript of college record, CPR certification, health exam, high school biology, high school chemistry, 3 years high school math, high school transcript, immunizations, minimum high school rank 78%. Transfer students are accepted.

Advanced Placement Credit by examination available. Credit given for nursing courses completed elsewhere dependent upon specific evaluations.

Contact ***Telephone:*** 403-220-4636. *Fax:* 403-284-4803.

GRADUATE PROGRAMS

Contact ***Telephone:*** 403-220-6241. *Fax:* 403-284-4803.

MASTER'S DEGREE PROGRAM

Degree MN

Available Programs Master's; RN to Master's.

Concentrations Available *Clinical nurse specialist programs in:* acute care, adult health, cardiovascular, community health, critical care, family health, gerontology, maternity-newborn, medical-surgical, parent-child, pediatric, perinatal, psychiatric/mental health, public health, rehabilitation, women's health. *Nurse practitioner programs in:* acute care, adult health, neonatal health.

Study Options Full-time and part-time.

Program Entrance Requirements Clinical experience, computer literacy, minimum overall college GPA of 3.0, transcript of college record, CPR certification, written essay, 3 letters of recommendation, nursing research course, statistics course.

Advanced Placement Credit given for nursing courses completed elsewhere dependent upon specific evaluations.

Degree Requirements 30 total credit hours, thesis or project, comprehensive exam.

POST-MASTER'S PROGRAM

Areas of Study *Nurse practitioner programs in:* acute care, adult health, neonatal health.

DOCTORAL DEGREE PROGRAM

Degree PhD

Available Programs Doctorate; Doctorate for Nurses with Non-Nursing Degrees.

Areas of Study Advanced practice nursing, aging, clinical practice, community health, critical care, ethics, family health, gerontology, health promotion/disease prevention, health-care systems, human health and illness, illness and transition, individualized study, maternity-newborn, neuro-behavior, nursing research, women's health.

Program Entrance Requirements Clinical experience, minimum overall college GPA of 3.0, 3 letters of recommendation, MSN or equivalent, scholarly papers, statistics course, vita, writing sample.

Degree Requirements Dissertation, oral exam, written exam.

University of Lethbridge

School of Health Sciences

Lethbridge, Alberta

http://www.uleth.ca/healthsciences/

Founded in 1967

DEGREES • BN • M SC

Nursing Program Faculty 34 (15% with doctorates).

Baccalaureate Enrollment 679 **Women** 91% **Men** 9% **Part-time** 1%

Graduate Enrollment 14 **Women** 93% **Men** 7%

Nursing Student Activities Nursing club.

Nursing Student Resources Academic advising; academic or career counseling; assistance for students with disabilities; bookstore; campus computer network; computer lab; e-mail services; employment services for current students; housing assistance; interactive nursing skills videos; Internet; learning resource lab; library services; nursing audiovisuals; remedial services; resume preparation assistance; skills, simulation, or other laboratory; tutoring; unpaid internships.

Library Facilities 573,058 volumes (14,743 in health, 2,554 in nursing); 1,262 periodical subscriptions (11,168 health-care related).

BACCALAUREATE PROGRAMS

Degree BN

Available Programs Accelerated Baccalaureate for Second Degree; Accelerated RN Baccalaureate; Generic Baccalaureate; RN Baccalaureate.

Site Options Lethbridge, AB.

Study Options Full-time.

Program Entrance Requirements CPR certification, high school biology, high school chemistry, 3 years high school math, 3 years high school science, high school transcript, immunizations, minimum high school rank 70%. Transfer students are accepted. *Application deadline:* 3/1 (fall). *Application fee:* CAN$75.

Advanced Placement Credit given for nursing courses completed elsewhere dependent upon specific evaluations.

Financial Aid ***Gift aid (need-based):*** private, college/university gift aid from institutional funds. *Financial aid application deadline:* Continuous.

Contact Mrs. Sherry Hogeweide, Academic Advisor, School of Health Sciences, University of Lethbridge, 4401 University Drive, Lethbridge, AB T1K 3M4. *Telephone:* 403-329-2220. *Fax:* 403-329-2668. *E-mail:* health.sciences@uleth.ca.

GRADUATE PROGRAMS

Contact Dr. David Gregory, Grad Studies Coordinator, School of Health Sciences, University of Lethbridge, 4401 University Drive, Lethbridge, AB T1K 3M4. *Telephone:* 403-329-2432. *Fax:* 403-329-2668. *E-mail:* health.sciences@uleth.ca.

MASTER'S DEGREE PROGRAM

Degree M Sc

Available Programs Master's.

Study Options Full-time and part-time.

Program Entrance Requirements Clinical experience; minimum overall college GPA of 3.0, transcript of college record, CPR certification, immunizations, interview. *Application deadline:* 3/1 (fall).

Advanced Placement Credit given for nursing courses completed elsewhere dependent upon specific evaluations.

Degree Requirements Thesis or project, comprehensive exam.

BRITISH COLUMBIA

British Columbia Institute of Technology

School of Health Sciences

Burnaby, British Columbia

http://www.health.bcit.ca/nursing/

Founded in 1964

DEGREE • BSN

Nursing Program Faculty 88

Baccalaureate Enrollment 492 **Women** 90% **Men** 10%

Distance Learning Courses Available.

Nursing Student Activities Student Nurses' Association.

Nursing Student Resources Academic advising; academic or career counseling; assistance for students with disabilities; bookstore; campus computer network; computer lab; computer-assisted instruction; e-mail services; housing assistance; interactive nursing skills videos; Internet; learning resource lab; library services; nursing audiovisuals; paid internships; resume preparation assistance; skills, simulation, or other laboratory; tutoring; unpaid internships.

Library Facilities 169,404 volumes (10,000 in health, 2,600 in nursing); 1,080 periodical subscriptions (110 health-care related).

BACCALAUREATE PROGRAMS

Degree BSN

Available Programs RN Baccalaureate; RPN to Baccalaureate.

Study Options Full-time.

Program Entrance Requirements Transcript of college record, CPR certification, written essay, high school biology, high school chemistry, 11 years high school math, 12 years high school science, high school transcript, immunizations, 2 letters of recommendation, prerequisite course work. Transfer students are accepted. *Application deadline:* 1/31 (fall), 8/31 (winter). *Application fee:* CAN$60.

Advanced Placement Credit given for nursing courses completed elsewhere dependent upon specific evaluations.

Expenses (2010-11) *Tuition, area resident:* full-time CAN$5510. *Required fees:* full-time CAN$520.

Financial Aid 70% of baccalaureate students in nursing programs received some form of financial aid in 2009-10. *Financial aid application deadline:* Continuous.

Contact Ms. Loreen Martin, Administrative Coordinator, School of Health Sciences, British Columbia Institute of Technology, 3700 Willingdon Avenue, SE12, Room 418, Burnaby, BC V5G 3H2. *Telephone:* 604-432-8884. *Fax:* 604-436-9590. *E-mail:* loreen_martin@bcit.ca.

CONTINUING EDUCATION PROGRAM

Contact Ms. Pauline O'Reilly, Program Head, School of Health Sciences, British Columbia Institute of Technology, 3700 Willingdon Avenue, SE12, Room 328, Burnaby, BC V5G 3H2. *Telephone:* 604-451-7115. *E-mail:* pauline_o'reilly@bcit.ca.

Kwantlen Polytechnic University

Faculty of Community and Health Sciences

Surrey, British Columbia

http://www.kwantlen.ca

Founded in 1981

DEGREE • BSN

Nursing Program Faculty 60 (13% with doctorates).

Baccalaureate Enrollment 360 **Women** 90% **Men** 10% **Part-time** 13%

Nursing Student Activities Student Nurses' Association.

Nursing Student Resources Academic advising; academic or career counseling; assistance for students with disabilities; bookstore; campus computer network; career placement assistance; computer lab; computer-assisted instruction; e-mail services; employment services for current students; interactive nursing skills videos; Internet; learning resource lab; library services; nursing audiovisuals; remedial services; resume preparation assistance; skills, simulation, or other laboratory.

BACCALAUREATE PROGRAMS

Degree BSN
Available Programs Generic Baccalaureate; RN Baccalaureate.
Study Options Full-time.
Program Entrance Requirements CPR certification, health insurance, high school biology, high school chemistry, high school math, 2 years high school science, high school transcript, immunizations. Transfer students are accepted.
Advanced Placement Credit given for nursing courses completed elsewhere dependent upon specific evaluations.
Financial Aid ***Gift aid (need-based):*** college/university gift aid from institutional funds. *Loans:* provincial loans.
Contact Ms. Theresa Abraniuk, Admissions Assistant, Faculty of Community and Health Sciences, Kwantlen Polytechnic University, 12666 72nd Avenue, Surrey, BC V3W 2M8. *Telephone:* 604-599-2317. *E-mail:* theresa.abraniuk@kwantlen.ca.

Thompson Rivers University
School of Nursing
Kamloops, British Columbia

http://www.cariboo.bc.ca/nursing/index.html
Founded in 1970

DEGREE • BSN
Nursing Program Faculty 56
Library Facilities 273,900 volumes (7,326 in health, 2,275 in nursing); 13,709 periodical subscriptions (89 health-care related).

BACCALAUREATE PROGRAMS

Degree BSN
Study Options Full-time and part-time.
Program Entrance Requirements Minimum overall college GPA of 2.7, transcript of college record, CPR certification, health exam, high school biology, high school chemistry, high school foreign language, high school math, high school science, high school transcript, immunizations, interview, 2 letters of recommendation, minimum high school GPA of 2.3, minimum GPA in nursing prerequisites of 2.3. Transfer students are accepted.
Advanced Placement Credit given for nursing courses completed elsewhere dependent upon specific evaluations.
Contact ***Telephone:*** 250-828-5435. *Fax:* 250-828-5450.

CONTINUING EDUCATION PROGRAM

Contact ***Telephone:*** 250-828-5210. *Fax:* 250-371-5510.

Trinity Western University
Department of Nursing
Langley, British Columbia

http://www.twu.ca/
Founded in 1962

DEGREES • BSCN • MSN
Nursing Program Faculty 10 (50% with doctorates).
Baccalaureate Enrollment 174 **Women** 95% **Men** 5% **Minority** 15.2% **International** 11.6%
Graduate Enrollment 43 **Women** 98% **Men** 2% **Minority** 32% **Part-time** 91%
Distance Learning Courses Available.
Nursing Student Activities Student Nurses' Association.
Nursing Student Resources Academic advising; academic or career counseling; assistance for students with disabilities; bookstore; campus computer network; career placement assistance; computer lab; computer-assisted instruction; e-mail services; employment services for current students; housing assistance; interactive nursing skills videos; Internet; learning resource lab; library services; nursing audiovisuals; remedial services; resume preparation assistance; skills, simulation, or other laboratory; tutoring.
Library Facilities 190,565 volumes (2,500 in health, 800 in nursing); 11,000 periodical subscriptions (369 health-care related).

BACCALAUREATE PROGRAMS

Degree BScN
Available Programs Generic Baccalaureate.
Study Options Full-time.
Program Entrance Requirements Minimum overall college GPA of 2.0, CPR certification, health insurance, high school biology, high school chemistry, 1 year of high school math, 2 years high school science, high school transcript, immunizations, 2 letters of recommendation, minimum high school GPA of 2.7, minimum GPA in nursing prerequisites of 2.3. Transfer students are accepted. *Application deadline:* 2/28 (fall).
Advanced Placement Credit given for nursing courses completed elsewhere dependent upon specific evaluations.
Financial Aid 70% of baccalaureate students in nursing programs received some form of financial aid in 2009-10. *Gift aid (need-based):* private, college/university gift aid from institutional funds. *Loans:* federal and provincial loans. *Financial aid application deadline (priority):* 2/28.
Contact Dr. Landa Terblanche, Dean, Department of Nursing, Trinity Western University, 7600 Glover Road, Langley, BC V2Y 1Y1. *Telephone:* 604-888-7511 Ext. 3268. *Fax:* 604-513-2018. *E-mail:* landa.terblanche@twu.ca.

GRADUATE PROGRAMS

Expenses (2010-11) *Tuition:* full-time CAN$9900; part-time CAN$660 per credit hour. *Required fees:* part-time CAN$3 per credit.
Financial Aid 25% of graduate students in nursing programs received some form of financial aid in 2009-10.
Contact Ms. Guelda Redman, MSN Faculty Assistant, Department of Nursing, Trinity Western University, 7600 Glover Road, Langley, BC V2Y 1Y1. *Telephone:* 604-888-7511 Ext. 3270. *Fax:* 604-513-2012. *E-mail:* guelda.redman@twu.ca.

MASTER'S DEGREE PROGRAM

Degree MSN
Available Programs Accelerated Master's; Master's.
Concentrations Available Clinical nurse leader; health-care administration; nursing administration; nursing education. *Clinical nurse specialist programs in:* gerontology. *Nurse practitioner programs in:* gerontology.
Study Options Full-time and part-time.
Program Entrance Requirements Minimum overall college GPA of 3.0, transcript of college record, written essay, 3 letters of recommendation, resume, statistics course. *Application deadline:* 5/1 (summer).
Advanced Placement Credit given for nursing courses completed elsewhere dependent upon specific evaluations.
Degree Requirements 30 total credit hours, thesis or project.

The University of British Columbia
Program in Nursing
Vancouver, British Columbia

http://www.nursing.ubc.ca/
Founded in 1915

DEGREES • BSN • MA/MSM • MSN • PHD
Nursing Program Faculty 48 (60% with doctorates).
Baccalaureate Enrollment 300
Graduate Enrollment 250
Nursing Student Activities Nursing Honor Society, Sigma Theta Tau, Student Nurses' Association.
Nursing Student Resources Academic advising; academic or career counseling; assistance for students with disabilities; bookstore; campus computer network; career placement assistance; computer lab; computer-assisted instruction; daycare for children of students; e-mail services; employment services for current students; housing assistance; interactive nursing skills videos; Internet; learning resource lab; library services; nursing audiovisuals; skills, simulation, or other laboratory.
Library Facilities 6.4 million volumes; 778,063 periodical subscriptions.

BACCALAUREATE PROGRAMS

Degree BSN
Available Programs Accelerated Baccalaureate; Accelerated Baccalaureate for Second Degree.
Study Options Full-time.
Program Entrance Requirements Minimum overall college GPA of 3.6, transcript of college record, CPR certification, written essay, health

exam, health insurance, high school transcript, immunizations, interview, professional liability insurance/malpractice insurance, prerequisite course work.
Contact Nursing Programs, Program in Nursing, The University of British Columbia, T201-2211 Wesbrook Mall, Vancouver, BC V6T 2B5. *Telephone:* 604-822-7420. *Fax:* 604-822-7466. *E-mail:* information@nursing.ubc.ca.

GRADUATE PROGRAMS

Financial Aid 10% of graduate students in nursing programs received some form of financial aid in 2009-10. 4 fellowships (averaging $8,000 per year), 14 research assistantships (averaging $800 per year), 3 teaching assistantships were awarded.
Contact Peggy Faulkner, Graduate Records Officer, Program in Nursing, The University of British Columbia, T201-2211 Wesbrook Mall, Vancouver, BC V6T 2B5. *Telephone:* 604-822-7446. *Fax:* 604-822-7466. *E-mail:* gro@nursing.ubc.ca.

MASTER'S DEGREE PROGRAM

Degrees MA/MSM; MSN
Available Programs Master's.
Concentrations Available Nursing administration; nursing education. *Clinical nurse specialist programs in:* adult health, community health, family health, psychiatric/mental health, public health. *Nurse practitioner programs in:* family health, primary care.
Site Options Kamloops, BC.
Study Options Full-time and part-time.
Program Entrance Requirements Computer literacy, minimum overall college GPA of 3.3, transcript of college record, 3 letters of recommendation, resume, GRE.
Advanced Placement Credit given for nursing courses completed elsewhere dependent upon specific evaluations.
Degree Requirements 33 total credit hours, thesis or project.

DOCTORAL DEGREE PROGRAM

Degree PhD
Available Programs Doctorate.
Areas of Study Addiction/substance abuse, advanced practice nursing, aging, clinical practice, community health, ethics, faculty preparation, family health, gerontology, health policy, health promotion/disease prevention, health-care systems, human health and illness, illness and transition, individualized study, information systems, maternity-newborn, nursing administration, nursing education, nursing policy, nursing research, nursing science, oncology, urban health, women's health.
Program Entrance Requirements interview, 3 letters of recommendation, MSN or equivalent, vita, writing sample, GRE. Application deadline: 2/1 (fall). Applications may be processed on a rolling basis for some programs.
Degree Requirements 18 total credit hours, dissertation, oral exam, written exam, residency.

POSTDOCTORAL PROGRAM

Areas of Study Addiction/substance abuse, adolescent health, aging, cancer care, chronic illness, community health, family health, gerontology, health promotion/disease prevention, individualized study, infection prevention/skin care, information systems, neuro-behavior, nursing informatics, nursing interventions, nursing research, nursing science, outcomes, self-care, vulnerable population, women's health.
Postdoctoral Program Contact Dr. Colleen Varcoe, Associate Director, Research, Program in Nursing, The University of British Columbia, T201-2211 Wesbrook Mall, Vancouver, BC V6T 2B5. *Telephone:* 604-827-3121. *Fax:* 604-822-7466. *E-mail:* colleen.varcoe@nursing.ubc.ca.

University of Northern British Columbia

Nursing Programme
Prince George, British Columbia

http://www.unbc.ca/nursing/
Founded in 1994

DEGREES • BSCN • M SC N
Nursing Program Faculty 40 (18% with doctorates).
Baccalaureate Enrollment 600
Graduate Enrollment 60
Distance Learning Courses Available.
Nursing Student Activities Student Nurses' Association.
Nursing Student Resources Academic advising; academic or career counseling; assistance for students with disabilities; bookstore; campus computer network; computer lab; computer-assisted instruction; e-mail services; employment services for current students; externships; Internet; learning resource lab; library services; nursing audiovisuals; skills, simulation, or other laboratory.
Library Facilities 310,433 volumes (4,000 in health, 2,000 in nursing); 19,570 periodical subscriptions (300 health-care related).

BACCALAUREATE PROGRAMS

Degree BScN
Available Programs Generic Baccalaureate; RN Baccalaureate.
Site Options Prince George, BC; Quesnel, BC; Terrace, BC.
Study Options Full-time.
Program Entrance Requirements Minimum overall college GPA of 2.33, transcript of college record, CPR certification, health exam, high school biology, high school chemistry, 1 year of high school math, 4 years high school science, high school transcript, immunizations, minimum high school GPA of 2.3, minimum high school rank 65%, minimum GPA in nursing prerequisites of 2.0, professional liability insurance/malpractice insurance. Transfer students are accepted. *Application deadline:* 3/31 (fall). *Application fee:* CAN$35.
Advanced Placement Credit given for nursing courses completed elsewhere dependent upon specific evaluations.
Contact ***Telephone:*** 250-960-5645.

GRADUATE PROGRAMS

Contact ***Telephone:*** 250-960-5848. *Fax:* 250-960-6410.

MASTER'S DEGREE PROGRAM

Degree M Sc N
Available Programs Master's.
Concentrations Available *Nurse practitioner programs in:* family health.
Study Options Full-time and part-time.
Program Entrance Requirements Clinical experience, minimum overall college GPA of 3.0, transcript of college record, CPR certification, written essay, 3 letters of recommendation, nursing research course, professional liability insurance/malpractice insurance, prerequisite course work. *Application deadline:* 2/15 (fall). *Application fee:* CAN$75.
Advanced Placement Credit given for nursing courses completed elsewhere dependent upon specific evaluations.
Degree Requirements 51 total credit hours, thesis or project.

POSTDOCTORAL PROGRAM

Areas of Study Chronic illness, community health, family health, health promotion/disease prevention, individualized study, nursing interventions, nursing research, nursing science, outcomes, vulnerable population.
Postdoctoral Program Contact ***Telephone:*** 250-960-6507. *Fax:* 250-960-6410.

University of Victoria

School of Nursing
Victoria, British Columbia

http://web.uvic.ca/nurs/
Founded in 1963

DEGREES • BSN • MN • PHD
Nursing Program Faculty 21 (95% with doctorates).
Baccalaureate Enrollment 1,100 **Women** 95% **Men** 5% **Part-time** 50%
Nursing Student Activities Student Nurses' Association.
Nursing Student Resources Academic advising; assistance for students with disabilities; bookstore; campus computer network; computer lab; e-mail services; employment services for current students; interactive nursing skills videos; Internet; library services; nursing audiovisuals; remedial services; resume preparation assistance; unpaid internships.
Library Facilities 1.8 million volumes; 14,000 periodical subscriptions.

BACCALAUREATE PROGRAMS

Degree BSN
Site Options Vancouver, BC.

Program Entrance Requirements Minimum overall college GPA of 3.5, transcript of college record, CPR certification, high school transcript, immunizations, prerequisite course work. Transfer students are accepted.
Contact *Telephone:* 250-721-7961. *Fax:* 250-721-6231.

GRADUATE PROGRAMS

Contact *Telephone:* 250-721-7961. *Fax:* 250-721-6231.

MASTER'S DEGREE PROGRAM

Degree MN
Available Programs Master's.
Site Options Victoria.
Study Options Full-time and part-time.
Program Entrance Requirements Clinical experience, transcript of college record, letters of recommendation.
Advanced Placement Credit given for nursing courses completed elsewhere dependent upon specific evaluations.
Degree Requirements 18 total credit hours, thesis or project.

DOCTORAL DEGREE PROGRAM

Degree PhD
Program Entrance Requirements Clinical experience, MSN or equivalent.
Degree Requirements Dissertation.

Vancouver Island University

Department of Nursing
Nanaimo, British Columbia

http://www.mala.bc.ca/www/discover/health/index.htm
Founded in 1969

DEGREE • BSCN

Nursing Program Faculty 34 (10% with doctorates).
Baccalaureate Enrollment 275 **Women** 92% **Men** 8% **Minority** 6%
Nursing Student Activities Student Nurses' Association.
Nursing Student Resources Academic advising; academic or career counseling; assistance for students with disabilities; bookstore; campus computer network; computer lab; computer-assisted instruction; e-mail services; employment services for current students; housing assistance; interactive nursing skills videos; Internet; learning resource lab; library services; nursing audiovisuals; remedial services; resume preparation assistance; skills, simulation, or other laboratory; tutoring; unpaid internships.
Library Facilities 9,475 volumes in health, 1,299 volumes in nursing; 800 periodical subscriptions health-care related.

BACCALAUREATE PROGRAMS

Degree BScN
Available Programs Generic Baccalaureate.
Study Options Full-time.
Program Entrance Requirements CPR certification, written essay, health insurance, high school biology, high school chemistry, 11 years high school math, high school transcript, immunizations, minimum GPA in nursing prerequisites of 3.0, prerequisite course work, RN licensure. Transfer students are accepted. *Application deadline:* 2/28 (fall). *Application fee:* CAN$35.
Advanced Placement Credit given for nursing courses completed elsewhere dependent upon specific evaluations.
Expenses (2010-11) *Tuition:* full-time CAN$19,685. *Room and board:* room only: CAN$3500 per academic year.
Financial Aid 53% of baccalaureate students in nursing programs received some form of financial aid in 2009-10. *Gift aid (need-based):* private, college/university gift aid from institutional funds. *Loans:* government student loans.
Contact Dr. France Bouthillette, Chair of Bachelor of Science in Nursing Programs, Department of Nursing, Vancouver Island University, 900 Fifth Street, Nanaimo, BC V9R 5S5. *Telephone:* 250-740-6260. *Fax:* 250-740-6468. *E-mail:* france.bouthillette@viu.ca.

MANITOBA

Brandon University

School of Health Studies
Brandon, Manitoba

http://www.brandonu.ca/academic/health studies
Founded in 1899

DEGREE • BN

Nursing Program Faculty 20 (40% with doctorates).
Baccalaureate Enrollment 480 **Women** 95% **Men** 5% **Minority** 10% **Part-time** 25%
Distance Learning Courses Available.
Nursing Student Activities Nursing Honor Society, Sigma Theta Tau, Student Nurses' Association.
Nursing Student Resources Academic advising; academic or career counseling; assistance for students with disabilities; bookstore; campus computer network; career placement assistance; computer lab; computer-assisted instruction; e-mail services; employment services for current students; housing assistance; interactive nursing skills videos; Internet; library services; resume preparation assistance; skills, simulation, or other laboratory; tutoring.
Library Facilities 238,816 volumes; 1,699 periodical subscriptions.

BACCALAUREATE PROGRAMS

Degree BN
Available Programs Baccalaureate for Second Degree; Generic Baccalaureate; LPN to Baccalaureate; RN Baccalaureate.
Site Options Winnipeg, MB.
Study Options Full-time and part-time.
Program Entrance Requirements Minimum overall college GPA of 2.0, CPR certification, immunizations, minimum GPA in nursing prerequisites of 2.0, prerequisite course work. Transfer students are accepted. *Application deadline:* 5/1 (fall).
Advanced Placement Credit given for nursing courses completed elsewhere dependent upon specific evaluations.
Expenses (2009-10) *Tuition, area resident:* full-time CAN$3000. *Room and board:* CAN$3200 per academic year. *Required fees:* full-time CAN$3000.
Financial Aid 30% of baccalaureate students in nursing programs received some form of financial aid in 2008-09. *Gift aid (need-based):* college/university gift aid from institutional funds. *Loans:* provincial and federal student loans. *Financial aid application deadline (priority):* 6/30.
Contact Ms. Tracey Collyer, Instructional Associate/Student Advisor, School of Health Studies, Brandon University, 270 18th Street, Brandon, MB R7A 6A9. *Telephone:* 204-571-8567. *Fax:* 204-571-8568. *E-mail:* collyert@brandonu.ca.

University of Manitoba

Faculty of Nursing
Winnipeg, Manitoba

http://www.umanitoba.ca/faculties/nursing/
Founded in 1877

DEGREES • BN • MN • PHD

Nursing Program Faculty 54 (50% with doctorates).
Baccalaureate Enrollment 1,016 **Women** 88% **Men** 12% **Part-time** 19%
Graduate Enrollment 80 **Women** 94% **Men** 6% **Part-time** 55%
Distance Learning Courses Available.
Nursing Student Activities Nursing Honor Society, Sigma Theta Tau, Student Nurses' Association.
Nursing Student Resources Academic advising; academic or career counseling; assistance for students with disabilities; bookstore; campus computer network; computer lab; computer-assisted instruction; daycare for children of students; e-mail services; employment services for current students; housing assistance; interactive nursing skills videos; Internet; learning resource lab; library services; skills, simulation, or other laboratory; unpaid internships.
Library Facilities 2 million volumes (137,100 in health, 5,000 in nursing); 43,782 periodical subscriptions (2,208 health-care related).

BACCALAUREATE PROGRAMS

Degree BN
Available Programs Baccalaureate for Second Degree; Generic Baccalaureate; RN Baccalaureate.
Site Options The Pas, MB; Thompson, MB.
Study Options Full-time and part-time.
Program Entrance Requirements Minimum overall college GPA of 2.5, transcript of college record, CPR certification, high school chemistry, high school math, high school science, high school transcript, immunizations, minimum high school GPA of 2.5, prerequisite course work. Transfer students are accepted. *Application deadline:* 4/1 (fall).
Advanced Placement Credit given for nursing courses completed elsewhere dependent upon specific evaluations.
Expenses (2010-11) *Tuition, state resident:* part-time CAN$120 per credit. *Tuition, nonresident:* part-time CAN$120 per credit.
Financial Aid ***Gift aid (need-based):*** state, private, college/university gift aid from institutional funds. *Loans:* Federal Direct (Subsidized and Unsubsidized Stafford PLUS), Perkins, state, college/university, TERI Loans. *Work-study:* part-time campus jobs. *Financial aid application deadline (priority):* 10/1.
Contact Dr. Marion McKay, Associate Dean, Undergraduate Program, Faculty of Nursing, University of Manitoba, 277 Helen Glass Centre for Nursing, Winnipeg, MB R3T 2N2. *Telephone:* 204-474-6220. *Fax:* 204-474-7682. *E-mail:* marion_mckay@umanitoba.ca.

GRADUATE PROGRAMS

Expenses (2010-11) *Tuition, state resident:* full-time CAN$4124. *Tuition, nonresident:* full-time CAN$4124.
Contact Dr. Judith Scanlan, Associate Dean, Graduate Programs, Faculty of Nursing, University of Manitoba, 281-89 Curry Place, Winnipeg, MB R3T 2N2. *Telephone:* 204-474-9317. *Fax:* 204-474-7682. *E-mail:* judith_scanlan@umanitoba.ca.

MASTER'S DEGREE PROGRAM

Degree MN
Available Programs Master's.
Concentrations Available Nursing administration. *Clinical nurse specialist programs in:* acute care, family health, gerontology, perinatal, women's health. *Nurse practitioner programs in:* primary care.
Study Options Full-time and part-time.
Program Entrance Requirements Clinical experience, minimum overall college GPA of 3.0, transcript of college record, written essay, 3 letters of recommendation, nursing research course, resume, statistics course. *Application deadline:* 4/1 (fall).
Advanced Placement Credit given for nursing courses completed elsewhere dependent upon specific evaluations.
Degree Requirements 27 total credit hours, thesis or project, comprehensive exam.

DOCTORAL DEGREE PROGRAM

Degree PhD
Available Programs Doctorate.
Areas of Study Oncology.
Program Entrance Requirements Clinical experience, letters of recommendation, MSN or equivalent.
Degree Requirements 21 total credit hours, dissertation.

CONTINUING EDUCATION PROGRAM

Contact Dr. Dauna Crooks, Professor, Faculty of Nursing, University of Manitoba, 293 Helen Glass Centre for Nursing, Winnipeg, MB R3T 2N2. *Telephone:* 204-474-9201. *Fax:* 204-474-7500. *E-mail:* dauna_crooks@umanitoba.ca.

NEW BRUNSWICK

Université de Moncton
School of Nursing
Moncton, New Brunswick

Founded in 1963

DEGREES • BSCN • M SC N

Nursing Program Faculty 24 (25% with doctorates).
Baccalaureate Enrollment 570 **Women** 90% **Men** 10% **International** 1%
Graduate Enrollment 8
Nursing Student Activities Student Nurses' Association.
Nursing Student Resources Academic or career counseling; assistance for students with disabilities; bookstore; campus computer network; career placement assistance; computer lab; computer-assisted instruction; daycare for children of students; e-mail services; externships; housing assistance; Internet; library services; nursing audiovisuals; placement services for program completers; resume preparation assistance; unpaid internships.
Library Facilities 789,046 volumes; 2,059 periodical subscriptions.

BACCALAUREATE PROGRAMS

Degree BScN
Available Programs RN Baccalaureate.
Site Options Moncton, NB; Edmundston, NB; Bathurst, NB.
Study Options Full-time and part-time.
Program Entrance Requirements Transcript of college record, CPR certification, high school biology, high school chemistry, 12 years high school math, high school science, high school transcript, immunizations, minimum high school rank 65%. Transfer students are accepted.
Advanced Placement Credit given for nursing courses completed elsewhere dependent upon specific evaluations.
Contact ***Telephone:*** 506-858-4443. *Fax:* 506-858-4544.

GRADUATE PROGRAMS

Contact ***Telephone:*** 506-858-4443. *Fax:* 506-858-4544.

MASTER'S DEGREE PROGRAM

Degree M Sc N
Available Programs Master's; RN to Master's.
Concentrations Available Health-care administration; nurse case management; nursing administration; nursing education. *Clinical nurse specialist programs in:* community health, family health, home health care, occupational health, pediatric, psychiatric/mental health, public health, school health. *Nurse practitioner programs in:* adult health, community health, family health, oncology, primary care.
Site Options Moncton, NB.
Study Options Full-time and part-time.
Program Entrance Requirements Minimum overall college GPA of 3.0, transcript of college record, CPR certification, written essay, 2 letters of recommendation, resume, statistics course.
Advanced Placement Credit given for nursing courses completed elsewhere dependent upon specific evaluations.
Degree Requirements 45 total credit hours, thesis or project.

CONTINUING EDUCATION PROGRAM

Contact ***Telephone:*** 506-858-4121.

University of New Brunswick Fredericton
Faculty of Nursing
Fredericton, New Brunswick

http://www.unbf.ca/nursing/
Founded in 1785

DEGREES • BN • MN

Nursing Program Faculty 75 (17% with doctorates).
Baccalaureate Enrollment 674
Graduate Enrollment 53 **Women** 96% **Men** 4% **Part-time** 30%
Distance Learning Courses Available.
Nursing Student Activities Student Nurses' Association, nursing club.
Nursing Student Resources Academic advising; academic or career counseling; assistance for students with disabilities; bookstore; campus computer network; computer lab; computer-assisted instruction; daycare for children of students; e-mail services; interactive nursing skills videos; Internet; learning resource lab; library services; nursing audiovisuals; resume preparation assistance; skills, simulation, or other laboratory; tutoring.
Library Facilities 1.3 million volumes (12,547 in health, 1,910 in nursing); 22,767 periodical subscriptions (250 health-care related).

BACCALAUREATE PROGRAMS

Degree BN

Available Programs Accelerated Baccalaureate; Generic Baccalaureate.

Site Options Bathurst, NB; Moncton, NB.

Study Options Full-time.

Program Entrance Requirements Minimum overall college GPA of 3.0, transcript of college record, CPR certification, written essay, health exam, high school biology, high school chemistry, 60 years high school math, high school transcript, immunizations, interview, minimum high school rank 70%, prerequisite course work. Transfer students are accepted. *Application deadline:* 3/31 (winter). *Application fee:* CAN$45.

Advanced Placement Credit given for nursing courses completed elsewhere dependent upon specific evaluations.

Expenses (2010-11) *Tuition:* full-time CAN$5482. *Room and board:* CAN$9352 per academic year.

Financial Aid 50% of baccalaureate students in nursing programs received some form of financial aid in 2009-10.

Contact Mr. Lee Heenan, Administrative Assistant, Faculty of Nursing, University of New Brunswick Fredericton, PO Box 4400, Fredericton, NB E3B 5A3. *Telephone:* 506-458-7670. *Fax:* 506-447-3374. *E-mail:* lheenan@unb.ca.

GRADUATE PROGRAMS

Expenses (2010-11) *Tuition:* full-time CAN$5947. *Required fees:* part-time CAN$928 per term.

Financial Aid 10% of graduate students in nursing programs received some form of financial aid in 2009-10.

Contact Mr. Francis Perry, Graduate Assistant, Faculty of Nursing, University of New Brunswick Fredericton, PO Box 4400, Fredericton, NB E3B 5A3. *Telephone:* 506-451-6844. *Fax:* 506-447-3374. *E-mail:* fperry@unb.ca.

MASTER'S DEGREE PROGRAM

Degree MN

Available Programs Master's.

Concentrations Available Nurse case management; nursing administration; nursing education; nursing informatics. *Clinical nurse specialist programs in:* acute care, adult health, cardiovascular, community health, critical care, family health, gerontology, maternity-newborn, medical-surgical, oncology, parent-child, pediatric, psychiatric/mental health, public health, school health, women's health. *Nurse practitioner programs in:* acute care, adult health, community health, family health, gerontology, neonatal health, pediatric, primary care, psychiatric/mental health, women's health.

Study Options Full-time and part-time.

Program Entrance Requirements Clinical experience, computer literacy, minimum overall college GPA of 3.3, transcript of college record, written essay, 3 letters of recommendation, nursing research course, physical assessment course, prerequisite course work, statistics course. *Application deadline:* 1/2 (winter). *Application fee:* CAN$50.

Advanced Placement Credit given for nursing courses completed elsewhere dependent upon specific evaluations.

Degree Requirements 27 total credit hours, thesis or project.

CONTINUING EDUCATION PROGRAM

Contact Mr. Lee Heenan, Administrative Assistant, Faculty of Nursing, University of New Brunswick Fredericton, PO Box 4400, Fredericton, NB E3B 5A3. *Telephone:* 506-458-7625. *Fax:* 506-447-3057. *E-mail:* nursing@unb.ca.

NEWFOUNDLAND AND LABRADOR

Memorial University of Newfoundland

School of Nursing
St. John's, Newfoundland and Labrador

http://www.nurs.mun.ca/
Founded in 1925

DEGREES • BN • MN

Nursing Program Faculty 42 (30% with doctorates).
Baccalaureate Enrollment 642 **Women** 92% **Men** 8% **International** 2% **Part-time** 50%
Graduate Enrollment 100 **Women** 91% **Men** 9% **International** 1% **Part-time** 82%
Distance Learning Courses Available.
Nursing Student Activities Student Nurses' Association.
Nursing Student Resources Academic advising; academic or career counseling; assistance for students with disabilities; bookstore; campus computer network; computer lab; computer-assisted instruction; daycare for children of students; e-mail services; employment services for current students; externships; interactive nursing skills videos; Internet; learning resource lab; library services; nursing audiovisuals; remedial services; skills, simulation, or other laboratory; tutoring.
Library Facilities 1.9 million volumes (40,000 in health, 5,000 in nursing); 17,170 periodical subscriptions (3,800 health-care related).

BACCALAUREATE PROGRAMS

Degree BN
Available Programs Accelerated Baccalaureate; Generic Baccalaureate; LPN to Baccalaureate; RN Baccalaureate.
Study Options Full-time.
Program Entrance Requirements Minimum overall college GPA of 3.0, transcript of college record, written essay, high school biology, high school chemistry, high school foreign language, high school math, high school science, high school transcript, 2 letters of recommendation, minimum high school rank 80%. Transfer students are accepted. *Application deadline:* 3/1 (fall).
Financial Aid ***Loans:*** college/university. *Financial aid application deadline:* Continuous.
Contact Ms. Lena Clark, Consortium Coordinator, School of Nursing, Memorial University of Newfoundland, Registrar's Office, PO Box 4200, St. John's, NF A1C 5S7. *Telephone:* 709-737-6871. *Fax:* 709-737-3890. *E-mail:* nursingadmissions@mun.ca.

GRADUATE PROGRAMS

Financial Aid 25% of graduate students in nursing programs received some form of financial aid in 2009-10. Fellowships, research assistantships, teaching assistantships available. *Financial aid application deadline:* 12/31.
Contact Dr. Shirley Solberg, Associate Director, Graduate Program and Research, School of Nursing, Memorial University of Newfoundland, 300 Prince Philip Drive, St. John's, NF A1B 3V6. *Telephone:* 709-777-6679. *Fax:* 709-777-7037. *E-mail:* ssolberg@mun.ca.

MASTER'S DEGREE PROGRAM

Degree MN
Available Programs Master's.
Concentrations Available Nursing education. *Nurse practitioner programs in:* acute care.
Study Options Full-time and part-time.
Online Degree Options Yes (online only).
Program Entrance Requirements Clinical experience, minimum overall college GPA of 3.0, transcript of college record, written essay, 2 letters of recommendation, nursing research course, professional liability insurance/malpractice insurance, prerequisite course work, resume, statistics course. *Application deadline:* 2/15 (fall). *Application fee:* CAN$40.
Advanced Placement Credit given for nursing courses completed elsewhere dependent upon specific evaluations.
Degree Requirements 28 total credit hours, thesis or project.

POST-MASTER'S PROGRAM

Areas of Study *Nurse practitioner programs in:* acute care.

NOVA SCOTIA

Dalhousie University

School of Nursing
Halifax, Nova Scotia

http://www.dal.ca/nursing
Founded in 1818

DEGREES • BSCN • MN • MN/MHSA • PHD

Nursing Program Faculty 60 (38% with doctorates).
Baccalaureate Enrollment 658 **Women** 95% **Men** 5% **Minority** 7%
Graduate Enrollment 105 **Women** 96% **Men** 4% **International** 2% **Part-time** 58%
Distance Learning Courses Available.
Nursing Student Activities Nursing Honor Society, Sigma Theta Tau, Student Nurses' Association.
Nursing Student Resources Academic advising; academic or career counseling; assistance for students with disabilities; bookstore; campus computer network; computer lab; computer-assisted instruction; daycare for children of students; e-mail services; employment services for current students; externships; housing assistance; interactive nursing skills videos; Internet; learning resource lab; library services; nursing audiovisuals; resume preparation assistance; skills, simulation, or other laboratory; tutoring.
Library Facilities 164 periodical subscriptions.

BACCALAUREATE PROGRAMS

Degree BScN
Available Programs Accelerated Baccalaureate; Accelerated Baccalaureate for Second Degree; Baccalaureate for Second Degree; Generic Baccalaureate; LPN to Baccalaureate; RN Baccalaureate.
Site Options Yarmouth, NS.
Study Options Full-time.
Online Degree Options Yes.
Program Entrance Requirements Minimum overall college GPA of 2.5, transcript of college record, high school biology, high school chemistry, 3 years high school math, high school transcript, immunizations, minimum high school rank 70%, minimum GPA in nursing prerequisites of 2.5, prerequisite course work. Transfer students are accepted. *Application deadline:* 3/15 (fall). Applications may be processed on a rolling basis for some programs. *Application fee:* CAN$65.
Advanced Placement Credit given for nursing courses completed elsewhere dependent upon specific evaluations.
Expenses (2010-11) *Tuition, area resident:* full-time CAN$7853. *International tuition:* CAN$15,759 full-time. *Room and board:* CAN$8700 per academic year. *Required fees:* full-time CAN$1000.
Financial Aid ***Gift aid (need-based):*** private, college/university gift aid from institutional funds, Vermont grants, Rhode Island grants. *Loans:* Canadian loans, private bank loans. *Financial aid application deadline:* Continuous.
Contact Dr. Susan French, Associate Director, Undergraduate Program Planning and Development (Acting), School of Nursing, Dalhousie University, 5869 University Avenue, Halifax, NS B3H 3J5. *Telephone:* 902-494-2423. *Fax:* 902-494-3487. *E-mail:* sudon.french@ns.sympatico.ca.

GRADUATE PROGRAMS

Expenses (2010-11) *Tuition, area resident:* full-time CAN$7892. *International tuition:* CAN$17,798 full-time. *Room and board:* CAN$8700 per academic year. *Required fees:* full-time CAN$1000.
Financial Aid Fellowships, research assistantships, teaching assistantships available.
Contact Dr. Ruth Martin Misener, Associate Director, Graduate Programs, School of Nursing, Dalhousie University, 5869 University Avenue, Halifax, NS B3H 3J5. *Telephone:* 902-494-2250. *Fax:* 902-494-3487. *E-mail:* ruth.martin-misener@dal.ca.

MASTER'S DEGREE PROGRAM

Degrees MN; MN/MHSA
Available Programs Master's.
Concentrations Available *Clinical nurse specialist programs in:* adult health, community health, family health, maternity-newborn, parent-child, pediatric, psychiatric/mental health, public health. *Nurse practitioner programs in:* adult health, family health, neonatal health, primary care.
Study Options Full-time and part-time.
Program Entrance Requirements Clinical experience, minimum overall college GPA of 3.0, transcript of college record, immunizations, interview, 3 letters of recommendation, nursing research course, prerequisite course work, statistics course. *Application deadline:* 2/1 (fall).
Degree Requirements 36 total credit hours, thesis or project.

POST-MASTER'S PROGRAM

Areas of Study *Nurse practitioner programs in:* adult health, family health, neonatal health, primary care.

DOCTORAL DEGREE PROGRAM

Degree PhD
Available Programs Doctorate.
Areas of Study Advanced practice nursing, aging, community health, family health, health policy, health promotion/disease prevention, human health and illness, illness and transition, maternity-newborn, nursing policy, nursing research, nursing science, oncology, women's health.
Program Entrance Requirements Clinical experience, minimum overall college GPA of 3.3, interview by faculty committee, interview, 3 letters of recommendation, MSN or equivalent, vita, writing sample. Application deadline: 2/1 (fall). Application fee: CAN$70.
Degree Requirements 27 total credit hours, dissertation, oral exam, residency.

St. Francis Xavier University

Department of Nursing
Antigonish, Nova Scotia

http://www.stfx.ca
Founded in 1853

DEGREE • BSCN

Nursing Program Faculty 67 (10% with doctorates).
Baccalaureate Enrollment 1,067 **Women** 90% **Men** 10% **Minority** 5% **International** 1% **Part-time** 40%
Nursing Student Activities Student Nurses' Association, nursing club.
Nursing Student Resources Academic advising; academic or career counseling; assistance for students with disabilities; bookstore; campus computer network; career placement assistance; computer lab; computer-assisted instruction; daycare for children of students; e-mail services; employment services for current students; externships; housing assistance; interactive nursing skills videos; Internet; learning resource lab; library services; nursing audiovisuals; other; paid internships; placement services for program completers; remedial services; resume preparation assistance; skills, simulation, or other laboratory; tutoring; unpaid internships.
Library Facilities 323,636 volumes (4,000 in health, 4,000 in nursing); 17,721 periodical subscriptions (1,015 health-care related).

BACCALAUREATE PROGRAMS

Degree BScN
Available Programs Accelerated Baccalaureate; Accelerated Baccalaureate for Second Degree; Accelerated LPN to Baccalaureate; Generic Baccalaureate; RN Baccalaureate.
Site Options Sydney, NS.
Study Options Full-time.
Program Entrance Requirements Transcript of college record, CPR certification, health exam, high school biology, high school chemistry, 2 years high school math, 2 years high school science, high school transcript, immunizations, minimum high school GPA, prerequisite course work. Transfer students are accepted.
Advanced Placement Credit given for nursing courses completed elsewhere dependent upon specific evaluations.
Contact ***Telephone:*** 902-867-5386. *Fax:* 902-867-2329.

CONTINUING EDUCATION PROGRAM

Contact ***Telephone:*** 902-867-5186. *Fax:* 902-867-5154.

ONTARIO

Brock University

Department of Nursing
St. Catharines, Ontario

http://www.brocku.ca/nursing/
Founded in 1964

DEGREE • BSCN

Nursing Program Faculty 27
Nursing Student Activities Student Nurses' Association, nursing club.
Nursing Student Resources Academic advising; academic or career counseling; assistance for students with disabilities; bookstore; campus computer network; computer lab; computer-assisted instruction; daycare for children of students; e-mail services; employment services for current students; housing assistance; interactive nursing skills videos; Internet; learning resource lab; library services; nursing audiovisuals; other; resume preparation assistance; skills, simulation, or other laboratory; tutoring.
Library Facilities 769,873 volumes.

BACCALAUREATE PROGRAMS

Degree BScN
Available Programs Generic Baccalaureate; RN Baccalaureate.
Study Options Full-time.
Program Entrance Requirements High school biology, high school chemistry.
Contact Dr. Lynn Rempel, Chair and Associate Professor, Department of Nursing, Brock University, 500 Glenridge Avenue, St. Catharines, ON L2S 3A1. *Telephone:* 905-688-5550 Ext. 4660. *E-mail:* lrempel@brocku.ca.

Lakehead University

School of Nursing
Thunder Bay, Ontario

http://www.lakeheadu.ca
Founded in 1965

DEGREE • BSCN

Nursing Program Faculty 15 (20% with doctorates).
Baccalaureate Enrollment 575 **Women** 82% **Men** 18%
Distance Learning Courses Available.
Nursing Student Activities Student Nurses' Association.
Nursing Student Resources Academic advising; academic or career counseling; assistance for students with disabilities; bookstore; campus computer network; career placement assistance; computer lab; daycare for children of students; e-mail services; employment services for current students; externships; housing assistance; interactive nursing skills videos; Internet; library services; nursing audiovisuals; resume preparation assistance; skills, simulation, or other laboratory; tutoring; unpaid internships.
Library Facilities 613,047 volumes; 33,396 periodical subscriptions.

BACCALAUREATE PROGRAMS

Degree BScN
Available Programs Accelerated Baccalaureate; Generic Baccalaureate; RN Baccalaureate.
Study Options Full-time and part-time.
Online Degree Options Yes.
Program Entrance Requirements Transcript of college record, CPR certification, health insurance, high school biology, high school chemistry, 4 years high school math, high school transcript, immunizations, minimum high school GPA. Transfer students are accepted. *Application deadline:* 1/12 (winter). Applications may be processed on a rolling basis for some programs.
Advanced Placement Credit given for nursing courses completed elsewhere dependent upon specific evaluations.
Contact *Telephone:* 807-343-8439. *Fax:* 807-343-8246.

Laurentian University

School of Nursing
Sudbury, Ontario

Founded in 1960

DEGREE • BSCN

Nursing Program Faculty 20 (20% with doctorates).
Nursing Student Resources Internet.

BACCALAUREATE PROGRAMS

Degree BScN
Study Options Full-time and part-time.
Program Entrance Requirements CPR certification, health exam, high school biology, high school chemistry, high school transcript, immunizations, prerequisite course work. Transfer students are accepted.
Advanced Placement Credit given for nursing courses completed elsewhere dependent upon specific evaluations.
Contact *Telephone:* 705-675-1151 Ext. 3808. *Fax:* 705-675-4861.

CONTINUING EDUCATION PROGRAM

Contact *Telephone:* 705-675-1151 Ext. 3808. *Fax:* 705-675-4861.

McMaster University

School of Nursing
Hamilton, Ontario

http://www.fhs.mcmaster.ca/nursing
Founded in 1887

DEGREES • BSCN • M SC • MSN/PHD • PHD

Nursing Program Faculty 53 (47% with doctorates).
Baccalaureate Enrollment 548 **Women** 90% **Men** 10% **Part-time** 20%
Nursing Student Activities Student Nurses' Association.
Nursing Student Resources Academic advising; academic or career counseling; assistance for students with disabilities; bookstore; campus computer network; career placement assistance; computer lab; daycare for children of students; e-mail services; employment services for current students; housing assistance; Internet; learning resource lab; library services; nursing audiovisuals; placement services for program completers; remedial services; resume preparation assistance; skills, simulation, or other laboratory; tutoring.
Library Facilities 1.7 million volumes (150,446 in health); 57,487 periodical subscriptions (89,267 health-care related).

BACCALAUREATE PROGRAMS

Degree BScN
Available Programs Baccalaureate for Second Degree; Generic Baccalaureate; RN Baccalaureate.
Site Options Kitchener, ON.
Study Options Full-time and part-time.
Program Entrance Requirements CPR certification, health exam, high school biology, high school chemistry, 4 years high school math, 4 years high school science, high school transcript, immunizations, minimum high school GPA of 3.0, minimum high school rank 75%. Transfer students are accepted.
Advanced Placement Credit by examination available. Credit given for nursing courses completed elsewhere dependent upon specific evaluations.
Contact *Telephone:* 905-525-9140 Ext. 22232. *Fax:* 905-528-4727.

GRADUATE PROGRAMS

Contact *Telephone:* 905-525-9140 Ext. 22982. *Fax:* 905-546-1129.

MASTER'S DEGREE PROGRAM

Degrees M Sc; MSN/PhD
Available Programs Master's.
Concentrations Available *Clinical nurse specialist programs in:* perinatal. *Nurse practitioner programs in:* neonatal health.
Study Options Full-time and part-time.
Program Entrance Requirements Transcript of college record, written essay, 2 letters of recommendation.
Advanced Placement Credit given for nursing courses completed elsewhere dependent upon specific evaluations.
Degree Requirements Thesis or project.

DOCTORAL DEGREE PROGRAM

Degree PhD
Available Programs Doctorate.
Program Entrance Requirements 2 letters of recommendation, MSN or equivalent, vita.
Degree Requirements Dissertation, oral exam.

Nipissing University

Nursing Department
North Bay, Ontario

http://www.nipissingu.ca/nursing/
Founded in 1992

DEGREE • BSCN

Nursing Program Faculty 12 (3% with doctorates).
Baccalaureate Enrollment 248 **Women** 92% **Men** 8%
Nursing Student Activities Student Nurses' Association.
Nursing Student Resources Academic advising; academic or career counseling; assistance for students with disabilities; bookstore; campus computer network; career placement assistance; computer lab; computer-assisted instruction; e-mail services; employment services for current students; housing assistance; interactive nursing skills videos; Internet; learning resource lab; library services; nursing audiovisuals; placement services for program completers; remedial services; resume preparation assistance; skills, simulation, or other laboratory; tutoring; unpaid internships.
Library Facilities 715,494 volumes (2,800 in health, 1,820 in nursing); 19,115 periodical subscriptions (2,430 health-care related).

BACCALAUREATE PROGRAMS

Degree BScN
Available Programs Generic Baccalaureate.
Study Options Full-time.
Program Entrance Requirements Minimum overall college GPA of 3.0, transcript of college record, high school biology, high school chemistry, high school transcript, immunizations, minimum high school rank 70%. Transfer students are accepted. *Application deadline:* Applications may be processed on a rolling basis for some programs.
Expenses (2009-10) *Tuition, area resident:* full-time CAN$4130. *International tuition:* CAN$10,000 full-time. *Room and board:* room only: CAN$5460 per academic year.
Financial Aid 44% of baccalaureate students in nursing programs received some form of financial aid in 2008-09.
Contact Registrar's Office, Nursing Department, Nipissing University, 100 College Drive, PO Box 5002, North Bay, ON P1B 8L7. *Telephone:* 705-474-3450 Ext. 4521. *E-mail:* registrar@nipssingu.ca.

Queen's University at Kingston

School of Nursing
Kingston, Ontario

http://nursing.queensu.ca/
Founded in 1841

DEGREES • BNSC • M SC • PHD

Nursing Program Faculty 20 (80% with doctorates).
Baccalaureate Enrollment 400 **Women** 95% **Men** 5% **Minority** 4% **International** 2%
Graduate Enrollment 51 **Women** 99% **Men** 1% **Minority** 5% **International** 5%
Distance Learning Courses Available.
Nursing Student Activities Student Nurses' Association.
Nursing Student Resources Academic advising; academic or career counseling; assistance for students with disabilities; bookstore; campus computer network; career placement assistance; computer lab; computer-assisted instruction; e-mail services; employment services for current students; housing assistance; interactive nursing skills videos; Internet; learning resource lab; library services; nursing audiovisuals; resume preparation assistance; skills, simulation, or other laboratory; tutoring; unpaid internships.
Library Facilities 3.5 million volumes (5,209 in health, 3,652 in nursing); 16,109 periodical subscriptions (1,054 health-care related).

BACCALAUREATE PROGRAMS

Degree BNSc
Available Programs Accelerated Baccalaureate; Generic Baccalaureate; RN Baccalaureate.
Study Options Full-time.
Program Entrance Requirements CPR certification, high school biology, high school chemistry, high school math, high school science, high school transcript, immunizations, minimum high school GPA, minimum high school rank. Transfer students are accepted. *Application deadline:* 2/1 (fall). *Application fee:* CAN$120.
Advanced Placement Credit given for nursing courses completed elsewhere dependent upon specific evaluations.
Expenses (2010-11) *Tuition, area resident:* full-time CAN$5461. *International tuition:* CAN$18,730 full-time. *Room and board:* CAN$11,275; room only: CAN$6217 per academic year. *Required fees:* full-time CAN$1079.
Financial Aid 41% of baccalaureate students in nursing programs received some form of financial aid in 2009-10. *Gift aid (need-based):* state, private, college/university gift aid from institutional funds. *Loans:* college/university, federal and provincial loans, alternative loans. *Work-study:* part-time campus jobs. *Financial aid application deadline (priority):* 7/1.
Contact Prof. Susan Laschinger, Chair, Admissions Committee, School of Nursing, Queen's University at Kingston, Cataraqui Building, 92 Barrie Street, Kingston, ON K7L 3N6. *Telephone:* 613-533-6000 Ext. 74743. *Fax:* 613-533-6770. *E-mail:* lasching@queensu.ca.

GRADUATE PROGRAMS

Expenses (2010-11) *Tuition, area resident:* full-time CAN$6258. *International tuition:* CAN$12,366 full-time. *Room and board:* room only: CAN$6217 per academic year. *Required fees:* full-time CAN$1002.
Financial Aid 100% of graduate students in nursing programs received some form of financial aid in 2009-10. 25 fellowships (averaging $6,636 per year), 4 research assistantships, 9 teaching assistantships (averaging $2,592 per year) were awarded; institutionally sponsored loans and scholarships also available. *Financial aid application deadline:* 2/1.
Contact Dr. Dana Edge, Graduate Coordinator, School of Nursing, Queen's University at Kingston, Cataraqui Building, 92 Barrie Street, Kingston, ON K7L 3N6. *Telephone:* 613-533-6000 Ext. 74765. *Fax:* 613-533-6770. *E-mail:* dana.edge@queensu.ca.

MASTER'S DEGREE PROGRAM

Degree M Sc
Available Programs Master's.
Concentrations Available *Nurse practitioner programs in:* primary care.
Study Options Full-time.
Program Entrance Requirements Minimum overall college GPA of 3.0, transcript of college record, 2 letters of recommendation, nursing research course, prerequisite course work, resume, statistics course. *Application deadline:* 2/1 (fall). *Application fee:* CAN$105.
Degree Requirements 15 total credit hours, thesis or project.

DOCTORAL DEGREE PROGRAM

Degree PhD
Available Programs Doctorate.
Areas of Study Illness and transition, nursing science.
Program Entrance Requirements Minimum overall college GPA of 3.2, 2 letters of recommendation, MSN or equivalent, statistics course, vita. Application deadline: 2/1 (fall). Application fee: CAN$105.
Degree Requirements 15 total credit hours, dissertation, oral exam, written exam, residency.

Ryerson University

Program in Nursing
Toronto, Ontario

http://www.ryerson.ca/nursing
Founded in 1948

DEGREES • BSCN • MN

Nursing Program Faculty 84 (34% with doctorates).
Baccalaureate Enrollment 2,754 **Women** 88% **Men** 12% **International** 1%
Graduate Enrollment 168 **Women** 93% **Men** 7% **Part-time** 54%
Distance Learning Courses Available.

Nursing Student Activities Sigma Theta Tau, Student Nurses' Association, nursing club.

Nursing Student Resources Academic advising; academic or career counseling; assistance for students with disabilities; bookstore; campus computer network; career placement assistance; computer lab; computer-assisted instruction; daycare for children of students; e-mail services; employment services for current students; housing assistance; interactive nursing skills videos; Internet; learning resource lab; library services; nursing audiovisuals; remedial services; resume preparation assistance; skills, simulation, or other laboratory; tutoring.

Library Facilities 487,361 volumes (29,163 in health, 4,963 in nursing); 28,075 periodical subscriptions (5,567 health-care related).

BACCALAUREATE PROGRAMS

Degree BScN

Available Programs Generic Baccalaureate; International Nurse to Baccalaureate; RN Baccalaureate; RPN to Baccalaureate.

Study Options Full-time.

Program Entrance Requirements Transcript of college record, CPR certification, health exam, health insurance, high school biology, high school chemistry, 3 years high school math, 4 years high school science, high school transcript, immunizations, minimum high school rank 78%. *Application deadline:* 3/1 (fall). *Application fee:* CAN$200.

Advanced Placement Credit given for nursing courses completed elsewhere dependent upon specific evaluations.

Expenses (2010-11) *Tuition, area resident:* full-time CAN$5963; part-time CAN$540 per unit. *International tuition:* CAN$17,540 full-time. *Room and board:* CAN$9745; room only: CAN$6625 per academic year.

Financial Aid 45% of baccalaureate students in nursing programs received some form of financial aid in 2009-10. *Gift aid (need-based):* college/university gift aid from institutional funds. *Loans:* Federal Direct (Subsidized and Unsubsidized Stafford). *Financial aid application deadline:* 1/15.

Contact Richard Perras, Student Affairs Coordinator, Program in Nursing, Ryerson University, 350 Victoria Street, Room POD-474, Toronto, ON M5B 2K3. *Telephone:* 416-979-5000 Ext. 6318. *Fax:* 416-979-5332. *E-mail:* rperras@ryerson.ca.

GRADUATE PROGRAMS

Expenses (2010-11) *Tuition, state resident:* full-time CAN$6000; part-time CAN$1100 per course.

Financial Aid 1% of graduate students in nursing programs received some form of financial aid in 2009-10.

Contact Mr. Gerry Warner, Program Administrator, Program in Nursing, Ryerson University, 350 Victoria Street, Toronto, ON M5B 2K3. *Telephone:* 416-979-5000 Ext. 7852. *Fax:* 416-979-5332. *E-mail:* gerry.warner@ryerson.ca.

MASTER'S DEGREE PROGRAM

Degree MN

Available Programs Master's.

Concentrations Available *Clinical nurse specialist programs in:* adult health, community health, family health, public health. *Nurse practitioner programs in:* primary care.

Study Options Full-time and part-time.

Program Entrance Requirements Minimum overall college GPA of 3.33, transcript of college record, written essay, 2 letters of recommendation, nursing research course, physical assessment course, resume. *Application deadline:* 3/31 (fall). Applications may be processed on a rolling basis for some programs. *Application fee:* CAN$100.

Advanced Placement Credit given for nursing courses completed elsewhere dependent upon specific evaluations.

Degree Requirements 11 total credit hours, thesis or project.

CONTINUING EDUCATION PROGRAM

Contact Paula Mastrilli, Program Manager, Program in Nursing, Ryerson University, 350 Victoria Street, POD481-D, Toronto, ON M5B 2K3. *Telephone:* 416-979-5178. *Fax:* 416-542-5878. *E-mail:* pmastril@gwemail.ryerson.ca.

Trent University
Nursing Program
Peterborough, Ontario

http://www.trentu.ca/nursing/
Founded in 1963

DEGREE • BSCN

Nursing Program Faculty 45 (10% with doctorates).
Baccalaureate Enrollment 523
Distance Learning Courses Available.
Nursing Student Activities Student Nurses' Association.
Nursing Student Resources Academic advising; academic or career counseling; assistance for students with disabilities; bookstore; campus computer network; computer lab; computer-assisted instruction; e-mail services; employment services for current students; housing assistance; interactive nursing skills videos; Internet; learning resource lab; library services; nursing audiovisuals; remedial services; resume preparation assistance; skills, simulation, or other laboratory; tutoring.
Library Facilities 740,653 volumes (6,393 in health, 1,281 in nursing); 1,464 periodical subscriptions (360 health-care related).

BACCALAUREATE PROGRAMS

Degree BScN
Available Programs Accelerated Baccalaureate; Generic Baccalaureate.
Site Options Peterborough, ON.
Study Options Full-time.
Program Entrance Requirements CPR certification, health exam, high school biology, high school chemistry, 4 years high school math, 4 years high school science, high school transcript, immunizations, minimum high school rank 70%. Transfer students are accepted.
Advanced Placement Credit given for nursing courses completed elsewhere dependent upon specific evaluations.
Contact *Telephone:* 705-748-1011 Ext. 7809. *Fax:* 705-748-1088.

University of Ottawa
School of Nursing
Ottawa, Ontario

http://www.health.uottawa.ca/sn/
Founded in 1848

DEGREES • BSCN • M SC N • PHD

Nursing Program Faculty 150 (23% with doctorates).
Baccalaureate Enrollment 1,748 **Women** 94% **Men** 6% **Part-time** 21%
Graduate Enrollment 200 **Women** 90% **Men** 10% **Part-time** 55%
Distance Learning Courses Available.
Nursing Student Activities Sigma Theta Tau, Student Nurses' Association.
Nursing Student Resources Academic advising; academic or career counseling; assistance for students with disabilities; bookstore; campus computer network; career placement assistance; computer lab; computer-assisted instruction; e-mail services; employment services for current students; housing assistance; interactive nursing skills videos; Internet; learning resource lab; library services; nursing audiovisuals; remedial services; resume preparation assistance; skills, simulation, or other laboratory; tutoring.
Library Facilities 3.3 million volumes (54,000 in health, 7,000 in nursing); 50,059 periodical subscriptions (1,050 health-care related).

BACCALAUREATE PROGRAMS

Degree BScN
Available Programs Baccalaureate for Second Degree; Generic Baccalaureate; International Nurse to Baccalaureate; LPN to Baccalaureate; RN Baccalaureate; RPN to Baccalaureate.
Site Options Montreal, QC; Pembroke, ON; Montreal , QC.
Study Options Full-time.
Program Entrance Requirements Transcript of college record, CPR certification, high school biology, high school chemistry, high school math, high school transcript, immunizations, minimum high school rank 70%. Transfer students are accepted. *Application deadline:* 2/15 (winter).
Advanced Placement Credit given for nursing courses completed elsewhere dependent upon specific evaluations.
Expenses (2010-11) *Tuition, area resident:* full-time CAN$6000; part-time CAN$600 per course. *International tuition:* CAN$12,000 full-time.

Financial Aid ***Gift aid (need-based):*** state, private, college/university gift aid from institutional funds. *Work-study:* part-time campus jobs. *Financial aid application deadline:* 1/31.

Contact Ms. Suzanne Biag, Academic Advisor, School of Nursing, University of Ottawa, 451 Smyth Road, Ottawa, ON K1H 8M5. *Telephone:* 613-562-5800 Ext. 5404. *Fax:* 613-562-5470. *E-mail:* sbiage@uottawa.ca.

GRADUATE PROGRAMS

Expenses (2010-11) *Tuition, area resident:* full-time CAN$6400; part-time CAN$630 per course. *International tuition:* CAN$16,000 full-time. *Required fees:* full-time CAN$850.

Financial Aid Fellowships, research assistantships, teaching assistantships, career-related internships or fieldwork, Federal Work-Study, scholarships, traineeships, tuition waivers (full and partial), and unspecified assistantships available.

Contact Dr. Jocelyn Tourigny, Assistant Director of Graduate Program, School of Nursing, University of Ottawa, 451 Smyth Road, Ottawa, ON K1H 8M5. *Telephone:* 613-562-5800 Ext. 8422. *Fax:* 613-562-5473. *E-mail:* jtourign@uottawa.ca.

MASTER'S DEGREE PROGRAM

Degree M Sc N

Available Programs Master's.

Concentrations Available *Clinical nurse specialist programs in:* acute care, community health. *Nurse practitioner programs in:* primary care.

Study Options Full-time and part-time.

Program Entrance Requirements Clinical experience, minimum overall college GPA of 3.0, transcript of college record, written essay, immunizations, 3 letters of recommendation, nursing research course, physical assessment course, prerequisite course work, resume, statistics course. *Application deadline:* 2/15 (winter).

Advanced Placement Credit given for nursing courses completed elsewhere dependent upon specific evaluations.

Degree Requirements 24 total credit hours, thesis or project.

DOCTORAL DEGREE PROGRAM

Degree PhD

Available Programs Doctorate; Doctorate for Nurses with Non-Nursing Degrees.

Areas of Study Health promotion/disease prevention, health-care systems, nursing policy, nursing research, nursing science.

Program Entrance Requirements Minimum overall college GPA of 3.5, 3 letters of recommendation, MSN or equivalent, statistics course, vita, writing sample.

Degree Requirements 18 total credit hours, dissertation, oral exam, written exam, residency.

POSTDOCTORAL PROGRAM

Areas of Study Community health, nursing interventions.

Postdoctoral Program Contact Dr. Jocelyn Tourigny, Assistant Director of Graduate Program, School of Nursing, University of Ottawa, 451 Smyth Road, Ottawa, ON K1H 8M5. *Telephone:* 613-562-5800. *E-mail:* jtourign@uottawa.ca.

University of Toronto

Faculty of Nursing
Toronto, Ontario

http://bloomberg.nursing.utoronto.ca/

Founded in 1827

DEGREES • BSCN • MN • PHD

Nursing Program Faculty 200 (50% with doctorates).

Baccalaureate Enrollment 320 **Women** 80% **Men** 20% **International** 15%

Graduate Enrollment 360 **Part-time** 10%

Distance Learning Courses Available.

Nursing Student Activities Student Nurses' Association, nursing club.

Nursing Student Resources Academic advising; academic or career counseling; assistance for students with disabilities; bookstore; campus computer network; career placement assistance; computer lab; computer-assisted instruction; daycare for children of students; e-mail services; employment services for current students; externships; housing assistance; interactive nursing skills videos; Internet; learning resource lab; library services; nursing audiovisuals; paid internships; remedial services; resume preparation assistance; skills, simulation, or other laboratory.

Library Facilities 13.4 million volumes; 75,545 periodical subscriptions.

BACCALAUREATE PROGRAMS

Degree BScN

Available Programs Accelerated Baccalaureate; Accelerated Baccalaureate for Second Degree; Accelerated RN Baccalaureate; Baccalaureate for Second Degree.

Study Options Full-time.

Program Entrance Requirements Minimum overall college GPA of 3.0, CPR certification, written essay, immunizations, 2 letters of recommendation, minimum GPA in nursing prerequisites of 3.0, prerequisite course work. *Application deadline:* 2/1 (fall).

Financial Aid 40% of baccalaureate students in nursing programs received some form of financial aid in 2009-10. *Work-study:* Federal Work-Study.

Contact Student Services, Faculty of Nursing, University of Toronto, 155 College Street, Toronto, ON M5T 1P8. *Telephone:* 416-978-2392. *Fax:* 416-978-8222. *E-mail:* inquiry.nursing@utoronto.ca.

GRADUATE PROGRAMS

Financial Aid 60% of graduate students in nursing programs received some form of financial aid in 2009-10.

Contact Student Services, Faculty of Nursing, University of Toronto, 155 College Street, Toronto, ON M5T 1P8. *Telephone:* 416-978-2392. *Fax:* 416-978-8222. *E-mail:* inquiry.nursing@utoronto.ca.

MASTER'S DEGREE PROGRAM

Degree MN

Available Programs Master's.

Concentrations Available Clinical nurse leader; health-care administration; nurse anesthesia; nursing administration; nursing education. *Clinical nurse specialist programs in:* acute care, adult health, community health, critical care, family health, gerontology, maternity-newborn, oncology, pediatric, psychiatric/mental health, public health, school health, women's health. *Nurse practitioner programs in:* acute care, adult health, family health, pediatric.

Study Options Full-time and part-time.

Online Degree Options Yes.

Program Entrance Requirements Clinical experience, minimum overall college GPA of 3.0, transcript of college record, CPR certification, written essay, 2 letters of recommendation, prerequisite course work, resume, statistics course.

Degree Requirements 9 total credit hours, thesis or project.

POST-MASTER'S PROGRAM

Areas of Study *Clinical nurse specialist programs in:* acute care, adult health, maternity-newborn, pediatric. *Nurse practitioner programs in:* acute care, adult health, pediatric.

DOCTORAL DEGREE PROGRAM

Degree PhD

Available Programs Doctorate.

Areas of Study Community health, ethics, family health, health policy, health-care systems, human health and illness, information systems, maternity-newborn, nursing administration, nursing education, nursing policy, nursing research, nursing science, oncology, women's health.

Program Entrance Requirements Minimum overall college GPA of 3.3, 2 letters of recommendation, MSN or equivalent, scholarly papers, statistics course, vita, writing sample.

Degree Requirements Dissertation, oral exam.

POSTDOCTORAL PROGRAM

Postdoctoral Program Contact Graduate Department, Faculty of Nursing, University of Toronto, 50 St. George Street, Toronto, ON M5S 3H4. *Telephone:* 416-978-8069.

CONTINUING EDUCATION PROGRAM

Contact The Bloomberg Centre for Advanced Studies in Professional Practice, Faculty of Nursing, University of Toronto, 155 College Street, Suite 130, Toronto, ON M5T 1P8. *E-mail:* caspp.nursing@utoronto.ca.

The University of Western Ontario

School of Nursing
London, Ontario

http://www.uwo.ca/fhs/nursing
Founded in 1878

DEGREES • BSCN • M SC N • PHD

Nursing Program Faculty 101 (18% with doctorates).
Baccalaureate Enrollment 1,153 **Women** 93.24% **Men** 6.76% **Part-time** 13.53%
Graduate Enrollment 54 **Women** 89% **Men** 11% **Part-time** 28%
Nursing Student Activities Nursing Honor Society, Sigma Theta Tau, Student Nurses' Association.
Nursing Student Resources Academic advising; academic or career counseling; assistance for students with disabilities; bookstore; campus computer network; computer lab; computer-assisted instruction; daycare for children of students; e-mail services; employment services for current students; housing assistance; interactive nursing skills videos; Internet; learning resource lab; library services; nursing audiovisuals; resume preparation assistance; unpaid internships.
Library Facilities 3.6 million volumes (357,263 in health, 40 in nursing); 74,274 periodical subscriptions (250 health-care related).

BACCALAUREATE PROGRAMS

Degree BScN
Available Programs Accelerated Baccalaureate; Generic Baccalaureate; RN Baccalaureate.
Study Options Full-time.
Program Entrance Requirements CPR certification, high school biology, high school chemistry, 4 years high school math, high school science, high school transcript, immunizations, minimum high school rank 80%. Transfer students are accepted.
Advanced Placement Credit given for nursing courses completed elsewhere dependent upon specific evaluations.
Contact ***Telephone:*** 519-661-2111 Ext. 86564. *Fax:* 519-661-3928.

GRADUATE PROGRAMS

Contact ***Telephone:*** 519-661-3409. *Fax:* 519-661-3928.

MASTER'S DEGREE PROGRAM

Degree M Sc N
Available Programs Master's.
Concentrations Available Health-care administration; nursing administration; nursing education. *Clinical nurse specialist programs in:* acute care, adult health, community health, psychiatric/mental health, public health, women's health. *Nurse practitioner programs in:* community health.
Study Options Full-time and part-time.
Program Entrance Requirements Minimum overall college GPA of 3.5, transcript of college record, written essay, interview, 2 letters of recommendation, nursing research course, prerequisite course work, resume, statistics course.
Advanced Placement Credit given for nursing courses completed elsewhere dependent upon specific evaluations.
Degree Requirements 7 total credit hours, thesis or project.

DOCTORAL DEGREE PROGRAM

Degree PhD
Available Programs Doctorate.
Areas of Study Addiction/substance abuse, advanced practice nursing, aging, clinical practice, community health, faculty preparation, health policy, health promotion/disease prevention, health-care systems, human health and illness, individualized study, nurse case management, nursing administration, nursing education, nursing research, nursing science, women's health.
Program Entrance Requirements Clinical experience, minimum overall college GPA of 3.5, interview by faculty committee, interview, 2 letters of recommendation, MSN or equivalent, scholarly papers, statistics course, vita, writing sample.
Degree Requirements 4 total credit hours, dissertation, written exam.

POSTDOCTORAL PROGRAM

Areas of Study Addiction/substance abuse, community health, health promotion/disease prevention, vulnerable population, women's health.
Postdoctoral Program Contact ***Telephone:*** 519-661-2111 Ext. 86573.

University of Windsor

Faculty of Nursing
Windsor, Ontario

http://www.uwindsor.ca/nursing
Founded in 1857

DEGREES • BSCN • M SC

Nursing Program Faculty 152 (10% with doctorates).
Baccalaureate Enrollment 917 **Women** 83% **Men** 17% **International** 6.5% **Part-time** 10%
Graduate Enrollment 62 **Women** 90% **Men** 10% **International** 1.6% **Part-time** 59.7%
Distance Learning Courses Available.
Nursing Student Activities Nursing Honor Society, Sigma Theta Tau, Student Nurses' Association, nursing club.
Nursing Student Resources Academic advising; academic or career counseling; assistance for students with disabilities; bookstore; campus computer network; career placement assistance; computer lab; computer-assisted instruction; e-mail services; employment services for current students; externships; interactive nursing skills videos; Internet; learning resource lab; library services; nursing audiovisuals; remedial services; resume preparation assistance; skills, simulation, or other laboratory; tutoring.
Library Facilities 2.8 million volumes (64,552 in nursing); 25,458 periodical subscriptions.

BACCALAUREATE PROGRAMS

Degree BScN
Available Programs Generic Baccalaureate.
Site Options Windsor, ON.
Study Options Full-time.
Program Entrance Requirements CPR certification, health exam, health insurance, high school biology, high school chemistry, high school math, 4 years high school science, high school transcript, immunizations, minimum high school rank 75%. Transfer students are accepted. *Application deadline:* 1/14 (fall). *Application fee:* CAN$125.
Advanced Placement Credit given for nursing courses completed elsewhere dependent upon specific evaluations.
Expenses (2010-11) *Tuition, area resident:* full-time CAN$5090; part-time CAN$509 per course. *International tuition:* CAN$17,950 full-time. *Room and board:* CAN$10,340; room only: CAN$7238 per academic year. *Required fees:* full-time CAN$800; part-time CAN$17 per credit; part-time CAN$255 per term.
Financial Aid 27% of baccalaureate students in nursing programs received some form of financial aid in 2009-10. *Gift aid (need-based):* college/university gift aid from institutional funds. *Loans:* Federal Direct (Subsidized and Unsubsidized Stafford PLUS). *Work-study:* part-time campus jobs. *Financial aid application deadline:* 6/15.
Contact Nursing Contact, Faculty of Nursing, University of Windsor, 401 Sunset Avenue, Windsor, ON N9B 3P4. *Telephone:* 519-253-3000 Ext. 2258. *Fax:* 519-973-7084. *E-mail:* nurse@uwindsor.ca.

GRADUATE PROGRAMS

Expenses (2010-11) *Tuition, area resident:* full-time CAN$4680; part-time CAN$1170 per term. *International tuition:* CAN$10,570 full-time. *Room and board:* CAN$10,340; room only: CAN$7238 per academic year. *Required fees:* full-time CAN$944; part-time CAN$13 per credit; part-time CAN$82 per term.
Financial Aid 23% of graduate students in nursing programs received some form of financial aid in 2009-10.
Contact Dr. Debbie Kane, Graduate Coordinator, Faculty of Nursing, University of Windsor, 401 Sunset Avenue, Windsor, ON N9B 3P4. *Telephone:* 519-253-3000 Ext. 2268. *Fax:* 519-973-7084. *E-mail:* dkane@uwindsor.ca.

MASTER'S DEGREE PROGRAM

Degree M Sc
Available Programs Master's.
Study Options Full-time and part-time.
Program Entrance Requirements Minimum overall college GPA of 3.0, transcript of college record, written essay, 3 letters of recommendation, nursing research course, physical assessment course, statistics course. *Application deadline:* 2/15 (fall). *Application fee:* CAN$85.

Advanced Placement Credit given for nursing courses completed elsewhere dependent upon specific evaluations.
Degree Requirements 10 total credit hours, thesis or project.

CONTINUING EDUCATION PROGRAM

Contact Nursing Main Office, Faculty of Nursing, University of Windsor, 401 Sunset Avenue, Windsor, ON N9B 3P4. *Telephone:* 519-253-3000 Ext. 2258. *Fax:* 519-973-7084. *E-mail:* nurse@uwindsor.ca.

York University
School of Nursing
Toronto, Ontario

Founded in 1959

DEGREE • BSCN

Nursing Program Faculty 19 (79% with doctorates).
Baccalaureate Enrollment 850 **Women** 96% **Men** 4% **Minority** 30% **International** 1% **Part-time** 15%
Nursing Student Resources Academic advising; academic or career counseling; assistance for students with disabilities; bookstore; campus computer network; career placement assistance; computer lab; computer-assisted instruction; daycare for children of students; e-mail services; employment services for current students; housing assistance; interactive nursing skills videos; Internet; learning resource lab; library services; nursing audiovisuals; skills, simulation, or other laboratory; unpaid internships.
Library Facilities 6.5 million volumes; 540,000 periodical subscriptions.

BACCALAUREATE PROGRAMS

Degree BScN
Available Programs Generic Baccalaureate; RN Baccalaureate.
Site Options King City, ON; Barrie, ON; Oshawa, ON.
Study Options Full-time and part-time.
Program Entrance Requirements CPR certification, written essay, health exam, high school biology, high school chemistry, high school math, high school science, high school transcript, immunizations, 1 letter of recommendation, minimum high school GPA, minimum GPA in nursing prerequisites. Transfer students are accepted.
Advanced Placement Credit by examination available. Credit given for nursing courses completed elsewhere dependent upon specific evaluations.
Contact ***Telephone:*** 416-736-5271 Ext. 66351. *Fax:* 416-736-5714.

CONTINUING EDUCATION PROGRAM

Contact ***Telephone:*** 416-736-5271. *Fax:* 416-736-5714.

PRINCE EDWARD ISLAND

University of Prince Edward Island
School of Nursing
Charlottetown, Prince Edward Island

Founded in 1834

DEGREE • BSCN

Nursing Program Faculty 10 (2% with doctorates).
Baccalaureate Enrollment 211 **Women** 97% **Men** 3% **International** 1%
Nursing Student Activities Nursing Honor Society, Student Nurses' Association, nursing club.
Nursing Student Resources Academic advising; academic or career counseling; assistance for students with disabilities; bookstore; campus computer network; career placement assistance; computer lab; computer-assisted instruction; daycare for children of students; e-mail services; employment services for current students; housing assistance; interactive nursing skills videos; Internet; learning resource lab; library services; nursing audiovisuals; placement services for program completers; remedial services; resume preparation assistance; skills, simulation, or other laboratory; tutoring.
Library Facilities 402,808 volumes; 26,196 periodical subscriptions.

BACCALAUREATE PROGRAMS

Degree BScN
Available Programs Generic Baccalaureate.
Study Options Full-time and part-time.
Program Entrance Requirements Transcript of college record, CPR certification, high school chemistry, high school math, high school science, high school transcript, immunizations, minimum high school GPA of 3.0, minimum high school rank 75%, minimum GPA in nursing prerequisites of 3.0, prerequisite course work. Transfer students are accepted.
Advanced Placement Credit given for nursing courses completed elsewhere dependent upon specific evaluations.
Contact ***Telephone:*** 902-566-0733. *Fax:* 902-566-0777.

QUEBEC

McGill University
School of Nursing
Montréal, Quebec

http://www.nursing.mcgill.ca
Founded in 1821

DEGREES • BSCN • M SC • PHD

Nursing Program Faculty 163 (13% with doctorates).
Baccalaureate Enrollment 438 **Women** 90% **Men** 10% **International** 2% **Part-time** 25%
Graduate Enrollment 93 **Women** 90% **Men** 10% **International** 5% **Part-time** 26%
Nursing Student Activities Student Nurses' Association.
Nursing Student Resources Academic advising; academic or career counseling; assistance for students with disabilities; bookstore; campus computer network; career placement assistance; computer lab; e-mail services; Internet; learning resource lab; library services; nursing audiovisuals; skills, simulation, or other laboratory; tutoring; unpaid internships.
Library Facilities 4.2 million volumes; 49,433 periodical subscriptions.

BACCALAUREATE PROGRAMS

Degree BScN
Available Programs Accelerated RN Baccalaureate; Generic Baccalaureate; RN Baccalaureate.
Study Options Full-time.
Program Entrance Requirements Minimum overall college GPA of 3.0, transcript of college record, high school chemistry, 4 years high school math, 4 years high school science, high school transcript, minimum high school GPA of 3.3, minimum high school rank 25%. Transfer students are accepted. *Application deadline:* 1/15 (fall), 11/1 (winter). *Application fee:* CAN$85.
Advanced Placement Credit given for nursing courses completed elsewhere dependent upon specific evaluations.
Expenses (2009-10) *Tuition, state resident:* full-time CAN$1968; part-time CAN$66 per credit. *Tuition, nonresident:* full-time CAN$5501; part-time CAN$183 per credit. *International tuition:* CAN$15,420 full-time. *Room and board:* CAN$11,000 per academic year. *Required fees:* full-time CAN$1420.
Financial Aid ***Gift aid (need-based):*** state, private, college/university gift aid from institutional funds, Canadian (Federal and Provincial) Student Assistance. *Loans:* college/university, alternative loans. *Work-study:* part-time campus jobs. *Financial aid application deadline:* 6/30.
Contact Ms. Celine Arseneault, Student Affairs Coordinator, Undergraduate Programs, School of Nursing, McGill University, 3506 University Street, Wilson Hall Building, Room 203, Montreal, QC H3A 2A7. *Telephone:* 514-398-3784. *Fax:* 514-398-8455. *E-mail:* undergraduate.nursing@mcgill.ca.

GRADUATE PROGRAMS

Expenses (2009-10) *Tuition, state resident:* full-time CAN$1968; part-time CAN$66 per credit. *Tuition, nonresident:* full-time CAN$5500;

part-time CAN$183 per credit. *International tuition:* CAN$13,444 full-time. *Required fees:* full-time CAN$1534.
Contact Ms. Anna Santandrea, Students Affairs Coordinator, Graduate and Post-Doctoral Studies, School of Nursing, McGill University, 3506 University Street, Montreal, QC H3A 2A7. *Telephone:* 514-398-4151. *Fax:* 514-398-8455. *E-mail:* anna.santandrea@mcgill.ca.

MASTER'S DEGREE PROGRAM

Degree M Sc
Available Programs Master's; Master's for Non-Nursing College Graduates.
Concentrations Available Nursing administration. *Clinical nurse specialist programs in:* acute care, adult health, cardiovascular, community health, critical care, family health, gerontology, home health care, maternity-newborn, medical-surgical, oncology, parent-child, pediatric, perinatal, psychiatric/mental health, public health, rehabilitation, women's health. *Nurse practitioner programs in:* neonatal health, primary care.
Study Options Full-time.
Program Entrance Requirements Clinical experience, minimum overall college GPA of 3.0, transcript of college record, CPR certification, written essay, immunizations, interview, 3 letters of recommendation, resume, statistics course. *Application deadline:* 1/15 (fall). *Application fee:* CAN$85.
Degree Requirements 53 total credit hours, thesis or project.

DOCTORAL DEGREE PROGRAM

Degree PhD
Available Programs Doctorate; Post-Baccalaureate Doctorate.
Areas of Study Family health, health-care systems, human health and illness, nursing administration, nursing research, oncology.
Program Entrance Requirements Minimum overall college GPA of 3.3, interview, 2 letters of recommendation, MSN or equivalent, statistics course, vita, writing sample. Application deadline: 1/15 (fall). Application fee: CAN$85.
Degree Requirements 90 total credit hours, dissertation, oral exam, written exam, residency.

POSTDOCTORAL PROGRAM

Areas of Study Cancer care, chronic illness.
Postdoctoral Program Contact Dr. C. Celeste Johnston, Associate Director, Research, School of Nursing, McGill University, 3506 University Street, Montreal, QC H3A 2A7. *Telephone:* 514-398-4157. *Fax:* 514-398-8455. *E-mail:* celeste.johnston@mcgill.ca.

Université de Montréal
Faculty of Nursing
Montréal, Quebec

http://www.scinf.umontreal.ca/
Founded in 1920

DEGREES • BSCN • M SC • PHD

Nursing Program Faculty 54 (90% with doctorates).
Baccalaureate Enrollment 780 **Women** 70% **Men** 30% **Minority** 30% **International** 3% **Part-time** 20%
Graduate Enrollment 326 **Women** 75% **Men** 25% **Minority** 20% **International** 3%
Distance Learning Courses Available.
Nursing Student Activities Student Nurses' Association.
Nursing Student Resources Academic advising; academic or career counseling; assistance for students with disabilities; bookstore; campus computer network; career placement assistance; computer lab; computer-assisted instruction; daycare for children of students; e-mail services; employment services for current students; externships; housing assistance; interactive nursing skills videos; Internet; learning resource lab; library services; nursing audiovisuals; other; placement services for program completers; remedial services; resume preparation assistance; skills, simulation, or other laboratory; tutoring.
Library Facilities 4 million volumes (32,536 in health, 32,536 in nursing); 18,330 periodical subscriptions (1,319 health-care related).

BACCALAUREATE PROGRAMS

Degree BScN
Available Programs RN Baccalaureate.
Study Options Full-time and part-time.
Program Entrance Requirements Transcript of college record, CPR certification, high school biology, high school chemistry, immunizations, minimum high school GPA. Transfer students are accepted. *Application deadline:* 3/1 (fall). *Application fee:* CAN$85.
Advanced Placement Credit given for nursing courses completed elsewhere dependent upon specific evaluations.
Expenses (2010-11) *Tuition, state resident:* full-time CAN$2068. *Tuition, nonresident:* full-time CAN$5668. *International tuition:* CAN$16,160 full-time.
Contact Catherine Sarrazin, Assistant to Vice Dean, Faculty of Nursing, Université de Montréal, Pav. Marg. d'Youville, CP 6128 Succursale Centre-Ville, Montreal, QC H3C 3J7. *Telephone:* 514-343-6439. *Fax:* 514-343-2306. *E-mail:* catherine.sarrazin@umontreal.ca.

GRADUATE PROGRAMS

Expenses (2010-11) *Tuition, area resident:* full-time CAN$3102. *Tuition, state resident:* full-time CAN$8501. *International tuition:* CAN$21,693 full-time.
Financial Aid 30% of graduate students in nursing programs received some form of financial aid in 2009-10. Fellowships, research assistantships, teaching assistantships, career-related internships or fieldwork, Federal Work-Study, and institutionally sponsored loans available.
Contact Suzanne Pinel, Assistant to the Vice Dean of Studies, Faculty of Nursing, Université de Montréal, Pav. Marg. d'Youville, CP 6128 Succursale Centre-Ville, Montreal, QC H3C 3J7. *Telephone:* 514-343-6111 Ext. 7098. *Fax:* 514-343-6111 Ext. 2705. *E-mail:* suzanne.pinel@umontreal.ca.

MASTER'S DEGREE PROGRAM

Degree M Sc
Available Programs Master's; RN to Master's.
Concentrations Available *Clinical nurse specialist programs in:* acute care, adult health, cardiovascular, community health, family health, gerontology, maternity-newborn, medical-surgical, occupational health, oncology, palliative care, parent-child, psychiatric/mental health, public health, rehabilitation, women's health. *Nurse practitioner programs in:* acute care, family health, primary care.
Study Options Full-time and part-time.
Program Entrance Requirements Transcript of college record, nursing research course, statistics course. *Application deadline:* 3/1 (fall). *Application fee:* CAN$85.
Degree Requirements 45 total credit hours, thesis or project.

POST-MASTER'S PROGRAM

Areas of Study *Nurse practitioner programs in:* acute care, family health, primary care.

DOCTORAL DEGREE PROGRAM

Degree PhD
Available Programs Doctorate.
Areas of Study Addiction/substance abuse, aging, bio-behavioral research, clinical practice, community health, critical care, family health, gerontology, health policy, health promotion/disease prevention, health-care systems, human health and illness, illness and transition, maternity-newborn, neuro-behavior, nursing administration, nursing education, nursing policy, nursing research, nursing science, oncology, urban health, women's health.
Program Entrance Requirements letters of recommendation, MSN or equivalent, statistics course. Application deadline: 3/1 (fall). Application fee: CAN$85.
Degree Requirements 90 total credit hours, dissertation, oral exam.

POSTDOCTORAL PROGRAM

Areas of Study Adolescent health, aging, cancer care, chronic illness, community health, family health, gerontology, health promotion/disease prevention, individualized study, neuro-behavior, nursing informatics, nursing interventions, nursing research, nursing science, outcomes, self-care, vulnerable population, women's health.
Postdoctoral Program Contact Ms. Chantal Cara, Vice Dean, Research, Faculty of Nursing, Université de Montréal, Pav. Marg. d'Youville, CP 6128 Succursale Centre-Ville, Montreal, QC H3C 3J7. *Telephone:* 514-343-5835. *Fax:* 514-343-2306. *E-mail:* chantal.cara@umontreal.ca.

CONTINUING EDUCATION PROGRAM

Contact Ms. Jocelyne Labarre, Program Coordinator, Faculty of Nursing, Université de Montréal, Pav. Marg. d'Youville, CP 6128 Succursale Centre-Ville, Montreal, QC H3C 3J7. *Telephone:* 514-343-7723. *Fax:* 514-343-2306. *E-mail:* jocyelyne.labarre@umontreal.ca.

Université de Sherbrooke

Department of Nursing
Sherbrooke, Quebec

http://www.usherbrooke.ca/scinf/
Founded in 1954

DEGREES • BSCN • M SC • PHD

Nursing Program Faculty 17 (76% with doctorates).

Baccalaureate Enrollment 482 **Women** 90% **Men** 10% **Minority** .5% **Part-time** 30%

Graduate Enrollment 61 **Women** 95% **Men** 5% **Part-time** 50%

Nursing Student Activities Student Nurses' Association.

Nursing Student Resources Academic advising; academic or career counseling; assistance for students with disabilities; bookstore; computer lab; computer-assisted instruction; e-mail services; externships; housing assistance; Internet; learning resource lab; library services; nursing audiovisuals; tutoring.

Library Facilities 1.2 million volumes (40,000 in health, 4,000 in nursing); 5,937 periodical subscriptions (3,000 health-care related).

BACCALAUREATE PROGRAMS

Degree BScN

Available Programs RN Baccalaureate.

Site Options Longueuil, QC.

Study Options Full-time and part-time.

Program Entrance Requirements Transcript of college record, high school chemistry, 4 years high school math, immunizations, professional liability insurance/malpractice insurance, RN licensure. Transfer students are accepted.

Advanced Placement Credit given for nursing courses completed elsewhere dependent upon specific evaluations.

Contact ***Telephone:*** 819-563-5355. *Fax:* 819-820-6816.

GRADUATE PROGRAMS

Contact ***Telephone:*** 819-564-5354. *Fax:* 819-820-6816.

MASTER'S DEGREE PROGRAM

Degree M Sc

Available Programs Master's.

Concentrations Available *Clinical nurse specialist programs in:* acute care, community health, family health, gerontology.

Site Options Longueuil, QC.

Study Options Full-time and part-time.

Program Entrance Requirements Transcript of college record, interview, 3 letters of recommendation, nursing research course, professional liability insurance/malpractice insurance, resume.

Degree Requirements 45 total credit hours, thesis or project.

DOCTORAL DEGREE PROGRAM

Degree PhD

Available Programs Doctorate.

Areas of Study Advanced practice nursing, aging, biology of health and illness, clinical practice, community health, critical care, family health, gerontology, health promotion/disease prevention, human health and illness, illness and transition, information systems, maternity-newborn, neuro-behavior, nurse case management, nursing administration, nursing education, nursing policy, nursing research, nursing science, oncology, women's health.

Site Options Longueuil, QC.

Program Entrance Requirements Clinical experience, interview, 3 letters of recommendation, MSN or equivalent, statistics course, vita, writing sample.

Degree Requirements 90 total credit hours, dissertation, oral exam, written exam.

POSTDOCTORAL PROGRAM

Postdoctoral Program Contact *Telephone:* 819-564-5355. *Fax:* 819-820-6816.

Université du Québec à Chicoutimi

Program in Nursing
Chicoutimi, Quebec

Founded in 1969

DEGREES • BNSC • MS/MPH • MSN

Nursing Program Faculty 10 (30% with doctorates).

Baccalaureate Enrollment 600 **Women** 90% **Men** 10% **Minority** 5% **Part-time** 75%

Graduate Enrollment 30 **Women** 90% **Men** 10% **Minority** 2% **Part-time** 80%

Distance Learning Courses Available.

Nursing Student Activities Nursing Honor Society, Student Nurses' Association.

Nursing Student Resources Academic advising; academic or career counseling; assistance for students with disabilities; bookstore; campus computer network; computer lab; computer-assisted instruction; e-mail services; employment services for current students; externships; housing assistance; interactive nursing skills videos; Internet; learning resource lab; library services; nursing audiovisuals; resume preparation assistance; skills, simulation, or other laboratory; tutoring; unpaid internships.

Library Facilities 689,214 volumes (6,300 in nursing); 5,092 periodical subscriptions (5,250 health-care related).

BACCALAUREATE PROGRAMS

Degree BNSc

Available Programs Accelerated RN Baccalaureate; RN Baccalaureate.

Site Options St. Felicien, QC; Alma, QC; Sept-Iles, QC.

Study Options Full-time and part-time.

Program Entrance Requirements Transcript of college record, health exam, high school biology, high school chemistry, high school math, immunizations, interview. Transfer students are accepted. *Application deadline:* 3/1 (winter). *Application fee:* CAN$30.

Advanced Placement Credit given for nursing courses completed elsewhere dependent upon specific evaluations.

Expenses (2010-11) *Tuition, area resident:* part-time CAN$310 per course. *Required fees:* part-time CAN$100 per credit.

Financial Aid 5% of baccalaureate students in nursing programs received some form of financial aid in 2009-10. *Gift aid (need-based):* private, college/university gift aid from institutional funds. *Loans:* college/university. *Work-study:* part-time campus jobs.

Contact Mme. Anna Gauthier, Secretary, Program in Nursing, Université du Québec à Chicoutimi, 555 Boulevard de l'Universite, Chicoutimi, QC G7H 2B1. *Telephone:* 418-545-5011 Ext. 5315. *Fax:* 418-615-1205. *E-mail:* anna_gauthier@uqac.ca.

GRADUATE PROGRAMS

Expenses (2010-11) *Tuition, area resident:* part-time CAN$310 per course. *Required fees:* part-time CAN$100 per credit.

Financial Aid 2% of graduate students in nursing programs received some form of financial aid in 2009-10.

Contact Mrs. Francoise Courville, Director of Masters Degree Program, Program in Nursing, Université du Québec à Chicoutimi, 555 Boulevard de l'Universit, Chicoutimi, QC G7H 2B1. *Telephone:* 418-545-5011 Ext. 2374. *Fax:* 418-545-5012. *E-mail:* francoise_courville@uqac.ca.

MASTER'S DEGREE PROGRAM

Degrees MS/MPH; MSN

Available Programs Accelerated RN to Master's; Master's; RN to Master's.

Concentrations Available *Clinical nurse specialist programs in:* acute care, adult health, cardiovascular, community health, critical care, family health, gerontology, home health care, maternity-newborn, medical-surgical, occupational health, oncology, parent-child, pediatric, perinatal, psychiatric/mental health, public health, rehabilitation, school health, women's health. *Nurse practitioner programs in:* primary care.

Site Options St. Felicien, QC; Alma, QC; Sept-Iles, QC.

Study Options Full-time and part-time.

Program Entrance Requirements Clinical experience, minimum overall college GPA of 3.2, transcript of college record, written essay, interview, 3 letters of recommendation, nursing research course, professional liability insurance/malpractice insurance, resume, statistics course. *Application deadline:* 3/1 (fall), 11/1 (winter). *Application fee:* CAN$30.

Advanced Placement Credit given for nursing courses completed elsewhere dependent upon specific evaluations.
Degree Requirements 45 total credit hours, thesis or project, comprehensive exam.

Université du Québec à Rimouski
Program in Nursing
Rimouski, Quebec

http://www.uquebec.ca/mscinf/
Founded in 1973

DEGREES • BSCN • M SC N
Nursing Program Faculty 17 (53% with doctorates).
Baccalaureate Enrollment 750 **Women** 90% **Men** 10% **Part-time** 74%
Graduate Enrollment 24 **Women** 96% **Men** 4% **Part-time** 92%
Distance Learning Courses Available.
Nursing Student Activities Student Nurses' Association.
Nursing Student Resources Academic advising; academic or career counseling; assistance for students with disabilities; bookstore; campus computer network; career placement assistance; computer lab; daycare for children of students; e-mail services; employment services for current students; housing assistance; Internet; learning resource lab; library services; nursing audiovisuals; other; placement services for program completers; resume preparation assistance; skills, simulation, or other laboratory; tutoring.
Library Facilities 263,142 volumes (5,200 in health, 1,100 in nursing); 3,951 periodical subscriptions (1,300 health-care related).

BACCALAUREATE PROGRAMS

Degree BScN
Available Programs RN Baccalaureate.
Site Options Rimouski, QC; Lvis, QC.
Study Options Full-time and part-time.
Program Entrance Requirements Transcript of college record, professional liability insurance/malpractice insurance, prerequisite course work. Transfer students are accepted.
Advanced Placement Credit by examination available.
Financial Aid 8% of baccalaureate students in nursing programs received some form of financial aid in 2008-09. *Loans:* college/university.
Contact Mr. Mario Dube, Directeur du module des sciences de la sante, Program in Nursing, Université du Québec à Rimouski, 300, allee des Ursulines, Rimouski, QC G5L 3A1. *Telephone:* 418-723-1986 Ext. 1568. *Fax:* 418-724-1450. *E-mail:* Mario_Dube@uqar.qc.ca.

GRADUATE PROGRAMS

Financial Aid 17% of graduate students in nursing programs received some form of financial aid in 2008-09.
Contact Dr. Guy Belanger, Directeur, Program in Nursing, Université du Québec à Rimouski, 300, allee des Ursulines, Rimouski, QC G5L 3A1. *Telephone:* 418-723-1986 Ext. 1345. *Fax:* 418-724-1450. *E-mail:* Guy_Belanger@uqar.qc.ca.

MASTER'S DEGREE PROGRAM

Degree M Sc N
Available Programs Master's.
Concentrations Available *Clinical nurse specialist programs in:* community health, critical care, gerontology, psychiatric/mental health.
Site Options Rimouski, QC; Lvis, QC.
Study Options Full-time and part-time.
Program Entrance Requirements Clinical experience, transcript of college record, interview, 3 letters of recommendation, nursing research course, prerequisite course work, statistics course.
Advanced Placement Credit given for nursing courses completed elsewhere dependent upon specific evaluations.
Degree Requirements 45 total credit hours, thesis or project.

CONTINUING EDUCATION PROGRAM

Contact Mr. Richard Tremblay, Coordonnateur, Program in Nursing, Université du Québec à Rimouski, 300, allee des Ursulines, Rimouski, QC G5L 3A1. *Telephone:* 418-723-1986 Ext. 1818. *Fax:* 418-724-1525. *E-mail:* formationcontinue@uqar.qc.ca.

Université du Québec à Trois-Rivières
Program in Nursing
Trois-Rivières, Quebec

Founded in 1969

DEGREES • BSN • MSN
Nursing Program Faculty 28 (30% with doctorates).
Baccalaureate Enrollment 180 **Women** 95% **Men** 5% **Minority** 5% **International** 1% **Part-time** 75%
Graduate Enrollment 50 **Women** 97% **Men** 3% **Minority** 1% **Part-time** 90%
Distance Learning Courses Available.
Nursing Student Activities Student Nurses' Association.
Nursing Student Resources Academic advising; academic or career counseling; assistance for students with disabilities; bookstore; campus computer network; career placement assistance; computer lab; computer-assisted instruction; daycare for children of students; e-mail services; employment services for current students; externships; interactive nursing skills videos; Internet; learning resource lab; library services; nursing audiovisuals; placement services for program completers; resume preparation assistance; skills, simulation, or other laboratory; tutoring; unpaid internships.
Library Facilities 464,338 volumes (2,000 in health, 500 in nursing); 2,000 periodical subscriptions health-care related.

BACCALAUREATE PROGRAMS

Degree BSN
Available Programs Generic Baccalaureate; RN Baccalaureate.
Study Options Full-time and part-time.
Program Entrance Requirements Transcript of college record, CPR certification, high school biology, high school chemistry, prerequisite course work, RN licensure. Transfer students are accepted. *Application deadline:* 3/1 (fall). Applications may be processed on a rolling basis for some programs. *Application fee:* CAN$30.
Advanced Placement Credit given for nursing courses completed elsewhere dependent upon specific evaluations.
Contact *Telephone:* 819-376-5011 Ext. 3471. *Fax:* 819-376-5048.

GRADUATE PROGRAMS

Contact *Telephone:* 819-376-5011 Ext. 3460.

MASTER'S DEGREE PROGRAM

Degree MSN
Available Programs Master's.
Concentrations Available *Clinical nurse specialist programs in:* acute care, adult health, community health, critical care, family health, home health care, maternity-newborn, medical-surgical, pediatric, perinatal, psychiatric/mental health, public health. *Nurse practitioner programs in:* primary care.
Study Options Full-time and part-time.
Program Entrance Requirements Minimum overall college GPA of 3, transcript of college record, CPR certification, immunizations, 3 letters of recommendation, nursing research course, physical assessment course, prerequisite course work, statistics course. *Application deadline:* 8/29 (fall), 11/29 (winter), 4/29 (spring). Applications may be processed on a rolling basis for some programs. *Application fee:* CAN$30.
Advanced Placement Credit by examination available.
Degree Requirements 45 total credit hours, thesis or project.

Université du Québec en Abitibi-Témiscamingue
Département des sciences sociales et de la santé
Rouyn-Noranda, Quebec

http://www.uqat.uquebec.ca/gestac/prg/7855.asp
Founded in 1983

DEGREE • BN
Nursing Program Faculty 12
Baccalaureate Enrollment 78 **Women** 95% **Men** 5% **Part-time** 64%
Nursing Student Resources Academic advising; assistance for students with disabilities; bookstore; campus computer network; computer lab;

computer-assisted instruction; housing assistance; Internet; library services; resume preparation assistance; skills, simulation, or other laboratory.
Library Facilities 135,882 volumes (3,239 in health, 715 in nursing); 302 periodical subscriptions (17 health-care related).

BACCALAUREATE PROGRAMS

Degree BN
Program Entrance Requirements Transfer students are accepted.
Contact ***Telephone:*** 819-762-0971 Ext. 2370. *Fax:* 819-797-4727.

Université du Québec en Outaouais

Département des Sciences Infirmières
Gatineau, Quebec

Founded in 1981

DEGREES • BSCN • M SC N
Nursing Program Faculty 13 (38% with doctorates).
Baccalaureate Enrollment 700 **Women** 90% **Men** 10% **Minority** 20% **Part-time** 40%
Graduate Enrollment 40 **Women** 99% **Men** 1% **Minority** 6% **Part-time** 100%
Nursing Student Activities Student Nurses' Association.
Nursing Student Resources Academic advising; academic or career counseling; bookstore; campus computer network; computer lab; daycare for children of students; e-mail services; employment services for current students; externships; housing assistance; Internet; learning resource lab; library services; nursing audiovisuals; placement services for program completers; skills, simulation, or other laboratory.
Library Facilities 230,910 volumes; 12,351 periodical subscriptions.

BACCALAUREATE PROGRAMS

Degree BScN
Available Programs Generic Baccalaureate; RN Baccalaureate.
Site Options St. Jerome, QC.
Study Options Full-time and part-time.
Program Entrance Requirements CPR certification, high school chemistry, immunizations, interview, RN licensure. Transfer students are accepted. *Application deadline:* 3/1 (fall). *Application fee:* CAN$30.
Advanced Placement Credit by examination available. Credit given for nursing courses completed elsewhere dependent upon specific evaluations.
Financial Aid ***Loans:*** college/university.
Contact Ms. Chantal Saint-Pierre, Directrice, Département des Sciences Infirmières, Université du Québec en Outaouais, Office D-0414, Hull, QC J8X 3X7. *Telephone:* 819-595-3900 Ext. 2345. *Fax:* 819-595-3801. *E-mail:* chantal.st-pierre@uqo.ca.

GRADUATE PROGRAMS

Contact Ms. Chantal Saint-Pierre, Directrice, Département des Sciences Infirmières, Université du Québec en Outaouais, CP 1250, Succursale Hull, Gatineau, QC J8X 3X7. *Telephone:* 819-595-3900 Ext. 2347. *Fax:* 819-595-2202. *E-mail:* chantal.st-pierre@uqo.ca.

MASTER'S DEGREE PROGRAM

Degree M Sc N
Available Programs Master's.
Concentrations Available Health-care administration. *Clinical nurse specialist programs in:* community health, critical care, psychiatric/mental health, rehabilitation. *Nurse practitioner programs in:* primary care.
Site Options St. Jerome, QC.
Study Options Full-time and part-time.
Program Entrance Requirements Computer literacy, 3 letters of recommendation, nursing research course, resume, statistics course. *Application deadline:* 5/1 (fall), 11/1 (winter), 3/1 (spring). *Application fee:* CAN$30.
Advanced Placement Credit given for nursing courses completed elsewhere dependent upon specific evaluations.
Degree Requirements 45 total credit hours, thesis or project.

Université Laval

Faculty of Nursing
Québec, Quebec

http://www.fsi.ulaval.ca
Founded in 1852

DEGREES • BSCN • MSN • PHD
Nursing Program Faculty 25 (64% with doctorates).
Baccalaureate Enrollment 798 **Women** 94% **Men** 6% **Minority** 18% **International** 12% **Part-time** 32%
Graduate Enrollment 116 **Women** 72% **Men** 28% **Minority** 32% **International** 24% **Part-time** 22%
Distance Learning Courses Available.
Nursing Student Activities Student Nurses' Association, nursing club.
Nursing Student Resources Academic advising; academic or career counseling; assistance for students with disabilities; bookstore; campus computer network; career placement assistance; computer lab; computer-assisted instruction; daycare for children of students; e-mail services; employment services for current students; externships; housing assistance; interactive nursing skills videos; Internet; learning resource lab; library services; nursing audiovisuals; placement services for program completers; resume preparation assistance; skills, simulation, or other laboratory; tutoring.
Library Facilities 3 million volumes (118,994 in health, 3,781 in nursing); 13,928 periodical subscriptions (624 health-care related).

BACCALAUREATE PROGRAMS

Degree BScN
Available Programs Accelerated Baccalaureate; Accelerated RN Baccalaureate; Generic Baccalaureate; RN Baccalaureate.
Study Options Full-time and part-time.
Program Entrance Requirements Transcript of college record, high school biology, high school chemistry, 5 years high school math, high school transcript, immunizations, minimum high school GPA. Transfer students are accepted.
Advanced Placement Credit given for nursing courses completed elsewhere dependent upon specific evaluations.
Contact ***Telephone:*** 418-656-2131 Ext. 7930. *Fax:* 418-656-7747.

GRADUATE PROGRAMS

Contact ***Telephone:*** 418-656-3356. *Fax:* 418-656-7304.

MASTER'S DEGREE PROGRAM

Degree MSN
Available Programs Accelerated Master's; Master's.
Concentrations Available Clinical nurse leader; health-care administration; nursing administration. *Clinical nurse specialist programs in:* acute care, adult health, cardiovascular, community health, critical care, family health, gerontology, oncology, palliative care, parent-child, pediatric, perinatal, psychiatric/mental health, public health, rehabilitation. *Nurse practitioner programs in:* adult health, primary care.
Study Options Full-time and part-time.
Program Entrance Requirements Clinical experience, transcript of college record, 2 letters of recommendation, nursing research course, resume, statistics course, French exam.
Advanced Placement Credit given for nursing courses completed elsewhere dependent upon specific evaluations.
Degree Requirements 45 total credit hours, thesis or project.

POST-MASTER'S PROGRAM

Areas of Study *Clinical nurse specialist programs in:* acute care, adult health, cardiovascular, community health, critical care, family health, gerontology, oncology, palliative care, parent-child, pediatric, perinatal, psychiatric/mental health, public health, rehabilitation. *Nurse practitioner programs in:* adult health, primary care.

DOCTORAL DEGREE PROGRAM

Degree PhD
Available Programs Doctorate.
Areas of Study Community health, nursing science.
Program Entrance Requirements Clinical experience, interview, 2 letters of recommendation, MSN or equivalent, scholarly papers, statistics course, vita, writing sample.
Degree Requirements 96 total credit hours, dissertation, oral exam, written exam.

POSTDOCTORAL PROGRAM

Areas of Study Aging, cancer care, community health, gerontology, health promotion/disease prevention, nursing interventions, nursing research, nursing science, outcomes.
Postdoctoral Program Contact ***Telephone:*** 418-656-3356. *Fax:* 418-656-7747.

CONTINUING EDUCATION PROGRAM

Contact ***Telephone:*** 418-656-2131 Ext. 6712. *Fax:* 418-656-7747.

SASKATCHEWAN

University of Saskatchewan
College of Nursing
Saskatoon, Saskatchewan

http://www.usask.ca/nursing/
Founded in 1907

DEGREES • BSN • MN • PHD

Nursing Program Faculty 134 (20% with doctorates).
Baccalaureate Enrollment 1,678 **Women** 93% **Men** 7% **Minority** 5% **Part-time** 17%
Graduate Enrollment 50 **Women** 94% **Men** 6% **Minority** 2% **Part-time** 62%
Distance Learning Courses Available.
Nursing Student Activities Student Nurses' Association.
Nursing Student Resources Academic advising; academic or career counseling; assistance for students with disabilities; bookstore; campus computer network; computer lab; computer-assisted instruction; daycare for children of students; e-mail services; employment services for current students; interactive nursing skills videos; Internet; learning resource lab; library services; nursing audiovisuals; other; remedial services; resume preparation assistance; skills, simulation, or other laboratory; tutoring.
Library Facilities 2 million volumes (92,505 in health, 3,932 in nursing); 444,519 periodical subscriptions (3,069 health-care related).

BACCALAUREATE PROGRAMS

Degree BSN
Available Programs Accelerated Baccalaureate; Accelerated RN Baccalaureate; Baccalaureate for Second Degree; Generic Baccalaureate; RN Baccalaureate.
Site Options Regina , SK; Prince Albert, SK; Saskatoon , SK.
Study Options Full-time and part-time.
Program Entrance Requirements Transcript of college record, CPR certification, high school biology, high school chemistry, 4 years high school math, 4 years high school science, high school transcript, immunizations, minimum high school GPA of 2.0. Transfer students are accepted. *Application deadline:* 1/15 (fall). *Application fee:* CAN$90.
Advanced Placement Credit given for nursing courses completed elsewhere dependent upon specific evaluations.
Expenses (2009-10) *Tuition, area resident:* full-time CAN$5099; part-time CAN$168 per credit hour. *Required fees:* full-time CAN$695; part-time CAN$159 per credit.
Financial Aid 75% of baccalaureate students in nursing programs received some form of financial aid in 2008-09. *Gift aid (need-based):* private, college/university gift aid from institutional funds. *Loans:* college/university, Canadian student loans, provincial loans. *Financial aid application deadline:* 3/15(priority: 2/15).
Contact Ms. Shelley Bueckert, Academic Advisor and Admissions Officer, College of Nursing, University of Saskatchewan, 107 Wiggins Road, Saskatoon, SK S7N 5E5. *Telephone:* 306-966-6231. *Fax:* 306-966-6621. *E-mail:* shelley.bueckert@usask.ca.

GRADUATE PROGRAMS

Expenses (2009-10) *Tuition, area resident:* part-time CAN$500 per course. *Room and board:* room only: CAN$8151 per academic year. *Required fees:* part-time CAN$61 per credit.
Financial Aid 30% of graduate students in nursing programs received some form of financial aid in 2008-09. Fellowships, research assistantships, teaching assistantships available. *Financial aid application deadline:* 1/31.
Contact Dr. Lynnette Stamler, Assistant Dean, Graduate Studies, Continuing Education, and Information Technology, College of Nursing, University of Saskatchewan, 107 Wiggins Road, Saskatoon, SK S7N 5E5. *Telephone:* 306-966-1477. *Fax:* 306-966-6703. *E-mail:* lynnette.stamler@usask.ca.

MASTER'S DEGREE PROGRAM

Degree MN
Available Programs Master's.
Concentrations Available Nursing education. *Nurse practitioner programs in:* primary care.
Site Options Saskatoon , SK.
Study Options Full-time and part-time.
Program Entrance Requirements Minimum overall college GPA of 2.5, transcript of college record, 3 letters of recommendation, nursing research course, statistics course. *Application deadline:* 11/15 (fall). *Application fee:* CAN$75.
Advanced Placement Credit given for nursing courses completed elsewhere dependent upon specific evaluations.
Degree Requirements 24 total credit hours, thesis or project.

POST-MASTER'S PROGRAM

Areas of Study *Nurse practitioner programs in:* primary care.

DOCTORAL DEGREE PROGRAM

Degree PhD
Available Programs Doctorate.
Areas of Study Individualized study.
Site Options Saskatoon , SK.
Program Entrance Requirements Minimum overall college GPA of 4, 3 letters of recommendation, MSN or equivalent, statistics course, vita. Application deadline: 11/15 (fall). Application fee: CAN$75.
Degree Requirements 18 total credit hours, dissertation, oral exam, written exam.

CONTINUING EDUCATION PROGRAM

Contact Prof. Patricia Wall, Coordinator, College of Nursing, University of Saskatchewan, Continuing Nursing Education, Box 6000, RPO, Saskatoon, SK S7N 4J8. *Telephone:* 306-966-6261. *Fax:* 306-966-7673. *E-mail:* pat.wall@usask.ca.

TWO-PAGE DESCRIPTIONS

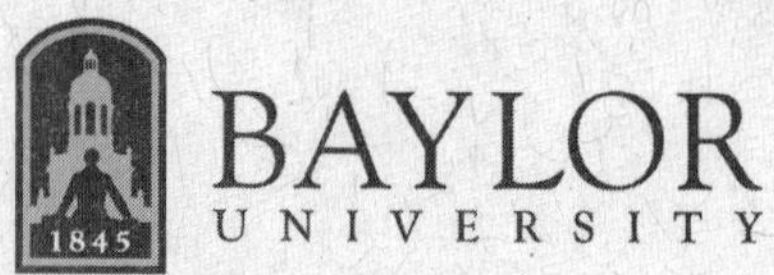

Louise Herrington School of Nursing

Learn. Lead. Serve.

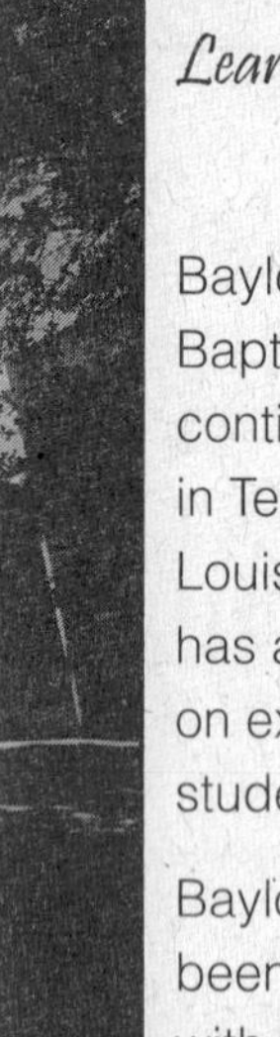

The Louise Herrington School of Nursing.

Baylor University is the world's largest Baptist university and is the oldest continuously operating university in Texas. Established in 1909, the Louise Herrington School of Nursing has an outstanding reputation based on excellent faculty, curriculum, and students.

Baylor School of Nursing has always been committed to providing students with premier education and clinical experience in a faith-based environment. Baylor's curriculum challenges students to think and act like nurses long before they graduate.

The undergraduate program consists of 131 semester hours and awards the Bachelor Science in Nursing (B.S.N.) degree. This includes 66 semester hours of prerequisites, which may be taken on the Baylor-Waco campus or at any other accredited college or university. The upper-level (junior and senior years) of the program consists of 65 semester hours completed on the School of Nursing campus in Dallas. Baylor's FastBacc is a twelve-month accelerated track that is designed for individuals who have already completed a bachelor's degree in a non-nursing discipline. It is an intensive full-time program that begins each summer with a combination of teaching methodologies, including traditional classroom, online course component, clinical and lab experiences, and hybrid interactive learning courses.

Baylor's graduate studies program is ranked nationally by *US News & World Report* for its academic reputation and offers part- or full-time study in one of three advanced practice majors: Family Nurse Practitioner (FNP), Neonatal Nursing (NNP) and Midwifery (CNM). Students completing the Nurse-Midwife track are awarded a Doctor of Nursing Practice (DNP) degree. Caring for the medically underserved is a special focus for the Baylor graduate program.

The School and all its programs have received full, national accreditation by the Commission on Collegiate Nursing Education (CCNE) and are approved by the Texas Board of Nurses. The Accreditation Commission for Midwifery Education (ACME) accredits the Midwifery program.

At the heart of the Louise Herrington School of Nursing is an exceptional faculty, each member committed to the success of Baylor's students. The faculty is a unique group—researchers, authors, winners of countless national awards, presidents of national organizations, former missionaries and administrators, and experts in their specialties. Faculty members are always accessible and are always focused on the needs of their students.

Located on the Baylor University Medical Center campus near downtown Dallas, the four-story complex includes a student computer lab (open 24 hours a day, 7 days a week), spacious classrooms wired for multimedia and video presentations, quiet study lounges, and the high-fidelity Don A. and Ruth Buchholz Patient Simulation Lab.

The Learning Resource Center, staffed by professional medical librarians, provides support services exclusively to Baylor's students and faculty members. The Barnabas Student Success Center, Student Ministry, and other student organizations are here to provide students with all the tools and resources they need to succeed in their education.

Classes are small and clinical experiences individualized to student needs. Financial support often is available. The School offers a comprehensive program that includes merit-based and need-based scholarships as well as grants, loans and part-time employment to ease the financial burdens of undergraduate nursing students.

The need is great. A career in nursing is one in which you choose to make a difference. You choose to serve. You choose to care. You have the potential to do extraordinary good, to make the world a better place. Our goal is to prepare the next generation of nurses. There's never been a more exciting time in medicine or health care. There's never been a greater need for the best and the brightest. Join us, and through a life of leadership and service, become an unstoppable force for good. When you are ready, Baylor is the next step in your calling to Learn, Lead, and Serve.

- *2010–11 GRADUATE TUITION & FEES:*

  Tuition: $1124 per semester hour

  General Student Fee (12 hours or more per semester): $1379

  General Student Fee (less than 12 hours): $155 per semester hour

  Course Fees: (varies) minimum $50

  For more information: http://bit.ly/BaylorNursing_grad_tuition_fees

- *APPLICATION DEADLINES:*

  Traditional Baccalaureate: January 15 (Fall semester); May 1 (Spring semester)

  FastBacc Track: November 1

  Graduate Program: April 15 (fall admission only); February 1 (F.N.P. early admit); NNP and N-M programs will make exceptions on deadlines on a case-by-case basis.

- *FACULTY INFORMATION: http://bit.ly/BaylorNursing_faculty*

CONTACT INFORMATION

Rebecca A. Robbins
Louise Herrington School of Nursing
Baylor University
3700 Worth Street
Dallas, Texas 75246
Phone: 214-820-3361
Fax: 214-820-3835
E-mail: BU_Nursing@baylor.edu
Web site: http://www.baylor.edu/Nursing

Undergraduate Program
Student Services Department
Louise Herrington School of Nursing
Phone 214-820-4160
Fax: 214-820-3835

Graduate Program
Louise Herrington School of Nursing
Phone 214-820-41111
Fax: 214-820-3375

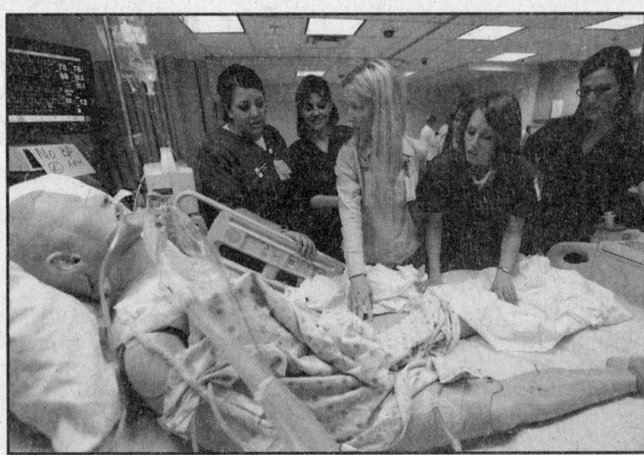

Students and instructor in the Simulation Lab.

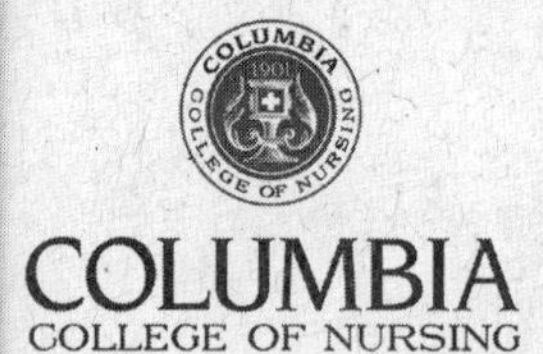

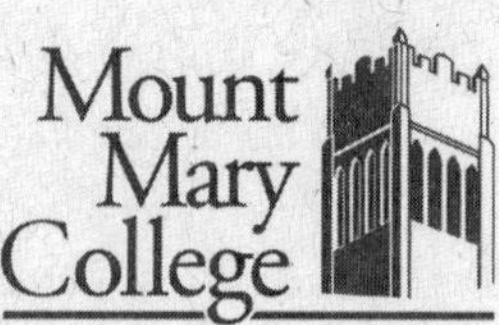

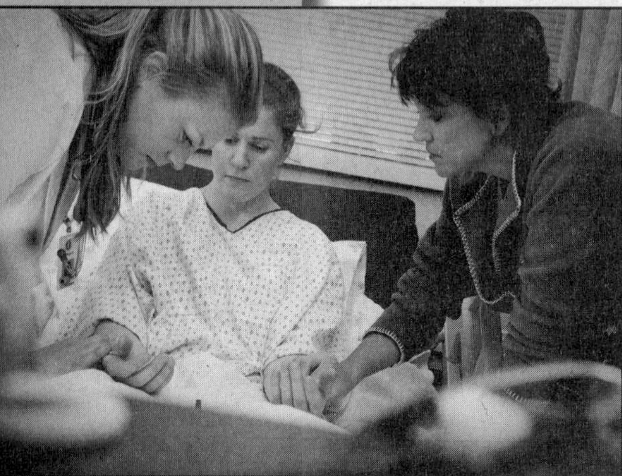

Promise . . .
Possibilities . . .
Success

Caring faculty members work with students throughout their learning process.

Mission: To prepare competent, compassionate health-care professionals distinguished by liberal arts education, evidence-based practice, clinical reasoning, safe patient care, and commitment to social justice.

Columbia College of Nursing (CCON) and Mount Mary College (MMC) offer a unique intercollegiate program leading to a Bachelor of Science in Nursing (B.S.N.) degree. For students who are registered nurses and have an associate degree or diploma in nursing, a degree completion program leading to a B.S.N. degree is also available.

The combination of Columbia's history of excellence with Mount Mary's highly respected tradition of a liberal arts–based education offers students the highest caliber of preparation for a career in nursing. Nursing students combine nursing instruction with clinical placements, enabling them to meet the challenges of health care today and into the future.

Affiliations between CCON and southeastern Wisconsin community clinical sites further guarantee that students, while experiencing the latest advances in nursing education, also remain on the cutting edge of today's changing health-care environment.

Graduates of the nursing program have found jobs in a variety of places within the health-care field including Milwaukee-area acute-care hospitals (Columbia–St. Mary's, Aurora St. Luke's, Community Memorial Hospital, Children's Hospital of Wisconsin, Waukesha Memorial, and Froedtert Hospital), long-term care facilities, community health agencies, clinics, and schools.

Columbia College of Nursing and Mount Mary encourage students to take advantage of a variety of study-abroad opportunities. In recent years, Mount Mary has sponsored programs to China, England, France, Guatemala, Ireland, Italy, Nicaragua, and Peru. Mount Mary also maintains affiliate relationships with international colleges and universities, including the American College, Dublin, Ireland; the American Intercontinental University, London and Dubai; Nanzan College, Japan; Universidad Cathólica de Santa Maria (UCSM), Arequipa, Peru; and Notre Dame College, Kyoto, Japan.

In its new location on Milwaukee's north side, CCON is easily accessible from the Interstate, is served by most of the city's major bus routes, and is near a diverse assortment of shops, restaurants, and recreational facilities. Mount Mary College is located on Milwaukee's northwest side, on 80 acres that provide a park-like campus in a residential area.

More than 95 percent of full-time students receive some form of financial assistance. For more information, contact the Admission

Office or visit the Mount Mary Financial Aid Web page at www.mtmary.edu/aid.htm.

The nursing program is open to both men and women. There are multiple entry points into the major. All students must first apply and be accepted to Mount Mary College as pre-nursing students. A population of students will be **directly admitted** into the nursing program. Another population will be admitted to Mount Mary College as pre-nursing students (Standard Admission). Standard Admission to Columbia College of Nursing is a two-step process. Student applications are evaluated individually, in conjunction with the Columbia College of Nursing faculty.

International students must take the Test of English as a Foreign Language (TOEFL). Mount Mary College has a rolling admissions policy, offers Early Acceptance, and honors Advanced Placement.

The nursing program is approved by the Wisconsin State Board of Nursing and the National League for Nursing Accrediting Commission and is a member of American Association of Colleges of Nursing. Both colleges are fully accredited by the North Central Association of Colleges and Schools.

Columbia College of Nursing and Mount Mary College do not discriminate against any individual for reasons of race, color, religion, age, disability, or national or ethnic origin.

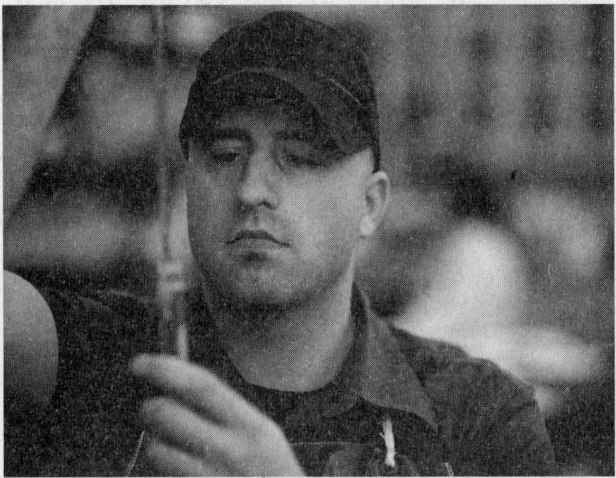

Science lab work is a critical part of the nursing student's education.

- *2010–11 UNDERGRADUATE TUITION & FEES: Full-time (12–18 credits), per year: $21,668; Full-time (12–18 credits), per semester: $10,834; Per Credit: $648; Nursing Tuition, per credit: $648; Accelerated Programs Tuition, per credit: $598; Tuition deposit: $200; For more information: www.mtmary.edu/pdfs/academics/nursing/nursing-tuition.pdf*
- *APPLICATION DEADLINES: Visit the http://www.mtmary.edu/nursing_fy.htm for complete admission details and to download he admission policy.*
- *FACULTY INFORMATION: http://www.ccon.edu/Faculty/faculty.htm*
- *MULTIMEDIA: For blogs and social media, visit www.mtmary.edu/blogs.htm*

CONTACT INFORMATION

Admissions Department
Columbia College of Nursing/Mount Mary College
2900 N. Menomonee River Parkway
Milwaukee, Wisconsin 53222-4597
Phone: 414-256-1219
800-321-6265 (toll-free)
E-mail: Kurtza@mtmary.edu
Web sites: www.ccon.edu
www.mtmary.edu
www.mtmary.edu/dept_nursing.htm

Find us on Facebook®: www.facebook.com/mountmary?v=wall
Follow us on Twitter™: http://twitter.com/MountMary

Columbia University

School of Nursing

A tradition of excellence in nursing leadership, practice, and research that spans more than a century.

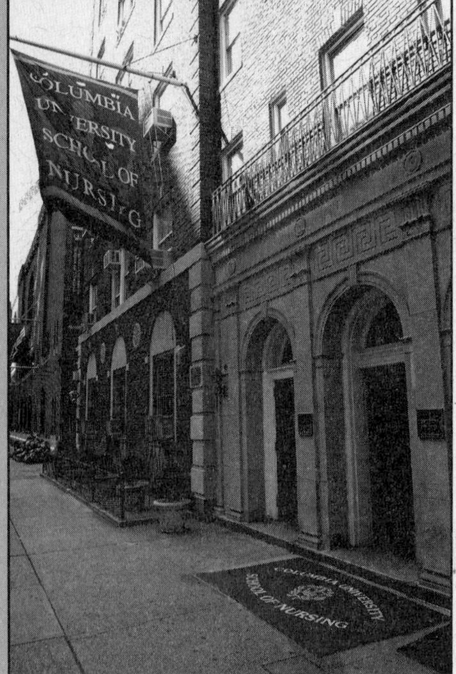

School of Nursing—located in the heart of Washington Heights, New York City.

Founded in 1892 as the Presbyterian Hospital School of Nursing, the School first offered the baccalaureate degree when it joined Columbia University. In 1956, it became the first nursing program in the country to award a master's degree in a clinical nursing specialty. Today, the primary focus of the School is to educate advanced practice nurses—nurse practitioners, nurse midwives, and nurse anesthetists. This is done through the academic program at the graduate, advanced certificate, and doctoral levels.

The curriculum is focused on preparing professional nurses who think critically, exercise technical competence, and make socially significant contributions to society through theory-based practice. Faculty members endeavor to provide knowledge, stimulate learning, define issues, and serve as resource persons, clinicians, administrators, leaders, and innovators in nursing. A major strength of the School is that the faculty members maintain clinical practices in their advanced roles and incorporate students into these settings. One of these practices, Columbia Advanced Practice Nurse Associates (CAPNA), has gained national exposure as an innovative model of primary-care delivery by advanced practice nurses who are on the primary provider panels of several major managed-care organizations.

In addition to these programs, the School contains five academic centers: the Center for AIDS Research, the Center for Health Policy and Health Services Research, the Center for Evidence-Based Practice, the Center for Interdisciplinary Research to Reduce Antimicrobial Resistance, and the World Health Organization Collaborating Center for International Nursing Development in Advanced Practice. Columbia was the first nursing school to be awarded this World Health Organization designation, which makes the School an active participant in international exchange and collaborative research in advanced practice and health services research. It also facilitates the development of international study opportunities for its students.

The School of Nursing offers four levels of educational programs. The Combined B.S./M.S. (Entry to Practice) Program is an accelerated combined-degree program (B.S./M.S.) for non-nurse baccalaureate-prepared graduates, designed to prepare the student for a career as an advanced practice nurse. Academic studies are closely integrated with clinical experience. Upon completion, the student is eligible to take the professional nurse licensure examination in any state.

The Graduate Program, leading to the M.S. degree, affords registered nurses with a bachelor's degree the opportunity to increase their knowledge in advanced nursing practice. The School currently offers nine graduate majors: anesthesia, acute care, neonatal, psychiatric mental health nursing, midwifery, the primary-care specialties (adult, family, and pediatric), and women's health. Joint degrees are available with the Schools of Public Health and Business.

The Advanced Certificate Program allows RNs with a master's degree in nursing to pursue an advanced practice program as a nurse practitioner.

The Ph.D. in Nursing Program is designed to prepare clinical nurse scholars to examine, shape, and refine the health-care delivery system.

The Doctor of Nursing Practice Program prepares nurses with the knowledge, skills, and attributes necessary for fully accountable practice with patients across sites and over time. The D.N.P. is the natural evolution and needed expansion of existing clinical degrees in nursing, the basic B.S. and the site-specific M.S. degree.

The School of Nursing building houses two Technology Learning Centers (TLCs), which include a mock hospital unit containing several patient units and an ambulatory-care area for practicing primary-care skills. The TLCs are used by graduate and undergraduate students for skills development, including physical assessment and state-of-the-art monitoring technology. There are also two informatics laboratories available to School of Nursing students.

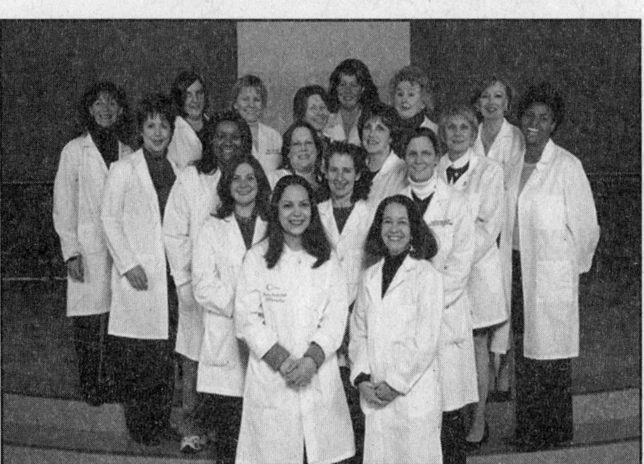

First DNP Cohort, which graduated in 2005.

The School of Nursing is part of the Columbia University Medical Center, a 20-acre campus overlooking the Hudson River on Manhattan's Upper West Side. Students can avail themselves of the recreational, cultural, and educational events and entertainment that have made New York City famous.

- *2010–11 UNDERGRADUATE TUITION & FEES: $1152 per credit*
- *2010–11 GRADUATE TUITION & FEES: $1212 per credit*
- *APPLICATION DEADLINES:*

  Combined B.S./M.S. Program (ETP): November 15

  Master's and Post Master's Certificate Nurse Anesthesia Program: November 1

  Master's Programs Summer Applicants: December 15

  Ph.D. Program: February 1

  Doctor of Nursing Practice (D.N.P.) Programs: March 1

  Master's Program Fall Applicants (Only Part-Time Status): April 1

- *FACULTY: http://www.cumc.columbia.edu/dept/nursing/faculty/index.html*

CONTACT INFORMATION

Judy Wolfe
Senior Director of Admissions and Financial Aid
Columbia University School of Nursing
617 West 168th Street
New York, New York 10463
Phone: 212-305-5756
800-899-8895 (toll-free)
Fax: 212-305-3680
E-mail: nursing@columbia.edu
Web site: http://www.nursing.columbia.edu

Find us on Facebook®: http://www.facebook.com/ColumbiaNursing

Duke University School of Nursing

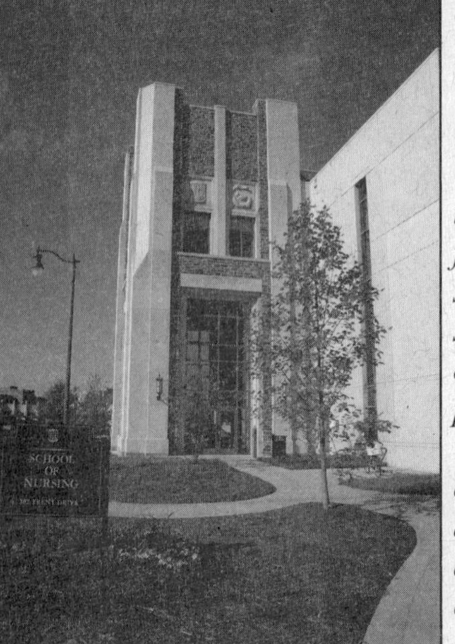

Since 1931, the Duke University School of Nursing remains on the forefront of nursing education, practice, and research.

Transforming care. Touching lives.

The mission of the Duke University School of Nursing is to create a center of excellence for the advancement of nursing science, the promotion of clinical scholarship, and the education of clinical leaders, advanced practitioners, and researchers. Through nursing research, education, and practice, students and faculty seek to enhance the quality of life for people of all cultures, economic levels, and geographic locations.

In support of James Duke's original vision, the School of Nursing has maintained a commitment to achieving excellence. Since the first nursing students were admitted to a three-year diploma program in 1931, the School remains on the forefront of nursing education, practice, and research. Historically, the School has been a health-care leader by first awarding baccalaureate degrees in 1938, establishing the Bachelor of Science in Nursing degree in 1953, and beginning one of the first nursing graduate programs in 1958.

Today, offering the Accelerated Bachelor of Science in Nursing degree, the Master of Science in Nursing degree, the Post-Master's Certificate in Nursing, the Doctorate of Nursing Practice (D.N.P.) program, and the Ph.D. program, the Duke University School of Nursing (DUSON) remains a national leader in nursing education. Through innovative teaching strategies, the incorporation of advanced technology, and collegial faculty-to-student relationships, the School remains dedicated to improving access to care, providing high-quality cost-effective care, and preparing health-care leaders for today and tomorrow.

The Duke University School of Nursing provides leadership in the health care of people through education, research, and health-care delivery. The School provides advanced and comprehensive education to prepare students for a lifetime of learning and for careers as leaders, practitioners, or researchers. As a result of the School's academic programs, Duke's faculty members, students, and graduates are constantly shaping the future of professional nursing practice. Faculty and students conduct research that adds to our understanding of health promotion and illness prevention, human responses to illness, and systems of care that facilitate better patient outcomes. For most programs, the curriculum allows students to customize learning opportunities to fit their goals and needs in collaboration with faculty advisors. Full-time and part-time options are available.

In January 2006, the School of Nursing established The Office of Global and Community Health Initiatives (OGACHI), which is allied with the Duke Global Health Institute. The overall goal of OGACHI is to address health disparities locally and abroad through the promotion of academic enrichment, service-learning, and research pertaining to issues of global health. The Office serves as a clearing house and catalyst for the development, facilitation, and monitoring of local, regional, and international activities of students and faculty as related to improving health around the world. It also cultivates and promotes interdisciplinary linkages across the campus and externally with other organizations, agencies, and communities in responding to disparate health outcomes of the poor and underserved. In addition, OGACHI seeks to increase diversity in nursing through special initiatives and programs, often in partnership with other institutions.

Using a student-centered approach, the Center for Nursing Discovery (CND) provides a variety of avenues of instructional methodology, including simulation using high fidelity (or "lifelike") adult and pediatric mannequins, role playing, faculty-assisted instruction, procedural task trainers to develop specific hands-on skills, standardized patients (trained actors), and the use of innovative, state-of-the-art multimedia. Practice in the CND, along with their clinical experiences, helps students move toward developing their own evidence-based nursing practice, achieving the ultimate goal of becoming clinical leaders in providing excellent patient care.

Duke Nurses are distinguished by their critical thinking skills, autonomy, and dedication to the highest standards in patient care, research, and education. With a focus on nursing education, innovations in research and health care, and finding ways to bring better care to people, the Duke School of Nursing looks for students who are mature and enthusiastic—students who care as much about people as they do about leading nursing in the new century. The Admissions staff is available to help and welcomes prospective students' e-mail, phone calls, and personal visits.

The Duke University School of Nursing is accredited by the Commission of Collegiate Nursing Education. In addition, the North Carolina Board of Nursing has approved the Accelerated Bachelor of Science in Nursing degree program.

- *2011–12 UNDERGRADUATE TUITION & FEES:*

  Tuition: $1010 per credit hour; fees vary by program

- *2011–12 GRADUATE TUITION & FEES:*

  Tuition: $1295 per credit hour; fees vary by program

- *APPLICATION DEADLINES:*

  Accelerated Bachelor of Science in Nursing (B.S.N.): July 1 for Spring enrollment; December 1 for Fall enrollment

  Master of Science in Nursing (M.S.N.)/Post-Master's Certificate: August 1 for Fall enrollment; December 1 for Spring enrollment; April 2 for Summer enrollment

  Doctor of Nursing Practice (D.N.P.): Post-master's D.N.P. applicants—February 1 for Fall enrollment

  Post-bachelor's D.N.P. applicants—September 1 for Spring enrollment; May 1 for Fall enrollment

  Ph.D. Program: December 8

- *FACULTY INFORMATION:*

  http://fds.duke.edu/db/nurse/faculty

CONTACT INFORMATION

Office of Admissions and Student Services
Duke University School of Nursing
Duke University
307 Trent Drive
Durham, North Carolina 27710
Phone: 919-684-4248
877-415-3853 (toll-free)
Fax: (919) 668-4693
E-mail: SONAdmissions@mc.duke.edu
Web site: http://www.nursing.duke.edu

UNDERGRADUATE NURSING PROGRAM:
Accelerated B.S.N. Admissions
DUMC 3322, 307 Trent Drive
Durham, North Carolina 27710
Phone: 919 684-4248
Fax: 919-668-4693
E-mail: SONAdmissions@mc.duke.edu

GRADUATE NURSING PROGRAM:
M.S.N., Post-Master's Certificate, and D.N.P. Admissions
DUMC 3322, 307 Trent Drive
Durham, North Carolina 27710
Phone: 919-684-4248
Fax: 919-668-4693
E-mail: SONAdmissions@mc.duke.edu

Ph.D. Program
Duke University Graduate School
2127 Campus Drive
Box 90065
Durham, North Carolina 27708
Phone: 919-684-3913
Fax: 919-684-2277
E-mail: grad-admissions-center@duke.edu

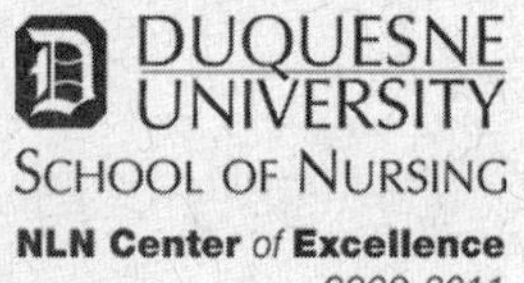

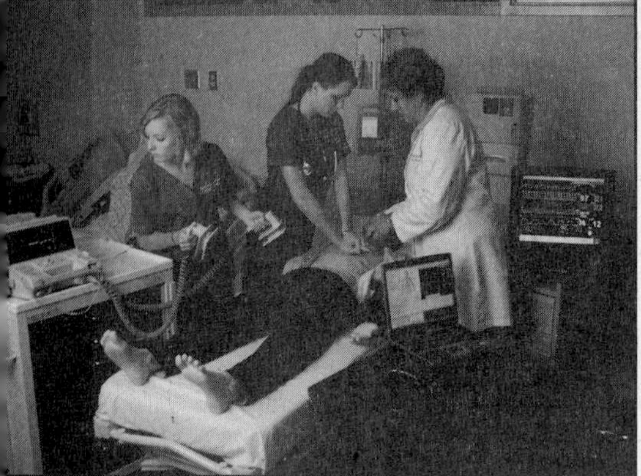

In the instructive environment of Duquesne's high-tech nursing labs, students acquire clinical knowledge and decision-making skills.

The Duquesne University School of Nursing was the first nursing school in Pennsylvania to offer a Bachelor of Science in Nursing degree and the first in the nation with an entirely online doctorate in nursing program.

Recognized as a National League for Nursing Center of Excellence, the School of Nursing is accredited by the Commission on Collegiate Nursing Education and the Pennsylvania State Board of Nursing.

Since its founding in 1878, Duquesne University has earned a reputation for academic excellence and having a faculty that is committed to teaching and to helping students succeed. Today, Duquesne is experiencing an exciting period of growth and increased recognition:

- Our graduate program in nursing has been nationally ranked by *US News & World Report*.
- We are sixteenth in the nation among small research universities, according to a *Chronicle of Higher Education* index that measured faculty productivity among more than 7,300 doctoral programs.
- We are one of the 2011 Princeton Review's "The Best 373 Colleges," a list that comprises only 15 percent of schools in the United States and Canada.

From the beginning, Duquesne has worked diligently to improve the quality of life for the people of Pittsburgh. To that end the School of Nursing operates a Nurse-Managed Wellness Center for underserved communities, where nurses and other health-care providers promote health and wellness and monitor chronic medical conditions. These clinics offer students an invaluable learning experience as well as an opportunity for community service. The School of Nursing is also home to the Center for Nursing Research, which supports qualitative and quantitative inquiry in areas related to health disparities, cultural competence, and chronic deviations from health.

Duquesne's green, self-contained, 49-acre campus—centrally located in a city with an international reputation for leadership in medicine and technology—has superb recreational facilities and student services and is only minutes away from Pittsburgh's rich cultural, sports, and entertainment offerings.

Bachelor of Science in Nursing (B.S.N.) Program

Clinical experiences, which begin in the sophomore year, create a strong foundation for nursing practice, and Duquesne's students complete over 1,170 clinical hours in hospitals and community health facilities. The clinical faculty-to-student ratio is 1:8.

Duquesne's nursing labs have the latest nursing simulators for helping students gain patient-care skills in a controlled environment designed to improve decision making and develop teamwork, communications, and leadership skills.

Nursing students can add international perspectives by participating in faculty-led, summertime study-abroad programs or for-credit learning experiences in Nicaragua during spring break. The University offers semester-long programs at a satellite campus in Italy and at an International Study Center in Ireland.

Second Degree B.S.N. Program

The Second Degree Bachelor of Science in Nursing (B.S.N.) program enables the non-nurse with a baccalaureate degree to obtain a B.S.N. in twelve months, after which the NCLEX-RN licensure examination can be taken. The program includes three semesters of course work and over 850 hours of clinical experience.

Graduate Programs

All graduate nursing programs are offered exclusively online in a user-friendly, asynchronous format. Online learning provides flexibility for professional nurses with busy schedules and permits students to earn degrees in a reasonable length of time. Course work is highly interactive, so students communicate often with instructors and classmates. Online flexibility plus academic rigor make the Duquesne University School of Nursing the ideal choice for graduate nursing education.

Master of Science in Nursing (M.S.N.)

Family Nurse Practitioner (FNP)
Forensic Nursing
Nursing Education

Post-Master's Certificates

Family Nurse Practitioner (FNP)
Forensic Nursing
Nursing Education
Transcultural/International Nursing

Ph.D. in Nursing

Doctor of Nursing Practice (D.N.P.)

Visit www.duq.edu/nursing for complete admission requirements and application instructions, or call 412-396-6050 or e-mail nursing@duq.edu.

- *2010–11 FULL-TIME UNDERGRADUATE TUITION & FEES: $27,502 (full-time)/$910 (per credit)*
- *2010–11 FULL-TIME GRADUATE TUITION & FEES: $991 per credit*
- *APPLICATION DEADLINES:*

  B.S.N.: May 1

  B.S.N. (transfer students): April 1 (fall admission); November 1 (spring admission)

  Second Degree B.S.N.: December 1

  M.S.N.: March 1

  Ph.D.: January 15

  D.N.P.: February 1

  Visit www.duq.edu/nursing for complete admission requirements and application instructions.
- *FACULTY INFORMATION: www.duq.edu/nursing*

CONTACT INFORMATION

Susan Hardner, Nurse Recruiter
545-A Fisher Hall
Duquesne University
600 Forbes Avenue
Pittsburgh, Pennsylvania 15282
Phone: 412-396-4945
Fax: 412-396-6346
E-mail: nursing@duq.edu
Web site: http://www.duq.edu/nursing

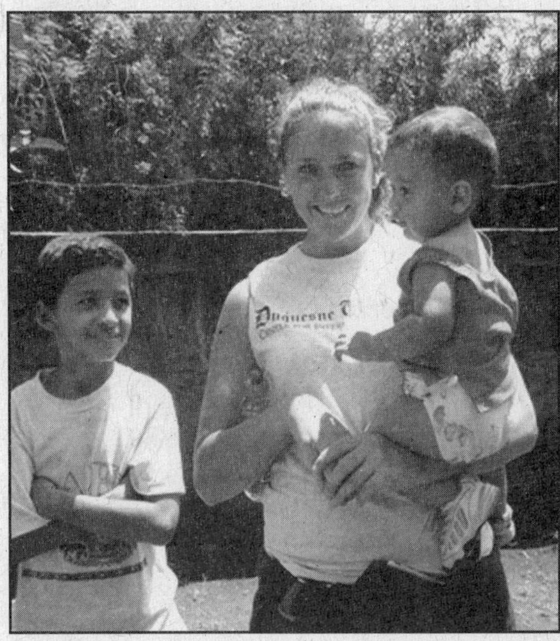

A Duquesne nursing student with Nicaraguan children during her international nursing experience.

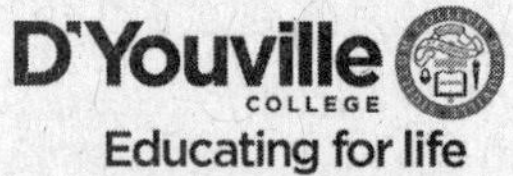

School of Nursing

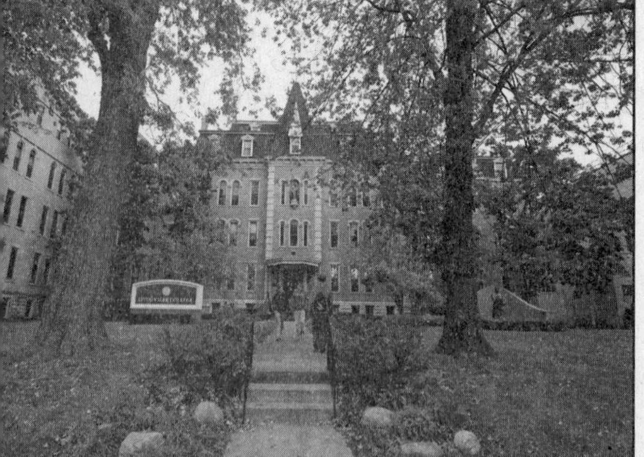

Educating competent, compassionate, knowledgeable, professional nurses.

The Koessler Administration Building dates back to 1872 when it was the home of Holy Angels Academy, a private boarding school for young ladies in elementary and secondary grades. In 1908, a charter established D'Youville College and the Academy of the Holy Angels. As the College grew, the Academy moved to another location in Buffalo in 1930. Today, the landmark building houses the President's suite and other administrative offices.

D'Youville College is a private, coeducational liberal arts and professional college offering students a high-quality education in more than thirty undergraduate and graduate degree programs. Founded in 1908 by the Grey Nuns as the first college for women in western New York to offer baccalaureate degrees to women, it was named for their founder, Saint Marguerite D'Youville. The current enrollment is 3,100 men and women. Students' learning is facilitated by the low 14:1 student-faculty ratio. The College is committed to helping its students grow not only academically but also in the social and personal areas of their college experience.

D'Youville College has been educating and preparing professional nurses for careers since 1942; the first Bachelor of Science in Nursing (B.S.N.) class graduated in 1946. In 1957, the RN to B.S.N. degree program was initiated, offering a specialized curriculum for the working professional nurse. All programs offered by the nursing department are fully accredited by the Commission on Collegiate Nursing Education (CCNE) and approved by the New York State Education Department.

The nursing faculty members are committed, dedicated educators who pride themselves on providing individual attention. Faculty members, the majority of whom are prepared at the doctoral level, represent diverse backgrounds, both clinically and educationally, providing numerous specialty areas for the students to draw upon.

D'Youville College has been growing and attracting students from all over the world since 1908, playing a leadership role in the areas of professional health training. D'Youville offers a four-year Bachelor of Science in Nursing degree program, and students who are interested in pursuing careers in nursing also have the option of completing a dual-degree, five-year sequence to graduate with both a baccalaureate and a master's degree. It is a direct-entry program in which accepted students do not have to reapply or re-qualify for upper-division courses.

The B.S.N. degree program combines a liberal arts foundation with professional nursing course work. Students begin their clinical experiences at area hospitals and health facilities in their sophomore year. Areas of clinical experience include geriatrics, pediatrics, OB/maternity, and medical/surgical nursing. To hone their clinical and research skills, students participate in internships during the summer of their junior year. The two-year RN to B.S.N. degree program includes an RN to B.S.N. option and a RN to B.S.N./M.S in nursing with a choice of clinical focus, in which RNs complete an additional year of study and graduate with both degrees. Convenient class scheduling provides working nursing professionals with the opportunity to study full-time by attending only two days a week. This alternative scheduling allows students to continue working in their professions while earning their degrees.

At the graduate level, nursing programs include the Master of Science (M.S.) in community health nursing, with concentrations in holistic nursing, hospice and palliative-care nursing, nursing management, and nursing education; the M.S. in nursing, with choice of clinical focus; and the Master of Science in family nurse practitioner studies as sell as a post-master's certificate in family nurse practitioner studies.

Specific facilities with which D'Youville has affiliations include Catholic Health System, which encompasses Mercy Hospital of Buffalo and Kenmore Mercy Hospital; Erie County Medical Center; WNY's Level 1 Trauma and Burn Center; Buffalo Psychiatric Center, Kaleida Health Care System, which comprises Women and Children's Hospital of Buffalo, Buffalo General Hospital, Millard Fillmore Hospital, and the Visiting Nurses Association of Western New York; BryLin Hospital; and the world-renowned Roswell Park Cancer Institute.

D'Youville College admits students on a rolling admissions basis but recommends students submit applications well before the start of the semester. Applications are reviewed as they are received by the Admissions Office. Undergraduate applicants must submit a completed application; official high school transcripts, and SAT or ACT scores. Transfer students must also submit official transcripts from all colleges previously attended.

Applicants to the master's program must present a baccalaureate degree in nursing from an accredited college or university program.

- *2011–12 UNDERGRADUATE TUITION & FEES: Full-time: $21,450*
  Room and Board: $10,000 per year
- *2011–12 GRADUATE TUITION & FEES: $790 per credit*
- *APPLICATION DEADLINES: Rolling admissions*
- *FACULTY: http://www.dyc.edu/academics/nursing/faculty.asp*

CONTACT INFORMATION

Dr. Judith Lewis
School of Nursing
D'Youville College
320 Porter Avenue
Buffalo, New York 14201
Phone: 716-829-7600
800-777-3921 (toll-free)
Fax: 716-829-7900
E-mail: admissions@dyc.edu
Web site: http://www.dyc.edu/academics/nursing/

UNDERGRADUATE NURSING PROGRAM

Dr. Steve Smith, Director of Admissions
Phone: 716-829-7600
E-mail: admissions@dyc.edu

GRADUATE NURSING PROGRAM

Linda Fisher, Director of Graduate Admissions
Phone: 716-829-8400
E-mail: graduateadmissions@dyc.edu

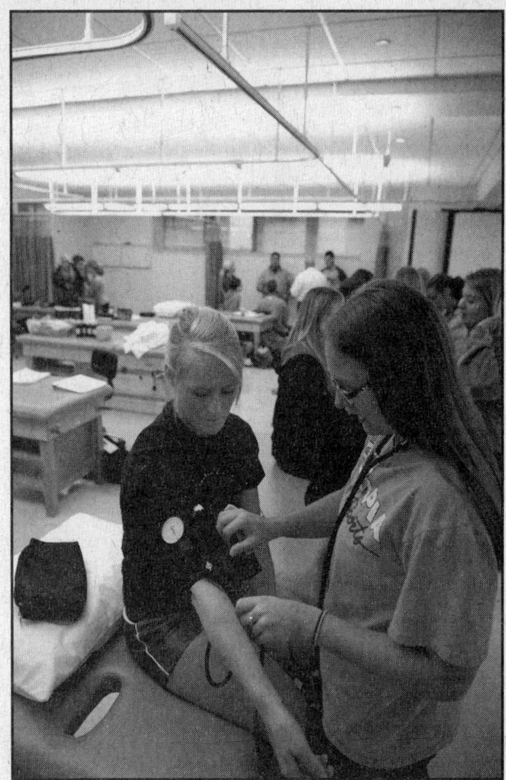

D'Youville College is internationally known for its wide array of health-care academic offerings. Majors include nursing, physician assistant, occupational and physical therapy, pharmacy, chiropractic, and dietetics. All majors include a strong liberal arts component.

Find us on Facebook®: http://www.dyc.edu/facebook
Follow us on Twitter™: http://www.dyc.edu/twitter

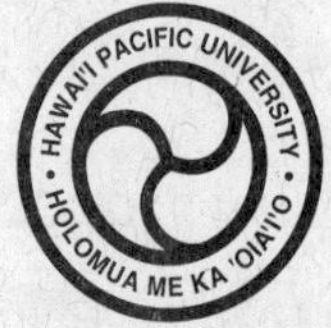

Hawai'i Pacific University College of Nursing and Health Sciences

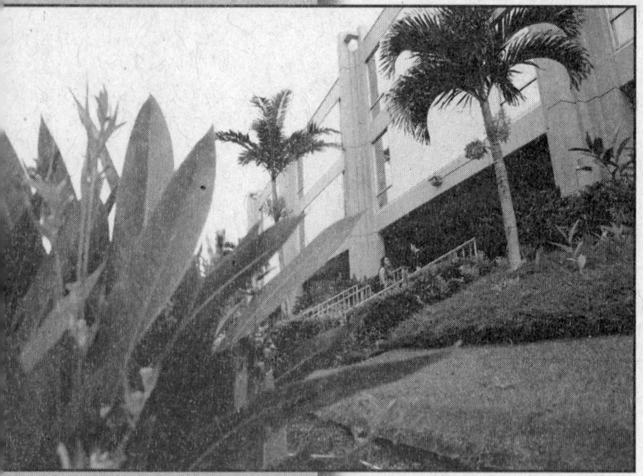

Nursing courses are taught at the Academic Center on the Hawai'i Loa campus.

Individual Attention & Extensive Resources

At HPU, students enjoy all of the technological and academic resources expected at a large university, delivered within the atmosphere of a small school. Our College of Nursing and Health Sciences has the largest nursing enrollment in the state of Hawai'i, with more than 1,300 students in its baccalaureate and master's degree programs. At the same time, HPU prides itself offering small nursing classes (24 to 32 students) and clinical groups (8 to 10 students) and providing individual attention to students.

HPU's Nursing Programs are built upon a strong foundation of liberal arts to prepare students to practice as professional nurses. HPU's liberally-educated baccalaureate nurse has the ability to analyze, think critically, and yet express the compassion needed in today's ever-changing health care environment. HPU's Nursing Programs also focus on developing cultural competency so nurses are ready to serve in the multicultural environment of our global community.

The College of Nursing and Health Sciences' challenging curriculum and competent, caring faculty guide students in learning the skills and knowledge necessary to care for individuals of all ages, their families and their communities. HPU partners with facilities all over the island of O'ahu so that students have many different options for gaining hands-on clinical experiences. Students have the opportunity to apply classroom and laboratory concepts, theories, and skills in a wide range of clinical settings, as well as in the University's own extensive simulation lab.

The baccalaureate nursing program offers four pathways toward a Bachelor of Science in Nursing (B.S.N.) degree:

- Basic Pathway—for the beginning or transfer student with fewer than 45 college credits.
- LPN to B.S.N. Pathway—for U.S. licensed practical nurses
- RN to B.S.N. Pathway—for licensed registered nurses from associate degree or diploma programs
- International Nurse Pathway—for those who have graduated from a nursing program in another country and are not licensed in the United States

Students are accepted directly into the College of Nursing and Health Sciences when they apply to the University. Nursing students must first complete General Common Core courses and Nursing prerequisites with a minimum 2.75 GPA before progressing into entry-level nursing courses. Once these prerequisite courses are completed, the student's portfolio is reviewed again, and students are admitted into entry-level nursing courses based on cumulative GPA, Science GPA, TEAS scores, and completed HPU credits. HPU's Nursing program offers 100–140 new seats in entry-level nursing courses each fall and each spring (up to 280 seats per year).

HPU also offers a graduate nursing program that brings together theory and community-based practice. The Master of Science in Nursing (M.S.N.) program enables the registered nurse the opportunity to advance as a family nurse practitioner (FNP) or a community clinical nurse specialist (CNS). The RN to M.S.N. Pathway allows registered nurses without baccalaureate degrees in nursing to make the transition into the M.S.N. program. Students in the Pathway program are granted provisional admission status until all prerequisites are completed. Students interested in gaining a solid foundation in current business and management practice may pursue a joint M.S.N./M.B.A. degree program.

A post-master's family nurse practitioner certificate is also possible for nurses with master's degrees seeking to expand their practice. A nurse educator certificate program can be taken as part of the CNS concentration or as a stand-alone certificate. Certificates in transcultural nursing and forensics are also available.

Hawai'i Pacific University offers several institutional scholarships and assistantships to U.S. citizens, permanent residents, and international applicants. Qualified applicants with demonstrated financial need may apply.

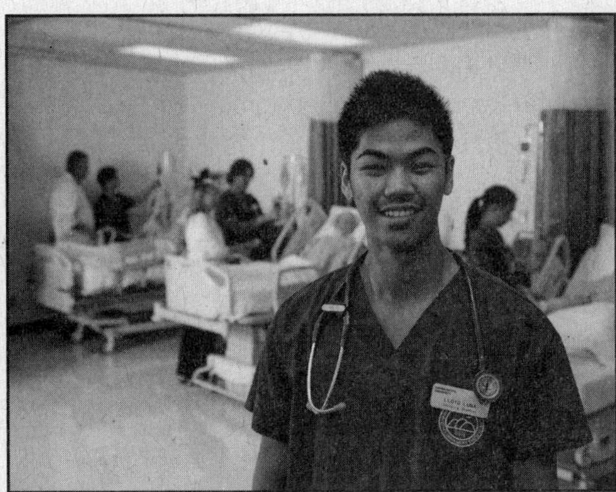

Lloyd Luna and other nursing students practice techniques on simulation mannequins in HPU's nursing simulation lab.

Please visit www.hpu.edu/scholarship for deadlines and an application.

- *2010–11 UNDERGRADUATE TUITION & FEES:*

  Part-time (freshmen and sophomores): $330 per credit (1–7 credits); $655 per credit (8+ credits, including first 7 credits)

  Part-time (juniors and seniors): $955 per credit

  Full-time: $7860 per semester (freshmen and sophomores); $11,460 per semester (juniors and seniors)

  Room and Board: $11,648 per year

- *2010–11 M.S.N. TUITION & FEES:*

  Full-time tuition (minimum 9 credits): $12,600 per semester (includes technology fee)

  Part-time tuition: $700 per credit

  Health insurance: $880

  Housing expense (off-campus): $11,094

  Books, supplies, transportation: $1885

- *APPLICATION DEADLINES:*

  B.S.N. programs: Rolling admissions

  M.S.N. and Graduate Certificate programs: Rolling admissions

- *FACULTY INFORMATION: www.hpu.edu/nursingfaculty (full-time)*
- *MULTIMEDIA: www.hpu.edu/virtualtour (virtual tour of HPU)*

CONTACT INFORMATION

Office of Admissions
Hawai'i Pacific University
1164 Bishop Street, Suite 200
Honolulu, Hawaii 96813
Phone: 808-544-0238
866-CALL-HPU (toll-free)
Fax: 808-544-1136
E-mail: admissions@hpu.edu
graduate@hpu.edu (graduate admissions)
Web site: http://www.hpu.edu/Petersons

Find us on Facebook®: www.facebook.com/hawaiipacific
Follow us on Twitter™: www.twitter.com/HPU

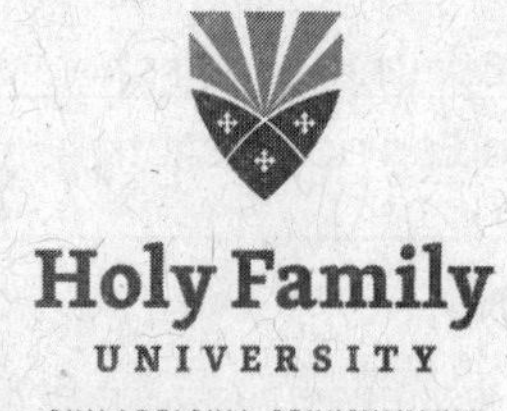

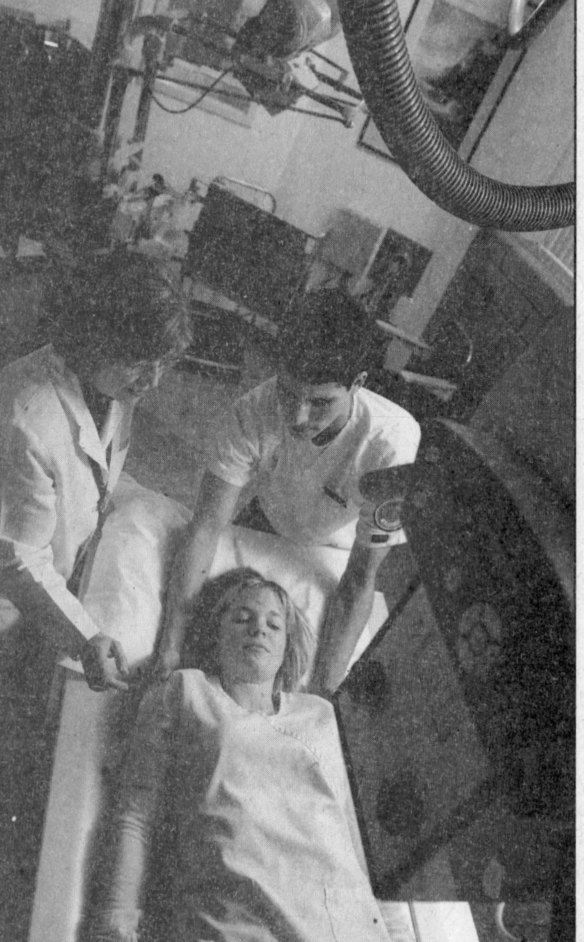

School of Nursing and Allied Health Professions

Patient Care from Spiritual, Ethical, and Moral Perspectives

Holy Family's nursing programs and state-of-the-art facilities fully prepare students for the environments and technologies they will encounter after graduation.

Since its founding more than half a century ago, Holy Family University has been a regional leader in the education of registered nurses (RNs). Building on this impressive legacy, the University now offers bachelor's and master's degrees in nursing, associate and bachelor's degrees in radiologic science, and certificate programs.

Offered through Holy Family's School of Nursing and Allied Health Professions, these programs approach patient care from spiritual, ethical, and moral perspectives.

Options abound for students enrolled in the School of Nursing and Allied Health Professions. The Bachelor of Science in Nursing (B.S.N.) degree is offered in traditional and accelerated formats. The Master of Science in Nursing (M.S.N.) program includes concentrations in community health nursing, nursing administration, and nursing education. Two post-master's certificate programs are offered—one in nursing education and one in nursing administration. The requirement for admission to these programs is the same as for the M.S.N. program.

Modern facilities in Holy Family's Nurse Education Building fully prepare students for the environments and technologies they're likely to encounter after graduating. Nursing students gain hands-on experience in a nursing simulation center and a newly renovated nursing practice lab. Low student-to-faculty ratios in classrooms and clinical settings ensure that students receive a personalized education.

Graduates of the pre-licensure baccalaureate nursing program are eligible for licensure in every state in the United States. Satisfactory performance on the National Council Licensure Examination for Registered Nurses (NCLEX-RN), as prescribed by the respective state, results in the graduate being known as a registered nurse (RN), and success on the NCLEX-RN in any state entitles the RN to apply for licensure in every other state.

Program approvals and accreditation have come from the State Board of Nursing, the Commission on Collegiate Nursing Education, and the Pennsylvania Department of Education.

In addition to its nursing programs, the School of Nursing and Allied Health Professionals offers bachelor's and associate degrees in radiologic science. As with nursing, Holy Family's Radiologic Science programs offer plenty of options for students to work in a fully energized X-ray lab, which offers computed radiography imaging.

Undergraduate applicants to Holy Family University must submit a completed application along with a $25 fee; offer proof of graduation from an accredited high school or equivalent; record acceptable scores on the SAT or ACT; and complete a full year of Algebra I and II and Geometry. Nursing applicants are expected to have completed biology, chemistry, a science elective, and 3 units of social studies.

Applicants to the master's program must possess a B.S.N. from an NLNAC-accredited or CCNE-accredited nursing program at a regionally accredited institution or an RN from an NLNAC-accredited program with a B.S. or B.A. degree in a related area; have completed an undergraduate statistics course with a grade of C or better and attained an undergraduate grade point average of 3.0 or above on a 4.0 scale; hold licensure as a registered nurse in the United States; and present two professional references, an application along with the $25 fee, official transcripts from all colleges or universities attended, a 250- to 500-word personal statement concerning the student's interest and reason for applying, and a resume.

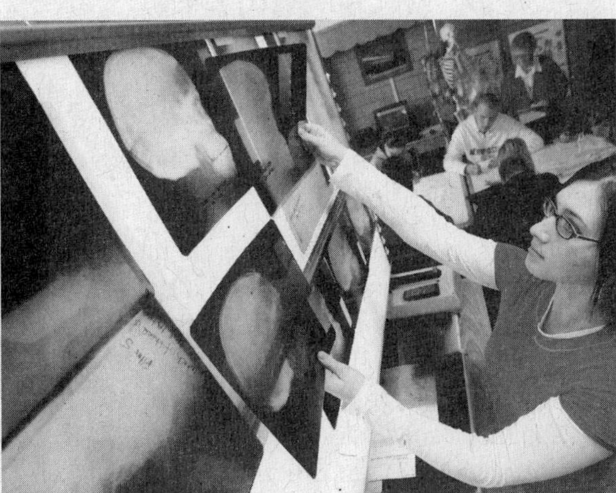

The low student-to-faculty ratios in Holy Family classrooms and clinical settings ensure that students receive a personalized education.

CONTACT INFORMATION

School of Nursing and Allied Health Professions
Holy Family University
9801 Frankford Avenue
Philadelphia, Pennsylvania 19114
Phone: 215-341-3293 (undergraduate)
267-341-3327 (graduate)
Fax: 215-281-1022 (undergraduate)
215-637-1478 (graduate)
E-mail: admissions@holyfamily.edu
gradstudy@holyfamily.edu
Web site: http://www.holyfamily.edu/sn/index.shtml

UNDERGRADUATE NURSING PROGRAM:
Karen A. Montalto, Ph.D., RN
Phone: 267-341-3603
E-mail: kmontalto10@holyfamily.edu

GRADUATE NURSING PROGRAM:
Ana Maria Catanzaro, Ph.D., RN
Phone: 267-341-3374
E-mail: acatanzaro@holyfamily.edu

- *2010–11 UNDERGRADUATE TUITION & FEES: $11,435 per full-time semester; $490 per part-time credit hour*

  General fee: $325 full-time; $60 part-time. Malpractice fee: $40
- *2010–11 GRADUATE TUITION & FEES: $600 per credit hour; $655 per credit hour for clinical courses; $85 general fee per semester*
- *APPLICATION DEADLINES: No deadlines; rolling admissions until nursing enrollment capacity is met*
- *FACULTY INFORMATION: http://www.holyfamily.edu/sn/faculty.shtml*

Find us on Facebook®: http://www.facebook.com/HolyFamilyUniversity
Follow us on Twitter™: http://www.twitter.com/holyfamilyu

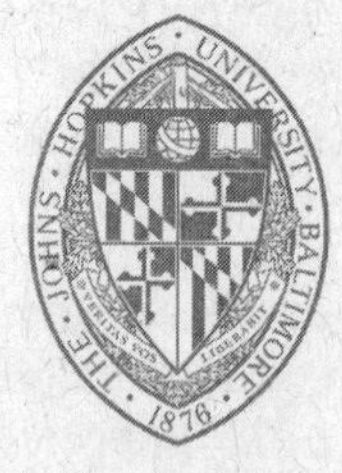

JOHNS HOPKINS

SCHOOL OF NURSING

People. Places. Possibilities.

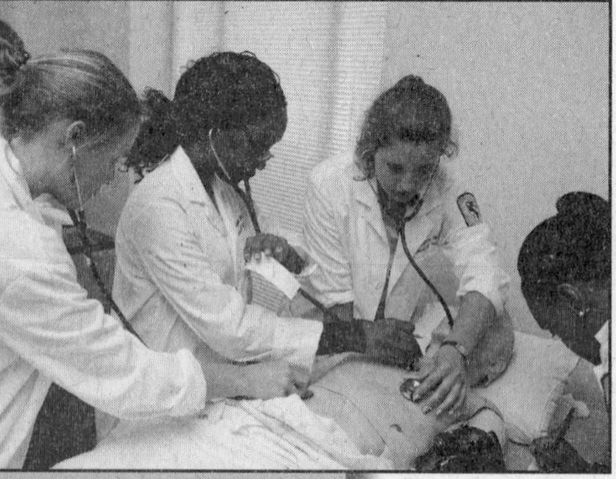

Students engage the "SimMan," a universal patient simulator.

The Johns Hopkins University School of Nursing is a place where exceptional people discover possibilities that forever change their lives and the world. With more than a century of established excellence in connection with The Johns Hopkins Hospital and the University, the School of Nursing is both connected to the past and focused on the future. It attracts students and faculty from around the world to collaborate, research, and learn the best practices to advance the science and art of nursing. Hopkins students enjoy the advantages of an education at an institution with a worldwide reputation and an outstanding network of alumni who are willing to serve as guides and mentors. A rigorous academic curriculum, which includes a strong scientific orientation, gives students the background to understand the health-care decisions they will make as professionals.

Recognized as a leader by its peers, the School of Nursing ranked second in the nation for Community Health Nursing Programs and fourth overall for Graduate Programs in the 2008 edition of *U.S. News & World Report*. The School is ranked fourth among nursing schools in the United States in the National Institutes of Health (NIH) research funding. Named a Center of Excellence in Nursing Education in 2010 by the National League for Nursing, the School is located adjacent to the top-ranked Johns Hopkins University schools of Medicine and Public Health and to The Johns Hopkins Hospital, the nation's No. 1 hospital.

Johns Hopkins University is accredited by Middle States Commission on Higher Education. The baccalaureate and master's programs of the School of Nursing are fully accredited by the National League for Nursing Accrediting Commission (NLNAC) and the Commission on Collegiate Nursing Education (CCNE). In addition, the baccalaureate and master's programs are approved by the Maryland State Board of Examiners of Nurses. The baccalaureate, master's, and doctoral programs are endorsed by the Maryland State Board for Higher Education. The School's Doctor of Nursing Practice (D.N.P.) program went through the accreditation process with the Commission on Collegiate Nursing Education (CCNE) in fall 2009 and received full accreditation until 2015. The School is also proud to be the only Peace Corps Fellows Program in nursing.

A complete baccalaureate and master's application consists of an application form and a nonrefundable $75 application fee. Doctoral applicants pay an application fee of $100. Applicants to the baccalaureate program are required to have three recommendations, official college- or university-level transcripts, an official high school transcript (unless the applicant has already completed a college degree), and SAT or ACT scores, if they are not more than five years old and the student does not already hold a bachelor's degree. A grade point average (GPA) above 3.0 (on a 4.0 scale) is recommended. Personal interviews may be requested.

Applicants to the master's program are required to have graduated from a baccalaureate or master's degree program in nursing with a GPA above 3.0 (on a 4.0 scale), a current Maryland state nursing license, academic and professional references, written expression of goals, and official transcripts from all previous colleges/universities attended. Personal interviews may be requested.

- *2010–11 UNDERGRADUATE TUITION & FEES:*

  Traditional Bachelor's Program: *Tuition: $33,168 (full-time—12 credit hours/semester); $1382 per credit (part-time). Housing, food, books, fees, and other costs: $19,671*

  Accelerated Bachelor's Program: *Tuition: $62,223 (full-time). Housing, food, books, fees, and other costs: $30,376*

- *2010–11 GRADUATE TUITION & FEES:*

  M.S.N. Program: *Tuition: $31,416 (full-time—9 credit hours/semester); $1309 per credit (part-time). Housing, food, books, fees, and other costs: $16,450*

  M.S.N./M.P.H. Program: *Tuition: $49,134 (full-time—16 credit hours/semester); $1293 per credit (part-time). Housing, food, books, fees, and other costs: $23,894*

  Ph.D. Program: *Tuition: $40,626 (full-time—9 credit hours/semester); $2257 per credit (part-time). Housing, food, books, fees, and other costs: $19,681*

  D.N.P. Program: *Tuition: $22,990 (full-time—9 credit hours/semester); $1277 per credit (part-time). Housing, food, books, fees, and other costs: $19,681*

- *APPLICATION DEADLINES:*

  Baccalaureate Program: *Early Decision: November 1 (accelerated and traditional options); Regular Decision: November 15 (accelerated option); January 15 (traditional option); Special deadline: Accelerated B.S. to M.S.N. with Clinical Residency: To Be Announced*

  Master's Program: *June 1(Fall entry); November 1 (Spring entry); March 1 (Summer entry)*

- *SPECIAL DEADLINES:*

  M.S.N./M.P.H.: December 1 (July enrollment)

  Clinical Nurse Specialist Women's Health/Nurse Midwifery: February 15 (Fall enrollment)

  M.S.N. Primary Care Nurse Practitioner (Adult, Family, Pediatric): February 15 (Fall enrollment)

  Note: B.S. to M.S.N. students who are enrolled in the Baccalaureate portion of the program must confirm their planned fall enrollment in the M.S.N. program by February 1.

- *Post-Degree Options*

  Post Master's Primary Care Nurse Practitioner (Adult, Family, and Pediatric): February 15 (full-time enrollment)

  Applied Health Informatics: June 1 (February 15 for tuition support)

  For all other post-degree programs, admission is on a rolling basis. On average, it takes the Admissions Committee approximately one month to six weeks to reach a decision upon receipt of a completed application.

  Ph.D. Program: Year-round, rolling admissions for September, January, and June start dates; scholarship consideration is given to those who apply by January 15.

  D.N.P. Program: March 1 (Fall entry)

- *FACULTY INFORMATION: www.nursing.jhu.edu/academics/faculty/*

- *MULTIMEDIA: www.nursing.jhu.edu/campus_life/*

CONTACT INFORMATION

Admissions and Student Services
School of Nursing
The Johns Hopkins University
525 North Wolfe Street
Baltimore, Maryland 21205
Phone: 410-955-7548
Fax: 410-614-7086
E-mail: jhuson@son.jhmi.edu
Web site: www.nursing.jhu.edu

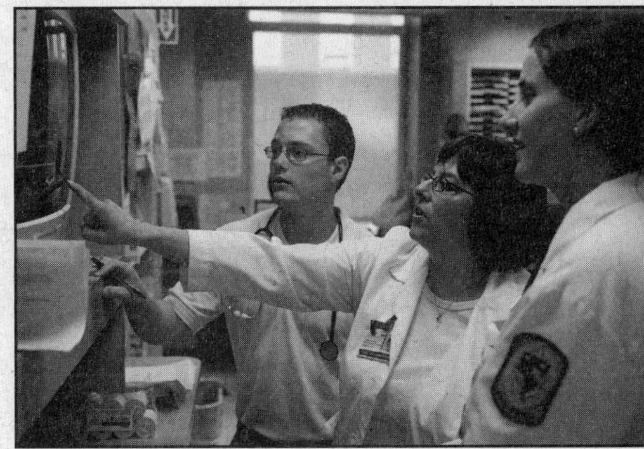

Students work closely with clinical instructor at The Johns Hopkins Hospital.

Find us on Facebook®: www.facebook.com/jhunursing
Follow us on Twitter™: twitter.com/JHUNursing

College of Nursing

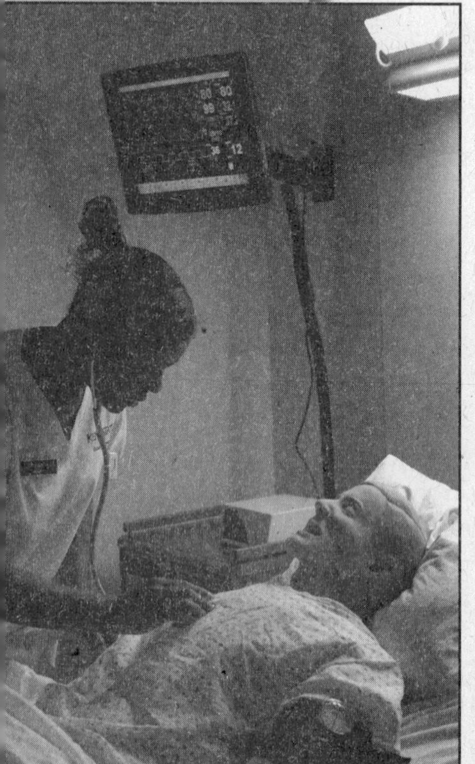

Advancing nursing and changing lives through academic distinction, knowledge creation and application, and recognized leadership.

In the Olga A. Mural Simulation Laboratory, students practice and improve patient care delivery with the help of realistically simulated illnesses and responses. The cutting-edge patient care complex emulates realistic scenarios so that students may learn critical thinking skills in a safe and controlled environment.

The College of Nursing was established in 1967 and is the largest nursing program in the state of Ohio, ranking in the 98th percentile in size in the United States. In addition, *Modern Healthcare* ranks the program as the fourth largest in the nation. Kent State University is the known as largest public research university in Northeast Ohio and is ranked among the top 200 universities in the world.

The nursing faculty comprises scholars and researchers who possess strong clinical skills and are active, creative contributors to the advancement of nursing knowledge. Through teaching, research, and service activities at the local, regional, national, and international levels, faculty members have worked to improve the delivery of health care.

The College's Center of Nursing Research and Scholarship is committed to the growth and development of faculty research, advancing innovative interdisciplinary academic and community-based collaborations to build nursing and health-care science. Strong community-based health-care collaborations, spanning several counties across Northeast Ohio, serve as a platform for building, translating, and applying knowledge for practice. There is a proud history inspired by research, as well as by academic and service leaders who advance nursing and change lives.

Kent State nursing students are supported by an academic atmosphere of intellectual curiosity resulting in a long-standing reputation for excellent academic performance, clinical knowledge, and leadership in the professional practice.

Students benefit from top-notch educational opportunities, including cutting-edge simulated experience opportunities that hone students' clinical competencies and strengthen their critical analysis skills. A comprehensive nursing program prepares students for the B.S.N. degree and beyond, with options for masters, post-certificate programs, Ph.D. in nursing, and most recently the D.N.P. degree.

Kent State University College of Nursing programs are comprehensive and growing:

- B.S.N.
- RN to B.S.N. Online
- Accelerated Second Degree B.S.N. Program for College Graduates
- Graduate and Advanced Practice concentrations, as well as Dual Degrees (M.S.N./M.B.A., M.S.N./M.P.A.)
- Doctoral Degrees
  - Ph.D. in Nursing
  - D.N.P. (Doctorate of Nursing Practice)
- Post-Master's Clinical and Education Certificates
- A.D.N.

A nursing degree from Kent State University College of Nursing provides something more than a diploma—it provides nursing excellence in practice and leadership. Kent State is known for its nursing leaders who lead professional organizations and hold key positions in nursing such as CEOs of nursing associations and commanders of hospitals. From charge nurses and directors of nursing development, chief nursing officers to directors of nursing research, Kent State lays the foundation for advancing in the nursing profession.

Recent nurse leaders who are Kent State alumni include Rebecca M. Patton, *Immediate Past President of the American Nurses Association* (serving two consecutive terms); Dr. Linda Q. Everett, *Past President of the National Organization of Nurse Executives;* Dr. Barbara L. Drew, *Past President of the American Psychiatric Nurses Association;* Colonel Nancy J. Hughes, *First Hospital Commander at Moncrief Army Community Hospital;* and Claire M. Zangerle, *President and Chief Executive Officer of the Visiting Nurse Association of Ohio.*

For details on tuition & fees, application deadlines, and further information, please visit the Kent State University College of Nursing Web site: www.kent.edu/nursing.

- *FACULTY: http://www.Kent.edu/nursing/facstaff/bio/*

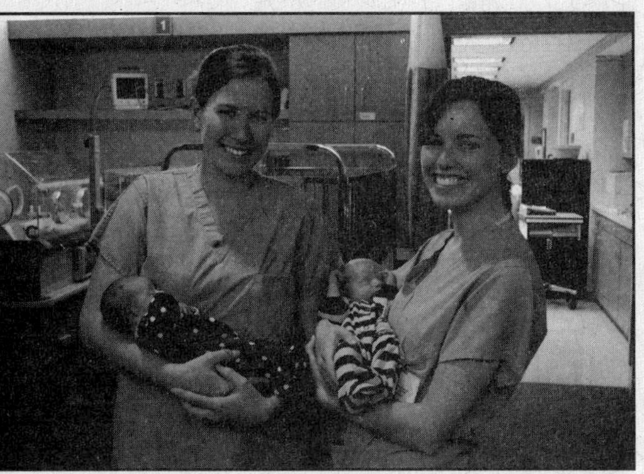

Students are eager to learn and make a difference in the lives of their patients. Here, 2 recent graduates pose for a picture with the babies they helped deliver.

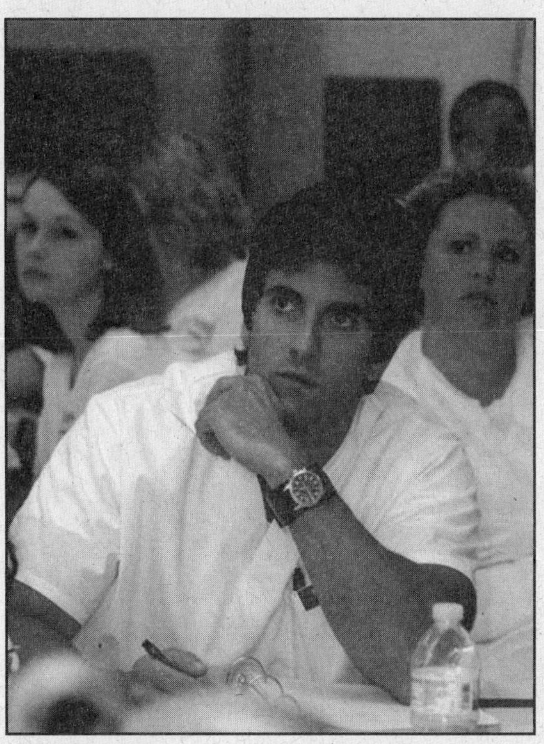

The Second-degree Accelerated B.S.N. program allows students with non-nursing bachelor's degrees to complete a nursing degree in 14 months. The intense and challenging program has more than quadrupled in size over the past several years and is helping to address the nursing shortage.

CONTACT INFORMATION

Laura Dzurec, Dean
Kent State University College of Nursing
Kent State University
113 Henderson Hall
Kent, Ohio 44242
Phone: 330-672-8790 (Undergraduate program)
330-672-8761 (Graduate program)
800-672-3000 (toll-free)
Web site: www.kent.edu/nursing

Find us on Facebook®: http://www.facebook.com/kentstate

LUTHER COLLEGE

Department of Nursing

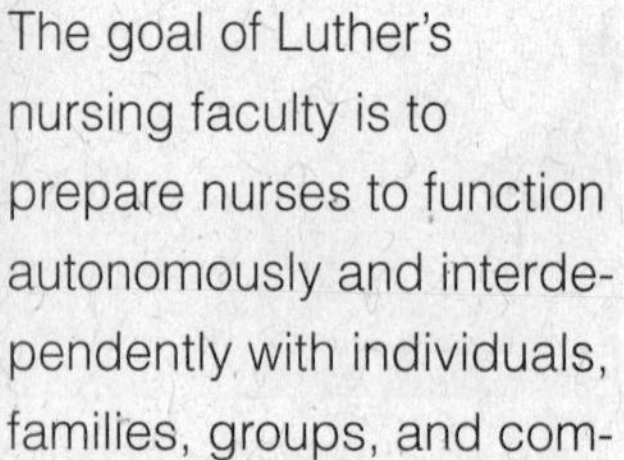

The Luther Bell and Dahl Centennial Union on the campus of Luther College.

The goal of Luther's nursing faculty is to prepare nurses to function autonomously and interdependently with individuals, families, groups, and communities to promote, maintain, and restore optimal health in a variety of health-care settings. The nursing major, therefore, offers an integrated program of liberal arts and 14 professional nursing courses. The program gives students a broad approach to nursing, providing a base for graduate study or immediate entry into the nursing profession.

Following graduation, Luther nursing students may take the National Council Licensure Examination for Registered Nurses (NCLEX-RN). Luther College also offers a baccalaureate completion program for registered nurses. More information is available upon request.

The first year at Luther provides a foundation in the liberal arts and sciences. All nursing majors are assigned a faculty adviser to help each student decide whether to pursue a nursing curriculum plan. All students interested in nursing are invited to participate in the nursing student club (PRN).

Clinical nursing courses begin in the fall of the sophomore year. Nursing courses at this level emphasize health assessment and fundamental skills throughout the life span in a variety of settings. These learning experiences develop new communication and interpersonal skills.

Third-year students experience a concentrated study of nursing concepts by caring for children and adults with physical and emotional problems. The sites for this clinical experience are Rochester Methodist Hospital and St. Mary's Hospital, affiliates of Mayo Clinic; the Federal Medical Center; and a variety of community-based health-care agencies in Rochester, Minnesota.

The senior year provides final preparation for entry into the practice of professional nursing. Courses focus on promoting health and preventing illness in childbearing families and in community groups. Students further develop leadership management and research skills through selected areas of nursing.

Minimum academic requirements must be met to be considered for enrollment in nursing courses. However, meeting the minimum requirements does not guarantee placement in the courses. Decisions affecting progression in the major are made at the end of each semester.

The study of nursing at Luther incorporates academic classroom learning, based in the newly renovated Valders Hall of Science, and clinical experience in several community facilities. These include Winneshiek Medical Center; the Decorah Free Clinic; Mayo Clinic: Methodist Hospital and Mayo Clinic: Saint Mary's Hospital; the Federal Medical Center; and a variety of community-based health-care agencies in Decorah, Iowa and Rochester, Minnesota.

Nursing scholarships are available to incoming students on a competitive basis upon admission. Selection of recipients is based on academic information submitted on the application and the high school transcript. Scholarship renewal is based on satisfactory academic and clinical performance in the major.

All nursing students benefit from the Bernice Fischer Cross and Bert S. Cross Perpetual Endowment for the Luther College Mayo Nursing Program and Health Sciences Program. This is used for equal-share assistance for the Luther College nursing students enrolled in the curriculum provided at Mayo Clinic in Rochester, Minnesota. The endowment is not a need-based scholarship.

Located in the small northeast Iowa town of Decorah (resident population: 8,100), Luther College is an undergraduate liberal arts institution of about 2,500 students that is affiliated with the Lutheran church (ELCA). The Upper Iowa River—the only waterway in the state designated as wild and scenic—flows through the lower portion of Luther's 200-acre central campus and borders Decorah's business district. Decorah is known nationwide for its recreational opportunities, numerous cultural heritage events and festivals, pedestrian-friendly village center, and its conscious efforts to thrive as a small town. Public transportation includes commercial airports in Rochester (Minnesota), Waterloo (Iowa), and La Crosse (Wisconsin); a municipal airport in Decorah; and train and bus depots in La Crosse, Wisconsin.

- *2011–12 UNDERGRADUATE TUITION & FEES: The comprehensive fee is $40,585 ($34,735 tuition, $2780 room, $3070 board).*
- *APPLICATION DEADLINES: Luther College operates on rolling admission. There is no application deadline.*
- *FACULTY INFORMATION: http://www.luther.edu/nursing/faculty/*
- *MULTIMEDIA: http://www.luther.edu/video/*

CONTACT INFORMATION

Dr. Sheryl A. Juve
Department of Nursing
Luther College
700 College Drive
Decorah, Iowa 52101
Phone: 563-387-1057
800-458-8437 (toll-free)
E-mail: juvesh01@luther.edu
Web site: http://www.luther.edu/nursing/

Find us on Facebook®: http://www.facebook.com/luthercollege1861
Follow us on Twitter™: www.twitter.com/luthercollege

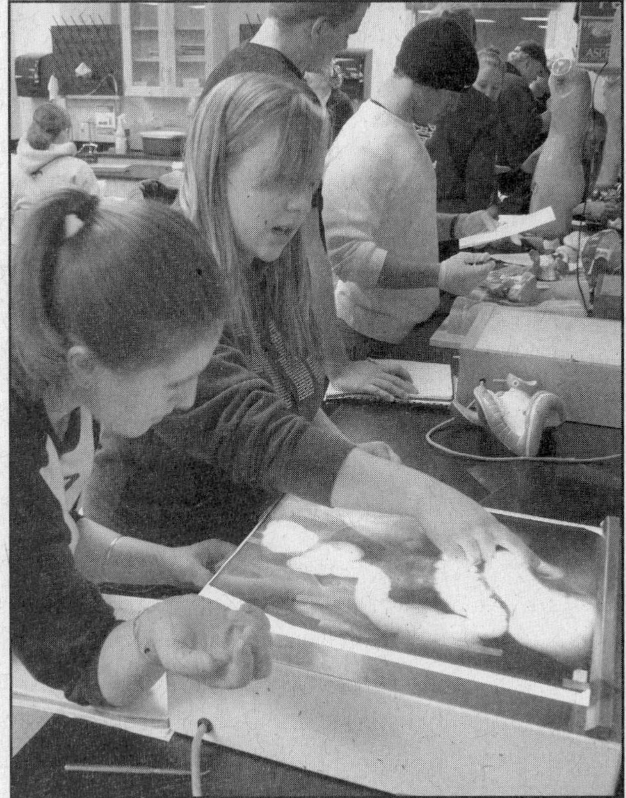

Luther nursing students studying human anatomy in state-of-the-art laboratories and facilities.

Marquette University College of Nursing

75 Years of Caring

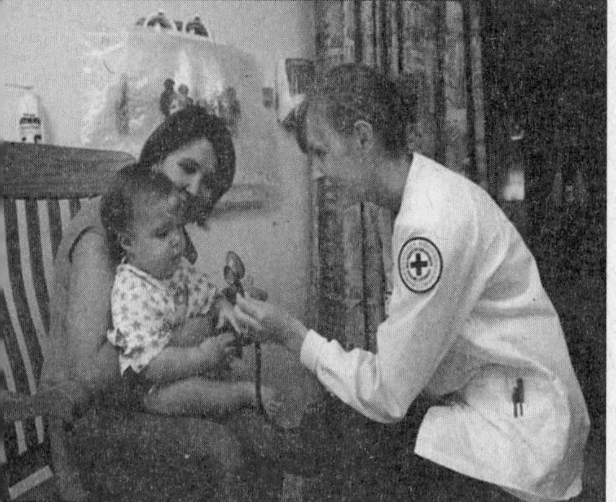

Pediatric care experience.

The four-year Bachelor of Science in Nursing (B.S.N.) degree program at Marquette University provides a strong academic foundation in nursing, natural and social science, and humanities. Preparation for a professional nursing role is emphasized through the development of clinical, cognitive, and leadership skills and personal and professional values. Students are admitted directly as freshmen into the College of Nursing, which assures placement in clinical nursing courses. Nursing courses begin on the first day of enrollment. Clinical reasoning, introduced in the second year through clinical laboratory and simulation experiences, are developed through seven clinical rotations in health-care agencies in the junior and senior years. A low student-teacher ratio (8:1) affords personal attention in all clinical rotations, including adult care, maternity, mental health, pediatric, and community health and a synthesis course in a setting of the student's area of interest.

The 128-credit B.S.N. program includes courses in the humanities, physical-biological sciences, and social-behavioral sciences as well as electives and courses in the nursing major. A University Core of Common Studies is foundational for all majors at Marquette University. Lower-division nursing courses are Dimensions of Professional Nursing, Health Assessment, Foundations of Nursing Practice, Pathophysiology 1 and 2, and Pharmacotherapeutics. Upper-division courses include Nursing Research, Care of Adults*, Childbearing Family Nursing*, Mental Health Nursing*, Primary Health Care Concepts, Gerontological Nursing, Family Centered Nursing of Children*, Nursing of Communities*, Care of Acutely Ill Adults*, Nursing Synthesis*, and Nursing Leadership. The asterisk (*) denotes clinical practice courses.

Marquette University College of Nursing offers the Master of Science in Nursing (M.S.N.) degree and post-master's certificates that prepare graduates for advanced practice roles or leadership roles within health-care systems. Individuals may enter through four pathways: post-B.S.N.; Direct Entry (DE), a combined RN and M.S.N. for those with non-nursing bachelor's degrees; and ADN-prepared nurses with bachelor's degrees in other disciplines. Graduates are academically eligible to seek formal professional certification as nurse practitioners, clinical nurse specialists, nurse midwives, or nurse administrators. Seven specialty options are available: health-care systems leadership, clinical nurse leader, and advanced practice programs in nurse midwifery, pediatrics, adults, older adults, and acute adult and pediatric care. Full-time students complete the 33–45 credit programs in four semesters.

At the Ph.D. program level, a 69 credit B.S.N. to Ph.D. program and a 51-credit post-M.S.N./Ph.D. program to prepare teachers/scholars focus on knowledge generation related to vulnerable populations.

A Doctor of Nursing Practice (D.N.P.) program began in fall 2008. The D.N.P. is another route to advanced practice or nursing administration and emphasizes translational research, epidemiology, informatics, health policy, statistics, and professional issues. All students complete a two-semester capstone clinical project. A residency course is also required.

The College is affiliated with more than eighty health-care agencies in Wisconsin and the surrounding states. These agencies include hospitals, clinics, home care facilities, public health departments, schools, parishes, long-term-care facilities, hospice, and clinics. Many of these agencies offer excellent student employment opportunities as well as financial aid and loan forgiveness programs once students graduate from the program.

Marquette is located on an 80-acre campus with excellent facilities. The College of Nursing has many technology-enhanced classrooms and a well-equipped Simulation Technology and Learning Resource Center (STLRC), including SIM-MAN G, a birthing simulator, and many other advanced simulation technology models for student learning. The STLRC provides computer access, media resources, and practice labs supplied with state-of-the-art models and equipment necessary to develop a solid foundation for clinical practice. Students participate in simulation exercises that are videotaped for maximal learning before entering into complex health-care systems.

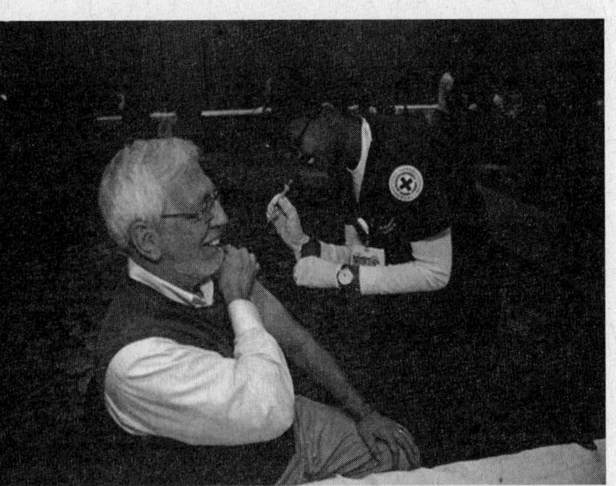

H1N1 flu clinic work.

- *2011–12 UNDERGRADUATE TUITION & FEES:*

  Full-time tuition: $31,400

  Typical room and board: $10,370; Fees: $422

  Part-time (non-part-time studies program): $875 per credit

- *2011–12 GRADUATE TUITION & FEES:*

  $905 per credit hour

  Nursing programs: $15,700 per term

- *APPLICATION DEADLINES:*

  Undergraduate: December 1

  Graduate and Post-Grad: August 1 for fall; November 1 for spring

  D.N.P.: February 15

  Direct Entry (DE) Master's: December 30 for May start

- *FACULTY INFORMATION:*

  http://www.mu.edu/facstaff

- *MULTIMEDIA: http://www.mu.edu/nursing*

CONTACT INFORMATION

Bridget O'Meara
Program & Communication Coordinator
College of Nursing
Marquette University
P.O. Box 1881
Milwaukee, Wisconsin 53233
Phone: 414-288-3869
Fax: 414-288-1939
E-mail: bridget.omeara@mu.edu
Web site: http://www.mu.edu/nursing

Undergraduate Nursing Program:
Harry Kraemer
Undergraduate Program Assistant
Phone: 414-288-3809
E-mail: Harry.kraemer@mu.edu

Graduate Nursing Program:
Karen Nest
Graduate Program Coordinator
Phone: 414-288- 3810
E-mail: Karen.nest@mu.edu

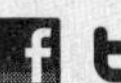

Find us on Facebook®: http://www.facebook.com/MarquetteU
Follow us on Twitter™: http://www.twitter.com/marquetteu

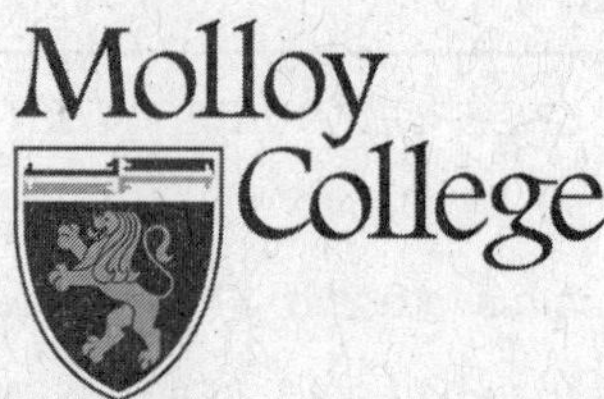

Division of Nursing

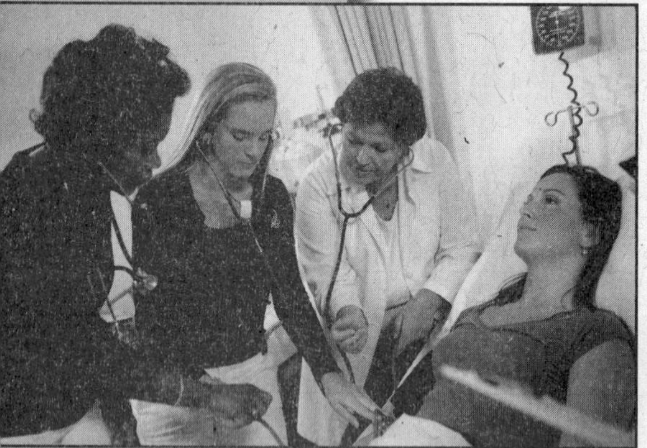

Molloy's undergraduate nursing program is the sixth largest in the United States, and the College also offers multiple graduate programs, including a Ph.D. in Nursing.

An Emphasis on Human Compassion, Dignity, and Respect

At Molloy, nursing is both art and science. One of the country's largest and most respected programs, Molloy's Nursing Division curriculum immerses students in clinical practice with an emphasis on human compassion, dignity, and respect for the patient. Molloy's programs proactively respond to the changing needs of today's health-care environment, providing students with individualized attention from an expert faculty that is easily accessible and always committed to students' success.

From Molloy's fully equipped, state-of-the-art learning laboratory to its innovative clinical practice opportunities, at Molloy students can find all the resources and support they need to become an effective, humanistic health-care provider—whether students are just beginning their nursing education or are professionals who are ready to take their career to the next level. At Molloy, students benefit from a comprehensive array of:

- Undergraduate programs. Offering a wealth of hands-on clinical experiences beginning in a student's sophomore year, Molloy's bachelor's degree program prepares students for a vital role in health care. Already working in health care or in another career? Consider one of Molloy's dual-degree programs, the degree completion program for registered nurses, the LPN to B.S./RN career mobility program, or the accelerated dual-degree program for second degree students holding a non-nursing baccalaureate or higher degree.
- Graduate programs. Focused on advanced theory and its application in a selected area of nursing, Molloy offers seven distinct tracks leading to master's degrees and nine master's certificates concentrating on advanced clinical practice, administrative and informatics expertise, and specialty training in education. Nurse Practitioner tracks are available in Pediatrics, Adult, Family or Psychiatry, Clinical Nurse Specialist (CNS), Adult Health, Nursing Education or Nursing Administration.
- Doctoral program. Molloy's first doctoral program is designed to prepare doctoral students to become leaders, advancing the profession of nursing through research, education, administration, and health policy.

Molloy College launched its first doctoral program, a Ph.D. in Nursing, in fall 2010. According to Veronica Feeg, Ph.D., RN, FAAN, Associate Dean and Director of the Doctoral Program, "Doctoral education is important for our profession and the Ph.D. at Molloy will produce the researchers and scholars who will lead the discipline."

"2010 was the International Year of the Nurse, so the timing was ideal for launching our

Nursing Ph.D. program," said Jeannine D. Muldoon, Ph.D., RN, Dean of the Division of Nursing. "We expect that our Ph.D. graduates will leave Molloy prepared to serve our communities, develop the next generation of nursing leaders and have a strong voice in health policy decisions that affect us all."

"This milestone event further demonstrates the College's commitment to academic excellence," said Valerie H. Collins, Ph.D., Vice President of Academic Affairs and Dean of Faculty. "Molloy's Nursing programs have always been among the finest in the country—the undergraduate program is the sixth largest in the United States—so we are pleased that the College's first doctoral program comes from this Division."

A Ph.D. from Molloy prepares nurses for leadership roles in academia, health policy formulation, health-care administration, and clinical practice. The curriculum focuses on theory, research, the humanities, and methodology. Essential elements of the curriculum feature leadership through caring, both in educational and organizational/policy settings, as well as theory and research in the nursing profession. Students are required to complete 45 credits of course work and a dissertation.

- *2010–11 UNDERGRADUATE TUITION & FEES:*

  Tuition: $21,170

  Fees: $960

- *2010–11 GRADUATE TUITION & FEES:*

  Master's program:
  Tuition: $810 per credit

  Fees: $830 (if taking more than 4 credits); $690 (less than 4 credits)

  Ph.D. program: $950/credit; fees same as for Master's program

- *APPLICATION DEADLINES:*

  Undergraduate: Rolling admissions

  Master's program: Rolling admissions

  Ph.D. program: February 1

CONTACT INFORMATION

Molloy College
1000 Hempstead Avenue
Rockville Centre, New York 11571
Phone: 888-4-MOLLOY (toll-free)
Web site: http://www.molloy.edu

Undergraduate Admissions
Phone: 516-678-5000, Ext. 6230
E-mail: admissions@molloy.edu

Graduate and Ph.D. Admissions
Alina Haitz
Phone: 516-678-5000, Ext. 6399
E-mail: ahaitz@molloy.edu

Find us on Facebook®: http://www.facebook.com/GoMolloy
Follow us on Twitter™: http://www.twitter.com/MolloyCollege

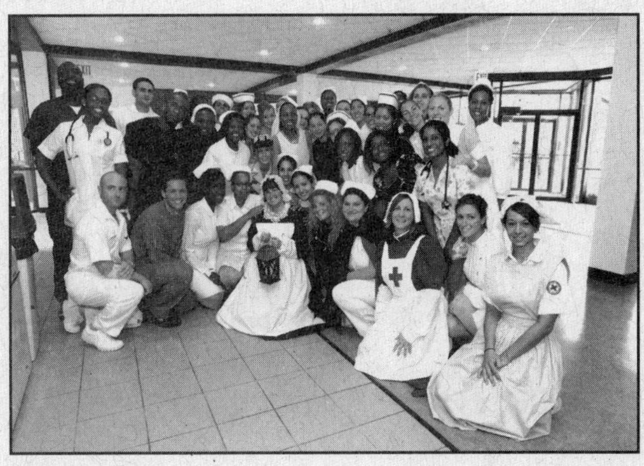

Molloy College recently celebrated the launch of its new Ph.D. program with a series of lectures and a "nursing fashion show" that featured students wearing uniforms from various decades.

QUINNIPIAC UNIVERSITY

School of Nursing

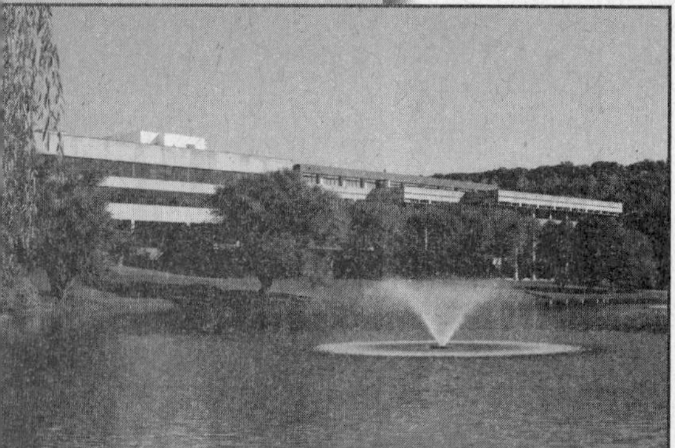

Education with a Personal Touch.

Professional nursing courses take place in the Graduate and Health Sciences building on Quinnipiac's 104-acre North Haven campus.

Quinnipiac University (QU), located in Hamden, Connecticut, just 8 miles from New Haven and midway between New York City and Boston, has 5,900 undergraduate and 2,000 graduate students. QU offers the B.S. in Nursing, an accelerated B.S.N. for those who hold a non-nursing college degree, and the graduate D.N.P. Doctorate of Nursing Practice plus two post-master's tracks.

Accredited by the National League for Nursing Accrediting Commission (NLNAC), Quinnipiac's bachelor's degree program in nursing offers the theoretical and clinical education students need to enter professional nursing practice. Graduates of the program are eligible to take the NCLEX-RN exam and are well prepared for graduate study in nursing. The nursing curriculum fosters professional socialization for future roles and responsibilities within the profession. Graduates of the program are prepared as generalists to begin the practice of holistic professional nursing, with sound theoretical foundations and more than 800 hours of diverse clinical practice experiences. In addition to the traditional four-year program, an innovative accelerated option is available to non-nurse college graduates.

The graduate nursing program prepares professional nurses at an advanced theoretical and clinical practice level in order to address present and potential societal health needs. The program commences a clinical doctorate resulting in the Doctorate of Nursing Practice (D.N.P.) degree. Three available tracks are Adult Nurse Practitioner, Women's Health Nurse Practitioner, and Family Nurse Practitioner. The following Post-master's tracks are also available: the Care of Individuals (for licensed APRNs) and the Care of Populations (for master's prepared nurses who are not APRNs). The graduate nursing program includes core courses that cover advanced concepts and theoretical foundations of nursing, epidemiology, and health-care policy and economics.

Quinnipiac's strong affiliates with health-care providers in the area allow students to complete clinical work at such institutions as Yale-New Haven Hospital, Connecticut Children's Medical Center, the Hospital of St. Raphael, and MidState Medical Center as well as in private practices, clinics, and other health-care centers.

Quinnipiac's Mount Carmel Campus is the main location for housing, recreation, and course work for undergraduates in their first two years. Starting in the junior year, the professional courses in nursing take place on the nearby 104-acre North Haven campus in the Graduate and Health Sciences building, which houses a remarkable facility with state-of-the-art technologies to prepare health-care professionals in a variety of fields. The Clinical Simulation Labs house "patients" that are lifelike simulation mannequins. Cameras capture the simulation for student assessment. The Pediatric/Neonatal Lab is filled with infant mannequins and introduces students to this special area of health care in the acute setting. The Clinical Skills labs and the Intensive Care Unit create real-world conditions to prepare students for clinical training assignments. The Physical Diagnosis Lab, Physical Exam Suite, and Health Assessment Lab duplicate care in an outpatient primary care setting, such as an emergency room or doctor's office. For more on the North Haven campus, see http://www.quinnipiac.edu/northhaven.xml.

Students applying as freshmen into the nursing program should file their application for admission by November 1. Information regarding admission requirements can be found at http://www.quinnipiac.edu/apply. Transfer students must have a minimum 3.0 GPA and are considered on a space-available basis.

The accelerated (second degree) nursing program begins at the end of May; a complete application and all supporting documents must be filed by October 1. See https://www.quinnipiac.edu/x756.xml for details.

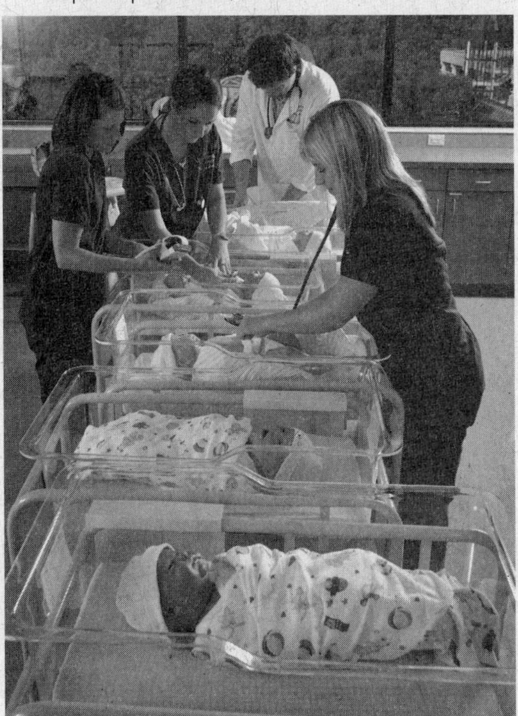

In the pediatric's maternity lab, students learn about fetal development and birthing. Students are taught to bathe and swaddle infants as well as how to educate new mothers about infant care.

Graduate admission information for the D.N.P. and the post-master's tracks can be found at https://www.quinnipiac.edu/x797.xml.

- *2011–12 UNDERGRADUATE TUITION & FEES:*

  Full-time: $36,130 (tuition); $13,430 (room and board)

  Part-time: $835 per credit
- *2011–12 GRADUATE TUITION: $855 per credit plus $35 per credit student fee.*
- *APPLICATION DEADLINES: Undergraduate applicants should apply by Nov. 1 for fall admission*

  Graduate students should contact the Office of Graduate Admissions for deadline information
- *FACULTY INFORMATION:*

  http://www.quinnipiac.edu/x1532.xml
- *MULTIMEDIA:*

  http://www.quinnipiac.edu/x4581.xml

CONTACT INFORMATION

Joan Isaac Mohr, VP and Dean of Admissions
Admissions Office
Quinnipiac University
275 Mt. Carmel Avenue
Hamden, Connecticut 06518
Phone: 203-582-8600
800 462 1944 (toll-free)
Fax: 203 582 8906
E-mail: admissions@quinnipiac.edu
Web site: http://www.quinnipiac.edu

Undergraduate Nursing Program:
Office of Undergraduate Admissions
Phone: 203-582-8600
E-mail: admissions@quinnipiac.edu

Graduate Nursing Program:
Office of Graduate Admissions
Phone: 203-582-8672
E-mail: graduate@quinnipiac.edu

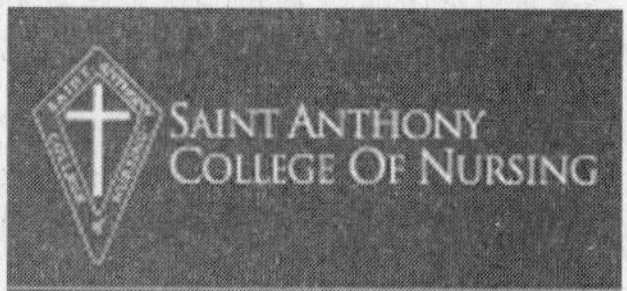

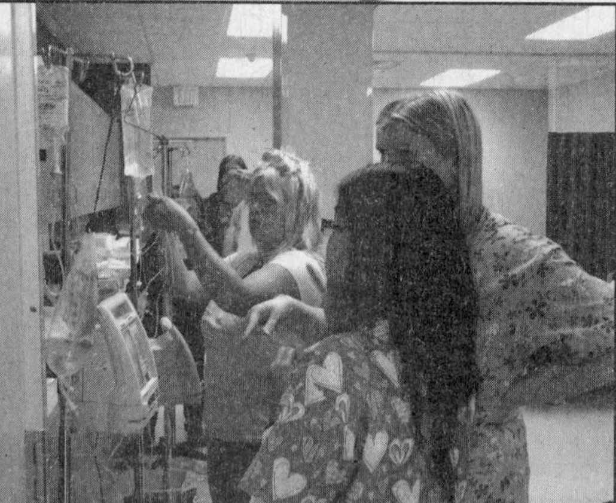

Personal, individualized attention in a caring environment.

SACN students attain a broad spectrum of scientific, critical thinking, humanistic, communication, and leadership concepts and experiences expected of today's medical professionals.

Saint Anthony College of Nursing (SACN) is a specialized college granting the Bachelor of Science in Nursing (B.S.N.) and Master of Science in Nursing (M.S.N.) degrees. The College is located in Rockford, Illinois, in the north-central part of the state. The surrounding area provides much to see and do. Students receive excellent academic instruction along with abundant clinical experience.

Striving for excellence in nursing education, SACN's upper-division baccalaureate nursing program integrates Christian ideals, values, and practices, while building on a broad foundation of general education courses in the humanities and sciences.

SACN students are admitted as juniors, entering with the prerequisite credits from another regionally accredited college or university. They complete the last two years of a four-year Bachelor of Science in Nursing (B.S.N.) degree, which provides a broad spectrum of scientific, critical thinking, humanistic, communication, and leadership concepts and experiences expected of today's medical professionals. These last two years build on the broad base of two academic years (64 semester hours) transferred from another regionally accredited college or university. To this end, cooperative agreements have been reached with several of the community colleges in the area. Prospective students are encouraged to work with the SACN admissions office at the beginning of their college career to ensure transfer of credits.

Clinical sites for B.S.N. students include Carrie Lynn Children's Center, Malik Eye Institute, Northern Illinois Hospice, Rockford Memorial Hospital, Rockford Public Schools, OSF Saint Anthony Medical Center, H. Douglas Singer Mental Health Center, Visiting Nurses Association, and many other institutions.

In response to national trends and health-care demands, the College implemented an additional degree program, a Master of Science in Nursing (M.S.N.), in August 2006. This program, designed for the part-time student to complete within three or four years, leads to a Master of Science in Nursing degree for nurse educators, clinical nurse leaders, clinical nurse specialists in adult health concepts, and family nurse practitioners. The faculty and staff members are well known for their ability to provide personal, individualized attention in a caring environment. Classes are generally held one night per week, with additional work done online.

Students entering the master's program must enter with a bachelor's degree. Students may present with a baccalaureate degree in nursing (B.S.N.) or a baccalaureate in a field other than nursing. Licensure as a registered nurse is required for the state in which they will partake of their clinical practicum. If the student's baccalaureate degree is not in nursing, he or she must successfully complete an undergraduate nursing concepts course and nursing research course from a regionally accredited college or university prior to enrolling in the master's-level nursing concepts course or nursing research course.

A post-master's certificate is available for those who already have earned an M.S.N. degree but would like to take courses toward eligibility for the Nurse Educator Certificate. Student-at-Large status is available for graduate students. Interested students should contact the Graduate Affairs Office for details.

The student-to-faculty ratio at SACN is less than 8:1, and the NCLEX-RN pass rate for 2010 was 94 percent. In addition, 96 percent of all undergraduate students applied for and received financial aid. Because SACN is a nonresidential facility, students commute from their homes or find a residence in the Rockford area.

Saint Anthony College of Nursing is accredited by the Higher Learning Commission, member of the North Central Association of Colleges and Schools (NCA). The B.S.N. and M.S.N. programs are accredited by the Commission on Collegiate Nursing Education.

- *2010–11 UNDERGRADUATE TUITION & FEES*

  Full-time: $9443 per semester

  Part-time: $590 per credit

  Testing fees vary from $93–$107

  Supplies fee: $60 (first semester)

  Graduation fee: $160

- *2010–11 GRADUATE TUITION & FEES:*
  $719 per credit

- *APPLICATION DEADLINES:*

  Undergraduate students: September 15 (spring admission); February 15 (fall admission)

  Graduate students: April 1

- *FACULTY INFORMATION:*
  http://www.sacn.edu/contact/

- *MULTIMEDIA:*
  http://www.sacn.edu

CONTACT INFORMATION

Nancy Sanders, Associate Dean
Saint Anthony College of Nursing
5658 E. State Street
Rockford, Illinois 61108-2468
Phone: 815-395-5100
Fax: 815-227-2730
E-mail: admissions@sacn.edu
Web site: http://www.sacn.edu

UNDERGRADUATE NURSING PROGRAM:
Cheryl Delgado
Supervisor of Enrollment Management
Phone: 815-227-2141
E-mail: cheryldelgado@sacn.edu

GRADUATE NURSING PROGRAM:
Melissa Wrolstad
Student Affairs Specialist–Graduate Affairs
Phone: 815-395-5476
E-mail: melissawrolstad@sacn.edu

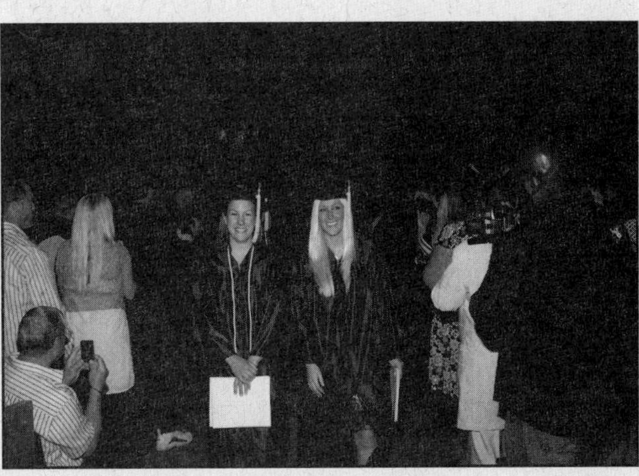

Saint Anthony College of Nursing students have a high graduation rate—92 percent of all students who attend the first day of class (full-time and part-time) will graduate.

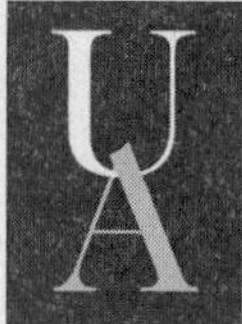

The University of Akron

College of Nursing

Nursing Transforms

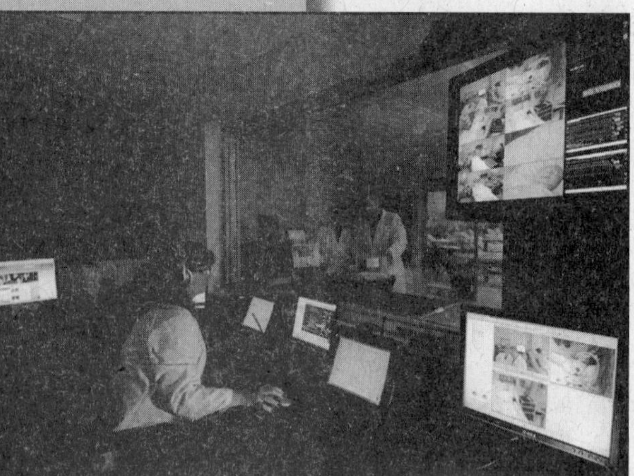

Transforming Lives through Caring, Competence, and Commitment

Our state-of-the-art simulation lab allows students to practice on high fidelity simulators and critique their recorded performance with their instructors.

Founded in 1967, the College of Nursing at The University of Akron (UA) offers multiple programs for students aspiring to become professional nurses and practicing nurses seeking career and professional advancement. Approved by the Ohio Board of Nursing and fully accredited by the Commission on Collegiate Nursing Education (CCNE), the College employs faculty members with a broad range of research and clinical backgrounds.

The basic Baccalaureate program is a four-year program. Clinical experiences are required in each semester of the program after the first year. The senior year features a senior practicum designed to give the student greater depth in an area of the student's choosing. A fifteen-month Accelerated B.S.N. program is open to students who hold a bachelor's degree.

The LPN/B.S.N. for the licensed LPN features testing for advanced placement. The LPN can finish the B.S.N. in five semesters.

The RN/B.S.N. sequence for the registered nurse (RN) features a full-time or part-time option, flexible hours for clinical requirements, and classroom time one day per week. An outreach RN/B.S.N. sequence is offered at the Lorain County Community College campus, Wayne College, and Medina County University Center (MCUC).

The Master of Science in Nursing (M.S.N.) program prepares graduates for advanced practice or administration. Students may choose adult/gerontological health nursing, behavioral health nursing, child and adolescent health nursing, or nurse anesthesia tracks. Advanced practice options include nurse practitioner (NP) or clinical nurse specialist (CNS).

The RN/M.S.N. sequence is designed for RNs who meet graduate admission criteria. Students take three years to complete both the B.S.N. and master's course work.

The University of Akron and Kent State University offer a Joint Ph.D. in Nursing (JPDN) program. A Doctor of Nursing Practice (D.N.P.) program is currently under review.

The College has a state-of-the-art Learning Resources Center (LRC) that includes simulated patient-care areas and a computer laboratory. The simulation area includes a birthing suite, an advanced clinical unit, and a control room providing video capture for students to review their work with faculty members.

The Nursing Center for Community Health links the College to the community and is used by the underinsured and medically vulnerable populations in the area for health-care services and by the faculty and students as a practice and research site.

Students applying for all baccalaureate programs must have completed prerequisite college/university courses. Basic B.S.N. candidates must have earned at least a 2.75 grade point average (GPA) in prerequisite and science courses. Course work begins in the fall.

Students entering the LPN/B.S.N. sequence must hold a current Ohio LPN license with a minimum prerequisite and science GPA of 2.75. Course work begins in January.

Requirements for the RN/B.S.N. sequence include a prerequisite GPA of 2.75 (or 3.0 for RN/M.S.N.) and current Ohio RN licensure. Course work begins in May.

Students applying to the M.S.N. program must hold a baccalaureate degree in nursing from an NLNAC-accredited nursing program; complete prerequisite courses; submit scores from the GRE taken within the last five years (CRNA program only), an essay, and three letters of reference; and hold a current Ohio RN license.

- *2010–11 UNDERGRADUATE TUITION & FEES (full year): $10,300 (Ohio Resident/full-time); $5260 (Ohio Resident/part-time); $17,950 (Nonresident/full-time); $9100 (Nonresident/part-time)*
- *2010–11 GRADUATE TUITION & FEES (full year): $8065 (Ohio Resident/full-time); $4140 (Ohio Resident/part-time); $12,900 (Nonresident/full-time); $5920 (Nonresident/part-time)*
- *APPLICATION DEADLINES: The University of Akron has rolling admissions year round. Contact the appropriate Admissions Office for specific deadlines for each semester: http://www.uakron.edu/admissions/.*
- *FACULTY INFORMATION: http://www.uakron.edu/nursing/about-us/faculty-profiles.dot*
- *MULTIMEDIA: http://www.uakron.edu/nursing/*

CONTACT INFORMATION

Rita A. Klein, Ed.D.
Director, Office of Student Affairs
College of Nursing
The University of Akron
302 Buchtel Common
Akron, Ohio 44325-3701
Phone: 330-972-5103
888-477-7887 (toll-free)
Fax: 330-972-5493
E-mail: rklein@uakron.edu
Web site: www.uakron.edu/nursing

Graduate Nursing Program:
Marlene Huff, Associate Professor
Phone: 330-972-5930
888-477-7887 (toll-free)
Fax: 330-972-5493
E-mail: mhuff@uakron.edu
Web site: www.uakron.edu/nursing

Find us on Facebook®: http://www.facebook.com/uanursing
Follow us on Twitter™: http://twitter.com/uanursing

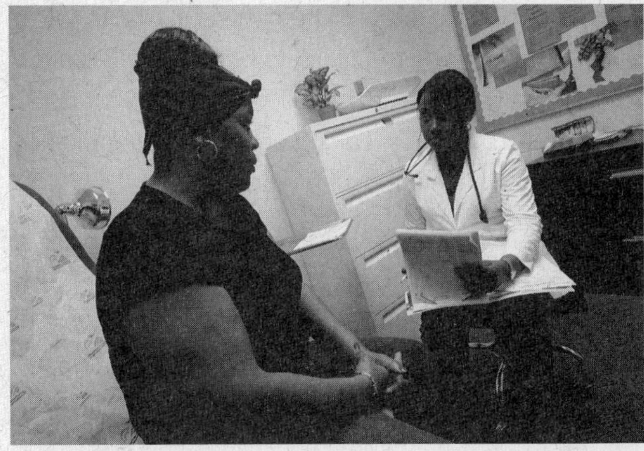

UA students have the unique advantage of experiencing direct patient care in our nurse-managed clinic.

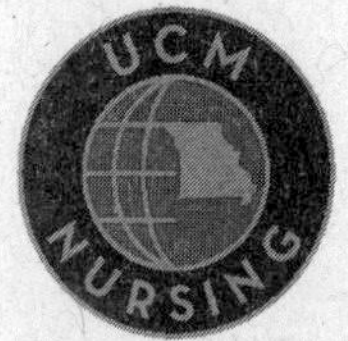

University of Central Missouri Department of Nursing

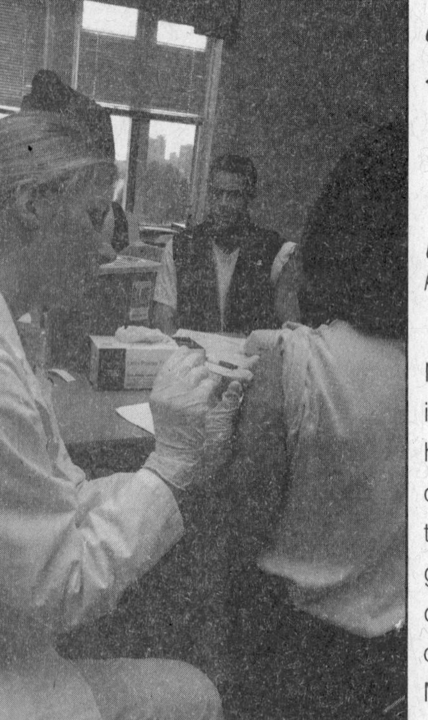

Celebrating 50+ Years of Nursing Excellence.

UCM Senior Nursing student participating in a shot clinic.

It's something everyone has in common: the need for health care. Health care is one of the only segments of the U.S. economy that is still growing. Nurses are in critical demand, and graduates of the University of Central Missouri's (UCM) Department of Nursing have achieved a 100 percent employment placement rate. UCM's Nursing program celebrated its 50th Anniversary in 2009 and is always looking ahead to better meet the needs of nursing students.

Through the "Caring for Missourians" initiative, the Department of Nursing has been able to expand the staff by 3 faculty members and 1 staff member, remodel the nursing lab and faculty offices, update office equipment, and purchase a SimMan 3G simulation system to provide students with a more realistic tool for clinical scenarios. Central Missouri's nursing program is nationally accredited at both the undergraduate and graduate levels by the Commission on Collegiate Nursing Education (CCNE).

Central Missouri's undergraduate nursing students have the unique opportunity to have clinical experiences in both urban and rural communities. One year of rural clinical nursing practice is followed by a year of urban clinical nursing practice and course work at Central Summit Center. Each day brings diverse opportunities for students to use intellect, skill, and compassion. Registered nurses face increasingly complex demands that require a broad-based bachelor's degree preparation. UCM's Bachelor of Science in Nursing (B.S.N.) includes general education credits and nursing prerequisites and an introduction to other disciplines, as well as a major focus on nursing.

Registered nurses with associate degrees in nursing can give their careers a profitable and professional boost by obtaining a bachelor's degree with UCM's RN to Baccalaureate program. The use of innovative online instruction provides a multitude of learning opportunities to improve critical thinking skills while gaining a deeper understanding of professional nursing. Students' schedules are flexible, and they proceed at their own pace, which enables them to maintain a work schedule as well as family time. Students can complete their degree in as little as one year (assuming all other prerequisites are met) with this 30-credit-hour program. Upon earning the Bachelor of Science degree, students are eligible to continue their education at the master's degree level, further enhancing their career opportunities.

UCM's Master of Science in Nursing (M.S.N.) program is the area's only graduate program designed to investigate the specialized practice and unique challenges of rural nursing. This is an excellent opportunity to research or become published in the rapidly growing rural family nursing field. Although students have the opportunity to become knowledgeable about rural nursing, they are prepared to practice in both urban and rural settings. Two M.S.N. tracks (Family Nurse Practitioner and Nurse Educator) are available to those wanting a foundation for advanced practice, specialty practice, and advanced study at the doctoral level. Online classes provide "anytime, anywhere" access and expand technological skills, making students more valuable in the workplace. A faculty advisor is available to help students plan a course of study to fit their individual needs and interests.

Please contact us today!

- *2010–11 UNDERGRADUATE TUITION & FEES:*

  Missouri Resident: $195.30 per credit hour

  Non-Resident: $390.60 per credit hour

  Online: $243.10 per credit hour
- *2010–11 GRADUATE TUITION & FEES:*

  Missouri Resident: $253.15 per credit hour

  Non-Resident: $506.30 per credit hour

  Online: $296.40 per credit hour

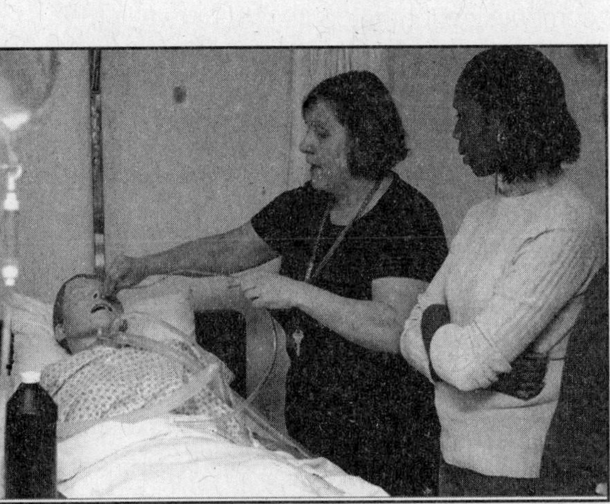

UCM Nursing students in a simulation lab.

- *APPLICATION DEADLINES: January 1 for Fall undergraduate admission; July 1 for Spring undergraduate admission*
- *FACULTY INFORMATION: http://www.ucmo.edu/nursing/facstaff.cfm*

CONTACT INFORMATION

Dr. Julie Clawson
Department of Nursing
University of Central Missouri
600 South College, UHC 106
Warrensburg, Missouri 64093
Phone: 660-543-4775
Fax: 660-543-8304
E-mail: clawson@ucmo.edu
Web site: http://www.ucmo.edu/nursing

UNDERGRADUATE NURSING PROGRAM:
Dr. Julie Clawson, Department Chair
Phone: 660-543-4775
E-mail: clawson@ucmo.edu

GRADUATE NURSING PROGRAM:
Dr. Linda Mulligan, Graduate Program Coordinator
Phone: 816-282-1100
E-mail: mulligan@ucmo.edu

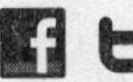

Find us on Facebook®: http://www.facebook.com/UCentralMO
Follow us on Twitter™: http://twitter.com/UCentralMo

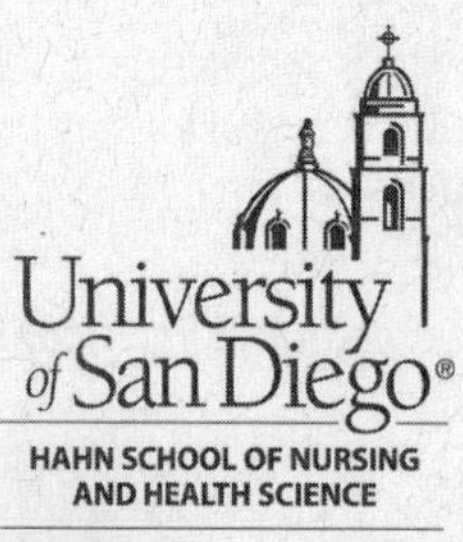

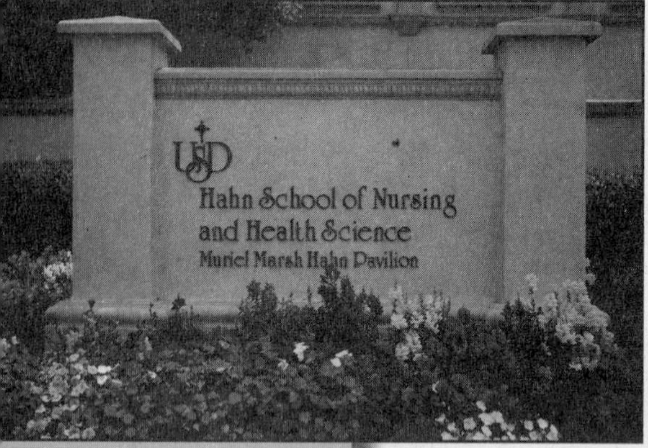

A Private School with a Public Conscience

Excellence in Nursing.

Since 1974, the University of San Diego's Hahn School of Nursing and Health Science has provided high-quality education to more than 1,600 alumni and 190 doctorally prepared nurse scientists. With an impressive global network of clinical partners, preceptors, and granting agencies, the School consistently ranks in the top tier of graduate nursing programs nationwide.

Faculty members prepare nurse scientists and leaders in education and practice in a research-intensive community of progressive scholars. The School seeks to deepen its commitment to social justice and health care as a human right by influencing health policy and promoting an ethical approach to nursing characterized by compassion and respect for the dignity of the individual.

International clinical, research, and cultural immersion experiences are available in Mexico, the Dominican Republic, India, and Pacific Rim countries. Participating students are accompanied by faculty members who are experts in international health.

The Hahn School of Nursing offers the Doctor of Philosophy (Ph.D.) and Doctor of Nursing Practice (D.N.P.) degrees as well as the Master of Science in Nursing (M.S.N.) degree for RNs. For those with a non-nursing degree (baccalaureate or higher), the School offers a Master's Entry Program in Nursing (MEPN). In addition, the School offers a Post-BSN-DNP program for RNs who desire preparation in primary care as a Family, Dual Pediatric/Family, or Dual Adult/ Family Nurse Practitioner, in Psychiatric-Mental Health as a Nurse Practitioner or dual preparation as a Nurse Practitioner/Clinical Nurse Specialist, and preparation in Adult-Gerontology as a Clinical Nurse Specialist.

Classes are offered in traditional fifteen-week semesters in spring and fall and also in concentrated intersession and summer semesters.

The School provides mentoring in a research-intensive environment and specializes in personalized attention and small classes, labs, and clinical practicums taught by doctorally prepared and/or clinically certified faculty members. The students—women and men who represent many faiths, ethnic groups, and geographical regions—share in common intellectual curiosity, critical thinking skills, and compassion for their patients.

The Hahn School of Nursing and Health Science occupies a recently renovated 18,000-square-foot, two-story building and the newly renovated and equipped 5,000-square-foot Simulation and Standardized Patient Nursing Laboratory, a unique educational resource in Southern California. With a trauma center, birthing area, and nursing station, this state-of-the art facility uses trained "patient" actors and programmed robotic equipment to simulate primary-care, acute-care, and emergency situations to ensure that students develop the full range of clinical skills. Student performances are digitally recorded and evaluated by peers and the clinical instructors.

The School is one of the few nursing schools in the country with the Standardized Patient Program.

The School is affiliated with a wide variety of clinical resources, including UCSD Medical Center, Sharp Health Care (Hospitals and Clinics), Palomar Pomerado Health Care System, Scripps Health (Hospitals and Clinics), Children's Hospital, Veterans Administration Hospital, Kaiser Permanente, and Balboa Naval Hospital. Many community agencies are also utilized, including schools, home health agencies, the San Diego Department of Health Services, HMOs, and community clinics.

The University of San Diego, a Catholic institution of higher learning chartered in 1949, enrolls some 7,800 undergraduate and graduate students and is known for its commitment to teaching, the liberal arts, the formation of values and community service.

Nursing programs are fully accredited by the Commission on Collegiate Nursing Education (CCNE) and the California Board of Registered Nursing.

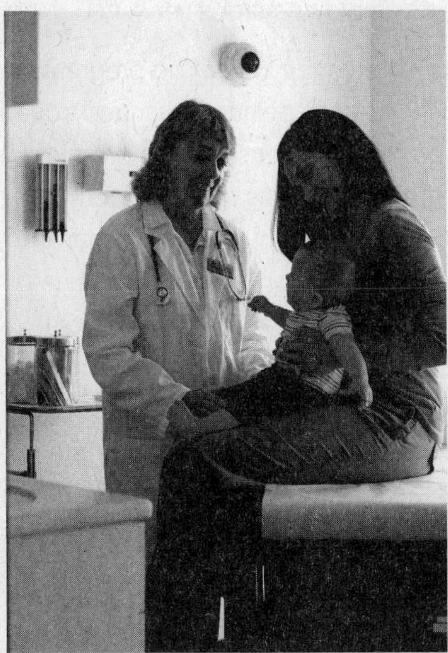

The University of San Diego provides excellent and diverse clinical/research experiences.

- *2010–11 GRADUATE TUITION & FEES*
  Master's Programs: $1215 per unit
  Doctoral Programs: $1245 per unit
  Living Expenses: Approximately $15,000 per year
  Other Educational Expenses: Approximately $5000 per year
- *FOR MORE INFORMATION: http://www.sandiego.edu/academics/nursing*
- *APPLICATION DEADLINES*
  D.N.P and Ph.D.: March 1
  Master's Entry Program in Nursing: November 1
  M.S.N. Programs: March 1 (fall entry); November 1 (spring entry) [Note: Spring entry is not available for Dual Adult/Family Nurse Practitioner, Family Nurse Practitioner, Dual Pediatric/Family Nurse Practitioner, and Psychiatric-Mental Health Nurse Practitioner programs]
- *FACULTY INFORMATION: http://www.sandiego.edu/academics/nursing/dir.php*
- *MULTIMEDIA: http://www.sandiego.edu/academics/nursing/news_video.php*

CONTACT INFORMATION

Hahn School of Nursing and Health Sciences
University of San Diego
5998 Alcala Park
San Diego, California 92110-2492
Phone: 619-260-4548
Fax: 619-260-4163
Web site:
http://www.sandiego.edu/academics/nursing

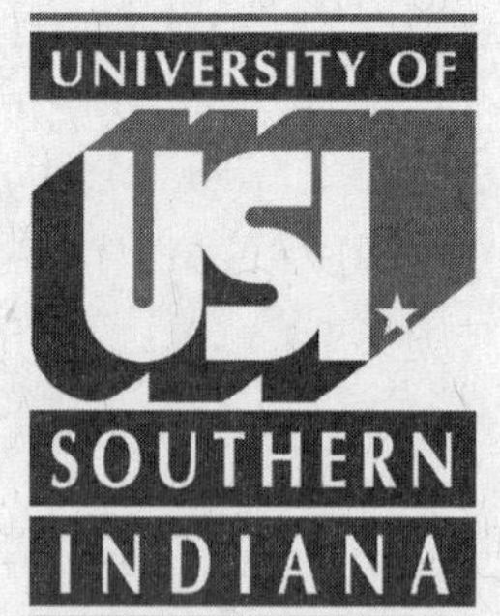

School of Nursing

Education That Begins with You

USI Health Professions Center.

The School of Nursing at the University of Southern Indiana (USI) was founded in 1988 as the first state-supported baccalaureate nursing program in southern Indiana. In 1996, the School initiated a master's degree program in nursing. A Doctor in Nursing Practice (DNP) program was implemented August 2008.

Recognizing the complexity of health care, the School of Nursing has developed undergraduate and graduate nursing curricula designed to prepare students for evidence-based practice, with an emphasis on clinical nursing competence. The baccalaureate and graduate nursing programs are fully accredited by the Commission on Collegiate Nursing Education. The 25 members of the nursing faculty represent diverse areas of teaching, practice, and research. Faculty members have expertise and strong clinical practice backgrounds in their areas of teaching. The School of Nursing is a leader in the development of distance education courses and programs. The RN-BSN, RN-MSN, and MSN nursing programs may be completed online. The DNP program combines on-campus intensives with online courses.

The Bachelor of Science in Nursing (BSN) program is designed to prepare the professional nurse to plan, implement, and evaluate health care for individuals, families, and groups in institutional and community settings. The nursing program is based on a planned progression of courses arranged to build upon previous knowledge and to develop skills and performance at an increasing level of competence. The 128 credits required for the degree include the University core curriculum courses supportive to the nursing major and 69 hours of nursing courses.

Registered nurses with an associate degree or diploma may obtain a baccalaureate and/or master's degree in nursing through the RN completion program. The flexibility of this program provides nurses with the opportunity to complete the course requirements in their own communities and on their own schedule with reasonable costs while receiving a high-quality education. No further testing of prior knowledge is required for nurses who hold a valid RN license and are in good standing in their current employment position.

The Master of Science in Nursing program is offered for nurses seeking advanced education in professional nursing. The graduate program prepares nurses for advanced practice as acute care nurse practitioners, family nurse practitioners, nurse educators, and nurse managers/leaders. The graduate degree is awarded upon the completion of 39 to 42 credits, depending on the graduate nursing specialty. Post-master's certificate programs are available for nurse practitioner, nursing management and leadership, and nursing education.

The Doctor of Nursing Practice (DNP) program is a 78-credit-hour post-master's program. A maximum of 42 credit hours from the M.S.N. may be applied to the D.N.P. degree. The DNP program prepares experts in advanced nursing with emphasis placed on innovative, evidence-based practice that reflects the application of credible research findings. The expanded knowledge base in nursing will broaden the DNP graduate's ability to translate that knowledge quickly and effectively to benefit patients, improve outcomes, and contribute to the profession. The curriculum consists of two to three years of doctoral-level course work, which culminates in the completion of an evidence-based capstone project.

The Charles E. Day Learning Resource Center, located in the College of Nursing and Health Professions, includes a learning laboratory with the latest technology. The state-of-the art Clinical Simulation Center provides students with hands-on learning prior to practice in hospitals and community settings and advance clinical decision making for acute care patients.

The University of Southern Indiana is a regionally responsive, needs-driven, comprehensive public university in the model of the "new American college." USI's appeal to students is found in its size, the accessibility of professors, its beautiful environment and innovative housing, its proximity to an urban center, and the friendliness of students, employees, and the community. Located in Evansville, Indiana, USI is an easy drive from Indianapolis, Nashville, and St. Louis.

- *2010–11 UNDERGRADUATE TUITION & FEES: Undergraduate tuition for in-state students was $185 per credit hour or $2775 per semester for full-time study (15 hours). Nonresident tuition was $277 per credit hour or $4155 for full-time study (15 hours). University fees ranged from $200–$400 per semester. Other fees and housing costs are determined on an individual basis.*
- *2010–11 GRADUATE TUITION & FEES: Graduate tuition was $270 per credit or $2430 per semester for full-time study (9 hours). (All students pay in-state tuition because the programs are online.) University fees ranged from $200–$400 per semester. Other fees and housing costs are determined on an individual basis*
- *APPLICATION DEADLINES: BSN Program: August 1; MSN Program: February 1 (fall), October 1 (spring); DNP Program: January 15*
- *FACULTY INFORMATION: http://health.usi.edu*
- *MULTIMEDIA: http://health.usi.edu/acadprog/nursing/default.asp*

CONTACT INFORMATION

Admissions and Advising Coordinator
College of Nursing and Health Professions
University of Southern Indiana
8600 University Blvd.
Evansville, Indiana 47712
Phone: 812-465-1150
E-mail: cnhpadmissions@usi.edu
kmwalker4@usi.edu
Web site: http://health.usi.edu

Undergraduate Nursing Program:
Dr. Jeri Burger, Program Director
Phone: 812 461-5340
E-mail: jlburger2@usi.edu

Graduate Nursing Program:
Dr. Mayola Rowser, Program Director
Phone: 812 461-5257
E-mail: mrowser@usi.edu

Find us on Facebook®: http://on.fb.me/UofSouthernIndiana_NursingHealthProfs

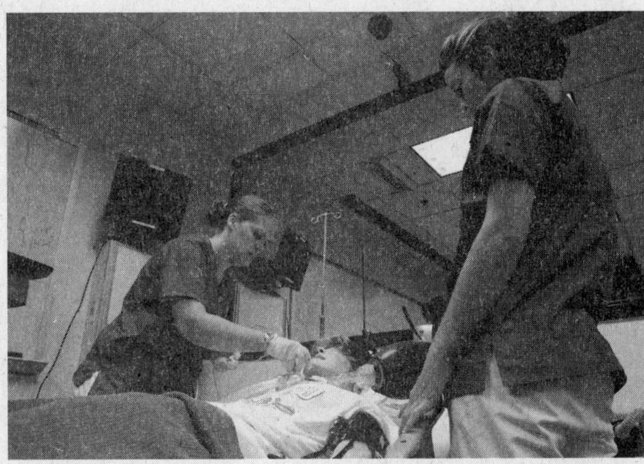

State-of-the-Art Simulation Center.

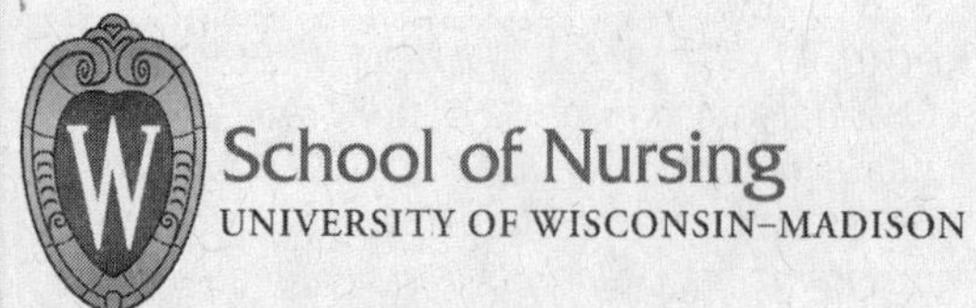

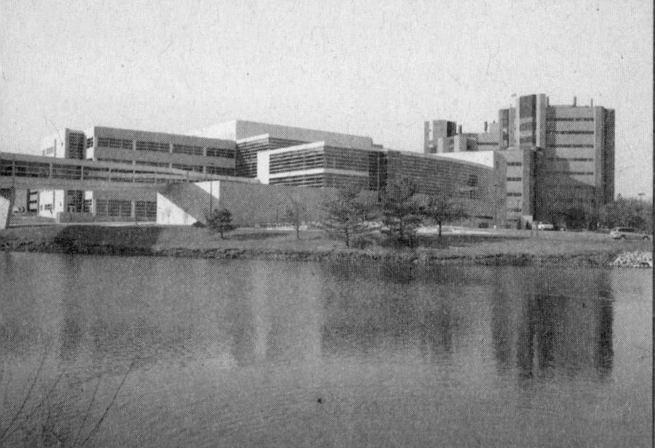

The Science of Nursing. The Future of Care.

Mission: To prepare leaders in nursing research, education, practice, and service.

The Health Sciences Learning Center on the UW–Madison campus.

The University of Wisconsin–Madison School of Nursing, established in 1924, is the leading nursing research institution in Wisconsin and a crucial part of the state's health-care system. As an integral academic partner situated in the health sciences sector of the campus with the School of Medicine and Public Health and the School of Pharmacy, the School of Nursing collaborates with scientists and renowned researchers across the UW–Madison campus, the nation, and the world. The school's research is translational in nature and grounded in practical application—the work being done has an immediate impact on Wisconsin's communities, hospitals, clinics, schools, and homes.

The School of Nursing is currently ranked among the top 20 nursing schools in the United States in National Institutes of Health (NIH) research funding and by the quality of its graduate programs. It has an enrollment of more than 500 students; offering the Bachelor of Science in Nursing (B.S.), Doctor of Nursing Practice (D.N.P.), and Doctor of Philosophy in Nursing (Ph.D.) degrees. Postdoctoral training opportunities are also available.

Facilities for clinical practice and research are extensive both in and outside of Madison. These include University of Wisconsin Hospital and Clinics, American Family Children's Hospital, and UW Carbone Cancer Center; hospitals and clinics in urban and rural settings; nursing homes; day-care centers; and public health agencies. On campus, the Health Sciences Learning Center (HSLC) brings together students in nursing, medicine, and pharmacy. State-of-the-art classrooms, computer resources, distance education facilities, and the Ebling Library are housed in the HSLC.

Advancing the science of nursing through research and scholarship is a strategic priority of the School of Nursing. To this end, nursing faculty members are expert scholars, clinicians, and teachers. Many have postdoctoral experience in nursing and related disciplines. Many have competed successfully for prestigious federal and private research and training awards and are well-known for their expertise in the university, local, national, and international communities.

Faculty members who teach in the clinical component are prepared in cutting-edge technology for education and practice; many are board-certified practitioners who maintain an active clinical practice in addition to their teaching roles.

Faculty and staff members and students affiliated with the University of Wisconsin–Madison School of Nursing are actively engaged in partnerships with a wide variety of community groups, governmental agencies, voluntary organizations, educational institutions, and health services organizations. These partnerships allow the School of

Nursing to contribute in unique ways to coordinated action directed at health improvement and the management of health problems.

The new Nursing Science Center, scheduled to open in 2013, is designed to be an educational facility that will provide an extraordinary and exciting opportunity for students of all levels to get involved in shaping the future of nursing education at the University of Wisconsin-Madison School of Nursing.

The baccalaureate degree program in nursing is accredited by the Commission on Collegiate Nursing Education (CCNE).

The University of Wisconsin–Madison is the second largest research university in the country and is a world-class university, nationally and internationally recognized for academic excellence. Located in Wisconsin's capital city, the campus includes thirteen academic schools and colleges and enrolls more than 40,000 students annually.

- *2010–11 FULL-TIME UNDERGRADUATE TUITION & FEES: $8986 (Residents); $24,236 (Nonresidents)*
- *2010–11 FULL-TIME GRADUATE TUITION & FEES: $10,940 (Residents); $25,106 (Nonresidents)*
- *APPLICATION DEADLINES: Undergraduate and Graduate: February 1*
- *FACULTY INFORMATION: http://www.son.wisc.edu/people/faculty.html*
- *MULTIMEDIA: http://www.son.wisc.edu/*

CONTACT INFORMATION

Academic Programs Office
School of Nursing
University of Wisconsin–Madison
600 Highland Ave; K6/146
Madison, Wisconsin 53792
Phone: 608-263-5202
Fax: 608-263-5296
Web site: http://www.son.wisc.edu/

Undergraduate Nursing Programs Office:
Phone: 608-263-5202
E-mail: ugadmit@son.wisc.edu

Graduate Nursing Programs Office:
Phone: 608-263-5180
E-mail: gradadmit@son.wisc.edu

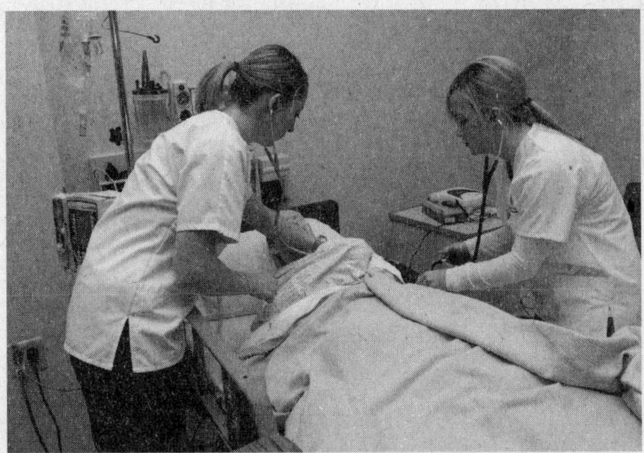

Nursing students have access to state-of-the-art simulation labs at the University of Wisconsin–Madison School of Nursing.

Find us on Facebook®: http://on.fb.me/UWiscMadison_SON

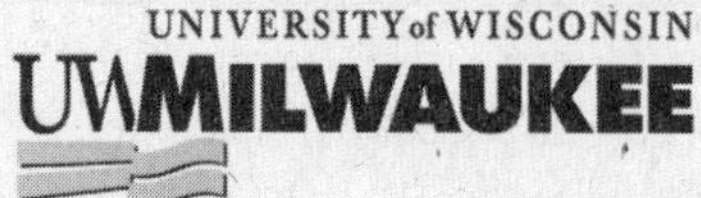

College of Nursing

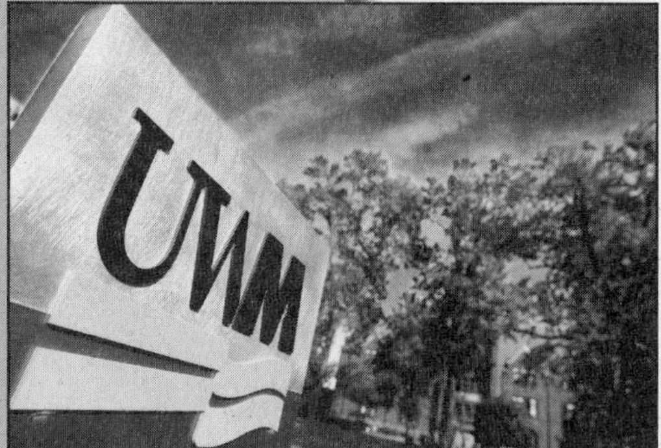

IDEAS: Innovation. Discovery. Engagement. Solutions.

UW–Milwaukee campus sign in front of Chapman Hall. (Photo by Peter Amland.)

Since its inception in 1965, the University of Wisconsin–Milwaukee (UWM) College of Nursing has been dedicated to providing academic programs of the highest quality that are at the forefront of nursing. The College is a vibrant, innovative environment for teaching, research, practice, and service to the community and the profession. The largest nursing school in Wisconsin, the College is one of three institutions in the state to offer students the full range of nursing degrees: Bachelor of Science in Nursing (B.S.), Master's of Nursing (M.N.), Doctor of Philosophy in Nursing (Ph.D.) and Doctor of Nursing Practice (D.N.P.). The College of Nursing has an enrollment of 1,166 undergraduate students as well as 279 graduate students.

The College of Nursing's faculty members create innovative classroom environments and provide the latest technological teaching tools. Consistently ranked for its academic excellence by U.S. News and World Report, the College gained the 28th position of nursing colleges receiving National Institutes of Health (NIH) funding. Faculty members also embrace practice by engaging regional and global communities in developing solutions to improve health.

The College enjoys clinical practice and research partnerships with over 150 clinical facilities throughout Southeastern Wisconsin and beyond. The College's Community Nursing Centers address the health needs of at-risk urban populations, engaging with community members to establish health-care solutions to fit their needs. Nationally recognized initiatives include the Collaborative for Intelligent Health Information Systems Initiative (CIHISI), a research center dedicated to creating health information technology solutions that improve the access, quality, and costs of health care. The Pediatric Nursing Research Consortium, a partnership with Children's Hospital of Wisconsin, the Medical College of Wisconsin, and Marquette University, combines the resources of clinical and academic researchers to create translational research in the care of children and families. The NIH-funded Self Management Science Center expands research aimed at enhancing the science of the self-management in individuals and families. Faculty members have also extended the scope of international research to health care in rural Malawi and Kenya. The College also maintains a close relationship with two sister nursing schools in South Korea.

The baccalaureate, master's, and doctorate in nursing practice programs are accredited by the Commission on Collegiate Nursing Education. The College of Nursing is also affiliated with Sigma Theta Tau International, Eta Nu Chapter, and the Nursing Centers Research Network.

The undergraduate nursing program is built upon a rigorous science-based curriculum and requires a dedication to scholarship and a passion for health care. Individuals may be considered for admission as pre-nursing students in the fall and spring as beginning freshmen or transfer students. Admission to the clinical major occurs in the junior year. Admission to the nursing major is highly competitive; the minimum GPA required can be significantly higher than the stated minimum GPA of 2.75 needed for application to the nursing major.

The College of Nursing continues to expand and enhance its graduate opportunities. The College offers multiple avenues by which to earn a master's degree: Advanced Generalist Masters, Family Nurse Practitioner, Clinical Nurse Specialist, and M.S./M.B.A. programs. Doctoral studies are available in face-to-face and online formats.

Graduate program application deadlines depend on the program of interest. Generally, applications are due to the UWM Graduate School by January 1 and to the College by February 1 for fall enrollment and to the UWM Graduate School by September 1 and to the College by October 1 for spring semester enrollment. Prospective students are encouraged to visit the College Web site for more detailed information about admission requirements.

- *2010–11 UNDERGRADUATE TUITION & FEES: Annual Full-time: $8154 (residents); $17,880 (nonresidents)*

  Additional tuition differential fee of $30 per credit is due upon admission to the clinical major.
- *2010–11 GRADUATE TUITION & FEES: Annual Full-time: $10,446 (residents); $23,734 (nonresidents)*
- *APPLICATION DEADLINES: Undergraduate: August 15 for spring admission to clinical major; January 15 for fall admission to clinical major.*

  Graduate: February 1 for fall admission; October 1 for spring admission
- *FACULTY INFORMATION: http://www4.uwm.edu/nursing/faculty_staff/*

CONTACT INFORMATION

Robin Jens, Director of Student Services
University of Wisconsin–Milwaukee College of Nursing
1921 East Hartford Avenue
P.O. Box 413
Milwaukee, Wisconsin 53201
Phone: 414-229-5047
Fax: 414-229-5554
E-mail: www.asknursing@uwm.edu
Web site: http://www.nursing.uwm.edu

UNDERGRADUATE NURSING PROGRAM:
Donna Wier, Senior Advisor
Undergraduate Admissions
Student Affairs Office
Room 129-Cunningham Hall
Phone: 414-229-5481
E-mail: ddw@uwm.edu

GRADUATE NURSING PROGRAM:
Sylvia Forbes, Advisor
Graduate Admissions
Student Affairs Office
Room 129-Cunningham Hall
Phone: 414-229-4662
E-mail: forbes@uwm.edu

f

Find us on Facebook®: http://on.fb.me/UWM_Nursing

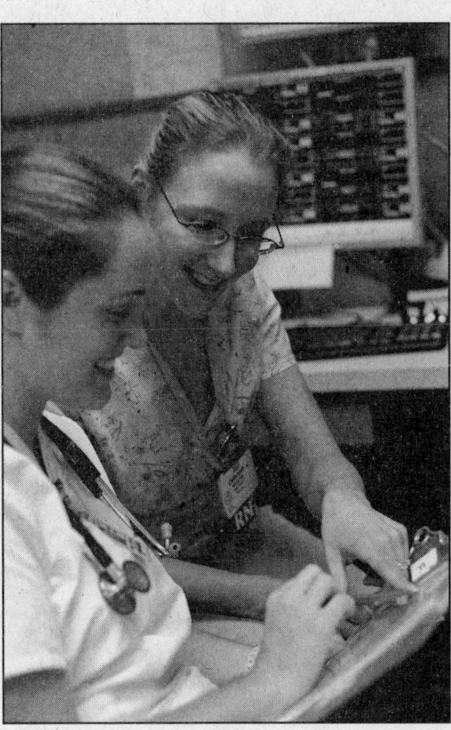

A UW–Milwaukee College of Nursing student working at St. Luke's Hospital in Milwaukee. Nursing students in clinical training get hands-on medical experience and the chance to work with real patients in a supervised setting. (Photo by Peter Jakubowski.)

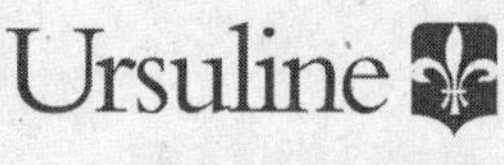

VALUES·VOICE·VISION

Breen School of Nursing

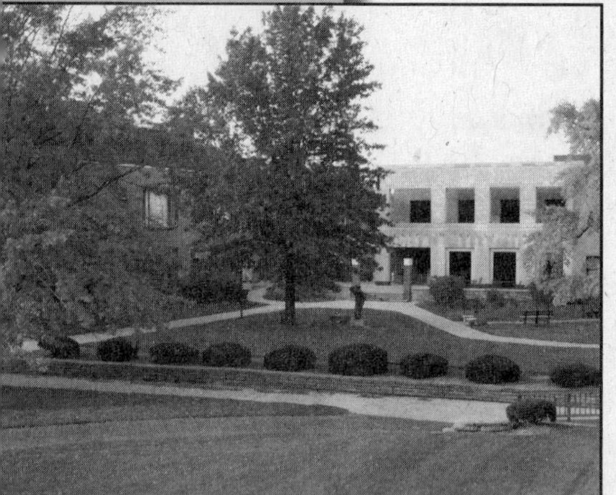

Transforming health through reflection and healing.

Located on a beautiful, 100-acre wooded campus in Pepper Pike, Ohio, just 15 miles east of Cleveland, Ursuline's campus is safe, intimate, and easily accessible.

Nursing has been a vital program at Ursuline College since 1975. Today, the Breen School of Nursing has the largest academic program on campus. An individualized approach enables students to enjoy personalized instruction while learning the material in greater depth by gaining experience in a wide variety of health-care environments. Breen School graduates are highly sought by employers who find them to be well prepared and flexible in adapting to new settings.

The Breen School of Nursing offers the Bachelor of Science in Nursing (B.S.N.), Master of Science in Nursing (M.S.N.), and Doctor of Nursing Practice (D.N.P.) degree programs, as well as post-master's certificates. The total nursing enrollment is approximately 600 students per year. B.S.N. graduates typically score higher than the national average on the NCLEX-RN exam. The M.S.N. program offers the following Advanced Practice Registered Nurse (APRN) role and population-focused education tracks: Adult Health Clinical Nurse Specialist, Adult Nurse Practitioner, and Family Nurse Practitioner. Nursing education and palliative care are also offered as additional subspecialty components to the M.S.N. or D.N.P. tracks. The focus of the post-M.S.N. and D.N.P. degree is leadership in evidence-based practice and policy development.

The B.S.N. and M.S.N. programs are accredited by the Commission on Collegiate Nursing Education (CCNE). The D.N.P. program, which was initiated in fall 2010, is approved by the Ohio Board of Regents and accredited by the Higher Learning Commission of North Central Association of Colleges and Schools; CCNE-accreditation visits will be made in November 2011 to review the D.N.P. program.

The Breen School of Nursing is affiliated with numerous internationally renowned health-care agencies that include the Cleveland Clinic Health Care System and the University Case Medical Center and Health System. M.S.N. and D.N.P. students may elect to complete their practicum and capstone experiences in another state or country.

The School's Nursing Resource Center (NRC) lab has four mid-fidelity manikins and four low-fidelity manikins for practicing skills, vital signs, health assessment, and simulation. The lab has a virtual IV computer that enables students to train on intravenous catheter insertion with a variety of scenarios as well as to complete an IV competency. Individual workstations allow nursing students to practice skills such as intramuscular, intravenous, and subcutaneous injections.

Undergraduate and graduate applications are accepted on a rolling basis. In addition to meeting the criteria for clear admission to the College, applicants seeking admission to the B.S.N. program directly from high school need to have a GPA of 2.75 or higher and minimum ACT scores of 20 or SAT composite scores of 1000. Students must also demonstrate proficiency by achieving a grade of at least C+ in algebra, biology with lab, and chemistry with lab. Transfer students need a strong recommendation from a counselor or teacher and at least a 2.5 cumulative GPA average in all completed college work. Applicants who have attended or are currently attending other nursing programs must also submit a letter of good standing from the program's dean or director.

Students applying to the RN to B.S.N. program must meet the criteria for clear admission to the College, have graduated from an accredited associate or diploma program, and hold an active RN license in the state of Ohio. Students applying to the LPN to B.S.N. program must meet the criteria for clear admission to the College, have graduated from an accredited LPN program, and hold an active LPN license in the state of Ohio. Second Degree Accelerated B.S.N. students must be accepted to Ursuline College, supply proof of a degree from an accredited college or university, and have earned a minimum GPA of 2.5 in their first degree program.

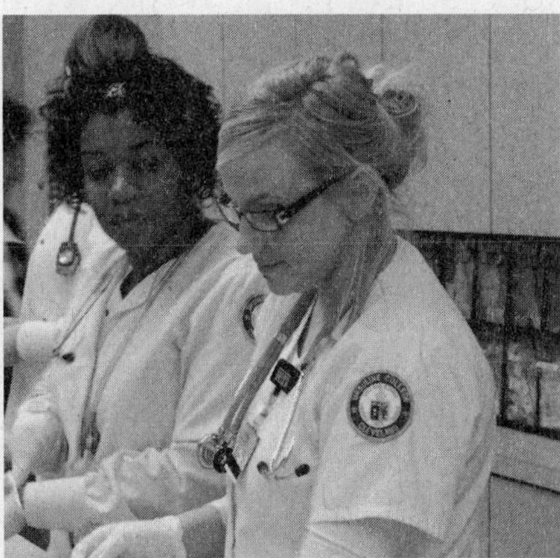

Ursuline College graduates are aggressively recruited by top Cleveland hospitals because of their caring and values-based approach to nursing.

- *2010–11 UNDERGRADUATE TUITION & FEES:*

  Generic B.S.N.: Resident/nonresident full-time tuition: $790 per credit hour

  Accelerated Second Degree B.S.N.: Resident/ nonresident full-time tuition: $632 per credit hour

- *2010–11 GRADUATE (M.S.N. and D.N.P.) NURSING TUITION & FEES:*

  Resident/nonresident full-time tuition: $841 per credit hour

- *APPLICATION DEADLINES*

  B.S.N. programs: Rolling admissions

  M.S.N. and D.N.P. programs: Mid-July (fall semester); mid-November (spring semester)

- *FACULTY INFORMATION: http://www.ursuline.edu/Academics/Nursing/Faculty/index.html*

CONTACT INFORMATION
Breen School of Nursing
Ursuline College
2550 Lander Road
Pepper Pike, Ohio 44124-4398
Phone: 440-646-8166
888-URSULINE (toll-free)
Fax: 440-449-4267
Web site: http://www.ursuline.edu/Academics/Nursing/index.html

Undergraduate Nursing Program:
B.S.N. Enrollment Coordinator
Undergraduate Nursing Program
Phone: 440-646-8171

Graduate Nursing Program:
Barbara Dussing, Administrative Assistant
Graduate Nursing Program
Phone: 440-684-6051
E-mail: bdussing@ursuline.edu

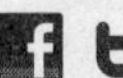

Find us on Facebook®:
Undergraduate: http://on.fb.me/ursuline_college
Graduate: http://on.fb.me/Ursuline_Coll_gradadmit

Follow us on Twitter™:
Undergraduate: http://twitter.com/UrsulineAdmit
Graduate: http://twitter.com/UrsulineGradStu

SCHOOL OF NURSING
VANDERBILT UNIVERSITY

Where Tradition Meets Innovation

Vanderbilt University School of Nursing is pioneering the use of smart phones as teaching tools. The School is one of the first in the nation to use a new application that transforms wireless devices, including Blackberry, iPod, iTouch, and laptops into classroom response devices for enhanced learning.

For over 100 years, Vanderbilt University School of Nursing (VUSN) has been providing innovative educational opportunities for its students. The School is currently ranked among the top 20 nursing schools in the United States and has an enrollment of more than 900 students. Vanderbilt offers the Master of Science in Nursing (M.S.N.), Doctor of Nursing Practice (D.N.P.), and Doctor of Philosophy in Nursing Science (Ph.D.) degrees. Postdoctoral training opportunities are also available. The M.S.N. program is accredited by the National League for Nursing Accreditation Commission (NLNAC).

The M.S.N. program has multiple entry options and accepts applicants with a Bachelor of Science in Nursing, an associate degree in nursing, a diploma in nursing, or a bachelor's degree in another field. The length of the program of studies depends on the applicant's prior educational background and selected specialty. The M.S.N. degree is offered in nine nurse practitioner specialties (acute care, adult, emergency, family, neonatal, pediatric acute or primary care, psychiatric-mental health, women's health) and also in health systems management, nursing informatics, nurse midwifery and nurse midwifery/family dual focus.

The specialty component of the M.S.N. program is delivered in a modified distance format to accommodate individuals who work full-time and/or maintain residence outside middle Tennessee and includes the following:

- Courses offered in concentrated blocks of time on campus
- Distributed course delivery methods, which allow for continued faculty contact in between on-campus sessions
- Clinical placement at student's home site with a Vanderbilt-approved preceptor

The Doctor of Nursing Practice (D.N.P.) program is built upon the school's internationally recognized advanced practice nursing programs and provides an alternative to a research-focused doctorate with education in evidence-based practice, quality improvement, and systems thinking. D.N.P. courses have an intensive experience on-campus in Nashville for approximately one week each semester to facilitate mentoring by faculty members and interaction with nursing Ph.D. students. A variety of online and distance learning technologies allows other course work, scholarly interaction, and clinical application to take place in the student's home location, without the need to relocate or give up employment. Students may enter with either a B.S.N. or M.S.N. degree.

The Ph.D. in Nursing Science program prepares scholars for research and teaching careers at major universities and for research positions in public or private sectors of health care. Graduates of the program conduct and disseminate research that addresses regional and national needs and extends the knowledge base in the discipline of nursing.

Two tracks of study are available: clinical research and health services research.

The Vanderbilt Medical Center maintains a reputation for excellence in teaching, practice, and research and provides students with a tertiary academic setting, where patients receive exemplary care from creative health-care teachers and scholars. Vanderbilt University is located on a 333-acre park-like campus approximately 1½ miles from downtown Nashville, providing a peaceful setting within an urban environment.

Financial aid is available from several sources for M.S.N., D.N.P, and Ph.D. students. All students who wish to apply for financial aid and scholarships must apply to the School of Nursing no later than March 15 for the next academic year. Information about financial aid can be obtained from the School of Nursing Admissions Office Web site, http://www.nursing.vanderbilt.edu/msn/admissions/financial_aid.html.

- *2010–11 GRADUATE TUITION & FEES:*

  M.S.N. and D.N.P. program tuition: $1051 per credit hour

  Ph.D. program tuition: $1623 per credit hour

- *APPLICATION DEADLINES:*

  M.S.N. program: Priority review deadline is December 1, with rolling admissions

  D.N.P. and Ph.D. programs: Application due date is January 15. Applications are accepted until programs are full.

- *FACULTY INFORMATION: http://www.nursing.vanderbilt.edu/facultystaff/*

- *MULTIMEDIA: http://bit.ly/VanderbiltNursing_multimedia*

CONTACT INFORMATION

Colleen Conway-Welch Ph.D., CNM, FAAN
Dean, Vanderbilt School of Nursing
Vanderbilt University
461 21st Avenue South
Nashville, Tennessee 37240
Phone: 615-322-3800
888-333-9192 (toll-free)
Fax: 615-343-0333
E-mail: vusn-admissions@vanderbilt.edu
Web site: www.nursing.vanderbilt.edu

Graduate Nursing Program:
Patricia A. Peerman, M.S., RN
Assistant Dean for Enrollment Management
Phone: 615-322-3800
Fax: 615-322-1708
E-mail: paddy.peerman@vanderbilt.edu

Find us on Facebook®: http://www.facebook.com/vanderbiltschoolofnursing
Follow us on Twitter™: http://twitter.com/VanderbiltNurse

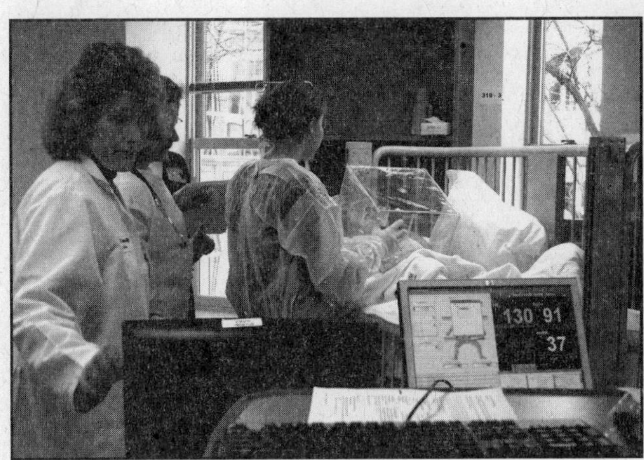

Vanderbilt University School of Nursing's Clinical Simulation Lab is a designated Laerdal Center of Excellence—one of only sixteen educational institutions in the nation to receive this honor. The designation is awarded to educational centers that have demonstrated excellence in educational philosophy and designed programs to help save lives.

INDEXES

BACCALAUREATE PROGRAMS

ACCELERATED BACCALAUREATE

U.S. AND U.S. TERRITORIES

Alabama

University of South Alabama, College of Nursing, *Mobile (BSN)*

Arizona

Chamberlain College of Nursing, *Phoenix (BSN)*

University of Phoenix, Online Campus, *Phoenix (BSN)*

University of Phoenix–Phoenix Campus, College of Nursing, *Phoenix (BSN)*

University of Phoenix–Southern Arizóna Campus, College of Social Sciences, *Tucson (BSN)*

California

Azusa Pacific University, School of Nursing, *Azusa (BSN)*

California State University, East Bay, Department of Nursing and Health Sciences, *Hayward (BS)*

California State University, Long Beach, Department of Nursing, *Long Beach (BSN)*

California State University, Northridge, Nursing Program, *Northridge (BSN)*

California State University, San Marcos, School of Nursing, *San Marcos (BSN)*

Mount St. Mary's College, Department of Nursing, *Los Angeles (BSN, BSc PN)*

National University, Department of Nursing, *La Jolla (BSN)*

Samuel Merritt University, School of Nursing, *Oakland (BSN)*

University of Phoenix–Bay Area Campus, College of Health and Human Services, *Pleasanton (BSN)*

University of Phoenix–Sacramento Valley Campus, College of Nursing, *Sacramento (BSN)*

University of Phoenix–San Diego Campus, College of Nursing, *San Diego (BSN)*

University of Phoenix–Southern California Campus, College of Nursing, *Costa Mesa (BSN)*

Colorado

Platt College, School of Nursing, *Aurora (BSN)*

Regis University, School of Nursing, *Denver (BSN)*

University of Northern Colorado, School of Nursing, *Greeley (BS)*

University of Phoenix–Denver Campus, College of Nursing, *Lone Tree (BSN)*

Connecticut

Southern Connecticut State University, Department of Nursing, *New Haven (BS)*

District of Columbia

The Catholic University of America, School of Nursing, *Washington (BSN)*

Florida

Barry University, School of Nursing, *Miami Shores (BSN)*

Florida State University, College of Nursing, *Tallahassee (BSN)*

Jacksonville University, School of Nursing, *Jacksonville (BSN)*

Miami Dade College, School of Nursing, *Miami (BSN)*

University of Phoenix–Central Florida Campus, College of Nursing, *Maitland (BSN)*

University of Phoenix–North Florida Campus, College of Nursing, *Jacksonville (BSN)*

University of Phoenix–West Florida Campus, College of Nursing, *Temple Terrace (BSN)*

Georgia

Emory University, Nell Hodgson Woodruff School of Nursing, *Atlanta (BSN)*

Kennesaw State University, School of Nursing, *Kennesaw (BSN)*

Hawaii

University of Phoenix–Hawaii Campus, College of Nursing, *Honolulu (BSN)*

Illinois

Loyola University Chicago, Marcella Niehoff School of Nursing, *Maywood (BSN)*

Resurrection University, *Oak Park (BSN)*

Southern Illinois University Edwardsville, School of Nursing, *Edwardsville (BS)*

Indiana

Saint Mary's College, Department of Nursing, *Notre Dame (BS)*

Valparaiso University, College of Nursing, *Valparaiso (BSN)*

Iowa

Allen College, Program in Nursing, *Waterloo (BSN)*

Kansas

MidAmerica Nazarene University, Division of Nursing, *Olathe (BSN)*

Wichita State University, School of Nursing, *Wichita (BSN)*

Louisiana

University of Louisiana at Monroe, Nursing, *Monroe (BS)*

University of Phoenix–Louisiana Campus, College of Nursing, *Metairie (BSN)*

Maine

University of Maine at Fort Kent, Department of Nursing, *Fort Kent (BSN)*

Maryland

Bowie State University, Department of Nursing, *Bowie (BSN)*

Massachusetts

Massachusetts College of Pharmacy and Health Sciences, School of Nursing, *Boston (BSN)*

MGH Institute of Health Professions, School of Nursing, *Boston (BSN)*

Regis College, School of Nursing and Health Professions, *Weston (BSN)*

Simmons College, Department of Nursing, *Boston (BS)*

Michigan

Northern Michigan University, College of Nursing and Allied Health Science, *Marquette (BSN)*

University of Phoenix–Metro Detroit Campus, College of Nursing, *Southfield (BSN)*

Missouri

Cox College, Department of Nursing, *Springfield (BSN)*

Goldfarb School of Nursing at Barnes-Jewish College, *St. Louis (BSN)*

Graceland University, School of Nursing, *Independence (BSN)*

Maryville University of Saint Louis, Nursing Program, School of Health Professions, *St. Louis (BSN)*

Missouri Southern State University, Department of Nursing, *Joplin (BSN)*

Research College of Nursing, College of Nursing, *Kansas City (BSN)*

Saint Louis University, School of Nursing, *St. Louis (BSN)*

University of Missouri, Sinclair School of Nursing, *Columbia (BSN)*

University of Missouri–Kansas City, School of Nursing, *Kansas City (BSN)*

University of Missouri–St. Louis, College of Nursing, *St. Louis (BSN)*

William Jewell College, Department of Nursing, *Liberty (BS)*

Montana

Montana State University, College of Nursing, *Bozeman (BSN)*

Nebraska

University of Nebraska Medical Center, College of Nursing, *Omaha (BSN)*

Nevada

Touro University, School of Nursing, *Henderson (BSN)*

University of Nevada, Las Vegas, School of Nursing, *Las Vegas (BSN)*

University of Nevada, Reno, Orvis School of Nursing, *Reno (BSN)*

University of Southern Nevada, College of Nursing, *Henderson (BSN)*

New Mexico

University of Phoenix–New Mexico Campus, College of Nursing, *Albuquerque (BSN)*

New York

Adelphi University, School of Nursing, *Garden City (BS)*

Columbia University, School of Nursing, *New York (BS)*

Hartwick College, Department of Nursing, *Oneonta (BS)*

Long Island University, Brooklyn Campus, School of Nursing, *Brooklyn (BS)*

Mount Saint Mary College, Division of Nursing, *Newburgh (BSN)*

New York University, College of Nursing, *New York (BS)*

The Sage Colleges, Department of Nursing, *Troy (BS)*

Stony Brook University, State University of New York, School of Nursing, *Stony Brook (BS)*

North Carolina

Queens University of Charlotte, Presbyterian School of Nursing, *Charlotte (BSN)*

Western Carolina University, School of Nursing, *Cullowhee (BSN)*

North Dakota

University of North Dakota, College of Nursing, *Grand Forks (BSN)*

Ohio

Chamberlain College of Nursing, *Columbus (BSN)*

Kent State University, College of Nursing, *Kent (BSN)*

University of Phoenix–Cleveland Campus, College of Nursing, *Independence (BSN)*

Walsh University, Department of Nursing, *North Canton (BSN)*

Oklahoma

Northwestern Oklahoma State University, Division of Nursing, *Alva (BSN)*

Oregon

Oregon Health & Science University, School of Nursing, *Portland (BS)*

Pennsylvania

DeSales University, Department of Nursing and Health, *Center Valley (BSN)*

Edinboro University of Pennsylvania, Department of Nursing, *Edinboro (BS)*

Holy Family University, School of Nursing and Allied Health Professions, *Philadelphia (BSN)*

Thomas Jefferson University, Department of Nursing, *Philadelphia (BSN)*

University of Pennsylvania, School of Nursing, *Philadelphia (BSN)*

Waynesburg University, Department of Nursing, *Waynesburg (BSN)*

Puerto Rico

Inter American University of Puerto Rico, Metropolitan Campus, Carmen Torres de Tiburcio School of Nursing, *San Juan (BSN)*

South Carolina

Lander University, School of Nursing, *Greenwood (BSN)*

Medical University of South Carolina, College of Nursing, *Charleston (BSN)*

South Dakota

South Dakota State University, College of Nursing, *Brookings (BS)*

Tennessee

Belmont University, School of Nursing, *Nashville (BSN)*

Carson-Newman College, Department of Nursing, *Jefferson City (BSN)*

Cumberland University, Rudy School of Nursing and Health Professions, *Lebanon (BSN)*

University of Memphis, Loewenberg School of Nursing, *Memphis (BSN)*

The University of Tennessee, College of Nursing, *Knoxville (BSN)*

Texas

The University of Texas at Arlington, College of Nursing, *Arlington (BSN)*

The University of Texas at El Paso, School of Nursing, *El Paso (BSN)*

Utah

University of Utah, College of Nursing, *Salt Lake City (BS)*

Weber State University, Program in Nursing, *Ogden (BSN)*

Virginia

Hampton University, School of Nursing, *Hampton (BS)*

Lynchburg College, School of Health Sciences and Human Performance, *Lynchburg (BS)*

Old Dominion University, Department of Nursing, *Norfolk (BSN)*

Washington

University of Washington, School of Nursing, *Seattle (BSN)*

West Virginia

West Virginia University, School of Nursing, *Morgantown (BSN)*

Wisconsin

Bellin College, Nursing Program, *Green Bay (BSN)*

University of Wisconsin–Oshkosh, College of Nursing, *Oshkosh (BSN)*

CANADA

Alberta

University of Calgary, Faculty of Nursing, *Calgary (BN)*

British Columbia

The University of British Columbia, Program in Nursing, *Vancouver (BSN)*

New Brunswick

University of New Brunswick Fredericton, Faculty of Nursing, *Fredericton (BN)*

Newfoundland and Labrador

Memorial University of Newfoundland, School of Nursing, *St. John's (BN)*

Nova Scotia

Dalhousie University, School of Nursing, *Halifax (BScN)*

St. Francis Xavier University, Department of Nursing, *Antigonish (BScN)*

Ontario

Lakehead University, School of Nursing, *Thunder Bay (BScN)*

Queen's University at Kingston, School of Nursing, *Kingston (BNSc)*

Trent University, Nursing Program, *Peterborough (BScN)*

University of Toronto, Faculty of Nursing, *Toronto (BScN)*

The University of Western Ontario, School of Nursing, *London (BScN)*

Quebec

Université Laval, Faculty of Nursing, *Québec (BScN)*

Saskatchewan

University of Saskatchewan, College of Nursing, *Saskatoon (BSN)*

ACCELERATED BACCALAUREATE FOR SECOND DEGREE

U.S. AND U.S. TERRITORIES

Arizona

Arizona State University at the Downtown Phoenix Campus, College of Nursing, *Phoenix (BSN)*

Chamberlain College of Nursing, *Phoenix (BSN)*

Northern Arizona University, School of Nursing, *Flagstaff (BSN)*

California

Concordia University, Bachelor of Science in Nursing Program, *Irvine (BSN)*

Loma Linda University, School of Nursing, *Loma Linda (BS)*

Colorado

Colorado State University–Pueblo, Department of Nursing, *Pueblo (BSN)*

University of Colorado at Colorado Springs, Beth-El College of Nursing and Health Sciences, *Colorado Springs (BSN)*

Connecticut

Fairfield University, School of Nursing, *Fairfield (BS)*

Quinnipiac University, Department of Nursing, *Hamden (BSN)*

Delaware

University of Delaware, School of Nursing, *Newark (BSN)*

District of Columbia

The Catholic University of America, School of Nursing, *Washington (BSN)*

Georgetown University, School of Nursing and Health Studies, *Washington (BSN)*

The George Washington University, Department of Nursing Education, *Washington (BSN)*

Howard University, Division of Nursing, *Washington (BSN)*

Florida

Barry University, School of Nursing, *Miami Shores (BSN)*

Florida Atlantic University, Christine E. Lynn College of Nursing, *Boca Raton (BS)*

Florida International University, Nursing Program, *Miami (BSN)*

Jacksonville University, School of Nursing, *Jacksonville (BSN)*

University of Central Florida, College of Nursing, *Orlando (BSN)*

University of Florida, College of Nursing, *Gainesville (BSN)*

University of Miami, School of Nursing and Health Studies, *Coral Gables (BSN)*

University of North Florida, School of Nursing, *Jacksonville (BSN)*

University of South Florida, College of Nursing, *Tampa (BS)*

Georgia

Albany State University, College of Sciences and Health Professions, *Albany (BSN)*

Georgia Southwestern State University, School of Nursing, *Americus (BSN)*

Kennesaw State University, School of Nursing, *Kennesaw (BSN)*

Idaho

Idaho State University, Department of Nursing, *Pocatello (BSN)*

Illinois

Blessing–Rieman College of Nursing, *Quincy (BSN)*
Bradley University, Department of Nursing, *Peoria (BSN, BSc PN)*
Illinois State University, Mennonite College of Nursing, *Normal (BSN)*
Lewis University, Program in Nursing, *Romeoville (BSN)*
Methodist College of Nursing, *Peoria (BSN)*
Resurrection University, *Oak Park (BSN)*
Trinity College of Nursing and Health Sciences, *Rock Island (BSN)*

Indiana

Ball State University, School of Nursing, *Muncie (BS)*
Indiana University–Purdue University Indianapolis, School of Nursing, *Indianapolis (BSN)*
Indiana University South Bend, Division of Nursing and Health Professions, *South Bend (BSN)*
Indiana Wesleyan University, School of Nursing, *Marion (BSN)*
Marian University, Department of Nursing and Nutritional Science, *Indianapolis (BSN)*
Purdue University, School of Nursing, *West Lafayette (BS)*
Purdue University Calumet, School of Nursing, *Hammond (BS)*
University of Indianapolis, School of Nursing, *Indianapolis (BSN)*

Iowa

Allen College, Program in Nursing, *Waterloo (BSN)*

Kansas

MidAmerica Nazarene University, Division of Nursing, *Olathe (BSN)*
Wichita State University, School of Nursing, *Wichita (BSN)*

Kentucky

Bellarmine University, Donna and Allan Lansing School of Nursing and Health Sciences, *Louisville (BSN)*
Northern Kentucky University, Department of Nursing, *Highland Heights (BSN)*
Spalding University, School of Nursing, *Louisville (BSN)*
University of Louisville, School of Nursing, *Louisville (BSN)*

Louisiana

Louisiana State University Health Sciences Center, School of Nursing, *New Orleans (BSN)*
Southeastern Louisiana University, School of Nursing, *Hammond (BS)*
University of Louisiana at Lafayette, College of Nursing, *Lafayette (BSN)*

Maine

University of Southern Maine, College of Nursing and Health Professions, *Portland (BS)*

Maryland

The Johns Hopkins University, School of Nursing, *Baltimore (BS)*
Salisbury University, Program in Nursing, *Salisbury (BS)*
Stevenson University, Nursing Division, *Stevenson (BS)*

Massachusetts

Curry College, Division of Nursing, *Milton (BS)*
Massachusetts College of Pharmacy and Health Sciences, School of Nursing, *Boston (BSN)*
Regis College, School of Nursing and Health Professions, *Weston (BSN)*
Salem State University, Program in Nursing, *Salem (BSN)*
Simmons College, Department of Nursing, *Boston (BS)*
University of Massachusetts Amherst, School of Nursing, *Amherst (BS)*
University of Massachusetts Boston, College of Nursing and Health Sciences, *Boston (BS)*

Michigan

Ferris State University, School of Nursing, *Big Rapids (BSN)*
Grand Valley State University, Kirkhof College of Nursing, *Allendale (BSN)*
Michigan State University, College of Nursing, *East Lansing (BSN)*
Saginaw Valley State University, Crystal M. Lange College of Nursing and Health Sciences, *University Center (BSN)*
University of Detroit Mercy, McAuley School of Nursing, *Detroit (BSN)*
University of Michigan, School of Nursing, *Ann Arbor (BSN)*
University of Michigan–Flint, Department of Nursing, *Flint (BSN)*
Wayne State University, College of Nursing, *Detroit (BSN)*

Minnesota

The College of St. Scholastica, Department of Nursing, *Duluth (BS)*
Concordia College, Department of Nursing, *Moorhead (BA)*
Minnesota State University Mankato, School of Nursing, *Mankato (BS)*

Mississippi

University of Mississippi Medical Center, Program in Nursing, *Jackson (BSN)*

Missouri

Cox College, Department of Nursing, *Springfield (BSN)*
Goldfarb School of Nursing at Barnes-Jewish College, *St. Louis (BSN)*
Research College of Nursing, College of Nursing, *Kansas City (BSN)*
Saint Louis University, School of Nursing, *St. Louis (BSN)*
Southeast Missouri State University, Department of Nursing, *Cape Girardeau (BSN)*
University of Missouri, Sinclair School of Nursing, *Columbia (BSN)*

Nebraska

Creighton University, School of Nursing, *Omaha (BSN)*
Nebraska Methodist College, Department of Nursing, *Omaha (BSN)*
University of Nebraska Medical Center, College of Nursing, *Omaha (BSN)*

Nevada

Nevada State College at Henderson, Nursing Program, *Henderson (BSN)*
Touro University, School of Nursing, *Henderson (BSN)*

New Jersey

Fairleigh Dickinson University, Metropolitan Campus, Henry P. Becton School of Nursing and Allied Health, *Teaneck (BSN)*
Felician College, Division of Nursing and Health Management, *Lodi (BSN)*
New Jersey City University, Department of Nursing, *Jersey City (BSN)*
Rutgers, The State University of New Jersey, College of Nursing, *Newark (BS)*
Seton Hall University, College of Nursing, *South Orange (BSN)*
University of Medicine and Dentistry of New Jersey, School of Nursing, *Newark (BSN)*
William Paterson University of New Jersey, Department of Nursing, *Wayne (BSN)*

New Mexico

New Mexico State University, School of Nursing, *Las Cruces (BSN)*
University of New Mexico, College of Nursing, *Albuquerque (BSN)*

New York

Adelphi University, School of Nursing, *Garden City (BS)*
The College of New Rochelle, School of Nursing, *New Rochelle (BSN)*
Columbia University, School of Nursing, *New York (BS)*
Concordia College–New York, Nursing Program, *Bronxville (BS)*
Dominican College, Department of Nursing, *Orangeburg (BSN)*
Hartwick College, Department of Nursing, *Oneonta (BS)*
Lehman College of the City University of New York, Department of Nursing, *Bronx (BS)*
Molloy College, Division of Nursing, *Rockville Centre (BS)*
New York University, College of Nursing, *New York (BS)*
Pace University, Lienhard School of Nursing, *New York (BS)*
The Sage Colleges, Department of Nursing, *Troy (BS)*
State University of New York Downstate Medical Center, College of Nursing, *Brooklyn (BS)*
University at Buffalo, the State University of New York, School of Nursing, *Buffalo (BS)*
University of Rochester, School of Nursing, *Rochester (BS)*

North Carolina

Duke University, School of Nursing, *Durham (BSN)*
Queens University of Charlotte, Presbyterian School of Nursing, *Charlotte (BSN)*
The University of North Carolina at Chapel Hill, School of Nursing, *Chapel Hill (BSN)*

North Dakota

University of North Dakota, College of Nursing, *Grand Forks (BSN)*

Ohio

Ashland University, Dwight Schar College of Nursing, *Ashland (BSN)*

Capital University, School of Nursing, *Columbus (BSN)*

Chamberlain College of Nursing, *Columbus (BSN)*

Cleveland State University, School of Nursing, *Cleveland (BSN)*

Kent State University, College of Nursing, *Kent (BSN)*

Mount Carmel College of Nursing, Nursing Programs, *Columbus (BSN)*

The University of Akron, College of Nursing, *Akron (BSN)*

University of Cincinnati, College of Nursing, *Cincinnati (BSN)*

Ursuline College, The Breen School of Nursing, *Pepper Pike (BSN)*

Walsh University, Department of Nursing, *North Canton (BSN)*

Wright State University, College of Nursing and Health, *Dayton (BSN)*

Oklahoma

Oklahoma City University, Kramer School of Nursing, *Oklahoma City (BSN)*

University of Oklahoma Health Sciences Center, College of Nursing, *Oklahoma City (BSN)*

Oregon

Linfield College, School of Nursing, *McMinnville (BSN)*

Pennsylvania

Duquesne University, School of Nursing, *Pittsburgh (BSN)*

Edinboro University of Pennsylvania, Department of Nursing, *Edinboro (BS)*

Gannon University, Villa Maria School of Nursing, *Erie (BSN)*

Thomas Jefferson University, Department of Nursing, *Philadelphia (BSN)*

University of Pennsylvania, School of Nursing, *Philadelphia (BSN)*

University of Pittsburgh, School of Nursing, *Pittsburgh (BSN)*

Villanova University, College of Nursing, *Villanova (BSN)*

Waynesburg University, Department of Nursing, *Waynesburg (BSN)*

West Chester University of Pennsylvania, Department of Nursing, *West Chester (BSN)*

Wilkes University, Department of Nursing, *Wilkes-Barre (BS)*

South Carolina

Lander University, School of Nursing, *Greenwood (BSN)*

Medical University of South Carolina, College of Nursing, *Charleston (BSN)*

Tennessee

Belmont University, School of Nursing, *Nashville (BSN)*

Carson-Newman College, Department of Nursing, *Jefferson City (BSN)*

Cumberland University, Rudy School of Nursing and Health Professions, *Lebanon (BSN)*

East Tennessee State University, College of Nursing, *Johnson City (BSN)*

Union University, School of Nursing, *Jackson (BSN)*

University of Memphis, Loewenberg School of Nursing, *Memphis (BSN)*

Texas

Angelo State University, Department of Nursing, *San Angelo (BSN)*

Baylor University, Louise Herrington School of Nursing, *Dallas (BSN)*

Texas A&M Health Science Center, College of Nursing, *College Station (BSN)*

Texas A&M University–Corpus Christi, School of Nursing and Health Sciences, *Corpus Christi (BSN)*

Texas Christian University, Harris College of Nursing, *Fort Worth (BSN)*

Texas Tech University Health Sciences Center, School of Nursing, *Lubbock (BSc PN)*

Texas Woman's University, College of Nursing, *Denton (BS)*

University of Houston–Victoria, School of Nursing, *Victoria (BSN)*

The University of Texas at Arlington, College of Nursing, *Arlington (BSN)*

The University of Texas Health Science Center at Houston, School of Nursing, *Houston (BSN)*

The University of Texas Health Science Center at San Antonio, School of Nursing, *San Antonio (BSN)*

The University of Texas Medical Branch, School of Nursing, *Galveston (BSN)*

Virginia

George Mason University, College of Health and Human Services, *Fairfax (BSN)*

Marymount University, School of Health Professions, *Arlington (BSN)*

Norfolk State University, Department of Nursing, *Norfolk (BSN)*

Shenandoah University, Division of Nursing, *Winchester (BSN)*

Virginia Commonwealth University, School of Nursing, *Richmond (BS)*

West Virginia

West Virginia University, School of Nursing, *Morgantown (BSN)*

Wheeling Jesuit University, Department of Nursing, *Wheeling (BSN)*

Wisconsin

Bellin College, Nursing Program, *Green Bay (BSN)*

Edgewood College, Program in Nursing, *Madison (BS)*

University of Wisconsin–Eau Claire, College of Nursing and Health Sciences, *Eau Claire (BSN)*

University of Wisconsin–Oshkosh, College of Nursing, *Oshkosh (BSN)*

Wyoming

University of Wyoming, Fay W. Whitney School of Nursing, *Laramie (BSN)*

CANADA

Alberta

University of Alberta, Faculty of Nursing, *Edmonton (BScN)*

University of Calgary, Faculty of Nursing, *Calgary (BN)*

University of Lethbridge, School of Health Sciences, *Lethbridge (BN)*

British Columbia

The University of British Columbia, Program in Nursing, *Vancouver (BSN)*

Nova Scotia

Dalhousie University, School of Nursing, *Halifax (BScN)*

St. Francis Xavier University, Department of Nursing, *Antigonish (BScN)*

Ontario

University of Toronto, Faculty of Nursing, *Toronto (BScN)*

ACCELERATED LPN TO BACCALAUREATE

U.S. AND U.S. TERRITORIES

California

San Francisco State University, School of Nursing, *San Francisco (BSN)*

Kansas

MidAmerica Nazarene University, Division of Nursing, *Olathe (BSN)*

New York

Dominican College, Department of Nursing, *Orangeburg (BSN)*

Ohio

Ursuline College, The Breen School of Nursing, *Pepper Pike (BSN)*

Oklahoma

Northwestern Oklahoma State University, Division of Nursing, *Alva (BSN)*

Pennsylvania

Wilkes University, Department of Nursing, *Wilkes-Barre (BS)*

South Dakota

Mount Marty College, Nursing Program, *Yankton (BSN)*

Virginia

Norfolk State University, Department of Nursing, *Norfolk (BSN)*

CANADA

Nova Scotia

St. Francis Xavier University, Department of Nursing, *Antigonish (BScN)*

ACCELERATED RN BACCALAUREATE

U.S. AND U.S. TERRITORIES

Arizona

Arizona State University at the Downtown Phoenix Campus, College of Nursing, *Phoenix (BSN)*

Arkansas
University of Arkansas for Medical Sciences, College of Nursing, *Little Rock (BSN)*

California
Azusa Pacific University, School of Nursing, *Azusa (BSN)*
Loma Linda University, School of Nursing, *Loma Linda (BS)*
West Coast University, Nursing Programs, *North Hollywood (BSN)*

Colorado
Colorado State University–Pueblo, Department of Nursing, *Pueblo (BSN)*

Delaware
Wilmington University, College of Health Professions, *New Castle (BSN)*

Florida
Northwest Florida State College, RN to BSN Degree Program, *Niceville (BSN)*
Remington College of Nursing, *Lake Mary (BSN)*

Georgia
Albany State University, College of Sciences and Health Professions, *Albany (BSN)*
Thomas University, Division of Nursing, *Thomasville (BSN)*

Idaho
Boise State University, Department of Nursing, *Boise (BS)*

Illinois
Benedictine University, Department of Nursing, *Lisle (BSN)*
DePaul University, Department of Nursing, *Chicago (BS)*
Lakeview College of Nursing, *Danville (BSN)*
Lewis University, Program in Nursing, *Romeoville (BSN)*
Olivet Nazarene University, Division of Nursing, *Bourbonnais (BSN)*
Resurrection University, *Oak Park (BSN)*
University of St. Francis, College of Nursing and Allied Health, *Joliet (BSN)*

Indiana
Indiana University Kokomo, Indiana University School of Nursing, *Kokomo (BSN)*
Purdue University Calumet, School of Nursing, *Hammond (BS)*
University of Evansville, Department of Nursing, *Evansville (BSN)*

Iowa
Allen College, Program in Nursing, *Waterloo (BSN)*
Mount Mercy University, Department of Nursing, *Cedar Rapids (BSN)*

Kansas
MidAmerica Nazarene University, Division of Nursing, *Olathe (BSN)*
Southwestern College, Nursing Program, *Winfield (BSN)*
Tabor College, Department of Nursing, *Hillsboro (BSN)*

Kentucky
Bellarmine University, Donna and Allan Lansing School of Nursing and Health Sciences, *Louisville (BSN)*
Eastern Kentucky University, Department of Baccalaureate and Graduate Nursing, *Richmond (BSN)*
Midway College, Program in Nursing (Baccalaureate), *Midway (BSN)*
Spalding University, School of Nursing, *Louisville (BSN)*

Maine
University of New England, Department of Nursing, *Biddeford (BSN)*

Maryland
College of Notre Dame of Maryland, Department of Nursing, *Baltimore (BS)*
Coppin State University, Helene Fuld School of Nursing, *Baltimore (BSN)*
Stevenson University, Nursing Division, *Stevenson (BS)*
Washington Adventist University, Nursing Department, *Takoma Park (BS)*

Massachusetts
Regis College, School of Nursing and Health Professions, *Weston (BSN)*
University of Massachusetts Amherst, School of Nursing, *Amherst (BS)*

Michigan
Ferris State University, School of Nursing, *Big Rapids (BSN)*

Missouri
Chamberlain College of Nursing, *St. Louis (BSN)*
Maryville University of Saint Louis, Nursing Program, School of Health Professions, *St. Louis (BSN)*
Missouri State University, Department of Nursing, *Springfield (BSN)*

Nebraska
Clarkson College, Master of Science in Nursing Program, *Omaha (BSN)*
Nebraska Wesleyan University, Department of Nursing, *Lincoln (BSN)*
University of Nebraska Medical Center, College of Nursing, *Omaha (BSN)*

Nevada
Touro University, School of Nursing, *Henderson (BSN)*

New Jersey
College of Saint Elizabeth, Department of Nursing, *Morristown (BSN)*
Rutgers, The State University of New Jersey, Camden College of Arts and Sciences, Department of Nursing, *Camden (BS)*

New York
The College of New Rochelle, School of Nursing, *New Rochelle (BSN)*
Daemen College, Department of Nursing, *Amherst (BS)*
Dominican College, Department of Nursing, *Orangeburg (BSN)*
Keuka College, Division of Nursing, *Keuka Park (BS)*
Lehman College of the City University of New York, Department of Nursing, *Bronx (BS)*
Medgar Evers College of the City University of New York, Department of Nursing, *Brooklyn (BSN)*
Mercy College, Program in Nursing, *Dobbs Ferry (BS)*
Molloy College, Division of Nursing, *Rockville Centre (BS)*
Mount Saint Mary College, Division of Nursing, *Newburgh (BSN)*
New York University, College of Nursing, *New York (BS)*
Roberts Wesleyan College, Division of Nursing, *Rochester (BScN)*
St. John Fisher College, Advanced Practice Nursing Program, *Rochester (BS)*
State University of New York at Binghamton, Decker School of Nursing, *Binghamton (BS)*
State University of New York Institute of Technology, School of Nursing and Health Systems, *Utica (BS)*
University of Rochester, School of Nursing, *Rochester (BS)*

North Carolina
Winston-Salem State University, Department of Nursing, *Winston-Salem (BSN)*

Ohio
Ashland University, Dwight Schar College of Nursing, *Ashland (BSN)*
College of Mount St. Joseph, Department of Nursing, *Cincinnati (BSN)*
Kent State University, College of Nursing, *Kent (BSN)*
Otterbein University, Department of Nursing, *Westerville (BSN)*
Ursuline College, The Breen School of Nursing, *Pepper Pike (BSN)*

Oklahoma
Bacone College, Department of Nursing, *Muskogee (BSN)*
Northeastern State University, Department of Nursing, *Tahlequah (BSN)*
Northwestern Oklahoma State University, Division of Nursing, *Alva (BSN)*
Oklahoma Wesleyan University, School of Nursing, *Bartlesville (BSN)*

Pennsylvania
Carlow University, School of Nursing, *Pittsburgh (BSN)*
DeSales University, Department of Nursing and Health, *Center Valley (BSN)*
Eastern University, Program in Nursing, *St. Davids (BSN)*
Gwynedd-Mercy College, School of Nursing, *Gwynedd Valley (BSN)*
Immaculata University, Department of Nursing, *Immaculata (BSN)*
La Roche College, Department of Nursing and Nursing Management, *Pittsburgh (BSN)*
Misericordia University, Department of Nursing, *Dallas (BSN)*
Mount Aloysius College, Division of Nursing, *Cresson (BSN)*
Thomas Jefferson University, Department of Nursing, *Philadelphia (BSN)*
University of Pennsylvania, School of Nursing, *Philadelphia (BSN)*
West Chester University of Pennsylvania, Department of Nursing, *West Chester (BSN)*
Wilkes University, Department of Nursing, *Wilkes-Barre (BS)*

South Carolina

Lander University, School of Nursing, *Greenwood (BSN)*

Tennessee

East Tennessee State University, College of Nursing, *Johnson City (BSN)*

King College, School of Nursing, *Bristol (BSN)*

University of Memphis, Loewenberg School of Nursing, *Memphis (BSN)*

The University of Tennessee, College of Nursing, *Knoxville (BSN)*

Texas

Texas Tech University Health Sciences Center, School of Nursing, *Lubbock (BSc PN)*

The University of Texas at Arlington, College of Nursing, *Arlington (BSN)*

The University of Texas at Tyler, Program in Nursing, *Tyler (BSN)*

Virginia

James Madison University, Department of Nursing, *Harrisonburg (BSN)*

Marymount University, School of Health Professions, *Arlington (BSN)*

West Virginia

Fairmont State University, School of Nursing and Allied Health Administration, *Fairmont (BSN)*

Marshall University, College of Health Professions, *Huntington (BSN)*

West Liberty University, Department of Health Sciences, *West Liberty (BSN)*

Wisconsin

University of Wisconsin–Oshkosh, College of Nursing, *Oshkosh (BSN)*

CANADA

Alberta

University of Lethbridge, School of Health Sciences, *Lethbridge (BN)*

Ontario

University of Toronto, Faculty of Nursing, *Toronto (BScN)*

Quebec

McGill University, School of Nursing, *Montréal (BScN)*

Université du Québec à Chicoutimi, Program in Nursing, *Chicoutimi (BNSc)*

Université Laval, Faculty of Nursing, *Québec (BScN)*

Saskatchewan

University of Saskatchewan, College of Nursing, *Saskatoon (BSN)*

ADN TO BACCALAUREATE

U.S. AND U.S. TERRITORIES

Alabama

Tuskegee University, Program in Nursing, *Tuskegee (BSN)*

University of Mobile, School of Nursing, *Mobile (BSN)*

University of South Alabama, College of Nursing, *Mobile (BSN)*

Arizona

Grand Canyon University, College of Nursing and Health Sciences, *Phoenix (BSN)*

Arkansas

Arkansas Tech University, Program in Nursing, *Russellville (BSN)*

Harding University, College of Nursing, *Searcy (BSN)*

Henderson State University, Department of Nursing, *Arkadelphia (BSN)*

Southern Arkansas University–Magnolia, Department of Nursing, *Magnolia (BSN)*

University of Arkansas at Fort Smith, Carol McKelvey Moore School of Nursing, *Fort Smith (BSN)*

University of Arkansas at Monticello, School of Nursing, *Monticello (BSN)*

University of Arkansas for Medical Sciences, College of Nursing, *Little Rock (BSN)*

University of Central Arkansas, Department of Nursing, *Conway (BSN)*

California

Azusa Pacific University, School of Nursing, *Azusa (BSN)*

Biola University, Department of Nursing, *La Mirada (BSN)*

California Baptist University, School of Nursing, *Riverside (BSN)*

California State University, Bakersfield, Program in Nursing, *Bakersfield (BSN)*

California State University, Chico, School of Nursing, *Chico (BSN)*

California State University, East Bay, Department of Nursing and Health Sciences, *Hayward (BS)*

California State University, Fresno, Department of Nursing, *Fresno (BSN)*

California State University, Fullerton, Department of Nursing, *Fullerton (BSN)*

California State University, Long Beach, Department of Nursing, *Long Beach (BSN)*

California State University, Northridge, Nursing Program, *Northridge (BSN)*

California State University, Sacramento, Division of Nursing, *Sacramento (BSN)*

California State University, Stanislaus, Department of Nursing, *Turlock (BSN)*

Humboldt State University, Department of Nursing, *Arcata (BSN)*

Loma Linda University, School of Nursing, *Loma Linda (BS)*

Mount St. Mary's College, Department of Nursing, *Los Angeles (BSN, BSc PN)*

Pacific Union College, Department of Nursing, *Angwin (BSN)*

Point Loma Nazarene University, School of Nursing, *San Diego (BSN)*

San Diego State University, School of Nursing, *San Diego (BSN)*

San Francisco State University, School of Nursing, *San Francisco (BSN)*

Sonoma State University, Department of Nursing, *Rohnert Park (BSN)*

Colorado

Colorado State University–Pueblo, Department of Nursing, *Pueblo (BSN)*

Mesa State College, Department of Nursing and Radiologic Sciences, *Grand Junction (BSN)*

Metropolitan State College of Denver, Department of Health Professions, *Denver (BS)*

Connecticut

Sacred Heart University, Program in Nursing, *Fairfield (BS)*

Southern Connecticut State University, Department of Nursing, *New Haven (BS)*

University of Hartford, College of Education, Nursing, and Health Professions, *West Hartford (BSN)*

Florida

Barry University, School of Nursing, *Miami Shores (BSN)*

Florida Gulf Coast University, School of Nursing, *Fort Myers (BSN)*

Florida Southern College, Department of Nursing, *Lakeland (BSN)*

Jacksonville University, School of Nursing, *Jacksonville (BSN)*

Northwest Florida State College, RN to BSN Degree Program, *Niceville (BSN)*

St. Petersburg College, Department of Nursing, *St. Petersburg (BSN)*

University of South Florida, College of Nursing, *Tampa (BS)*

The University of Tampa, Department of Nursing, *Tampa (BSN)*

University of West Florida, Department of Nursing, *Pensacola (BSN)*

Georgia

Albany State University, College of Sciences and Health Professions, *Albany (BSN)*

Armstrong Atlantic State University, Program in Nursing, *Savannah (BSN)*

Brenau University, School of Health and Science, *Gainesville (BSN)*

Georgia Southern University, School of Nursing, *Statesboro (BSN)*

Kennesaw State University, School of Nursing, *Kennesaw (BSN)*

Macon State College, School of Nursing and Health Sciences, *Macon (BSN)*

North Georgia College & State University, Department of Nursing, *Dahlonega (BSN)*

Thomas University, Division of Nursing, *Thomasville (BSN)*

Guam

University of Guam, School of Nursing and Health Sciences, *Mangilao (BSN)*

Hawaii

University of Hawaii at Hilo, Department in Nursing, *Hilo (BSN)*

University of Hawaii at Manoa, School of Nursing and Dental Hygiene, *Honolulu (BSN)*

Idaho

Idaho State University, Department of Nursing, *Pocatello (BSN)*

Lewis-Clark State College, Division of Nursing and Health Sciences, *Lewiston (BSN)*

Illinois

Blessing–Rieman College of Nursing, *Quincy (BSN)*

Bradley University, Department of Nursing, *Peoria (BSN, BSc PN)*

MacMurray College, Department of Nursing, *Jacksonville (BSN)*

McKendree University, Department of Nursing, *Lebanon (BSN)*

Northern Illinois University, School of Nursing and Health Studies, *De Kalb (BS)*

Resurrection University, *Oak Park (BSN)*

Rockford College, Department of Nursing, *Rockford (BSN)*

Southern Illinois University Edwardsville, School of Nursing, *Edwardsville (BS)*

Trinity College of Nursing and Health Sciences, *Rock Island (BSN)*

University of Illinois at Chicago, College of Nursing, *Chicago (BSN)*

Indiana

Anderson University, School of Nursing, *Anderson (BSN)*

Bethel College, Department of Nursing, *Mishawaka (BSN)*

Indiana State University, Department of Nursing, *Terre Haute (BS)*

Indiana University East, School of Nursing, *Richmond (BSN)*

Indiana University–Purdue University Indianapolis, School of Nursing, *Indianapolis (BSN)*

Purdue University, School of Nursing, *West Lafayette (BS)*

Purdue University North Central, Department of Nursing, *Westville (BS)*

University of Indianapolis, School of Nursing, *Indianapolis (BSN)*

Iowa

Allen College, Program in Nursing, *Waterloo (BSN)*

Briar Cliff University, Department of Nursing, *Sioux City (BSN)*

Iowa Wesleyan College, Division of Health and Natural Sciences, *Mount Pleasant (BSN)*

Luther College, Department of Nursing, *Decorah (BA)*

Mercy College of Health Sciences, Division of Nursing, *Des Moines (BSN)*

Kansas

Emporia State University, Newman Division of Nursing, *Emporia (BSN)*

Kansas Wesleyan University, Department of Nursing Education, *Salina (BSN)*

MidAmerica Nazarene University, Division of Nursing, *Olathe (BSN)*

Tabor College, Department of Nursing, *Hillsboro (BSN)*

The University of Kansas, School of Nursing, *Kansas City (BSN)*

Washburn University, School of Nursing, *Topeka (BSN)*

Wichita State University, School of Nursing, *Wichita (BSN)*

Kentucky

Kentucky State University, School of Nursing, *Frankfort (BSN)*

Midway College, Program in Nursing (Baccalaureate), *Midway (BSN)*

Morehead State University, Department of Nursing, *Morehead (BSN)*

Louisiana

McNeese State University, College of Nursing, *Lake Charles (BSN)*

Northwestern State University of Louisiana, College of Nursing, *Shreveport (BSN)*

Southeastern Louisiana University, School of Nursing, *Hammond (BS)*

University of Louisiana at Lafayette, College of Nursing, *Lafayette (BSN)*

University of Louisiana at Monroe, Nursing, *Monroe (BS)*

Maine

University of Southern Maine, College of Nursing and Health Professions, *Portland (BS)*

Maryland

Salisbury University, Program in Nursing, *Salisbury (BS)*

Stevenson University, Nursing Division, *Stevenson (BS)*

Massachusetts

Anna Maria College, Department of Nursing, *Paxton (BSN)*

Atlantic Union College, Department of Nursing, *South Lancaster (BS)*

Fitchburg State University, Department of Nursing, *Fitchburg (BS)*

Framingham State University, Department of Nursing, *Framingham (BS)*

Northeastern University, School of Nursing, *Boston (BSN)*

Regis College, School of Nursing and Health Professions, *Weston (BSN)*

Salem State University, Program in Nursing, *Salem (BSN)*

Simmons College, Department of Nursing, *Boston (BS)*

Michigan

Andrews University, Department of Nursing, *Berrien Springs (BS)*

Davenport University, Division of Nursing, *Grand Rapids (BSN)*

Grand Valley State University, Kirkhof College of Nursing, *Allendale (BSN)*

Lake Superior State University, Department of Nursing, *Sault Sainte Marie (BSN)*

Madonna University, College of Nursing and Health, *Livonia (BSN)*

Spring Arbor University, Program in Nursing, *Spring Arbor (BSN)*

Western Michigan University, College of Health and Human Services, *Kalamazoo (BSN)*

Minnesota

Augsburg College, Program in Nursing, *Minneapolis (BS)*

The College of St. Scholastica, Department of Nursing, *Duluth (BS)*

Minnesota State University Moorhead, School of Nursing and Healthcare Leadership, *Moorhead (BSN)*

Mississippi

Delta State University, School of Nursing, *Cleveland (BSN)*

Mississippi University for Women, College of Nursing and Speech Language Pathology, *Columbus (BSN)*

University of Southern Mississippi, School of Nursing, *Hattiesburg (BSN)*

William Carey University, School of Nursing, *Hattiesburg (BSN)*

Missouri

Chamberlain College of Nursing, *St. Louis (BSN)*

Cox College, Department of Nursing, *Springfield (BSN)*

Goldfarb School of Nursing at Barnes-Jewish College, *St. Louis (BSN)*

Graceland University, School of Nursing, *Independence (BSN)*

Missouri Southern State University, Department of Nursing, *Joplin (BSN)*

Missouri State University, Department of Nursing, *Springfield (BSN)*

Missouri Western State University, Department of Nursing, *St. Joseph (BSN)*

University of Central Missouri, Department of Nursing, *Warrensburg (BS)*

University of Missouri, Sinclair School of Nursing, *Columbia (BSN)*

Webster University, Department of Nursing, *St. Louis (BSN)*

Montana

Montana State University–Northern, College of Nursing, *Havre (BSN)*

Nebraska

Clarkson College, Master of Science in Nursing Program, *Omaha (BSN)*

College of Saint Mary, Division of Health Care Professions, *Omaha (BSN)*

Midland Lutheran College, Department of Nursing, *Fremont (BSN)*

Nebraska Methodist College, Department of Nursing, *Omaha (BSN)*

Nebraska Wesleyan University, Department of Nursing, *Lincoln (BSN)*

Union College, Division of Health Sciences, *Lincoln (BSN)*

University of Nebraska Medical Center, College of Nursing, *Omaha (BSN)*

Nevada

Touro University, School of Nursing, *Henderson (BSN)*

University of Nevada, Reno, Orvis School of Nursing, *Reno (BSN)*

New Hampshire

Franklin Pierce University, Master of Science in Nursing, *Rindge (BS)*

Rivier College, Division of Nursing, *Nashua (BS)*

New Jersey

College of Saint Elizabeth, Department of Nursing, *Morristown (BSN)*

Kean University, Department of Nursing, *Union (BSN)*

Monmouth University, Marjorie K. Unterberg School of Nursing, *West Long Branch (BSN)*

Saint Peter's College, Nursing Program, *Jersey City (BSN)*

William Paterson University of New Jersey, Department of Nursing, *Wayne (BSN)*

New York

Adelphi University, School of Nursing, *Garden City (BS)*

The College at Brockport, State University of New York, Department of Nursing, *Brockport (BSN)*

Daemen College, Department of Nursing, *Amherst (BS)*

Elmira College, Program in Nursing Education, *Elmira (BS)*

Lehman College of the City University of New York, Department of Nursing, *Bronx (BS)*

Le Moyne College, Nursing Programs, *Syracuse (BS)*

Medgar Evers College of the City University of New York, Department of Nursing, *Brooklyn (BSN)*

Molloy College, Division of Nursing, *Rockville Centre (BS)*

The Sage Colleges, Department of Nursing, *Troy (BS)*

St. Francis College, Department of Nursing, *Brooklyn Heights (BS)*

St. John Fisher College, Advanced Practice Nursing Program, *Rochester (BS)*

State University of New York at Plattsburgh, Department of Nursing, *Plattsburgh (BS)*

State University of New York Institute of Technology, School of Nursing and Health Systems, *Utica (BS)*

State University of New York Upstate Medical University, College of Nursing, *Syracuse (BS)*

University of Rochester, School of Nursing, *Rochester (BS)*

York College of the City University of New York, Program in Nursing, *Jamaica (BS)*

North Carolina

Barton College, School of Nursing, *Wilson (BSN)*

East Carolina University, College of Nursing, *Greenville (BSN)*

Lees-McRae College, Nursing Program, *Banner Elk (BSN)*

Lenoir-Rhyne University, Program in Nursing, *Hickory (BS)*

Queens University of Charlotte, Presbyterian School of Nursing, *Charlotte (BSN)*

The University of North Carolina at Chapel Hill, School of Nursing, *Chapel Hill (BSN)*

The University of North Carolina at Charlotte, School of Nursing, *Charlotte (BSN)*

The University of North Carolina at Greensboro, School of Nursing, *Greensboro (BSN)*

Winston-Salem State University, Department of Nursing, *Winston-Salem (BSN)*

North Dakota

Dickinson State University, Department of Nursing, *Dickinson (BSN)*

North Dakota State University, Department of Nursing, *Fargo (BSN)*

University of North Dakota, College of Nursing, *Grand Forks (BSN)*

Ohio

Ashland University, Dwight Schar College of Nursing, *Ashland (BSN)*

Capital University, School of Nursing, *Columbus (BSN)*

Case Western Reserve University, Frances Payne Bolton School of Nursing, *Cleveland (BSN)*

Kent State University, College of Nursing, *Kent (BSN)*

Malone University, School of Nursing, *Canton (BSN)*

Mercy College of Northwest Ohio, Division of Nursing, *Toledo (BSN)*

Miami University, Department of Nursing, *Hamilton (BSN)*

Shawnee State University, Department of Nursing, *Portsmouth (BSN)*

The University of Akron, College of Nursing, *Akron (BSN)*

University of Cincinnati, College of Nursing, *Cincinnati (BSN)*

The University of Toledo, College of Nursing, *Toledo (BSN)*

Oklahoma

East Central University, Department of Nursing, *Ada (BS)*

Northwestern Oklahoma State University, Division of Nursing, *Alva (BSN)*

Oklahoma Baptist University, School of Nursing, *Shawnee (BSN)*

Oklahoma City University, Kramer School of Nursing, *Oklahoma City (BSN)*

Oklahoma Panhandle State University, Bachelor of Science in Nursing Program, *Goodwell (BSN)*

Oklahoma Wesleyan University, School of Nursing, *Bartlesville (BSN)*

Oral Roberts University, Anna Vaughn School of Nursing, *Tulsa (BSN)*

Rogers State University, Nursing Program, *Claremore (BSN)*

Southern Nazarene University, School of Nursing, *Bethany (BS)*

Southwestern Oklahoma State University, Division of Nursing, *Weatherford (BSN)*

University of Oklahoma Health Sciences Center, College of Nursing, *Oklahoma City (BSN)*

Oregon

Linfield College, School of Nursing, *McMinnville (BSN)*

Pennsylvania

Bloomsburg University of Pennsylvania, Department of Nursing, *Bloomsburg (BSN)*

Clarion University of Pennsylvania, School of Nursing, *Oil City (BSN)*

DeSales University, Department of Nursing and Health, *Center Valley (BSN)*

Drexel University, College of Nursing and Health Professions, *Philadelphia (BSN)*

Edinboro University of Pennsylvania, Department of Nursing, *Edinboro (BS)*

Gannon University, Villa Maria School of Nursing, *Erie (BSN)*

Gwynedd-Mercy College, School of Nursing, *Gwynedd Valley (BSN)*

Holy Family University, School of Nursing and Allied Health Professions, *Philadelphia (BSN)*

Marywood University, Department of Nursing, *Scranton (BSN)*

Mount Aloysius College, Division of Nursing, *Cresson (BSN)*

Neumann University, Program in Nursing and Health Sciences, *Aston (BS)*

Penn State University Park, School of Nursing, *University Park (BS)*

Slippery Rock University of Pennsylvania, Department of Nursing, *Slippery Rock (BSN)*

Thomas Jefferson University, Department of Nursing, *Philadelphia (BSN)*

University of Pennsylvania, School of Nursing, *Philadelphia (BSN)*

Villanova University, College of Nursing, *Villanova (BSN)*

Widener University, School of Nursing, *Chester (BSN)*

Wilkes University, Department of Nursing, *Wilkes-Barre (BS)*

Puerto Rico

Inter American University of Puerto Rico, Metropolitan Campus, Carmen Torres de Tiburcio School of Nursing, *San Juan (BSN)*

University of Puerto Rico, Medical Sciences Campus, School of Nursing, *San Juan (BSN)*

Rhode Island

University of Rhode Island, College of Nursing, *Kingston (BS)*

South Carolina

Charleston Southern University, Wingo School of Nursing, *Charleston (BSN)*

Francis Marion University, Department of Nursing, *Florence (BSN)*

University of South Carolina Aiken, School of Nursing, *Aiken (BSN)*

South Dakota

Mount Marty College, Nursing Program, *Yankton (BSN)*

Presentation College, Department of Nursing, *Aberdeen (BSN)*

Tennessee

Belmont University, School of Nursing, *Nashville (BSN)*

Cumberland University, Rudy School of Nursing and Health Professions, *Lebanon (BSN)*

East Tennessee State University, College of Nursing, *Johnson City (BSN)*

Milligan College, Department of Nursing, *Milligan College (BSN)*

Southern Adventist University, School of Nursing, *Collegedale (BS)*

Tennessee Technological University, Whitson-Hester School of Nursing, *Cookeville (BSN)*

Tennessee Wesleyan College, Fort Sanders Nursing Department, *Knoxville (BSN)*

University of Memphis, Loewenberg School of Nursing, *Memphis (BSN)*

The University of Tennessee at Chattanooga, School of Nursing, *Chattanooga (BSN)*

The University of Tennessee at Martin, Department of Nursing, *Martin (BSN)*

Texas

Lamar University, Department of Nursing, *Beaumont (BSN)*

Midwestern State University, Nursing Program, *Wichita Falls (BSN)*

Southwestern Adventist University, Department of Nursing, *Keene (BS)*

Tarleton State University, Department of Nursing, *Stephenville (BSN)*

Texas A&M University–Corpus Christi, School of Nursing and Health Sciences, *Corpus Christi (BSN)*

Texas A&M University–Texarkana, Nursing Department, *Texarkana (BSN)*

University of Mary Hardin-Baylor, College of Nursing, *Belton (BSN)*

The University of Texas at Brownsville, Department of Nursing, *Brownsville (BSN)*

The University of Texas at Tyler, Program in Nursing, *Tyler (BSN)*
The University of Texas Health Science Center at Houston, School of Nursing, *Houston (BSN)*
The University of Texas Health Science Center at San Antonio, School of Nursing, *San Antonio (BSN)*
The University of Texas–Pan American, Department of Nursing, *Edinburg (BSN)*
University of the Incarnate Word, Program in Nursing, *San Antonio (BSN)*
West Texas A&M University, Division of Nursing, *Canyon (BSN)*

Utah

Utah Valley University, Department of Nursing, *Orem (BSN)*
Weber State University, Program in Nursing, *Ogden (BSN)*

Vermont

Norwich University, Department of Nursing, *Northfield (BSN)*
Southern Vermont College, Department of Nursing, *Bennington (BSN)*
University of Vermont, Department of Nursing, *Burlington (BS)*

Virgin Islands

University of the Virgin Islands, Division of Nursing, *Saint Thomas (BSN)*

Virginia

Eastern Mennonite University, Department of Nursing, *Harrisonburg (BSN)*
Jefferson College of Health Sciences, Nursing Education Program, *Roanoke (BSN)*
Marymount University, School of Health Professions, *Arlington (BSN)*
Shenandoah University, Division of Nursing, *Winchester (BSN)*
University of Virginia, School of Nursing, *Charlottesville (BSN)*
The University of Virginia's College at Wise, Department of Nursing, *Wise (BSN)*
Virginia Commonwealth University, School of Nursing, *Richmond (BS)*

Washington

Pacific Lutheran University, School of Nursing, *Tacoma (BSN)*
University of Washington, School of Nursing, *Seattle (BSN)*
Walla Walla University, School of Nursing, *College Place (BS)*

West Virginia

Bluefield State College, Program in Nursing, *Bluefield (BSN)*
Fairmont State University, School of Nursing and Allied Health Administration, *Fairmont (BSN)*
Shepherd University, Department of Nursing Education, *Shepherdstown (BSN)*
West Virginia University, School of Nursing, *Morgantown (BSN)*

Wisconsin

Alverno College, Division of Nursing, *Milwaukee (BSN)*
Cardinal Stritch University, Ruth S. Coleman College of Nursing, *Milwaukee (BSN)*
Carroll University, Nursing Program, *Waukesha (BSN)*
Concordia University Wisconsin, Program in Nursing, *Mequon (BSN)*
Marian University, School of Nursing, *Fond du Lac (BSN)*
Silver Lake College, Nursing Program, *Manitowoc (BSN)*
University of Wisconsin–Eau Claire, College of Nursing and Health Sciences, *Eau Claire (BSN)*

Wyoming

University of Wyoming, Fay W. Whitney School of Nursing, *Laramie (BSN)*

BACCALAUREATE FOR SECOND DEGREE

U.S. AND U.S. TERRITORIES

Alabama

Samford University, Ida V. Moffett School of Nursing, *Birmingham (BSN)*
Spring Hill College, Division of Nursing, *Mobile (BSN)*
The University of Alabama, Capstone College of Nursing, *Tuscaloosa (BSN)*
The University of Alabama at Birmingham, School of Nursing, *Birmingham (BSN)*
The University of Alabama in Huntsville, College of Nursing, *Huntsville (BSN)*

Arizona

Arizona State University at the Downtown Phoenix Campus, College of Nursing, *Phoenix (BSN)*

Arkansas

University of Arkansas for Medical Sciences, College of Nursing, *Little Rock (BSN)*

California

California State University, Chico, School of Nursing, *Chico (BSN)*
California State University, Dominguez Hills, Program in Nursing, *Carson (BSN)*
California State University, Fullerton, Department of Nursing, *Fullerton (BSN)*
California State University, Long Beach, Department of Nursing, *Long Beach (BSN)*
California State University, Sacramento, Division of Nursing, *Sacramento (BSN)*
Dominican University of California, Program in Nursing, *San Rafael (BSN)*
Humboldt State University, Department of Nursing, *Arcata (BSN)*
Sonoma State University, Department of Nursing, *Rohnert Park (BSN)*
University of San Francisco, School of Nursing, *San Francisco (BSN)*

Colorado

Colorado State University–Pueblo, Department of Nursing, *Pueblo (BSN)*

Connecticut

Saint Joseph College, Department of Nursing, *West Hartford (BS)*

District of Columbia

Howard University, Division of Nursing, *Washington (BSN)*

Florida

Barry University, School of Nursing, *Miami Shores (BSN)*
Jacksonville University, School of Nursing, *Jacksonville (BSN)*
University of Miami, School of Nursing and Health Studies, *Coral Gables (BSN)*

Georgia

Albany State University, College of Sciences and Health Professions, *Albany (BSN)*
Armstrong Atlantic State University, Program in Nursing, *Savannah (BSN)*
Emory University, Nell Hodgson Woodruff School of Nursing, *Atlanta (BSN)*
Georgia Southwestern State University, School of Nursing, *Americus (BSN)*
Kennesaw State University, School of Nursing, *Kennesaw (BSN)*

Illinois

MacMurray College, Department of Nursing, *Jacksonville (BSN)*
Methodist College of Nursing, *Peoria (BSN)*
Resurrection University, *Oak Park (BSN)*
Saint Anthony College of Nursing, *Rockford (BSN)*
University of Illinois at Chicago, College of Nursing, *Chicago (BSN)*
Western Illinois University, School of Nursing, *Macomb (BSN)*

Indiana

Ball State University, School of Nursing, *Muncie (BS)*
Indiana University Bloomington, Department of Nursing–Bloomington Division, *Bloomington (BSN)*
Indiana University Northwest, School of Nursing and Health Professions, *Gary (BSN)*
Purdue University, School of Nursing, *West Lafayette (BS)*

Iowa

Allen College, Program in Nursing, *Waterloo (BSN)*
Clarke University, Department of Nursing and Health, *Dubuque (BS)*
Iowa Wesleyan College, Division of Health and Natural Sciences, *Mount Pleasant (BSN)*
Morningside College, Department of Nursing Education, *Sioux City (BSN)*

Kansas

Washburn University, School of Nursing, *Topeka (BSN)*

Kentucky

Bellarmine University, Donna and Allan Lansing School of Nursing and Health Sciences, *Louisville (BSN)*
Eastern Kentucky University, Department of Baccalaureate and Graduate Nursing, *Richmond (BSN)*
University of Kentucky, Graduate School Programs in the College of Nursing, *Lexington (BSN)*

Maryland

Coppin State University, Helene Fuld School of Nursing, *Baltimore (BSN)*
The Johns Hopkins University, School of Nursing, *Baltimore (BS)*

Massachusetts

Regis College, School of Nursing and Health Professions, *Weston (BSN)*

Simmons College, Department of Nursing, *Boston (BS)*

Michigan

Eastern Michigan University, School of Nursing, *Ypsilanti (BSN)*

Grand Valley State University, Kirkhof College of Nursing, *Allendale (BSN)*

Saginaw Valley State University, Crystal M. Lange College of Nursing and Health Sciences, *University Center (BSN)*

Minnesota

St. Catherine University, Department of Nursing, *St. Paul (BS)*

Missouri

Cox College, Department of Nursing, *Springfield (BSN)*

Missouri Southern State University, Department of Nursing, *Joplin (BSN)*

Research College of Nursing, College of Nursing, *Kansas City (BSN)*

University of Missouri–St. Louis, College of Nursing, *St. Louis (BSN)*

Nebraska

Clarkson College, Master of Science in Nursing Program, *Omaha (BSN)*

University of Nebraska Medical Center, College of Nursing, *Omaha (BSN)*

Nevada

Touro University, School of Nursing, *Henderson (BSN)*

New Jersey

Rutgers, The State University of New Jersey, College of Nursing, *Newark (BS)*

Seton Hall University, College of Nursing, *South Orange (BSN)*

New York

Adelphi University, School of Nursing, *Garden City (BS)*

College of Mount Saint Vincent, Department of Nursing, *Riverdale (BS)*

The College of New Rochelle, School of Nursing, *New Rochelle (BSN)*

Lehman College of the City University of New York, Department of Nursing, *Bronx (BS)*

Molloy College, Division of Nursing, *Rockville Centre (BS)*

New York University, College of Nursing, *New York (BS)*

The Sage Colleges, Department of Nursing, *Troy (BS)*

St. John Fisher College, Advanced Practice Nursing Program, *Rochester (BS)*

Wagner College, Department of Nursing, *Staten Island (BS)*

North Carolina

Queens University of Charlotte, Presbyterian School of Nursing, *Charlotte (BSN)*

The University of North Carolina at Greensboro, School of Nursing, *Greensboro (BSN)*

Winston-Salem State University, Department of Nursing, *Winston-Salem (BSN)*

North Dakota

University of North Dakota, College of Nursing, *Grand Forks (BSN)*

Ohio

Ashland University, Dwight Schar College of Nursing, *Ashland (BSN)*

Kent State University, College of Nursing, *Kent (BSN)*

Wright State University, College of Nursing and Health, *Dayton (BSN)*

Oklahoma

Northwestern Oklahoma State University, Division of Nursing, *Alva (BSN)*

Oklahoma Baptist University, School of Nursing, *Shawnee (BSN)*

Oklahoma Wesleyan University, School of Nursing, *Bartlesville (BSN)*

Southern Nazarene University, School of Nursing, *Bethany (BS)*

Oregon

Linfield College, School of Nursing, *McMinnville (BSN)*

Pennsylvania

Bloomsburg University of Pennsylvania, Department of Nursing, *Bloomsburg (BSN)*

Carlow University, School of Nursing, *Pittsburgh (BSN)*

Cedar Crest College, Department of Nursing, *Allentown (BS)*

DeSales University, Department of Nursing and Health, *Center Valley (BSN)*

Eastern University, Program in Nursing, *St. Davids (BSN)*

Edinboro University of Pennsylvania, Department of Nursing, *Edinboro (BS)*

Gannon University, Villa Maria School of Nursing, *Erie (BSN)*

Indiana University of Pennsylvania, Department of Nursing and Allied Health, *Indiana (BSN)*

La Salle University, School of Nursing and Health Sciences, *Philadelphia (BSN)*

Misericordia University, Department of Nursing, *Dallas (BSN)*

Neumann University, Program in Nursing and Health Sciences, *Aston (BS)*

Robert Morris University, School of Nursing and Health Sciences, *Moon Township (BSN)*

Thomas Jefferson University, Department of Nursing, *Philadelphia (BSN)*

University of Pennsylvania, School of Nursing, *Philadelphia (BSN)*

The University of Scranton, Department of Nursing, *Scranton (BS)*

Villanova University, College of Nursing, *Villanova (BSN)*

Rhode Island

Rhode Island College, Department of Nursing, *Providence (BSN)*

South Carolina

Lander University, School of Nursing, *Greenwood (BSN)*

South Dakota

Presentation College, Department of Nursing, *Aberdeen (BSN)*

Tennessee

Belmont University, School of Nursing, *Nashville (BSN)*

Cumberland University, Rudy School of Nursing and Health Professions, *Lebanon (BSN)*

Milligan College, Department of Nursing, *Milligan College (BSN)*

Tennessee Technological University, Whitson-Hester School of Nursing, *Cookeville (BSN)*

University of Memphis, Loewenberg School of Nursing, *Memphis (BSN)*

The University of Tennessee at Chattanooga, School of Nursing, *Chattanooga (BSN)*

Texas

Texas A&M University–Corpus Christi, School of Nursing and Health Sciences, *Corpus Christi (BSN)*

Texas Woman's University, College of Nursing, *Denton (BS)*

The University of Texas at Arlington, College of Nursing, *Arlington (BSN)*

University of the Incarnate Word, Program in Nursing, *San Antonio (BSN)*

Utah

Westminster College, School of Nursing and Health Sciences, *Salt Lake City (BSN)*

Virginia

Eastern Mennonite University, Department of Nursing, *Harrisonburg (BSN)*

Marymount University, School of Health Professions, *Arlington (BSN)*

Radford University, School of Nursing, *Radford (BSN)*

Washington

Seattle University, College of Nursing, *Seattle (BSN)*

Wisconsin

Alverno College, Division of Nursing, *Milwaukee (BSN)*

Bellin College, Nursing Program, *Green Bay (BSN)*

Columbia College of Nursing/Mount Mary College Nursing Program, *Milwaukee (BSN)*

Edgewood College, Program in Nursing, *Madison (BS)*

University of Wisconsin–Oshkosh, College of Nursing, *Oshkosh (BSN)*

CANADA

Alberta

University of Alberta, Faculty of Nursing, *Edmonton (BScN)*

University of Calgary, Faculty of Nursing, *Calgary (BN)*

Manitoba

Brandon University, School of Health Studies, *Brandon (BN)*

University of Manitoba, Faculty of Nursing, *Winnipeg (BN)*

Nova Scotia

Dalhousie University, School of Nursing, *Halifax (BScN)*

Ontario

McMaster University, School of Nursing, *Hamilton (BScN)*

University of Ottawa, School of Nursing, *Ottawa (BScN)*
University of Toronto, Faculty of Nursing, *Toronto (BScN)*

Saskatchewan

University of Saskatchewan, College of Nursing, *Saskatoon (BSN)*

GENERIC BACCALAUREATE

U.S. AND U.S. TERRITORIES

Alabama

Auburn University, School of Nursing, *Auburn University (BSN)*
Auburn University Montgomery, School of Nursing, *Montgomery (BSN)*
Jacksonville State University, College of Nursing and Health Sciences, *Jacksonville (BSN)*
Oakwood University, Department of Nursing, *Huntsville (BS)*
Samford University, Ida V. Moffett School of Nursing, *Birmingham (BSN)*
Spring Hill College, Division of Nursing, *Mobile (BSN)*
Troy University, School of Nursing, *Troy (BSN)*
Tuskegee University, Program in Nursing, *Tuskegee (BSN)*
The University of Alabama, Capstone College of Nursing, *Tuscaloosa (BSN)*
The University of Alabama at Birmingham, School of Nursing, *Birmingham (BSN)*
The University of Alabama in Huntsville, College of Nursing, *Huntsville (BSN)*
University of Mobile, School of Nursing, *Mobile (BSN)*
University of North Alabama, College of Nursing and Allied Health, *Florence (BSN)*
University of South Alabama, College of Nursing, *Mobile (BSN)*

Alaska

University of Alaska Anchorage, School of Nursing, *Anchorage (BS)*

Arizona

Arizona State University at the Downtown Phoenix Campus, College of Nursing, *Phoenix (BSN)*
Northern Arizona University, School of Nursing, *Flagstaff (BSN)*
The University of Arizona, College of Nursing, *Tucson (BSN)*

Arkansas

Arkansas State University - Jonesboro, Department of Nursing, *State University (BSN)*
Arkansas Tech University, Program in Nursing, *Russellville (BSN)*
Harding University, College of Nursing, *Searcy (BSN)*
Henderson State University, Department of Nursing, *Arkadelphia (BSN)*
Southern Arkansas University–Magnolia, Department of Nursing, *Magnolia (BSN)*
University of Arkansas, Eleanor Mann School of Nursing, *Fayetteville (BSN)*
University of Arkansas at Fort Smith, Carol McKelvey Moore School of Nursing, *Fort Smith (BSN)*
University of Arkansas at Monticello, School of Nursing, *Monticello (BSN)*
University of Arkansas at Pine Bluff, Department of Nursing, *Pine Bluff (BSN)*
University of Arkansas for Medical Sciences, College of Nursing, *Little Rock (BSN)*
University of Central Arkansas, Department of Nursing, *Conway (BSN)*

California

Azusa Pacific University, School of Nursing, *Azusa (BSN)*
Biola University, Department of Nursing, *La Mirada (BSN)*
California Baptist University, School of Nursing, *Riverside (BSN)*
California State University, Bakersfield, Program in Nursing, *Bakersfield (BSN)*
California State University Channel Islands, Nursing Program, *Camarillo (BSN)*
California State University, Chico, School of Nursing, *Chico (BSN)*
California State University, East Bay, Department of Nursing and Health Sciences, *Hayward (BS)*
California State University, Fresno, Department of Nursing, *Fresno (BSN)*
California State University, Fullerton, Department of Nursing, *Fullerton (BSN)*
California State University, Long Beach, Department of Nursing, *Long Beach (BSN)*
California State University, Los Angeles, School of Nursing, *Los Angeles (BSN)*
California State University, Sacramento, Division of Nursing, *Sacramento (BSN)*
California State University, San Bernardino, Department of Nursing, *San Bernardino (BSN)*
California State University, San Marcos, School of Nursing, *San Marcos (BSN)*
California State University, Stanislaus, Department of Nursing, *Turlock (BSN)*
Dominican University of California, Program in Nursing, *San Rafael (BSN)*
Humboldt State University, Department of Nursing, *Arcata (BSN)*
Loma Linda University, School of Nursing, *Loma Linda (BS)*
Mount St. Mary's College, Department of Nursing, *Los Angeles (BSN, BSc PN)*
National University, Department of Nursing, *La Jolla (BSN)*
Point Loma Nazarene University, School of Nursing, *San Diego (BSN)*
Samuel Merritt University, School of Nursing, *Oakland (BSN)*
San Diego State University, School of Nursing, *San Diego (BSN)*
San Francisco State University, School of Nursing, *San Francisco (BSN)*
San Jose State University, The Valley Foundation School of Nursing, *San Jose (BS)*
Sonoma State University, Department of Nursing, *Rohnert Park (BSN)*
University of California, Irvine, Program in Nursing Science, *Irvine (BS)*
University of California, Los Angeles, School of Nursing, *Los Angeles (BS)*
University of San Francisco, School of Nursing, *San Francisco (BSN)*

Colorado

Adams State College, Nursing Program, *Alamosa (BSN)*
Colorado State University–Pueblo, Department of Nursing, *Pueblo (BSN)*
Denver College of Nursing, *Denver (BSN)*
Mesa State College, Department of Nursing and Radiologic Sciences, *Grand Junction (BSN)*
Regis University, School of Nursing, *Denver (BSN)*
University of Colorado at Colorado Springs, Beth-El College of Nursing and Health Sciences, *Colorado Springs (BSN)*
University of Colorado Denver, College of Nursing, *Denver (BS)*
University of Northern Colorado, School of Nursing, *Greeley (BS)*

Connecticut

Central Connecticut State University, Department of Nursing, *New Britain (BSN)*
Fairfield University, School of Nursing, *Fairfield (BS)*
Quinnipiac University, Department of Nursing, *Hamden (BSN)*
Sacred Heart University, Program in Nursing, *Fairfield (BS)*
Saint Joseph College, Department of Nursing, *West Hartford (BS)*
Southern Connecticut State University, Department of Nursing, *New Haven (BS)*
University of Connecticut, School of Nursing, *Storrs (BS)*
Western Connecticut State University, Department of Nursing, *Danbury (BS)*

Delaware

Delaware State University, Department of Nursing, *Dover (BSN)*
University of Delaware, School of Nursing, *Newark (BSN)*
Wesley College, Nursing Program, *Dover (BSN)*

District of Columbia

The Catholic University of America, School of Nursing, *Washington (BSN)*
Georgetown University, School of Nursing and Health Studies, *Washington (BSN)*
Howard University, Division of Nursing, *Washington (BSN)*
Trinity (Washington) University, Nursing Program, *Washington (BSN)*

Florida

Barry University, School of Nursing, *Miami Shores (BSN)*
Bethune-Cookman University, School of Nursing, *Daytona Beach (BSN)*
Florida Agricultural and Mechanical University, School of Nursing, *Tallahassee (BSN)*
Florida Atlantic University, Christine E. Lynn College of Nursing, *Boca Raton (BS)*
Florida Gulf Coast University, School of Nursing, *Fort Myers (BSN)*
Florida Hospital College of Health Sciences, Department of Nursing, *Orlando (BS)*
Florida International University, Nursing Program, *Miami (BSN)*
Florida Southern College, Department of Nursing, *Lakeland (BSN)*

Florida State University, College of Nursing, *Tallahassee (BSN)*

Jacksonville University, School of Nursing, *Jacksonville (BSN)*

Kaplan University Online, The School of Nursing Online, *Fort Lauderdale (BSN)*

Miami Dade College, School of Nursing, *Miami (BSN)*

Nova Southeastern University, College of Allied Health and Nursing, *Fort Lauderdale (BSN)*

South University, Nursing Program, *Royal Palm Beach (BSN)*

University of Central Florida, College of Nursing, *Orlando (BSN)*

University of Florida, College of Nursing, *Gainesville (BSN)*

University of Miami, School of Nursing and Health Studies, *Coral Gables (BSN)*

University of North Florida, School of Nursing, *Jacksonville (BSN)*

University of South Florida, College of Nursing, *Tampa (BS)*

The University of Tampa, Department of Nursing, *Tampa (BSN)*

University of West Florida, Department of Nursing, *Pensacola (BSN)*

Georgia

Albany State University, College of Sciences and Health Professions, *Albany (BSN)*

Armstrong Atlantic State University, Program in Nursing, *Savannah (BSN)*

Augusta State University, Department of Nursing, *Augusta (BSN)*

Brenau University, School of Health and Science, *Gainesville (BSN)*

Clayton State University, Department of Nursing, *Morrow (BSN)*

College of Coastal Georgia, Department of Nursing and Health Sciences, *Brunswick (BS)*

Columbus State University, Nursing Program, *Columbus (BSN)*

Emory University, Nell Hodgson Woodruff School of Nursing, *Atlanta (BSN)*

Georgia Baptist College of Nursing of Mercer University, Department of Nursing, *Atlanta (BSN)*

Georgia College & State University, College of Health Sciences, *Milledgeville (BSN)*

Georgia Health Sciences University, School of Nursing, *Augusta (BSN)*

Georgia Southern University, School of Nursing, *Statesboro (BSN)*

Georgia Southwestern State University, School of Nursing, *Americus (BSN)*

Georgia State University, Byrdine F. Lewis School of Nursing, *Atlanta (BS)*

Kennesaw State University, School of Nursing, *Kennesaw (BSN)*

LaGrange College, Department of Nursing, *LaGrange (BSN)*

Macon State College, School of Nursing and Health Sciences, *Macon (BSN)*

Piedmont College, School of Nursing, *Demorest (BSN)*

University of West Georgia, School of Nursing, *Carrollton (BSN)*

Valdosta State University, College of Nursing, *Valdosta (BSN)*

Guam

University of Guam, School of Nursing and Health Sciences, *Mangilao (BSN)*

Hawaii

Hawai`i Pacific University, College of Nursing and Health Sciences, *Honolulu (BSN)*

University of Hawaii at Hilo, Department in Nursing, *Hilo (BSN)*

University of Hawaii at Manoa, School of Nursing and Dental Hygiene, *Honolulu (BSN)*

Idaho

Boise State University, Department of Nursing, *Boise (BS)*

Idaho State University, Department of Nursing, *Pocatello (BSN)*

Lewis-Clark State College, Division of Nursing and Health Sciences, *Lewiston (BSN)*

Northwest Nazarene University, School of Health and Science, *Nampa (BSN)*

Illinois

Aurora University, School of Nursing, *Aurora (BSN)*

Blessing–Rieman College of Nursing, *Quincy (BSN)*

Bradley University, Department of Nursing, *Peoria (BSN, BSc PN)*

Chicago State University, Department of Nursing, *Chicago (BSN)*

Elmhurst College, Deicke Center for Nursing Education, *Elmhurst (BS)*

Illinois State University, Mennonite College of Nursing, *Normal (BSN)*

Illinois Wesleyan University, School of Nursing, *Bloomington (BSN)*

Lakeview College of Nursing, *Danville (BSN)*

Lewis University, Program in Nursing, *Romeoville (BSN)*

Loyola University Chicago, Marcella Niehoff School of Nursing, *Maywood (BSN)*

MacMurray College, Department of Nursing, *Jacksonville (BSN)*

Methodist College of Nursing, *Peoria (BSN)*

Millikin University, School of Nursing, *Decatur (BSN)*

Northern Illinois University, School of Nursing and Health Studies, *De Kalb (BS)*

North Park University, School of Nursing, *Chicago (BS)*

Olivet Nazarene University, Division of Nursing, *Bourbonnais (BSN)*

Rockford College, Department of Nursing, *Rockford (BSN)*

Saint Anthony College of Nursing, *Rockford (BSN)*

Saint Francis Medical Center College of Nursing, Baccalaureate Nursing Program, *Peoria (BSN)*

St. John's College, Department of Nursing, *Springfield (BSN)*

Saint Xavier University, School of Nursing, *Chicago (BSN)*

Southern Illinois University Edwardsville, School of Nursing, *Edwardsville (BS)*

Trinity Christian College, Department of Nursing, *Palos Heights (BSN)*

Trinity College of Nursing and Health Sciences, *Rock Island (BSN)*

University of Illinois at Chicago, College of Nursing, *Chicago (BSN)*

University of St. Francis, College of Nursing and Allied Health, *Joliet (BSN)*

Western Illinois University, School of Nursing, *Macomb (BSN)*

Indiana

Anderson University, School of Nursing, *Anderson (BSN)*

Ball State University, School of Nursing, *Muncie (BS)*

Bethel College, Department of Nursing, *Mishawaka (BSN)*

Goshen College, Department of Nursing, *Goshen (BSN)*

Indiana State University, Department of Nursing, *Terre Haute (BS)*

Indiana University Bloomington, Department of Nursing–Bloomington Division, *Bloomington (BSN)*

Indiana University East, School of Nursing, *Richmond (BSN)*

Indiana University Kokomo, Indiana University School of Nursing, *Kokomo (BSN)*

Indiana University Northwest, School of Nursing and Health Professions, *Gary (BSN)*

Indiana University–Purdue University Fort Wayne, Department of Nursing, *Fort Wayne (BS)*

Indiana University–Purdue University Indianapolis, School of Nursing, *Indianapolis (BSN)*

Indiana University South Bend, Division of Nursing and Health Professions, *South Bend (BSN)*

Indiana University Southeast, Division of Nursing, *New Albany (BSN)*

Indiana Wesleyan University, School of Nursing, *Marion (BSN)*

Marian University, Department of Nursing and Nutritional Science, *Indianapolis (BSN)*

Purdue University, School of Nursing, *West Lafayette (BS)*

Purdue University Calumet, School of Nursing, *Hammond (BS)*

Saint Mary's College, Department of Nursing, *Notre Dame (BS)*

University of Evansville, Department of Nursing, *Evansville (BSN)*

University of Indianapolis, School of Nursing, *Indianapolis (BSN)*

University of Saint Francis, Department of Nursing, *Fort Wayne (BSN)*

University of Southern Indiana, College of Nursing and Health Professions, *Evansville (BSN)*

Valparaiso University, College of Nursing, *Valparaiso (BSN)*

Iowa

Allen College, Program in Nursing, *Waterloo (BSN)*

Briar Cliff University, Department of Nursing, *Sioux City (BSN)*

Clarke University, Department of Nursing and Health, *Dubuque (BS)*

Coe College, Department of Nursing, *Cedar Rapids (BSN)*

Dordt College, Nursing Program, *Sioux Center (BSN)*

Grand View University, Division of Nursing, *Des Moines (BSN)*

Iowa Wesleyan College, Division of Health and Natural Sciences, *Mount Pleasant (BSN)*

Luther College, Department of Nursing, *Decorah (BA)*

Morningside College, Department of Nursing Education, *Sioux City (BSN)*

Mount Mercy University, Department of Nursing, *Cedar Rapids (BSN)*

Northwestern College, Nursing Program, *Orange City (BSN)*

St. Ambrose University, Program in Nursing (BSN), *Davenport (BSN)*

The University of Iowa, College of Nursing, *Iowa City (BSN)*

Kansas

Baker University, School of Nursing, *Topeka (BSN)*

Bethel College, Department of Nursing, *North Newton (BSN)*

Emporia State University, Newman Division of Nursing, *Emporia (BSN)*

Fort Hays State University, Department of Nursing, *Hays (BSN)*

Kansas Wesleyan University, Department of Nursing Education, *Salina (BSN)*

MidAmerica Nazarene University, Division of Nursing, *Olathe (BSN)*

Newman University, Division of Nursing, *Wichita (BSN)*

Pittsburg State University, Department of Nursing, *Pittsburg (BSN)*

Southwestern College, Nursing Program, *Winfield (BSN)*

The University of Kansas, School of Nursing, *Kansas City (BSN)*

University of Saint Mary, Bachelor of Science in Nursing Program, *Leavenworth (BSN)*

Washburn University, School of Nursing, *Topeka (BSN)*

Wichita State University, School of Nursing, *Wichita (BSN)*

Kentucky

Bellarmine University, Donna and Allan Lansing School of Nursing and Health Sciences, *Louisville (BSN)*

Berea College, Department of Nursing, *Berea (BSN)*

Eastern Kentucky University, Department of Baccalaureate and Graduate Nursing, *Richmond (BSN)*

Kentucky Christian University, School of Nursing, *Grayson (BSN)*

Morehead State University, Department of Nursing, *Morehead (BSN)*

Murray State University, Program in Nursing, *Murray (BSN)*

Northern Kentucky University, Department of Nursing, *Highland Heights (BSN)*

Spalding University, School of Nursing, *Louisville (BSN)*

Thomas More College, Program in Nursing, *Crestview Hills (BSN)*

University of Kentucky, Graduate School Programs in the College of Nursing, *Lexington (BSN)*

University of Louisville, School of Nursing, *Louisville (BSN)*

Louisiana

Dillard University, Division of Nursing, *New Orleans (BSN)*

Grambling State University, School of Nursing, *Grambling (BSN)*

Louisiana College, Department of Nursing, *Pineville (BSN)*

Louisiana State University Health Sciences Center, School of Nursing, *New Orleans (BSN)*

McNeese State University, College of Nursing, *Lake Charles (BSN)*

Nicholls State University, Department of Nursing, *Thibodaux (BSN)*

Northwestern State University of Louisiana, College of Nursing, *Shreveport (BSN)*

Our Lady of Holy Cross College, Division of Nursing, *New Orleans (BSN)*

Southeastern Louisiana University, School of Nursing, *Hammond (BS)*

Southern University and Agricultural and Mechanical College, School of Nursing, *Baton Rouge (BSN)*

University of Louisiana at Lafayette, College of Nursing, *Lafayette (BSN)*

University of Louisiana at Monroe, Nursing, *Monroe (BS)*

Maine

Husson University, School of Nursing, *Bangor (BSN)*

Saint Joseph's College of Maine, Department of Nursing, *Standish (BSN)*

University of Maine, School of Nursing, *Orono (BSN)*

University of Maine at Fort Kent, Department of Nursing, *Fort Kent (BSN)*

University of New England, Department of Nursing, *Biddeford (BSN)*

University of Southern Maine, College of Nursing and Health Professions, *Portland (BS)*

Maryland

Bowie State University, Department of Nursing, *Bowie (BSN)*

Coppin State University, Helene Fuld School of Nursing, *Baltimore (BSN)*

The Johns Hopkins University, School of Nursing, *Baltimore (BS)*

Salisbury University, Program in Nursing, *Salisbury (BS)*

Stevenson University, Nursing Division, *Stevenson (BS)*

Towson University, Department of Nursing, *Towson (BS)*

University of Maryland, Baltimore, Master's Program in Nursing, *Baltimore (BSN)*

Washington Adventist University, Nursing Department, *Takoma Park (BS)*

Massachusetts

American International College, Division of Nursing, *Springfield (BSN)*

Boston College, William F. Connell School of Nursing, *Chestnut Hill (BS)*

Curry College, Division of Nursing, *Milton (BS)*

Elms College, Division of Nursing, *Chicopee (BS)*

Endicott College, Major in Nursing, *Beverly (BS)*

Northeastern University, School of Nursing, *Boston (BSN)*

Regis College, School of Nursing and Health Professions, *Weston (BSN)*

Salem State University, Program in Nursing, *Salem (BSN)*

Simmons College, Department of Nursing, *Boston (BS)*

University of Massachusetts Amherst, School of Nursing, *Amherst (BS)*

University of Massachusetts Boston, College of Nursing and Health Sciences, *Boston (BS)*

University of Massachusetts Dartmouth, College of Nursing, *North Dartmouth (BSN)*

University of Massachusetts Lowell, Department of Nursing, *Lowell (BS)*

Worcester State College, Department of Nursing, *Worcester (BS)*

Michigan

Andrews University, Department of Nursing, *Berrien Springs (BS)*

Calvin College, Department of Nursing, *Grand Rapids (BSN)*

Davenport University, Division of Nursing, *Grand Rapids (BSN)*

Davenport University, Bachelor of Science in Nursing Program, *Kalamazoo (BSN)*

Eastern Michigan University, School of Nursing, *Ypsilanti (BSN)*

Ferris State University, School of Nursing, *Big Rapids (BSN)*

Finlandia University, College of Professional Studies, *Hancock (BSN)*

Grand Valley State University, Kirkhof College of Nursing, *Allendale (BSN)*

Hope College, Department of Nursing, *Holland (BSN)*

Lake Superior State University, Department of Nursing, *Sault Sainte Marie (BSN)*

Madonna University, College of Nursing and Health, *Livonia (BSN)*

Michigan State University, College of Nursing, *East Lansing (BSN)*

Northern Michigan University, College of Nursing and Allied Health Science, *Marquette (BSN)*

Oakland University, School of Nursing, *Rochester (BSN)*

Saginaw Valley State University, Crystal M. Lange College of Nursing and Health Sciences, *University Center (BSN)*

Siena Heights University, Nursing Program, *Adrian (BSN)*

University of Detroit Mercy, McAuley School of Nursing, *Detroit (BSN)*

University of Michigan, School of Nursing, *Ann Arbor (BSN)*

University of Michigan–Flint, Department of Nursing, *Flint (BSN)*

Wayne State University, College of Nursing, *Detroit (BSN)*

Western Michigan University, College of Health and Human Services, *Kalamazoo (BSN)*

Minnesota

Bemidji State University, Department of Nursing, *Bemidji (BS)*

Bethel University, Department of Nursing, *St. Paul (BSN)*

College of Saint Benedict, Department of Nursing, *Saint Joseph (BS)*

The College of St. Scholastica, Department of Nursing, *Duluth (BS)*

Concordia College, Department of Nursing, *Moorhead (BA)*

Crown College, Nursing Department, *St. Bonifacius (BSN)*

Globe University, Bachelor of Science in Nursing, *Woodbury (BS)*
Gustavus Adolphus College, Department of Nursing, *St. Peter (BA)*
Minnesota Intercollegiate Nursing Consortium, *Northfield (BA)*
Minnesota State University Mankato, School of Nursing, *Mankato (BS)*
Minnesota State University Moorhead, School of Nursing and Healthcare Leadership, *Moorhead (BSN)*
St. Catherine University, Department of Nursing, *St. Paul (BS)*
St. Cloud State University, Department of Nursing Science, *St. Cloud (BS)*
St. Olaf College, Department of Nursing, *Northfield (BA)*
University of Minnesota, Twin Cities Campus, School of Nursing, *Minneapolis (BSN)*
Winona State University, College of Nursing and Health Sciences, *Winona (BS)*

Mississippi

Alcorn State University, School of Nursing, *Natchez (BSN)*
Delta State University, School of Nursing, *Cleveland (BSN)*
Mississippi College, School of Nursing, *Clinton (BSN)*
Mississippi University for Women, College of Nursing and Speech Language Pathology, *Columbus (BSN)*
University of Mississippi Medical Center, Program in Nursing, *Jackson (BSN)*
University of Southern Mississippi, School of Nursing, *Hattiesburg (BSN)*
William Carey University, School of Nursing, *Hattiesburg (BSN)*

Missouri

Avila University, School of Nursing, *Kansas City (BSN)*
Central Methodist University, College of Liberal Arts and Sciences, *Fayette (BN)*
Chamberlain College of Nursing, *St. Louis (BSN)*
Cox College, Department of Nursing, *Springfield (BSN)*
Goldfarb School of Nursing at Barnes-Jewish College, *St. Louis (BSN)*
Graceland University, School of Nursing, *Independence (BSN)*
Maryville University of Saint Louis, Nursing Program, School of Health Professions, *St. Louis (BSN)*
Missouri Southern State University, Department of Nursing, *Joplin (BSN)*
Missouri State University, Department of Nursing, *Springfield (BSN)*
Missouri Western State University, Department of Nursing, *St. Joseph (BSN)*
Research College of Nursing, College of Nursing, *Kansas City (BSN)*
Saint Louis University, School of Nursing, *St. Louis (BSN)*
Saint Luke's College, Nursing College, *Kansas City (BSN)*
Southeast Missouri State University, Department of Nursing, *Cape Girardeau (BSN)*
Truman State University, Program in Nursing, *Kirksville (BSN)*
University of Central Missouri, Department of Nursing, *Warrensburg (BS)*
University of Missouri, Sinclair School of Nursing, *Columbia (BSN)*
University of Missouri–Kansas City, School of Nursing, *Kansas City (BSN)*
University of Missouri–St. Louis, College of Nursing, *St. Louis (BSN)*
William Jewell College, Department of Nursing, *Liberty (BS)*

Montana

Carroll College, Department of Nursing, *Helena (BSN)*
Montana State University, College of Nursing, *Bozeman (BSN)*

Nebraska

BryanLGH College of Health Sciences, School of Nursing, *Lincoln (BSN)*
Clarkson College, Master of Science in Nursing Program, *Omaha (BSN)*
College of Saint Mary, Division of Health Care Professions, *Omaha (BSN)*
Creighton University, School of Nursing, *Omaha (BSN)*
Midland Lutheran College, Department of Nursing, *Fremont (BSN)*
Nebraska Methodist College, Department of Nursing, *Omaha (BSN)*
Union College, Division of Health Sciences, *Lincoln (BSN)*
University of Nebraska Medical Center, College of Nursing, *Omaha (BSN)*

Nevada

Nevada State College at Henderson, Nursing Program, *Henderson (BSN)*
Touro University, School of Nursing, *Henderson (BSN)*
University of Nevada, Las Vegas, School of Nursing, *Las Vegas (BSN)*
University of Nevada, Reno, Orvis School of Nursing, *Reno (BSN)*
University of Southern Nevada, College of Nursing, *Henderson (BSN)*

New Hampshire

Colby-Sawyer College, Department of Nursing, *New London (BSN)*
Rivier College, Division of Nursing, *Nashua (BS)*
University of New Hampshire, Department of Nursing, *Durham (BS)*

New Jersey

Bloomfield College, Division of Nursing, *Bloomfield (BS)*
The College of New Jersey, School of Nursing, Health and Exercise Science, *Ewing (BSN)*
Fairleigh Dickinson University, Metropolitan Campus, Henry P. Becton School of Nursing and Allied Health, *Teaneck (BSN)*
Felician College, Division of Nursing and Health Management, *Lodi (BSN)*
Ramapo College of New Jersey, Master of Science in Nursing Program, *Mahwah (BSN)*
Rutgers, The State University of New Jersey, Camden College of Arts and Sciences, Department of Nursing, *Camden (BS)*
Rutgers, The State University of New Jersey, College of Nursing, *Newark (BS)*
Saint Peter's College, Nursing Program, *Jersey City (BSN)*
Seton Hall University, College of Nursing, *South Orange (BSN)*
Thomas Edison State College, School of Nursing, *Trenton (BSN)*
William Paterson University of New Jersey, Department of Nursing, *Wayne (BSN)*

New Mexico

New Mexico State University, School of Nursing, *Las Cruces (BSN)*
University of New Mexico, College of Nursing, *Albuquerque (BSN)*

New York

Adelphi University, School of Nursing, *Garden City (BS)*
The College at Brockport, State University of New York, Department of Nursing, *Brockport (BSN)*
College of Mount Saint Vincent, Department of Nursing, *Riverdale (BS)*
The College of New Rochelle, School of Nursing, *New Rochelle (BSN)*
Concordia College–New York, Nursing Program, *Bronxville (BS)*
Dominican College, Department of Nursing, *Orangeburg (BSN)*
D'Youville College, Department of Nursing, *Buffalo (BSN)*
Elmira College, Program in Nursing Education, *Elmira (BS)*
Farmingdale State College, Nursing Department, *Farmingdale (BS)*
Hartwick College, Department of Nursing, *Oneonta (BS)*
Hunter College of the City University of New York, Hunter-Bellevue School of Nursing, *New York (BS)*
Lehman College of the City University of New York, Department of Nursing, *Bronx (BS)*
Long Island University, Brooklyn Campus, School of Nursing, *Brooklyn (BS)*
Molloy College, Division of Nursing, *Rockville Centre (BS)*
Mount Saint Mary College, Division of Nursing, *Newburgh (BSN)*
Nazareth College of Rochester, Department of Nursing, *Rochester (BS)*
New York Institute of Technology, Department of Nursing, *Old Westbury (BSN)*
New York University, College of Nursing, *New York (BS)*
Pace University, Lienhard School of Nursing, *New York (BS)*
Roberts Wesleyan College, Division of Nursing, *Rochester (BScN)*
The Sage Colleges, Department of Nursing, *Troy (BS)*
St. John Fisher College, Advanced Practice Nursing Program, *Rochester (BS)*
State University of New York at Binghamton, Decker School of Nursing, *Binghamton (BS)*
State University of New York at Plattsburgh, Department of Nursing, *Plattsburgh (BS)*
Stony Brook University, State University of New York, School of Nursing, *Stony Brook (BS)*
University at Buffalo, the State University of New York, School of Nursing, *Buffalo (BS)*
Utica College, Department of Nursing, *Utica (BS)*
Wagner College, Department of Nursing, *Staten Island (BS)*

North Carolina

Appalachian State University, Department of Nursing, *Boone (BSN)*

Barton College, School of Nursing, *Wilson (BSN)*

East Carolina University, College of Nursing, *Greenville (BSN)*

Fayetteville State University, Program in Nursing, *Fayetteville (BS)*

Lenoir-Rhyne University, Program in Nursing, *Hickory (BS)*

North Carolina Agricultural and Technical State University, School of Nursing, *Greensboro (BSN)*

North Carolina Central University, Department of Nursing, *Durham (BSN)*

Queens University of Charlotte, Presbyterian School of Nursing, *Charlotte (BSN)*

The University of North Carolina at Chapel Hill, School of Nursing, *Chapel Hill (BSN)*

The University of North Carolina at Charlotte, School of Nursing, *Charlotte (BSN)*

The University of North Carolina at Greensboro, School of Nursing, *Greensboro (BSN)*

The University of North Carolina at Pembroke, Nursing Program, *Pembroke (BSN)*

The University of North Carolina Wilmington, School of Nursing, *Wilmington (BS)*

Western Carolina University, School of Nursing, *Cullowhee (BSN)*

Winston-Salem State University, Department of Nursing, *Winston-Salem (BSN)*

North Dakota

Minot State University, Department of Nursing, *Minot (BSN)*

North Dakota State University, Department of Nursing, *Fargo (BSN)*

University of Mary, Division of Nursing, *Bismarck (BS)*

University of North Dakota, College of Nursing, *Grand Forks (BSN)*

Ohio

Capital University, School of Nursing, *Columbus (BSN)*

Case Western Reserve University, Frances Payne Bolton School of Nursing, *Cleveland (BSN)*

Cleveland State University, School of Nursing, *Cleveland (BSN)*

College of Mount St. Joseph, Department of Nursing, *Cincinnati (BSN)*

Defiance College, Bachelor's Degree in Nursing, *Defiance (BSN)*

Franciscan University of Steubenville, Department of Nursing, *Steubenville (BSN)*

Hiram College, Nursing Department, *Hiram (BSN)*

Kent State University, College of Nursing, *Kent (BSN)*

Kettering College of Medical Arts, Division of Nursing, *Kettering (BSN)*

Lourdes College, School of Nursing, *Sylvania (BSN)*

Malone University, School of Nursing, *Canton (BSN)*

Mercy College of Northwest Ohio, Division of Nursing, *Toledo (BSN)*

Miami University, Department of Nursing, *Hamilton (BSN)*

Miami University Hamilton, Bachelor of Science in Nursing Program, *Hamilton (BSN)*

Mount Carmel College of Nursing, Nursing Programs, *Columbus (BSN)*

Muskingum University, Department of Nursing, *New Concord (BSN)*

Notre Dame College, Nursing Department, *South Euclid (BSN)*

The Ohio State University, College of Nursing, *Columbus (BSN)*

Ohio University, School of Nursing, *Athens (BSN)*

Otterbein University, Department of Nursing, *Westerville (BSN)*

The University of Akron, College of Nursing, *Akron (BSN)*

University of Cincinnati, College of Nursing, *Cincinnati (BSN)*

The University of Toledo, College of Nursing, *Toledo (BSN)*

Ursuline College, The Breen School of Nursing, *Pepper Pike (BSN)*

Walsh University, Department of Nursing, *North Canton (BSN)*

Wright State University, College of Nursing and Health, *Dayton (BSN)*

Xavier University, School of Nursing, *Cincinnati (BSN)*

Oklahoma

East Central University, Department of Nursing, *Ada (BS)*

Langston University, School of Nursing and Health Professions, *Langston (BSN)*

Northwestern Oklahoma State University, Division of Nursing, *Alva (BSN)*

Oklahoma Baptist University, School of Nursing, *Shawnee (BSN)*

Oklahoma Christian University, Nursing Program, *Oklahoma City (BSN)*

Oklahoma City University, Kramer School of Nursing, *Oklahoma City (BSN)*

Oklahoma Wesleyan University, School of Nursing, *Bartlesville (BSN)*

Oral Roberts University, Anna Vaughn School of Nursing, *Tulsa (BSN)*

Southern Nazarene University, School of Nursing, *Bethany (BS)*

Southwestern Oklahoma State University, Division of Nursing, *Weatherford (BSN)*

University of Central Oklahoma, Department of Nursing, *Edmond (BSN)*

University of Oklahoma Health Sciences Center, College of Nursing, *Oklahoma City (BSN)*

University of Tulsa, School of Nursing, *Tulsa (BSN)*

Oregon

Concordia University, Nursing Program, *Portland (BSN)*

George Fox University, Nursing Department, *Newberg (BSN)*

Linfield College, School of Nursing, *McMinnville (BSN)*

Oregon Health & Science University, School of Nursing, *Portland (BS)*

University of Portland, School of Nursing, *Portland (BSN)*

Pennsylvania

Alvernia University, Nursing, *Reading (BSN)*

Bloomsburg University of Pennsylvania, Department of Nursing, *Bloomsburg (BSN)*

Carlow University, School of Nursing, *Pittsburgh (BSN)*

Cedar Crest College, Department of Nursing, *Allentown (BS)*

DeSales University, Department of Nursing and Health, *Center Valley (BSN)*

Drexel University, College of Nursing and Health Professions, *Philadelphia (BSN)*

Duquesne University, School of Nursing, *Pittsburgh (BSN)*

Eastern University, Program in Nursing, *St. Davids (BSN)*

East Stroudsburg University of Pennsylvania, Department of Nursing, *East Stroudsburg (BS)*

Edinboro University of Pennsylvania, Department of Nursing, *Edinboro (BS)*

Gannon University, Villa Maria School of Nursing, *Erie (BSN)*

Holy Family University, School of Nursing and Allied Health Professions, *Philadelphia (BSN)*

Immaculata University, Department of Nursing, *Immaculata (BSN)*

Indiana University of Pennsylvania, Department of Nursing and Allied Health, *Indiana (BSN)*

La Salle University, School of Nursing and Health Sciences, *Philadelphia (BSN)*

Mansfield University of Pennsylvania, Department of Health Sciences–Nursing, *Mansfield (BSN)*

Marywood University, Department of Nursing, *Scranton (BSN)*

Messiah College, Department of Nursing, *Grantham (BSN)*

Misericordia University, Department of Nursing, *Dallas (BSN)*

Moravian College, St. Luke's School of Nursing, *Bethlehem (BS)*

Neumann University, Program in Nursing and Health Sciences, *Aston (BS)*

Penn State University Park, School of Nursing, *University Park (BS)*

Robert Morris University, School of Nursing and Health Sciences, *Moon Township (BSN)*

Saint Francis University, Department of Nursing, *Loretto (BSN)*

Temple University, Department of Nursing, *Philadelphia (BSN)*

Thomas Jefferson University, Department of Nursing, *Philadelphia (BSN)*

University of Pennsylvania, School of Nursing, *Philadelphia (BSN)*

University of Pittsburgh, School of Nursing, *Pittsburgh (BSN)*

University of Pittsburgh at Bradford, Department of Nursing, *Bradford (BSN)*

The University of Scranton, Department of Nursing, *Scranton (BS)*

Villanova University, College of Nursing, *Villanova (BSN)*

Waynesburg University, Department of Nursing, *Waynesburg (BSN)*

West Chester University of Pennsylvania, Department of Nursing, *West Chester (BSN)*

Widener University, School of Nursing, *Chester (BSN)*

Wilkes University, Department of Nursing, *Wilkes-Barre (BS)*

York College of Pennsylvania, Department of Nursing, *York (BS)*

Puerto Rico

Inter American University of Puerto Rico, Arecibo Campus, Nursing Program, *Arecibo (BS)*
Inter American University of Puerto Rico, Metropolitan Campus, Carmen Torres de Tiburcio School of Nursing, *San Juan (BSN)*
Pontifical Catholic University of Puerto Rico, Department of Nursing, *Ponce (BSN)*
Universidad Adventista de las Antillas, Department of Nursing, *Mayagüez (BSN)*
Universidad del Turabo, Nursing Program, *Gurabo (BS)*
University of Puerto Rico at Arecibo, Department of Nursing, *Arecibo (BSN)*
University of Puerto Rico at Humacao, Department of Nursing, *Humacao (BS)*
University of Puerto Rico, Mayagüez Campus, Department of Nursing, *Mayagüez (BSN)*
University of Puerto Rico, Medical Sciences Campus, School of Nursing, *San Juan (BSN)*
University of the Sacred Heart, Program in Nursing, *San Juan (BSN)*

Rhode Island

Rhode Island College, Department of Nursing, *Providence (BSN)*
Salve Regina University, Department of Nursing, *Newport (BS)*
University of Rhode Island, College of Nursing, *Kingston (BS)*

South Carolina

Charleston Southern University, Wingo School of Nursing, *Charleston (BSN)*
Clemson University, School of Nursing, *Clemson (BS)*
Francis Marion University, Department of Nursing, *Florence (BSN)*
Lander University, School of Nursing, *Greenwood (BSN)*
South Carolina State University, Department of Nursing, *Orangeburg (BSN)*
University of South Carolina, College of Nursing, *Columbia (BSN)*
University of South Carolina Aiken, School of Nursing, *Aiken (BSN)*
University of South Carolina Beaufort, Nursing Program, *Bluffton (BSN)*
University of South Carolina Upstate, Mary Black School of Nursing, *Spartanburg (BSN)*

South Dakota

Augustana College, Department of Nursing, *Sioux Falls (BA)*
Mount Marty College, Nursing Program, *Yankton (BSN)*
National American University, School of Nursing, *Rapid City (BSN)*
Presentation College, Department of Nursing, *Aberdeen (BSN)*
South Dakota State University, College of Nursing, *Brookings (BS)*

Tennessee

Austin Peay State University, School of Nursing, *Clarksville (BSN)*
Baptist College of Health Sciences, Nursing Division, *Memphis (BSN)*
Belmont University, School of Nursing, *Nashville (BSN)*
Bethel University, Nursing Program, *McKenzie (BSN)*
Carson-Newman College, Department of Nursing, *Jefferson City (BSN)*
Cumberland University, Rudy School of Nursing and Health Professions, *Lebanon (BSN)*
East Tennessee State University, College of Nursing, *Johnson City (BSN)*
King College, School of Nursing, *Bristol (BSN)*
Lipscomb University, Department of Nursing, *Nashville (BSN)*
Martin Methodist College, Division of Nursing, *Pulaski (BSN)*
Middle Tennessee State University, School of Nursing, *Murfreesboro (BSN)*
Milligan College, Department of Nursing, *Milligan College (BSN)*
South College, Department of Nursing, *Knoxville (BSN)*
Tennessee State University, School of Nursing, *Nashville (BSN)*
Tennessee Technological University, Whitson-Hester School of Nursing, *Cookeville (BSN)*
Tennessee Wesleyan College, Fort Sanders Nursing Department, *Knoxville (BSN)*
Union University, School of Nursing, *Jackson (BSN)*
University of Memphis, Loewenberg School of Nursing, *Memphis (BSN)*
The University of Tennessee, College of Nursing, *Knoxville (BSN)*
The University of Tennessee at Chattanooga, School of Nursing, *Chattanooga (BSN)*
The University of Tennessee at Martin, Department of Nursing, *Martin (BSN)*

Texas

Baylor University, Louise Herrington School of Nursing, *Dallas (BSN)*
East Texas Baptist University, Department of Nursing, *Marshall (BSN)*
Lamar University, Department of Nursing, *Beaumont (BSN)*
Midwestern State University, Nursing Program, *Wichita Falls (BSN)*
Patty Hanks Shelton School of Nursing, *Abilene (BSN)*
Prairie View A&M University, College of Nursing, *Houston (BSN)*
Southwestern Adventist University, Department of Nursing, *Keene (BS)*
Tarleton State University, Department of Nursing, *Stephenville (BSN)*
Texas A&M Health Science Center, College of Nursing, *College Station (BSN)*
Texas A&M International University, Canseco School of Nursing, *Laredo (BSN)*
Texas A&M University–Corpus Christi, School of Nursing and Health Sciences, *Corpus Christi (BSN)*
Texas Christian University, Harris College of Nursing, *Fort Worth (BSN)*
Texas Tech University Health Sciences Center, School of Nursing, *Lubbock (BSc PN)*
Texas Woman's University, College of Nursing, *Denton (BS)*
University of Mary Hardin-Baylor, College of Nursing, *Belton (BSN)*
The University of Texas at Arlington, College of Nursing, *Arlington (BSN)*
The University of Texas at Austin, School of Nursing, *Austin (BSN)*
The University of Texas at El Paso, School of Nursing, *El Paso (BSN)*
The University of Texas at Tyler, Program in Nursing, *Tyler (BSN)*
The University of Texas Health Science Center at Houston, School of Nursing, *Houston (BSN)*
The University of Texas Health Science Center at San Antonio, School of Nursing, *San Antonio (BSN)*
The University of Texas Medical Branch, School of Nursing, *Galveston (BSN)*
The University of Texas–Pan American, Department of Nursing, *Edinburg (BSN)*
University of the Incarnate Word, Program in Nursing, *San Antonio (BSN)*
West Texas A&M University, Division of Nursing, *Canyon (BSN)*

Utah

Southern Utah University, Department of Nursing, *Cedar City (BSN)*
University of Utah, College of Nursing, *Salt Lake City (BS)*
Westminster College, School of Nursing and Health Sciences, *Salt Lake City (BSN)*

Vermont

Norwich University, Department of Nursing, *Northfield (BSN)*
University of Vermont, Department of Nursing, *Burlington (BS)*

Virgin Islands

University of the Virgin Islands, Division of Nursing, *Saint Thomas (BSN)*

Virginia

Eastern Mennonite University, Department of Nursing, *Harrisonburg (BSN)*
George Mason University, College of Health and Human Services, *Fairfax (BSN)*
Hampton University, School of Nursing, *Hampton (BS)*
James Madison University, Department of Nursing, *Harrisonburg (BSN)*
Jefferson College of Health Sciences, Nursing Education Program, *Roanoke (BSN)*
Liberty University, Department of Nursing, *Lynchburg (BSN)*
Lynchburg College, School of Health Sciences and Human Performance, *Lynchburg (BS)*
Marymount University, School of Health Professions, *Arlington (BSN)*
Old Dominion University, Department of Nursing, *Norfolk (BSN)*
Radford University, School of Nursing, *Radford (BSN)*
Shenandoah University, Division of Nursing, *Winchester (BSN)*
University of Virginia, School of Nursing, *Charlottesville (BSN)*
The University of Virginia's College at Wise, Department of Nursing, *Wise (BSN)*
Virginia Commonwealth University, School of Nursing, *Richmond (BS)*

Washington

Gonzaga University, Department of Nursing, *Spokane (BSN)*
Northwest University, The Mark and Huldah Buntain School of Nursing, *Kirkland (BS)*

Pacific Lutheran University, School of Nursing, *Tacoma (BSN)*

Seattle Pacific University, School of Health Sciences, *Seattle (BS)*

Seattle University, College of Nursing, *Seattle (BSN)*

University of Washington, School of Nursing, *Seattle (BSN)*

Walla Walla University, School of Nursing, *College Place (BS)*

Washington State University College of Nursing and Consortium, *Spokane (BSN)*

West Virginia

Alderson-Broaddus College, Department of Nursing, *Philippi (BSN)*

Marshall University, College of Health Professions, *Huntington (BSN)*

Mountain State University, College of Nursing, *Beckley (BSN)*

Shepherd University, Department of Nursing Education, *Shepherdstown (BSN)*

University of Charleston, Department of Nursing, *Charleston (BSN)*

West Liberty University, Department of Health Sciences, *West Liberty (BSN)*

West Virginia University, School of Nursing, *Morgantown (BSN)*

West Virginia Wesleyan College, School of Nursing, *Buckhannon (BSN)*

Wheeling Jesuit University, Department of Nursing, *Wheeling (BSN)*

Wisconsin

Alverno College, Division of Nursing, *Milwaukee (BSN)*

Bellin College, Nursing Program, *Green Bay (BSN)*

Carroll University, Nursing Program, *Waukesha (BSN)*

Columbia College of Nursing/Mount Mary College Nursing Program, *Milwaukee (BSN)*

Concordia University Wisconsin, Program in Nursing, *Mequon (BSN)*

Edgewood College, Program in Nursing, *Madison (BS)*

Marian University, School of Nursing, *Fond du Lac (BSN)*

Marquette University, College of Nursing, *Milwaukee (BSN)*

Milwaukee School of Engineering, School of Nursing, *Milwaukee (BSN)*

University of Wisconsin–Eau Claire, College of Nursing and Health Sciences, *Eau Claire (BSN)*

University of Wisconsin–Madison, School of Nursing, *Madison (BS)*

University of Wisconsin–Milwaukee, College of Nursing, *Milwaukee (BSN)*

University of Wisconsin–Oshkosh, College of Nursing, *Oshkosh (BSN)*

Viterbo University, School of Nursing, *La Crosse (BSN)*

Wisconsin Lutheran College, Nursing Program, *Milwaukee (BSN)*

Wyoming

University of Wyoming, Fay W. Whitney School of Nursing, *Laramie (BSN)*

CANADA

Alberta

Athabasca University, Centre for Nursing and Health Studies, *Athabasca (BN)*

University of Alberta, Faculty of Nursing, *Edmonton (BScN)*

University of Calgary, Faculty of Nursing, *Calgary (BN)*

University of Lethbridge, School of Health Sciences, *Lethbridge (BN)*

British Columbia

Kwantlen Polytechnic University, Faculty of Community and Health Sciences, *Surrey (BSN)*

Trinity Western University, Department of Nursing, *Langley (BScN)*

University of Northern British Columbia, Nursing Programme, *Prince George (BScN)*

Vancouver Island University, Department of Nursing, *Nanaimo (BScN)*

Manitoba

Brandon University, School of Health Studies, *Brandon (BN)*

University of Manitoba, Faculty of Nursing, *Winnipeg (BN)*

New Brunswick

University of New Brunswick Fredericton, Faculty of Nursing, *Fredericton (BN)*

Newfoundland and Labrador

Memorial University of Newfoundland, School of Nursing, *St. John's (BN)*

Nova Scotia

Dalhousie University, School of Nursing, *Halifax (BScN)*

St. Francis Xavier University, Department of Nursing, *Antigonish (BScN)*

Ontario

Brock University, Department of Nursing, *St. Catharines (BScN)*

Lakehead University, School of Nursing, *Thunder Bay (BScN)*

McMaster University, School of Nursing, *Hamilton (BScN)*

Nipissing University, Nursing Department, *North Bay (BScN)*

Queen's University at Kingston, School of Nursing, *Kingston (BNSc)*

Ryerson University, Program in Nursing, *Toronto (BScN)*

Trent University, Nursing Program, *Peterborough (BScN)*

University of Ottawa, School of Nursing, *Ottawa (BScN)*

The University of Western Ontario, School of Nursing, *London (BScN)*

University of Windsor, Faculty of Nursing, *Windsor (BScN)*

York University, School of Nursing, *Toronto (BScN)*

Prince Edward Island

University of Prince Edward Island, School of Nursing, *Charlottetown (BScN)*

Quebec

McGill University, School of Nursing, *Montréal (BScN)*

Université du Québec à Trois-Rivières, Program in Nursing, *Trois-Rivières (BSN)*

Université du Québec en Outaouais, Département des Sciences Infirmières, *Gatineau (BScN)*

Université Laval, Faculty of Nursing, *Québec (BScN)*

Saskatchewan

University of Saskatchewan, College of Nursing, *Saskatoon (BSN)*

INTERNATIONAL NURSE TO BACCALAUREATE

U.S. AND U.S. TERRITORIES

Delaware

Wesley College, Nursing Program, *Dover (BSN)*

Wilmington University, College of Health Professions, *New Castle (BSN)*

Hawaii

Hawai`i Pacific University, College of Nursing and Health Sciences, *Honolulu (BSN)*

Iowa

Morningside College, Department of Nursing Education, *Sioux City (BSN)*

Massachusetts

Salem State University, Program in Nursing, *Salem (BSN)*

Nebraska

Nebraska Wesleyan University, Department of Nursing, *Lincoln (BSN)*

University of Nebraska Medical Center, College of Nursing, *Omaha (BSN)*

New Jersey

College of Saint Elizabeth, Department of Nursing, *Morristown (BSN)*

New York

College of Mount Saint Vincent, Department of Nursing, *Riverdale (BS)*

Daemen College, Department of Nursing, *Amherst (BS)*

Lehman College of the City University of New York, Department of Nursing, *Bronx (BS)*

Long Island University, Brooklyn Campus, School of Nursing, *Brooklyn (BS)*

The Sage Colleges, Department of Nursing, *Troy (BS)*

St. Francis College, Department of Nursing, *Brooklyn Heights (BS)*

North Dakota

University of North Dakota, College of Nursing, *Grand Forks (BSN)*

Oklahoma

Oklahoma Wesleyan University, School of Nursing, *Bartlesville (BSN)*

Pennsylvania

Eastern University, Program in Nursing, *St. Davids (BSN)*

Edinboro University of Pennsylvania, Department of Nursing, *Edinboro (BS)*

Gannon University, Villa Maria School of Nursing, *Erie (BSN)*

Holy Family University, School of Nursing and Allied Health Professions, *Philadelphia (BSN)*
Marywood University, Department of Nursing, *Scranton (BSN)*
Neumann University, Program in Nursing and Health Sciences, *Aston (BS)*
Villanova University, College of Nursing, *Villanova (BSN)*

South Carolina
University of South Carolina Aiken, School of Nursing, *Aiken (BSN)*

South Dakota
Mount Marty College, Nursing Program, *Yankton (BSN)*

Texas
The University of Texas at Tyler, Program in Nursing, *Tyler (BSN)*

CANADA

Ontario
Ryerson University, Program in Nursing, *Toronto (BScN)*
University of Ottawa, School of Nursing, *Ottawa (BScN)*

LPN TO BACCALAUREATE

U.S. AND U.S. TERRITORIES

Arizona
University of Phoenix–Phoenix Campus, College of Nursing, *Phoenix (BSN)*
University of Phoenix–Southern Arizona Campus, College of Social Sciences, *Tucson (BSN)*

Arkansas
Arkansas State University - Jonesboro, Department of Nursing, *State University (BSN)*
Arkansas Tech University, Program in Nursing, *Russellville (BSN)*
Harding University, College of Nursing, *Searcy (BSN)*
Henderson State University, Department of Nursing, *Arkadelphia (BSN)*
University of Arkansas, Eleanor Mann School of Nursing, *Fayetteville (BSN)*
University of Arkansas at Monticello, School of Nursing, *Monticello (BSN)*
University of Arkansas for Medical Sciences, College of Nursing, *Little Rock (BSN)*
University of Central Arkansas, Department of Nursing, *Conway (BSN)*

California
Biola University, Department of Nursing, *La Mirada (BSN)*
California State University, Long Beach, Department of Nursing, *Long Beach (BSN)*
California State University, San Bernardino, Department of Nursing, *San Bernardino (BSN)*
California State University, Stanislaus, Department of Nursing, *Turlock (BSN)*
Loma Linda University, School of Nursing, *Loma Linda (BS)*
National University, Department of Nursing, *La Jolla (BSN)*
University of Phoenix–Sacramento Valley Campus, College of Nursing, *Sacramento (BSN)*

Colorado
Colorado State University–Pueblo, Department of Nursing, *Pueblo (BSN)*
Mesa State College, Department of Nursing and Radiologic Sciences, *Grand Junction (BSN)*
University of Phoenix–Denver Campus, College of Nursing, *Lone Tree (BSN)*

Delaware
Delaware State University, Department of Nursing, *Dover (BSN)*
Wesley College, Nursing Program, *Dover (BSN)*

District of Columbia
Howard University, Division of Nursing, *Washington (BSN)*

Florida
Barry University, School of Nursing, *Miami Shores (BSN)*

Georgia
Armstrong Atlantic State University, Program in Nursing, *Savannah (BSN)*
Augusta State University, Department of Nursing, *Augusta (BSN)*
Piedmont College, School of Nursing, *Demorest (BSN)*

Hawaii
Hawai`i Pacific University, College of Nursing and Health Sciences, *Honolulu (BSN)*
University of Phoenix–Hawaii Campus, College of Nursing, *Honolulu (BSN)*

Idaho
Boise State University, Department of Nursing, *Boise (BS)*
Idaho State University, Department of Nursing, *Pocatello (BSN)*
Lewis-Clark State College, Division of Nursing and Health Sciences, *Lewiston (BSN)*

Illinois
Bradley University, Department of Nursing, *Peoria (BSN, BSc PN)*
Chicago State University, Department of Nursing, *Chicago (BSN)*

Indiana
Ball State University, School of Nursing, *Muncie (BS)*
Indiana State University, Department of Nursing, *Terre Haute (BS)*
Marian University, Department of Nursing and Nutritional Science, *Indianapolis (BSN)*
Purdue University Calumet, School of Nursing, *Hammond (BS)*

Iowa
Allen College, Program in Nursing, *Waterloo (BSN)*
Briar Cliff University, Department of Nursing, *Sioux City (BSN)*
Iowa Wesleyan College, Division of Health and Natural Sciences, *Mount Pleasant (BSN)*
Morningside College, Department of Nursing Education, *Sioux City (BSN)*

Kansas
Bethel College, Department of Nursing, *North Newton (BSN)*
Emporia State University, Newman Division of Nursing, *Emporia (BSN)*
Newman University, Division of Nursing, *Wichita (BSN)*
Southwestern College, Nursing Program, *Winfield (BSN)*
Washburn University, School of Nursing, *Topeka (BSN)*

Louisiana
McNeese State University, College of Nursing, *Lake Charles (BSN)*
Nicholls State University, Department of Nursing, *Thibodaux (BSN)*
Northwestern State University of Louisiana, College of Nursing, *Shreveport (BSN)*
Southeastern Louisiana University, School of Nursing, *Hammond (BS)*
University of Louisiana at Lafayette, College of Nursing, *Lafayette (BSN)*
University of Louisiana at Monroe, Nursing, *Monroe (BS)*
University of Phoenix–Louisiana Campus, College of Nursing, *Metairie (BSN)*

Massachusetts
Salem State University, Program in Nursing, *Salem (BSN)*
Simmons College, Department of Nursing, *Boston (BS)*

Michigan
Lake Superior State University, Department of Nursing, *Sault Sainte Marie (BSN)*
Madonna University, College of Nursing and Health, *Livonia (BSN)*
Northern Michigan University, College of Nursing and Allied Health Science, *Marquette (BSN)*

Missouri
Cox College, Department of Nursing, *Springfield (BSN)*
Maryville University of Saint Louis, Nursing Program, School of Health Professions, *St. Louis (BSN)*
Missouri Southern State University, Department of Nursing, *Joplin (BSN)*
Missouri State University, Department of Nursing, *Springfield (BSN)*

Montana
Montana State University, College of Nursing, *Bozeman (BSN)*

Nebraska
Clarkson College, Master of Science in Nursing Program, *Omaha (BSN)*
Nebraska Methodist College, Department of Nursing, *Omaha (BSN)*
Union College, Division of Health Sciences, *Lincoln (BSN)*
University of Nebraska Medical Center, College of Nursing, *Omaha (BSN)*

New Hampshire
Rivier College, Division of Nursing, *Nashua (BS)*

New Jersey
William Paterson University of New Jersey, Department of Nursing, *Wayne (BSN)*

New York

Adelphi University, School of Nursing, *Garden City (BS)*
College of Mount Saint Vincent, Department of Nursing, *Riverdale (BS)*
Dominican College, Department of Nursing, *Orangeburg (BSN)*
Molloy College, Division of Nursing, *Rockville Centre (BS)*
Nazareth College of Rochester, Department of Nursing, *Rochester (BS)*
The Sage Colleges, Department of Nursing, *Troy (BS)*

North Carolina

North Carolina Agricultural and Technical State University, School of Nursing, *Greensboro (BSN)*
The University of North Carolina at Greensboro, School of Nursing, *Greensboro (BSN)*
Winston-Salem State University, Department of Nursing, *Winston-Salem (BSN)*

North Dakota

Dickinson State University, Department of Nursing, *Dickinson (BSN)*
North Dakota State University, Department of Nursing, *Fargo (BSN)*
University of Mary, Division of Nursing, *Bismarck (BS)*
University of North Dakota, College of Nursing, *Grand Forks (BSN)*

Ohio

Kent State University, College of Nursing, *Kent (BSN)*
Lourdes College, School of Nursing, *Sylvania (BSN)*
Otterbein University, Department of Nursing, *Westerville (BSN)*
The University of Akron, College of Nursing, *Akron (BSN)*

Oklahoma

Langston University, School of Nursing and Health Professions, *Langston (BSN)*
Northwestern Oklahoma State University, Division of Nursing, *Alva (BSN)*
Oklahoma Baptist University, School of Nursing, *Shawnee (BSN)*
Oklahoma Wesleyan University, School of Nursing, *Bartlesville (BSN)*
Southern Nazarene University, School of Nursing, *Bethany (BS)*
University of Central Oklahoma, Department of Nursing, *Edmond (BSN)*

Pennsylvania

Alvernia University, Nursing, *Reading (BSN)*
Cedar Crest College, Department of Nursing, *Allentown (BS)*
Holy Family University, School of Nursing and Allied Health Professions, *Philadelphia (BSN)*
Indiana University of Pennsylvania, Department of Nursing and Allied Health, *Indiana (BSN)*
La Salle University, School of Nursing and Health Sciences, *Philadelphia (BSN)*
Marywood University, Department of Nursing, *Scranton (BSN)*
Waynesburg University, Department of Nursing, *Waynesburg (BSN)*

South Carolina

University of South Carolina Aiken, School of Nursing, *Aiken (BSN)*

South Dakota

Mount Marty College, Nursing Program, *Yankton (BSN)*

Tennessee

Baptist College of Health Sciences, Nursing Division, *Memphis (BSN)*
Cumberland University, Rudy School of Nursing and Health Professions, *Lebanon (BSN)*
East Tenhessee State University, College of Nursing, *Johnson City (BSN)*
Milligan College, Department of Nursing, *Milligan College (BSN)*
Tennessee State University, School of Nursing, *Nashville (BSN)*
Union University, School of Nursing, *Jackson (BSN)*

Texas

Prairie View A&M University, College of Nursing, *Houston (BSN)*
Southwestern Adventist University, Department of Nursing, *Keene (BS)*
Tarleton State University, Department of Nursing, *Stephenville (BSN)*
The University of Texas at Tyler, Program in Nursing, *Tyler (BSN)*
West Texas A&M University, Division of Nursing, *Canyon (BSN)*

Utah

Southern Utah University, Department of Nursing, *Cedar City (BSN)*

Virgin Islands

University of the Virgin Islands, Division of Nursing, *Saint Thomas (BSN)*

Virginia

Eastern Mennonite University, Department of Nursing, *Harrisonburg (BSN)*
Hampton University, School of Nursing, *Hampton (BS)*
Shenandoah University, Division of Nursing, *Winchester (BSN)*

Washington

Pacific Lutheran University, School of Nursing, *Tacoma (BSN)*
Walla Walla University, School of Nursing, *College Place (BS)*

Wisconsin

Alverno College, Division of Nursing, *Milwaukee (BSN)*

CANADA

Manitoba

Brandon University, School of Health Studies, *Brandon (BN)*

Newfoundland and Labrador

Memorial University of Newfoundland, School of Nursing, *St. John's (BN)*

Nova Scotia

Dalhousie University, School of Nursing, *Halifax (BScN)*

Ontario

University of Ottawa, School of Nursing, *Ottawa (BScN)*

LPN TO RN BACCALAUREATE

U.S. AND U.S. TERRITORIES

Arkansas

Harding University, College of Nursing, *Searcy (BSN)*
University of Arkansas, Eleanor Mann School of Nursing, *Fayetteville (BSN)*
University of Central Arkansas, Department of Nursing, *Conway (BSN)*

California

California State University, Chico, School of Nursing, *Chico (BSN)*
California State University, Los Angeles, School of Nursing, *Los Angeles (BSN)*
California State University, Sacramento, Division of Nursing, *Sacramento (BSN)*
Holy Names University, Department of Nursing, *Oakland (BSN)*
Point Loma Nazarene University, School of Nursing, *San Diego (BSN)*

Colorado

Colorado State University–Pueblo, Department of Nursing, *Pueblo (BSN)*
Mesa State College, Department of Nursing and Radiologic Sciences, *Grand Junction (BSN)*

Florida

Barry University, School of Nursing, *Miami Shores (BSN)*

Georgia

Georgia Southern University, School of Nursing, *Statesboro (BSN)*
Georgia Southwestern State University, School of Nursing, *Americus (BSN)*

Illinois

MacMurray College, Department of Nursing, *Jacksonville (BSN)*
Saint Xavier University, School of Nursing, *Chicago (BSN)*

Indiana

Indiana State University, Department of Nursing, *Terre Haute (BS)*
Indiana University–Purdue University Fort Wayne, Department of Nursing, *Fort Wayne (BS)*

Iowa

Iowa Wesleyan College, Division of Health and Natural Sciences, *Mount Pleasant (BSN)*

Kansas

Wichita State University, School of Nursing, *Wichita (BSN)*

Louisiana

Dillard University, Division of Nursing, *New Orleans (BSN)*
Grambling State University, School of Nursing, *Grambling (BSN)*
McNeese State University, College of Nursing, *Lake Charles (BSN)*
Southeastern Louisiana University, School of Nursing, *Hammond (BS)*

University of Louisiana at Monroe, Nursing, *Monroe (BS)*

Massachusetts

Salem State University, Program in Nursing, *Salem (BSN)*

Michigan

Lake Superior State University, Department of Nursing, *Sault Sainte Marie (BSN)*

Mississippi

Alcorn State University, School of Nursing, *Natchez (BSN)*

Missouri

Chamberlain College of Nursing, *St. Louis (BSN)*

Cox College, Department of Nursing, *Springfield (BSN)*

Nebraska

Clarkson College, Master of Science in Nursing Program, *Omaha (BSN)*

Midland Lutheran College, Department of Nursing, *Fremont (BSN)*

University of Nebraska Medical Center, College of Nursing, *Omaha (BSN)*

New Hampshire

Rivier College, Division of Nursing, *Nashua (BS)*

New York

Adelphi University, School of Nursing, *Garden City (BS)*

College of Mount Saint Vincent, Department of Nursing, *Riverdale (BS)*

Molloy College, Division of Nursing, *Rockville Centre (BS)*

North Carolina

North Carolina Agricultural and Technical State University, School of Nursing, *Greensboro (BSN)*

The University of North Carolina at Greensboro, School of Nursing, *Greensboro (BSN)*

North Dakota

Dickinson State University, Department of Nursing, *Dickinson (BSN)*

Oklahoma

Northwestern Oklahoma State University, Division of Nursing, *Alva (BSN)*

University of Oklahoma Health Sciences Center, College of Nursing, *Oklahoma City (BSN)*

University of Tulsa, School of Nursing, *Tulsa (BSN)*

Pennsylvania

Alvernia University, Nursing, *Reading (BSN)*

Bloomsburg University of Pennsylvania, Department of Nursing, *Bloomsburg (BSN)*

Gannon University, Villa Maria School of Nursing, *Erie (BSN)*

Holy Family University, School of Nursing and Allied Health Professions, *Philadelphia (BSN)*

Neumann University, Program in Nursing and Health Sciences, *Aston (BS)*

The University of Scranton, Department of Nursing, *Scranton (BS)*

Wilkes University, Department of Nursing, *Wilkes-Barre (BS)*

York College of Pennsylvania, Department of Nursing, *York (BS)*

South Dakota

Mount Marty College, Nursing Program, *Yankton (BSN)*

Presentation College, Department of Nursing, *Aberdeen (BSN)*

Tennessee

Belmont University, School of Nursing, *Nashville (BSN)*

Carson-Newman College, Department of Nursing, *Jefferson City (BSN)*

Cumberland University, Rudy School of Nursing and Health Professions, *Lebanon (BSN)*

Middle Tennessee State University, School of Nursing, *Murfreesboro (BSN)*

Milligan College, Department of Nursing, *Milligan College (BSN)*

The University of Tennessee at Martin, Department of Nursing, *Martin (BSN)*

Texas

The University of Texas at Tyler, Program in Nursing, *Tyler (BSN)*

Virginia

Hampton University, School of Nursing, *Hampton (BS)*

Shenandoah University, Division of Nursing, *Winchester (BSN)*

West Virginia

Alderson-Broaddus College, Department of Nursing, *Philippi (BSN)*

Fairmont State University, School of Nursing and Allied Health Administration, *Fairmont (BSN)*

Wisconsin

Concordia University Wisconsin, Program in Nursing, *Mequon (BSN)*

CANADA

Alberta

Athabasca University, Centre for Nursing and Health Studies, *Athabasca (BN)*

RN BACCALAUREATE

U.S. AND U.S. TERRITORIES

Alabama

Auburn University Montgomery, School of Nursing, *Montgomery (BSN)*

Jacksonville State University, College of Nursing and Health Sciences, *Jacksonville (BSN)*

Oakwood University, Department of Nursing, *Huntsville (BS)*

Stillman College, Nursing Major, *Tuscaloosa (BSN)*

Troy University, School of Nursing, *Troy (BSN)*

Tuskegee University, Program in Nursing, *Tuskegee (BSN)*

The University of Alabama, Capstone College of Nursing, *Tuscaloosa (BSN)*

The University of Alabama at Birmingham, School of Nursing, *Birmingham (BSN)*

The University of Alabama in Huntsville, College of Nursing, *Huntsville (BSN)*

University of Mobile, School of Nursing, *Mobile (BSN)*

University of North Alabama, College of Nursing and Allied Health, *Florence (BSN)*

University of South Alabama, College of Nursing, *Mobile (BSN)*

Alaska

University of Alaska Anchorage, School of Nursing, *Anchorage (BS)*

Arizona

Arizona State University at the Downtown Phoenix Campus, College of Nursing, *Phoenix (BSN)*

Chamberlain College of Nursing, *Phoenix (BSN)*

Grand Canyon University, College of Nursing and Health Sciences, *Phoenix (BSN)*

Northern Arizona University, School of Nursing, *Flagstaff (BSN)*

Arkansas

Arkansas State University - Jonesboro, Department of Nursing, *State University (BSN)*

Arkansas Tech University, Program in Nursing, *Russellville (BSN)*

Harding University, College of Nursing, *Searcy (BSN)*

Southern Arkansas University–Magnolia, Department of Nursing, *Magnolia (BSN)*

University of Arkansas, Eleanor Mann School of Nursing, *Fayetteville (BSN)*

University of Arkansas at Little Rock, BSN Programs, *Little Rock (BSN)*

University of Arkansas at Monticello, School of Nursing, *Monticello (BSN)*

University of Arkansas for Medical Sciences, College of Nursing, *Little Rock (BSN)*

University of Central Arkansas, Department of Nursing, *Conway (BSN)*

California

Biola University, Department of Nursing, *La Mirada (BSN)*

California Baptist University, School of Nursing, *Riverside (BSN)*

California State University Channel Islands, Nursing Program, *Camarillo (BSN)*

California State University, Chico, School of Nursing, *Chico (BSN)*

California State University, Dominguez Hills, Program in Nursing, *Carson (BSN)*

California State University, Los Angeles, School of Nursing, *Los Angeles (BSN)*

California State University, San Bernardino, Department of Nursing, *San Bernardino (BSN)*

Concordia University, Bachelor of Science in Nursing Program, *Irvine (BSN)*

Dominican University of California, Program in Nursing, *San Rafael (BSN)*

Fresno Pacific University, RN to BSN Program, *Fresno (BSN)*

Holy Names University, Department of Nursing, *Oakland (BSN)*

Humboldt State University, Department of Nursing, *Arcata (BSN)*

Loma Linda University, School of Nursing, *Loma Linda (BS)*

National University, Department of Nursing, *La Jolla (BSN)*
Point Loma Nazarene University, School of Nursing, *San Diego (BSN)*
San Diego State University, School of Nursing, *San Diego (BSN)*
San Francisco State University, School of Nursing, *San Francisco (BSN)*
Sonoma State University, Department of Nursing, *Rohnert Park (BSN)*
University of Phoenix–Central Valley Campus, College of Health and Human Services, *Fresno (BSN)*
Vanguard University of Southern California, Nursing Program, *Costa Mesa (BSN)*
West Coast University, Nursing Programs, *North Hollywood (BSN)*

Colorado

Adams State College, Nursing Program, *Alamosa (BSN)*
American Sentinel University, RN to Bachelor of Science Nursing, *Aurora (BSN)*
Colorado State University–Pueblo, Department of Nursing, *Pueblo (BSN)*
Denver College of Nursing, *Denver (BSN)*
Mesa State College, Department of Nursing and Radiologic Sciences, *Grand Junction (BSN)*
Metropolitan State College of Denver, Department of Health Professions, *Denver (BS)*
Regis University, School of Nursing, *Denver (BSN)*
University of Colorado at Colorado Springs, Beth-El College of Nursing and Health Sciences, *Colorado Springs (BSN)*
University of Colorado Denver, College of Nursing, *Denver (BS)*
University of Northern Colorado, School of Nursing, *Greeley (BS)*

Connecticut

Central Connecticut State University, Department of Nursing, *New Britain (BSN)*
Fairfield University, School of Nursing, *Fairfield (BS)*
Sacred Heart University, Program in Nursing, *Fairfield (BS)*
Saint Joseph College, Department of Nursing, *West Hartford (BS)*
Southern Connecticut State University, Department of Nursing, *New Haven (BS)*
University of Hartford, College of Education, Nursing, and Health Professions, *West Hartford (BSN)*
Western Connecticut State University, Department of Nursing, *Danbury (BS)*

Delaware

University of Delaware, School of Nursing, *Newark (BSN)*
Wilmington University, College of Health Professions, *New Castle (BSN)*

District of Columbia

Howard University, Division of Nursing, *Washington (BSN)*
Trinity (Washington) University, Nursing Program, *Washington (BSN)*
University of the District of Columbia, Nursing Education Program, *Washington (BSN)*

Florida

Barry University, School of Nursing, *Miami Shores (BSN)*
Bethune-Cookman University, School of Nursing, *Daytona Beach (BSN)*
Florida Atlantic University, Christine E. Lynn College of Nursing, *Boca Raton (BS)*
Florida Hospital College of Health Sciences, Department of Nursing, *Orlando (BS)*
Florida International University, Nursing Program, *Miami (BSN)*
Florida State College at Jacksonville, Nursing Department, *Jacksonville (BSN)*
Florida State University, College of Nursing, *Tallahassee (BSN)*
Indian River State College, Bachelor of Science in Nursing Program, *Fort Pierce (BSN)*
Miami Dade College, School of Nursing, *Miami (BSN)*
Northwest Florida State College, RN to BSN Degree Program, *Niceville (BSN)*
Nova Southeastern University, College of Allied Health and Nursing, *Fort Lauderdale (BSN)*
Palm Beach Atlantic University, School of Nursing, *West Palm Beach (BSN)*
St. Petersburg College, Department of Nursing, *St. Petersburg (BSN)*
South University, Nursing Program, *Royal Palm Beach (BSN)*
South University, College of Nursing, *Tampa (BSN)*
University of Central Florida, College of Nursing, *Orlando (BSN)*
University of Miami, School of Nursing and Health Studies, *Coral Gables (BSN)*
University of North Florida, School of Nursing, *Jacksonville (BSN)*
University of Phoenix–South Florida Campus, College of Nursing, *Fort Lauderdale (BSN)*
The University of Tampa, Department of Nursing, *Tampa (BSN)*

Georgia

Albany State University, College of Sciences and Health Professions, *Albany (BSN)*
Armstrong Atlantic State University, Program in Nursing, *Savannah (BSN)*
Augusta State University, Department of Nursing, *Augusta (BSN)*
Brenau University, School of Health and Science, *Gainesville (BSN)*
Clayton State University, Department of Nursing, *Morrow (BSN)*
College of Coastal Georgia, Department of Nursing and Health Sciences, *Brunswick (BS)*
Columbus State University, Nursing Program, *Columbus (BSN)*
Georgia Baptist College of Nursing of Mercer University, Department of Nursing, *Atlanta (BSN)*
Georgia College & State University, College of Health Sciences, *Milledgeville (BSN)*
Georgia Southwestern State University, School of Nursing, *Americus (BSN)*
Gordon College, Division of Nursing and Health Sciences, *Barnesville (BSN)*
Kennesaw State University, School of Nursing, *Kennesaw (BSN)*
LaGrange College, Department of Nursing, *LaGrange (BSN)*
Piedmont College, School of Nursing, *Demorest (BSN)*
Thomas University, Division of Nursing, *Thomasville (BSN)*
University of West Georgia, School of Nursing, *Carrollton (BSN)*
Valdosta State University, College of Nursing, *Valdosta (BSN)*

Guam

University of Guam, School of Nursing and Health Sciences, *Mangilao (BSN)*

Hawaii

Hawai`i Pacific University, College of Nursing and Health Sciences, *Honolulu (BSN)*
University of Hawaii at Hilo, Department in Nursing, *Hilo (BSN)*
University of Hawaii at Manoa, School of Nursing and Dental Hygiene, *Honolulu (BSN)*

Idaho

Boise State University, Department of Nursing, *Boise (BS)*
Brigham Young University–Idaho, Department of Nursing, *Rexburg (BSN)*

Illinois

Aurora University, School of Nursing, *Aurora (BSN)*
Blessing–Rieman College of Nursing, *Quincy (BSN)*
Bradley University, Department of Nursing, *Peoria (BSN; BSc PN)*
Chicago State University, Department of Nursing, *Chicago (BSN)*
Eastern Illinois University, Nursing Program, *Charleston (BSN)*
Elmhurst College, Deicke Center for Nursing Education, *Elmhurst (BS)*
Governors State University, College of Health and Human Services, *University Park (BS)*
Illinois State University, Mennonite College of Nursing, *Normal (BSN)*
Lakeview College of Nursing, *Danville (BSN)*
Loyola University Chicago, Marcella Niehoff School of Nursing, *Maywood (BSN)*
MacMurray College, Department of Nursing, *Jacksonville (BSN)*
Methodist College of Nursing, *Peoria (BSN)*
Millikin University, School of Nursing, *Decatur (BSN)*
Northern Illinois University, School of Nursing and Health Studies, *De Kalb (BS)*
North Park University, School of Nursing, *Chicago (BS)*
Resurrection University, *Oak Park (BSN)*
Rockford College, Department of Nursing, *Rockford (BSN)*
Saint Anthony College of Nursing, *Rockford (BSN)*
Saint Francis Medical Center College of Nursing, Baccalaureate Nursing Program, *Peoria (BSN)*
Trinity Christian College, Department of Nursing, *Palos Heights (BSN)*
Trinity College of Nursing and Health Sciences, *Rock Island (BSN)*
University of Illinois at Chicago, College of Nursing, *Chicago (BSN)*
Western Illinois University, School of Nursing, *Macomb (BSN)*

Indiana

Ball State University, School of Nursing, *Muncie (BS)*

Bethel College, Department of Nursing, *Mishawaka (BSN)*

Goshen College, Department of Nursing, *Goshen (BSN)*

Huntington University, Department of Nursing, *Huntington (BSN)*

Indiana State University, Department of Nursing, *Terre Haute (BS)*

Indiana University Bloomington, Department of Nursing–Bloomington Division, *Bloomington (BSN)*

Indiana University East, School of Nursing, *Richmond (BSN)*

Indiana University Northwest, School of Nursing and Health Professions, *Gary (BSN)*

Indiana University–Purdue University Fort Wayne, Department of Nursing, *Fort Wayne (BS)*

Indiana University–Purdue University Indianapolis, School of Nursing, *Indianapolis (BSN)*

Indiana University South Bend, Division of Nursing and Health Professions, *South Bend (BSN)*

Indiana University Southeast, Division of Nursing, *New Albany (BSN)*

Indiana Wesleyan University, School of Nursing, *Marion (BSN)*

Marian University, Department of Nursing and Nutritional Science, *Indianapolis (BSN)*

Purdue University, School of Nursing, *West Lafayette (BS)*

Purdue University Calumet, School of Nursing, *Hammond (BS)*

Purdue University North Central, Department of Nursing, *Westville (BS)*

University of Evansville, Department of Nursing, *Evansville (BSN)*

University of Saint Francis, Department of Nursing, *Fort Wayne (BSN)*

University of Southern Indiana, College of Nursing and Health Professions, *Evansville (BSN)*

Valparaiso University, College of Nursing, *Valparaiso (BSN)*

Vincennes University, Department of Nursing, *Vincennes (BSN)*

Iowa

Allen College, Program in Nursing, *Waterloo (BSN)*

Briar Cliff University, Department of Nursing, *Sioux City (BSN)*

Clarke University, Department of Nursing and Health, *Dubuque (BS)*

Coe College, Department of Nursing, *Cedar Rapids (BSN)*

Grand View University, Division of Nursing, *Des Moines (BSN)*

Iowa Wesleyan College, Division of Health and Natural Sciences, *Mount Pleasant (BSN)*

Morningside College, Department of Nursing Education, *Sioux City (BSN)*

St. Ambrose University, Program in Nursing (BSN), *Davenport (BSN)*

University of Dubuque, School of Professional Programs, *Dubuque (BSN)*

The University of Iowa, College of Nursing, *Iowa City (BSN)*

Upper Iowa University, RN-BSN Nursing Program, *Fayette (BSN)*

Kansas

Baker University, School of Nursing, *Topeka (BSN)*

Bethel College, Department of Nursing, *North Newton (BSN)*

Emporia State University, Newman Division of Nursing, *Emporia (BSN)*

Fort Hays State University, Department of Nursing, *Hays (BSN)*

Kansas Wesleyan University, Department of Nursing Education, *Salina (BSN)*

MidAmerica Nazarene University, Division of Nursing, *Olathe (BSN)*

Newman University, Division of Nursing, *Wichita (BSN)*

Pittsburg State University, Department of Nursing, *Pittsburg (BSN)*

Southwestern College, Nursing Program, *Winfield (BSN)*

The University of Kansas, School of Nursing, *Kansas City (BSN)*

University of Saint Mary, Bachelor of Science in Nursing Program, *Leavenworth (BSN)*

Washburn University, School of Nursing, *Topeka (BSN)*

Wichita State University, School of Nursing, *Wichita (BSN)*

Kentucky

Bellarmine University, Donna and Allan Lansing School of Nursing and Health Sciences, *Louisville (BSN)*

Eastern Kentucky University, Department of Baccalaureate and Graduate Nursing, *Richmond (BSN)*

Midway College, Program in Nursing (Baccalaureate), *Midway (BSN)*

Morehead State University, Department of Nursing, *Morehead (BSN)*

Murray State University, Program in Nursing, *Murray (BSN)*

Northern Kentucky University, Department of Nursing, *Highland Heights (BSN)*

University of Kentucky, Graduate School Programs in the College of Nursing, *Lexington (BSN)*

University of Louisville, School of Nursing, *Louisville (BSN)*

Louisiana

Dillard University, Division of Nursing, *New Orleans (BSN)*

Grambling State University, School of Nursing, *Grambling (BSN)*

Louisiana State University Health Sciences Center, School of Nursing, *New Orleans (BSN)*

Loyola University New Orleans, School of Nursing, *New Orleans (BSN)*

Nicholls State University, Department of Nursing, *Thibodaux (BSN)*

Northwestern State University of Louisiana, College of Nursing, *Shreveport (BSN)*

Our Lady of the Lake College, Division of Nursing, *Baton Rouge (BSN)*

Southeastern Louisiana University, School of Nursing, *Hammond (BS)*

University of Louisiana at Monroe, Nursing, *Monroe (BS)*

Maine

Saint Joseph's College of Maine, Department of Nursing, *Standish (BSN)*

University of Maine, School of Nursing, *Orono (BSN)*

University of Maine at Fort Kent, Department of Nursing, *Fort Kent (BSN)*

University of New England, Department of Nursing, *Biddeford (BSN)*

University of Southern Maine, College of Nursing and Health Professions, *Portland (BS)*

Maryland

Bowie State University, Department of Nursing, *Bowie (BSN)*

College of Notre Dame of Maryland, Department of Nursing, *Baltimore (BS)*

Coppin State University, Helene Fuld School of Nursing, *Baltimore (BSN)*

The Johns Hopkins University, School of Nursing, *Baltimore (BS)*

Salisbury University, Program in Nursing, *Salisbury (BS)*

Stevenson University, Nursing Division, *Stevenson (BS)*

Towson University, Department of Nursing, *Towson (BS)*

University of Maryland, Baltimore, Master's Program in Nursing, *Baltimore (BSN)*

Massachusetts

American International College, Division of Nursing, *Springfield (BSN)*

Anna Maria College, Department of Nursing, *Paxton (BSN)*

Atlantic Union College, Department of Nursing, *South Lancaster (BS)*

Curry College, Division of Nursing, *Milton (BS)*

Elms College, Division of Nursing, *Chicopee (BS)*

Emmanuel College, Department of Nursing, *Boston (BSN)*

Endicott College, Major in Nursing, *Beverly (BS)*

Fitchburg State University, Department of Nursing, *Fitchburg (BS)*

Northeastern University, School of Nursing, *Boston (BSN)*

Regis College, School of Nursing and Health Professions, *Weston (BSN)*

Simmons College, Department of Nursing, *Boston (BS)*

University of Massachusetts Boston, College of Nursing and Health Sciences, *Boston (BS)*

University of Massachusetts Dartmouth, College of Nursing, *North Dartmouth (BSN)*

University of Massachusetts Lowell, Department of Nursing, *Lowell (BS)*

Worcester State College, Department of Nursing, *Worcester (BS)*

Michigan

Davenport University, Division of Nursing, *Grand Rapids (BSN)*

Davenport University, Bachelor of Science in Nursing Program, *Kalamazoo (BSN)*

Eastern Michigan University, School of Nursing, *Ypsilanti (BSN)*

Ferris State University, School of Nursing, *Big Rapids (BSN)*

Finlandia University, College of Professional Studies, *Hancock (BSN)*

Grand Valley State University, Kirkhof College of Nursing, *Allendale (BSN)*

Lake Superior State University, Department of Nursing, *Sault Sainte Marie (BSN)*

Madonna University, College of Nursing and Health, *Livonia (BSN)*

Michigan State University, College of Nursing, *East Lansing (BSN)*

Northern Michigan University, College of Nursing and Allied Health Science, *Marquette (BSN)*

Oakland University, School of Nursing, *Rochester (BSN)*

Saginaw Valley State University, Crystal M. Lange College of Nursing and Health Sciences, *University Center (BSN)*

Siena Heights University, Nursing Program, *Adrian (BSN)*

University of Detroit Mercy, McAuley School of Nursing, *Detroit (BSN)*

University of Michigan, School of Nursing, *Ann Arbor (BSN)*

University of Michigan–Flint, Department of Nursing, *Flint (BSN)*

Minnesota

Bemidji State University, Department of Nursing, *Bemidji (BS)*

Bethel University, Department of Nursing, *St. Paul (BSN)*

Minnesota State University Mankato, School of Nursing, *Mankato (BS)*

Minnesota State University Moorhead, School of Nursing and Healthcare Leadership, *Moorhead (BSN)*

St. Catherine University, Department of Nursing, *St. Paul (BS)*

Walden University, Nursing Programs, *Minneapolis (BSN)*

Winona State University, College of Nursing and Health Sciences, *Winona (BS)*

Mississippi

Alcorn State University, School of Nursing, *Natchez (BSN)*

Mississippi College, School of Nursing, *Clinton (BSN)*

Missouri

Chamberlain College of Nursing, *St. Louis (BSN)*

College of the Ozarks, Armstrong McDonald School of Nursing, *Point Lookout (BSN)*

Cox College, Department of Nursing, *Springfield (BSN)*

Goldfarb School of Nursing at Barnes-Jewish College, *St. Louis (BSN)*

Graceland University, School of Nursing, *Independence (BSN)*

Grantham University, Nursing Programs, *Kansas City (BSN)*

Lincoln University, Department of Nursing, *Jefferson City (BSN)*

Maryville University of Saint Louis, Nursing Program, School of Health Professions, *St. Louis (BSN)*

Missouri Southern State University, Department of Nursing, *Joplin (BSN)*

Missouri State University, Department of Nursing, *Springfield (BSN)*

Saint Louis University, School of Nursing, *St. Louis (BSN)*

Southeast Missouri State University, Department of Nursing, *Cape Girardeau (BSN)*

Southwest Baptist University, College of Nursing, *Bolivar (BSN)*

University of Central Missouri, Department of Nursing, *Warrensburg (BS)*

University of Missouri, Sinclair School of Nursing, *Columbia (BSN)*

University of Missouri–Kansas City, School of Nursing, *Kansas City (BSN)*

University of Missouri–St. Louis, College of Nursing, *St. Louis (BSN)*

Webster University, Department of Nursing, *St. Louis (BSN)*

Montana

Montana State University–Northern, College of Nursing, *Havre (BSN)*

Salish Kootenai College, Nursing Department, *Pablo (BS)*

Nebraska

BryanLGH College of Health Sciences, School of Nursing, *Lincoln (BSN)*

Clarkson College, Master of Science in Nursing Program, *Omaha (BSN)*

Creighton University, School of Nursing, *Omaha (BSN)*

Midland Lutheran College, Department of Nursing, *Fremont (BSN)*

Nebraska Wesleyan University, Department of Nursing, *Lincoln (BSN)*

University of Nebraska Medical Center, College of Nursing, *Omaha (BSN)*

Nevada

Great Basin College, BSN Program, *Elko (BSN)*

Nevada State College at Henderson, Nursing Program, *Henderson (BSN)*

Touro University, School of Nursing, *Henderson (BSN)*

University of Nevada, Reno, Orvis School of Nursing, *Reno (BSN)*

New Hampshire

Franklin Pierce University, Master of Science in Nursing, *Rindge (BS)*

Rivier College, Division of Nursing, *Nashua (BS)*

Saint Anselm College, Department of Nursing, *Manchester (BSN)*

University of New Hampshire, Department of Nursing, *Durham (BS)*

New Jersey

Bloomfield College, Division of Nursing, *Bloomfield (BS)*

College of Saint Elizabeth, Department of Nursing, *Morristown (BSN)*

Fairleigh Dickinson University, Metropolitan Campus, Henry P. Becton School of Nursing and Allied Health, *Teaneck (BSN)*

Kean University, Department of Nursing, *Union (BSN)*

Monmouth University, Marjorie K. Unterberg School of Nursing, *West Long Branch (BSN)*

New Jersey City University, Department of Nursing, *Jersey City (BSN)*

Ramapo College of New Jersey, Master of Science in Nursing Program, *Mahwah (BSN)*

The Richard Stockton College of New Jersey, Program in Nursing, *Pomona (BSN)*

Rutgers, The State University of New Jersey, Camden College of Arts and Sciences, Department of Nursing, *Camden (BS)*

Rutgers, The State University of New Jersey, College of Nursing, *Newark (BS)*

Saint Peter's College, Nursing Program, *Jersey City (BSN)*

Seton Hall University, College of Nursing, *South Orange (BSN)*

University of Medicine and Dentistry of New Jersey, School of Nursing, *Newark (BSN)*

William Paterson University of New Jersey, Department of Nursing, *Wayne (BSN)*

New Mexico

New Mexico Highlands University, Department of Nursing, *Las Vegas (BSN)*

New Mexico State University, School of Nursing, *Las Cruces (BSN)*

University of New Mexico, College of Nursing, *Albuquerque (BSN)*

Western New Mexico University, Nursing Department, *Silver City (BSN)*

New York

Adelphi University, School of Nursing, *Garden City (BS)*

The College of New Rochelle, School of Nursing, *New Rochelle (BSN)*

College of Staten Island of the City University of New York, Department of Nursing, *Staten Island (BS)*

Daemen College, Department of Nursing, *Amherst (BS)*

Dominican College, Department of Nursing, *Orangeburg (BSN)*

D'Youville College, Department of Nursing, *Buffalo (BSN)*

Elmira College, Program in Nursing Education, *Elmira (BS)*

Excelsior College, School of Nursing, *Albany (BS)*

Farmingdale State College, Nursing Department, *Farmingdale (BS)*

Hartwick College, Department of Nursing, *Oneonta (BS)*

Hunter College of the City University of New York, Hunter-Bellevue School of Nursing, *New York (BS)*

Lehman College of the City University of New York, Department of Nursing, *Bronx (BS)*

Le Moyne College, Nursing Programs, *Syracuse (BS)*

Long Island University, Brooklyn Campus, School of Nursing, *Brooklyn (BS)*

Long Island University, C.W. Post Campus, Department of Nursing, *Brookville (BS)*

Mercy College, Program in Nursing, *Dobbs Ferry (BS)*

Molloy College, Division of Nursing, *Rockville Centre (BS)*

Mount Saint Mary College, Division of Nursing, *Newburgh (BSN)*

Nazareth College of Rochester, Department of Nursing, *Rochester (BS)*

New York City College of Technology of the City University of New York, Department of Nursing, *Brooklyn (BS)*

New York University, College of Nursing, *New York (BS)*

Niagara University, Department of Nursing, *Niagara University (BS)*

Roberts Wesleyan College, Division of Nursing, *Rochester (BScN)*

The Sage Colleges, Department of Nursing, *Troy (BS)*

St. John Fisher College, Advanced Practice Nursing Program, *Rochester (BS)*

St. Joseph's College, New York, Department of Nursing, *Brooklyn (BSN)*

State University of New York at Plattsburgh, Department of Nursing, *Plattsburgh (BS)*

State University of New York College of Agriculture and Technology at Morrisville, Division of Nursing, *Morrisville (BS)*

State University of New York College of Technology at Delhi, Bachelor of Science in Nursing Program, *Delhi (BSN)*

State University of New York Downstate Medical Center, College of Nursing, *Brooklyn (BS)*

State University of New York Empire State College, Bachelor of Science in Nursing Program, *Saratoga Springs (BS)*

State University of New York Institute of Technology, School of Nursing and Health Systems, *Utica (BS)*

Stony Brook University, State University of New York, School of Nursing, *Stony Brook (BS)*

University of Rochester, School of Nursing, *Rochester (BS)*

Utica College, Department of Nursing, *Utica (BS)*

York College of the City University of New York, Program in Nursing, *Jamaica (BS)*

North Carolina

Appalachian State University, Department of Nursing, *Boone (BSN)*

Barton College, School of Nursing, *Wilson (BSN)*

Cabarrus College of Health Sciences, Louise Harkey School of Nursing, *Concord (BSN)*

Fayetteville State University, Program in Nursing, *Fayetteville (BS)*

Gardner-Webb University, School of Nursing, *Boiling Springs (BSN)*

North Carolina Agricultural and Technical State University, School of Nursing, *Greensboro (BSN)*

Queens University of Charlotte, Presbyterian School of Nursing, *Charlotte (BSN)*

The University of North Carolina at Chapel Hill, School of Nursing, *Chapel Hill (BSN)*

The University of North Carolina at Charlotte, School of Nursing, *Charlotte (BSN)*

The University of North Carolina at Greensboro, School of Nursing, *Greensboro (BSN)*

The University of North Carolina at Pembroke, Nursing Program, *Pembroke (BSN)*

The University of North Carolina Wilmington, School of Nursing, *Wilmington (BS)*

Western Carolina University, School of Nursing, *Cullowhee (BSN)*

Winston-Salem State University, Department of Nursing, *Winston-Salem (BSN)*

North Dakota

Dickinson State University, Department of Nursing, *Dickinson (BSN)*

Medcenter One College of Nursing, *Bismarck (BSN)*

Minot State University, Department of Nursing, *Minot (BSN)*

University of Mary, Division of Nursing, *Bismarck (BS)*

University of North Dakota, College of Nursing, *Grand Forks (BSN)*

Ohio

Ashland University, Dwight Schar College of Nursing, *Ashland (BSN)*

Capital University, School of Nursing, *Columbus (BSN)*

Case Western Reserve University, Frances Payne Bolton School of Nursing, *Cleveland (BSN)*

Cedarville University, Department of Nursing, *Cedarville (BSN)*

Chamberlain College of Nursing, *Columbus (BSN)*

Cleveland State University, School of Nursing, *Cleveland (BSN)*

Defiance College, Bachelor's Degree in Nursing, *Defiance (BSN)*

Franciscan University of Steubenville, Department of Nursing, *Steubenville (BSN)*

Kent State University, College of Nursing, *Kent (BSN)*

Kettering College of Medical Arts, Division of Nursing, *Kettering (BSN)*

Lourdes College, School of Nursing, *Sylvania (BSN)*

Malone University, School of Nursing, *Canton (BSN)*

Mercy College of Northwest Ohio, Division of Nursing, *Toledo (BSN)*

Miami University, Department of Nursing, *Hamilton (BSN)*

Miami University Hamilton, Bachelor of Science in Nursing Program, *Hamilton (BSN)*

Mount Carmel College of Nursing, Nursing Programs, *Columbus (BSN)*

Mount Vernon Nazarene University, School of Nursing and Health Sciences, *Mount Vernon (BSN)*

Notre Dame College, Nursing Department, *South Euclid (BSN)*

Ohio Northern University, Nursing Program, *Ada (BSN)*

The Ohio State University, College of Nursing, *Columbus (BSN)*

Ohio University, School of Nursing, *Athens (BSN)*

Otterbein University, Department of Nursing, *Westerville (BSN)*

Shawnee State University, Department of Nursing, *Portsmouth (BSN)*

The University of Akron, College of Nursing, *Akron (BSN)*

University of Cincinnati, College of Nursing, *Cincinnati (BSN)*

University of Rio Grande, Holzer School of Nursing, *Rio Grande (BSN)*

Urbana University, BSN Completion Program, *Urbana (BSN)*

Walsh University, Department of Nursing, *North Canton (BSN)*

Wright State University, College of Nursing and Health, *Dayton (BSN)*

Oklahoma

Langston University, School of Nursing and Health Professions, *Langston (BSN)*

Northeastern State University, Department of Nursing, *Tahlequah (BSN)*

Northwestern Oklahoma State University, Division of Nursing, *Alva (BSN)*

Oklahoma Baptist University, School of Nursing, *Shawnee (BSN)*

Oklahoma Wesleyan University, School of Nursing, *Bartlesville (BSN)*

Oral Roberts University, Anna Vaughn School of Nursing, *Tulsa (BSN)*

Southwestern Oklahoma State University, Division of Nursing, *Weatherford (BSN)*

University of Central Oklahoma, Department of Nursing, *Edmond (BSN)*

University of Tulsa, School of Nursing, *Tulsa (BSN)*

Oregon

Oregon Health & Science University, School of Nursing, *Portland (BS)*

Pennsylvania

Alvernia University, Nursing, *Reading (BSN)*

Bloomsburg University of Pennsylvania, Department of Nursing, *Bloomsburg (BSN)*

California University of Pennsylvania, Department of Nursing, *California (BSN)*

Cedar Crest College, Department of Nursing, *Allentown (BS)*

Clarion University of Pennsylvania, School of Nursing, *Oil City (BSN)*

DeSales University, Department of Nursing and Health, *Center Valley (BSN)*

Drexel University, College of Nursing and Health Professions, *Philadelphia (BSN)*

East Stroudsburg University of Pennsylvania, Department of Nursing, *East Stroudsburg (BS)*

Gannon University, Villa Maria School of Nursing, *Erie (BSN)*

Gwynedd-Mercy College, School of Nursing, *Gwynedd Valley (BSN)*

Holy Family University, School of Nursing and Allied Health Professions, *Philadelphia (BSN)*

Indiana University of Pennsylvania, Department of Nursing and Allied Health, *Indiana (BSN)*

La Roche College, Department of Nursing and Nursing Management, *Pittsburgh (BSN)*

La Salle University, School of Nursing and Health Sciences, *Philadelphia (BSN)*

Mansfield University of Pennsylvania, Department of Health Sciences–Nursing, *Mansfield (BSN)*

Marywood University, Department of Nursing, *Scranton (BSN)*

Millersville University of Pennsylvania, Department of Nursing, *Millersville (BSN)*

Misericordia University, Department of Nursing, *Dallas (BSN)*

Moravian College, St. Luke's School of Nursing, *Bethlehem (BS)*

Neumann University, Program in Nursing and Health Sciences, *Aston (BS)*

Penn State University Park, School of Nursing, *University Park (BS)*

Pennsylvania College of Technology, School of Health Sciences, *Williamsport (BSN)*

Saint Francis University, Department of Nursing, *Loretto (BSN)*
Slippery Rock University of Pennsylvania, Department of Nursing, *Slippery Rock (BSN)*
Temple University, Department of Nursing, *Philadelphia (BSN)*
Thomas Jefferson University, Department of Nursing, *Philadelphia (BSN)*
University of Pennsylvania, School of Nursing, *Philadelphia (BSN)*
University of Pittsburgh, School of Nursing, *Pittsburgh (BSN)*
University of Pittsburgh at Bradford, Department of Nursing, *Bradford (BSN)*
The University of Scranton, Department of Nursing, *Scranton (BS)*
Villanova University, College of Nursing, *Villanova (BSN)*
Widener University, School of Nursing, *Chester (BSN)*
Wilkes University, Department of Nursing, *Wilkes-Barre (BS)*
York College of Pennsylvania, Department of Nursing, *York (BS)*

Puerto Rico

Universidad Adventista de las Antillas, Department of Nursing, *Mayagüez (BSN)*

Rhode Island

Rhode Island College, Department of Nursing, *Providence (BSN)*
Salve Regina University, Department of Nursing, *Newport (BS)*
University of Rhode Island, College of Nursing, *Kingston (BS)*

South Carolina

Charleston Southern University, Wingo School of Nursing, *Charleston (BSN)*
Clemson University, School of Nursing, *Clemson (BS)*
Lander University, School of Nursing, *Greenwood (BSN)*
South Carolina State University, Department of Nursing, *Orangeburg (BSN)*
University of South Carolina Aiken, School of Nursing, *Aiken (BSN)*
University of South Carolina Beaufort, Nursing Program, *Bluffton (BSN)*
University of South Carolina Upstate, Mary Black School of Nursing, *Spartanburg (BSN)*

South Dakota

Dakota Wesleyan University, Nursing Department, *Mitchell (BA)*
Mount Marty College, Nursing Program, *Yankton (BSN)*
Presentation College, Department of Nursing, *Aberdeen (BSN)*
South Dakota State University, College of Nursing, *Brookings (BS)*

Tennessee

Aquinas College, Department of Nursing, *Nashville (BSN)*
Austin Peay State University, School of Nursing, *Clarksville (BSN)*
Baptist College of Health Sciences, Nursing Division, *Memphis (BSN)*
Belmont University, School of Nursing, *Nashville (BSN)*
Carson-Newman College, Department of Nursing, *Jefferson City (BSN)*
Cumberland University, Rudy School of Nursing and Health Professions, *Lebanon (BSN)*
East Tennessee State University, College of Nursing, *Johnson City (BSN)*
Lincoln Memorial University, Caylor School of Nursing, *Harrogate (BSN)*
Middle Tennessee State University, School of Nursing, *Murfreesboro (BSN)*
Milligan College, Department of Nursing, *Milligan College (BSN)*
Tennessee State University, School of Nursing, *Nashville (BSN)*
Tennessee Technological University, Whitson-Hester School of Nursing, *Cookeville (BSN)*
Tennessee Wesleyan College, Fort Sanders Nursing Department, *Knoxville (BSN)*
Union University, School of Nursing, *Jackson (BSN)*
University of Memphis, Loewenberg School of Nursing, *Memphis (BSN)*

Texas

Angelo State University, Department of Nursing, *San Angelo (BSN)*
Lamar University, Department of Nursing, *Beaumont (BSN)*
Lubbock Christian University, Department of Nursing, *Lubbock (BSN)*
Midwestern State University, Nursing Program, *Wichita Falls (BSN)*
Patty Hanks Shelton School of Nursing, *Abilene (BSN)*
Prairie View A&M University, College of Nursing, *Houston (BSN)*
Stephen F. Austin State University, Richard and Lucille Dewitt School of Nursing, *Nacogdoches (BSN)*
Texas A&M Health Science Center, College of Nursing, *College Station (BSN)*
Texas A&M International University, Canseco School of Nursing, *Laredo (BSN)*
Texas A&M University–Corpus Christi, School of Nursing and Health Sciences, *Corpus Christi (BSN)*
Texas Woman's University, College of Nursing, *Denton (BS)*
University of Houston–Victoria, School of Nursing, *Victoria (BSN)*
The University of Texas at Arlington, College of Nursing, *Arlington (BSN)*
The University of Texas at Austin, School of Nursing, *Austin (BSN)*
The University of Texas at El Paso, School of Nursing, *El Paso (BSN)*
The University of Texas at Tyler, Program in Nursing, *Tyler (BSN)*
The University of Texas Medical Branch, School of Nursing, *Galveston (BSN)*
The University of Texas–Pan American, Department of Nursing, *Edinburg (BSN)*
Wayland Baptist University, Bachelor of Science in Nursing Program, *Plainview (BSN)*

Utah

Brigham Young University, College of Nursing, *Provo (BS)*
Dixie State College of Utah, Nursing Department, *St. George (BSN)*
Southern Utah University, Department of Nursing, *Cedar City (BSN)*
University of Utah, College of Nursing, *Salt Lake City (BS)*
Western Governors University, Online College of Health Professions, *Salt Lake City (BS)*
Westminster College, School of Nursing and Health Sciences, *Salt Lake City (BSN)*

Vermont

Norwich University, Department of Nursing, *Northfield (BSN)*
Southern Vermont College, Department of Nursing, *Bennington (BSN)*

Virgin Islands

University of the Virgin Islands, Division of Nursing, *Saint Thomas (BSN)*

Virginia

Eastern Mennonite University, Department of Nursing, *Harrisonburg (BSN)*
ECPI College of Technology, BSN Program, *Virginia Beach (BSN)*
George Mason University, College of Health and Human Services, *Fairfax (BSN)*
Hampton University, School of Nursing, *Hampton (BS)*
Jefferson College of Health Sciences, Nursing Education Program, *Roanoke (BSN)*
Liberty University, Department of Nursing, *Lynchburg (BSN)*
Marymount University, School of Health Professions, *Arlington (BSN)*
Norfolk State University, Department of Nursing, *Norfolk (BSN)*
Old Dominion University, Department of Nursing, *Norfolk (BSN)*
Radford University, School of Nursing, *Radford (BSN)*
Shenandoah University, Division of Nursing, *Winchester (BSN)*
University of Virginia, School of Nursing, *Charlottesville (BSN)*
The University of Virginia's College at Wise, Department of Nursing, *Wise (BSN)*

Washington

Olympic College, Nursing Programs, *Bremerton (BSN)*
Seattle Pacific University, School of Health Sciences, *Seattle (BS)*
Walla Walla University, School of Nursing, *College Place (BS)*
Washington State University College of Nursing and Consortium, *Spokane (BSN)*

West Virginia

Alderson-Broaddus College, Department of Nursing, *Philippi (BSN)*
Bluefield State College, Program in Nursing, *Bluefield (BSN)*
Fairmont State University, School of Nursing and Allied Health Administration, *Fairmont (BSN)*
Mountain State University, College of Nursing, *Beckley (BSN)*
Shepherd University, Department of Nursing Education, *Shepherdstown (BSN)*
West Virginia University, School of Nursing, *Morgantown (BSN)*
Wheeling Jesuit University, Department of Nursing, *Wheeling (BSN)*

Wisconsin

Alverno College, Division of Nursing, *Milwaukee (BSN)*

Columbia College of Nursing/Mount Mary College Nursing Program, *Milwaukee (BSN)*

Concordia University Wisconsin, Program in Nursing, *Mequon (BSN)*

Maranatha Baptist Bible College, Nursing Department, *Watertown (BSN)*

Milwaukee School of Engineering, School of Nursing, *Milwaukee (BSN)*

University of Phoenix–Milwaukee Campus, College of Health and Human Services, *Milwaukee (BSN)*

University of Wisconsin–Eau Claire, College of Nursing and Health Sciences, *Eau Claire (BSN)*

University of Wisconsin–Green Bay, BSN–LINC Online RN–BSN Program, *Green Bay (BSN)*

University of Wisconsin–Madison, School of Nursing, *Madison (BS)*

University of Wisconsin–Milwaukee, College of Nursing, *Milwaukee (BSN)*

University of Wisconsin–Oshkosh, College of Nursing, *Oshkosh (BSN)*

Viterbo University, School of Nursing, *La Crosse (BSN)*

CANADA

Alberta

Athabasca University, Centre for Nursing and Health Studies, *Athabasca (BN)*

University of Alberta, Faculty of Nursing, *Edmonton (BScN)*

University of Calgary, Faculty of Nursing, *Calgary (BN)*

University of Lethbridge, School of Health Sciences, *Lethbridge (BN)*

British Columbia

British Columbia Institute of Technology, School of Health Sciences, *Burnaby (BSN)*

Kwantlen Polytechnic University, Faculty of Community and Health Sciences, *Surrey (BSN)*

University of Northern British Columbia, Nursing Programme, *Prince George (BScN)*

Manitoba

Brandon University, School of Health Studies, *Brandon (BN)*

University of Manitoba, Faculty of Nursing, *Winnipeg (BN)*

New Brunswick

Université de Moncton, School of Nursing, *Moncton (BScN)*

Newfoundland and Labrador

Memorial University of Newfoundland, School of Nursing, *St. John's (BN)*

Nova Scotia

Dalhousie University, School of Nursing, *Halifax (BScN)*

St. Francis Xavier University, Department of Nursing, *Antigonish (BScN)*

Ontario

Brock University, Department of Nursing, *St. Catharines (BScN)*

Lakehead University, School of Nursing, *Thunder Bay (BScN)*

McMaster University, School of Nursing, *Hamilton (BScN)*

Queen's University at Kingston, School of Nursing, *Kingston (BNSc)*

Ryerson University, Program in Nursing, *Toronto (BScN)*

University of Ottawa, School of Nursing, *Ottawa (BScN)*

The University of Western Ontario, School of Nursing, *London (BScN)*

York University, School of Nursing, *Toronto (BScN)*

Quebec

McGill University, School of Nursing, *Montréal (BScN)*

Université de Montréal, Faculty of Nursing, *Montréal (BScN)*

Université de Sherbrooke, Department of Nursing, *Sherbrooke (BScN)*

Université du Québec à Chicoutimi, Program in Nursing, *Chicoutimi (BNSc)*

Université du Québec à Rimouski, Program in Nursing, *Rimouski (BScN)*

Université du Québec à Trois-Rivières, Program in Nursing, *Trois-Rivières (BSN)*

Université du Québec en Outaouais, Département des Sciences Infirmières, *Gatineau (BScN)*

Université Laval, Faculty of Nursing, *Québec (BScN)*

Saskatchewan

University of Saskatchewan, College of Nursing, *Saskatoon (BSN)*

RPN TO BACCALAUREATE

U.S. AND U.S. TERRITORIES

California

San Jose State University, The Valley Foundation School of Nursing, *San Jose (BS)*

Massachusetts

Curry College, Division of Nursing, *Milton (BS)*

Michigan

Lake Superior State University, Department of Nursing, *Sault Sainte Marie (BSN)*

Nebraska

University of Nebraska Medical Center, College of Nursing, *Omaha (BSN)*

New Mexico

Eastern New Mexico University, Department of Allied Health–Nursing, *Portales (BSN)*

New York

St. Francis College, Department of Nursing, *Brooklyn Heights (BS)*

Ohio

Franciscan University of Steubenville, Department of Nursing, *Steubenville (BSN)*

CANADA

Alberta

University of Alberta, Faculty of Nursing, *Edmonton (BScN)*

British Columbia

British Columbia Institute of Technology, School of Health Sciences, *Burnaby (BSN)*

Ontario

Ryerson University, Program in Nursing, *Toronto (BScN)*

University of Ottawa, School of Nursing, *Ottawa (BScN)*

MASTER'S DEGREE PROGRAMS

ACCELERATED AD/RN TO MASTER'S

U.S. AND U.S. TERRITORIES

Alabama

Spring Hill College, Division of Nursing, *Mobile (MSN)*

California

California State University, Fullerton, Department of Nursing, *Fullerton (MSN)*
University of San Francisco, School of Nursing, *San Francisco (MSN)*
Western University of Health Sciences, College of Graduate Nursing, *Pomona (MSN)*

Delaware

Wesley College, Nursing Program, *Dover (MSN)*
Wilmington University, College of Health Professions, *New Castle (MSN, MSN/MBA, MSN/MS)*

Florida

Florida International University, Nursing Program, *Miami (MSN)*
Florida Southern College, Department of Nursing, *Lakeland (MSN, MSN/MBA)*

Georgia

Albany State University, College of Sciences and Health Professions, *Albany (MSN)*
Brenau University, School of Health and Science, *Gainesville (MSN)*

Idaho

Idaho State University, Department of Nursing, *Pocatello (MS)*

Kentucky

Frontier School of Midwifery and Family Nursing, Nursing Degree Programs, *Hyden (MSN)*

Massachusetts

Regis College, School of Nursing and Health Professions, *Weston (MSN)*
Simmons College, Department of Nursing, *Boston (MS)*

Michigan

Ferris State University, School of Nursing, *Big Rapids (MSN, MSN/MBA)*
University of Detroit Mercy, McAuley School of Nursing, *Detroit (MSN)*

Mississippi

University of Mississippi Medical Center, Program in Nursing, *Jackson (MSN)*

Missouri

Missouri State University, Department of Nursing, *Springfield (MSN)*

Nebraska

Nebraska Wesleyan University, Department of Nursing, *Lincoln (MSN)*

New York

Daemen College, Department of Nursing, *Amherst (MS)*
State University of New York Institute of Technology, School of Nursing and Health Systems, *Utica (MS)*
University of Rochester, School of Nursing, *Rochester (MS, MSN/PhD)*

Ohio

Case Western Reserve University, Frances Payne Bolton School of Nursing, *Cleveland (MSN, MSN/MA, MSN/MBA, MSN/MPH)*

Pennsylvania

DeSales University, Department of Nursing and Health, *Center Valley (MSN, MSN/MBA)*
Gannon University, Villa Maria School of Nursing, *Erie (MSN)*
University of Pennsylvania, School of Nursing, *Philadelphia (MSN, MSN/MPH, MSN/PhD)*
The University of Scranton, Department of Nursing, *Scranton (MSN)*
Wilkes University, Department of Nursing, *Wilkes-Barre (MS)*

Tennessee

Middle Tennessee State University, School of Nursing, *Murfreesboro (MSN)*
Vanderbilt University, School of Nursing, *Nashville (MSN, MSN/MDIV, MSN/MTS)*

Texas

Texas A&M University–Corpus Christi, School of Nursing and Health Sciences, *Corpus Christi (MSN)*
The University of Texas at Tyler, Program in Nursing, *Tyler (MSN, MSN/MBA)*
University of the Incarnate Word, Program in Nursing, *San Antonio (MSN)*

West Virginia

West Virginia University, School of Nursing, *Morgantown (MSN)*

ACCELERATED MASTER'S

U.S. AND U.S. TERRITORIES

Alabama

University of South Alabama, College of Nursing, *Mobile (MSN)*

California

California State University, Fresno, Department of Nursing, *Fresno (MSN)*
California State University, Long Beach, Department of Nursing, *Long Beach (MSN, MSN/MHeA)*
University of Phoenix–Sacramento Valley Campus, College of Nursing, *Sacramento (MSN, MSN/MHA)*
Western University of Health Sciences, College of Graduate Nursing, *Pomona (MSN)*

Georgia

Albany State University, College of Sciences and Health Professions, *Albany (MSN)*
Georgia Health Sciences University, School of Nursing, *Augusta (MSN)*
Thomas University, Division of Nursing, *Thomasville (MSN, MSN/MBA)*

Hawaii

University of Hawaii at Manoa, School of Nursing and Dental Hygiene, *Honolulu (MS, MSN/MBA)*

Illinois

Benedictine University, Department of Nursing, *Lisle (MSN)*
Lewis University, Program in Nursing, *Romeoville (MSN, MSN/MBA)*

Massachusetts

Boston College, William F. Connell School of Nursing, *Chestnut Hill (MS, MSN/MA, MSN/MBA, MSN/PhD)*
Regis College, School of Nursing and Health Professions, *Weston (MSN)*
Simmons College, Department of Nursing, *Boston (MS)*
University of Massachusetts Lowell, Department of Nursing, *Lowell (MS)*

Nebraska

Nebraska Wesleyan University, Department of Nursing, *Lincoln (MSN)*

New York

Roberts Wesleyan College, Division of Nursing, *Rochester (M Sc N)*
The Sage Colleges, Department of Nursing, *Troy (MS, MS/MBA)*

Ohio

Ursuline College, The Breen School of Nursing, *Pepper Pike (MSN)*

Oklahoma

Southern Nazarene University, School of Nursing, *Bethany (MS)*

Pennsylvania

Carlow University, School of Nursing, *Pittsburgh (MSN)*
Thomas Jefferson University, Department of Nursing, *Philadelphia (MSN)*
Villanova University, College of Nursing, *Villanova (MSN)*
Waynesburg University, Department of Nursing, *Waynesburg (MSN, MSN/MBA)*

Tennessee

Vanderbilt University, School of Nursing, *Nashville (MSN, MSN/MDIV, MSN/MTS)*

Washington

Pacific Lutheran University, School of Nursing, *Tacoma (MSN, MSN/MBA)*

West Virginia

West Virginia University, School of Nursing, *Morgantown (MSN)*

Wisconsin

Cardinal Stritch University, Ruth S. Coleman College of Nursing, *Milwaukee (MSN)*

CANADA

British Columbia

Trinity Western University, Department of Nursing, *Langley (MSN)*

Quebec

Université Laval, Faculty of Nursing, *Québec (MSN)*

ACCELERATED MASTER'S FOR NON-NURSING COLLEGE GRADUATES

U.S. AND U.S. TERRITORIES

Alabama

The University of Alabama at Birmingham, School of Nursing, *Birmingham (MSN, MSN/MPH)*

Arizona

The University of Arizona, College of Nursing, *Tucson (MS)*

California

Azusa Pacific University, School of Nursing, *Azusa (MSN)*
California Baptist University, School of Nursing, *Riverside (MSN)*
California State University, Fullerton, Department of Nursing, *Fullerton (MSN)*
San Francisco State University, School of Nursing, *San Francisco (MSN)*
Sonoma State University, Department of Nursing, *Rohnert Park (MSN)*
University of San Diego, Hahn School of Nursing and Health Science, *San Diego (MSN)*
University of San Francisco, School of Nursing, *San Francisco (MSN)*
Western University of Health Sciences, College of Graduate Nursing, *Pomona (MSN)*

Georgia

Georgia Health Sciences University, School of Nursing, *Augusta (MSN)*

Illinois

Millikin University, School of Nursing, *Decatur (MSN)*

Indiana

University of Indianapolis, School of Nursing, *Indianapolis (MSN, MSN/MBA)*

Maryland

University of Maryland, Baltimore, Master's Program in Nursing, *Baltimore (MS, MSN/MBA, MSN/MPH, MSN/JD)*

Massachusetts

Boston College, William F. Connell School of Nursing, *Chestnut Hill (MS, MSN/MA, MSN/MBA, MSN/PhD)*
Northeastern University, School of Nursing, *Boston (MS, MSN/MBA)*
Regis College, School of Nursing and Health Professions, *Weston (MSN)*
Salem State University, Program in Nursing, *Salem (MSN, MSN/MBA)*
Simmons College, Department of Nursing, *Boston (MS)*
University of Massachusetts Worcester, Graduate School of Nursing, *Worcester (MS)*

Missouri

Saint Louis University, School of Nursing, *St. Louis (MSN)*

New York

Columbia University, School of Nursing, *New York (MS, MSN/MBA, MSN/MPH)*
Mercy College, Program in Nursing, *Dobbs Ferry (MS)*
University of Rochester, School of Nursing, *Rochester (MS, MSN/PhD)*

North Carolina

East Carolina University, College of Nursing, *Greenville (MSN)*

Ohio

College of Mount St. Joseph, Department of Nursing, *Cincinnati (MN)*
The Ohio State University, College of Nursing, *Columbus (MS, MS/MPH)*
University of Cincinnati, College of Nursing, *Cincinnati (MSN, MSN/MBA, MSN/PhD)*

Oregon

Oregon Health & Science University, School of Nursing, *Portland (MS, MN/MPH)*

Pennsylvania

University of Pennsylvania, School of Nursing, *Philadelphia (MSN, MSN/MPH, MSN/PhD)*

Tennessee

The University of Tennessee Health Science Center, College of Nursing, *Memphis (MSN)*
Vanderbilt University, School of Nursing, *Nashville (MSN, MSN/MDIV, MSN/MTS)*

Virginia

Virginia Commonwealth University, School of Nursing, *Richmond (MS)*

ACCELERATED MASTER'S FOR NURSES WITH NON-NURSING DEGREES

U.S. AND U.S. TERRITORIES

California

Azusa Pacific University, School of Nursing, *Azusa (MSN)*
California State University, Los Angeles, School of Nursing, *Los Angeles (MSN)*
San Francisco State University, School of Nursing, *San Francisco (MSN)*

Connecticut

University of Connecticut, School of Nursing, *Storrs (MS, MS/MBA)*

Illinois

Bradley University, Department of Nursing, *Peoria (MSN)*
Lewis University, Program in Nursing, *Romeoville (MSN, MSN/MBA)*
Resurrection University, *Oak Park (MSN)*

Massachusetts

Boston College, William F. Connell School of Nursing, *Chestnut Hill (MS, MSN/MA, MSN/MBA, MSN/PhD)*
Regis College, School of Nursing and Health Professions, *Weston (MSN)*
Simmons College, Department of Nursing, *Boston (MS)*

Mississippi

Delta State University, School of Nursing, *Cleveland (MSN)*

New Jersey

Kean University, Department of Nursing, *Union (MSN, MSN/MPA)*
Seton Hall University, College of Nursing, *South Orange (MSN, MSN/MA, MSN/MBA)*

New York

Mercy College, Program in Nursing, *Dobbs Ferry (MS)*
Roberts Wesleyan College, Division of Nursing, *Rochester (M Sc N)*

North Carolina

East Carolina University, College of Nursing, *Greenville (MSN)*

Ohio

The Ohio State University, College of Nursing, *Columbus (MS, MS/MPH)*

Oklahoma

Southern Nazarene University, School of Nursing, *Bethany (MS)*

Pennsylvania

Waynesburg University, Department of Nursing, *Waynesburg (MSN, MSN/MBA)*

Tennessee

University of Memphis, Loewenberg School of Nursing, *Memphis (MSN)*
The University of Tennessee, College of Nursing, *Knoxville (MSN)*

Washington

Seattle University, College of Nursing, *Seattle (MSN)*
Washington State University College of Nursing and Consortium, *Spokane (MN)*

ACCELERATED RN TO MASTER'S

U.S. AND U.S. TERRITORIES

Arizona

The University of Arizona, College of Nursing, *Tucson (MS)*

California

California State University, Los Angeles, School of Nursing, *Los Angeles (MSN)*

Delaware

Wesley College, Nursing Program, *Dover (MSN)*

Georgia

Brenau University, School of Health and Science, *Gainesville (MSN)*

Illinois

Lewis University, Program in Nursing, *Romeoville (MSN, MSN/MBA)*
Saint Francis Medical Center College of Nursing, Baccalaureate Nursing Program, *Peoria (MSN)*

Iowa

The University of Iowa, College of Nursing, *Iowa City (MSN, MSN/MBA, MSN/MPH)*

Kentucky

Spalding University, School of Nursing, *Louisville (MSN)*

Massachusetts

Regis College, School of Nursing and Health Professions, *Weston (MSN)*

Simmons College, Department of Nursing, *Boston (MS)*

University of Massachusetts Lowell, Department of Nursing, *Lowell (MS)*

Michigan

University of Michigan, School of Nursing, *Ann Arbor (MS, MSN/MBA, MSN/MPH)*

University of Michigan–Flint, Department of Nursing, *Flint (MSN)*

Minnesota

Minnesota State University Mankato, School of Nursing, *Mankato (MSN, MSN/MS)*

Missouri

Maryville University of Saint Louis, Nursing Program, School of Health Professions, *St. Louis (MSN)*

Nebraska

Nebraska Wesleyan University, Department of Nursing, *Lincoln (MSN)*

New Jersey

Fairleigh Dickinson University, Metropolitan Campus, Henry P. Becton School of Nursing and Allied Health, *Teaneck (MSN)*

Felician College, Division of Nursing and Health Management, *Lodi (MSN, MA/MSM)*

New York

Daemen College, Department of Nursing, *Amherst (MS)*

Mercy College, Program in Nursing, *Dobbs Ferry (MS)*

The Sage Colleges, Department of Nursing, *Troy (MS, MS/MBA)*

State University of New York Institute of Technology, School of Nursing and Health Systems, *Utica (MS)*

State University of New York Upstate Medical University, College of Nursing, *Syracuse (MS)*

University of Rochester, School of Nursing, *Rochester (MS, MSN/PhD)*

Ohio

Kent State University, College of Nursing, *Kent (MSN, MSN/MBA, MSN/MPA)*

Pennsylvania

Gannon University, Villa Maria School of Nursing, *Erie (MSN)*

Thomas Jefferson University, Department of Nursing, *Philadelphia (MSN)*

University of Pennsylvania, School of Nursing, *Philadelphia (MSN, MSN/MPH, MSN/PhD)*

The University of Scranton, Department of Nursing, *Scranton (MSN)*

Waynesburg University, Department of Nursing, *Waynesburg (MSN, MSN/MBA)*

Wilkes University, Department of Nursing, *Wilkes-Barre (MS)*

Tennessee

King College, School of Nursing, *Bristol (MSN, MSN/MBA)*

Southern Adventist University, School of Nursing, *Collegedale (MSN, MSN/MBA)*

The University of Tennessee, College of Nursing, *Knoxville (MSN)*

Vanderbilt University, School of Nursing, *Nashville (MSN, MSN/MDIV, MSN/MTS)*

Texas

Texas A&M University–Corpus Christi, School of Nursing and Health Sciences, *Corpus Christi (MSN)*

The University of Texas at Tyler, Program in Nursing, *Tyler (MSN, MSN/MBA)*

Washington

Gonzaga University, Department of Nursing, *Spokane (MSN)*

Washington State University College of Nursing and Consortium, *Spokane (MN)*

West Virginia

West Virginia University, School of Nursing, *Morgantown (MSN)*

CANADA

Quebec

Université du Québec à Chicoutimi, Program in Nursing, *Chicoutimi (MSN, MS/MPH)*

JOINT DEGREES

U.S. AND U.S. TERRITORIES

Alabama

Samford University, Ida V. Moffett School of Nursing, *Birmingham (MSN, MSN/MBA)*

The University of Alabama, Capstone College of Nursing, *Tuscaloosa (MSN, MSN/MA, MSN/Ed D)*

The University of Alabama at Birmingham, School of Nursing, *Birmingham (MSN, MSN/MPH)*

Arizona

Arizona State University at the Downtown Phoenix Campus, College of Nursing, *Phoenix (MS, MS/MPH)*

Grand Canyon University, College of Nursing and Health Sciences, *Phoenix (MS, MSN/MBA)*

University of Phoenix, Online Campus, *Phoenix (MSN, MSN/MBA, MSN/MHA)*

University of Phoenix–Phoenix Campus, College of Nursing, *Phoenix (MSN, MSN/MBA, MSN/MHA)*

California

California State University, Long Beach, Department of Nursing, *Long Beach (MSN, MSN/MHeA)*

Holy Names University, Department of Nursing, *Oakland (MSN, MSN/MBA)*

University of California, Los Angeles, School of Nursing, *Los Angeles (MSN, MSN/MBA)*

University of Phoenix–Bay Area Campus, College of Health and Human Services, *Pleasanton (MSN, MSN/MBA, MSN/MHA)*

University of Phoenix–Sacramento Valley Campus, College of Nursing, *Sacramento (MSN, MSN/MHA)*

University of Phoenix–Southern California Campus, College of Nursing, *Costa Mesa (MSN, MSN/MBA, MSN/MHA)*

Colorado

University of Phoenix–Denver Campus, College of Nursing, *Lone Tree (MSN, MSN/MHA, MSN/Ed D)*

Connecticut

University of Connecticut, School of Nursing, *Storrs (MS, MS/MBA)*

University of Hartford, College of Education, Nursing, and Health Professions, *West Hartford (MSN, MSN/MSOB)*

Yale University, School of Nursing, *New Haven (MSN, MSN/MPH, MSN/MDIV)*

Delaware

Wilmington University, College of Health Professions, *New Castle (MSN, MSN/MBA, MSN/MS)*

District of Columbia

The Catholic University of America, School of Nursing, *Washington (MSN, MA/MSM)*

Florida

Barry University, School of Nursing, *Miami Shores (MSN, MSN/MBA)*

Florida Atlantic University, Christine E. Lynn College of Nursing, *Boca Raton (MS, MSN/MBA)*

Florida Southern College, Department of Nursing, *Lakeland (MSN, MSN/MBA)*

Jacksonville University, School of Nursing, *Jacksonville (MSN, MSN/MBA)*

Nova Southeastern University, College of Allied Health and Nursing, *Fort Lauderdale (MSN, MSN/MBA)*

University of Florida, College of Nursing, *Gainesville (MSN, MSN/PhD)*

University of Phoenix–North Florida Campus, College of Nursing, *Jacksonville (MSN, MSN/MHA, MSN/Ed D)*

University of Phoenix–South Florida Campus, College of Nursing, *Fort Lauderdale (MSN, MSN/MBA, MSN/MHA)*

University of South Florida, College of Nursing, *Tampa (MS, MS/MPH)*

Georgia

Armstrong Atlantic State University, Program in Nursing, *Savannah (MSN, MS/MHSA)*

Emory University, Nell Hodgson Woodruff School of Nursing, *Atlanta (MSN, MSN/MPH)*

Georgia College & State University, College of Health Sciences, *Milledgeville (MSN, MSN/MBA)*

Thomas University, Division of Nursing, *Thomasville (MSN, MSN/MBA)*

Hawaii

Hawai`i Pacific University, College of Nursing and Health Sciences, *Honolulu (MSN, MSN/MBA)*

University of Hawaii at Manoa, School of Nursing and Dental Hygiene, *Honolulu (MS, MSN/MBA)*

Idaho

Boise State University, Department of Nursing, *Boise (MSN, MSN/MS)*

Illinois

Elmhurst College, Deicke Center for Nursing Education, *Elmhurst (MS, MSN/MBA)*

Lewis University, Program in Nursing, *Romeoville (MSN, MSN/MBA)*

Loyola University Chicago, Marcella Niehoff School of Nursing, *Maywood (MSN, MSN/MBA, MSN/MDIV)*

Northern Illinois University, School of Nursing and Health Studies, *De Kalb (MS, MSN/MPH)*

North Park University, School of Nursing, *Chicago (MS, MSN/MA, MSN/MBA, MSN/MM)*

Saint Xavier University, School of Nursing, *Chicago (MSN, MSN/MBA)*

University of Illinois at Chicago, College of Nursing, *Chicago (MS, MS/MBA, MS/MPH)*

Indiana

Anderson University, School of Nursing, *Anderson (MSN, MSN/MBA)*

Indiana University–Purdue University Indianapolis, School of Nursing, *Indianapolis (MSN, MSN/MPH)*

University of Indianapolis, School of Nursing, *Indianapolis (MSN, MSN/MBA)*

Valparaiso University, College of Nursing, *Valparaiso (MSN, MSN/MBA)*

Iowa

The University of Iowa, College of Nursing, *Iowa City (MSN, MSN/MBA, MSN/MPH)*

Kansas

The University of Kansas, School of Nursing, *Kansas City (MS, MS/MHSA, MS/MPH)*

Wichita State University, School of Nursing, *Wichita (MSN, MSN/MBA)*

Kentucky

Bellarmine University, Donna and Allan Lansing School of Nursing and Health Sciences, *Louisville (MSN, MSN/MBA)*

Maine

Saint Joseph's College of Maine, Department of Nursing, *Standish (MSN, MSN/MHA)*

University of Southern Maine, College of Nursing and Health Professions, *Portland (MS, MS/MBA)*

Maryland

The Johns Hopkins University, School of Nursing, *Baltimore (MSN, MSN/MBA, MSN/MPH, MSN/PhD)*

University of Maryland, Baltimore, Master's Program in Nursing, *Baltimore (MS, MSN/MBA, MSN/MPH, MSN/JD)*

Massachusetts

Boston College, William F. Connell School of Nursing, *Chestnut Hill (MS, MSN/MA, MSN/MBA, MSN/PhD)*

Northeastern University, School of Nursing, *Boston (MS, MSN/MBA)*

Salem State University, Program in Nursing, *Salem (MSN, MSN/MBA)*

Michigan

Ferris State University, School of Nursing, *Big Rapids (MSN, MSN/MBA)*

Madonna University, College of Nursing and Health, *Livonia (M Sc N, MSN/MBA)*

Spring Arbor University, Program in Nursing, *Spring Arbor (MSN, MSN/MBA)*

University of Michigan, School of Nursing, *Ann Arbor (MS, MSN/MBA, MSN/MPH)*

Minnesota

Minnesota State University Mankato, School of Nursing, *Mankato (MSN, MSN/MS)*

University of Minnesota, Twin Cities Campus, School of Nursing, *Minneapolis (MS, MS/MPH)*

Missouri

University of Missouri, Sinclair School of Nursing, *Columbia (MSN, MSN/PhD)*

Nevada

University of Nevada, Reno, Orvis School of Nursing, *Reno (MSN, MSN/MPH)*

New Jersey

Felician College, Division of Nursing and Health Management, *Lodi (MSN, MA/MSM)*

Kean University, Department of Nursing, *Union (MSN, MSN/MPA)*

Rutgers, The State University of New Jersey, College of Nursing, *Newark (MS, MS/MPH)*

Seton Hall University, College of Nursing, *South Orange (MSN, MSN/MA, MSN/MBA)*

New Mexico

University of New Mexico, College of Nursing, *Albuquerque (MSN, MSN/MALAS, MSN/MPA, MSN/MPH)*

New York

Adelphi University, School of Nursing, *Garden City (MS, MS/MBA)*

Columbia University, School of Nursing, *New York (MS, MSN/MBA, MSN/MPH)*

Hunter College of the City University of New York, Hunter-Bellevue School of Nursing, *New York (MS, MS/MPH)*

New York University, College of Nursing, *New York (MS, MS/MPH)*

The Sage Colleges, Department of Nursing, *Troy (MS, MS/MBA)*

State University of New York Downstate Medical Center, College of Nursing, *Brooklyn (MS, MS/MPH)*

University of Rochester, School of Nursing, *Rochester (MS, MSN/PhD)*

North Carolina

Duke University, School of Nursing, *Durham (MSN, MSN/MBA)*

Gardner-Webb University, School of Nursing, *Boiling Springs (MSN, MSN/MBA)*

Queens University of Charlotte, Presbyterian School of Nursing, *Charlotte (MSN, MSN/MBA)*

The University of North Carolina at Greensboro, School of Nursing, *Greensboro (MSN, MSN/MBA)*

North Dakota

University of Mary, Division of Nursing, *Bismarck (MSN, MSN/MBA)*

Ohio

Capital University, School of Nursing, *Columbus (MSN, MN/MBA, MSN/JD, MSN/MDIV)*

Case Western Reserve University, Frances Payne Bolton School of Nursing, *Cleveland (MSN, MSN/MA, MSN/MBA, MSN/MPH)*

Cleveland State University, School of Nursing, *Cleveland (MSN, MSN/MBA)*

Kent State University, College of Nursing, *Kent (MSN, MSN/MBA, MSN/MPA)*

The Ohio State University, College of Nursing, *Columbus (MS, MS/MPH)*

University of Cincinnati, College of Nursing, *Cincinnati (MSN, MSN/MBA, MSN/PhD)*

Wright State University, College of Nursing and Health, *Dayton (MS, MS/MBA)*

Xavier University, School of Nursing, *Cincinnati (MSN, MSN/MBA)*

Oklahoma

Oklahoma City University, Kramer School of Nursing, *Oklahoma City (MSN, MSN/MBA)*

Oregon

Oregon Health & Science University, School of Nursing, *Portland (MS, MN/MPH)*

Pennsylvania

Bloomsburg University of Pennsylvania, Department of Nursing, *Bloomsburg (MSN, MSN/MBA)*

DeSales University, Department of Nursing and Health, *Center Valley (MSN, MSN/MBA)*

La Salle University, School of Nursing and Health Sciences, *Philadelphia (MSN, MSN/MBA)*

Marywood University, Department of Nursing, *Scranton (MSN, MSN/MPH)*

Penn State University Park, School of Nursing, *University Park (MS, MSN/PhD)*

University of Pennsylvania, School of Nursing, *Philadelphia (MSN, MSN/MPH, MSN/PhD)*

Waynesburg University, Department of Nursing, *Waynesburg (MSN, MSN/MBA)*

Widener University, School of Nursing, *Chester (MSN, MSN/PhD)*

Tennessee

King College, School of Nursing, *Bristol (MSN, MSN/MBA)*

Southern Adventist University, School of Nursing, *Collegedale (MSN, MSN/MBA)*

Vanderbilt University, School of Nursing, *Nashville (MSN, MSN/MDIV, MSN/MTS)*

Texas

Lamar University, Department of Nursing, *Beaumont (MSN, MSN/MBA)*

Midwestern State University, Nursing Program, *Wichita Falls (MSN, MN/MHSA, MSN/MHA)*

Texas Woman's University, College of Nursing, *Denton (MS, MSN/MHA)*

The University of Texas at Arlington, College of Nursing, *Arlington (MSN, MSN/MBA, MSN/MHA, MSN/MPH)*

The University of Texas at Austin, School of Nursing, *Austin (MSN, MSN/MBA)*

The University of Texas at Tyler, Program in Nursing, *Tyler (MSN, MSN/MBA)*

The University of Texas Health Science Center at Houston, School of Nursing, *Houston (MSN, MSN/MPH)*

The University of Texas Health Science Center at San Antonio, School of Nursing, *San Antonio (MSN, MSN/MPH)*

Utah

University of Utah, College of Nursing, *Salt Lake City (MS, MSN/MPH)*

Virginia

Lynchburg College, School of Health Sciences and Human Performance, *Lynchburg (MSN, MSN/MBA)*

University of Virginia, School of Nursing, *Charlottesville (MSN, MSN/MBA, MSN/PhD)*

Washington

Pacific Lutheran University, School of Nursing, *Tacoma (MSN, MSN/MBA)*

University of Washington, School of Nursing, *Seattle (MN, MN/MPH)*

Wisconsin

Edgewood College, Program in Nursing, *Madison (MS, MSN/MBA)*

Marquette University, College of Nursing, *Milwaukee (MSN, MSN/MBA)*

University of Wisconsin–Milwaukee, College of Nursing, *Milwaukee (MN, MSN/MBA)*

CANADA

Alberta

Athabasca University, Centre for Nursing and Health Studies, *Athabasca (MN, MN/MHSA, MN/MBA)*

British Columbia

The University of British Columbia, Program in Nursing, *Vancouver (MSN, MA/MSM)*

Nova Scotia

Dalhousie University, School of Nursing, *Halifax (MN, MN/MHSA)*

Ontario

McMaster University, School of Nursing, *Hamilton (M Sc, MSN/PhD)*

Quebec

Université du Québec à Chicoutimi, Program in Nursing, *Chicoutimi (MSN, MS/MPH)*

MASTER'S

U.S. AND U.S. TERRITORIES

Alabama

Auburn University, School of Nursing, *Auburn University (MSN)*

Auburn University Montgomery, School of Nursing, *Montgomery (MSN)*

Jacksonville State University, College of Nursing and Health Sciences, *Jacksonville (MSN)*

Samford University, Ida V. Moffett School of Nursing, *Birmingham (MSN, MSN/MBA)*

Spring Hill College, Division of Nursing, *Mobile (MSN)*

Troy University, School of Nursing, *Troy (MSN)*

The University of Alabama, Capstone College of Nursing, *Tuscaloosa (MSN, MSN/MA, MSN/Ed D)*

The University of Alabama at Birmingham, School of Nursing, *Birmingham (MSN, MSN/MPH)*

The University of Alabama in Huntsville, College of Nursing, *Huntsville (MSN)*

University of Mobile, School of Nursing, *Mobile (MSN)*

University of North Alabama, College of Nursing and Allied Health, *Florence (MSN)*

University of South Alabama, College of Nursing, *Mobile (MSN)*

Alaska

University of Alaska Anchorage, School of Nursing, *Anchorage (MS)*

Arizona

Arizona State University at the Downtown Phoenix Campus, College of Nursing, *Phoenix (MS, MS/MPH)*

Chamberlain College of Nursing, *Phoenix (MSN)*

Grand Canyon University, College of Nursing and Health Sciences, *Phoenix (MS, MSN/MBA)*

Northern Arizona University, School of Nursing, *Flagstaff (MS)*

The University of Arizona, College of Nursing, *Tucson (MS)*

University of Phoenix, Online Campus, *Phoenix (MSN, MSN/MBA, MSN/MHA)*

University of Phoenix–Phoenix Campus, College of Nursing, *Phoenix (MSN, MSN/MBA, MSN/MHA)*

University of Phoenix–Southern Arizona Campus, College of Social Sciences, *Tucson (MSN)*

Arkansas

Arkansas State University - Jonesboro, Department of Nursing, *State University (MSN)*

Arkansas Tech University, Program in Nursing, *Russellville (MSN)*

University of Arkansas, Eleanor Mann School of Nursing, *Fayetteville (MSN)*

University of Arkansas for Medical Sciences, College of Nursing, *Little Rock (MN Sc)*

University of Central Arkansas, Department of Nursing, *Conway (MSN)*

California

Azusa Pacific University, School of Nursing, *Azusa (MSN)*

California Baptist University, School of Nursing, *Riverside (MSN)*

California State University, Chico, School of Nursing, *Chico (MSN)*

California State University, Dominguez Hills, Program in Nursing, *Carson (MSN)*

California State University, Fresno, Department of Nursing, *Fresno (MSN)*

California State University, Fullerton, Department of Nursing, *Fullerton (MSN)*

California State University, Long Beach, Department of Nursing, *Long Beach (MSN, MSN/MHeA)*

California State University, Los Angeles, School of Nursing, *Los Angeles (MSN)*

California State University, Sacramento, Division of Nursing, *Sacramento (MS)*

California State University, San Bernardino, Department of Nursing, *San Bernardino (MSN)*

Dominican University of California, Program in Nursing, *San Rafael (MSN)*

Holy Names University, Department of Nursing, *Oakland (MSN, MSN/MBA)*

Loma Linda University, School of Nursing, *Loma Linda (MS)*

Mount St. Mary's College, Department of Nursing, *Los Angeles (MSN)*

Point Loma Nazarene University, School of Nursing, *San Diego (MSN)*

Samuel Merritt University, School of Nursing, *Oakland (MSN)*

San Diego State University, School of Nursing, *San Diego (MSN)*

San Francisco State University, School of Nursing, *San Francisco (MSN)*

San Jose State University, The Valley Foundation School of Nursing, *San Jose (MS)*

Sonoma State University, Department of Nursing, *Rohnert Park (MSN)*

University of California, Irvine, Program in Nursing Science, *Irvine (MS)*

University of California, Los Angeles, School of Nursing, *Los Angeles (MSN, MSN/MBA)*

University of California, San Francisco, School of Nursing, *San Francisco (MS)*

University of Phoenix–Bay Area Campus, College of Health and Human Services, *Pleasanton (MSN, MSN/MBA, MSN/MHA)*

University of Phoenix–San Diego Campus, College of Nursing, *San Diego (MSN, MSN/Ed D)*

University of Phoenix–Southern California Campus, College of Nursing, *Costa Mesa (MSN, MSN/MBA, MSN/MHA)*

University of San Diego, Hahn School of Nursing and Health Science, *San Diego (MSN)*

Western University of Health Sciences, College of Graduate Nursing, *Pomona (MSN)*

Colorado

American Sentinel University, RN to Bachelor of Science Nursing, *Aurora (MSN)*

Colorado State University–Pueblo, Department of Nursing, *Pueblo (MS)*

Regis University, School of Nursing, *Denver (MS)*

University of Colorado at Colorado Springs, Beth-El College of Nursing and Health Sciences, *Colorado Springs (MSN)*

University of Colorado Denver, College of Nursing, *Denver (MS)*

University of Northern Colorado, School of Nursing, *Greeley (MS)*

University of Phoenix–Denver Campus, College of Nursing, *Lone Tree (MSN, MSN/MHA, MSN/Ed D)*

Connecticut

Fairfield University, School of Nursing, *Fairfield (MSN)*

Quinnipiac University, Department of Nursing, *Hamden (MSN)*

Sacred Heart University, Program in Nursing, *Fairfield (MSN)*

Saint Joseph College, Department of Nursing, *West Hartford (MS)*

Southern Connecticut State University, Department of Nursing, *New Haven (MSN)*

University of Connecticut, School of Nursing, *Storrs (MS, MS/MBA)*

University of Hartford, College of Education, Nursing, and Health Professions, *West Hartford (MSN, MSN/MSOB)*

Western Connecticut State University, Department of Nursing, *Danbury (MS)*

Yale University, School of Nursing, *New Haven (MSN, MSN/MPH, MSN/MDIV)*

Delaware

University of Delaware, School of Nursing, *Newark (MSN)*

Wesley College, Nursing Program, *Dover (MSN)*

Wilmington University, College of Health Professions, *New Castle (MSN, MSN/MBA, MSN/MS)*

District of Columbia

The Catholic University of America, School of Nursing, *Washington (MSN, MA/MSM)*
Georgetown University, School of Nursing and Health Studies, *Washington (MS)*
The George Washington University, Department of Nursing Education, *Washington (MSN)*
Howard University, Division of Nursing, *Washington (MSN)*

Florida

Barry University, School of Nursing, *Miami Shores (MSN, MSN/MBA)*
Florida Agricultural and Mechanical University, School of Nursing, *Tallahassee (MSN)*
Florida Atlantic University, Christine E. Lynn College of Nursing, *Boca Raton (MS, MSN/MBA)*
Florida Gulf Coast University, School of Nursing, *Fort Myers (MSN)*
Florida International University, Nursing Program, *Miami (MSN)*
Florida Southern College, Department of Nursing, *Lakeland (MSN, MSN/MBA)*
Florida State University, College of Nursing, *Tallahassee (MSN)*
Jacksonville University, School of Nursing, *Jacksonville (MSN, MSN/MBA)*
Kaplan University Online, The School of Nursing Online, *Fort Lauderdale (MSN)*
Nova Southeastern University, College of Allied Health and Nursing, *Fort Lauderdale (MSN, MSN/MBA)*
South University, Nursing Program, *Royal Palm Beach (MSN)*
South University, College of Nursing, *Tampa (MS)*
University of Central Florida, College of Nursing, *Orlando (MSN)*
University of Florida, College of Nursing, *Gainesville (MSN, MSN/PhD)*
University of Miami, School of Nursing and Health Studies, *Coral Gables (MSN)*
University of North Florida, School of Nursing, *Jacksonville (MSN)*
University of Phoenix–Central Florida Campus, College of Nursing, *Maitland (MSN, MSN/Ed D)*
University of Phoenix–North Florida Campus, College of Nursing, *Jacksonville (MSN, MSN/MHA, MSN/Ed D)*
University of Phoenix–South Florida Campus, College of Nursing, *Fort Lauderdale (MSN, MSN/MBA, MSN/MHA)*
University of South Florida, College of Nursing, *Tampa (MS, MS/MPH)*
The University of Tampa, Department of Nursing, *Tampa (MSN)*

Georgia

Albany State University, College of Sciences and Health Professions, *Albany (MSN)*
Armstrong Atlantic State University, Program in Nursing, *Savannah (MSN, MS/MHSA)*
Brenau University, School of Health and Science, *Gainesville (MSN)*
Clayton State University, Department of Nursing, *Morrow (MSN)*
Emory University, Nell Hodgson Woodruff School of Nursing, *Atlanta (MSN, MSN/MPH)*
Georgia Baptist College of Nursing of Mercer University, Department of Nursing, *Atlanta (MSN)*
Georgia College & State University, College of Health Sciences, *Milledgeville (MSN, MSN/MBA)*
Georgia Health Sciences University, School of Nursing, *Augusta (MSN)*
Georgia Southern University, School of Nursing, *Statesboro (MSN)*
Georgia State University, Byrdine F. Lewis School of Nursing, *Atlanta (MSN)*
Kennesaw State University, School of Nursing, *Kennesaw (MSN)*
North Georgia College & State University, Department of Nursing, *Dahlonega (MS)*
Thomas University, Division of Nursing, *Thomasville (MSN, MSN/MBA)*
University of West Georgia, School of Nursing, *Carrollton (MSN)*
Valdosta State University, College of Nursing, *Valdosta (MSN)*

Hawaii

Hawai`i Pacific University, College of Nursing and Health Sciences, *Honolulu (MSN, MSN/MBA)*
University of Hawaii at Manoa, School of Nursing and Dental Hygiene, *Honolulu (MS, MSN/MBA)*
University of Phoenix–Hawaii Campus, College of Nursing, *Honolulu (MSN, MSN/Ed D)*

Idaho

Boise State University, Department of Nursing, *Boise (MSN, MSN/MS)*
Idaho State University, Department of Nursing, *Pocatello (MS)*
Northwest Nazarene University, School of Health and Science, *Nampa (MSN)*

Illinois

Aurora University, School of Nursing, *Aurora (MSN)*
Benedictine University, Department of Nursing, *Lisle (MSN)*
Blessing–Rieman College of Nursing, *Quincy (MSN)*
Bradley University, Department of Nursing, *Peoria (MSN)*
DePaul University, Department of Nursing, *Chicago (MS)*
Elmhurst College, Deicke Center for Nursing Education, *Elmhurst (MS, MSN/MBA)*
Governors State University, College of Health and Human Services, *University Park (MS)*
Illinois State University, Mennonite College of Nursing, *Normal (MSN)*
Loyola University Chicago, Marcella Niehoff School of Nursing, *Maywood (MSN, MSN/MBA, MSN/MDIV)*
McKendree University, Department of Nursing, *Lebanon (MSN)*
Millikin University, School of Nursing, *Decatur (MSN)*
Northern Illinois University, School of Nursing and Health Studies, *De Kalb (MS, MSN/MPH)*
North Park University, School of Nursing, *Chicago (MS, MSN/MA, MSN/MBA, MSN/MM)*
Olivet Nazarene University, Division of Nursing, *Bourbonnais (MSN)*
Resurrection University, *Oak Park (MSN)*
Rush University, College of Nursing, *Chicago (MSN)*
Saint Anthony College of Nursing, *Rockford (MSN)*
Saint Francis Medical Center College of Nursing, Baccalaureate Nursing Program, *Peoria (MSN)*
Saint Xavier University, School of Nursing, *Chicago (MSN, MSN/MBA)*
Southern Illinois University Edwardsville, School of Nursing, *Edwardsville (MS)*
University of Illinois at Chicago, College of Nursing, *Chicago (MS, MS/MBA, MS/MPH)*
University of St. Francis, College of Nursing and Allied Health, *Joliet (MSN)*

Indiana

Anderson University, School of Nursing, *Anderson (MSN, MSN/MBA)*
Ball State University, School of Nursing, *Muncie (MS)*
Bethel College, Department of Nursing, *Mishawaka (MSN)*
Indiana State University, Department of Nursing, *Terre Haute (MSN)*
Indiana University–Purdue University Fort Wayne, Department of Nursing, *Fort Wayne (MS)*
Indiana University–Purdue University Indianapolis, School of Nursing, *Indianapolis (MSN, MSN/MPH)*
Indiana University South Bend, Division of Nursing and Health Professions, *South Bend (MSN)*
Indiana Wesleyan University, School of Nursing, *Marion (MSN)*
Purdue University, School of Nursing, *West Lafayette (MS)*
Purdue University Calumet, School of Nursing, *Hammond (MS)*
University of Indianapolis, School of Nursing, *Indianapolis (MSN, MSN/MBA)*
University of Saint Francis, Department of Nursing, *Fort Wayne (MSN)*
University of Southern Indiana, College of Nursing and Health Professions, *Evansville (MSN)*
Valparaiso University, College of Nursing, *Valparaiso (MSN, MSN/MBA)*

Iowa

Allen College, Program in Nursing, *Waterloo (MSN)*
Briar Cliff University, Department of Nursing, *Sioux City (MSN)*
Clarke University, Department of Nursing and Health, *Dubuque (MSN)*
Grand View University, Division of Nursing, *Des Moines (MS)*
Mount Mercy University, Department of Nursing, *Cedar Rapids (MSN)*
St. Ambrose University, Program in Nursing (BSN), *Davenport (MSN)*

The University of Iowa, College of Nursing, *Iowa City (MSN, MSN/MBA, MSN/MPH)*

Kansas

Fort Hays State University, Department of Nursing, *Hays (MSN)*

Pittsburg State University, Department of Nursing, *Pittsburg (MSN)*

The University of Kansas, School of Nursing, *Kansas City (MS, MS/MHSA, MS/MPH)*

Washburn University, School of Nursing, *Topeka (MSN)*

Wichita State University, School of Nursing, *Wichita (MSN, MSN/MBA)*

Kentucky

Bellarmine University, Donna and Allan Lansing School of Nursing and Health Sciences, *Louisville (MSN, MSN/MBA)*

Eastern Kentucky University, Department of Baccalaureate and Graduate Nursing, *Richmond (MSN)*

Murray State University, Program in Nursing, *Murray (MSN)*

Northern Kentucky University, Department of Nursing, *Highland Heights (MSN)*

Spalding University, School of Nursing, *Louisville (MSN)*

University of Kentucky, Graduate School Programs in the College of Nursing, *Lexington (MSN)*

University of Louisville, School of Nursing, *Louisville (MSN)*

Louisiana

Grambling State University, School of Nursing, *Grambling (MSN)*

Louisiana State University Health Sciences Center, School of Nursing, *New Orleans (MN)*

Loyola University New Orleans, School of Nursing, *New Orleans (MSN)*

McNeese State University, College of Nursing, *Lake Charles (MSN)*

Northwestern State University of Louisiana, College of Nursing, *Shreveport (MSN)*

Our Lady of the Lake College, Division of Nursing, *Baton Rouge (MSN)*

Southeastern Louisiana University, School of Nursing, *Hammond (MSN)*

Southern University and Agricultural and Mechanical College, School of Nursing, *Baton Rouge (MSN)*

University of Louisiana at Lafayette, College of Nursing, *Lafayette (MSN)*

Maine

Husson University, School of Nursing, *Bangor (MSN)*

Saint Joseph's College of Maine, Department of Nursing, *Standish (MSN, MSN/MHA)*

University of Maine, School of Nursing, *Orono (MSN)*

University of Southern Maine, College of Nursing and Health Professions, *Portland (MS, MS/MBA)*

Maryland

Bowie State University, Department of Nursing, *Bowie (MSN)*

Coppin State University, Helene Fuld School of Nursing, *Baltimore (MSN)*

The Johns Hopkins University, School of Nursing, *Baltimore (MSN, MSN/MBA, MSN/MPH, MSN/PhD)*

Salisbury University, Program in Nursing, *Salisbury (MS)*

Towson University, Department of Nursing, *Towson (MS)*

University of Maryland, Baltimore, Master's Program in Nursing, *Baltimore (MS, MSN/MBA, MSN/MPH, MSN/JD)*

Massachusetts

American International College, Division of Nursing, *Springfield (MSN)*

Boston College, William F. Connell School of Nursing, *Chestnut Hill (MS, MSN/MA, MSN/MBA, MSN/PhD)*

Curry College, Division of Nursing, *Milton (MSN)*

Elms College, Division of Nursing, *Chicopee (MSN)*

Emmanuel College, Department of Nursing, *Boston (MS)*

Endicott College, Major in Nursing, *Beverly (MSN)*

Fitchburg State University, Department of Nursing, *Fitchburg (M Sc N)*

Framingham State University, Department of Nursing, *Framingham (MSN)*

MGH Institute of Health Professions, School of Nursing, *Boston (MS)*

Northeastern University, School of Nursing, *Boston (MS, MSN/MBA)*

Regis College, School of Nursing and Health Professions, *Weston (MSN)*

Salem State University, Program in Nursing, *Salem (MSN, MSN/MBA)*

Simmons College, Department of Nursing, *Boston (MS)*

University of Massachusetts Amherst, School of Nursing, *Amherst (MS)*

University of Massachusetts Boston, College of Nursing and Health Sciences, *Boston (MS)*

University of Massachusetts Dartmouth, College of Nursing, *North Dartmouth (MS)*

University of Massachusetts Lowell, Department of Nursing, *Lowell (MS)*

University of Massachusetts Worcester, Graduate School of Nursing, *Worcester (MS)*

Worcester State College, Department of Nursing, *Worcester (MS)*

Michigan

Andrews University, Department of Nursing, *Berrien Springs (MS)*

Eastern Michigan University, School of Nursing, *Ypsilanti (MSN)*

Ferris State University, School of Nursing, *Big Rapids (MSN, MSN/MBA)*

Grand Valley State University, Kirkhof College of Nursing, *Allendale (MSN)*

Madonna University, College of Nursing and Health, *Livonia (M Sc N, MSN/MBA)*

Michigan State University, College of Nursing, *East Lansing (MSN)*

Northern Michigan University, College of Nursing and Allied Health Science, *Marquette (MSN)*

Oakland University, School of Nursing, *Rochester (MSN)*

Saginaw Valley State University, Crystal M. Lange College of Nursing and Health Sciences, *University Center (MSN)*

Spring Arbor University, Program in Nursing, *Spring Arbor (MSN, MSN/MBA)*

University of Detroit Mercy, McAuley School of Nursing, *Detroit (MSN)*

University of Michigan, School of Nursing, *Ann Arbor (MS, MSN/MBA, MSN/MPH)*

University of Phoenix–Metro Detroit Campus, College of Nursing, *Southfield (MSN)*

Wayne State University, College of Nursing, *Detroit (MSN)*

Western Michigan University, College of Health and Human Services, *Kalamazoo (MSN)*

Minnesota

Augsburg College, Program in Nursing, *Minneapolis (MA)*

Bethel University, Department of Nursing, *St. Paul (MA)*

The College of St. Scholastica, Department of Nursing, *Duluth (MA)*

Concordia College, Department of Nursing, *Moorhead (MS)*

Minnesota State University Mankato, School of Nursing, *Mankato (MSN, MSN/MS)*

Minnesota State University Moorhead, School of Nursing and Healthcare Leadership, *Moorhead (MS)*

St. Catherine University, Department of Nursing, *St. Paul (MA)*

University of Minnesota, Twin Cities Campus, School of Nursing, *Minneapolis (MS, MS/MPH)*

Walden University, Nursing Programs, *Minneapolis (MSN)*

Winona State University, College of Nursing and Health Sciences, *Winona (MS)*

Mississippi

Alcorn State University, School of Nursing, *Natchez (MSN)*

Delta State University, School of Nursing, *Cleveland (MSN)*

Mississippi University for Women, College of Nursing and Speech Language Pathology, *Columbus (MSN)*

University of Mississippi Medical Center, Program in Nursing, *Jackson (MSN)*

University of Southern Mississippi, School of Nursing, *Hattiesburg (MSN)*

William Carey University, School of Nursing, *Hattiesburg (MSN)*

Missouri

Central Methodist University, College of Liberal Arts and Sciences, *Fayette (MSN)*

Goldfarb School of Nursing at Barnes-Jewish College, *St. Louis (MSN)*

Graceland University, School of Nursing, *Independence (MSN)*

Grantham University, Nursing Programs, *Kansas City (MSN)*

Maryville University of Saint Louis, Nursing Program, School of Health Professions, *St. Louis (MSN)*

Missouri Southern State University, Department of Nursing, *Joplin (MSN)*

Missouri State University, Department of Nursing, *Springfield (MSN)*

Missouri Western State University, Department of Nursing, *St. Joseph (MSN)*

Research College of Nursing, College of Nursing, *Kansas City (MSN)*

Saint Louis University, School of Nursing, *St. Louis (MSN)*

Southeast Missouri State University, Department of Nursing, *Cape Girardeau (MSN)*

University of Central Missouri, Department of Nursing, *Warrensburg (MS)*

University of Missouri, Sinclair School of Nursing, *Columbia (MSN, MSN/PhD)*

University of Missouri–Kansas City, School of Nursing, *Kansas City (MSN)*

University of Missouri–St. Louis, College of Nursing, *St. Louis (MSN)*

Webster University, Department of Nursing, *St. Louis (MSN)*

Montana

Montana State University, College of Nursing, *Bozeman (MN)*

Nebraska

BryanLGH College of Health Sciences, School of Nursing, *Lincoln (MS)*

Clarkson College, Master of Science in Nursing Program, *Omaha (MSN)*

Creighton University, School of Nursing, *Omaha (MSN)*

Nebraska Methodist College, Department of Nursing, *Omaha (MSN)*

Nebraska Wesleyan University, Department of Nursing, *Lincoln (MSN)*

University of Nebraska Medical Center, College of Nursing, *Omaha (MSN)*

Nevada

Touro University, School of Nursing, *Henderson (MSN)*

University of Nevada, Las Vegas, School of Nursing, *Las Vegas (MSN)*

University of Nevada, Reno, Orvis School of Nursing, *Reno (MSN, MSN/MPH)*

New Hampshire

Franklin Pierce University, Master of Science in Nursing, *Rindge (MSN)*

Rivier College, Division of Nursing, *Nashua (MS)*

University of New Hampshire, Department of Nursing, *Durham (MS)*

New Jersey

The College of New Jersey, School of Nursing, Health and Exercise Science, *Ewing (MSN)*

Fairleigh Dickinson University, Metropolitan Campus, Henry P. Becton School of Nursing and Allied Health, *Teaneck (MSN)*

Felician College, Division of Nursing and Health Management, *Lodi (MSN, MA/MSM)*

Kean University, Department of Nursing, *Union (MSN, MSN/MPA)*

Monmouth University, Marjorie K. Unterberg School of Nursing, *West Long Branch (MSN)*

Ramapo College of New Jersey, Master of Science in Nursing Program, *Mahwah (MSN)*

Rutgers, The State University of New Jersey, College of Nursing, *Newark (MS, MS/MPH)*

Saint Peter's College, Nursing Program, *Jersey City (MSN)*

Seton Hall University, College of Nursing, *South Orange (MSN, MSN/MA, MSN/MBA)*

Thomas Edison State College, School of Nursing, *Trenton (MSN)*

University of Medicine and Dentistry of New Jersey, School of Nursing, *Newark (MSN)*

William Paterson University of New Jersey, Department of Nursing, *Wayne (MSN)*

New Mexico

New Mexico State University, School of Nursing, *Las Cruces (MSN)*

University of New Mexico, College of Nursing, *Albuquerque (MSN, MSN/MALAS, MSN/MPA, MSN/MPH)*

University of Phoenix–New Mexico Campus, College of Nursing, *Albuquerque (MSN, MSN/Ed D)*

New York

Adelphi University, School of Nursing, *Garden City (MS, MS/MBA)*

College of Mount Saint Vincent, Department of Nursing, *Riverdale (MSN)*

The College of New Rochelle, School of Nursing, *New Rochelle (MS)*

College of Staten Island of the City University of New York, Department of Nursing, *Staten Island (MS)*

Columbia University, School of Nursing, *New York (MS, MSN/MBA, MSN/MPH)*

Daemen College, Department of Nursing, *Amherst (MS)*

Dominican College, Department of Nursing, *Orangeburg (M Sc N)*

D'Youville College, Department of Nursing, *Buffalo (MS)*

Excelsior College, School of Nursing, *Albany (MS)*

Hunter College of the City University of New York, Hunter-Bellevue School of Nursing, *New York (MS, MS/MPH)*

Lehman College of the City University of New York, Department of Nursing, *Bronx (MS)*

Le Moyne College, Nursing Programs, *Syracuse (MS)*

Long Island University, Brooklyn Campus, School of Nursing, *Brooklyn (MS)*

Long Island University, C.W. Post Campus, Department of Nursing, *Brookville (MS)*

Mercy College, Program in Nursing, *Dobbs Ferry (MS)*

Molloy College, Division of Nursing, *Rockville Centre (MS)*

Mount Saint Mary College, Division of Nursing, *Newburgh (MS)*

Nazareth College of Rochester, Department of Nursing, *Rochester (MS)*

New York University, College of Nursing, *New York (MS, MS/MPH)*

Pace University, Lienhard School of Nursing, *New York (MS)*

The Sage Colleges, Department of Nursing, *Troy (MS, MS/MBA)*

St. John Fisher College, Advanced Practice Nursing Program, *Rochester (MS)*

St. Joseph's College, New York, Department of Nursing, *Brooklyn (MS)*

State University of New York at Binghamton, Decker School of Nursing, *Binghamton (MS)*

State University of New York Downstate Medical Center, College of Nursing, *Brooklyn (MS, MS/MPH)*

State University of New York Institute of Technology, School of Nursing and Health Systems, *Utica (MS)*

State University of New York Upstate Medical University, College of Nursing, *Syracuse (MS)*

Stony Brook University, State University of New York, School of Nursing, *Stony Brook (MS)*

University at Buffalo, the State University of New York, School of Nursing, *Buffalo (MS)*

University of Rochester, School of Nursing, *Rochester (MS, MSN/PhD)*

North Carolina

Duke University, School of Nursing, *Durham (MSN, MSN/MBA)*

East Carolina University, College of Nursing, *Greenville (MSN)*

Gardner-Webb University, School of Nursing, *Boiling Springs (MSN, MSN/MBA)*

Queens University of Charlotte, Presbyterian School of Nursing, *Charlotte (MSN, MSN/MBA)*

The University of North Carolina at Chapel Hill, School of Nursing, *Chapel Hill (MSN)*

The University of North Carolina at Charlotte, School of Nursing, *Charlotte (MSN)*

The University of North Carolina at Greensboro, School of Nursing, *Greensboro (MSN, MSN/MBA)*

The University of North Carolina Wilmington, School of Nursing, *Wilmington (MSN)*

Western Carolina University, School of Nursing, *Cullowhee (MS)*

Winston-Salem State University, Department of Nursing, *Winston-Salem (MSN)*

North Dakota

North Dakota State University, Department of Nursing, *Fargo (MS)*

University of Mary, Division of Nursing, *Bismarck (MSN, MSN/MBA)*

University of North Dakota, College of Nursing, *Grand Forks (MS)*

Ohio

Capital University, School of Nursing, *Columbus (MSN, MN/MBA, MSN/JD, MSN/MDIV)*

Case Western Reserve University, Frances Payne Bolton School of Nursing, *Cleveland (MSN, MSN/MA, MSN/MBA, MSN/MPH)*

Chamberlain College of Nursing, *Columbus (MSN)*

Cleveland State University, School of Nursing, *Cleveland (MSN, MSN/MBA)*

Franciscan University of Steubenville, Department of Nursing, *Steubenville (MSN)*

Kent State University, College of Nursing, *Kent (MSN, MSN/MBA, MSN/MPA)*

Malone University, School of Nursing, *Canton (MSN)*

Mount Carmel College of Nursing, Nursing Programs, *Columbus (MS)*

The Ohio State University, College of Nursing, *Columbus (MS, MS/MPH)*

Ohio University, School of Nursing, *Athens (MSN)*

Otterbein University, Department of Nursing, *Westerville (MSN)*

The University of Akron, College of Nursing, *Akron (MSN)*

University of Cincinnati, College of Nursing, *Cincinnati (MSN, MSN/MBA, MSN/PhD)*

University of Phoenix–Cleveland Campus, College of Nursing, *Independence (MSN)*

The University of Toledo, College of Nursing, *Toledo (MSN)*

Urbana University, BSN Completion Program, *Urbana (MSN)*

Ursuline College, The Breen School of Nursing, *Pepper Pike (MSN)*

Wright State University, College of Nursing and Health, *Dayton (MS, MS/MBA)*

Xavier University, School of Nursing, *Cincinnati (MSN, MSN/MBA)*

Oklahoma

Northeastern State University, Department of Nursing, *Tahlequah (MSN)*

Oklahoma Baptist University, School of Nursing, *Shawnee (MSN)*

Oklahoma City University, Kramer School of Nursing, *Oklahoma City (MSN, MSN/MBA)*

University of Oklahoma Health Sciences Center, College of Nursing, *Oklahoma City (MS)*

Oregon

Oregon Health & Science University, School of Nursing, *Portland (MS, MN/MPH)*

University of Portland, School of Nursing, *Portland (MS)*

Pennsylvania

Bloomsburg University of Pennsylvania, Department of Nursing, *Bloomsburg (MSN, MSN/MBA)*

Carlow University, School of Nursing, *Pittsburgh (MSN)*

Cedar Crest College, Department of Nursing, *Allentown (MSN)*

Chatham University, Program in Nursing, *Pittsburgh (MSN)*

Clarion University of Pennsylvania, School of Nursing, *Oil City (MSN)*

DeSales University, Department of Nursing and Health, *Center Valley (MSN, MSN/MBA)*

Drexel University, College of Nursing and Health Professions, *Philadelphia (MSN)*

Duquesne University, School of Nursing, *Pittsburgh (MSN)*

Gannon University, Villa Maria School of Nursing, *Erie (MSN)*

Gwynedd-Mercy College, School of Nursing, *Gwynedd Valley (MSN)*

Holy Family University, School of Nursing and Allied Health Professions, *Philadelphia (MSN)*

Immaculata University, Department of Nursing, *Immaculata (MSN)*

Indiana University of Pennsylvania, Department of Nursing and Allied Health, *Indiana (MS)*

La Roche College, Department of Nursing and Nursing Management, *Pittsburgh (MSN)*

La Salle University, School of Nursing and Health Sciences, *Philadelphia (MSN, MSN/MBA)*

Mansfield University of Pennsylvania, Department of Health Sciences–Nursing, *Mansfield (MSN)*

Marywood University, Department of Nursing, *Scranton (MSN, MSN/MPH)*

Millersville University of Pennsylvania, Department of Nursing, *Millersville (MSN)*

Misericordia University, Department of Nursing, *Dallas (MSN)*

Moravian College, St. Luke's School of Nursing, *Bethlehem (MS)*

Neumann University, Program in Nursing and Health Sciences, *Aston (MS)*

Penn State University Park, School of Nursing, *University Park (MS, MSN/PhD)*

Robert Morris University, School of Nursing and Health Sciences, *Moon Township (MSN)*

Temple University, Department of Nursing, *Philadelphia (MSN)*

Thomas Jefferson University, Department of Nursing, *Philadelphia (MSN)*

University of Pennsylvania, School of Nursing, *Philadelphia (MSN, MSN/MPH, MSN/PhD)*

University of Pittsburgh, School of Nursing, *Pittsburgh (MSN)*

The University of Scranton, Department of Nursing, *Scranton (MSN)*

Villanova University, College of Nursing, *Villanova (MSN)*

West Chester University of Pennsylvania, Department of Nursing, *West Chester (MSN)*

Widener University, School of Nursing, *Chester (MSN, MSN/PhD)*

Wilkes University, Department of Nursing, *Wilkes-Barre (MS)*

York College of Pennsylvania, Department of Nursing, *York (MS)*

Puerto Rico

University of Puerto Rico, Medical Sciences Campus, School of Nursing, *San Juan (MSN)*

University of the Sacred Heart, Program in Nursing, *San Juan (MSN)*

Rhode Island

Rhode Island College, Department of Nursing, *Providence (MSN)*

University of Rhode Island, College of Nursing, *Kingston (MS)*

South Carolina

Charleston Southern University, Wingo School of Nursing, *Charleston (MSN)*

Clemson University, School of Nursing, *Clemson (MS)*

Medical University of South Carolina, College of Nursing, *Charleston (MSN)*

University of South Carolina, College of Nursing, *Columbia (MSN)*

South Dakota

South Dakota State University, College of Nursing, *Brookings (MS)*

Tennessee

Belmont University, School of Nursing, *Nashville (MSN)*

Carson-Newman College, Department of Nursing, *Jefferson City (MSN)*

East Tennessee State University, College of Nursing, *Johnson City (MSN)*

King College, School of Nursing, *Bristol (MSN, MSN/MBA)*

Middle Tennessee State University, School of Nursing, *Murfreesboro (MSN)*

Southern Adventist University, School of Nursing, *Collegedale (MSN, MSN/MBA)*

Tennessee Technological University, Whitson-Hester School of Nursing, *Cookeville (MSN, M Sc N)*

Union University, School of Nursing, *Jackson (MSN)*

University of Memphis, Loewenberg School of Nursing, *Memphis (MSN)*

The University of Tennessee, College of Nursing, *Knoxville (MSN)*

The University of Tennessee at Chattanooga, School of Nursing, *Chattanooga (MSN)*

Vanderbilt University, School of Nursing, *Nashville (MSN, MSN/MDIV, MSN/MTS)*

Texas

Angelo State University, Department of Nursing, *San Angelo (MSN)*

Baylor University, Louise Herrington School of Nursing, *Dallas (MSN)*

Lamar University, Department of Nursing, *Beaumont (MSN, MSN/MBA)*

Midwestern State University, Nursing Program, *Wichita Falls (MSN, MN/MHSA, MSN/MHA)*

Patty Hanks Shelton School of Nursing, *Abilene (MSN)*

Prairie View A&M University, College of Nursing, *Houston (MSN)*

Texas A&M International University, Canseco School of Nursing, *Laredo (MSN)*

Texas A&M University–Corpus Christi, School of Nursing and Health Sciences, *Corpus Christi (MSN)*

Texas A&M University–Texarkana, Nursing Department, *Texarkana (MSN)*

Texas Christian University, Harris College of Nursing, *Fort Worth (MSN)*

Texas Tech University Health Sciences Center, School of Nursing, *Lubbock (MSN)*

Texas Woman's University, College of Nursing, *Denton (MS, MSN/MHA)*

University of Houston–Victoria, School of Nursing, *Victoria (MSN)*

University of Mary Hardin-Baylor, College of Nursing, *Belton (MSN)*

The University of Texas at Arlington, College of Nursing, *Arlington (MSN, MSN/MBA, MSN/MHA, MSN/MPH)*

The University of Texas at Austin, School of Nursing, *Austin (MSN, MSN/MBA)*

The University of Texas at Brownsville, Department of Nursing, *Brownsville (MSN)*

The University of Texas at El Paso, School of Nursing, *El Paso (MSN)*

The University of Texas at Tyler, Program in Nursing, *Tyler (MSN, MSN/MBA)*

The University of Texas Health Science Center at Houston, School of Nursing, *Houston (MSN, MSN/MPH)*

The University of Texas Health Science Center at San Antonio, School of Nursing, *San Antonio (MSN, MSN/MPH)*

The University of Texas Medical Branch, School of Nursing, *Galveston (MSN)*

The University of Texas–Pan American, Department of Nursing, *Edinburg (MSN)*

University of the Incarnate Word, Program in Nursing, *San Antonio (MSN)*

West Texas A&M University, Division of Nursing, *Canyon (MSN)*

Utah

Brigham Young University, College of Nursing, *Provo (MS)*

University of Utah, College of Nursing, *Salt Lake City (MS, MSN/MPH)*

Weber State University, Program in Nursing, *Ogden (MSN)*

Westminster College, School of Nursing and Health Sciences, *Salt Lake City (MSN)*

Vermont

University of Vermont, Department of Nursing, *Burlington (MS)*

Virginia

Eastern Mennonite University, Department of Nursing, *Harrisonburg (MSN)*
George Mason University, College of Health and Human Services, *Fairfax (MSN)*
Hampton University, School of Nursing, *Hampton (MS)*
James Madison University, Department of Nursing, *Harrisonburg (MSN)*
Jefferson College of Health Sciences, Nursing Education Program, *Roanoke (MSN)*
Liberty University, Department of Nursing, *Lynchburg (MSN)*
Lynchburg College, School of Health Sciences and Human Performance, *Lynchburg (MSN, MSN/MBA)*
Marymount University, School of Health Professions, *Arlington (MSN)*
Old Dominion University, Department of Nursing, *Norfolk (MSN)*
Shenandoah University, Division of Nursing, *Winchester (MSN)*
University of Virginia, School of Nursing, *Charlottesville (MSN, MSN/MBA, MSN/PhD)*
Virginia Commonwealth University, School of Nursing, *Richmond (MS)*

Washington

Gonzaga University, Department of Nursing, *Spokane (MSN)*
Pacific Lutheran University, School of Nursing, *Tacoma (MSN, MSN/MBA)*
Seattle Pacific University, School of Health Sciences, *Seattle (MSN)*
Seattle University, College of Nursing, *Seattle (MSN)*
University of Washington, School of Nursing, *Seattle (MN, MN/MPH)*
Washington State University College of Nursing and Consortium, *Spokane (MN)*

West Virginia

Marshall University, College of Health Professions, *Huntington (MSN)*
Mountain State University, College of Nursing, *Beckley (MSN)*
West Virginia University, School of Nursing, *Morgantown (MSN)*
West Virginia Wesleyan College, School of Nursing, *Buckhannon (MSN)*
Wheeling Jesuit University, Department of Nursing, *Wheeling (MSN)*

Wisconsin

Alverno College, Division of Nursing, *Milwaukee (MSN)*
Bellin College, Nursing Program, *Green Bay (MSN)*
Concordia University Wisconsin, Program in Nursing, *Mequon (MSN)*
Edgewood College, Program in Nursing, *Madison (MS, MSN/MBA)*
Marian University, School of Nursing, *Fond du Lac (MSN)*
Marquette University, College of Nursing, *Milwaukee (MSN, MSN/MBA)*
University of Phoenix–Milwaukee Campus, College of Health and Human Services, *Milwaukee (MSN)*
University of Wisconsin–Eau Claire, College of Nursing and Health Sciences, *Eau Claire (MSN)*
University of Wisconsin–Milwaukee, College of Nursing, *Milwaukee (MN, MSN/MBA)*
University of Wisconsin–Oshkosh, College of Nursing, *Oshkosh (MSN)*
Viterbo University, School of Nursing, *La Crosse (MSN)*

Wyoming

University of Wyoming, Fay W. Whitney School of Nursing, *Laramie (MS)*

CANADA

Alberta

Athabasca University, Centre for Nursing and Health Studies, *Athabasca (MN, MN/MHSA, MN/MBA)*
University of Alberta, Faculty of Nursing, *Edmonton (MN)*
University of Calgary, Faculty of Nursing, *Calgary (MN)*
University of Lethbridge, School of Health Sciences, *Lethbridge (M Sc)*

British Columbia

Trinity Western University, Department of Nursing, *Langley (MSN)*
The University of British Columbia, Program in Nursing, *Vancouver (MSN, MA/MSM)*
University of Northern British Columbia, Nursing Programme, *Prince George (M Sc N)*
University of Victoria, School of Nursing, *Victoria (MN)*

Manitoba

University of Manitoba, Faculty of Nursing, *Winnipeg (MN)*

New Brunswick

Université de Moncton, School of Nursing, *Moncton (M Sc N)*
University of New Brunswick Fredericton, Faculty of Nursing, *Fredericton (MN)*

Newfoundland and Labrador

Memorial University of Newfoundland, School of Nursing, *St. John's (MN)*

Nova Scotia

Dalhousie University, School of Nursing, *Halifax (MN, MN/MHSA)*

Ontario

McMaster University, School of Nursing, *Hamilton (M Sc, MSN/PhD)*
Queen's University at Kingston, School of Nursing, *Kingston (M Sc)*
Ryerson University, Program in Nursing, *Toronto (MN)*
University of Ottawa, School of Nursing, *Ottawa (M Sc N)*
University of Toronto, Faculty of Nursing, *Toronto (MN)*
The University of Western Ontario, School of Nursing, *London (M Sc N)*
University of Windsor, Faculty of Nursing, *Windsor (M Sc)*

Quebec

McGill University, School of Nursing, *Montréal (M Sc)*
Université de Montréal, Faculty of Nursing, *Montréal (M Sc)*
Université de Sherbrooke, Department of Nursing, *Sherbrooke (M Sc)*
Université du Québec à Chicoutimi, Program in Nursing, *Chicoutimi (MSN, MS/MPH)*
Université du Québec à Rimouski, Program in Nursing, *Rimouski (M Sc N)*
Université du Québec à Trois-Rivières, Program in Nursing, *Trois-Rivières (MSN)*
Université du Québec en Outaouais, Département des Sciences Infirmières, *Gatineau (M Sc N)*
Université Laval, Faculty of Nursing, *Québec (MSN)*

Saskatchewan

University of Saskatchewan, College of Nursing, *Saskatoon (MN)*

MASTER'S FOR NON-NURSING COLLEGE GRADUATES

U.S. AND U.S. TERRITORIES

California

California State University, Dominguez Hills, Program in Nursing, *Carson (MSN)*
California State University, Fullerton, Department of Nursing, *Fullerton (MSN)*
California State University, Long Beach, Department of Nursing, *Long Beach (MSN, MSN/MHeA)*
California State University, Los Angeles, School of Nursing, *Los Angeles (MSN)*
Samuel Merritt University, School of Nursing, *Oakland (MSN)*
San Francisco State University, School of Nursing, *San Francisco (MSN)*
University of California, Los Angeles, School of Nursing, *Los Angeles (MSN, MSN/MBA)*
University of California, San Francisco, School of Nursing, *San Francisco (MS)*

Connecticut

Yale University, School of Nursing, *New Haven (MSN, MSN/MPH, MSN/MDIV)*

District of Columbia

Georgetown University, School of Nursing and Health Studies, *Washington (MS)*

Florida

University of Miami, School of Nursing and Health Studies, *Coral Gables (MSN)*

Hawaii

University of Hawaii at Manoa, School of Nursing and Dental Hygiene, *Honolulu (MS, MSN/MBA)*

Illinois

DePaul University, Department of Nursing, *Chicago (MS)*
Rush University, College of Nursing, *Chicago (MSN)*
University of Illinois at Chicago, College of Nursing, *Chicago (MS, MS/MBA, MS/MPH)*

Maine

University of Southern Maine, College of Nursing and Health Professions, *Portland (MS, MS/MBA)*

Massachusetts

MGH Institute of Health Professions, School of Nursing, *Boston (MS)*

Northeastern University, School of Nursing, *Boston (MS, MSN/MBA)*

Regis College, School of Nursing and Health Professions, *Weston (MSN)*

Simmons College, Department of Nursing, *Boston (MS)*

Nebraska

University of Nebraska Medical Center, College of Nursing, *Omaha (MSN)*

New York

Columbia University, School of Nursing, *New York (MS, MSN/MBA, MSN/MPH)*

Mercy College, Program in Nursing, *Dobbs Ferry (MS)*

Ohio

The Ohio State University, College of Nursing, *Columbus (MS, MS/MPH)*

The University of Toledo, College of Nursing, *Toledo (MSN)*

Oklahoma

University of Oklahoma Health Sciences Center, College of Nursing, *Oklahoma City (MS)*

Oregon

University of Portland, School of Nursing, *Portland (MS)*

Pennsylvania

Immaculata University, Department of Nursing, *Immaculata (MSN)*

Thomas Jefferson University, Department of Nursing, *Philadelphia (MSN)*

Wilkes University, Department of Nursing, *Wilkes-Barre (MS)*

Tennessee

University of Memphis, Loewenberg School of Nursing, *Memphis (MSN)*

The University of Tennessee, College of Nursing, *Knoxville (MSN)*

Vanderbilt University, School of Nursing, *Nashville (MSN, MSN/MDIV, MSN/MTS)*

Texas

Angelo State University, Department of Nursing, *San Angelo (MSN)*

The University of Texas at Austin, School of Nursing, *Austin (MSN, MSN/MBA)*

Vermont

University of Vermont, Department of Nursing, *Burlington (MS)*

Virginia

University of Virginia, School of Nursing, *Charlottesville (MSN, MSN/MBA, MSN/PhD)*

Washington

Pacific Lutheran University, School of Nursing, *Tacoma (MSN, MSN/MBA)*

Wisconsin

Marquette University, College of Nursing, *Milwaukee (MSN, MSN/MBA)*

University of Wisconsin–Milwaukee, College of Nursing, *Milwaukee (MN, MSN/MBA)*

CANADA

Quebec

McGill University, School of Nursing, *Montréal (M Sc)*

MASTER'S FOR NURSES WITH NON-NURSING DEGREES

U.S. AND U.S. TERRITORIES

Alabama

University of South Alabama, College of Nursing, *Mobile (MSN)*

Arizona

University of Phoenix, Online Campus, *Phoenix (MSN, MSN/MBA, MSN/MHA)*

Arkansas

Arkansas Tech University, Program in Nursing, *Russellville (MSN)*

University of Arkansas for Medical Sciences, College of Nursing, *Little Rock (MN Sc)*

California

California State University, Dominguez Hills, Program in Nursing, *Carson (MSN)*

California State University, Fresno, Department of Nursing, *Fresno (MSN)*

Dominican University of California, Program in Nursing, *San Rafael (MSN)*

Holy Names University, Department of Nursing, *Oakland (MSN, MSN/MBA)*

Samuel Merritt University, School of Nursing, *Oakland (MSN)*

San Francisco State University, School of Nursing, *San Francisco (MSN)*

University of California, San Francisco, School of Nursing, *San Francisco (MS)*

University of San Diego, Hahn School of Nursing and Health Science, *San Diego (MSN)*

University of San Francisco, School of Nursing, *San Francisco (MSN)*

Connecticut

Fairfield University, School of Nursing, *Fairfield (MSN)*

Saint Joseph College, Department of Nursing, *West Hartford (MS)*

University of Hartford, College of Education, Nursing, and Health Professions, *West Hartford (MSN, MSN/MSOB)*

Yale University, School of Nursing, *New Haven (MSN, MSN/MPH, MSN/MDIV)*

Delaware

University of Delaware, School of Nursing, *Newark (MSN)*

Florida

Florida Atlantic University, Christine E. Lynn College of Nursing, *Boca Raton (MS, MSN/MBA)*

Florida International University, Nursing Program, *Miami (MSN)*

Florida Southern College, Department of Nursing, *Lakeland (MSN, MSN/MBA)*

University of South Florida, College of Nursing, *Tampa (MS, MS/MPH)*

Georgia

Thomas University, Division of Nursing, *Thomasville (MSN, MSN/MBA)*

Illinois

DePaul University, Department of Nursing, *Chicago (MS)*

Resurrection University, *Oak Park (MSN)*

Rush University, College of Nursing, *Chicago (MSN)*

Saint Francis Medical Center College of Nursing, Baccalaureate Nursing Program, *Peoria (MSN)*

Saint Xavier University, School of Nursing, *Chicago (MSN, MSN/MBA)*

University of Illinois at Chicago, College of Nursing, *Chicago (MS, MS/MBA, MS/MPH)*

University of St. Francis, College of Nursing and Allied Health, *Joliet (MSN)*

Indiana

University of Saint Francis, Department of Nursing, *Fort Wayne (MSN)*

Iowa

Allen College, Program in Nursing, *Waterloo (MSN)*

The University of Iowa, College of Nursing, *Iowa City (MSN, MSN/MBA, MSN/MPH)*

Kansas

Wichita State University, School of Nursing, *Wichita (MSN, MSN/MBA)*

Kentucky

Bellarmine University, Donna and Allan Lansing School of Nursing and Health Sciences, *Louisville (MSN, MSN/MBA)*

Louisiana

Loyola University New Orleans, School of Nursing, *New Orleans (MSN)*

Maine

Husson University, School of Nursing, *Bangor (MSN)*

Saint Joseph's College of Maine, Department of Nursing, *Standish (MSN, MSN/MHA)*

University of Southern Maine, College of Nursing and Health Professions, *Portland (MS, MS/MBA)*

Massachusetts

MGH Institute of Health Professions, School of Nursing, *Boston (MS)*

Regis College, School of Nursing and Health Professions, *Weston (MSN)*

Salem State University, Program in Nursing, *Salem (MSN, MSN/MBA)*

Simmons College, Department of Nursing, *Boston (MS)*

Worcester State College, Department of Nursing, *Worcester (MS)*

Michigan

University of Detroit Mercy, McAuley School of Nursing, *Detroit (MSN)*

Minnesota

Metropolitan State University, College of Nursing and Health Sciences, *St. Paul (MSN)*

Minnesota State University Mankato, School of Nursing, *Mankato (MSN, MSN/MS)*

Minnesota State University Moorhead, School of Nursing and Healthcare Leadership, *Moorhead (MS)*

Winona State University, College of Nursing and Health Sciences, *Winona (MS)*

Missouri

Saint Louis University, School of Nursing, *St. Louis (MSN)*

Nebraska

BryanLGH College of Health Sciences, School of Nursing, *Lincoln (MS)*

Nebraska Methodist College, Department of Nursing, *Omaha (MSN)*

Nevada

Touro University, School of Nursing, *Henderson (MSN)*

New Hampshire

Franklin Pierce University, Master of Science in Nursing, *Rindge (MSN)*

Rivier College, Division of Nursing, *Nashua (MS)*

University of New Hampshire, Department of Nursing, *Durham (MS)*

New Jersey

The College of New Jersey, School of Nursing, Health and Exercise Science, *Ewing (MSN)*

Fairleigh Dickinson University, Metropolitan Campus, Henry P. Becton School of Nursing and Allied Health, *Teaneck (MSN)*

Kean University, Department of Nursing, *Union (MSN, MSN/MPA)*

Monmouth University, Marjorie K. Unterberg School of Nursing, *West Long Branch (MSN)*

Saint Peter's College, Nursing Program, *Jersey City (MSN)*

Seton Hall University, College of Nursing, *South Orange (MSN, MSN/MA, MSN/MBA)*

University of Medicine and Dentistry of New Jersey, School of Nursing, *Newark (MSN)*

William Paterson University of New Jersey, Department of Nursing, *Wayne (MSN)*

New York

College of Mount Saint Vincent, Department of Nursing, *Riverdale (MSN)*

Daemen College, Department of Nursing, *Amherst (MS)*

Lehman College of the City University of New York, Department of Nursing, *Bronx (MS)*

Le Moyne College, Nursing Programs, *Syracuse (MS)*

Long Island University, C.W. Post Campus, Department of Nursing, *Brookville (MS)*

Mercy College, Program in Nursing, *Dobbs Ferry (MS)*

Pace University, Lienhard School of Nursing, *New York (MS)*

State University of New York Upstate Medical University, College of Nursing, *Syracuse (MS)*

North Carolina

The University of North Carolina at Chapel Hill, School of Nursing, *Chapel Hill (MSN)*

Ohio

The Ohio State University, College of Nursing, *Columbus (MS, MS/MPH)*

The University of Toledo, College of Nursing, *Toledo (MSN)*

Wright State University, College of Nursing and Health, *Dayton (MS, MS/MBA)*

Xavier University, School of Nursing, *Cincinnati (MSN, MSN/MBA)*

Pennsylvania

Bloomsburg University of Pennsylvania, Department of Nursing, *Bloomsburg (MSN, MSN/MBA)*

Drexel University, College of Nursing and Health Professions, *Philadelphia (MSN)*

Indiana University of Pennsylvania, Department of Nursing and Allied Health, *Indiana (MS)*

Thomas Jefferson University, Department of Nursing, *Philadelphia (MSN)*

Widener University, School of Nursing, *Chester (MSN, MSN/PhD)*

Tennessee

East Tennessee State University, College of Nursing, *Johnson City (MSN)*

Tennessee Technological University, Whitson-Hester School of Nursing, *Cookeville (MSN, M Sc N)*

University of Memphis, Loewenberg School of Nursing, *Memphis (MSN)*

The University of Tennessee, College of Nursing, *Knoxville (MSN)*

Texas

Texas A&M International University, Canseco School of Nursing, *Laredo (MSN)*

The University of Texas at Austin, School of Nursing, *Austin (MSN, MSN/MBA)*

Vermont

University of Vermont, Department of Nursing, *Burlington (MS)*

Virginia

Eastern Mennonite University, Department of Nursing, *Harrisonburg (MSN)*

Jefferson College of Health Sciences, Nursing Education Program, *Roanoke (MSN)*

University of Virginia, School of Nursing, *Charlottesville (MSN, MSN/MBA, MSN/PhD)*

Virginia Commonwealth University, School of Nursing, *Richmond (MS)*

Washington

Gonzaga University, Department of Nursing, *Spokane (MSN)*

Pacific Lutheran University, School of Nursing, *Tacoma (MSN, MSN/MBA)*

Seattle Pacific University, School of Health Sciences, *Seattle (MSN)*

University of Washington, School of Nursing, *Seattle (MN, MN/MPH)*

Wisconsin

Marquette University, College of Nursing, *Milwaukee (MSN, MSN/MBA)*

Wyoming

University of Wyoming, Fay W. Whitney School of Nursing, *Laramie (MS)*

CANADA

Alberta

Athabasca University, Centre for Nursing and Health Studies, *Athabasca (MN, MN/MHSA, MN/MBA)*

RN TO MASTER'S

U.S. AND U.S. TERRITORIES

Alabama

Samford University, Ida V. Moffett School of Nursing, *Birmingham (MSN, MSN/MBA)*

Spring Hill College, Division of Nursing, *Mobile (MSN)*

The University of Alabama, Capstone College of Nursing, *Tuscaloosa (MSN, MSN/MA, MSN/Ed D)*

The University of Alabama in Huntsville, College of Nursing, *Huntsville (MSN)*

Arkansas

Arkansas Tech University, Program in Nursing, *Russellville (MSN)*

University of Arkansas for Medical Sciences, College of Nursing, *Little Rock (MN Sc)*

University of Central Arkansas, Department of Nursing, *Conway (MSN)*

California

Dominican University of California, Program in Nursing, *San Rafael (MSN)*

Loma Linda University, School of Nursing, *Loma Linda (MS)*

Mount St. Mary's College, Department of Nursing, *Los Angeles (MSN)*

Point Loma Nazarene University, School of Nursing, *San Diego (MSN)*

University of San Francisco, School of Nursing, *San Francisco (MSN)*

Colorado

Regis University, School of Nursing, *Denver (MS)*

University of Colorado Denver, College of Nursing, *Denver (MS)*

Connecticut

Sacred Heart University, Program in Nursing, *Fairfield (MSN)*

Southern Connecticut State University, Department of Nursing, *New Haven (MSN)*

University of Connecticut, School of Nursing, *Storrs (MS, MS/MBA)*

Delaware

University of Delaware, School of Nursing, *Newark (MSN)*

Wesley College, Nursing Program, *Dover (MSN)*

Florida

Florida Atlantic University, Christine E. Lynn College of Nursing, *Boca Raton (MS, MSN/MBA)*

Florida Southern College, Department of Nursing, *Lakeland (MSN, MSN/MBA)*

Kaplan University Online, The School of Nursing Online, *Fort Lauderdale (MSN)*

South University, Nursing Program, *Royal Palm Beach (MSN)*

University of Central Florida, College of Nursing, *Orlando (MSN)*

University of North Florida, School of Nursing, *Jacksonville (MSN)*

University of South Florida, College of Nursing, *Tampa (MS, MS/MPH)*

The University of Tampa, Department of Nursing, *Tampa (MSN)*

Georgia

Albany State University, College of Sciences and Health Professions, *Albany (MSN)*

Armstrong Atlantic State University, Program in Nursing, *Savannah (MSN, MS/MHSA)*

Brenau University, School of Health and Science, *Gainesville (MSN)*

Clayton State University, Department of Nursing, *Morrow (MSN)*

Emory University, Nell Hodgson Woodruff School of Nursing, *Atlanta (MSN, MSN/MPH)*

Georgia College & State University, College of Health Sciences, *Milledgeville (MSN, MSN/MBA)*

Georgia Health Sciences University, School of Nursing, *Augusta (MSN)*

Georgia Southern University, School of Nursing, *Statesboro (MSN)*

Georgia State University, Byrdine F. Lewis School of Nursing, *Atlanta (MSN)*

Valdosta State University, College of Nursing, *Valdosta (MSN)*

Hawaii

Hawai`i Pacific University, College of Nursing and Health Sciences, *Honolulu (MSN, MSN/MBA)*

University of Hawaii at Manoa, School of Nursing and Dental Hygiene, *Honolulu (MS, MSN/MBA)*

Idaho

Northwest Nazarene University, School of Health and Science, *Nampa (MSN)*

Illinois

Bradley University, Department of Nursing, *Peoria (MSN)*

DePaul University, Department of Nursing, *Chicago (MS)*

Lewis University, Program in Nursing, *Romeoville (MSN, MSN/MBA)*

Loyola University Chicago, Marcella Niehoff School of Nursing, *Maywood (MSN, MSN/MBA, MSN/MDIV)*

McKendree University, Department of Nursing, *Lebanon (MSN)*

North Park University, School of Nursing, *Chicago (MS, MSN/MA, MSN/MBA, MSN/MM)*

Resurrection University, *Oak Park (MSN)*

Rush University, College of Nursing, *Chicago (MSN)*

Indiana

Anderson University, School of Nursing, *Anderson (MSN, MSN/MBA)*

Ball State University, School of Nursing, *Muncie (MS)*

Indiana University–Purdue University Indianapolis, School of Nursing, *Indianapolis (MSN, MSN/MPH)*

University of Southern Indiana, College of Nursing and Health Professions, *Evansville (MSN)*

Valparaiso University, College of Nursing, *Valparaiso (MSN, MSN/MBA)*

Iowa

Allen College, Program in Nursing, *Waterloo (MSN)*

Kansas

The University of Kansas, School of Nursing, *Kansas City (MS, MS/MHSA, MS/MPH)*

Wichita State University, School of Nursing, *Wichita (MSN, MSN/MBA)*

Kentucky

Bellarmine University, Donna and Allan Lansing School of Nursing and Health Sciences, *Louisville (MSN, MSN/MBA)*

University of Kentucky, Graduate School Programs in the College of Nursing, *Lexington (MSN)*

Louisiana

Loyola University New Orleans, School of Nursing, *New Orleans (MSN)*

University of Louisiana at Lafayette, College of Nursing, *Lafayette (MSN)*

Maine

Saint Joseph's College of Maine, Department of Nursing, *Standish (MSN, MSN/MHA)*

University of Maine, School of Nursing, *Orono (MSN)*

University of Southern Maine, College of Nursing and Health Professions, *Portland (MS, MS/MBA)*

Maryland

Salisbury University, Program in Nursing, *Salisbury (MS)*

University of Maryland, Baltimore, Master's Program in Nursing, *Baltimore (MS, MSN/MBA, MSN/MPH, MSN/JD)*

Massachusetts

Boston College, William F. Connell School of Nursing, *Chestnut Hill (MS, MSN/MA, MSN/MBA, MSN/PhD)*

Curry College, Division of Nursing, *Milton (MSN)*

Elms College, Division of Nursing, *Chicopee (MSN)*

MGH Institute of Health Professions, School of Nursing, *Boston (MS)*

Northeastern University, School of Nursing, *Boston (MS, MSN/MBA)*

Regis College, School of Nursing and Health Professions, *Weston (MSN)*

Salem State University, Program in Nursing, *Salem (MSN, MSN/MBA)*

Simmons College, Department of Nursing, *Boston (MS)*

Worcester State College, Department of Nursing, *Worcester (MS)*

Michigan

Saginaw Valley State University, Crystal M. Lange College of Nursing and Health Sciences, *University Center (MSN)*

University of Michigan, School of Nursing, *Ann Arbor (MS, MSN/MBA, MSN/MPH)*

Minnesota

Metropolitan State University, College of Nursing and Health Sciences, *St. Paul (MSN)*

Minnesota State University Mankato, School of Nursing, *Mankato (MSN, MSN/MS)*

Walden University, Nursing Programs, *Minneapolis (MSN)*

Winona State University, College of Nursing and Health Sciences, *Winona (MS)*

Mississippi

University of Mississippi Medical Center, Program in Nursing, *Jackson (MSN)*

University of Southern Mississippi, School of Nursing, *Hattiesburg (MSN)*

Missouri

Graceland University, School of Nursing, *Independence (MSN)*

Grantham University, Nursing Programs, *Kansas City (MSN)*

Maryville University of Saint Louis, Nursing Program, School of Health Professions, *St. Louis (MSN)*

Missouri State University, Department of Nursing, *Springfield (MSN)*

Saint Louis University, School of Nursing, *St. Louis (MSN)*

Webster University, Department of Nursing, *St. Louis (MSN)*

Nebraska

Clarkson College, Master of Science in Nursing Program, *Omaha (MSN)*

Nebraska Methodist College, Department of Nursing, *Omaha (MSN)*

Nebraska Wesleyan University, Department of Nursing, *Lincoln (MSN)*

University of Nebraska Medical Center, College of Nursing, *Omaha (MSN)*

New Hampshire

Franklin Pierce University, Master of Science in Nursing, *Rindge (MSN)*

Rivier College, Division of Nursing, *Nashua (MS)*

New Jersey

The College of New Jersey, School of Nursing, Health and Exercise Science, *Ewing (MSN)*

Fairleigh Dickinson University, Metropolitan Campus, Henry P. Becton School of Nursing and Allied Health, *Teaneck (MSN)*

Monmouth University, Marjorie K. Unterberg School of Nursing, *West Long Branch (MSN)*

Seton Hall University, College of Nursing, *South Orange (MSN, MSN/MA, MSN/MBA)*

Thomas Edison State College, School of Nursing, *Trenton (MSN)*

University of Medicine and Dentistry of New Jersey, School of Nursing, *Newark (MSN)*

New York

The College of New Rochelle, School of Nursing, *New Rochelle (MS)*

Daemen College, Department of Nursing, *Amherst (MS)*

D'Youville College, Department of Nursing, *Buffalo (MS)*

Excelsior College, School of Nursing, *Albany (MS)*

Long Island University, Brooklyn Campus, School of Nursing, *Brooklyn (MS)*

New York University, College of Nursing, *New York (MS, MS/MPH)*

St. John Fisher College, Advanced Practice Nursing Program, *Rochester (MS)*

State University of New York Upstate Medical University, College of Nursing, *Syracuse (MS)*

Stony Brook University, State University of New York, School of Nursing, *Stony Brook (MS)*

North Carolina

Duke University, School of Nursing, *Durham (MSN, MSN/MBA)*

East Carolina University, College of Nursing, *Greenville (MSN)*

Gardner-Webb University, School of Nursing, *Boiling Springs (MSN, MSN/MBA)*

Queens University of Charlotte, Presbyterian School of Nursing, *Charlotte (MSN, MSN/MBA)*

The University of North Carolina at Chapel Hill, School of Nursing, *Chapel Hill (MSN)*

The University of North Carolina at Charlotte, School of Nursing, *Charlotte (MSN)*

North Dakota

University of Mary, Division of Nursing, *Bismarck (MSN, MSN/MBA)*

University of North Dakota, College of Nursing, *Grand Forks (MS)*

Ohio

Capital University, School of Nursing, *Columbus (MSN, MN/MBA, MSN/JD, MSN/MDIV)*

Case Western Reserve University, Frances Payne Bolton School of Nursing, *Cleveland (MSN, MSN/MA, MSN/MBA, MSN/MPH)*

Franciscan University of Steubenville, Department of Nursing, *Steubenville (MSN)*

The University of Akron, College of Nursing, *Akron (MSN)*

Xavier University, School of Nursing, *Cincinnati (MSN, MSN/MBA)*

Oregon

University of Portland, School of Nursing, *Portland (MS)*

Pennsylvania

Bloomsburg University of Pennsylvania, Department of Nursing, *Bloomsburg (MSN, MSN/MBA)*

Carlow University, School of Nursing, *Pittsburgh (MSN)*

Clarion University of Pennsylvania, School of Nursing, *Oil City (MSN)*

DeSales University, Department of Nursing and Health, *Center Valley (MSN, MSN/MBA)*

Drexel University, College of Nursing and Health Professions, *Philadelphia (MSN)*

Gannon University, Villa Maria School of Nursing, *Erie (MSN)*

Gwynedd-Mercy College, School of Nursing, *Gwynedd Valley (MSN)*

La Roche College, Department of Nursing and Nursing Management, *Pittsburgh (MSN)*

La Salle University, School of Nursing and Health Sciences, *Philadelphia (MSN, MSN/MBA)*

Misericordia University, Department of Nursing, *Dallas (MSN)*

Neumann University, Program in Nursing and Health Sciences, *Aston (MS)*

Thomas Jefferson University, Department of Nursing, *Philadelphia (MSN)*

University of Pittsburgh, School of Nursing, *Pittsburgh (MSN)*

The University of Scranton, Department of Nursing, *Scranton (MSN)*

Villanova University, College of Nursing, *Villanova (MSN)*

Wilkes University, Department of Nursing, *Wilkes-Barre (MS)*

York College of Pennsylvania, Department of Nursing, *York (MS)*

Rhode Island

University of Rhode Island, College of Nursing, *Kingston (MS)*

South Carolina

Charleston Southern University, Wingo School of Nursing, *Charleston (MSN)*

Clemson University, School of Nursing, *Clemson (MS)*

South Dakota

South Dakota State University, College of Nursing, *Brookings (MS)*

Tennessee

Carson-Newman College, Department of Nursing, *Jefferson City (MSN)*

Tennessee State University, School of Nursing, *Nashville (MSN)*

The University of Tennessee, College of Nursing, *Knoxville (MSN)*

Vanderbilt University, School of Nursing, *Nashville (MSN, MSN/MDIV, MSN/MTS)*

Texas

Angelo State University, Department of Nursing, *San Angelo (MSN)*

Midwestern State University, Nursing Program, *Wichita Falls (MSN, MN/MHSA, MSN/MHA)*

Texas Tech University Health Sciences Center, School of Nursing, *Lubbock (MSN)*

Texas Woman's University, College of Nursing, *Denton (MS, MSN/MHA)*

University of Houston–Victoria, School of Nursing, *Victoria (MSN)*

The University of Texas at El Paso, School of Nursing, *El Paso (MSN)*

The University of Texas at Tyler, Program in Nursing, *Tyler (MSN, MSN/MBA)*

The University of Texas Health Science Center at San Antonio, School of Nursing, *San Antonio (MSN, MSN/MPH)*

West Texas A&M University, Division of Nursing, *Canyon (MSN)*

Utah

Western Governors University, Online College of Health Professions, *Salt Lake City (MS)*

Vermont

University of Vermont, Department of Nursing, *Burlington (MS)*

Virginia

George Mason University, College of Health and Human Services, *Fairfax (MSN)*

Hampton University, School of Nursing, *Hampton (MS)*

Old Dominion University, Department of Nursing, *Norfolk (MSN)*

Shenandoah University, Division of Nursing, *Winchester (MSN)*

Virginia Commonwealth University, School of Nursing, *Richmond (MS)*

West Virginia

West Virginia University, School of Nursing, *Morgantown (MSN)*

Wheeling Jesuit University, Department of Nursing, *Wheeling (MSN)*

Wisconsin

Marquette University, College of Nursing, *Milwaukee (MSN, MSN/MBA)*

University of Wisconsin–Eau Claire, College of Nursing and Health Sciences, *Eau Claire (MSN)*

CANADA

Alberta

University of Calgary, Faculty of Nursing, *Calgary (MN)*

New Brunswick

Université de Moncton, School of Nursing, *Moncton (M Sc N)*

Quebec

Université de Montréal, Faculty of Nursing, *Montréal (M Sc)*

Université du Québec à Chicoutimi, Program in Nursing, *Chicoutimi (MSN, MS/MPH)*

CONCENTRATIONS WITHIN MASTER'S DEGREE PROGRAMS

CASE MANAGEMENT

American Sentinel University, CO
Boise State University, ID
Carlow University, PA
DePaul University, IL
Duke University, NC
The Johns Hopkins University, MD
Lewis University, IL
Loyola University New Orleans, LA
Pacific Lutheran University, WA
Regis College, MA
Saint Peter's College, NJ
Samuel Merritt University, CA
San Francisco State University, CA
Seton Hall University, NJ
Shenandoah University, VA
Université de Moncton, NB
The University of Alabama, AL
University of Central Florida, FL
University of Kentucky, KY
University of Nebraska Medical Center, NE
University of New Brunswick Fredericton, NB
The University of North Carolina at Chapel Hill, NC
Ursuline College, OH
Valdosta State University, GA
Washington State University College of Nursing and Consortium, WA

CLINICAL NURSE LEADER

Boise State University, ID
Brenau University, GA
California Baptist University, CA
California State University, Dominguez Hills, CA
Cleveland State University, OH
Creighton University, NE
Curry College, MA
Dominican University of California, CA
East Tennessee State University, TN
Elmhurst College, IL
Fairfield University, CT
Florida Atlantic University, FL
The George Washington University, DC
Georgia Health Sciences University, GA
Grand Valley State University, MI
Grand View University, IA
Idaho State University, ID
Illinois State University, IL
James Madison University, VA
Lynchburg College, VA
Marquette University, WI
Millikin University, IL
Montana State University, MT
Moravian College, PA
The Ohio State University, OH
Pacific Lutheran University, WA
Pittsburg State University, KS
Queens University of Charlotte, NC
Regis College, MA
Resurrection University, IL
Rush University, IL
Sacred Heart University, CT
Saint Anthony College of Nursing, IL
Saint Francis Medical Center College of Nursing, IL
Saint Xavier University, IL
Salem State University, MA
Seton Hall University, NJ
South Dakota State University, SD
Southern Connecticut State University, CT
Spring Hill College, AL
Texas Christian University, TX
Touro University, NV
Trinity Western University, BC
Université Laval, QC
The University of Alabama, AL
The University of Alabama at Birmingham, AL
The University of Alabama in Huntsville, AL
University of California, Los Angeles, CA
University of Connecticut, CT
University of Florida, FL
University of Mary Hardin-Baylor, TX
University of Maryland, Baltimore, MD
University of Massachusetts Amherst, MA
University of Medicine and Dentistry of New Jersey, NJ
University of Nevada, Reno, NV
The University of North Carolina at Chapel Hill, NC
University of Oklahoma Health Sciences Center, OK
University of Pittsburgh, PA
University of Portland, OR
University of Rhode Island, RI
University of Rochester, NY
University of San Diego, CA
University of San Francisco, CA
University of Southern Maine, ME
University of South Florida, FL
The University of Tennessee Health Science Center, TN
University of the Incarnate Word, TX
The University of Toledo, OH
University of Toronto, ON
University of Utah, UT
University of Virginia, VA
University of West Georgia, GA
University of Wisconsin–Milwaukee, WI
University of Wisconsin–Oshkosh, WI
Virginia Commonwealth University, VA
Viterbo University, WI
Western Governors University, UT
Western University of Health Sciences, CA
Wright State University, OH
Xavier University, OH

CLINICAL NURSE SPECIALIST PROGRAMS

Acute Care

Arizona State University at the Downtown Phoenix Campus, AZ
California State University, Fresno, CA
Colorado State University–Pueblo, CO
George Mason University, VA
Georgetown University, DC
Georgia Baptist College of Nursing of Mercer University, GA
Indiana University–Purdue University Indianapolis, IN
The Johns Hopkins University, MD
King College, TN
Liberty University, VA
Loyola University Chicago, IL
McGill University, QC
MGH Institute of Health Professions, MA
Regis College, MA
Rhode Island College, RI
The Sage Colleges, NY
Seattle Pacific University, WA
Thomas Jefferson University, PA
Université de Montréal, QC
Université de Sherbrooke, QC
Université du Québec à Chicoutimi, QC
Université du Québec à Trois-Rivières, QC
Université Laval, QC
University of Arkansas, AR
University of Arkansas for Medical Sciences, AR
University of Calgary, AB
University of California, Los Angeles, CA
University of Central Florida, FL
University of Colorado Denver, CO
University of Connecticut, CT
University of Illinois at Chicago, IL
University of Kentucky, KY
University of Manitoba, MB
University of Maryland, Baltimore, MD
University of Massachusetts Boston, MA
University of Missouri, MO
University of Nebraska Medical Center, NE
University of New Brunswick Fredericton, NB
University of Oklahoma Health Sciences Center, OK
University of Ottawa, ON
University of San Diego, CA
University of South Alabama, AL
The University of Texas Health Science Center at Houston, TX
University of Toronto, ON
University of Virginia, VA
University of Washington, WA
The University of Western Ontario, ON
Virginia Commonwealth University, VA
Wayne State University, MI
Wichita State University, KS

Adult Health

Alverno College, WI
Angelo State University, TX
Arizona State University at the Downtown Phoenix Campus, AZ
Arkansas State University - Jonesboro, AR
Armstrong Atlantic State University, GA
Auburn University, AL
Auburn University Montgomery, AL
Azusa Pacific University, CA
Ball State University, IN
Bloomsburg University of Pennsylvania, PA
Boston College, MA
California Baptist University, CA
California State University, Chico, CA
California State University, Long Beach, CA
The Catholic University of America, DC
Clemson University, SC
The College of New Jersey, NJ
The College of St. Scholastica, MN
College of Staten Island of the City University of New York, NY
Creighton University, NE
Dalhousie University, NS
DeSales University, PA
East Carolina University, NC
Eastern Michigan University, MI
Florida Southern College, FL
George Mason University, VA

Georgia College & State University, GA
Georgia State University, GA
Governors State University, IL
Grambling State University, LA
Grand Canyon University, AZ
Idaho State University, ID
Indiana University–Purdue University Indianapolis, IN
The Johns Hopkins University, MD
Kennesaw State University, GA
Kent State University, OH
King College, TN
La Salle University, PA
Lehman College of the City University of New York, NY
Loma Linda University, CA
Long Island University, C.W. Post Campus, NY
Louisiana State University Health Sciences Center, LA
Madonna University, MI
Malone University, OH
Marquette University, WI
McGill University, QC
McNeese State University, LA
MGH Institute of Health Professions, MA
Michigan State University, MI
Minnesota State University Mankato, MN
Minnesota State University Moorhead, MN
Molloy College, NY
Mount Carmel College of Nursing, OH
Mount Saint Mary College, NY
Mount St. Mary's College, CA
Murray State University, KY
North Dakota State University, ND
Northern Illinois University, IL
Northwestern State University of Louisiana, LA
The Ohio State University, OH
Otterbein University, OH
Penn State University Park, PA
Purdue University Calumet, IN
Rhode Island College, RI
Rutgers, The State University of New Jersey, College of Nursing, NJ
Ryerson University, ON
The Sage Colleges, NY
Saint Anthony College of Nursing, IL
St. John Fisher College, NY
St. Joseph's College, New York, NY
Saint Louis University, MO
San Diego State University, CA
San Francisco State University, CA
Seattle Pacific University, WA
Southeastern Louisiana University, LA
Southeast Missouri State University, MO
State University of New York Downstate Medical Center, NY
Stony Brook University, State University of New York, NY
Texas A&M University–Corpus Christi, TX
Texas Christian University, TX
Texas Woman's University, TX
Thomas Jefferson University, PA
Troy University, AL
Union University, TN
Université de Montréal, QC
Université du Québec à Chicoutimi, QC
Université du Québec à Trois-Rivières, QC
Université Laval, QC
University at Buffalo, the State University of New York, NY
The University of Akron, OH
The University of Alabama at Birmingham, AL
The University of Alabama in Huntsville, AL
University of Arkansas for Medical Sciences, AR
The University of British Columbia, BC
University of Calgary, AB
University of California, Los Angeles, CA
University of Cincinnati, OH
University of Colorado at Colorado Springs, CO
University of Colorado Denver, CO
University of Delaware, DE
University of Illinois at Chicago, IL
The University of Iowa, IA
The University of Kansas, KS
University of Kentucky, KY
University of Louisiana at Lafayette, LA
University of Mary Hardin-Baylor, TX
University of Massachusetts Dartmouth, MA
University of Minnesota, Twin Cities Campus, MN
University of Missouri, MO
University of Nebraska Medical Center, NE
University of New Brunswick Fredericton, NB
University of New Hampshire, NH
University of North Florida, FL
University of Pennsylvania, PA
University of Puerto Rico, Medical Sciences Campus, PR
University of St. Francis, IL
University of San Diego, CA
The University of Scranton, PA
University of Southern Mississippi, MS
The University of Tennessee, TN
The University of Texas at Austin, TX
The University of Texas Health Science Center at Houston, TX
The University of Texas–Pan American, TX
University of the Incarnate Word, TX
The University of Toledo, OH
University of Toronto, ON
University of Virginia, VA
University of Washington, WA
The University of Western Ontario, ON
University of Wisconsin–Eau Claire, WI
Ursuline College, OH
Valdosta State University, GA
Valparaiso University, IN
Western Connecticut State University, CT
Widener University, PA
Winona State University, MN
Wright State University, OH
York College of Pennsylvania, PA

Cardiovascular

Creighton University, NE
George Mason University, VA
The Johns Hopkins University, MD
Loyola University Chicago, IL
McGill University, QC
The Ohio State University, OH
The Sage Colleges, NY
Université de Montréal, QC
Université du Québec à Chicoutimi, QC
Université Laval, QC
University of Calgary, AB
University of California, San Francisco, CA
University of Illinois at Chicago, IL
University of Missouri, MO
University of Nebraska Medical Center, NE
University of New Brunswick Fredericton, NB
University of North Florida, FL
University of Washington, WA
Yale University, CT

Community Health

Arizona State University at the Downtown Phoenix Campus, AZ
Augsburg College, MN
Bloomsburg University of Pennsylvania, PA
Boston College, MA
California State University, Fresno, CA
California State University, San Bernardino, CA
The Catholic University of America, DC
Cleveland State University, OH
Dalhousie University, NS
DePaul University, IL
D'Youville College, NY
Georgia Southern University, GA
Hawai`i Pacific University, HI
Holy Family University, PA
Hunter College of the City University of New York, NY
Indiana University–Purdue University Indianapolis, IN
Jacksonville State University, AL
The Johns Hopkins University, MD
Kean University, NJ
La Roche College, PA
Louisiana State University Health Sciences Center, LA
McGill University, QC
Mount St. Mary's College, CA
New Mexico State University, NM
Northern Illinois University, IL
North Park University, IL
The Ohio State University, OH
Penn State University Park, PA
Rhode Island College, RI
Rush University, IL
Rutgers, The State University of New Jersey, College of Nursing, NJ
Ryerson University, ON
The Sage Colleges, NY
Salem State University, MA
San Diego State University, CA
Seattle Pacific University, WA
Seattle University, WA
State University of New York at Binghamton, NY
Stony Brook University, State University of New York, NY
Thomas Jefferson University, PA
Université de Moncton, NB
Université de Montréal, QC
Université de Sherbrooke, QC
Université du Québec à Chicoutimi, QC
Université du Québec à Rimouski, QC
Université du Québec à Trois-Rivières, QC
Université du Québec en Outaouais, QC
Université Laval, QC
University of Alaska Anchorage, AK
The University of British Columbia, BC
University of Calgary, AB
University of California, San Francisco, CA
University of Illinois at Chicago, IL
The University of Iowa, IA
University of Kentucky, KY
University of Maryland, Baltimore, MD
University of Massachusetts Dartmouth, MA
University of Michigan, MI
University of Missouri, MO
University of Nebraska Medical Center, NE

University of New Brunswick Fredericton, NB
The University of North Carolina at Charlotte, NC
University of North Dakota, ND
University of North Florida, FL
University of Ottawa, ON
University of Puerto Rico, Medical Sciences Campus, PR
University of South Alabama, AL
University of Southern Mississippi, MS
The University of Texas at Austin, TX
University of Toronto, ON
University of Virginia, VA
University of Washington, WA
The University of Western Ontario, ON
Washington State University College of Nursing and Consortium, WA
Wayne State University, MI
Wesley College, DE
William Paterson University of New Jersey, NJ
Worcester State College, MA
Wright State University, OH

Critical Care

California State University, Fresno, CA
Duke University, NC
George Mason University, VA
Georgetown University, DC
Georgia Baptist College of Nursing of Mercer University, GA
Indiana University–Purdue University Indianapolis, IN
The Johns Hopkins University, MD
McGill University, QC
Murray State University, KY
Northwestern State University of Louisiana, LA
Purdue University Calumet, IN
Rush University, IL
The Sage Colleges, NY
San Diego State University, CA
Seattle Pacific University, WA
Stony Brook University, State University of New York, NY
Thomas Jefferson University, PA
Université du Québec à Chicoutimi, QC
Université du Québec à Rimouski, QC
Université du Québec à Trois-Rivières, QC
Université du Québec en Outaouais, QC
Université Laval, QC
University of Calgary, AB
University of California, San Francisco, CA
University of Central Florida, FL
University of Cincinnati, OH
University of Kentucky, KY
University of Maryland, Baltimore, MD
University of Massachusetts Boston, MA
University of Missouri, MO
University of Nebraska Medical Center, NE
University of New Brunswick Fredericton, NB
University of North Florida, FL
University of Puerto Rico, Medical Sciences Campus, PR
The University of Texas Health Science Center at Houston, TX
The University of Texas Health Science Center at San Antonio, TX
University of Toronto, ON
University of Virginia, VA
University of Washington, WA
Wayne State University, MI
Widener University, PA
Yale University, CT

Family Health

Creighton University, NE
Dalhousie University, NS
Florida Southern College, FL
The Johns Hopkins University, MD
Loma Linda University, CA
McGill University, QC
MGH Institute of Health Professions, MA
Minnesota State University Mankato, MN
Missouri Southern State University, MO
Pittsburg State University, KS
Point Loma Nazarene University, CA
Ryerson University, ON
The Sage Colleges, NY
Saint Joseph College, CT
Southern University and Agricultural and Mechanical College, LA
State University of New York at Binghamton, NY
Tennessee State University, TN
Université de Moncton, NB
Université de Montréal, QC
Université de Sherbrooke, QC
Université du Québec à Chicoutimi, QC
Université du Québec à Trois-Rivières, QC
Université Laval, QC
The University of British Columbia, BC
University of Calgary, AB
University of Illinois at Chicago, IL
University of Manitoba, MB
University of Nebraska Medical Center, NE
University of New Brunswick Fredericton, NB
University of Northern Colorado, CO
University of South Alabama, AL
University of Toronto, ON
Valdosta State University, GA
Webster University, MO

Forensic Nursing

Boston College, MA
Cleveland State University, OH
Duquesne University, PA
Fairleigh Dickinson University, Metropolitan Campus, NJ
Fitchburg State University, MA
The Johns Hopkins University, MD
Monmouth University, NJ
Xavier University, OH

Gerontology

Alverno College, WI
Auburn University, AL
Auburn University Montgomery, AL
Bloomsburg University of Pennsylvania, PA
Boston College, MA
California State University, Dominguez Hills, CA
Case Western Reserve University, OH
Clemson University, SC
The College of St. Scholastica, MN
College of Staten Island of the City University of New York, NY
Creighton University, NE
Duke University, NC
Florida Southern College, FL
Gwynedd-Mercy College, PA
The Johns Hopkins University, MD
Kent State University, OH
Lehman College of the City University of New York, NY
Marquette University, WI
McGill University, QC
MGH Institute of Health Professions, MA
Neumann University, PA
Penn State University Park, PA
Point Loma Nazarene University, CA
Rush University, IL
The Sage Colleges, NY
St. John Fisher College, NY
Saint Louis University, MO
San Diego State University, CA
San Jose State University, CA
Seattle Pacific University, WA
Southeastern Louisiana University, LA
State University of New York at Binghamton, NY
Trinity Western University, BC
Université de Montréal, QC
Université de Sherbrooke, QC
Université du Québec à Chicoutimi, QC
Université du Québec à Rimouski, QC
Université Laval, QC
The University of Akron, OH
University of Calgary, AB
University of California, Los Angeles, CA
University of California, San Francisco, CA
University of Cincinnati, OH
University of Illinois at Chicago, IL
The University of Iowa, IA
The University of Kansas, KS
University of Kentucky, KY
University of Manitoba, MB
University of Michigan, MI
University of Minnesota, Twin Cities Campus, MN
University of Nebraska Medical Center, NE
University of New Brunswick Fredericton, NB
University of North Dakota, ND
University of North Florida, FL
University of Puerto Rico, Medical Sciences Campus, PR
University of Rhode Island, RI
University of South Alabama, AL
The University of Texas Health Science Center at Houston, TX
University of Toronto, ON
University of Washington, WA
Valparaiso University, IN
Wilkes University, PA

Home Health Care

Carlow University, PA
McGill University, QC
Thomas Jefferson University, PA
Université de Moncton, NB
Université du Québec à Chicoutimi, QC
Université du Québec à Trois-Rivières, QC
University of Michigan, MI
University of Missouri, MO

Maternity-newborn

Clemson University, SC
Creighton University, NE
Dalhousie University, NS
Duke University, NC
Grambling State University, LA
The Johns Hopkins University, MD
Loma Linda University, CA
McGill University, QC
San Diego State University, CA
State University of New York Downstate Medical Center, NY
Troy University, AL

Université de Montréal, QC
Université du Québec à Chicoutimi, QC
Université du Québec à Trois-Rivières, QC
University of Calgary, AB
University of Connecticut, CT
University of Illinois at Chicago, IL
University of Missouri, MO
University of Nebraska Medical Center, NE
University of New Brunswick Fredericton, NB
University of North Florida, FL
University of Puerto Rico, Medical Sciences Campus, PR
University of South Alabama, AL
University of Toronto, ON
University of Washington, WA

Medical-surgical

Alverno College, WI
Angelo State University, TX
Azusa Pacific University, CA
Case Western Reserve University, OH
DePaul University, IL
George Mason University, VA
Hunter College of the City University of New York, NY
The Johns Hopkins University, MD
Loma Linda University, CA
Malone University, OH
McGill University, QC
Murray State University, KY
New Mexico State University, NM
Point Loma Nazarene University, CA
Rush University, IL
The Sage Colleges, NY
Saint Francis Medical Center College of Nursing, IL
Seattle Pacific University, WA
State University of New York Upstate Medical University, NY
Texas Christian University, TX
Thomas Jefferson University, PA
Université de Montréal, QC
Université du Québec à Chicoutimi, QC
Université du Québec à Trois-Rivières, QC
University of Arkansas, AR
University of Calgary, AB
University of Central Arkansas, AR
University of Cincinnati, OH
University of Illinois at Chicago, IL
University of Kentucky, KY
University of Michigan, MI
University of Nebraska Medical Center, NE
University of New Brunswick Fredericton, NB
University of North Florida, FL
University of Pittsburgh, PA
University of San Diego, CA
University of Southern Maine, ME
The University of Texas at Austin, TX
The University of Texas Health Science Center at San Antonio, TX
University of Virginia, VA
University of Washington, WA

Occupational Health

Université de Moncton, NB
Université de Montréal, QC
Université du Québec à Chicoutimi, QC
University of California, San Francisco, CA
University of Cincinnati, OH
University of Illinois at Chicago, IL
The University of Iowa, IA
University of Michigan, MI
University of Washington, WA

Oncology

Creighton University, NE
Duke University, NC
George Mason University, VA
Gwynedd-Mercy College, PA
Indiana University–Purdue University Indianapolis, IN
The Johns Hopkins University, MD
King College, TN
Loyola University Chicago, IL
McGill University, QC
The Ohio State University, OH
Rutgers, The State University of New Jersey, College of Nursing, NJ
The Sage Colleges, NY
Seattle Pacific University, WA
Thomas Jefferson University, PA
Université de Montréal, QC
Université du Québec à Chicoutimi, QC
Université Laval, QC
University of California, Los Angeles, CA
University of California, San Francisco, CA
University of Kentucky, KY
University of Missouri, MO
University of Nebraska Medical Center, NE
University of New Brunswick Fredericton, NB
University of Toronto, ON
University of Virginia, VA
University of Washington, WA
Yale University, CT

Palliative Care

Boston College, MA
Daemen College, NY
D'Youville College, NY
The Johns Hopkins University, MD
The Sage Colleges, NY
Seattle Pacific University, WA
Université de Montréal, QC
Université Laval, QC
University of Colorado Denver, CO
University of Missouri, MO
University of Virginia, VA
Ursuline College, OH

Parent-child

Azusa Pacific University, CA
California State University, Dominguez Hills, CA
Clemson University, SC
Dalhousie University, NS
Hunter College of the City University of New York, NY
The Johns Hopkins University, MD
Lehman College of the City University of New York, NY
Loma Linda University, CA
Louisiana State University Health Sciences Center, LA
McGill University, QC
Rutgers, The State University of New Jersey, College of Nursing, NJ
Seattle Pacific University, WA
Stony Brook University, State University of New York, NY
Université de Montréal, QC
Université du Québec à Chicoutimi, QC
Université Laval, QC
University of Calgary, AB
University of Kentucky, KY
University of Nebraska Medical Center, NE
University of New Brunswick Fredericton, NB
University of Washington, WA

Pediatric

Arizona State University at the Downtown Phoenix Campus, AZ
Auburn University, AL
Auburn University Montgomery, AL
Azusa Pacific University, CA
Boston College, MA
California State University, Fresno, CA
The Catholic University of America, DC
Clemson University, SC
Creighton University, NE
Dalhousie University, NS
Duke University, NC
Georgia State University, GA
Grambling State University, LA
Gwynedd-Mercy College, PA
Indiana University–Purdue University Indianapolis, IN
The Johns Hopkins University, MD
Kent State University, OH
Loma Linda University, CA
Marquette University, WI
McGill University, QC
MGH Institute of Health Professions, MA
Minnesota State University Mankato, MN
Rush University, IL
St. John Fisher College, NY
Saint Louis University, MO
Seattle Pacific University, WA
Stony Brook University, State University of New York, NY
Texas Christian University, TX
Texas Woman's University, TX
Thomas Jefferson University, PA
Union University, TN
Université de Moncton, NB
Université du Québec à Chicoutimi, QC
Université du Québec à Trois-Rivières, QC
Université Laval, QC
The University of Akron, OH
University of Arkansas for Medical Sciences, AR
University of Calgary, AB
University of California, Los Angeles, CA
University of California, San Francisco, CA
University of Delaware, DE
University of Illinois at Chicago, IL
University of Kentucky, KY
University of Minnesota, Twin Cities Campus, MN
University of Missouri, MO
University of Nebraska Medical Center, NE
University of New Brunswick Fredericton, NB
University of North Florida, FL
University of Pennsylvania, PA
University of Puerto Rico, Medical Sciences Campus, PR
University of South Alabama, AL
The University of Tennessee, TN
University of Toronto, ON
Wright State University, OH

Perinatal

Georgia State University, GA
The Johns Hopkins University, MD
McGill University, QC
McMaster University, ON
San Francisco State University, CA
Stony Brook University, State University of New York, NY
Université du Québec à Chicoutimi, QC
Université du Québec à Trois-Rivières, QC

Université Laval, QC
University of Calgary, AB
University of California, San Francisco, CA
University of Illinois at Chicago, IL
University of Kentucky, KY
University of Manitoba, MB
University of Nebraska Medical Center, NE
University of Washington, WA

Psychiatric/mental Health

Arizona State University at the Downtown Phoenix Campus, AZ
Boston College, MA
California State University, Fresno, CA
California State University, Los Angeles, CA
Case Western Reserve University, OH
Colorado State University–Pueblo, CO
Dalhousie University, NS
Georgia State University, GA
Gonzaga University, WA
Hunter College of the City University of New York, NY
Husson University, ME
Indiana University–Purdue University Indianapolis, IN
Kent State University, OH
Louisiana State University Health Sciences Center, LA
McGill University, QC
McNeese State University, LA
MGH Institute of Health Professions, MA
New Mexico State University, NM
Northeastern University, MA
The Ohio State University, OH
Point Loma Nazarene University, CA
Rivier College, NH
Rush University, IL
Rutgers, The State University of New Jersey, College of Nursing, NJ
The Sage Colleges, NY
Saint Joseph College, CT
Saint Louis University, MO
Shenandoah University, VA
Southeastern Louisiana University, LA
Stony Brook University, State University of New York, NY
Temple University, PA
Université de Moncton, NB
Université de Montréal, QC
Université du Québec à Chicoutimi, QC
Université du Québec à Rimouski, QC
Université du Québec à Trois-Rivières, QC
Université du Québec en Outaouais, QC
Université Laval, QC
The University of Akron, OH
University of Alaska Anchorage, AK
The University of British Columbia, BC
University of Calgary, AB
University of California, San Francisco, CA
University of Delaware, DE
University of Florida, FL
University of Hawaii at Manoa, HI
University of Illinois at Chicago, IL
The University of Iowa, IA
University of Kentucky, KY
University of Louisiana at Lafayette, LA
University of Louisville, KY
University of Maryland, Baltimore, MD
University of Massachusetts Lowell, MA
University of Medicine and Dentistry of New Jersey, NJ
University of Michigan, MI
University of Minnesota, Twin Cities Campus, MN
University of Nebraska Medical Center, NE
University of New Brunswick Fredericton, NB
The University of North Carolina at Chapel Hill, NC
University of North Dakota, ND
University of North Florida, FL
University of Pennsylvania, PA
University of Pittsburgh, PA
University of Puerto Rico, Medical Sciences Campus, PR
University of Rhode Island, RI
University of South Alabama, AL
University of Southern Maine, ME
University of Southern Mississippi, MS
The University of Tennessee, TN
The University of Toledo, OH
University of Toronto, ON
University of Utah, UT
University of Virginia, VA
The University of Western Ontario, ON
Valdosta State University, GA
Wayne State University, MI
Widener University, PA
Wilkes University, PA
Yale University, CT

Public Health

Bloomsburg University of Pennsylvania, PA
California State University, Fresno, CA
California State University, Long Beach, CA
Case Western Reserve University, OH
Dalhousie University, NS
Eastern Kentucky University, KY
Emory University, GA
The Johns Hopkins University, MD
La Salle University, PA
McGill University, QC
Mount Mercy University, IA
The Ohio State University, OH
Rush University, IL
Ryerson University, ON
Salem State University, MA
San Francisco State University, CA
Thomas Jefferson University, PA
Université de Moncton, NB
Université de Montréal, QC
Université du Québec à Chicoutimi, QC
Université du Québec à Trois-Rivières, QC
Université Laval, QC
The University of British Columbia, BC
University of Calgary, AB
University of Cincinnati, OH
University of Florida, FL
University of Hartford, CT
University of Illinois at Chicago, IL
University of Kentucky, KY
University of Missouri, MO
University of Nebraska Medical Center, NE
University of New Brunswick Fredericton, NB
University of North Dakota, ND
The University of Texas at Austin, TX
The University of Texas at Brownsville, TX
University of Toronto, ON
University of Virginia, VA
The University of Western Ontario, ON
West Chester University of Pennsylvania, PA
Worcester State College, MA
Wright State University, OH

Rehabilitation

McGill University, QC
Salem State University, MA
Université de Montréal, QC
Université du Québec à Chicoutimi, QC
Université du Québec en Outaouais, QC
Université Laval, QC
University of Calgary, AB
University of Missouri, MO

School Health

Azusa Pacific University, CA
Bloomsburg University of Pennsylvania, PA
California State University, Fullerton, CA
Kean University, NJ
Monmouth University, NJ
San Diego State University, CA
San Jose State University, CA
Seton Hall University, NJ
Université de Moncton, NB
Université du Québec à Chicoutimi, QC
University of Delaware, DE
University of Illinois at Chicago, IL
University of Missouri, MO
University of Nevada, Reno, NV
University of New Brunswick Fredericton, NB
University of Toronto, ON
Wright State University, OH
Xavier University, OH

WomensHealth'

Drexel University, PA
Georgia State University, GA
The Johns Hopkins University, MD
Kent State University, OH
McGill University, QC
St. John Fisher College, NY
San Diego State University, CA
Seattle Pacific University, WA
Stony Brook University, State University of New York, NY
Texas Woman's University, TX
Université de Montréal, QC
Université du Québec à Chicoutimi, QC
University of Calgary, AB
University of Illinois at Chicago, IL
University of Kentucky, KY
University of Manitoba, MB
University of Missouri, MO
University of Nebraska Medical Center, NE
University of New Brunswick Fredericton, NB
University of North Florida, FL
University of South Alabama, AL
University of Toronto, ON
The University of Western Ontario, ON
Valparaiso University, IN
Wesley College, DE

HEALTH-CARE ADMINISTRATION

Adelphi University, NY
Albany State University, GA
Boise State University, ID
California State University, Long Beach, CA
Clarkson College, NE
Cleveland State University, OH
The College of New Rochelle, NY
Daemen College, NY
Duke University, NC
Fairfield University, CT
Georgetown University, DC
The George Washington University, DC
Goldfarb School of Nursing at Barnes-Jewish College, MO

Gonzaga University, WA
Hampton University, VA
Holy Family University, PA
The Johns Hopkins University, MD
Kaplan University Online, FL
Kean University, NJ
Kent State University, OH
La Roche College, PA
Loma Linda University, CA
Louisiana State University Health Sciences Center, LA
Loyola University New Orleans, LA
McNeese State University, LA
Mercy College, NY
Midwestern State University, TX
Missouri Western State University, MO
The Ohio State University, OH
Pacific Lutheran University, WA
Quinnipiac University, CT
Regis College, MA
Regis University, CO
Resurrection University, IL
The Sage Colleges, NY
Salisbury University, MD
Seton Hall University, NJ
Southern Illinois University Edwardsville, IL
Southern University and Agricultural and Mechanical College, LA
Tennessee Technological University, TN
Thomas University, GA
Towson University, MD
Trinity Western University, BC
Université de Moncton, NB
Université du Québec en Outaouais, QC
Université Laval, QC
The University of Alabama at Birmingham, AL
The University of Alabama in Huntsville, AL
University of Alaska Anchorage, AK
University of Delaware, DE
University of Illinois at Chicago, IL
The University of Kansas, KS
University of Louisiana at Lafayette, LA
University of Maine, ME
University of Michigan, MI
University of Nebraska Medical Center, NE
University of Oklahoma Health Sciences Center, OK
University of Pennsylvania, PA
University of Phoenix, AZ
University of Phoenix–Bay Area Campus, CA
University of Phoenix–Hawaii Campus, HI
University of Phoenix–Metro Detroit Campus, MI
University of Phoenix–North Florida Campus, FL
University of Phoenix–Phoenix Campus, AZ
University of Phoenix–Sacramento Valley Campus, CA
University of Phoenix–San Diego Campus, CA
University of Phoenix–Southern Arizona Campus, AZ
University of Phoenix–Southern California Campus, CA
University of Phoenix–South Florida Campus, FL
University of Rochester, NY
The University of Texas at Arlington, TX
University of Toronto, ON
The University of Western Ontario, ON
Vanderbilt University, TN
Villanova University, PA
Wright State University, OH

LEGAL NURSE CONSULTANT

Capital University, OH
Cleveland State University, OH
Wilmington University, DE

NURSE ANESTHESIA

Arkansas State University - Jonesboro, AR
Bloomsburg University of Pennsylvania, PA
Boston College, MA
Bradley University, IL
BryanLGH College of Health Sciences, NE
California State University, Fullerton, CA
Case Western Reserve University, OH
Clarkson College, NE
Columbia University, NY
DePaul University, IL
Drexel University, PA
Duke University, NC
East Carolina University, NC
Fairfield University, CT
Florida Gulf Coast University, FL
Florida International University, FL
Gannon University, PA
Georgetown University, DC
Georgia Health Sciences University, GA
Goldfarb School of Nursing at Barnes-Jewish College, MO
La Salle University, PA
Loma Linda University, CA
Louisiana State University Health Sciences Center, LA
Michigan State University, MI
Millikin University, IL
Mountain State University, WV
Murray State University, KY
Northeastern University, MA
Oakland University, MI
Old Dominion University, VA
Oregon Health & Science University, OR
Our Lady of the Lake College, LA
Rush University, IL
Samford University, AL
Samuel Merritt University, CA
Southern Illinois University Edwardsville, IL
State University of New York Downstate Medical Center, NY
Texas Christian University, TX
Thomas Jefferson University, PA
Union University, TN
University at Buffalo, the State University of New York, NY
The University of Akron, OH
University of Cincinnati, OH
The University of Iowa, IA
University of Maryland, Baltimore, MD
University of Medicine and Dentistry of New Jersey, NJ
University of Miami, FL
University of Michigan–Flint, MI
University of Minnesota, Twin Cities Campus, MN
The University of North Carolina at Charlotte, NC
The University of North Carolina at Greensboro, NC
University of North Dakota, ND
University of Pennsylvania, PA
University of Pittsburgh, PA
University of Puerto Rico, Medical Sciences Campus, PR
The University of Scranton, PA
University of South Florida, FL
The University of Tennessee, TN
The University of Tennessee at Chattanooga, TN
The University of Texas Health Science Center at Houston, TX
University of Toronto, ON
Villanova University, PA
Western Carolina University, NC
York College of Pennsylvania, PA
Youngstown State University, OH

NURSE-MIDWIFERY

California State University, Fullerton, CA
Case Western Reserve University, OH
Columbia University, NY
East Carolina University, NC
Emory University, GA
Georgetown University, DC
James Madison University, VA
The Johns Hopkins University, MD
Loyola University Chicago, IL
Marquette University, WI
New York University, NY
The Ohio State University, OH
Old Dominion University, VA
Oregon Health & Science University, OR
San Diego State University, CA
Shenandoah University, VA
State University of New York Downstate Medical Center, NY
Stony Brook University, State University of New York, NY
Texas Tech University Health Sciences Center, TX
University of California, San Francisco, CA
University of Cincinnati, OH
University of Colorado Denver, CO
University of Florida, FL
University of Illinois at Chicago, IL
University of Indianapolis, IN
The University of Kansas, KS
University of Medicine and Dentistry of New Jersey, NJ
University of Miami, FL
University of Michigan, MI
University of Minnesota, Twin Cities Campus, MN
University of New Mexico, NM
University of Pennsylvania, PA
University of Utah, UT
University of Washington, WA
Vanderbilt University, TN
Wayne State University, MI
Wichita State University, KS
Yale University, CT

NURSE PRACTITIONER PROGRAMS

Acute Care

Allen College, IA
Arizona State University at the Downtown Phoenix Campus, AZ
Barry University, FL
California State University, Los Angeles, CA
Case Western Reserve University, OH
The Catholic University of America, DC
Colorado State University–Pueblo, CO
Columbia University, NY
Creighton University, NE
Drexel University, PA

Duke University, NC
Emory University, GA
Florida Gulf Coast University, FL
Georgetown University, DC
Goldfarb School of Nursing at Barnes-Jewish College, MO
Grand Canyon University, AZ
Indiana University–Purdue University Indianapolis, IN
The Johns Hopkins University, MD
Kent State University, OH
Loyola University Chicago, IL
Madonna University, MI
Marquette University, WI
Memorial University of Newfoundland, NL
MGH Institute of Health Professions, MA
New York University, NY
Northeastern University, MA
Northern Kentucky University, KY
Northwestern State University of Louisiana, LA
The Ohio State University, OH
Rhode Island College, RI
Rush University, IL
Rutgers, The State University of New Jersey, College of Nursing, NJ
The Sage Colleges, NY
Saint Louis University, MO
San Diego State University, CA
Southern Adventist University, TN
Texas Tech University Health Sciences Center, TX
Texas Woman's University, TX
Thomas Jefferson University, PA
Université de Montréal, QC
The University of Alabama at Birmingham, AL
The University of Alabama in Huntsville, AL
University of Arkansas for Medical Sciences, AR
University of Calgary, AB
University of California, Los Angeles, CA
University of California, San Francisco, CA
University of Connecticut, CT
University of Florida, FL
University of Illinois at Chicago, IL
University of Kentucky, KY
University of Maryland, Baltimore, MD
University of Massachusetts Worcester, MA
University of Medicine and Dentistry of New Jersey, NJ
University of Miami, FL
University of Michigan, MI
University of Mississippi Medical Center, MS
University of Nebraska Medical Center, NE
University of New Brunswick Fredericton, NB
University of New Mexico, NM
University of Pennsylvania, PA
University of Pittsburgh, PA
University of Rochester, NY
University of South Alabama, AL
University of South Carolina, SC
University of Southern Indiana, IN
The University of Texas at Arlington, TX
The University of Texas at Tyler, TX
The University of Texas Health Science Center at Houston, TX
The University of Texas Health Science Center at San Antonio, TX
University of Toronto, ON
University of Virginia, VA
University of Washington, WA
Vanderbilt University, TN
Virginia Commonwealth University, VA
Wayne State University, MI
Wichita State University, KS
Wright State University, OH
Yale University, CT

Adult Health

Adelphi University, NY
Allen College, IA
Arizona State University at the Downtown Phoenix Campus, AZ
Armstrong Atlantic State University, GA
Azusa Pacific University, CA
Ball State University, IN
Bloomsburg University of Pennsylvania, PA
Boston College, MA
California State University, Long Beach, CA
California State University, Los Angeles, CA
Case Western Reserve University, OH
The Catholic University of America, DC
Clarkson College, NE
Clemson University, SC
College of Mount Saint Vincent, NY
The College of St. Scholastica, MN
College of Staten Island of the City University of New York, NY
Columbia University, NY
Creighton University, NE
Daemen College, NY
Dalhousie University, NS
DePaul University, IL
Duke University, NC
East Carolina University, NC
East Tennessee State University, TN
Emory University, GA
Fairleigh Dickinson University, Metropolitan Campus, NJ
Felician College, NJ
Florida Agricultural and Mechanical University, FL
Florida Atlantic University, FL
Florida Gulf Coast University, FL
Florida International University, FL
George Mason University, VA
The George Washington University, DC
Georgia State University, GA
Goldfarb School of Nursing at Barnes-Jewish College, MO
Gwynedd-Mercy College, PA
Hunter College of the City University of New York, NY
Indiana University–Purdue University Fort Wayne, IN
Indiana University–Purdue University Indianapolis, IN
James Madison University, VA
The Johns Hopkins University, MD
Kaplan University Online, FL
Kennesaw State University, GA
Kent State University, OH
La Salle University, PA
Lewis University, IL
Loma Linda University, CA
Long Island University, Brooklyn Campus, NY
Loyola University Chicago, IL
Loyola University New Orleans, LA
Madonna University, MI
Marian University, WI
Marquette University, WI
Maryville University of Saint Louis, MO
McNeese State University, LA
Medical University of South Carolina, SC
Metropolitan State University, MN
MGH Institute of Health Professions, MA
Michigan State University, MI
Molloy College, NY
Monmouth University, NJ
Mount Saint Mary College, NY
Neumann University, PA
Northeastern University, MA
Northern Illinois University, IL
Northern Kentucky University, KY
North Park University, IL
Oakland University, MI
The Ohio State University, OH
Otterbein University, OH
Penn State University Park, PA
Purdue University, IN
Quinnipiac University, CT
Regis College, MA
Research College of Nursing, MO
Rhode Island College, RI
The Richard Stockton College of New Jersey, NJ
Rush University, IL
Rutgers, The State University of New Jersey, College of Nursing, NJ
The Sage Colleges, NY
St. Catherine University, MN
Saint Louis University, MO
Saint Peter's College, NJ
San Diego State University, CA
Seattle Pacific University, WA
Seattle University, WA
Seton Hall University, NJ
Southeastern Louisiana University, LA
Southern Adventist University, TN
Spalding University, KY
Spring Arbor University, MI
State University of New York Institute of Technology, NY
State University of New York Upstate Medical University, NY
Stony Brook University, State University of New York, NY
Temple University, PA
Texas Woman's University, TX
Thomas Jefferson University, PA
Université de Moncton, NB
Université Laval, QC
University at Buffalo, the State University of New York, NY
The University of Akron, OH
The University of Alabama at Birmingham, AL
University of Alberta, AB
University of Calgary, AB
University of California, Irvine, CA
University of California, Los Angeles, CA
University of California, San Francisco, CA
University of Central Arkansas, AR
University of Central Florida, FL
University of Cincinnati, OH
University of Colorado at Colorado Springs, CO
University of Colorado Denver, CO
University of Delaware, DE
University of Florida, FL
University of Hawaii at Manoa, HI
University of Illinois at Chicago, IL
The University of Iowa, IA
The University of Kansas, KS
University of Kentucky, KY
University of Louisiana at Lafayette, LA
University of Louisville, KY

University of Maryland, Baltimore, MD
University of Massachusetts Boston, MA
University of Massachusetts Dartmouth, MA
University of Medicine and Dentistry of New Jersey, NJ
University of Miami, FL
University of Michigan, MI
University of Michigan–Flint, MI
University of Missouri–Kansas City, MO
University of Missouri–St. Louis, MO
University of Nebraska Medical Center, NE
University of New Brunswick Fredericton, NB
University of New Hampshire, NH
The University of North Carolina at Chapel Hill, NC
The University of North Carolina at Charlotte, NC
The University of North Carolina at Greensboro, NC
University of Oklahoma Health Sciences Center, OK
University of Pennsylvania, PA
University of Pittsburgh, PA
University of Rochester, NY
University of St. Francis, IL
University of San Diego, CA
University of Southern Maine, ME
University of South Florida, FL
The University of Tampa, FL
The University of Tennessee, TN
The University of Texas at Arlington, TX
The University of Texas at Tyler, TX
The University of Texas Health Science Center at Houston, TX
The University of Toledo, OH
University of Toronto, ON
University of Vermont, VT
University of Washington, WA
University of Wisconsin–Eau Claire, WI
University of Wisconsin–Oshkosh, WI
Ursuline College, OH
Vanderbilt University, TN
Villanova University, PA
Virginia Commonwealth University, VA
Viterbo University, WI
Washburn University, KS
Western Connecticut State University, CT
William Paterson University of New Jersey, NJ
Wilmington University, DE
Winona State University, MN
Yale University, CT
York College of Pennsylvania, PA

Community Health

Athabasca University, AB
DePaul University, IL
The Ohio State University, OH
The Sage Colleges, NY
State University of New York at Binghamton, NY
Université de Moncton, NB
University of Hawaii at Manoa, HI
University of Medicine and Dentistry of New Jersey, NJ
University of Nebraska Medical Center, NE
University of New Brunswick Fredericton, NB
University of Saint Francis, IN
University of Virginia, VA
The University of Western Ontario, ON

Family Health

Albany State University, GA
Alcorn State University, MS
Allen College, IA
Angelo State University, TX
Arizona State University at the Downtown Phoenix Campus, AZ
Athabasca University, AB
Azusa Pacific University, CA
Ball State University, IN
Barry University, FL
Baylor University, TX
Belmont University, TN
Boston College, MA
Bowie State University, MD
Brenau University, GA
Briar Cliff University, IA
Brigham Young University, UT
California State University, Dominguez Hills, CA
California State University, Fresno, CA
California State University, Long Beach, CA
California State University, Los Angeles, CA
California State University, Sacramento, CA
Carlow University, PA
Carson-Newman College, TN
Case Western Reserve University, OH
The Catholic University of America, DC
Clarion University of Pennsylvania, PA
Clarke University, IA
Clarkson College, NE
Clemson University, SC
College of Mount Saint Vincent, NY
The College of New Jersey, NJ
The College of New Rochelle, NY
The College of St. Scholastica, MN
Colorado State University–Pueblo, CO
Columbia University, NY
Concordia University Wisconsin, WI
Coppin State University, MD
Creighton University, NE
Dalhousie University, NS
Delta State University, MS
DePaul University, IL
DeSales University, PA
Dominican College, NY
Drexel University, PA
Duke University, NC
Duquesne University, PA
D'Youville College, NY
East Carolina University, NC
Eastern Kentucky University, KY
East Tennessee State University, TN
Emory University, GA
Fairfield University, CT
Fairleigh Dickinson University, Metropolitan Campus, NJ
Felician College, NJ
Florida Atlantic University, FL
Florida Gulf Coast University, FL
Florida International University, FL
Florida State University, FL
Fort Hays State University, KS
Franciscan University of Steubenville, OH
Gannon University, PA
George Mason University, VA
Georgetown University, DC
The George Washington University, DC
Georgia College & State University, GA
Georgia Health Sciences University, GA
Georgia Southern University, GA
Georgia State University, GA
Gonzaga University, WA
Graceland University, IA
Grambling State University, LA
Grand Canyon University, AZ
Hampton University, VA
Hawai`i Pacific University, HI
Holy Names University, CA
Howard University, DC
Husson University, ME
Idaho State University, ID
Illinois State University, IL
Indiana State University, IN
Indiana University–Purdue University Indianapolis, IN
Indiana University South Bend, IN
Indiana Wesleyan University, IN
Jacksonville University, FL
James Madison University, VA
The Johns Hopkins University, MD
Kaplan University Online, FL
Kennesaw State University, GA
Kent State University, OH
La Salle University, PA
Lehman College of the City University of New York, NY
Loma Linda University, CA
Long Island University, Brooklyn Campus, NY
Long Island University, C.W. Post Campus, NY
Loyola University Chicago, IL
Loyola University New Orleans, LA
Malone University, OH
Marshall University, WV
Marymount University, VA
Maryville University of Saint Louis, MO
Medical University of South Carolina, SC
Metropolitan State University, MN
MGH Institute of Health Professions, MA
Michigan State University, MI
Middle Tennessee State University, TN
Midwestern State University, TX
Millersville University of Pennsylvania, PA
Minnesota State University Mankato, MN
Misericordia University, PA
Mississippi University for Women, MS
Missouri State University, MO
Molloy College, NY
Monmouth University, NJ
Montana State University, MT
Mountain State University, WV
Mount Carmel College of Nursing, OH
Murray State University, KY
North Dakota State University, ND
Northeastern University, MA
Northern Arizona University, AZ
Northern Illinois University, IL
Northern Kentucky University, KY
Northern Michigan University, MI
North Georgia College & State University, GA
North Park University, IL
Northwestern State University of Louisiana, LA
Oakland University, MI
The Ohio State University, OH
Ohio University, OH
Old Dominion University, VA
Oregon Health & Science University, OR
Otterbein University, OH
Pace University, NY
Pacific Lutheran University, WA
Patty Hanks Shelton School of Nursing, TX
Penn State University Park, PA
Pittsburg State University, KS
Prairie View A&M University, TX
Purdue University Calumet, IN
Quinnipiac University, CT

Regis College, MA
Regis University, CO
Research College of Nursing, MO
Rivier College, NH
Rush University, IL
Rutgers, The State University of New Jersey, College of Nursing, NJ
Sacred Heart University, CT
The Sage Colleges, NY
Saginaw Valley State University, MI
Saint Anthony College of Nursing, IL
St. John Fisher College, NY
Saint Joseph College, CT
Saint Louis University, MO
Saint Xavier University, IL
Salisbury University, MD
Samford University, AL
Samuel Merritt University, CA
San Francisco State University, CA
San Jose State University, CA
Seattle Pacific University, WA
Seattle University, WA
Shenandoah University, VA
Simmons College, MA
Sonoma State University, CA
South Dakota State University, SD
Southeast Missouri State University, MO
Southern Adventist University, TN
Southern Connecticut State University, CT
Southern Illinois University Edwardsville, IL
Southern University and Agricultural and Mechanical College, LA
Spalding University, KY
State University of New York at Binghamton, NY
State University of New York Downstate Medical Center, NY
State University of New York Institute of Technology, NY
State University of New York Upstate Medical University, NY
Temple University, PA
Tennessee State University, TN
Tennessee Technological University, TN
Texas A&M International University, TX
Texas A&M University–Corpus Christi, TX
Texas Tech University Health Sciences Center, TX
Texas Woman's University, TX
Thomas Jefferson University, PA
Touro University, NV
Troy University, AL
Union University, TN
Université de Moncton, NB
Université de Montréal, QC
University at Buffalo, the State University of New York, NY
The University of Alabama at Birmingham, AL
The University of Alabama in Huntsville, AL
University of Alaska Anchorage, AK
University of Arkansas for Medical Sciences, AR
The University of British Columbia, BC
University of California, Irvine, CA
University of California, Los Angeles, CA
University of California, San Francisco, CA
University of Central Arkansas, AR
University of Central Florida, FL
University of Central Missouri, MO
University of Cincinnati, OH
University of Colorado at Colorado Springs, CO
University of Colorado Denver, CO
University of Delaware, DE
University of Detroit Mercy, MI
University of Florida, FL
University of Hawaii at Manoa, HI
University of Illinois at Chicago, IL
University of Indianapolis, IN
The University of Iowa, IA
The University of Kansas, KS
University of Kentucky, KY
University of Louisville, KY
University of Maine, ME
University of Mary, ND
University of Maryland, Baltimore, MD
University of Massachusetts Boston, MA
University of Massachusetts Lowell, MA
University of Massachusetts Worcester, MA
University of Medicine and Dentistry of New Jersey, NJ
University of Memphis, TN
University of Miami, FL
University of Michigan, MI
University of Michigan–Flint, MI
University of Minnesota, Twin Cities Campus, MN
University of Mississippi Medical Center, MS
University of Missouri, MO
University of Missouri–Kansas City, MO
University of Missouri–St. Louis, MO
University of Nebraska Medical Center, NE
University of Nevada, Las Vegas, NV
University of Nevada, Reno, NV
University of New Brunswick Fredericton, NB
University of New Hampshire, NH
University of New Mexico, NM
The University of North Carolina at Chapel Hill, NC
The University of North Carolina at Charlotte, NC
The University of North Carolina Wilmington, NC
University of North Dakota, ND
University of Northern British Columbia, BC
University of Northern Colorado, CO
University of North Florida, FL
University of Oklahoma Health Sciences Center, OK
University of Pennsylvania, PA
University of Phoenix, AZ
University of Phoenix–Hawaii Campus, HI
University of Phoenix–Phoenix Campus, AZ
University of Phoenix–Sacramento Valley Campus, CA
University of Phoenix–Southern Arizona Campus, AZ
University of Phoenix–Southern California Campus, CA
University of Pittsburgh, PA
University of Rhode Island, RI
University of Rochester, NY
University of St. Francis, IL
University of Saint Francis, IN
University of San Diego, CA
The University of Scranton, PA
University of South Alabama, AL
University of South Carolina, SC
University of Southern Indiana, IN
University of Southern Maine, ME
University of Southern Mississippi, MS
University of South Florida, FL
The University of Tampa, FL
The University of Tennessee, TN
The University of Tennessee at Chattanooga, TN
The University of Texas at Arlington, TX
The University of Texas at Austin, TX
The University of Texas at El Paso, TX
The University of Texas at Tyler, TX
The University of Texas Health Science Center at Houston, TX
The University of Texas Health Science Center at San Antonio, TX
The University of Texas Medical Branch, TX
The University of Texas–Pan American, TX
The University of Toledo, OH
University of Toronto, ON
University of Vermont, VT
University of Virginia, VA
University of Washington, WA
University of Wisconsin–Eau Claire, WI
University of Wisconsin–Oshkosh, WI
University of Wyoming, WY
Ursuline College, OH
Vanderbilt University, TN
Villanova University, PA
Virginia Commonwealth University, VA
Viterbo University, WI
Wagner College, NY
Washburn University, KS
Washington State University College of Nursing and Consortium, WA
Western Carolina University, NC
Western University of Health Sciences, CA
Westminster College, UT
West Texas A&M University, TX
West Virginia University, WV
Wheeling Jesuit University, WV
Wichita State University, KS
Widener University, PA
William Paterson University of New Jersey, NJ
Wilmington University, DE
Winona State University, MN
Winston-Salem State University, NC
Wright State University, OH
Yale University, CT

Gerontology

Allen College, IA
Bloomsburg University of Pennsylvania, PA
Boston College, MA
California State University, Long Beach, CA
Case Western Reserve University, OH
The Catholic University of America, DC
Clemson University, SC
The College of St. Scholastica, MN
College of Staten Island of the City University of New York, NY
Columbia University, NY
Concordia University Wisconsin, WI
Creighton University, NE
Delta State University, MS
Duke University, NC
East Tennessee State University, TN
Emory University, GA
Florida Agricultural and Mechanical University, FL
Florida Atlantic University, FL
Hampton University, VA
Hunter College of the City University of New York, NY
James Madison University, VA
Kent State University, OH
Long Island University, Brooklyn Campus, NY
Marquette University, WI

MGH Institute of Health Professions, MA
Michigan State University, MI
Mississippi University for Women, MS
Nazareth College of Rochester, NY
Neumann University, PA
New York University, NY
Oakland University, MI
Rush University, IL
The Sage Colleges, NY
St. Catherine University, MN
Saint Louis University, MO
San Diego State University, CA
Seton Hall University, NJ
Southeastern Louisiana University, LA
Spring Arbor University, MI
State University of New York at Binghamton, NY
Texas Tech University Health Sciences Center, TX
Trinity Western University, BC
The University of Akron, OH
The University of Alabama at Birmingham, AL
University of Alberta, AB
University of Arkansas for Medical Sciences, AR
University of California, Irvine, CA
University of California, Los Angeles, CA
University of California, San Francisco, CA
University of Hawaii at Manoa, HI
University of Illinois at Chicago, IL
University of Indianapolis, IN
The University of Iowa, IA
The University of Kansas, KS
University of Kentucky, KY
University of Maryland, Baltimore, MD
University of Massachusetts Boston, MA
University of Massachusetts Lowell, MA
University of Massachusetts Worcester, MA
University of Medicine and Dentistry of New Jersey, NJ
University of Michigan, MI
University of Minnesota, Twin Cities Campus, MN
University of Mississippi Medical Center, MS
University of Missouri, MO
University of Nebraska Medical Center, NE
University of New Brunswick Fredericton, NB
The University of North Carolina at Chapel Hill, NC
The University of North Carolina at Greensboro, NC
University of North Dakota, ND
University of Pennsylvania, PA
University of Rhode Island, RI
University of Rochester, NY
University of South Alabama, AL
The University of Texas at Arlington, TX
The University of Texas at Tyler, TX
The University of Texas Health Science Center at Houston, TX
The University of Texas Medical Branch, TX
University of Utah, UT
University of Wisconsin–Eau Claire, WI
Vanderbilt University, TN
Villanova University, PA
Wayne State University, MI
West Virginia University, WV
Wilmington University, DE
Yale University, CT

Neonatal Health

Arizona State University at the Downtown Phoenix Campus, AZ
Baylor University, TX
Case Western Reserve University, OH
The College of New Jersey, NJ
Columbia University, NY
Creighton University, NE
Dalhousie University, NS
Duke University, NC
East Carolina University, NC
Indiana University–Purdue University Indianapolis, IN
Louisiana State University Health Sciences Center, LA
McGill University, QC
McMaster University, ON
Northeastern University, MA
Northwestern State University of Louisiana, LA
The Ohio State University, OH
Regis University, CO
Rush University, IL
St. Catherine University, MN
Saint Francis Medical Center College of Nursing, IL
South Dakota State University, SD
Stony Brook University, State University of New York, NY
Thomas Jefferson University, PA
The University of Alabama at Birmingham, AL
University of Calgary, AB
University of California, San Francisco, CA
University of Cincinnati, OH
University of Connecticut, CT
University of Florida, FL
The University of Iowa, IA
University of Louisville, KY
University of Missouri–Kansas City, MO
University of Missouri–St. Louis, MO
University of Nebraska Medical Center, NE
University of New Brunswick Fredericton, NB
University of Oklahoma Health Sciences Center, OK
University of Pennsylvania, PA
University of Pittsburgh, PA
University of Rochester, NY
University of South Alabama, AL
The University of Texas at Arlington, TX
The University of Texas Medical Branch, TX
University of Washington, WA
Vanderbilt University, TN
Wayne State University, MI
West Virginia University, WV

Occupational Health

The University of Alabama at Birmingham, AL
University of California, Los Angeles, CA
University of California, San Francisco, CA
University of Cincinnati, OH
University of Illinois at Chicago, IL
University of South Florida, FL
University of the Sacred Heart, PR

Oncology

Case Western Reserve University, OH
Columbia University, NY
Creighton University, NE
Duke University, NC
Thomas Jefferson University, PA
Université de Moncton, NB
University of California, Los Angeles, CA
University of Nebraska Medical Center, NE
The University of North Carolina at Chapel Hill, NC
University of South Florida, FL
University of Virginia, VA
Yale University, CT

Pediatric

Arizona State University at the Downtown Phoenix Campus, AZ
Azusa Pacific University, CA
Boston College, MA
California State University, Fresno, CA
California State University, Long Beach, CA
California State University, Los Angeles, CA
Case Western Reserve University, OH
The Catholic University of America, DC
The College of St. Scholastica, MN
Colorado State University–Pueblo, CO
Columbia University, NY
Creighton University, NE
DePaul University, IL
Drexel University, PA
Duke University, NC
Emory University, GA
Florida International University, FL
Georgia Health Sciences University, GA
Georgia State University, GA
Grambling State University, LA
Gwynedd-Mercy College, PA
Hampton University, VA
Hunter College of the City University of New York, NY
Indiana University–Purdue University Indianapolis, IN
The Johns Hopkins University, MD
Kent State University, OH
Lehman College of the City University of New York, NY
Loma Linda University, CA
Loyola University Chicago, IL
Marquette University, WI
Medical University of South Carolina, SC
MGH Institute of Health Professions, MA
Mississippi University for Women, MS
Molloy College, NY
New York University, NY
Northeastern University, MA
Northern Kentucky University, KY
Northwestern State University of Louisiana, LA
The Ohio State University, OH
Purdue University, IN
Regis College, MA
Rush University, IL
Rutgers, The State University of New Jersey, College of Nursing, NJ
St. Catherine University, MN
Saint Louis University, MO
Seton Hall University, NJ
Spalding University, KY
State University of New York Upstate Medical University, NY
Stony Brook University, State University of New York, NY
Temple University, PA
Texas Tech University Health Sciences Center, TX
Texas Woman's University, TX
Thomas Jefferson University, PA
The University of Akron, OH
The University of Alabama at Birmingham, AL

University of Arkansas for Medical Sciences, AR
University of California, Los Angeles, CA
University of California, San Francisco, CA
University of Central Florida, FL
University of Cincinnati, OH
University of Colorado Denver, CO
University of Florida, FL
University of Hawaii at Manoa, HI
University of Illinois at Chicago, IL
The University of Iowa, IA
University of Kentucky, KY
University of Maryland, Baltimore, MD
University of Michigan, MI
University of Minnesota, Twin Cities Campus, MN
University of Missouri, MO
University of Missouri–Kansas City, MO
University of Missouri–St. Louis, MO
University of Nebraska Medical Center, NE
University of New Brunswick Fredericton, NB
University of New Mexico, NM
The University of North Carolina at Chapel Hill, NC
University of Oklahoma Health Sciences Center, OK
University of Pennsylvania, PA
University of Pittsburgh, PA
University of Rochester, NY
University of San Diego, CA
University of South Alabama, AL
University of South Florida, FL
The University of Tennessee, TN
The University of Texas at Arlington, TX
The University of Texas at Austin, TX
The University of Texas at Tyler, TX
The University of Texas Health Science Center at Houston, TX
The University of Texas Health Science Center at San Antonio, TX
The University of Texas–Pan American, TX
The University of Toledo, OH
University of Toronto, ON
University of Virginia, VA
University of Washington, WA
Vanderbilt University, TN
Villanova University, PA
Virginia Commonwealth University, VA
Wayne State University, MI
West Virginia University, WV
Wichita State University, KS
Wright State University, OH
Yale University, CT

Primary Care

Arkansas State University - Jonesboro, AR
Athabasca University, AB
Auburn University Montgomery, AL
Azusa Pacific University, CA
California State University, Los Angeles, CA
California State University, Sacramento, CA
Dalhousie University, NS
Duke University, NC
Emory University, GA
Florida Southern College, FL
George Mason University, VA
Gonzaga University, WA
Hampton University, VA
The Johns Hopkins University, MD
Kennesaw State University, GA
Kent State University, OH
Loma Linda University, CA
Louisiana State University Health Sciences Center, LA
Madonna University, MI
McGill University, QC
MGH Institute of Health Professions, MA
New York University, NY
Northeastern University, MA
The Ohio State University, OH
Queen's University at Kingston, ON
Regis College, MA
Ryerson University, ON
Samford University, AL
Simmons College, MA
State University of New York at Binghamton, NY
Université de Moncton, NB
Université de Montréal, QC
Université du Québec à Chicoutimi, QC
Université du Québec à Trois-Rivières, QC
Université du Québec en Outaouais, QC
Université Laval, QC
The University of Alabama at Birmingham, AL
The University of British Columbia, BC
University of Connecticut, CT
University of Manitoba, MB
University of Maryland, Baltimore, MD
University of Massachusetts Worcester, MA
University of Michigan, MI
University of Missouri, MO
University of Nebraska Medical Center, NE
University of New Brunswick Fredericton, NB
The University of North Carolina at Chapel Hill, NC
University of North Florida, FL
University of Ottawa, ON
University of Pennsylvania, PA
University of Saskatchewan, SK
University of Virginia, VA
University of Washington, WA
Virginia Commonwealth University, VA
Wayne State University, MI
Western Kentucky University, KY
Yale University, CT

Psychiatric/mental Health

Allen College, IA
Arizona State University at the Downtown Phoenix Campus, AZ
Boston College, MA
California State University, Long Beach, CA
California State University, Los Angeles, CA
Case Western Reserve University, OH
The College of St. Scholastica, MN
Columbia University, NY
Creighton University, NE
Delta State University, MS
Drexel University, PA
Eastern Kentucky University, KY
East Tennessee State University, TN
Fairfield University, CT
Fairleigh Dickinson University, Metropolitan Campus, NJ
Georgia State University, GA
Gonzaga University, WA
Kent State University, OH
Loma Linda University, CA
McNeese State University, LA
MGH Institute of Health Professions, MA
Mississippi University for Women, MS
Molloy College, NY
Monmouth University, NJ
Montana State University, MT
New Mexico State University, NM
New York University, NY
Northeastern University, MA
The Ohio State University, OH
Oregon Health & Science University, OR
Regis College, MA
Rivier College, NH
Rush University, IL
Rutgers, The State University of New Jersey, College of Nursing, NJ
The Sage Colleges, NY
Saint Louis University, MO
Seattle University, WA
Shenandoah University, VA
South Dakota State University, SD
Southeastern Louisiana University, LA
State University of New York Upstate Medical University, NY
Stony Brook University, State University of New York, NY
University at Buffalo, the State University of New York, NY
The University of Akron, OH
The University of Alabama at Birmingham, AL
University of Alaska Anchorage, AK
University of Arkansas for Medical Sciences, AR
University of California, San Francisco, CA
University of Colorado Denver, CO
University of Florida, FL
University of Illinois at Chicago, IL
The University of Iowa, IA
The University of Kansas, KS
University of Kentucky, KY
University of Louisiana at Lafayette, LA
University of Louisville, KY
University of Maryland, Baltimore, MD
University of Massachusetts Lowell, MA
University of Medicine and Dentistry of New Jersey, NJ
University of Michigan, MI
University of Michigan–Flint, MI
University of Mississippi Medical Center, MS
University of Missouri, MO
University of Nebraska Medical Center, NE
University of New Brunswick Fredericton, NB
The University of North Carolina at Chapel Hill, NC
University of North Dakota, ND
University of Pennsylvania, PA
University of Pittsburgh, PA
University of Rochester, NY
University of San Diego, CA
University of South Alabama, AL
University of Southern Maine, ME
University of Southern Mississippi, MS
The University of Tennessee, TN
The University of Texas at Arlington, TX
The University of Texas Health Science Center at Houston, TX
The University of Texas Health Science Center at San Antonio, TX
University of Utah, UT
University of Vermont, VT
University of Virginia, VA
University of Washington, WA
University of Wyoming, WY
Vanderbilt University, TN
Washington State University College of Nursing and Consortium, WA
Wayne State University, MI
Wichita State University, KS

Winston-Salem State University, NC
Yale University, CT

School Health

La Roche College, PA
Seton Hall University, NJ
University of Illinois at Chicago, IL

WomensHealth'

Arizona State University at the Downtown Phoenix Campus, AZ
Boston College, MA
California State University, Fullerton, CA
California State University, Long Beach, CA
Case Western Reserve University, OH
Columbia University, NY
DePaul University, IL
Drexel University, PA
Emory University, GA
Florida Agricultural and Mechanical University, FL
Georgetown University, DC
Georgia State University, GA
Hampton University, VA
Indiana University–Purdue University Fort Wayne, IN
Indiana University–Purdue University Indianapolis, IN
Kent State University, OH
Loyola University Chicago, IL
MGH Institute of Health Professions, MA
Northwestern State University of Louisiana, LA
The Ohio State University, OH
Old Dominion University, VA
Regis College, MA
Rutgers, The State University of New Jersey, College of Nursing, NJ
San Diego State University, CA
State University of New York Downstate Medical Center, NY
Stony Brook University, State University of New York, NY
Texas Woman's University, TX
The University of Alabama at Birmingham, AL
University of Arkansas for Medical Sciences, AR
University of Cincinnati, OH
University of Colorado Denver, CO
University of Illinois at Chicago, IL
University of Indianapolis, IN
University of Medicine and Dentistry of New Jersey, NJ
University of Minnesota, Twin Cities Campus, MN
University of Missouri–Kansas City, MO
University of Missouri–St. Louis, MO
University of Nebraska Medical Center, NE
University of New Brunswick Fredericton, NB
The University of North Carolina at Chapel Hill, NC
University of Pennsylvania, PA
University of South Alabama, AL
The University of Texas at Tyler, TX
The University of Texas Health Science Center at Houston, TX
Vanderbilt University, TN
Virginia Commonwealth University, VA
Wayne State University, MI
Wesley College, DE
West Virginia University, WV
Yale University, CT

NURSING ADMINISTRATION

Adelphi University, NY
Allen College, IA
American International College, MA
American Sentinel University, CO
Anderson University, IN
Arkansas Tech University, AR
Armstrong Atlantic State University, GA
Athabasca University, AB
Aurora University, IL
Azusa Pacific University, CA
Ball State University, IN
Barry University, FL
Bellarmine University, KY
Bellin College, WI
Bethel College, IN
Bethel University, MN
Blessing–Rieman College of Nursing, IL
Bloomsburg University of Pennsylvania, PA
Boise State University, ID
Bradley University, IL
California State University, Dominguez Hills, CA
California State University, Fullerton, CA
California State University, Los Angeles, CA
California State University, Sacramento, CA
California State University, San Bernardino, CA
Capital University, OH
Carlow University, PA
Chatham University, PA
Clarkson College, NE
Clayton State University, GA
Clemson University, SC
Cleveland State University, OH
College of Mount Saint Vincent, NY
The College of New Jersey, NJ
The College of New Rochelle, NY
The College of St. Scholastica, MN
Creighton University, NE
Delta State University, MS
DePaul University, IL
DeSales University, PA
Drexel University, PA
Duke University, NC
East Carolina University, NC
Eastern Mennonite University, VA
East Tennessee State University, TN
Edgewood College, WI
Elms College, MA
Emmanuel College, MA
Endicott College, MA
Excelsior College, NY
Fairleigh Dickinson University, Metropolitan Campus, NJ
Felician College, NJ
Ferris State University, MI
Florida Atlantic University, FL
Florida International University, FL
Florida Southern College, FL
Fort Hays State University, KS
Framingham State University, MA
Franklin Pierce University, NH
Gannon University, PA
Gardner-Webb University, NC
George Mason University, VA
The George Washington University, DC
Georgia College & State University, GA
Goldfarb School of Nursing at Barnes-Jewish College, MO
Gonzaga University, WA
Grand Canyon University, AZ
Hampton University, VA
Holy Names University, CA
Idaho State University, ID
Illinois State University, IL
Immaculata University, PA
Indiana State University, IN
Indiana University of Pennsylvania, PA
Indiana University–Purdue University Fort Wayne, IN
Indiana University–Purdue University Indianapolis, IN
Indiana Wesleyan University, IN
Jacksonville University, FL
James Madison University, VA
Jefferson College of Health Sciences, VA
The Johns Hopkins University, MD
Kean University, NJ
Kent State University, OH
Lamar University, TX
La Roche College, PA
La Salle University, PA
Lehman College of the City University of New York, NY
Le Moyne College, NY
Lewis University, IL
Loma Linda University, CA
Long Island University, Brooklyn Campus, NY
Louisiana State University Health Sciences Center, LA
Loyola University Chicago, IL
Madonna University, MI
Mansfield University of Pennsylvania, PA
Marquette University, WI
Marshall University, WV
Marywood University, PA
McGill University, QC
McKendree University, IL
McNeese State University, LA
Medical University of South Carolina, SC
Mercy College, NY
Metropolitan State University, MN
Middle Tennessee State University, TN
Midwestern State University, TX
Molloy College, NY
Monmouth University, NJ
Moravian College, PA
Mountain State University, WV
Mount Carmel College of Nursing, OH
Mount St. Mary's College, CA
Nebraska Methodist College, NE
Nebraska Wesleyan University, NE
New Mexico State University, NM
New York University, NY
Northeastern University, MA
Northern Kentucky University, KY
North Park University, IL
Northwestern State University of Louisiana, LA
Nova Southeastern University, FL
The Ohio State University, OH
Ohio University, OH
Oklahoma City University, OK
Old Dominion University, VA
Otterbein University, OH
Our Lady of the Lake College, LA
Pacific Lutheran University, WA
Patty Hanks Shelton School of Nursing, TX
Penn State University Park, PA
Pittsburg State University, KS
Prairie View A&M University, TX
Purdue University Calumet, IN
Queens University of Charlotte, NC

Regis College, MA
Regis University, CO
Research College of Nursing, MO
Resurrection University, IL
Roberts Wesleyan College, NY
Sacred Heart University, CT
The Sage Colleges, NY
Saginaw Valley State University, MI
St. Ambrose University, IA
Saint Joseph's College of Maine, ME
Saint Peter's College, NJ
Saint Xavier University, IL
Salem State University, MA
Samford University, AL
San Diego State University, CA
San Francisco State University, CA
San Jose State University, CA
Seattle Pacific University, WA
Seton Hall University, NJ
Simmons College, MA
Sonoma State University, CA
South Dakota State University, SD
Southeastern Louisiana University, LA
Southern Nazarene University, OK
Spalding University, KY
State University of New York at Binghamton, NY
State University of New York Institute of Technology, NY
Texas A&M University–Corpus Christi, TX
Texas A&M University–Texarkana, TX
Texas Tech University Health Sciences Center, TX
Texas Woman's University, TX
Thomas University, GA
Trinity Western University, BC
Troy University, AL
Union University, TN
Université de Moncton, NB
Université Laval, QC
The University of Akron, OH
The University of Alabama, AL
The University of Alabama at Birmingham, AL
University of Arkansas for Medical Sciences, AR
The University of British Columbia, BC
University of California, Los Angeles, CA
University of California, San Francisco, CA
University of Central Florida, FL
University of Cincinnati, OH
University of Colorado Denver, CO
University of Detroit Mercy, MI
University of Hartford, CT
University of Hawaii at Manoa, HI
University of Houston–Victoria, TX
University of Illinois at Chicago, IL
University of Indianapolis, IN
The University of Iowa, IA
The University of Kansas, KS
University of Kentucky, KY
University of Louisiana at Lafayette, LA
University of Manitoba, MB
University of Mary, ND
University of Maryland, Baltimore, MD
University of Memphis, TN
University of Michigan, MI
University of Minnesota, Twin Cities Campus, MN
University of Mississippi Medical Center, MS
University of Missouri, MO
University of Mobile, AL
University of Nebraska Medical Center, NE
University of New Brunswick Fredericton, NB
University of New Mexico, NM
University of North Alabama, AL
The University of North Carolina at Chapel Hill, NC
The University of North Carolina at Charlotte, NC
The University of North Carolina at Greensboro, NC
University of Pennsylvania, PA
University of Phoenix, AZ
University of Phoenix–Bay Area Campus, CA
University of Phoenix–Central Florida Campus, FL
University of Phoenix–Cleveland Campus, OH
University of Phoenix–Denver Campus, CO
University of Phoenix–Hawaii Campus, HI
University of Phoenix–Metro Detroit Campus, MI
University of Phoenix–New Mexico Campus, NM
University of Phoenix–North Florida Campus, FL
University of Phoenix–Phoenix Campus, AZ
University of Phoenix–Sacramento Valley Campus, CA
University of Phoenix–San Diego Campus, CA
University of Phoenix–Southern Arizona Campus, AZ
University of Phoenix–Southern California Campus, CA
University of Phoenix–South Florida Campus, FL
University of Pittsburgh, PA
University of Puerto Rico, Medical Sciences Campus, PR
University of Rhode Island, RI
University of San Diego, CA
University of South Alabama, AL
University of Southern Indiana, IN
University of Southern Mississippi, MS
The University of Tennessee, TN
The University of Texas at Arlington, TX
The University of Texas at Austin, TX
The University of Texas at Brownsville, TX
The University of Texas at El Paso, TX
The University of Texas at Tyler, TX
The University of Texas Health Science Center at Houston, TX
The University of Texas Health Science Center at San Antonio, TX
The University of Texas Medical Branch, TX
University of Toronto, ON
University of Vermont, VT
University of Virginia, VA
The University of Western Ontario, ON
University of West Georgia, GA
University of Wisconsin–Eau Claire, WI
Urbana University, OH
Valdosta State University, GA
Vanderbilt University, TN
Virginia Commonwealth University, VA
Walden University, MN
Washburn University, KS
Washington State University College of Nursing and Consortium, WA
Waynesburg University, PA
Weber State University, UT
Webster University, MO
Western Carolina University, NC
Western Kentucky University, KY
Western Michigan University, MI
Western University of Health Sciences, CA
West Texas A&M University, TX
West Virginia University, WV
West Virginia Wesleyan College, WV
Wheeling Jesuit University, WV
Wilkes University, PA
William Paterson University of New Jersey, NJ
Wilmington University, DE
Winona State University, MN
Wright State University, OH
Xavier University, OH
Yale University, CT
York College of Pennsylvania, PA

NURSING EDUCATION

Adelphi University, NY
Albany State University, GA
Alcorn State University, MS
Allen College, IA
Alverno College, WI
American International College, MA
American Sentinel University, CO
Anderson University, IN
Andrews University, MI
Angelo State University, TX
Arkansas State University - Jonesboro, AR
Athabasca University, AB
Auburn University, AL
Auburn University Montgomery, AL
Aurora University, IL
Azusa Pacific University, CA
Ball State University, IN
Barry University, FL
Bellarmine University, KY
Bellin College, WI
Belmont University, TN
Bethel College, IN
Bethel University, MN
Blessing–Rieman College of Nursing, IL
Boise State University, ID
Bowie State University, MD
Bradley University, IL
Brenau University, GA
Briar Cliff University, IA
California Baptist University, CA
California State University, Chico, CA
California State University, Dominguez Hills, CA
California State University, Fresno, CA
California State University, Fullerton, CA
California State University, Long Beach, CA
California State University, Los Angeles, CA
California State University, Sacramento, CA
California State University, San Bernardino, CA
Capital University, OH
Cardinal Stritch University, WI
Carlow University, PA
Carson-Newman College, TN
Charleston Southern University, SC
Chatham University, PA
Clarion University of Pennsylvania, PA
Clarke University, IA
Clarkson College, NE
Clayton State University, GA
Clemson University, SC
Cleveland State University, OH
College of Mount Saint Vincent, NY
The College of New Rochelle, NY
Colorado State University–Pueblo, CO
Concordia College, MN
Concordia University Wisconsin, WI

Creighton University, NE
Daemen College, NY
Delta State University, MS
DePaul University, IL
DeSales University, PA
Drexel University, PA
Duke University, NC
Duquesne University, PA
D'Youville College, NY
East Carolina University, NC
Eastern Kentucky University, KY
East Tennessee State University, TN
Edgewood College, WI
Elmhurst College, IL
Elms College, MA
Emmanuel College, MA
Endicott College, MA
Excelsior College, NY
Fairleigh Dickinson University, Metropolitan Campus, NJ
Felician College, NJ
Ferris State University, MI
Florida Atlantic University, FL
Florida Gulf Coast University, FL
Florida International University, FL
Florida Southern College, FL
Florida State University, FL
Fort Hays State University, KS
Framingham State University, MA
Franciscan University of Steubenville, OH
Franklin Pierce University, NH
Gardner-Webb University, NC
George Mason University, VA
Georgetown University, DC
Georgia Baptist College of Nursing of Mercer University, GA
Georgia College & State University, GA
Goldfarb School of Nursing at Barnes-Jewish College, MO
Gonzaga University, WA
Graceland University, IA
Grambling State University, LA
Grand Canyon University, AZ
Hampton University, VA
Hawai`i Pacific University, HI
Holy Family University, PA
Holy Names University, CA
Husson University, ME
Idaho State University, ID
Immaculata University, PA
Indiana State University, IN
Indiana University of Pennsylvania, PA
Indiana University–Purdue University Fort Wayne, IN
Indiana Wesleyan University, IN
Jacksonville University, FL
Jefferson College of Health Sciences, VA
Kaplan University Online, FL
Kent State University, OH
Lamar University, TX
La Roche College, PA
Lehman College of the City University of New York, NY
Le Moyne College, NY
Lewis University, IL
Liberty University, VA
Loma Linda University, CA
Long Island University, Brooklyn Campus, NY
Long Island University, C.W. Post Campus, NY
Louisiana State University Health Sciences Center, LA
Lynchburg College, VA
Mansfield University of Pennsylvania, PA
Marian University, WI
Marshall University, WV
Marymount University, VA
Maryville University of Saint Louis, MO
McKendree University, IL
McNeese State University, LA
Medical University of South Carolina, SC
Memorial University of Newfoundland, NL
Mercy College, NY
MGH Institute of Health Professions, MA
Middle Tennessee State University, TN
Midwestern State University, TX
Millersville University of Pennsylvania, PA
Millikin University, IL
Minnesota State University Mankato, MN
Minnesota State University Moorhead, MN
Misericordia University, PA
Missouri Southern State University, MO
Missouri State University, MO
Molloy College, NY
Monmouth University, NJ
Moravian College, PA
Mountain State University, WV
Mount Carmel College of Nursing, OH
Mount Mercy University, IA
Mount St. Mary's College, CA
Nebraska Methodist College, NE
Nebraska Wesleyan University, NE
Neumann University, PA
New York University, NY
North Dakota State University, ND
Northeastern State University, OK
Northern Arizona University, AZ
Northern Illinois University, IL
Northern Kentucky University, KY
North Georgia College & State University, GA
Northwestern State University of Louisiana, LA
Northwest Nazarene University, ID
Nova Southeastern University, FL
Oakland University, MI
Ohio University, OH
Oklahoma Baptist University, OK
Oklahoma City University, OK
Old Dominion University, VA
Oregon Health & Science University, OR
Otterbein University, OH
Our Lady of the Lake College, LA
Pace University, NY
Pacific Lutheran University, WA
Patty Hanks Shelton School of Nursing, TX
Pittsburg State University, KS
Point Loma Nazarene University, CA
Prairie View A&M University, TX
Queens University of Charlotte, NC
Ramapo College of New Jersey, NJ
Regis College, MA
Regis University, CO
Research College of Nursing, MO
Resurrection University, IL
Rivier College, NH
Robert Morris University, PA
Roberts Wesleyan College, NY
The Sage Colleges, NY
Saginaw Valley State University, MI
Saint Anthony College of Nursing, IL
St. Catherine University, MN
Saint Francis Medical Center College of Nursing, IL
St. John Fisher College, NY
Saint Joseph College, CT
St. Joseph's College, New York, NY
Saint Joseph's College of Maine, ME
Saint Louis University, MO
Salem State University, MA
Salisbury University, MD
Samford University, AL
San Diego State University, CA
San Jose State University, CA
Seattle Pacific University, WA
Seton Hall University, NJ
Sonoma State University, CA
South Dakota State University, SD
Southeastern Louisiana University, LA
Southeast Missouri State University, MO
Southern Adventist University, TN
Southern Connecticut State University, CT
Southern Illinois University Edwardsville, IL
Southern Nazarene University, OK
Southern University and Agricultural and Mechanical College, LA
South University, FL
Spalding University, KY
Spring Arbor University, MI
State University of New York at Binghamton, NY
Temple University, PA
Tennessee State University, TN
Tennessee Technological University, TN
Texas A&M University–Texarkana, TX
Texas Christian University, TX
Texas Tech University Health Sciences Center, TX
Texas Woman's University, TX
Thomas Jefferson University, PA
Thomas University, GA
Towson University, MD
Trinity Western University, BC
Troy University, AL
Union University, TN
Université de Moncton, NB
The University of Alabama, AL
The University of Alabama at Birmingham, AL
University of Alaska Anchorage, AK
University of Arkansas, AR
University of Arkansas for Medical Sciences, AR
The University of British Columbia, BC
University of Central Arkansas, AR
University of Central Florida, FL
University of Central Missouri, MO
University of Detroit Mercy, MI
University of Hartford, CT
University of Hawaii at Manoa, HI
University of Houston–Victoria, TX
University of Indianapolis, IN
The University of Iowa, IA
University of Louisiana at Lafayette, LA
University of Louisville, KY
University of Maine, ME
University of Mary, ND
University of Mary Hardin-Baylor, TX
University of Massachusetts Worcester, MA
University of Medicine and Dentistry of New Jersey, NJ
University of Memphis, TN
University of Miami, FL
University of Mississippi Medical Center, MS
University of Missouri, MO
University of Missouri–Kansas City, MO
University of Missouri–St. Louis, MO
University of Mobile, AL
University of Nebraska Medical Center, NE

University of Nevada, Las Vegas, NV
University of Nevada, Reno, NV
University of New Brunswick Fredericton, NB
University of New Mexico, NM
University of North Alabama, AL
The University of North Carolina at Chapel Hill, NC
The University of North Carolina at Charlotte, NC
The University of North Carolina at Greensboro, NC
The University of North Carolina Wilmington, NC
University of North Dakota, ND
University of Northern Colorado, CO
University of Oklahoma Health Sciences Center, OK
University of Phoenix, AZ
University of Phoenix–Bay Area Campus, CA
University of Phoenix–Central Florida Campus, FL
University of Phoenix–Denver Campus, CO
University of Phoenix–Hawaii Campus, HI
University of Phoenix–Metro Detroit Campus, MI
University of Phoenix–New Mexico Campus, NM
University of Phoenix–North Florida Campus, FL
University of Phoenix–Phoenix Campus, AZ
University of Phoenix–Sacramento Valley Campus, CA
University of Phoenix–San Diego Campus, CA
University of Phoenix–Southern Arizona Campus, AZ
University of Phoenix–Southern California Campus, CA
University of Phoenix–South Florida Campus, FL
University of Pittsburgh, PA
University of Puerto Rico, Medical Sciences Campus, PR
University of Rhode Island, RI
University of St. Francis, IL
University of San Diego, CA
University of Saskatchewan, SK
The University of Scranton, PA
University of South Alabama, AL
University of Southern Indiana, IN
University of South Florida, FL
The University of Texas at Arlington, TX
The University of Texas at Brownsville, TX
The University of Texas at El Paso, TX
The University of Texas at Tyler, TX
The University of Texas Health Science Center at Houston, TX
The University of Texas Health Science Center at San Antonio, TX
The University of Texas Medical Branch, TX
The University of Toledo, OH
University of Toronto, ON
University of Utah, UT
The University of Western Ontario, ON
University of West Georgia, GA
University of Wisconsin–Eau Claire, WI
University of Wisconsin–Oshkosh, WI
University of Wyoming, WY
Urbana University, OH
Valdosta State University, GA
Villanova University, PA
Virginia Commonwealth University, VA
Viterbo University, WI
Wagner College, NY
Walden University, MN
Washington State University College of Nursing and Consortium, WA
Waynesburg University, PA
Weber State University, UT
Webster University, MO
Western Carolina University, NC
Western Governors University, UT
Western Kentucky University, KY
Western Michigan University, MI
Westminster College, UT
West Texas A&M University, TX
West Virginia Wesleyan College, WV
Wheeling Jesuit University, WV
Widener University, PA
Wilkes University, PA
William Carey University, MS
William Paterson University of New Jersey, NJ
Wilmington University, DE
Winona State University, MN
Winston-Salem State University, NC
Worcester State College, MA
Xavier University, OH
York College of Pennsylvania, PA
Youngstown State University, OH

NURSING INFORMATICS

American Sentinel University, CO
Case Western Reserve University, OH
Duke University, NC
East Tennessee State University, TN
Excelsior College, NY
Fairleigh Dickinson University, Metropolitan Campus, NJ
Ferris State University, MI
Georgia College & State University, GA
Georgia State University, GA
Kaplan University Online, FL
Middle Tennessee State University, TN
Molloy College, NY
New York University, NY
Saginaw Valley State University, MI
Tennessee Technological University, TN
Thomas Jefferson University, PA
Troy University, AL
The University of Alabama at Birmingham, AL
University of Colorado Denver, CO
University of Illinois at Chicago, IL
The University of Iowa, IA
The University of Kansas, KS
University of Maryland, Baltimore, MD
University of Medicine and Dentistry of New Jersey, NJ
University of Michigan, MI
University of Nebraska Medical Center, NE
University of New Brunswick Fredericton, NB
The University of North Carolina at Chapel Hill, NC
University of Pittsburgh, PA
The University of Texas Health Science Center at San Antonio, TX
University of Utah, UT
University of Washington, WA
Vanderbilt University, TN
Walden University, MN
Xavier University, OH

Doctoral Programs

U.S. and U.S. Territories

Alabama

Samford University, Ida V. Moffett School of Nursing, *Birmingham (DNP)*
Troy University, School of Nursing, *Troy (DNP)*
The University of Alabama, Capstone College of Nursing, *Tuscaloosa (DNP)*
The University of Alabama at Birmingham, School of Nursing, *Birmingham (PhD)*
The University of Alabama in Huntsville, College of Nursing, *Huntsville (DNP)*

Arizona

Arizona State University at the Downtown Phoenix Campus, College of Nursing, *Phoenix (DNP)*
The University of Arizona, College of Nursing, *Tucson (PhD)*
University of Phoenix, Online Campus, *Phoenix (PhD)*

Arkansas

University of Arkansas for Medical Sciences, College of Nursing, *Little Rock (PhD)*.

California

Azusa Pacific University, School of Nursing, *Azusa (PhD)*
Loma Linda University, School of Nursing, *Loma Linda (PhD)*
University of California, Los Angeles, School of Nursing, *Los Angeles (PhD)*
University of California, San Francisco, School of Nursing, *San Francisco (PhD)*
University of San Diego, Hahn School of Nursing and Health Science, *San Diego (DNP, PhD)*
University of San Francisco, School of Nursing, *San Francisco (DNP)*
Western University of Health Sciences, College of Graduate Nursing, *Pomona (DNP)*

Colorado

University of Colorado at Colorado Springs, Beth-El College of Nursing and Health Sciences, *Colorado Springs (DNP)*
University of Colorado Denver, College of Nursing, *Denver (PhD)*
University of Northern Colorado, School of Nursing, *Greeley (PhD)*

Connecticut

Fairfield University, School of Nursing, *Fairfield (DNP)*
Sacred Heart University, Program in Nursing, *Fairfield (DNP)*
University of Connecticut, School of Nursing, *Storrs (PhD)*
Yale University, School of Nursing, *New Haven (PhD)*

District of Columbia

The Catholic University of America, School of Nursing, *Washington (DNP, PhD)*
The George Washington University, Department of Nursing Education, *Washington (DNP)*

Florida

Barry University, School of Nursing, *Miami Shores (PhD)*
Florida Agricultural and Mechanical University, School of Nursing, *Tallahassee (PhD)*
Florida Atlantic University, Christine E. Lynn College of Nursing, *Boca Raton (PhD)*
Florida International University, Nursing Program, *Miami (PhD)*
Florida State University, College of Nursing, *Tallahassee (DNP)*
University of Central Florida, College of Nursing, *Orlando (PhD)*
University of Florida, College of Nursing, *Gainesville (PhD)*
University of Miami, School of Nursing and Health Studies, *Coral Gables (PhD)*
University of South Florida, College of Nursing, *Tampa (PhD)*

Georgia

Emory University, Nell Hodgson Woodruff School of Nursing, *Atlanta (PhD)*
Georgia Baptist College of Nursing of Mercer University, Department of Nursing, *Atlanta (PhD)*
Georgia Health Sciences University, School of Nursing, *Augusta (PhD)*
Georgia Southern University, School of Nursing, *Statesboro (DNP)*
Georgia State University, Byrdine F. Lewis School of Nursing, *Atlanta (PhD)*

Hawaii

University of Hawaii at Manoa, School of Nursing and Dental Hygiene, *Honolulu (PhD)*

Illinois

Illinois State University, Mennonite College of Nursing, *Normal (PhD)*
Loyola University Chicago, Marcella Niehoff School of Nursing, *Maywood (PhD)*
Rush University, College of Nursing, *Chicago (DNP)*
Saint Francis Medical Center College of Nursing, Baccalaureate Nursing Program, *Peoria (DNP)*
Southern Illinois University Edwardsville, School of Nursing, *Edwardsville (DNP)*
University of Illinois at Chicago, College of Nursing, *Chicago (PhD)*
University of St. Francis, College of Nursing and Allied Health, *Joliet (DNP)*

Indiana

Ball State University, School of Nursing, *Muncie (DNP)*
Indiana State University, Department of Nursing, *Terre Haute (DNP)*
Indiana University–Purdue University Indianapolis, School of Nursing, *Indianapolis (PhD)*
Purdue University, School of Nursing, *West Lafayette (DNP)*
University of Southern Indiana, College of Nursing and Health Professions, *Evansville (DNP)*

Iowa

The University of Iowa, College of Nursing, *Iowa City (PhD)*

Kansas

The University of Kansas, School of Nursing, *Kansas City (PhD)*
Wichita State University, School of Nursing, *Wichita (DNP)*

Kentucky

Bellarmine University, Donna and Allan Lansing School of Nursing and Health Sciences, *Louisville (DNP)*
Frontier School of Midwifery and Family Nursing, Nursing Degree Programs, *Hyden (DNP)*
University of Kentucky, Graduate School Programs in the College of Nursing, *Lexington (PhD)*
University of Louisville, School of Nursing, *Louisville (PhD)*

Louisiana

Louisiana State University Health Sciences Center, School of Nursing, *New Orleans (DNS)*
Loyola University New Orleans, School of Nursing, *New Orleans (DNP)*
Southern University and Agricultural and Mechanical College, School of Nursing, *Baton Rouge (PhD)*

Maine

University of Southern Maine, College of Nursing and Health Professions, *Portland (DNP)*

Maryland

The Johns Hopkins University, School of Nursing, *Baltimore (PhD)*
University of Maryland, Baltimore, Master's Program in Nursing, *Baltimore (DNP)*

Massachusetts

Boston College, William F. Connell School of Nursing, *Chestnut Hill (PhD)*
MGH Institute of Health Professions, School of Nursing, *Boston (DNP)*
Northeastern University, School of Nursing, *Boston (DNP, PhD)*
Regis College, School of Nursing and Health Professions, *Weston (DNP)*
Simmons College, Department of Nursing, *Boston (DNP)*
University of Massachusetts Amherst, School of Nursing, *Amherst (PhD)*
University of Massachusetts Boston, College of Nursing and Health Sciences, *Boston (PhD)*
University of Massachusetts Dartmouth, College of Nursing, *North Dartmouth (PhD)*
University of Massachusetts Lowell, Department of Nursing, *Lowell (PhD)*
University of Massachusetts Worcester, Graduate School of Nursing, *Worcester (PhD)*

Michigan

Grand Valley State University, Kirkhof College of Nursing, *Allendale (DNP)*
Madonna University, College of Nursing and Health, *Livonia (DNP)*
Michigan State University, College of Nursing, *East Lansing (PhD)*
University of Michigan, School of Nursing, *Ann Arbor (PhD)*

University of Michigan–Flint, Department of Nursing, *Flint (DNP)*
Wayne State University, College of Nursing, *Detroit (DNP)*

Minnesota

The College of St. Scholastica, Department of Nursing, *Duluth (DNP)*
Minnesota State University Mankato, School of Nursing, *Mankato (DNP)*
Minnesota State University Moorhead, School of Nursing and Healthcare Leadership, *Moorhead (DNP)*
St. Catherine University, Department of Nursing, *St. Paul (DNP)*
University of Minnesota, Twin Cities Campus, School of Nursing, *Minneapolis (PhD)*
Winona State University, College of Nursing and Health Sciences, *Winona (DNP)*

Mississippi

University of Mississippi Medical Center, Program in Nursing, *Jackson (PhD)*
University of Southern Mississippi, School of Nursing, *Hattiesburg (PhD)*

Missouri

Goldfarb School of Nursing at Barnes-Jewish College, *St. Louis (PhD)*
Maryville University of Saint Louis, Nursing Program, School of Health Professions, *St. Louis (DNP)*
Saint Louis University, School of Nursing, *St. Louis (DNP, PhD)*
University of Missouri, Sinclair School of Nursing, *Columbia (PhD)*
University of Missouri–Kansas City, School of Nursing, *Kansas City (PhD)*
University of Missouri–St. Louis, College of Nursing, *St. Louis (DNP)*

Nebraska

Creighton University, School of Nursing, *Omaha (DNP)*
University of Nebraska Medical Center, College of Nursing, *Omaha (PhD)*

Nevada

Touro University, School of Nursing, *Henderson (DNP)*
University of Nevada, Las Vegas, School of Nursing, *Las Vegas (PhD)*

New Jersey

Fairleigh Dickinson University, Metropolitan Campus, Henry P. Becton School of Nursing and Allied Health, *Teaneck (DNP)*
Rutgers, The State University of New Jersey, College of Nursing, *Newark (PhD)*
Seton Hall University, College of Nursing, *South Orange (DNP)*
University of Medicine and Dentistry of New Jersey, School of Nursing, *Newark (DNP)*
William Paterson University of New Jersey, Department of Nursing, *Wayne (DNP)*

New Mexico

University of New Mexico, College of Nursing, *Albuquerque (PhD)*

New York

Adelphi University, School of Nursing, *Garden City (PhD)*
Columbia University, School of Nursing, *New York (PhD)*
Daemen College, Department of Nursing, *Amherst (DNP)*
Lehman College of the City University of New York, Department of Nursing, *Bronx (DNS)*
Molloy College, Division of Nursing, *Rockville Centre (PhD)*
New York University, College of Nursing, *New York (DNP, PhD)*
Pace University, Lienhard School of Nursing, *New York (DNP)*
The Sage Colleges, Department of Nursing, *Troy (DNS)*
St. John Fisher College, Advanced Practice Nursing Program, *Rochester (DNP)*
State University of New York at Binghamton, Decker School of Nursing, *Binghamton (PhD)*
Stony Brook University, State University of New York, School of Nursing, *Stony Brook (DNP)*
University at Buffalo, the State University of New York, School of Nursing, *Buffalo (PhD)*
University of Rochester, School of Nursing, *Rochester (DNP, PhD)*

North Carolina

Duke University, School of Nursing, *Durham (PhD)*
East Carolina University, College of Nursing, *Greenville (PhD)*
The University of North Carolina at Chapel Hill, School of Nursing, *Chapel Hill (PhD)*
The University of North Carolina at Greensboro, School of Nursing, *Greensboro (PhD)*

North Dakota

North Dakota State University, Department of Nursing, *Fargo (DNP)*
University of North Dakota, College of Nursing, *Grand Forks (PhD)*

Ohio

Case Western Reserve University, Frances Payne Bolton School of Nursing, *Cleveland (PhD)*
Kent State University, College of Nursing, *Kent (DNP, PhD)*
The Ohio State University, College of Nursing, *Columbus (DNP)*
The University of Akron, College of Nursing, *Akron (PhD)*
University of Cincinnati, College of Nursing, *Cincinnati (PhD)*
The University of Toledo, College of Nursing, *Toledo (DNP)*
Ursuline College, The Breen School of Nursing, *Pepper Pike (DNP)*
Wright State University, College of Nursing and Health, *Dayton (DNP)*

Oklahoma

Oklahoma City University, Kramer School of Nursing, *Oklahoma City (DNP, PhD)*
University of Oklahoma Health Sciences Center, College of Nursing, *Oklahoma City (PhD)*

Oregon

Oregon Health & Science University, School of Nursing, *Portland (PhD)*
University of Portland, School of Nursing, *Portland (DNP)*

Pennsylvania

Chatham University, Program in Nursing, *Pittsburgh (DNP)*
Drexel University, College of Nursing and Health Professions, *Philadelphia (Dr NP)*
Duquesne University, School of Nursing, *Pittsburgh (DNP, PhD)*
Indiana University of Pennsylvania, Department of Nursing and Allied Health, *Indiana (PhD)*
Penn State University Park, School of Nursing, *University Park (PhD)*
Robert Morris University, School of Nursing and Health Sciences, *Moon Township (DNP)*
Temple University, Department of Nursing, *Philadelphia (DNP)*
Thomas Jefferson University, Department of Nursing, *Philadelphia (DNP)*
University of Pennsylvania, School of Nursing, *Philadelphia (PhD)*
University of Pittsburgh, School of Nursing, *Pittsburgh (PhD)*
Villanova University, College of Nursing, *Villanova (PhD)*
Waynesburg University, Department of Nursing, *Waynesburg (DNP)*
Widener University, School of Nursing, *Chester (DNP, PhD)*

Rhode Island

University of Rhode Island, College of Nursing, *Kingston (PhD)*

South Carolina

Medical University of South Carolina, College of Nursing, *Charleston (PhD)*
University of South Carolina, College of Nursing, *Columbia (DNP, PhD)*

South Dakota

South Dakota State University, College of Nursing, *Brookings (PhD)*

Tennessee

East Tennessee State University, College of Nursing, *Johnson City (PhD)*
The University of Tennessee, College of Nursing, *Knoxville (PhD)*
The University of Tennessee at Chattanooga, School of Nursing, *Chattanooga (DNP)*
The University of Tennessee Health Science Center, College of Nursing, *Memphis (DNP)*
Vanderbilt University, School of Nursing, *Nashville (DNP, PhD)*

Texas

Baylor University, Louise Herrington School of Nursing, *Dallas (DNP)*
Texas Christian University, Harris College of Nursing, *Fort Worth (DNP)*
Texas Tech University Health Sciences Center, School of Nursing, *Lubbock (DNP)*
Texas Woman's University, College of Nursing, *Denton (PhD)*
The University of Texas at Arlington, College of Nursing, *Arlington (DNP, PhD)*
The University of Texas at Austin, School of Nursing, *Austin (PhD)*
The University of Texas at Tyler, Program in Nursing, *Tyler (DNS)*
The University of Texas Health Science Center at Houston, School of Nursing, *Houston (PhD)*

The University of Texas Health Science Center at San Antonio, School of Nursing, *San Antonio (PhD)*

The University of Texas Medical Branch, School of Nursing, *Galveston (PhD)*

Utah

University of Utah, College of Nursing, *Salt Lake City (DNP, DNP/MPH, PhD)*

Virginia

George Mason University, College of Health and Human Services, *Fairfax (PhD)*

Hampton University, School of Nursing, *Hampton (PhD)*

Marymount University, School of Health Professions, *Arlington (DNP)*

Old Dominion University, Department of Nursing, *Norfolk (DNP)*

Radford University, School of Nursing, *Radford (DNP)*

University of Virginia, School of Nursing, *Charlottesville (PhD)*

Virginia Commonwealth University, School of Nursing, *Richmond (PhD)*

Washington

University of Washington, School of Nursing, *Seattle (DNP, PhD)*

Washington State University College of Nursing and Consortium, *Spokane (PhD)*

West Virginia

West Virginia University, School of Nursing, *Morgantown (DNP, PhD)*

Wisconsin

Concordia University Wisconsin, Program in Nursing, *Mequon (DNP)*

Marquette University, College of Nursing, *Milwaukee (DNP, PhD)*

University of Phoenix–Milwaukee Campus, College of Health and Human Services, *Milwaukee (PhD)*

University of Wisconsin–Eau Claire, College of Nursing and Health Sciences, *Eau Claire (DNP)*

University of Wisconsin–Madison, School of Nursing, *Madison (PhD)*

University of Wisconsin–Milwaukee, College of Nursing, *Milwaukee (DNP, PhD)*

CANADA

Alberta

University of Alberta, Faculty of Nursing, *Edmonton (PhD)*

University of Calgary, Faculty of Nursing, *Calgary (PhD)*

British Columbia

The University of British Columbia, Program in Nursing, *Vancouver (PhD)*

University of Victoria, School of Nursing, *Victoria (PhD)*

Manitoba

University of Manitoba, Faculty of Nursing, *Winnipeg (PhD)*

Nova Scotia

Dalhousie University, School of Nursing, *Halifax (PhD)*

Ontario

McMaster University, School of Nursing, *Hamilton (PhD)*

Queen's University at Kingston, School of Nursing, *Kingston (PhD)*

University of Ottawa, School of Nursing, *Ottawa (PhD)*

University of Toronto, Faculty of Nursing, *Toronto (PhD)*

The University of Western Ontario, School of Nursing, *London (PhD)*

Quebec

McGill University, School of Nursing, *Montréal (PhD)*

Université de Montréal, Faculty of Nursing, *Montréal (PhD)*

Université de Sherbrooke, Department of Nursing, *Sherbrooke (PhD)*

Université Laval, Faculty of Nursing, *Québec (PhD)*

Saskatchewan

University of Saskatchewan, College of Nursing, *Saskatoon (PhD)*

Postdoctoral Programs

U.S. AND U.S. TERRITORIES

Arkansas

University of Arkansas for Medical Sciences, College of Nursing, *Little Rock*

California

University of California, Los Angeles, School of Nursing, *Los Angeles*

University of California, San Francisco, School of Nursing, *San Francisco*

Colorado

University of Colorado Denver, College of Nursing, *Denver*

Connecticut

Yale University, School of Nursing, *New Haven*

Illinois

University of Illinois at Chicago, College of Nursing, *Chicago*

Indiana

Indiana University–Purdue University Indianapolis, School of Nursing, *Indianapolis*

Iowa

The University of Iowa, College of Nursing, *Iowa City*

Kansas

The University of Kansas, School of Nursing, *Kansas City*

Kentucky

University of Louisville, School of Nursing, *Louisville*

Maryland

The Johns Hopkins University, School of Nursing, *Baltimore*

Massachusetts

University of Massachusetts Boston, College of Nursing and Health Sciences, *Boston*

Michigan

University of Michigan, School of Nursing, *Ann Arbor*

Wayne State University, College of Nursing, *Detroit*

Nebraska

University of Nebraska Medical Center, College of Nursing, *Omaha*

New York

Columbia University, School of Nursing, *New York*

University of Rochester, School of Nursing, *Rochester*

North Carolina

The University of North Carolina at Chapel Hill, School of Nursing, *Chapel Hill*

Ohio

Case Western Reserve University, Frances Payne Bolton School of Nursing, *Cleveland*

Oregon

Oregon Health & Science University, School of Nursing, *Portland*

Pennsylvania

Penn State University Park, School of Nursing, *University Park*

University of Pennsylvania, School of Nursing, *Philadelphia*

University of Pittsburgh, School of Nursing, *Pittsburgh*

South Carolina

Medical University of South Carolina, College of Nursing, *Charleston*

Tennessee

Vanderbilt University, School of Nursing, *Nashville*

Texas

The University of Texas at Austin, School of Nursing, *Austin*

Utah

University of Utah, College of Nursing, *Salt Lake City*

Virginia

University of Virginia, School of Nursing, *Charlottesville*

Virginia Commonwealth University, School of Nursing, *Richmond*

Washington

University of Washington, School of Nursing, *Seattle*

Wisconsin

University of Wisconsin–Madison, School of Nursing, *Madison*

CANADA

British Columbia

The University of British Columbia, Program in Nursing, *Vancouver*

University of Northern British Columbia, Nursing Programme, *Prince George*

Ontario

University of Ottawa, School of Nursing, *Ottawa*

The University of Western Ontario, School of Nursing, *London*

Quebec

McGill University, School of Nursing, *Montréal*

Université de Montréal, Faculty of Nursing, *Montréal*

Université de Sherbrooke, Department of Nursing, *Sherbrooke*

Université Laval, Faculty of Nursing, *Québec*

ONLINE BACCALAUREATE PROGRAMS

Albany State University, GA
Alcorn State University, MS
Angelo State University, TX
Arkansas Tech University, AR
Ashland University, OH
Ball State University, IN
Blessing–Rieman College of Nursing, IL
Boise State University, ID
Brenau University, GA
California State University, Dominguez Hills, CA
Carson-Newman College, TN
Chamberlain College of Nursing, MO
Clarion University of Pennsylvania, PA
Clarkson College, NE
Clayton State University, GA
Cleveland State University, OH
The College of St. Scholastica, MN
Columbus State University, GA
Creighton University, NE
Dalhousie University, NS
Davenport University, MI
Delta State University, MS
East Carolina University, NC
Eastern Illinois University, IL
Eastern New Mexico University, NM
East Tennessee State University, TN
ECPI College of Technology, VA
Ferris State University, MI
Finlandia University, MI
Florida International University, FL
Florida State University, FL
Fort Hays State University, KS
George Mason University, VA
Georgia Southern University, GA
Georgia Southwestern State University, GA
Grand Canyon University, AZ
Illinois State University, IL
Indiana State University, IN
Jacksonville State University, AL
Jacksonville University, FL
Kettering College of Medical Arts, OH
Lakehead University, ON
Lamar University, TX
Lander University, SC
Lehman College of the City University of New York, NY
Loyola University New Orleans, LA
Marymount University, VA
Mercy College, NY
Mercy College of Northwest Ohio, OH
Mesa State College, CO
Methodist College of Nursing, IL
Michigan State University, MI
Middle Tennessee State University, TN
Minot State University, ND
Mississippi College, MS
Mississippi University for Women, MS
Missouri State University, MO
Montana State University–Northern, MT
Morehead State University, KY
Mount Aloysius College, PA
Northeastern State University, OK
Northern Arizona University, AZ
North Georgia College & State University, GA
Northwestern State University of Louisiana, LA
Ohio University, OH
Oklahoma Panhandle State University, OK
Penn State University Park, PA
Pittsburg State University, KS
Presentation College, SD
Purdue University Calumet, IN
Queens University of Charlotte, NC
Radford University, VA
Ramapo College of New Jersey, NJ
Rivier College, NH
Roberts Wesleyan College, NY
St. Petersburg College, FL
San Diego State University, CA
Silver Lake College, WI
Slippery Rock University of Pennsylvania, PA
South Dakota State University, SD
Southeastern Louisiana University, LA
Southeast Missouri State University, MO
Southern Arkansas University–Magnolia, AR
South University, FL
South University, FL
Southwest Baptist University, MO
Southwestern College, KS
Southwestern Oklahoma State University, OK
State University of New York at Plattsburgh, NY
State University of New York College of Technology at Delhi, NY
State University of New York Empire State College, NY
Tabor College, KS
Texas A&M Health Science Center, TX
Texas A&M University–Corpus Christi, TX
Texas Tech University Health Sciences Center, TX
Texas Woman's University, TX
Touro University, NV
University of Arkansas at Fort Smith, AR
University of Arkansas for Medical Sciences, AR
University of Central Missouri, MO
University of Colorado at Colorado Springs, CO
University of Colorado Denver, CO
University of Illinois at Chicago, IL
University of Louisiana at Lafayette, LA
University of Louisiana at Monroe, LA
University of Louisville, KY
University of Maine at Fort Kent, ME
University of Mary, ND
University of Maryland, Baltimore, MD
University of Massachusetts Amherst, MA
University of Massachusetts Boston, MA
University of Michigan–Flint, MI
University of Missouri, MO
University of Missouri–St. Louis, MO
University of North Alabama, AL
The University of North Carolina at Chapel Hill, NC
The University of North Carolina Wilmington, NC
University of North Dakota, ND
University of Phoenix, AZ
University of Phoenix–Phoenix Campus, AZ
University of Phoenix–Sacramento Valley Campus, CA
University of Phoenix–Southern Arizona Campus, AZ
University of Phoenix–South Florida Campus, FL
University of Phoenix–West Florida Campus, FL
University of St. Francis, IL
University of Saint Mary, KS
University of South Carolina Aiken, SC
University of South Carolina Upstate, SC
University of Southern Indiana, IN
University of Southern Mississippi, MS
The University of Texas at Arlington, TX
The University of Texas at Tyler, TX
The University of Texas Medical Branch, TX
University of the Incarnate Word, TX
The University of Toledo, OH
University of West Florida, FL
University of Wisconsin–Green Bay, WI
University of Wisconsin–Oshkosh, WI
University of Wyoming, WY
Utica College, NY
Walden University, MN
Weber State University, UT
Western Carolina University, NC
Western Governors University, UT
Western Illinois University, IL
Wichita State University, KS
Wilmington University, DE

ONLINE ONLY BACCALAUREATE PROGRAMS

Angelo State University, TX
Ashland University, OH
Chamberlain College of Nursing, MO
Clarion University of Pennsylvania, PA
Eastern Illinois University, IL
Eastern New Mexico University, NM
Georgia Southwestern State University, GA
Kettering College of Medical Arts, OH
Loyola University New Orleans, LA
Methodist College of Nursing, IL
Montana State University–Northern, MT
Northeastern State University, OK
Northern Arizona University, AZ
North Georgia College & State University, GA
Oklahoma Panhandle State University, OK
Slippery Rock University of Pennsylvania, PA
State University of New York College of Technology at Delhi, NY
State University of New York Empire State College, NY
Tabor College, KS
Texas Tech University Health Sciences Center, TX
University of Arkansas at Fort Smith, AR
University of Louisiana at Monroe, LA
University of North Alabama, AL
The University of North Carolina at Chapel Hill, NC
University of Saint Mary, KS
The University of Texas at Tyler, TX
The University of Texas Medical Branch, TX
Walden University, MN

ONLINE MASTER'S DEGREE PROGRAMS

Albany State University, GA
Alcorn State University, MS
Allen College, IA
Angelo State University, TX
Athabasca University, AB
Ball State University, IN

Bellin College, WI
Benedictine University, IL
California State University, Chico, CA
California State University, Fullerton, CA
Charleston Southern University, SC
Clarkson College, NE
Clayton State University, GA
Cleveland State University, OH
Delta State University, MS
Drexel University, PA
Duke University, NC
Duquesne University, PA
East Carolina University, NC
Eastern Mennonite University, VA
East Tennessee State University, TN
Excelsior College, NY
Felician College, NJ
Ferris State University, MI
Fitchburg State University, MA
Florida Atlantic University, FL
Florida State University, FL
Fort Hays State University, KS
George Mason University, VA
Georgia Health Sciences University, GA
Gonzaga University, WA
Graceland University, IA
Grand Canyon University, AZ
Hampton University, VA
Idaho State University, ID
Indiana State University, IN
Indiana Wesleyan University, IN
Jacksonville State University, AL
Jacksonville University, FL
Lamar University, TX
La Roche College, PA
Lewis University, IL
Liberty University, VA
Loyola University New Orleans, LA
Mansfield University of Pennsylvania, PA
McKendree University, IL
McNeese State University, LA
Medical University of South Carolina, SC
Memorial University of Newfoundland, NL
Mercy College, NY
Michigan State University, MI
Middle Tennessee State University, TN
Missouri State University, MO
Nebraska Methodist College, NE
Northeastern State University, OK
Northern Arizona University, AZ
Northern Kentucky University, KY
Northwest Nazarene University, ID
Old Dominion University, VA
Pace University, NY
Penn State University Park, PA
Purdue University Calumet, IN
Ramapo College of New Jersey, NJ
Regis University, CO
Research College of Nursing, MO
Rush University, IL
Sacred Heart University, CT
Saint Francis Medical Center College of Nursing, IL
Saint Joseph's College of Maine, ME
Saint Louis University, MO
Saint Xavier University, IL
Samuel Merritt University, CA
Seton Hall University, NJ
South Dakota State University, SD
South University, FL
Spring Arbor University, MI
Spring Hill College, AL
Tennessee State University, TN
Tennessee Technological University, TN
Texas A&M University–Corpus Christi, TX
Texas Christian University, TX
Texas Tech University Health Sciences Center, TX
Texas Woman's University, TX
Touro University, NV
Troy University, AL
The University of Alabama, AL
The University of Alabama at Birmingham, AL
The University of Alabama in Huntsville, AL
University of Arkansas, AR
University of Central Arkansas, AR
University of Central Missouri, MO
University of Cincinnati, OH
University of Colorado at Colorado Springs, CO
University of Colorado Denver, CO
University of Florida, FL
University of Hawaii at Manoa, HI
University of Indianapolis, IN
The University of Kansas, KS
University of Louisiana at Lafayette, LA
University of Mary, ND
University of Maryland, Baltimore, MD
University of Massachusetts Amherst, MA
University of Medicine and Dentistry of New Jersey, NJ
University of Memphis, TN
University of Michigan–Flint, MI
University of Missouri, MO
University of Missouri–St. Louis, MO
University of Nevada, Las Vegas, NV
University of New Mexico, NM
University of North Alabama, AL
The University of North Carolina at Charlotte, NC
University of North Dakota, ND
University of Northern Colorado, CO
University of Oklahoma Health Sciences Center, OK
University of Phoenix, AZ
University of Phoenix–New Mexico Campus, NM
University of Phoenix–Phoenix Campus, AZ
University of Phoenix–Southern Arizona Campus, AZ
University of Phoenix–South Florida Campus, FL
University of Pittsburgh, PA
University of Rochester, NY
University of St. Francis, IL
University of Southern Indiana, IN
The University of Texas at Arlington, TX
The University of Texas at El Paso, TX
The University of Texas Medical Branch, TX
University of Toronto, ON
University of Wyoming, WY
Vanderbilt University, TN
Walden University, MN
Western Carolina University, NC
Western Governors University, UT
Western University of Health Sciences, CA
West Virginia University, WV
Wright State University, OH
Yale University, CT

ONLINE ONLY MASTER'S DEGREE PROGRAMS

Albany State University, GA
Angelo State University, TX
Ball State University, IN
Benedictine University, IL
California State University, Chico, CA
Charleston Southern University, SC
Clarkson College, NE
Clayton State University, GA
Cleveland State University, OH
Delta State University, MS
Duquesne University, PA
Eastern Mennonite University, VA
Excelsior College, NY
Ferris State University, MI
Fitchburg State University, MA
Florida State University, FL
George Mason University, VA
Gonzaga University, WA
Graceland University, IA
Idaho State University, ID
Indiana State University, IN
Jacksonville State University, AL
Lamar University, TX
La Roche College, PA
Lewis University, IL
Liberty University, VA
Mansfield University of Pennsylvania, PA
McNeese State University, LA
Medical University of South Carolina, SC
Memorial University of Newfoundland, NL
Missouri State University, MO
Nebraska Methodist College, NE
Northeastern State University, OK
Northern Arizona University, AZ
Northwest Nazarene University, ID
Old Dominion University, VA
Pace University, NY
Ramapo College of New Jersey, NJ
Saint Francis Medical Center College of Nursing, IL
Saint Joseph's College of Maine, ME
Saint Louis University, MO
Seton Hall University, NJ
Spring Arbor University, MI
Spring Hill College, AL
Tennessee Technological University, TN
Texas A&M University–Corpus Christi, TX
Texas Christian University, TX
Texas Tech University Health Sciences Center, TX
Touro University, NV
The University of Alabama, AL
The University of Alabama at Birmingham, AL
University of Central Arkansas, AR
University of Central Missouri, MO
University of Colorado at Colorado Springs, CO
University of Louisiana at Lafayette, LA
University of Maryland, Baltimore, MD
University of Massachusetts Amherst, MA
University of Missouri, MO
University of Nevada, Las Vegas, NV
University of New Mexico, NM
University of North Alabama, AL
University of Northern Colorado, CO
University of Southern Indiana, IN
The University of Texas at El Paso, TX
The University of Texas Medical Branch, TX
Walden University, MN
Western University of Health Sciences, CA
West Virginia University, WV

ONLINE DOCTORAL DEGREE PROGRAMS

Ball State University, IN
The Catholic University of America, DC
Chatham University, PA
Concordia University Wisconsin, WI
Duquesne University, PA
George Mason University, VA
Georgia Southern University, GA
Hampton University, VA
Indiana State University, IN
Loyola University New Orleans, LA
Medical University of South Carolina, SC
Minnesota State University Moorhead, MN
North Dakota State University, ND
Northeastern University, MA
Old Dominion University, VA
Radford University, VA
Rush University, IL
Saint Francis Medical Center College of Nursing, IL
Simmons College, MA
Texas Christian University, TX
Touro University, NV
Troy University, AL
The University of Alabama, AL
The University of Alabama in Huntsville, AL
The University of Arizona, AZ
University of Colorado at Colorado Springs, CO
University of Florida, FL
University of Hawaii at Manoa, HI
The University of Kansas, KS
University of Michigan–Flint, MI
University of Nevada, Las Vegas, NV
University of New Mexico, NM
University of North Dakota, ND
University of Northern Colorado, CO
University of Phoenix, AZ
University of St. Francis, IL
The University of Tennessee, TN
The University of Tennessee at Chattanooga, TN
The University of Tennessee Health Science Center, TN
The University of Texas Medical Branch, TX
The University of Toledo, OH
University of Wisconsin–Milwaukee, WI
Western University of Health Sciences, CA
West Virginia University, WV
Winona State University, MN
Wright State University, OH

ONLINE ONLY DOCTORAL DEGREE PROGRAMS

Ball State University, IN
Chatham University, PA
Concordia University Wisconsin, WI
Duquesne University, PA
George Mason University, VA
Georgia Southern University, GA
Hampton University, VA
Indiana State University, IN
Loyola University New Orleans, LA
Medical University of South Carolina, SC
Minnesota State University Moorhead, MN
Northeastern University, MA
Old Dominion University, VA
Radford University, VA
Rush University, IL
Saint Francis Medical Center College of Nursing, IL
Simmons College, MA
Texas Christian University, TX
Touro University, NV
Troy University, AL
The University of Alabama, AL
The University of Alabama in Huntsville, AL
The University of Arizona, AZ
University of Colorado at Colorado Springs, CO
University of Hawaii at Manoa, HI
University of Michigan–Flint, MI
University of Nevada, Las Vegas, NV
University of North Dakota, ND
University of Northern Colorado, CO
University of Phoenix, AZ
University of St. Francis, IL
The University of Tennessee, TN
The University of Tennessee at Chattanooga, TN
The University of Tennessee Health Science Center, TN
The University of Texas Medical Branch, TX
The University of Toledo, OH
Western University of Health Sciences, CA
West Virginia University, WV
Winona State University, MN
Wright State University, OH

CONTINUING EDUCATION PROGRAMS

U.S. AND U.S. TERRITORIES

Alabama

Auburn University, School of Nursing, *Auburn University*
Jacksonville State University, College of Nursing and Health Sciences, *Jacksonville*
Samford University, Ida V. Moffett School of Nursing, *Birmingham*
The University of Alabama in Huntsville, College of Nursing, *Huntsville*
University of Mobile, School of Nursing, *Mobile*
University of North Alabama, College of Nursing and Allied Health, *Florence*

Arizona

Arizona State University at the Downtown Phoenix Campus, College of Nursing, *Phoenix*
Grand Canyon University, College of Nursing and Health Sciences, *Phoenix*
University of Phoenix, Online Campus, *Phoenix*
University of Phoenix–Phoenix Campus, College of Nursing, *Phoenix*
University of Phoenix–Southern Arizona Campus, College of Social Sciences, *Tucson*

Arkansas

Harding University, College of Nursing, *Searcy*
University of Arkansas, Eleanor Mann School of Nursing, *Fayetteville*
University of Arkansas for Medical Sciences, College of Nursing, *Little Rock*

California

Azusa Pacific University, School of Nursing, *Azusa*
California State University, Bakersfield, Program in Nursing, *Bakersfield*
California State University, Chico, School of Nursing, *Chico*
California State University, Dominguez Hills, Program in Nursing, *Carson*
California State University, Fresno, Department of Nursing, *Fresno*
California State University, Fullerton, Department of Nursing, *Fullerton*
Pacific Union College, Department of Nursing, *Angwin*
Point Loma Nazarene University, School of Nursing, *San Diego*
San Diego State University, School of Nursing, *San Diego*
San Francisco State University, School of Nursing, *San Francisco*
University of California, Los Angeles, School of Nursing, *Los Angeles*
University of Phoenix–Sacramento Valley Campus, College of Nursing, *Sacramento*
University of Phoenix–Southern California Campus, College of Nursing, *Costa Mesa*

Colorado

University of Colorado at Colorado Springs, Beth-El College of Nursing and Health Sciences, *Colorado Springs*
University of Colorado Denver, College of Nursing, *Denver*

Connecticut

Fairfield University, School of Nursing, *Fairfield*
Quinnipiac University, Department of Nursing, *Hamden*
University of Connecticut, School of Nursing, *Storrs*
University of Hartford, College of Education, Nursing, and Health Professions, *West Hartford*

Delaware

Wesley College, Nursing Program, *Dover*

Florida

Florida Agricultural and Mechanical University, School of Nursing, *Tallahassee*
Florida Atlantic University, Christine E. Lynn College of Nursing, *Boca Raton*
Florida Gulf Coast University, School of Nursing, *Fort Myers*
St. Petersburg College, Department of Nursing, *St. Petersburg*
University of Miami, School of Nursing and Health Studies, *Coral Gables*
University of South Florida, College of Nursing, *Tampa*
The University of Tampa, Department of Nursing, *Tampa*

Georgia

Armstrong Atlantic State University, Program in Nursing, *Savannah*
Brenau University, School of Health and Science, *Gainesville*
Kennesaw State University, School of Nursing, *Kennesaw*
Valdosta State University, College of Nursing, *Valdosta*

Illinois

Lewis University, Program in Nursing, *Romeoville*
Olivet Nazarene University, Division of Nursing, *Bourbonnais*
Rush University, College of Nursing, *Chicago*
Saint Xavier University, School of Nursing, *Chicago*
Southern Illinois University Edwardsville, School of Nursing, *Edwardsville*
University of Illinois at Chicago, College of Nursing, *Chicago*

Indiana

Indiana State University, Department of Nursing, *Terre Haute*
Indiana University Kokomo, Indiana University School of Nursing, *Kokomo*
Indiana University–Purdue University Fort Wayne, Department of Nursing, *Fort Wayne*
Indiana University–Purdue University Indianapolis, School of Nursing, *Indianapolis*
Purdue University, School of Nursing, *West Lafayette*
University of Southern Indiana, College of Nursing and Health Professions, *Evansville*
Valparaiso University, College of Nursing, *Valparaiso*

Iowa

Allen College, Program in Nursing, *Waterloo*
Briar Cliff University, Department of Nursing, *Sioux City*
Clarke University, Department of Nursing and Health, *Dubuque*
Grand View University, Division of Nursing, *Des Moines*
Luther College, Department of Nursing, *Decorah*
Mount Mercy University, Department of Nursing, *Cedar Rapids*
St. Ambrose University, Program in Nursing (BSN), *Davenport*
The University of Iowa, College of Nursing, *Iowa City*

Kansas

MidAmerica Nazarene University, Division of Nursing, *Olathe*
Pittsburg State University, Department of Nursing, *Pittsburg*
The University of Kansas, School of Nursing, *Kansas City*
Washburn University, School of Nursing, *Topeka*

Kentucky

Bellarmine University, Donna and Allan Lansing School of Nursing and Health Sciences, *Louisville*
Kentucky Christian University, School of Nursing, *Grayson*
Midway College, Program in Nursing (Baccalaureate), *Midway*
Murray State University, Program in Nursing, *Murray*
Northern Kentucky University, Department of Nursing, *Highland Heights*
Spalding University, School of Nursing, *Louisville*
University of Kentucky, Graduate School Programs in the College of Nursing, *Lexington*
University of Louisville, School of Nursing, *Louisville*
Western Kentucky University, School of Nursing, *Bowling Green*

Louisiana

Louisiana State University Health Sciences Center, School of Nursing, *New Orleans*
McNeese State University, College of Nursing, *Lake Charles*
Nicholls State University, Department of Nursing, *Thibodaux*
Northwestern State University of Louisiana, College of Nursing, *Shreveport*
Our Lady of the Lake College, Division of Nursing, *Baton Rouge*
University of Louisiana at Lafayette, College of Nursing, *Lafayette*
University of Louisiana at Monroe, Nursing, *Monroe*

Maine

Saint Joseph's College of Maine, Department of Nursing, *Standish*
University of New England, Department of Nursing, *Biddeford*
University of Southern Maine, College of Nursing and Health Professions, *Portland*

Maryland

The Johns Hopkins University, School of Nursing, *Baltimore*

University of Maryland, Baltimore, Master's Program in Nursing, *Baltimore*

Massachusetts

Anna Maria College, Department of Nursing, *Paxton*

Boston College, William F. Connell School of Nursing, *Chestnut Hill*

Endicott College, Major in Nursing, *Beverly*

Framingham State University, Department of Nursing, *Framingham*

Massachusetts College of Pharmacy and Health Sciences, School of Nursing, *Boston*

Northeastern University, School of Nursing, *Boston*

Regis College, School of Nursing and Health Professions, *Weston*

Salem State University, Program in Nursing, *Salem*

University of Massachusetts Amherst, School of Nursing, *Amherst*

University of Massachusetts Boston, College of Nursing and Health Sciences, *Boston*

University of Massachusetts Dartmouth, College of Nursing, *North Dartmouth*

University of Massachusetts Worcester, Graduate School of Nursing, *Worcester*

Michigan

Grand Valley State University, Kirkhof College of Nursing, *Allendale*

Madonna University, College of Nursing and Health, *Livonia*

Michigan State University, College of Nursing, *East Lansing*

Northern Michigan University, College of Nursing and Allied Health Science, *Marquette*

Oakland University, School of Nursing, *Rochester*

Saginaw Valley State University, Crystal M. Lange College of Nursing and Health Sciences, *University Center*

Wayne State University, College of Nursing, *Detroit*

Western Michigan University, College of Health and Human Services, *Kalamazoo*

Minnesota

Bemidji State University, Department of Nursing, *Bemidji*

Minnesota State University Mankato, School of Nursing, *Mankato*

University of Minnesota, Twin Cities Campus, School of Nursing, *Minneapolis*

Mississippi

University of Mississippi Medical Center, Program in Nursing, *Jackson*

Missouri

Cox College, Department of Nursing, *Springfield*

Missouri State University, Department of Nursing, *Springfield*

Saint Louis University, School of Nursing, *St. Louis*

University of Missouri, Sinclair School of Nursing, *Columbia*

University of Missouri–Kansas City, School of Nursing, *Kansas City*

University of Missouri–St. Louis, College of Nursing, *St. Louis*

Nebraska

Clarkson College, Master of Science in Nursing Program, *Omaha*

Nebraska Methodist College, Department of Nursing, *Omaha*

University of Nebraska Medical Center, College of Nursing, *Omaha*

Nevada

Touro University, School of Nursing, *Henderson*

University of Nevada, Las Vegas, School of Nursing, *Las Vegas*

New Hampshire

Saint Anselm College, Department of Nursing, *Manchester*

New Jersey

College of Saint Elizabeth, Department of Nursing, *Morristown*

Fairleigh Dickinson University, Metropolitan Campus, Henry P. Becton School of Nursing and Allied Health, *Teaneck*

Monmouth University, Marjorie K. Unterberg School of Nursing, *West Long Branch*

Ramapo College of New Jersey, Master of Science in Nursing Program, *Mahwah*

Rutgers, The State University of New Jersey, College of Nursing, *Newark*

University of Medicine and Dentistry of New Jersey, School of Nursing, *Newark*

New Mexico

New Mexico State University, School of Nursing, *Las Cruces*

New York

Adelphi University, School of Nursing, *Garden City*

Columbia University, School of Nursing, *New York*

Elmira College, Program in Nursing Education, *Elmira*

Hunter College of the City University of New York, Hunter-Bellevue School of Nursing, *New York*

Lehman College of the City University of New York, Department of Nursing, *Bronx*

Molloy College, Division of Nursing, *Rockville Centre*

Nazareth College of Rochester, Department of Nursing, *Rochester*

New York University, College of Nursing, *New York*

The Sage Colleges, Department of Nursing, *Troy*

State University of New York at Binghamton, Decker School of Nursing, *Binghamton*

State University of New York Downstate Medical Center, College of Nursing, *Brooklyn*

State University of New York Institute of Technology, School of Nursing and Health Systems, *Utica*

State University of New York Upstate Medical University, College of Nursing, *Syracuse*

Stony Brook University, State University of New York, School of Nursing, *Stony Brook*

University of Rochester, School of Nursing, *Rochester*

North Carolina

Queens University of Charlotte, Presbyterian School of Nursing, *Charlotte*

The University of North Carolina at Chapel Hill, School of Nursing, *Chapel Hill*

The University of North Carolina Wilmington, School of Nursing, *Wilmington*

Winston-Salem State University, Department of Nursing, *Winston-Salem*

Ohio

Case Western Reserve University, Frances Payne Bolton School of Nursing, *Cleveland*

Cleveland State University, School of Nursing, *Cleveland*

Kent State University, College of Nursing, *Kent*

Mercy College of Northwest Ohio, Division of Nursing, *Toledo*

The Ohio State University, College of Nursing, *Columbus*

Otterbein University, Department of Nursing, *Westerville*

Shawnee State University, Department of Nursing, *Portsmouth*

The University of Akron, College of Nursing, *Akron*

University of Cincinnati, College of Nursing, *Cincinnati*

The University of Toledo, College of Nursing, *Toledo*

Wright State University, College of Nursing and Health, *Dayton*

Oklahoma

Oklahoma City University, Kramer School of Nursing, *Oklahoma City*

University of Oklahoma Health Sciences Center, College of Nursing, *Oklahoma City*

Oregon

Linfield College, School of Nursing, *McMinnville*

Oregon Health & Science University, School of Nursing, *Portland*

Pennsylvania

Alvernia University, Nursing, *Reading*

Bloomsburg University of Pennsylvania, Department of Nursing, *Bloomsburg*

Carlow University, School of Nursing, *Pittsburgh*

DeSales University, Department of Nursing and Health, *Center Valley*

Drexel University, College of Nursing and Health Professions, *Philadelphia*

Duquesne University, School of Nursing, *Pittsburgh*

Holy Family University, School of Nursing and Allied Health Professions, *Philadelphia*

La Roche College, Department of Nursing and Nursing Management, *Pittsburgh*

La Salle University, School of Nursing and Health Sciences, *Philadelphia*

Marywood University, Department of Nursing, *Scranton*

Millersville University of Pennsylvania, Department of Nursing, *Millersville*

Moravian College, St. Luke's School of Nursing, *Bethlehem*

Mount Aloysius College, Division of Nursing, *Cresson*

Penn State University Park, School of Nursing, *University Park*

Temple University, Department of Nursing, *Philadelphia*

Thomas Jefferson University, Department of Nursing, *Philadelphia*

University of Pennsylvania, School of Nursing, *Philadelphia*

University of Pittsburgh, School of Nursing, *Pittsburgh*

Villanova University, College of Nursing, *Villanova*

Widener University, School of Nursing, *Chester*

Wilkes University, Department of Nursing, *Wilkes-Barre*

Puerto Rico

Universidad Adventista de las Antillas, Department of Nursing, *Mayagüez*

University of Puerto Rico, Mayagüez Campus, Department of Nursing, *Mayagüez*

University of Puerto Rico, Medical Sciences Campus, School of Nursing, *San Juan*

Rhode Island

Salve Regina University, Department of Nursing, *Newport*

South Carolina

Clemson University, School of Nursing, *Clemson*

Medical University of South Carolina, College of Nursing, *Charleston*

University of South Carolina, College of Nursing, *Columbia*

South Dakota

South Dakota State University, College of Nursing, *Brookings*

Tennessee

East Tennessee State University, College of Nursing, *Johnson City*

Southern Adventist University, School of Nursing, *Collegedale*

Tennessee State University, School of Nursing, *Nashville*

Union University, School of Nursing, *Jackson*

The University of Tennessee, College of Nursing, *Knoxville*

The University of Tennessee at Chattanooga, School of Nursing, *Chattanooga*

The University of Tennessee at Martin, Department of Nursing, *Martin*

Texas

Lamar University, Department of Nursing, *Beaumont*

Midwestern State University, Nursing Program, *Wichita Falls*

Patty Hanks Shelton School of Nursing, *Abilene*

Tarleton State University, Department of Nursing, *Stephenville*

Texas A&M University–Corpus Christi, School of Nursing and Health Sciences, *Corpus Christi*

Texas Christian University, Harris College of Nursing, *Fort Worth*

Texas Tech University Health Sciences Center, School of Nursing, *Lubbock*

University of Mary Hardin-Baylor, College of Nursing, *Belton*

The University of Texas at Arlington, College of Nursing, *Arlington*

The University of Texas at Tyler, Program in Nursing, *Tyler*

The University of Texas Health Science Center at Houston, School of Nursing, *Houston*

The University of Texas Health Science Center at San Antonio, School of Nursing, *San Antonio*

Virginia

George Mason University, College of Health and Human Services, *Fairfax*

Jefferson College of Health Sciences, Nursing Education Program, *Roanoke*

Old Dominion University, Department of Nursing, *Norfolk*

Shenandoah University, Division of Nursing, *Winchester*

Washington

Pacific Lutheran University, School of Nursing, *Tacoma*

University of Washington, School of Nursing, *Seattle*

Washington State University College of Nursing and Consortium, *Spokane*

West Virginia

Fairmont State University, School of Nursing and Allied Health Administration, *Fairmont*

Shepherd University, Department of Nursing Education, *Shepherdstown*

West Virginia University, School of Nursing, *Morgantown*

Wisconsin

Alverno College, Division of Nursing, *Milwaukee*

University of Wisconsin–Eau Claire, College of Nursing and Health Sciences, *Eau Claire*

University of Wisconsin–Madison, School of Nursing, *Madison*

University of Wisconsin–Oshkosh, College of Nursing, *Oshkosh*

Viterbo University, School of Nursing, *La Crosse*

Wisconsin Lutheran College, Nursing Program, *Milwaukee*

CANADA

British Columbia

British Columbia Institute of Technology, School of Health Sciences, *Burnaby*

Thompson Rivers University, School of Nursing, *Kamloops*

Manitoba

University of Manitoba, Faculty of Nursing, *Winnipeg*

New Brunswick

Université de Moncton, School of Nursing, *Moncton*

University of New Brunswick Fredericton, Faculty of Nursing, *Fredericton*

Nova Scotia

St. Francis Xavier University, Department of Nursing, *Antigonish*

Ontario

Laurentian University, School of Nursing, *Sudbury*

Ryerson University, Program in Nursing, *Toronto*

University of Toronto, Faculty of Nursing, *Toronto*

University of Windsor, Faculty of Nursing, *Windsor*

York University, School of Nursing, *Toronto*

Quebec

Université de Montréal, Faculty of Nursing, *Montréal*

Université du Québec à Rimouski, Program in Nursing, *Rimouski*

Université Laval, Faculty of Nursing, *Québec*

Saskatchewan

University of Saskatchewan, College of Nursing, *Saskatoon*

ALPHABETICAL LISTING

SPECIAL ADVERTISING SECTION

Thomas Jefferson University School of Population Health

University of Medicine & Dentistry of New Jersey

Saint Louis University

St. Mary's University

The Winston Preparatory Schools